RESOURCE MANUAL FOR

NURSING RESEARCH

Generating and Assessing Evidence *for* Nursing Practice

NINTH EDITION

Denise F. Polit
Cheryl Tatano Beck

The perfect complement to the 9th edition of *Nursing Research: Generating and Assessing Evidence for Nursing Practice*, this knowledge builder strengthens the textbook in important ways. It reinforces the acquisition of basic research skills through systematic learning exercises, with an emphasis on careful reading and critiquing of actual studies—fundamental to designing and planning one's own study.

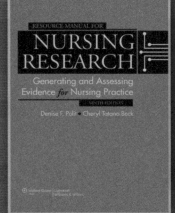

The Resource Manual includes:

- Full research reports and a grant application in 13 appendices, which represent a rich array of research endeavors, including quantitative and qualitative studies, an evidence-based practice project report, an instrument development paper, a meta-analysis, and a meta-synthesis.

- Full critiques of two of the research reports that serve as models for a comprehensive research critique

- A successful grant application that was funded by the National Institute of Nursing Research, together with the Study Section's summary sheet

The Resource Manual also includes the invaluable Toolkit, on CD and online, which offers important research resources to beginning and advanced researchers. The refined and easily adaptable research tools address a broad range of research situations, are available as editable Word files, and are offered to meet your specific needs.

ORDER TODAY!

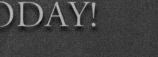
Wolters Kluwer | Lippincott
Health | Williams & Wilkins

the**Point**

ISBN: 978-1-6054-7782-4

Quick Guide to Bivariate Statistical Tests

Level of measurement of dependent variable	Group Comparisons: Number of groups (the independent variable)				Correlational analyses (To examine relationship strength)
	2 Groups		3+ Groups		
	Independent Groups Tests	Dependent Groups Tests	Independent Groups Tests	Dependent Groups Tests	
Nominal (Categorical)	χ^2 pp. 420–421 (or Fisher's exact test) p. 421	McNemar"s test p. 421	χ^2 pp. 420–421	Cochran's Q	Phi coefficient (dichotomous) or Cramér's V (not restricted to dichotomous) p. 422
Ordinal (Rank)	Mann-Whitney Test (or Median test) p. 416	Wilcoxon signed ranks test p. 416	Kruskal-Wallis H test p. 420	Friedman's test p. 420	Spearman's rho (or Kendall's tau) p. 422
Interval or Ratio (Continuous)*	Independent group *t test* pp. 413–415	Paired *t test* p. 415	ANOVA pp. 416–420	RM-ANOVA p. 420	Pearson's *r* pp. 421–422
	Multifactor ANOVA for 2+ independent variables p. 420				
	RM-ANOVA for 2+ groups x 2+ measurements over time p. 446				

*For distributions that are markedly nonnormal or samples that are small, the nonparametric tests in the row above may be needed.

Quick Guide to an Evidence Hierarchy of Designs for Cause-Probing Questions

Level I
a. Systematic review of RCTs
b. Systematic review of nonrandomized trials

Level II
a. Single RCT
b. Single nonrandomized trial

Level III
Systematic review of correlational/observational studies

Level IV
Single correlational/observational study

Level V
Systematic review of descriptive/qualitative/physiologic studies

Level VI
Single descriptive/qualitative/physiologic study

Level VII
Opinions of authorities, expert committees

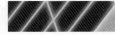

NURSING RESEARCH: GENERATING AND ASSESSING EVIDENCE FOR NURSING PRACTICE

Ninth Edition

Denise F. Polit, PhD, FAAN

President
Humanalysis, Inc.
Saratoga Springs, New York, *and*
Professor
Griffith University School of Nursing
Gold Coast, Australia
(www.denisepolit.com)

Cheryl Tatano Beck, DNSc, CNM, FAAN

Distinguished Professor
School of Nursing
University of Connecticut
Storrs, Connecticut

 Wolters Kluwer | Lippincott Williams & Wilkins
Health

Philadelphia • Baltimore • New York • London
Buenos Aires • Hong Kong • Sydney • Tokyo

Acquisitions Editor: Hilarie Surrena
Product Manager: Mary Kinsella
Editorial Assistant: Amanda Jordan
Design Coordinator: Joan Wendt
Manufacturing Coordinator: Karin Duffield
Prepress Vendor: Aptara, Inc.

Ninth edition

9 8 7 6 5

Printed in China

Library of Congress Cataloging-in-Publication Data
Polit, Denise F., author.
    Nursing research : generating and assessing evidence for nursing practice / Denise F. Polit, PhD, FAAN, President, Humanalysis, Inc., Saratoga Springs, New York and Professor, Griffith University School of Nursing, Gold Coast, Australia (www.denisepolit.com), Cheryl Tatano Beck, DNSc, CNM, FAAN, Distinguished Professor, School of Nursing, University of Connecticut, Storrs, Connecticut. – Ninth Edition.
        p. ; cm.
    Includes bibliographical references and index.
    Summary: "Thoroughly updated and revised to emphasize the link between research and evidence-based practice, this Ninth Edition of a classic textbook presents state-of-the-art methods for conducting high-quality studies. The ancillary Resource Manual includes application exercises, models of comprehensive research critiques, a full NINR grant application, and a Toolkit on a CD-ROM, containing exemplary research tools (e.g., consent forms, a demographic questionnaire, statistical table templates)—all in easily-adapted Word documents"—Provided by publisher.
    ISBN 978-1-60547-708-4 (hardback)
    1. Nursing—Research—Methodology.   I. Beck, Cheryl Tatano, author.
II. Title.
    [DNLM: 1. Nursing Research—methods. WY 20.5]
    RT81.5.P64 2012
    610.73072—dc22
                                                                                2010044281

LWW.com

TO

The memory of Pat Hungler (1931–2010)
who co-authored the first 6 editions of this book.

Acknowledgments

This ninth edition, like the previous eight editions, depended on the contribution of many individuals. Many faculty and students who used the text have made invaluable suggestions for its improvement, and to all of you we are very grateful. In addition to all those who assisted us during the past 30 years with the earlier editions, the following individuals deserve special mention.

We would like to acknowledge the comments of the reviewers of the previous edition, anonymous to us initially, whose feedback greatly influenced our revisions. Several of the comments triggered our work on the new chapters, and on the re-organization of content, and for this we are indebted.

Faculty at Griffith University in Australia made useful suggestions, and also inspired the inclusion of some new content in this edition. Valori Banfi, reference librarian at the University of Connecticut, provided ongoing assistance, and Dr. Mary Ann Cordeau helped with the section on historical research. We are also grateful for the insights of Dr. Robert Gable regarding instrument development in Chapter 15. Dr. Deborah Dillon McDonald was extraordinarily generous in giving us access to her NINR grant application and related material for the *Resource Manual*.

We also extend our thanks to those who helped to turn the manuscript into a finished product. The staff at Lippincott Williams & Wilkins has been of great assistance to us over the years. We are indebted to Hilarie Surrena, Mary Kinsella, Erika Kors, and all the others behind the scenes for their fine contributions. Special thanks also to Jeri Litteral of Aptara, Inc., who was extremely diligent and delightful.

Finally, we thank our family and friends. Our husbands Alan and Chuck have perhaps become accustomed to our demanding schedules, but we recognize that their support involves a high degree of patience and some sacrifices.

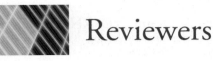

Reviewers

Jennifer Beck, PhD, RN, CNE
Interim Dean, School of Nursing
Our Lady of the Lake College
Baton Rouge, Louisiana

Diane M. Breckenridge, PhD, MSN, RN
Associate Professor
La Salle University
Nursing Research Director
Abington Memorial Hospital
Philadelphia, Pennsylvania

Lynn Clark Callister, RN, PhD, FAAN
Professor
Brigham Young University College of Nursing
Provo, Utah

Deborah J. Clark, RN, PhD, MSN, MBA
Director, BSN Program
ECPI, MCI, School of Health Science
Virginia Beach, Virginia

Bonnie S. Dean, PhD, RN
Assistant Professor
Duquesne University School of Nursing
Pittsburgh, Pennsylvania

Debbie R. Faulk, PhD, RN, CNE
Professor of Nursing
EARN Program Coordinator
Auburn Montgomery School of Nursing
Montgomery, Alabama

Betsy Frank, RN, PhD, ANEF
Professor
Indiana State University College of Nursing Health
    and Human Services
Department of Baccalaureate Nursing
    Completion
Terre Haute, Indiana

Sara L. Gill, PhD, RN, IBCLC
Associate Professor
University of Texas Health Science Center
San Antonio School of Nursing
San Antonio, Texas

Angela Gillis, PhD, RN
Professor and Former Chair
St. Francis Xavier University School of
    Nursing
Antigonish, Nova Scotia

Valerie J. Gooder, PhD, RN
Assistant Professor
Weber State University
Ogden, Utah

Beverly G. Hart, RN, PhD, PMHNP-BC
Professor of Baccalaureate and Graduate
    Nursing
Eastern Kentucky University
Richmond, Kentucky

Karen L. Hessler, PhD, FNP-C
Assistant Professor of Nursing
University of Northern Colorado
Greeley, Colorado

Rebecca Keele, PhD Nursing, PHCNS-BC
Associate Professor of Nursing
New Mexico State University
School of Nursing
College of Health and Social Services
Las Cruces, New Mexico

Margaret A. Louis, RN, PhD, CNE,
BC-Informatics
Associate Professor
School of Nursing
University of Nevada, Las Vegas

Carla L. Mueller, PhD, RN
Professor
Department of Nursing
University of Saint Francis
Fort Wayne, Indiana

Cynthia O'Neal, RN, PhD
Assistant Professor
Texas Tech University Health Sciences Center
Lubbock, Texas

Carolyn D. Pauling, RNC, PhD
Associate Professor of Nursing
Grand View University
Des Moines, Iowa

Michael Perlow, DNS, RN, BS, Biology;
BSN; MSN; DNS
Interim Dean
Murray State University
Murray, Kentucky

Janice M. Polizzi, MSN, RN
Associate Professor
Florida Hospital College of Health Sciences
Orlando, Florida

Laurel A. Quinn, ND, RN, CLNC, CNE
Chair, Department of Nursing
Trinity Christian College
Palos Heights, Illinois

Kathy Reavy, PhD, RN
Associate Professor
School of Nursing
Boise State University
Boise, Idaho

Mary Anne Hales Reynolds, RN, PhD,
ACNS-BC
Associate Clinical Professor
School of Nursing
Idaho State University
Pocatello, Idaho

Ratchneewan Ross, PhD, RN
Associate Professor
College of Nursing
Kent State University
Kent, Ohio

Marina Fowler Slemmons, PhD, CPNP
Professor
North Georgia College & State University
Dahlonega, Georgia

Amy Spurlock PhD, RN
Professor
Troy University
Troy, Alabama

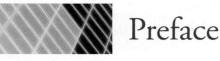

Preface

R esearch methodology is not a static enterprise. Even after writing eight editions of
this book, we continue to draw inspiration and new
material from ground-breaking advances in research
methods and in nurse researchers' use of those
methods. It is exciting and heartening to share many
of those advances, which we expect will be translated into powerful evidence for nursing practice.
We considered the 8th edition as a watershed edition
of a classic textbook, but we are persuaded that this
edition is even better. We have retained many features that made this book a classic, including its
focus on research as a support for evidence-based
nursing, but have introduced important innovations
that will help to shape the future of nursing research.

NEW TO THIS EDITION

New Organization of Qualitative and Quantitative Materials

In previous editions, we endeavored to balance
material on qualitative and quantitative methods to
ensure that both would be given similar emphasis.
This balance may have been obscured, however, by
intermingling content on both approaches within
chapters. In this edition, we have blended material
on qualitative and quantitative research mainly in
the early chapters—for example, in the chapters on

evidence-based practice and research ethics. Then,
we devoted an entire section of the book (Part III) to
methods in quantitative research and another section
(Part IV) to methods for qualitative inquiry. We
hope that this new organization will permit greater
continuity of ideas and will better meet the needs of
students and faculty.

New Chapters

We have added two chapters on mixed methods
research, which involves the integration of qualitative
and quantitative data in a single inquiry. These new
chapters represent a formal recognition of the tremendous methodologic refinements and the surge of interest in mixed methods research that have occurred in
the past decade. Chapter 25 describes basic strategies
in mixed methods design, sampling, and data analysis.
Chapter 26 describes the use of mixed methods
research in the development and testing of nursing
interventions. Many nursing studies—including many
doctoral inquiries—now use mixed methods, so we
think these additional chapters will provide useful
guidance to an emerging generation of scholars.

New Content

Throughout the book, we have included material on
methodologic innovations that have arisen in nursing, medicine, and the social sciences during the

past 4 to 5 years. A few of the many additions, which are too numerous to catalog here completely, include new models of generalizability, new or updated guidelines for reporting research in journals, technological advances in data collection, advances in dealing with the problem of missing data, new approaches to systematic reviews (includes mixed studies reviews), a revised model for developing and testing interventions (the 2008 Medical Research Council framework), and new guidelines for obtaining research funding from the National Institutes of Health (NIH).

ORGANIZATION OF THE TEXT

The content of this edition is organized into six main parts.

- **Part I—Foundations of Nursing Research and Evidence-Based Practice** introduces fundamental concepts in nursing research. Chapter 1 summarizes the history and future of nursing research, discusses the philosophical underpinnings of qualitative research versus quantitative research, and describes major purposes of nursing research. Chapter 2 offers guidance on utilizing research to build an evidence-based practice. Chapter 3 introduces readers to key research terms, and presents an overview of steps in the research process for both qualitative and quantitative studies.
- **Part II—Conceptualizing and Planning a Study to Generate Evidence** further sets the stage for learning about the research process by discussing issues relating to a study's conceptualization: the formulation of research questions and hypotheses (Chapter 4), the review of relevant research (Chapter 5), the development of theoretical and conceptual contexts (Chapter 6), and the fostering of ethically sound approaches in doing research (Chapter 7). Chapter 8 provides an overview of important issues that must be attended to during the planning of any type of study.
- **Part III—Designing and Conducting Quantitative Studies to Generate Evidence** presents material on undertaking quantitative nursing studies. Chapter 9 describes fundamental principles

and applications of quantitative research design, and Chapter 10 focuses on methods to enhance the rigor of a quantitative study, including mechanisms of research control. Chapter 11 examines research with different purposes, including surveys, outcomes research, and needs assessments. Chapter 12 presents strategies for sampling study participants in quantitative research. Chapter 13 describes using structured data collection methods that yield quantitative information. Chapter 14 discusses the concept of measurement, and then focuses on methods of assessing the quality of data from formal measuring instruments. Chapter 15 presents material on how to develop high-quality self-report instruments. Chapters 16, 17, and 18 present an overview of univariate, bivariate, and multivariate statistical analyses, respectively. Chapter 19 describes the development of an overall analytic strategy for quantitative studies, including new material on handling missing data and interpreting results.
- **Part IV—Designing and Conducting Qualitative Studies to Generate Evidence** presents material on undertaking qualitative nursing studies. Chapter 20 is devoted to research designs and approaches for qualitative studies, including material on critical theory, feminist, and participatory action research. Chapter 21 discusses strategies for sampling study participants in qualitative inquiries. Chapter 22 describes methods of gathering unstructured self-report and observational data for qualitative studies. Chapter 23 discusses methods of analyzing qualitative data, with specific information on grounded theory, phenomenologic, and ethnographic analyses. Chapter 24 elaborates on methods qualitative researchers can use to enhance (and assess) integrity and quality throughout their inquiries.
- **Part V—Designing and Conducting Mixed Methods Studies to Generate Evidence** presents new material on mixed methods nursing studies. Chapter 25 discusses a broad range of issues, including asking mixed methods questions, designing a study to address the questions, sampling participants in mixed methods research, and analyzing and integrating qualitative and quantitative data. Chapter 26 presents innovative information

about using mixed methods approaches in the development of nursing interventions.

- **Part VI—Building an Evidence Base for Nursing Practice** provides additional guidance on linking research and clinical practice. Chapter 27 offers an overview of methods of conducting systematic reviews that support EBP, with an emphasis on meta-analyses, metasyntheses, and mixed studies reviews. Chapter 28 discusses dissemination of evidence—how to prepare a research report (including theses and dissertations), and how to disseminate and publish research findings. The concluding chapter (Chapter 29) offers suggestions and guidelines on developing research proposals and getting financial support, and includes new information about applying for NIH grants and interpreting scores from NIH's new scoring system.

KEY FEATURES

This textbook was designed to be helpful to those who are learning how to do research, as well as to those who are learning to appraise research reports critically and to use research findings in practice. Many of the features successfully used in previous editions have been retained in this 9th edition. Among the basic principles that helped to shape this and earlier editions of this book are (1) an unswerving conviction that the development of research skills is critical to the nursing profession, (2) a fundamental belief that research is intellectually and professionally rewarding, and (3) faith in our opinion that learning about research methods need be neither intimidating nor dull. Consistent with these principles, we have tried to present the fundamentals of research methods in a way that both facilitates understanding and arouses curiosity and interest. Key features of our approach include the following:

- **Research Examples.** Each chapter concludes with one or two actual research examples designed to highlight critical points made in the chapter and to sharpen the reader's critical thinking skills. In addition, many research examples are used to illustrate key points in the text and to stimulate ideas for a study.

- **Critiquing Guidelines.** Most chapters include a section devoted to guidelines for conducting a critique of each aspect of a research report. These sections provide a list of questions to draw attention to specific aspects of a report that are amenable to appraisal.
- **Clear, "user friendly" style.** Our writing style is designed to be easily digestible and nonintimidating. Concepts are introduced carefully and systematically, difficult ideas are presented clearly, and readers are assumed to have no prior exposure to technical terms.
- **Specific practical tips on doing research.** The textbook is filled with practical guidance on how to translate the abstract notions of research methods into realistic strategies for conducting research. Every chapter includes several tips for applying the chapter's lessons to real-life situations. These suggestions are in recognition of the fact that there is often a large gap between what gets taught in research methods textbooks and what a researcher needs to know in conducting a study.
- **Aids to student learning.** Several features are used to enhance and reinforce learning and to help focus the student's attention on specific areas of text content, including the following: succinct, bulleted summaries at the end of each chapter; tables and figures that provide examples and graphic materials in support of the text discussion; study suggestions at the end of each chapter; a detailed glossary; and a comprehensive index for accessing information quickly.

TEACHING–LEARNING PACKAGE

Nursing Research: Generating and Assessing Evidence for Nursing Practice, 9th edition, has an ancillary package designed with both students and instructors in mind.

- **The *Resource Manual* augments the textbook in important ways. The manual itself provides students with exercises that correspond to each text chapter, with a focus on opportunities to critique actual studies. The appendix includes 12 research journal articles in their entirety, plus a successful grant application for a study funded by the National Institute of Nursing Research. The 12 reports cover a range of nursing research endeavors, including qualitative and quantitative studies, an instrument development study, an evidence-based practice translation project, and two systematic reviews. Full critiques of two of the reports are also included, and can serve as models for a comprehensive research critique.

- **The Toolkit to the *Resource Manual*** is a must-have innovation that will save considerable time for both students and seasoned researchers. Included on a CD-ROM, the Toolkit offers dozens of research resources in Word documents that can be downloaded and used directly or adapted. The resources reflect best-practice research material, most of which have been pretested and refined in our own research. The Toolkit originated with our realization that in our technologically advanced environment, it is possible to not only *illustrate* methodologic tools as graphics in the textbook but also to make them directly available for use and adaptation. Thus, we have included dozens of documents in Word files that can readily be used in research projects, without forcing researchers to "reinvent the wheel" or tediously retype material from the textbook. Examples include informed consent forms, a demographic questionnaire, content validity forms, and a coding sheet for a meta-analysis—to name only a few. The Toolkit also has lists of relevant and useful websites for each chapter, which can be "clicked" on directly without having to retype the URL and risk a typographical error.

- **The Instructor's Resource CD-ROM** includes a PowerPoint slides summarizing key points in each chapter, test questions that have been placed into a program that allows instructors to automatically generate a test and an image bank.

It is our hope that the content, style, and organization of this book continue to meet the needs of a broad spectrum of nursing students and nurse researchers. We also hope that the book will help to foster enthusiasm for the kinds of discoveries that research can produce, and for the knowledge that will help support an evidence-based nursing practice.

DENISE F. POLIT, PhD, FAAN

CHERYL TATANO BECK, DNSC, CNM, FAAN

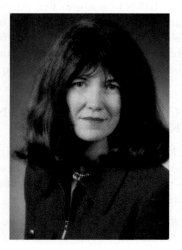

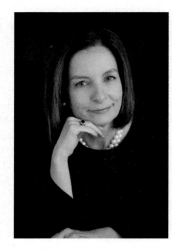

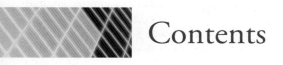

Contents

PART 4:   DESIGNING AND CONDUCTING QUALITATIVE STUDIES
TO GENERATE EVIDENCE FOR NURSING   486

PART 5:   DESIGNING AND CONDUCTING MIXED METHODS STUDIES
TO GENERATE EVIDENCE FOR NURSING   602

PART 6:   BUILDING AN EVIDENCE BASE FOR NURSING PRACTICE   652

PART 1

FOUNDATIONS OF NURSING RESEARCH

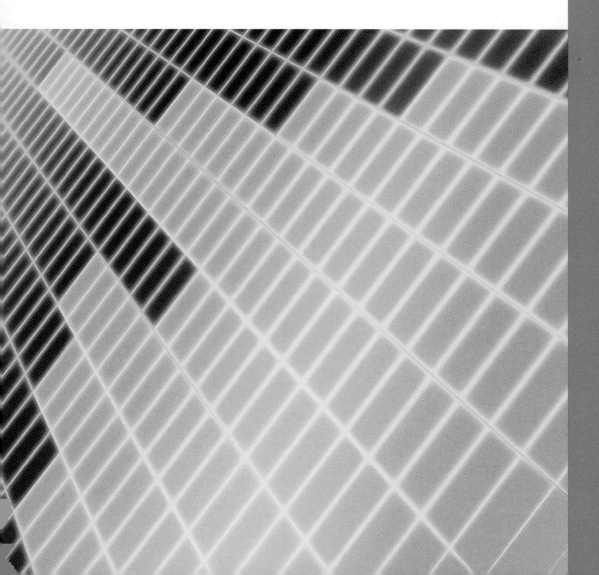

1 | Introduction to Nursing Research in an Evidence-Based Practice Environment

NURSING RESEARCH IN PERSPECTIVE

In all parts of the world, nursing has experienced a profound culture change. Nurses are increasingly expected to understand and conduct research, and to base their professional practice on research evidence—that is, to adopt an **evidence-based practice (EBP)**. EBP involves using the best evidence in making patient care decisions, and such evidence typically comes from research conducted by nurses and other healthcare professionals.

What Is Nursing Research?

Research is systematic inquiry that uses disciplined methods to answer questions or solve problems. The ultimate goal of research is to develop, refine, and expand knowledge.

Nurses are increasingly engaged in disciplined studies that benefit nursing and its clients, and that contribute to improvements in the entire healthcare system. **Nursing research** is systematic inquiry designed to develop trustworthy evidence about issues of importance to the nursing profession, including nursing practice, education, administration, and informatics. In this book, we emphasize **clinical nursing research**, that is, research designed to guide nursing practice and to improve the health and quality of life of nurses' clients.

Nursing research has experienced remarkable growth in the past three decades, providing nurses with a growing evidence base from which to practice. Yet many questions endure and much remains to be done to incorporate research innovations into nursing practice.

Examples of nursing research questions:

- What is the effect of increased body mass index on survival and complications following elective open heart surgery? (Barnett et al., 2010)
- What is it like for children with leukemia to experience cancer-related fatigue? (Wu et al., 2010)

The Importance of Research in Nursing

Although there is not a consensus about what types of "evidence" are appropriate for EBP, there is general agreement that research findings from rigorous studies provide especially strong evidence for informing nurses' decisions and actions. Nurses are accepting the need to base specific nursing actions and decisions on research evidence indicating that the actions are clinically appropriate, cost-effective, and result in positive outcomes for clients.

In the United States, research plays an important role in nursing in terms of credentialing and status. The American Nurses Credentialing Center (ANCC)—an arm of the American Nurses Association and the largest and most prestigious credentialing organization in the U.S.—developed a Magnet Recognition Program to acknowledge healthcare organizations that provide very high-quality nursing care, and to elevate the standards and reputation of the nursing profession. As noted by Turkel and her colleagues (2005), "To achieve Magnet status, the Chief Nurse Executive needs to create, foster, and sustain a practice environment where nursing research and evidence-based practice is integrated into both the delivery of nursing care and the framework for nursing administration decision making" (p. 254). In 2008, a new Magnet application process was instituted. A key component is "new knowledge, improvements, and innovations" that are viewed as affecting quality of care, which are represented by empirical (research-based) outcomes at the center of the model.

Changes to nursing practice now occur regularly because of EBP efforts. These practice changes often are local initiatives that are not publicized, but broader clinical changes are also occurring based on accumulating research evidence about beneficial practice innovations.

Example of EBP: Numerous clinical practice changes reflect the impact of research. For example, "kangaroo care" (the holding of diaper-clad preterm infants skin-to-skin by parents) is now widely practiced in neonatal intensive care units (NICUs) (Engler et al., 2002), but this is a new trend. As recently as the 1990s, only a minority of NICUs offered kangaroo care options. The adoption of this practice reflects mounting evidence that early skin-to-skin contact has benefits without negative side effects (e.g., Moore et al., 2007). Some of that evidence was developed in rigorous studies by nurse researchers in several countries (e.g., Chwo et al., 2002; Cong et al., 2009; Hake-Brooks & Anderson., 2008; Ludington-Hoe et al., 2004).

The Consumer–Producer Continuum in Nursing Research

With the current emphasis on EBP, every nurse has a responsibility to engage in one or more roles along a continuum of research participation. At one end of the continuum are **consumers of nursing research**, who read research reports or research summaries for relevant findings that might affect their practice. EBP depends on well-informed nursing research consumers.

At the other end of the continuum are **producers of nursing research**: nurses who actively participate in generating evidence by doing research. At one time, most nurse researchers were academics who taught in schools of nursing, but research is increasingly being conducted by practicing nurses who want to find what works best for their patients. Between these two points on the consumer-producer continuum lie a rich variety of research activities in which nurses may engage. These activities include:

- Participating in a **journal club** in a practice setting, which involves meetings among nurses to discuss and critique research articles
- Solving clinical problems and making clinical decisions based on rigorous research
- Collaborating in the development of an idea for a clinical study
- Reviewing a proposed research plan with respect to its feasibility in a clinical setting
- Recruiting potential study participants
- Collecting research information (e.g., distributing questionnaires to patients)
- Giving clients advice about participation in studies
- Discussing the implications and relevance of research findings with clients

In all the possible research-related activities, nurses with some research skills are equipped to make a contribution to nursing and to EBP. An understanding of nursing research can improve the depth and breadth of *every* nurse's professional practice.

NURSING RESEARCH: PAST, PRESENT, AND FUTURE

Nursing research has not always had the prominence and importance it enjoys today, but its interesting history portends a distinguished future. Table 1.1

TABLE 1.1	Historical Landmarks in Nursing Research

YEAR	EVENT
1859	Nightingale's *Notes on Nursing* is published
1900	*American Journal of Nursing* begins publication
1923	Columbia University establishes first doctoral program for nurses
	Goldmark Report with recommendations for nursing education is published
1936	Sigma Theta Tau awards first nursing research grant in the United States
1948	Brown publishes report on inadequacies of nursing education
1952	The journal *Nursing Research* begins publication
1955	Inception of the American Nurses' Foundation to sponsor nursing research
1957	Establishment of nursing research center at Walter Reed Army Institute of Research
1963	*International Journal of Nursing Studies* begins publication
1965	American Nurses' Association (ANA) sponsors nursing research conferences
1969	*Canadian Journal of Nursing Research* begins publication
1972	ANA establishes a Commission on Research and Council of Nurse Researchers
1976	Stetler and Marram publish guidelines on assessing research for use in practice
	Journal of Advanced Nursing begins publication
1978	*Research in Nursing & Health and Advances in Nursing Science* begin publication
1979	*Western Journal of Nursing Research* begins publication
1982	Conduct and Utilization of Research in Nursing (CURN) project publishes report
1983	*Annual Review of Nursing Research* begins publication
1985	ANA Cabinet on Nursing Research establishes research priorities
1986	National Center for Nursing Research (NCNR) is established within U.S. National Institutes of Health
1988	*Applied Nursing Research and Nursing Science Quarterly* begin publication; Conference on Research Priorities is convened by NCNR
1989	U.S. Agency for Health Care Policy and Research (AHCPR) is established
1993	NCNR becomes a full institute, the National Institute of Nursing Research (NINR)
	The Cochrane Collaboration is established
	Magnet Recognition Program® makes first awards
1994	*Qualitative Health Research* begins publication
1995	Joanna Briggs Institute, an international EBP collaborative, is established in Australia
1997	Canadian Health Services Research Foundation is established with federal funding
1999	AHCPR is renamed Agency for Healthcare Research and Quality (AHRQ)
2000	NINR's annual funding exceeds $100 million
	The Canadian Institute of Health Research is launched
	Council for the Advancement of Nursing Science (CANS) is established
2004	*Worldviews on Evidence-Based Nursing* begins publication
2006	NINR issues strategic plan for 2006–2010
2010	NINR budget exceeds $140 million

summarizes some of the key events in the historical evolution of nursing research.

The Early Years: From Nightingale to the 1960s

Most people would agree that research in nursing began with Florence Nightingale. Her landmark publication, *Notes on Nursing* (1859), described her early interest in environmental factors that promote physical and emotional well-being. Her most widely known research contribution involved an analysis of factors affecting soldier mortality and morbidity during the Crimean War. Based on her skillful analyses, she was successful in effecting some changes in nursing care—and, more generally, in public health.

Most studies in the early 1900s concerned nurses' education. For example, in 1923, a group called the Committee for the Study of Nursing Education studied the educational preparation of nurse teachers and administrators and the clinical experiences of nursing students. The committee issued the Goldmark Report, which identified educational inadequacies and concluded that advanced educational preparation was essential. As more nurses received university-based education, studies concerning nursing students—their characteristics, problems, and satisfactions—became more numerous.

Funding for independent research was all but nonexistent in the early years. However, signaling its enduring commitment to research, the nursing honor society Sigma Theta Tau (which became Sigma Theta Tau International in 1985) was the first organization to fund nursing research in the United States, awarding a $600 grant to Alice Crist Malone in 1936.

During the 1940s, government-initiated studies of nursing education continued, spurred on by the high demand for nursing personnel during World War II. For example, Brown (1948) reassessed nursing education in a study initiated at the request of the National Nursing Council for War Service. Brown recommended that nurses' education occur in collegiate settings. Many studies about nurses' roles and attitudes, hospital environments, and nurse–patient interactions stemmed from the Brown report.

Several forces in the 1950s put nursing research on a rapidly accelerating upswing in the United States. An increase in the number of nurses with advanced degrees, the establishment of a nursing research center at the Walter Reed Army Institute of Research, increased availability of funding, and the inception of the American Nurses' Foundation—which is devoted to the promotion of nursing research—provided impetus to nursing research during this period.

Until the 1950s, nurse researchers had few outlets for reporting their studies. The *American Journal of Nursing*, first published in 1900, began to publish a few studies in the 1930s. A surge in the number of studies being conducted in the 1950s, however, created the need for a new journal; thus, *Nursing Research* came into being in 1952. As shown in Table 1.1, dissemination opportunities in professional journals grew steadily thereafter.

In the 1960s, nursing leaders began to express concern about the dearth of research in nursing practice. Several professional nursing organizations, such as the Western Interstate Council for Higher Education in Nursing, established research priorities during this period, and practice-oriented research on various clinical topics began to emerge in the literature.

Example of nursing research breakthroughs in the 1960s: Jeanne Quint Benoliel began a program of research that had a major impact on medicine, medical sociology, and nursing. She explored the subjective experiences of patients after diagnosis with a life-threatening illness (1967). Of particular note, physicians in the early 1960s usually did not advise women that they had breast cancer, even after a mastectomy. Quint's (1962) seminal study of the personal experiences of women after radical mastectomy contributed to changes in communication and information control by physicians and nurses.

Nursing Research in the 1970s

By the 1970s, the growing number of nursing studies and discussions of theoretical and contextual issues created the need for additional communication outlets. Several journals that focus on nursing research were established in the 1970s, including *Advances in Nursing Science, Research in Nursing & Health*, and the *Western Journal of Nursing Research*.

During the 1970s, there was a change in emphasis in nursing research from areas such as teaching and nurses themselves to improvements in client care—signifying a growing awareness by nurses of the need for an evidence base from which to practice. Nurses also began to pay attention to the clinical utilization of research findings. A seminal article by Stetler and Marram (1976) offered guidance on assessing research for application in practice settings.

In the United States, research skills among nurses continued to improve in the 1970s, and the cadre of nurses with earned doctorates steadily increased. Nursing research also expanded internationally. For example, nurse researchers in Europe began efforts at greater collaboration. The Workgroup of European Nurse Researchers was established in 1978 to develop greater communication and opportunities for systematic partnerships among the 25 European National Nurses Associations involved (*www.wenr.org*).

Example of nursing research breakthroughs in the 1970s: Kathryn Barnard's research led to breakthroughs in the area of neonatal and young child development. Her research program focused on the identification and assessment of children at risk of developmental and health problems, such as abused and neglected children and failure-to-thrive children (Barnard, 1973, 1976; Barnard & Collar, 1973). Her research contributed to early interventions for children with disabilities, and to the field of developmental psychology.

Nursing Research in the 1980s

The 1980s brought nursing research to a new level of development. An increase in the number of qualified nurse researchers, the widespread availability of computers for the collection and analysis of information, and an ever-growing recognition that research is an integral part of professional nursing led nursing leaders to raise new issues and concerns. More attention was paid to the types of questions being asked, the methods of collecting and analyzing information being used, the linking of research to theory, and the utilization of research findings in practice.

Of particular importance in the United States was the establishment in 1986 of the National Center for Nursing Research (NCNR) at the National Institutes of Health (NIH) by congressional mandate, despite a presidential veto that was overridden largely as a result of nurse-scientists' successful lobbying efforts. The purpose of NCNR was to promote and financially support research projects and training relating to patient care. Funding for nursing research also became available in Canada in the 1980s through the National Health Research Development Program (NHRDP) and the Medical Research Council of Canada.

Several nursing groups developed priorities for nursing research during the 1980s. For example, in 1985, the American Nurses' Association Cabinet on Nursing Research established priorities that helped focus research more precisely on aspects of nursing practice. Nurses also began to conduct formal projects specifically designed to increase research utilization, such as the Conduct and Utilization of Research in Nursing (CURN) project.

Several forces outside of nursing in the late 1980s helped to shape today's nursing research landscape. A group from the McMaster Medical School in Canada designed a clinical learning strategy that was called evidence-based medicine (EBM). EBM, which promulgated the view that research findings were far superior to the opinions of authorities as a basis for clinical decisions, constituted a profound shift for medical education and practice, and has had a major effect on all healthcare professions.

In 1989, the U.S. government established the Agency for Health Care Policy and Research (AHCPR). AHCPR (which was renamed the Agency for Healthcare Research and Quality, or AHRQ, in 1999) is the federal agency that has been charged with supporting research specifically designed to improve the quality of healthcare, reduce health costs, and enhance patient safety, and thus plays a pivotal role in the expansion of EBP (*www.ahrq.gov*).

Example of nursing research breakthroughs in the 1980s: A research team headed by Dorothy Brooten conducted studies that led to the testing of a model of site transitional care. Brooten and her colleagues (1986, 1988), for example, conducted studies of nurse-managed follow-up services for very-low-birth-weight infants who were discharged early from the hospital, and demonstrated a significant cost savings, with comparable health outcomes. Brooten and colleagues expanded their research to other high-risk patients (1994). The site transitional care model has been used as a framework for patients who are at health risk as a result of early discharge from hospitals, and has been recognized by numerous healthcare disciplines.

Nursing Research in the 1990s

Nursing science came into its maturity in the United States during the 1990s. As but one example, nursing research was given more national visibility when NCNR was promoted to full institute status within the NIH: in 1993, the **National Institute of Nursing Research (NINR)** was launched. The birth of NINR helped put nursing research into the mainstream of research activities enjoyed by other health disciplines. Funding for nursing research has also grown. In 1986, NCNR had a budget of $16 million, but by fiscal year 1999, the budget for NINR had grown to about $70 million. Funding opportunities for nursing research expanded in other countries as well. For example, the Canadian Health Services Research Foundation (CHSRF) was established in 1997 with an endowment from federal funds, and plans for the Canadian Institute for Health Research got underway.

Several journals were established in the 1990s in response to the growth in clinically oriented research and interest in EBP, including *Clinical Nursing Research* and *Journal of Clinical Nursing*. Another new journal, *Qualitative Health Research*, signaled the emergence of in-depth studies using different methodologies than had typically been used in earlier research.

Major contributions to EBP occurred near the turn of the century. Of particular importance, the Cochrane Collaboration was inaugurated in 1993. This collaboration, an international network of institutions and individuals, maintains and updates systematic reviews of hundreds of clinical interventions to facilitate EBP (*www.cochrane.org*). In Australia, another international network devoted to the evaluation of evidence in health disciplines was established in 1995: The Joanna Briggs Institute has collaborating centers worldwide (*www.joannabriggs.edu.au*). International cooperation around the issue of EBP in nursing also began to develop in the 1990s. For example, Sigma Theta Tau International sponsored the first international research utilization conference in Toronto in 1998, and a few years later, it launched the journal *Worldviews of Evidence-Based Nursing*.

Example of nursing research breakthroughs in the 1990s: Many studies that Donaldson (2000) identified as *breakthroughs* in nursing research were conducted in the 1990s. This reflects, in part, the growth of **research programs** in which teams of researchers engage in a series of related studies, rather than discrete, unconnected studies. For example, several nurse researchers had breakthroughs in the area of psychoneuro-immunology, which has been adopted as the model of mind–body interactions. Swanson and Zeller, for example, conducted studies relating to HIV infection and neuropsychological function (Swanson et al., 1993; Swanson et al., 1998), which led to discoveries in environmental management as a means of improving immune system status.

Current and Future Directions for Nursing Research

Nursing research continues to develop at a rapid pace and will undoubtedly flourish in the 21st century. Funding continues to grow—for example, NINR funding in fiscal year 2010 was more than $140 million. Broadly speaking, the priority for future nursing research will be the promotion of excellence in nursing science. Toward this end, nurse researchers and practicing nurses will be sharpening their research skills, and using those skills to address emerging issues of importance to the profession and its clientele.

Among the trends we foresee for the early 21st century are the following:

- *Continued focus on EBP.* Encouragement for nurses to engage in evidence-based patient care is sure to continue. In turn, improvements will be needed both in the quality of studies and in nurses' skills in locating, understanding, critiquing, and using relevant study results. Relatedly, there is an emerging interest in **translational research**— research on how findings from studies can best be translated into nursing practice.
- *Development of a stronger evidence base through multiple, confirmatory strategies.* Practicing nurses are unlikely to adopt an innovation based on weakly designed or isolated studies. Strong research designs are essential, and confirmation is usually needed through the **replication** (i.e., the repeating) of studies with different clients, in different clinical settings, and at different times to ensure that the findings are robust.
- *Greater emphasis on systematic reviews.* **Systematic reviews** are a cornerstone of EBP, and will take on increased importance in all health disciplines. The purpose of a systematic review is to amass and integrate comprehensive research information on a topic, to draw conclusions about the state of evidence. Best practice clinical guidelines typically rely on such systematic reviews.
- *Expanded local research in healthcare settings.* In the current evidence-based environment, there is likely to be an increase of small, localized research designed to solve immediate problems. In the United States and in other countries where Magnet status has been awarded, this trend will be reinforced as more hospitals apply and are re-certified for Magnet status. Mechanisms will need to be developed to ensure that evidence from these small projects becomes available to others facing similar problems, such as communication within and between regional nursing research alliances.
- *Strengthening of interdisciplinary collaboration.* Collaboration of nurses with researchers in related fields (as well as intradisciplinary collaboration among nurse researchers) is likely to continue to expand in the 21st century as

researchers address fundamental problems at the biobehavioral and psychobiologic interface. In turn, such collaborative efforts could lead to nurse researchers playing a more prominent role in national and international healthcare policies.
- *Expanded dissemination of research findings.* The Internet and other electronic communication have a big impact on disseminating research information, which in turn helps to promote EBP. Through such technological advances as electronic location and retrieval of research articles; on-line publishing; online resources, such as Lippincott's NursingCenter.com; e-mail; and electronic mailing lists and listservs, information about innovations can be communicated more widely and more quickly than ever before.
- *Increasing the visibility of nursing research.* The 21st century is likely to witness efforts to increase the visibility of nursing research. Most people are unaware that nurses are scholars and researchers. Nurse researchers must market themselves and their research to professional organizations, consumer organizations, governments, and the corporate world to increase support for their research.
- *Increased focus on cultural issues and health disparities.* The issue of health disparities has emerged as a central concern in nursing and other health disciplines, and this in turn has raised consciousness about the ecological validity and cultural sensitivity of health interventions, and the cultural competence of healthcare workers. **Ecological validity** is the extent to which study designs and findings have relevance in a variety of real-world contexts. There is growing awareness that research must be sensitive to the health beliefs, behaviors, and values of culturally and linguistically diverse populations.
- *Shared decision making.* Another emerging issue in healthcare is shared decision making, which is a move toward putting patients in a more central role in their decision-making about healthcare (Barratt, 2008). A major challenge in the years ahead will involve getting both research evidence and patient preferences into clinical decisions, and designing research to study the process and the outcomes.

Research priorities for the near future have been articulated by NINR, by Sigma Theta Tau International, and by other nursing organizations. For example, NINR's 2010 budget request identified three areas of research emphasis: promoting health and preventing disease; symptom management, self-management, and caregiving; and end-of-life research (NINR website: *http://ninr.nih.gov/ninr/*). A 2006 survey of nurse executives from hospitals with Magnet recognition (Lundmark & Hickey, 2007) indicated a number of research priorities for a "national Magnet research agenda," including clinical outcomes (e.g., errors and adverse events), practice environment issues (e.g., failure to rescue), satisfaction (e.g., patient satisfaction with pain management), and human resource issues (e.g., nursing staff adequacy). Research priorities that have been expressed by Sigma Theta Tau International include: promotion of healthy communities through health promotion, disease prevention, and recognition of social, economic and political determinants; implementation of evidence-based practice; targeting the needs of vulnerable populations, such as the chronically ill and poor; and capacity development for research by nurses (Sigma Theta Tau International website: *www.nursingsociety.org*).

SOURCES OF EVIDENCE FOR NURSING PRACTICE

Nurses make clinical decisions based on a large repertoire of knowledge and information. Nursing students are taught how to practice nursing by nursing faculty. Nurses also learn from each other and from interactions with other healthcare professionals. Some of what students and nurses learn is based on systematic research, but much of it is not.

Information sources for clinical practice vary in dependability and validity. Increasingly, there are discussions of *evidence hierarchies* that acknowledge that certain types of evidence are better than others. A brief discussion of some alternative sources of evidence shows how research-based information is different.

Tradition and Authority

Many decisions are made based on customs or tradition. Within any culture, certain "truths" are accepted as given. For example, citizens of democratic societies typically accept, without *proof*, that democracy is the best form of government. This type of knowledge is so much a part of a common heritage that few seek verification. Tradition facilitates communication by providing a common foundation of accepted truth, but many traditions have never been evaluated for their validity. There is concern that many nursing interventions are based on tradition, customs, and "unit culture" rather than on sound evidence.

Another common source of information is an authority, a person with specialized expertise. We often make decisions about matters with which we have little experience; it seems natural to place our trust in the judgment of people with specialized training or experience. As a source of evidence, however, authority has shortcomings. Authorities are not infallible, particularly if their expertise is based primarily on personal experience; yet, like tradition, their knowledge often goes unchallenged.

Clinical Experience, Trial and Error, and Intuition

Clinical experience is a familiar, functional source of knowledge. The ability to generalize, to recognize regularities, and to make predictions is an important characteristic of the human mind. Nevertheless, personal experience is limited as a knowledge source because each nurse's experience is too narrow to be generally useful. A second limitation is that the same objective event is often experienced and perceived differently by two nurses.

A related method is trial and error in which alternatives are tried successively until a solution to a problem is found. We likely have all used this method in our professional work. For example, many patients dislike the taste of potassium chloride solution. Nurses try to disguise the taste of the medication in various ways until one method meets with the approval of the patient. Trial and error may offer a practical means of securing knowledge, but it is fallible because the solutions may be idiosyncratic.

Intuition is a knowledge source that cannot be explained based on reasoning or prior instruction. Although intuition and hunches undoubtedly play a role in nursing—as they do in the conduct of research—it is difficult to develop nursing policies and practices based on intuition.

Logical Reasoning

Solutions to some problems are developed by logical thought processes. Logical reasoning as a problem solving method combines experience, intellectual faculties, and formal systems of thought. **Inductive reasoning** is the process of developing generalizations from specific observations. For example, a nurse may observe the anxious behavior of (specific) hospitalized children and conclude that (in general) children's separation from their parents is stressful. **Deductive reasoning** is the process of developing specific predictions from general principles. For example, if we assume that separation anxiety occurs in hospitalized children (in general), then we might predict that (specific) children in a hospital whose parents do not room-in will manifest symptoms of stress.

Both systems of reasoning are useful as a means of understanding and organizing phenomena, and both play a role in research. Logical reasoning in and of itself, however, is limited because the validity of reasoning depends on the accuracy of the information (or premises) with which one starts.

Assembled Information

In making clinical decisions, healthcare professionals also rely on information that has been assembled for a variety of purposes. For example, local, national, and international *bench-marking data* provide information on such issues as the rates of using various procedures (e.g., rates of cesarean deliveries) or infection rates, and can facilitate evaluations of clinical practices. *Cost data*—information on the costs associated with certain procedures, policies,

or practices—are sometimes used as a factor in clinical decision-making. *Quality improvement and risk data*, such as medication error reports, can be used to assess the need for practice changes. Such sources are useful, but they do not provide a good mechanism for determining whether improvements in patient outcomes result from their use.

Disciplined Research

Research conducted in a disciplined framework is the most sophisticated method of acquiring knowledge. Nursing research combines logical reasoning with other features to create evidence that, although fallible, tends to be more reliable than other methods of acquiring evidence. Carefully synthesized findings from rigorous research are at the pinnacle of most evidence hierarchies. The current emphasis on EBP requires nurses to base their clinical practice to the greatest extent possible on research-based findings rather than on tradition, authority, intuition, or personal experience—although nursing will always remain a rich blend of art and science.

PARADIGMS FOR NURSING RESEARCH

A **paradigm** is a world view, a general perspective on the complexities of the world. Paradigms for human inquiry are often characterized in terms of the ways in which they respond to basic philosophical questions, such as, What is the nature of reality? (ontologic) and What is the relationship between the inquirer and those being studied? (epistemologic).

Disciplined inquiry in nursing has been conducted mainly within two broad paradigms, *positivism* and *constructivism*. This section describes these two paradigms and outlines the research methods associated with them. In later chapters, we describe the *transformative paradigm* that involves *critical theory research* (Chapter 20), and a *pragmatism paradigm* that involves *mixed methods research* (Chapters 25 and 26).

The Positivist Paradigm

The paradigm that dominated nursing research for decades is known as **positivism** (also called *logical positivism*). Positivism is rooted in 19th century thought, guided by such philosophers as Mill, Newton, and Locke. Positivism reflects a broader cultural phenomenon that, in the humanities, is referred to as **modernism**, which emphasizes the rational and the scientific.

As shown in Table 1.2, a fundamental assumption of positivists is that there is a reality *out there* that can be studied and known (an **assumption** is a basic principle that is believed to be true without proof or verification). Adherents of positivism assume that nature is basically ordered and regular and that an objective reality exists independent of human observation. In other words, the world is assumed not to be merely a creation of the human mind. The related assumption of **determinism** refers to the positivists' belief that phenomena are not haphazard, but rather have antecedent causes. If a person has a cerebrovascular accident, the scientist in a positivist tradition assumes that there must be one or more reasons that can be potentially identified. Within the **positivist paradigm**, much research activity is directed at understanding the underlying causes of phenomena.

Positivists value objectivity and attempt to hold personal beliefs and biases in check to avoid contaminating the phenomena under study. The positivists' scientific approach involves using orderly, disciplined procedures with tight controls of the research situation to test researchers' hunches about the phenomena being studied and relationships among them.

Strict positivist thinking has been challenged, and few researchers adhere to the tenets of pure positivism. In the **postpositivist paradigm**, there is still a belief in reality and a desire to understand it, but postpositivists recognize the impossibility of total objectivity. They do, however, see objectivity as a goal and strive to be as neutral as possible. Postpositivists also appreciate the impediments to knowing reality with certainty and therefore seek *probabilistic* evidence—i.e., learning what the true state of a phenomenon *probably* is, with a high degree of likelihood. This modified positivist position remains a dominant force in nursing research. For the sake of simplicity, we refer to it as positivism.

The Constructivist Paradigm

The **constructivist paradigm** (often called the **naturalistic paradigm**) began as a countermovement to positivism with writers such as Weber and Kant. Just as positivism reflects the cultural phenomenon of modernism that burgeoned after the industrial revolution, naturalism is an outgrowth of the cultural transformation called **postmodernism**. Postmodern thinking emphasizes the value of **deconstruction**—taking apart old ideas and structures—and **reconstruction**—putting ideas and structures together in new ways. The constructivist paradigm represents a major alternative system for conducting disciplined research in nursing. Table 1.2 compares the major assumptions of the positivist and constructivist paradigms.

For the naturalistic inquirer, reality is not a fixed entity but rather is a construction of the individuals participating in the research; reality exists within a context, and many constructions are possible. Naturalists thus take the position of relativism: If there are multiple interpretations of reality that exist in people's minds, then there is no process by which the ultimate truth or falsity of the constructions can be determined.

The constructivist paradigm assumes that knowledge is maximized when the distance between the inquirer and those under study is minimized. The voices and interpretations of study participants are crucial to understanding the phenomenon of interest, and subjective interactions are the primary way to access them. Findings from a constructivist inquiry are the product of the interaction between the inquirer and the participants.

Paradigms and Methods: Quantitative and Qualitative Research

Research methods are the techniques researchers use to structure a study and to gather and analyze information relevant to the research question. The two alternative paradigms correspond to different methods for developing evidence. A key methodologic distinction is between **quantitative research**,

TABLE 1.2	Major Assumptions of the Positivist and Constructivist Paradigms	
TYPE OF QUESTION	**POSITIVIST PARADIGM ASSUMPTION**	**CONSTRUCTIVIST PARADIGM ASSUMPTION**
Ontologic: What is the nature of reality?	Reality exists; there is a real world driven by real natural causes and ensuing effects	Reality is multiple and subjective, mentally constructed by individuals; simultaneous shaping, not cause and effect
Epistemologic: How is the inquirer related to those being researched?	The inquirer is independent from those being researched; findings are not influenced by the researcher	The inquirer interacts with those being researched; findings are the creation of the interactive process
Axiologic: What is the role of values in the inquiry?	Values and biases are to be held in check; objectivity is sought	Subjectivity and values are inevitable and desirable
Methodologic: How is evidence best obtained?	Deductive processes; theory verification Emphasis on discrete, specific concepts Focus on the objective and quantifiable Corroboration of researchers' predictions Outsider knowledge—researcher is external, separate Fixed, prespecified design Tight controls over context Large, representative samples Measured, quantitative information Statistical analysis Seeks generalizations Focus on the product	Inductive processes; theory generation Emphasis on entirety of some phenomena, holistic Focus on the subjective and nonquantifiable Emerging insight grounded in participants' experiences Insider knowledge—researcher is internal, part of process Flexible, emergent design Context-bound, contextualized Small, information-rich samples Narrative, unstructured information Qualitative analysis Seeks in-depth understanding Focus on the product and the process

which is most closely allied with positivism, and **qualitative research**, which is associated with constructivist inquiry—although positivists sometimes undertake qualitative studies, and constructivist researchers sometimes collect quantitative information. This section provides an overview of the methods associated with the two paradigms.

The Scientific Method and Quantitative Research

The traditional, positivist **scientific method** refers to a set of orderly, disciplined procedures used to acquire information. Quantitative researchers use deductive reasoning to generate predictions that are tested in the real world. They typically move in a systematic fashion from the definition of a problem and the selection of concepts on which to focus, to the solution of the problem. By **systematic**, we mean that the investigator progresses logically through a series of steps, according to a specified plan of action.

Quantitative researchers use various control strategies. **Control** involves imposing conditions on the research situation so that biases are minimized and precision and validity are maximized. Control mechanisms are discussed at length in this book.

Quantitative researchers gather **empirical evidence**—evidence that is rooted in objective reality and gathered through the senses. Empirical evidence, then, consists of observations gathered through sight, hearing, taste, touch, or smell. Observations of the presence or absence of skin inflammation, patients' anxiety level, or infant birth weight are all examples of empirical observations. The requirement to use empirical evidence means that findings are grounded in reality rather than in researchers' personal beliefs.

Evidence for a study in the positivist paradigm is gathered according to an established plan, using structured methods to collect needed information. Usually (but not always) the information gathered is **quantitative**—that is, numeric information that is obtained from a formal measurement and is analyzed statistically.

A traditional scientific study strives to go beyond the specifics of a research situation. For example, quantitative researchers are typically not as interested in understanding why a *particular* person has a stroke as in understanding what factors influence its occurrence in people generally. The degree to which research findings can be generalized to individuals other than those who participated in the study is called the study's **generalizability**.

The scientific method has enjoyed considerable stature as a method of inquiry, and has been used productively by nurse researchers studying a range of nursing problems. This is not to say, however, that this approach can solve all nursing problems. One important limitation—common to both quantitative and qualitative research—is that research cannot be used to answer moral or ethical questions. Many persistent, intriguing questions about human beings fall into this area—questions such as whether euthanasia should be practiced or abortion should be legal.

The traditional research approach also must contend with problems of *measurement*. To study a phenomenon, quantitative researchers attempt to measure it by attaching numeric values that express quantity. For example, if the phenomenon of interest

is patient morale, researchers might want to assess if morale is higher under certain conditions than under others. Although there are reasonably accurate measures of physiologic phenomena, such as blood pressure, comparably accurate measures of such psychological phenomena as morale or hope have not been developed.

Another issue is that nursing research focuses on humans, who are inherently complex and diverse. Traditional quantitative methods typically concentrate on a relatively small portion of the human experience (e.g., weight gain, depression) in a single study. Complexities tend to be controlled and, if possible, eliminated, rather than studied directly, and this narrowness of focus can sometimes obscure insights. Finally, quantitative research within the positivist paradigm has been accused of an inflexibility of vision that does not capture the full breadth of human experience.

Constructivist Methods and Qualitative Research

Researchers in constructivist traditions emphasize the inherent complexity of humans, their ability to shape and create their own experiences, and the idea that truth is a composite of realities. Consequently, constructivist studies are heavily focused on understanding the human experience as it is lived, usually through the careful collection and analysis of **qualitative** materials that are narrative and subjective.

Researchers who reject the traditional scientific method believe that it is overly *reductionist*—that is, it reduces human experience to the few concepts under investigation, and those concepts are defined in advance by the researcher rather than emerging from the experiences of those under study. Constructivist researchers tend to emphasize the dynamic, holistic, and individual aspects of human life and attempt to capture those aspects in their entirety, within the context of those who are experiencing them.

Flexible, evolving procedures are used to capitalize on findings that emerge in the course of the study. Constructivist inquiry usually takes place in the **field** (i.e., in naturalistic settings), often over an extended time period. In constructivist research, the collection of information and its analysis typically progress concurrently; as researchers sift through information, insights are gained, new questions emerge, and further evidence is sought to amplify or confirm the insights. Through an inductive process, researchers integrate information to develop a theory or description that helps illuminate the phenomenon under observation.

Constructivist studies yield rich, in-depth information that can elucidate varied dimensions of a complicated phenomenon. Findings from in-depth qualitative research are typically grounded in the real-life experiences of people with first-hand knowledge of a phenomenon. Nevertheless, the approach has several limitations. Human beings are used directly as the instrument through which information is gathered, and humans are extremely intelligent and sensitive—but fallible—tools. The subjectivity that enriches the analytic insights of skillful researchers can yield trivial and obvious "findings" among less competent ones.

Another potential limitation involves the subjectivity of constructivist inquiry, which sometimes raises concerns about the idiosyncratic nature of the conclusions. Would two constructivist researchers studying the same phenomenon in similar settings arrive at similar conclusions? The situation is further complicated by the fact that most constructivist studies involve a small group of participants. Thus, the generalizability of findings from constructivist inquiries is an issue of potential concern.

Multiple Paradigms and Nursing Research

Paradigms should be viewed as lenses that help to sharpen our focus on a phenomenon, not as blinders that limit intellectual curiosity. The emergence of alternative paradigms for studying nursing problems is, in our view, a healthy and desirable trend in the pursuit of evidence for practice. Although researchers' world view may be paradigmatic, knowledge itself is not. Nursing knowledge would be thin if there were not a rich array of methods available within the two paradigms—methods that

are often complementary in their strengths and limitations. We believe that intellectual pluralism should be encouraged.

We have emphasized differences between the two paradigms and associated methods so that distinctions would be easy to understand—although for many of the issues included in Table 1.2, differences are more on a continuum than they are a dichotomy. Subsequent chapters of this book elaborate further on differences in terminology, methods, and research products. It is equally important, however, to note that the two main paradigms have many features in common, only some of which are mentioned here:

- *Ultimate goals.* The ultimate aim of disciplined research, regardless of the underlying paradigm, is to gain understanding about phenomena. Both quantitative and qualitative researchers seek to capture the truth with regard to an aspect of the world in which they are interested, and both groups can make significant—and mutually beneficial—contributions to evidence for nursing practice.
- *External evidence.* Although the word *empiricism* has come to be allied with the classic scientific method, researchers in both traditions gather and analyze evidence empirically, that is, through their senses. Neither qualitative nor quantitative researchers are armchair analysts, depending on their own beliefs and world views to generate knowledge.
- *Reliance on human cooperation.* Because evidence for nursing research comes primarily from humans, human cooperation is essential. To understand people's characteristics and experiences, researchers must persuade them to participate in the investigation *and* to speak and act candidly.
- *Ethical constraints.* Research with human beings is guided by ethical principles that sometimes interfere with research goals. As discussed in Chapter 7, ethical dilemmas often confront researchers, regardless of paradigms or methods.
- *Fallibility of disciplined research.* Virtually all studies—in either paradigm—have some limitations. Every research question can be addressed

in many ways, and inevitably, there are trade-offs. The fallibility of any single study makes it important to understand and critique researchers' methodologic decisions when evaluating evidence quality.

Thus, despite philosophic and methodologic differences, researchers using traditional scientific methods or constructivist methods share overall goals and face many similar challenges. The selection of an appropriate method depends on researchers' personal philosophy, and also on the research question. If a researcher asks, "What are the effects of cryotherapy on nausea and oral mucositis in patients undergoing chemotherapy?" the researcher needs to examine the effects through the careful quantitative assessment of patients. On the other hand, if a researcher asks, "What is the process by which parents learn to cope with the death of a child?," the researcher would be hard pressed to quantify such a process. Personal world views of researchers help to shape their questions.

In reading about the alternative paradigms for nursing research, you likely were more attracted to one of the two paradigms. It is important, however, to learn about and respect both approaches to disciplined inquiry and to recognize their respective strengths and limitations. In this textbook, we describe methods associated with both qualitative and quantitative research in an effort to assist you in becoming *methodologically bilingual*. This is especially important because large numbers of nurse researchers are now undertaking mixed methods research that involves gathering and analyzing both qualitative and quantitative data (Chapters 25 and 26).

THE PURPOSES OF NURSING RESEARCH

The general purpose of nursing research is to answer questions or solve problems of relevance to nursing. Specific purposes can be classified in various ways. We present a few, primarily so that we can illustrate the range of questions that nurse researchers have addressed.

Applied and Basic Research

Sometimes a distinction is made between basic and applied research. As traditionally defined, **basic research** is undertaken to extend the base of knowledge in a discipline, or to formulate or refine a theory. For example, a researcher may perform an in-depth study to better understand normal grieving processes, without having *explicit* nursing applications in mind. Some types of basic research are called **bench research**, which is usually performed in a laboratory and focuses on the molecular and cellular mechanisms that underlie disease.

Example of basic nursing research: Using a mouse model of antiretroviral-induced painful peripheral neuropathy, Dorsey and colleagues (2009) conducted a whole-genome microassay screen to identify drug-induced regulation of the gene giant axonal neuropathy.

Applied research seeks solutions to existing problems and tends to be of greater immediate utility for EBP. Basic research is appropriate for discovering general principles of human behavior and biophysiologic processes; applied research is designed to indicate how these principles can be used to solve problems in nursing practice. In nursing, the findings from applied research may pose questions for basic research, and the results of basic research often suggest clinical applications.

Example of applied nursing research: Bingham and colleagues (2010) evaluated the effectiveness of a unit-specific intervention to reduce the probability of ventilator-associated pneumonia.

Research to Achieve Varying Levels of Explanation

Another way to classify research purposes concerns the extent to which studies provide explanatory information. Although specific study goals can range along an explanatory continuum, a fundamental distinction (relevant especially in quantitative research) is between studies whose primary intent is to *describe* phenomena, and those that are cause-probing—that is, designed to illuminate the underlying causes of phenomena.

Within a descriptive/explanatory framework, the specific purposes of nursing research include identification, description, exploration, prediction/control, and explanation. For each purpose, various types of question are addressed—some more amenable to qualitative than to quantitative inquiry, and vice versa.

Identification and Description

Qualitative researchers sometimes study phenomena about which little is known. In some cases, so little is known that the phenomenon has yet to be clearly identified or named or has been inadequately defined. The in-depth, probing nature of qualitative

research is well suited to the task of answering such questions as, "What is this phenomenon?" and "What is its name?" (Table 1.3). In quantitative research, by contrast, researchers begin with a phenomenon that has been previously studied or defined—sometimes in a qualitative study. Thus, in quantitative research, identification typically precedes the inquiry.

Qualitative example of identification:
Rosedale (2009) studied the experiences of women after breast cancer treatment. She identified, through in-depth conversations with 13 women, a unique description of intense loneliness that she called *survivor loneliness.*

TABLE 1.3	Research Purposes and Types of Research Questions	
PURPOSE	**TYPES OF QUESTIONS: QUANTITATIVE RESEARCH**	**TYPES OF QUESTIONS: QUALITATIVE RESEARCH**
Identification		What is this phenomenon? What is its name?
Description	How prevalent is the phenomenon? How often does the phenomenon occur? What are the characteristics of the phenomenon?	What are the dimensions of the phenomenon? What is important about the phenomenon?
Exploration	What factors are related to the phenomenon? What are the antecedents of the phenomenon?	What is the full nature of the phenomenon? What is really going on here? What is the process by which the phenomenon evolves or is experienced?
Explanation	What is the causal pathway through which the phenomenon unfolds? Does the theory explain the phenomenon?	How does the phenomenon work? Why does the phenomenon exist? What does the phenomenon mean? How did the phenomenon occur?
Prediction	What will happen if we alter a phenomenon or introduce an intervention? If phenomenon X occurs, will phenomenon Y follow?	
Control	How can we make the phenomenon happen or alter its prevalence? Can the occurrence of the phenomenon be prevented or controlled?	

Description is another important purpose of research. Examples of phenomena that nurse researchers have described include patients' stress, pain, confusion, and coping. Quantitative description focuses on the incidence, size, and measurable attributes of phenomena. Qualitative researchers, on the other hand, describe the dimensions, meanings, and importance of phenomena. Table 1.3 shows descriptive questions posed by quantitative and qualitative researchers.

Quantitative example of description: Amar and Alexy (2010) conducted a study to describe the prevalence among college students of having had a stalking experience and the frequency of using different coping strategies to manage stalking.

Qualitative example of description: Drageset and colleagues (2010) undertook an in-depth study to describe how women coped with breast cancer in the period between diagnosis and surgery.

Exploration

Exploratory research begins with a phenomenon of interest, but rather than simply observing and describing it, exploratory research investigates the full nature of the phenomenon, the manner in which it is manifested, and the other factors to which it is related. For example, a *descriptive* quantitative study of patients' preoperative stress might document the degree of stress patients feel before surgery and the percentage of patients who are stressed. An *exploratory* study might ask: What factors diminish or increase a patient's stress? Is a patient's stress related to behaviors of the nursing staff? Qualitative methods are especially useful for exploring the full nature of a little-understood phenomenon. Exploratory qualitative research is designed to shed light on the various ways in which a phenomenon is manifested and on underlying processes.

Quantitative example of exploration: Chang and colleagues (2010) explored the relationship between use of Sheng-Hua-Tang (a classic Chinese herbal formula believed to improve blood flow) and physical and emotional health in postpartum women in Taiwan.

Qualitative example of exploration: Through in-depth conversations and observations in the field, Watanabe and Inoue (2010) explored the transformational experiences in adult-to-adult living donor liver transplant recipients.

Explanation

The goals of explanatory research are to understand the underpinnings of natural phenomena and to explain systematic relationships among them. Explanatory research is often linked to **theories**, which are a method of integrating ideas about phenomena and their interrelationships. Whereas descriptive research provides new information and exploratory research provides promising insights, explanatory research attempts to offer understanding of the underlying causes or full nature of a phenomenon. In quantitative research, theories or prior findings are used deductively to generate hypothesized explanations that are then tested empirically. In qualitative studies, researchers search for explanations about how or why a phenomenon exists or what a phenomenon means as a basis for *developing* a theory that is grounded in rich, in-depth evidence.

Quantitative example of explanation: Munir and Nielsen (2009) tested a theoretical model to explain the effects of transformational leadership behaviors on sleep quality in Danish healthcare workers.

Qualitative example of explanation: Sparud-Lundin and colleagues (2010) conducted an in-depth study to develop a theoretical understanding of the process of transitioning to adult life among young adults with type 1 diabetes.

Prediction and Control

Many phenomena defy explanation, yet it is frequently possible to make predictions and to control phenomena based on research findings, even in the absence of complete understanding. For example, research has shown that the incidence of Down syndrome in infants increases with the age of the mother. We can predict that a woman aged 40 years is at higher risk of bearing a child with Down syndrome than is a woman aged 25 years. We can partially control the outcome by educating women about the risks and offering amniocentesis to women older than 35 years of age. Note, however, that the ability to predict and control does not depend on an explanation of *why* older women are at a higher risk of having an abnormal child. In many quantitative studies, prediction and control are key objectives. Although explanatory studies are powerful in an EBP environment, studies whose purpose is prediction and control are also critical in helping clinicians make decisions.

> **Quantitative example of prediction:** Kelly and colleagues (2010) studied the ability of community "social capital" factors (e.g., neighborhood block conditions, community integration) to predict attitudes about violence in a Mexican-American neighborhood.

Research Purposes Linked to EBP

The purpose of most nursing studies can be categorized on the descriptive–explanatory dimension just described, but some studies do not fall into such a system. For example, a study to develop and rigorously test a new method of measuring patient outcomes cannot easily be classified using this categorization.

In both nursing and medicine, several books have been written to facilitate evidence-based practice, and these books categorize studies in terms of the types of information needed by clinicians (DiCenso et al., 2005; Guyatt et al., 2008; Melnyk & Fineout-Overholt, 2011). These writers focus on several types of clinical concerns: treatment, therapy, or intervention; diagnosis and assessment; prognosis; prevention of harm; etiology; and meaning. Not all nursing studies have these purposes, but many of them do.

Treatment, Therapy, or Intervention
Nurse researchers undertake studies designed to help nurses make evidence-based treatment decisions about how to *prevent* a health problem or how to *address* an existing problem. Such studies range

from evaluations of highly specific treatments or therapies (e.g., comparing two types of cooling blankets for febrile patients) to complex multisession interventions designed to effect major behavioral changes (e.g., nurse-led smoking cessation interventions). Such **intervention research** plays a critical role in EBP.

> **Example of a study aimed at treatment/ therapy:** Liao and co-researchers (2010) tested the effectiveness of a supportive care program on the anxiety levels of women with suspected breast cancer.

Diagnosis and Assessment
A burgeoning number of nursing studies concern the rigorous development and evaluation of formal instruments to screen, diagnose, and assess patients and to measure important clinical outcomes. High-quality instruments with documented accuracy are essential both for clinical practice and for further research.

> **Example of a study aimed at diagnosis/ assessment:** Power and colleagues (2010) developed and explored the accuracy of an instrument designed to assess the impact and symptoms of hyperemesis gravidarum.

Prognosis
Studies of prognosis examine outcomes associated with a disease or health problem, estimate the probability they will occur, and indicate when (and for which types of people) the outcomes are most likely. Such studies facilitate the development of long-term care plans for patients. They provide valuable information for guiding patients to make lifestyle choices or to be vigilant for key symptoms. Prognostic studies can also play a role in resource allocation decisions.

> **Example of a study aimed at prognosis:** Li and colleagues (2010) studied the prognosis of children with cancer in terms of the impact of the disease on the children's physical, emotional, and psychosocial well-being.

Prevention of Harm

Nurses frequently encounter patients who face potentially harmful exposures—some as a result of healthcare factors, others because of environmental agents, and still others because of personal behaviors or characteristics. Providing useful information to patients about such harms and how best to avoid them, and taking appropriate prophylactic measures with patients in care, depends on the availability of accurate evidence.

Example of a study aimed at identifying and preventing harms: Williams and colleagues (2010) tested the effect of introducing a discharge plan on the occurrence of preventable adverse events within 72 hours of intensive care unit discharge.

Etiology or Causation

It is difficult, and sometimes impossible, to prevent harms or treat problems if we do not know what causes them. For example, there would be no smoking cessation programs if research had not provided firm evidence that smoking cigarettes causes or contributes to a wide range of health problems. Thus, identifying factors that affect or cause illness, mortality, or morbidity is an important purpose of many nursing studies.

Example of a study aimed at studying causation: Liaw and colleagues (2010) studied nurses' behaviors during the bathing of preterm infants. Behaviors that were viewed as potentially contributing to infant stress (or as reducing infant stress) were identified.

Meaning and Processes

Designing effective interventions, motivating people to comply with treatments and health promotion activities, and providing sensitive advice to patients are among the many healthcare activities that can greatly benefit from understanding the clients' perspectives. Research that provides evidence about what health and illness mean to clients, what barriers they face to positive health

practices, and what processes they experience in a transition through a healthcare crisis are important to evidence-based nursing practice.

Example of a study aimed at studying meaning: Forsner and colleagues (2009) conducted a study to illuminate the meaning of children's being afraid when in contact with medical care.

TIP: Most of these EBP-related purposes (except diagnosis and meaning) fundamentally call for cause-probing research. For example, research on interventions focuses on whether an intervention causes improvements in key outcomes. Prognosis research asks if a disease or health condition causes subsequent adverse outcomes. And etiology research seeks explanations about the underlying causes of health problems.

ASSISTANCE FOR USERS OF NURSING RESEARCH

This book is designed primarily to help you develop skills for conducting research, but in an environment that stresses EBP, it is extremely important to hone your skills in reading, evaluating, and using nursing studies. We provide specific guidance to consumers in most chapters by including guidelines for critiquing aspects of a study covered in the chapter. The questions in Box 1.1 are designed to assist you in using the information in this chapter in an overall preliminary assessment of a research report.

TIP: The *Resource Manual* that accompanies this book offers particularly rich opportunities to practice your critiquing skills. The Toolkit on the CD-ROM with the *Resource Manual* and on thePoint includes Box 1.1 as a Word document, which will allow you to adapt these questions, if desired, and to answer them directly into a Word document without having to retype the questions.

> ### BOX 1.1 Questions for a Preliminary Overview of a Research Report
>
> 1. How relevant is the research problem in this report to the actual practice of nursing? Does the study focus on a topic that is a priority area for nursing research?
> 2. Is the research quantitative or qualitative?
> 3. What is the underlying purpose (or purposes) of the study—identification, description, exploration, explanation, or prediction and control? Does the purpose correspond to an EBP focus such as treatment, diagnosis, prognosis, prevention of harm, etiology, or meaning?
> 4. Is this study fundamentally cause-probing?
> 5. What might be some clinical implications of this research? To what type of people and settings is the research most relevant? If the findings are accurate, how might the results of this study be used by *me*?

RESEARCH EXAMPLES

Each chapter of this book presents brief descriptions of studies conducted by nurse researchers, focusing on aspects emphasized in the chapter. A review of the full journal articles would prove useful for learning more about the studies, their methods, and the findings.

Research Example of a Quantitative Study

Study: A home-based nurse-coached inspiratory muscle training intervention in heart failure (Padula et al., 2009)

Study Purpose: The purpose of the study was to evaluate the effectiveness of a 12-week nurse-coached inspiratory muscle training (IMT) program for men and women with chronic heart failure. The home-based intervention was designed to increase respiratory muscle strength and endurance.

Study Methods: A total of 32 adults with heart failure were recruited to participate in the study. Some of the participants, at random, were put into a group that received the intervention, while others in a control group did not receive it, but they did receive an educational booklet. The intervention involved use of the Threshold Device for resistive IMT breathing training. Those in the intervention group trained 7 days a week for 10 to 20 minutes daily over the course of the 12 weeks. The researchers compared the two groups with regard to a variety of physiologic (e.g., maximum inspiratory pressure, dyspnea) and psychological

(self-efficacy, quality-of-life) outcomes. Outcome information was gathered during six home visits—at the outset of the study (prior to the intervention) and then 5 additional times.

Key Findings: The analysis suggested that the intervention was associated with several improved outcomes, such as higher values of PI_{max}, higher respiratory rate, and lower dyspnea.

Conclusions: Padula and her colleagues concluded that IMT is a safe, effective, and relatively low-cost intervention to improve respiratory muscle strength in patients with heart failure.

Research Example of a Qualitative Study

Study: The experiences of socioeconomically disadvantaged postpartum women in the first 4 weeks at home (Landy et al., 2009)

Study Purpose: The purpose of this study was to explore and describe the experiences of socioeconomically disadvantaged women in the first 4 weeks after postpartum hospital discharge.

Study Methods: Women who had had a vaginal delivery and who had low family income or social support were recruited from four Canadian hospitals. Women were interviewed in their homes, and responded conversationally to such broad questions as: What has life been like since you came home with your new baby? What kinds of concerns have you had about yourself and your baby? The audiotaped interviews lasted between 45 minutes and 3 hours.

Key Findings: The women's experiences in the first month after hospital discharge could be characterized by two overarching themes. The first was the ongoing burden of their day-to-day lives. This broad theme captured the context of the women's lives and included the subthemes of poverty and material deprivation, stigmatization as a result of living publicly examined lives, and precarious social support. The second broad theme was the women's ongoing struggles to adjust to changes resulting from the arrival of a new baby. The subthemes that emerged in this area included feeling out of control, the absence of help at home, and complex relationships with the baby's father. All of these themes were supported in the article with rich excerpts from the recorded interviews.

Conclusions: The researchers concluded that their study provided valuable insight into the spectrum of issues that contribute to health inequities resulting from socioeconomic disadvantage. They urged greater public policy focus on developing a comprehensive health disparities reduction strategy.

SUMMARY POINTS

- **Nursing research** is systematic inquiry to develop knowledge about issues of importance to nurses. Nurses are adopting an **evidence-based practice (EBP)** that incorporates research findings into their clinical decisions.
- Knowledge of nursing research enhances the professional practice of both **consumers of research** (who read and evaluate studies) and **producers of research** (who design and undertake studies).
- Nursing research began with Florence Nightingale but developed slowly until its rapid acceleration in the 1950s. Since the 1970s, nursing research has focused on problems relating to clinical practice.
- The **National Institute of Nursing Research** (NINR), established at the U.S. National Institutes of Health in 1993, affirms the stature of nursing research in the United States.
- Contemporary emphases in nursing research include EBP projects, **replications** of research, research integration through systematic reviews, multisite and interdisciplinary studies, expanded dissemination efforts, and increased focus on health disparities.

- Disciplined research is considered a better evidence source for nursing practice than other sources such as tradition, authority, personal experience, trial and error, intuition, and logical reasoning.
- Nursing research usually is conducted within one of two broad **paradigms**, which are world views with underlying **assumptions** about the complexities of reality: the positivist paradigm and the constructivist paradigm.
- In the **positivist paradigm**, it is assumed that there is an objective reality and that natural phenomena are regular and orderly. The related assumption of **determinism** is the belief that phenomena are not haphazard and result from prior causes.
- In the **constructivist (naturalistic) paradigm**, it is assumed that reality is not *fixed*, but is rather a construction of human minds; thus, "truth" is a composite of multiple constructions of reality.
- The positivist paradigm is associated with **quantitative research**—the collection and analysis of numeric information. Quantitative research is typically conducted within the traditional **scientific method**, which is a systematic, controlled process. Quantitative researchers gather and analyze **empirical evidence** (evidence collected through the human senses) and strive for **generalizability** of their findings beyond the study setting.
- Researchers within the constructivist paradigm emphasize understanding the human experience as it is lived through the collection and analysis of subjective, narrative materials using flexible procedures that evolve in the **field**; this paradigm is associated with **qualitative research**.
- **Basic research** is designed to extend the base of information for the sake of knowledge. **Applied research** focuses on discovering solutions to immediate problems.
- A fundamental distinction, especially relevant in quantitative research, is between studies whose primary intent is to *describe* phenomena and those that are **cause-probing**—that is, designed to illuminate underlying causes of phenomena.

Specific purposes on the description/explanation continuum include identification, description, exploration, prediction/control, and explanation.
- Many nursing studies can also be classified in terms of a key EBP aim: treatment/therapy/intervention; diagnosis and assessment; prognosis; harm and etiology; and meaning and process.

⬤◯⬤◯⬤◯⬤◯⬤◯⬤◯⬤◯⬤◯⬤◯⬤◯⬤◯⬤

STUDY ACTIVITIES

Chapter 1 of the *Resource Manual for Nursing Research: Generating and Assessing Evidence for Nursing Practice, 9th ed.*, offers study suggestions for reinforcing concepts presented in this chapter. In addition, the following questions can be addressed in classroom or online discussions:

1. Is your world view closer to the positivist or the constructivist paradigm? Explore the aspects of the two paradigms that are especially consistent with your world view.
2. Answer the questions in Box 1.1 about the Padula et al. (2009) study described at the end of this chapter. Could this study have been undertaken as a qualitative study? Why or why not?
3. Answer the questions in Box 1.1 about the Landy et al. (2009) study described at the end of this chapter. Could this study have been undertaken as a quantitative study? Why or why not?

◯⬤◯⬤◯⬤◯⬤◯⬤◯⬤◯⬤◯⬤◯⬤◯⬤◯⬤◯

STUDIES CITED IN CHAPTER 1

Amar, A., & Alexy, E. (2010). Coping with stalking. *Issues in Mental Health Nursing, 31*, 8–14.

Barnard, K. E. (1973). The effects of stimulation on the sleep behavior of the premature infant. In M. Batey (Ed.), *Communicating nursing research* (Vol. 6, pp. 12–33). Boulder, CO: WICHE.

Barnard, K. E. (1976). The state of the art: Nursing and early intervention with handicapped infants. In T. Tjossem (Ed.), *Proceedings of the 1974 President's Committee on Mental Retardation*. Baltimore: University Park Press.

Barnard, K. E., & Collar, B. S. (1973). Early diagnosis, interpretation, and intervention. *Annals of the New York Academy of Sciences, 205*, 373–382.

Barnett, S., Martin, L., & Halpin, L. (2010). Impact of body mass index on clinical outcome and health-related quality of life following open-heart surgery. *Journal of Nursing Care Quality, 25*, 65–72.

Bingham, M., Ashley, J., DeJong, M., & Swift, C. (2010). Implementing a unit-level intervention to reduce the probability of ventilator-associated pneumonia. *Nursing Research, 59*, S40–S47.

Brooten, D., Brown, L. P., Munro, B. H., York, R., Cohen, S., Roncoli, M., & Hollingsworth, A. (1988). Early discharge and specialist transitional care. *Image: Journal of Nursing Scholarship, 20*, 64–68.

Brooten, D., Kumar, S., Brown, L. P., Butts, P., Finkler, S., Bakewell-Sachs, S., Gibbons, S., & Delivoria-Papadopoulos, M. (1986). A randomized clinical trail of early hospital discharge and home follow-up of very low birthweight infants. *New England Journal of Medicine, 315*, 934–939.

Brooten, D., Roncoli, M., Finkler, S., Arnold, L., Cohen, A., & Mennuti, M. (1994). A randomized clinical trial of early hospital discharge and home follow-up of women having cesarean birth. *Obstetrics and Gynecology, 84*, 832–838.

Chang, P., Tseng, Y., Chuang, C., Chen, Y., Hsieh, W., Hurng, B., Lin, S, & Chen, P. (2010). Use of Sheng-Hua-Tang and health-related quality of life in postpartum women. *International Journal of Nursing Studies, 47*, 13–19.

Chwo, M. J., Anderson, G. C., Good, M., Dowling, D. A., Shiau, S. H., & Chu, D. M. (2002). A randomized controlled trial of early kangaroo care for preterm infants: Effects on temperature, weight, behavior, and acuity. *Journal of Nursing Research, 10*, 129–142.

Cong, X., Ludington-How, S., McCain, G., & Fu, P. (2009). Kangaroo care modifies preterm infant heart rate variability in response to heel stick pain. *Early Human Development, 85*, 561–567.

Dorsey, S., Leitch, C., Renn, C., Lessans, S., Smith, B., Wang, X., & Dionne, R. (2009). Genome-wide screen identifies drug-induced regulation of the gene giant axonal neuropathy (Gan) in a mouse model of antiretroviral-induced painful peripheral neuropathy. *Biological Research for Nursing, 11*, 7–16.

Drageset, S., Lindstrøm, C., & Underlid, K. (2010). Coping with breast cancer: Between diagnosis and surgery. *Journal of Advanced Nursing, 66*, 149–158.

Engler, A. J., Ludington-Hoe, S. M., Cusson, R. M., Adams, R., Bahnsen, M., Brumbaugh, E., Coates, P., Grieb, J., McHargue, L., Ryan, D. L., Settle, M., & Williams, D. (2002). Kangaroo care: National survey of practice, knowledge, barriers, and perceptions. *MCN: The American Journal of Maternal/Child Nursing, 27*, 146–153.

Forsner, M., Jansson, L., & Söderberg, A. (2009). Afraid of medical care: School-aged children's narratives about medical fear. *Journal of Pediatric Nursing, 24*, 519–528.

Hake-Brooks, S., & Anderson, G. (2008). Kangaroo care and breastfeeding of mother-preterm dyads 0-18 months: A randomized controlled trial. *Neonatal Network, 27,* 151–159.

Kelly, P., Rasu, R., Lesser, J., Oscos-Sanchez, M., Mancha, J., & Orriega, A. (2010). Mexican-American neighborhood's social capital and attitudes about violence. *Issues in Mental Health Nursing, 31,* 15–20.

Landy, C. K., Sword, W., & Valaitis, R. (2009). The experiences of socioeconomically disadvantaged postpartum women in the first 4 weeks at home. *Qualitative Health Research, 19,* 194–206.

Li, H., Chung, O., & Chiu, S. (2010). The impact of cancer on children's physical, emotional, and psychosocial well-being. *Cancer Nursing, 33,* 47–54.

Liao, M., Chen, P., Chen, M., & Chen, S. (2010). Effect of supportive care on the anxiety of women with suspected breast cancer. *Journal of Advanced Nursing, 66,* 49–59.

Liaw, J., Yang, L., Chou, H., Yang, M., & Chao, S. (2010). Relationships between nurse caregiving behaviours and preterm infant responses during bathing. *Journal of Clinical Nursing, 19,* 89–99.

Ludington-Hoe, S. M., Anderson, G. C., Swinth, J. Y., Thompson, C., & Hadeed, A. J. (2004). Randomized controlled trial of kangaroo care: Cardiorespiratory and thermal effects on healthy preterm infants. *Neonatal Network, 23,* 39–48.

Lundmark, V., & Hickey, J. (2007). The Magnet Recognition Program: Developing a national Magnet research agenda. *Journal of Nursing Care Quality, 22,* 195–198.

Moore, E., Anderson. G., & Bergman, N. (2007). Early skin-to-skin contact for mothers and their health newborn infants. *Cochrane Database of Systematic Reviews, 18,* CD0003519.

Munir, F., & Nielsen, K. (2009). Does self-efficacy mediate the relationship between transformational leadership behaviours and healthcare workers' sleep quality? *Journal of Advanced Nursing, 65,* 1833–1843.

Padula, C., Yeaw, E., Mistry, S. (2009). A home-based nurse-coached inspiratory muscle training intervention in heart failure. *Applied Nursing Research, 22,* 18–25.

Power, Z., Campbell, M., Kilcoyne, P., Kitchener, H., & Waterman, H. (2010). The Hyperemesis Impact of Symptoms Questionnaire: Development and validation of a clinical tool. *International Journal of Nursing Studies, 47,* 67–77.

Quint, J. C. (1962). Delineation of qualitative aspects of nursing care. *Nursing Research, 11,* 204–206.

Quint, J. C. (1967). *The nurse and the dying patient.* New York: Macmillan.

Rosedale, M. (2009). Survivor loneliness of women following breast cancer. *Oncology Nursing Forum, 36,* 175–183.

Sparud-Lundin, C., Ohm, I., & Danielson, E. (2010). Redefining relationships in young adults with type 1 diabetes. *Journal of Advanced Nursing, 66,* 128–138.

Swanson, B., Cronin-Stubbs, D., Zeller, J. M., Kessler, H. A., & Bielauskas, L. A. (1993). Characterizing the neuropsychological functioning of persons with human immunodeficiency virus infection. *Archives of Psychiatric Nursing, 7,* 82–90.

Swanson, B., Zeller, J. M., & Spear, G. (1998). Cortisol upregulates HIV p24 antigen in cultured human monocyte-derived macrophages. *Journal of the Association of Nurses in AIDS Care, 9,* 78–83.

Watanabe, A., & Inoue, T. (2010). Transformational experiences in adult-to-adult living donor transplant recipients. *Journal of Advanced Nursing, 66,* 69–91.

Williams, T., Gavin, L., Elliott, N., Brearley, L., & Dobb, G. (2010). Introduction of a discharge plan to reduce adverse events within 72 hours of discharge from the ICU. *Journal of Nursing Care Quality, 25,* 73–79.

Wu, M., Hsu, L., Zhang, B., Shen, N., Lu, H., & Li, S. (2010). The experiences of cancer-related fatigue among Chinese children with leukemia. *International Journal of Nursing Studies, 47,* 49–59.

Methodologic and nonresearch references cited in this chapter can be found in a separate section at the end of the book.

2 | Evidence-Based Nursing: Translating Research Evidence into Practice

This book will help you to develop the skills you need to generate and evaluate research evidence for nursing practice. Before we delve into methodologic techniques, we discuss key aspects of evidence-based practice (EBP) to clarify the key role that research plays in nursing.

BACKGROUND OF EVIDENCE-BASED NURSING PRACTICE

This section provides a context for understanding evidence-based nursing practice and a closely related concept, research utilization.

Definition of EBP

According to pioneer David Sackett, evidence-based practice "is the integration of best research evidence with clinical expertise and patient values" (Sackett et al., 2000, p. 1). Scott and McSherry (2008), in their review of evidence-based nursing concepts, identified 13 overlapping but distinct definitions of evidence-based nursing and EBP. The definition proposed by Sigma Theta Tau International (2008) captures current thinking about EBP within the nursing community: "The process of shared decision making between practitioner, patient, and others significant to them based on research evidence, the patient's experiences and preferences, clinical expertise or know-how, and other available robust sources of information." A key ingredient in EBP is the effort to personalize "best evidence" to a specific patient's needs within a particular clinical context.

A basic feature of EBP as a clinical problem-solving strategy is that it de-emphasizes decisions based on custom, authority, or ritual. The emphasis is on identifying the best available research evidence and *integrating* it with other factors. In many areas of clinical decision making, research has demonstrated that "tried and true" practices taught in basic nursing education are not always best. For example, although many nurses not so long ago were taught to place infants in the prone sleeping position to prevent aspiration, there is now persuasive evidence that the supine (back) sleeping position decreases the risk of sudden infant death syndrome (SIDS). Because research evidence can provide invaluable insights about human health and illness, nurses must be lifelong learners who have the skills to search for, understand, and evaluate new information about patient care—as well as the capacity to adapt to change.

Research Utilization and EBP

The terms *research utilization* and *evidence-based practice* are sometimes used synonymously. Although there is overlap between the two concepts, they are distinct. **Research utilization** (RU), the narrower of the two terms, is the use of findings from a study or set of studies in a practical application that is unrelated to the original research. In RU, the emphasis is on translating new knowledge into real-world applications.

EBP is broader than RU because it incorporates research findings with other factors, as just noted. Also, whereas RU begins with the research itself (how can I put this new knowledge to good use in my clinical setting?), the start-point in EBP is a clinical question (what does the evidence say is the best approach to solving this clinical problem?).

Research utilization was an important concept in nursing before the EBP movement took hold. This section provides a brief overview of research utilization in nursing.

The Research Utilization Continuum

The start-point of research utilization is the emergence of new knowledge and innovations. Research is conducted and, over time, evidence on a topic accumulates. The evidence works its way into use—to varying degrees and at differing rates.

Theorists who have studied knowledge development and the diffusion of ideas recognize a continuum in terms of how research findings are put to use. At one end of the continuum are clearly identifiable attempts to base actions on research findings (e.g., placing infants in supine instead of prone sleeping position). Research findings can, however, be used in a more diffuse manner—in a way that reflects awareness or enlightenment. Thus, a nurse may read a qualitative study describing *courage* among individuals with long-term health problems as a dynamic process that includes efforts to develop problem-solving skills. The study may make the nurse more observant and sensitive in working with patients with long-term illnesses, but it may not necessarily lead to formal changes in clinical actions.

Estabrooks (1999) studied research utilization in a sample of 600 Canadian nurses and identified three distinct types: (1) **indirect research utilization**, involving changes in nurses' thinking; (2) **direct**

research utilization, involving the direct use of findings in giving patient care; and (3) **persuasive utilization**, involving the use of findings to persuade others (typically those in decision-making positions) to make changes in nursing policies. These ways of thinking about research utilization suggest a role for both qualitative and quantitative research.

The History of Research Utilization in Nursing Practice

During the 1980s, *research utilization* emerged as an important buzz word. Changes in nursing education and research were prompted by the desire to develop a knowledge base for nursing practice. In education, nursing schools began to include courses on research methods so that students would become skillful research consumers. In research, there was a shift in focus toward clinical nursing problems.

Yet, concerns about the limited use of research evidence in the delivery of nursing care continued to mount. Such concerns were fuelled by studies suggesting that nurses were often unaware of research findings or did not incorporate evidence into their practice. The need to reduce the gap between research and practice led to formal RU projects, including the ground-breaking **Conduct and Utilization of Research in Nursing (CURN) Project**, a 5-year development project undertaken by the Michigan Nurses' Association in the 1970s. CURN's objectives were to increase the use of research findings in nurses' daily practice by disseminating current findings and facilitating organizational changes needed to implement innovations. CURN project staff saw RU as an organizational process, with the commitment of organizations that employ nurses as essential to its success (Horsley, Crane, & Bingle, 1978). The CURN project team concluded that RU by practicing nurses was feasible, but only if the research is relevant to practice and if the results are broadly disseminated.

During the 1980s and 1990s, RU projects were undertaken by numerous hospitals and organizations. These projects were institutional attempts to implement changes in nursing practice based on research findings. During the 1990s, however, the call for research utilization began to be superseded by the push for EBP.

EBP in Nursing

The EBP movement has both advocates and critics. Supporters argue that EBP offers a solution to improving health care quality in cost-constrained environments. EBP is viewed as a rational approach to providing the best possible care with the most cost-effective use of resources. Advocates also note that EBP provides a framework for self-directed lifelong learning that is essential in an era of rapid clinical advances and the information explosion. Critics worry that the advantages of EBP are exaggerated and that individual clinical judgments and patient inputs are being devalued. They are also concerned that, in the current EBP environment, insufficient attention is being paid to the role of qualitative research. Although there is a need for close scrutiny of how the EBP journey unfolds, an EBP path is the one that health care professions will almost surely follow in the years ahead.

Overview of the EBP Movement

One of the cornerstones of EBP is the Cochrane Collaboration, which was founded in the United Kingdom based on the work of British epidemiologist Archie Cochrane. Cochrane published an influential book in the 1970s that drew attention to the dearth of solid evidence about the effects of health care. He called for efforts to make research summaries of clinical trials available to health care providers. This eventually led to the development of the Cochrane Center in Oxford in 1993, and an international partnership called the Cochrane Collaboration, with centers established in over a dozen locations throughout the world. The aim of the collaboration is to help providers make good decisions about health care by preparing and disseminating systematic reviews of the effects of health care interventions.

At about the same time that the Cochrane Collaboration got under way, a group from McMaster Medical School in Canada (including Dr. David Sackett) developed a clinical learning strategy they called *evidence-based medicine*. The evidence-based medicine movement has shifted to a broader conception of using best evidence by all health care practitioners (not just physicians) in a multidisciplinary team.

EBP is considered a major shift for health care education and practice. In the EBP environment, a skillful clinician can no longer rely on a repository of memorized information, but rather must be adept in accessing, evaluating, and using new evidence that emerges in systematic research.

Types of Evidence and Evidence Hierarchies

There is no consensus about the definition of *evidence*, nor about what constitutes usable evidence for EBP, but there is broad agreement that findings from rigorous research are paramount. There is, however, debate about what constitutes "*rigorous*" research and what qualifies as "*best*" evidence.

At the outset of the EBP movement, there was a definite bias toward reliance on information from studies called *randomized controlled trials* (RCTs). This bias stemmed from the fact that the Cochrane Collaboration initially focused on the effectiveness of interventions, rather than on other aspects of health care practice. RCTs are, in fact, very well suited for drawing conclusions about the effects of health care interventions (Chapter 9). The bias in ranking sources of evidence, in terms of questions about effective treatments, led to some resistance to EBP by nurses who felt that evidence from qualitative and non-RCT studies would be ignored.

Positions about the contribution of various types of evidence are less rigid than previously. Nevertheless, most **evidence hierarchies**, which rank types of evidence sources according to the strength of the evidence they provide, look something like the one shown in Figure 2.1. This figure, adapted from schemes presented in several references on EBP (DiCenso et al., 2005; Melnyk & Fineout-Overholt, 2011) shows a 7-level hierarchy that has at its pinnacle systematic reviews of RCTs. That is, the strongest possible evidence according to this hierarchy comes from **systematic reviews** that integrate findings from multiple RCTs using rigorous, methodical procedures. The second rung of the

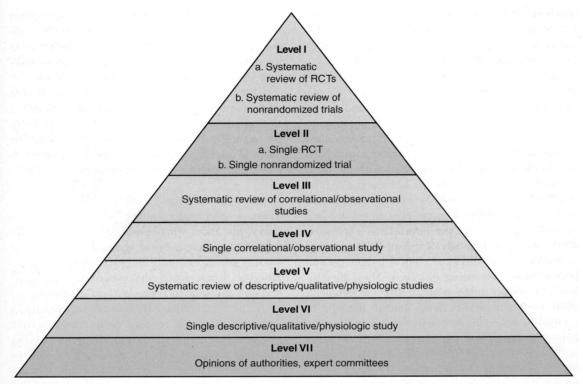

FIGURE 2.1 Evidence hierarchy: levels of evidence regarding the effectiveness of an intervention.

hierarchy is individual RCT studies, and so on (the terms in this hierarchy are explained in subsequent chapters of this book). At the bottom of this evidence hierarchy is opinions from experts.

We cannot emphasize too strongly that this evidence hierarchy is *not* universally appropriate—a point that is not always made sufficiently clear. This hierarchy has merit for ranking evidence for certain types of clinical questions, but not others: it is primarily appropriate with regard to questions about the effects of clinical interventions. For example, a question about the effect of massage therapy on pain in cancer patients would classify evidence according to this hierarchy, but many important questions would not. The hierarchy in Figure 2.1 would not be relevant for ranking evidence for such questions as: What is the experience of pain like for patients with cancer? What percentage of cancer patients experience intense pain, and for how long does the pain persist? Do men and

women with cancer experience similar levels of pain? Chapter 9 discusses different designs for various questions.

Thus, in nursing, *best evidence* refers to findings from research that is methodologically appropriate, rigorous, and clinically relevant for pressing clinical questions—questions not only about the efficacy, safety, and cost-effectiveness of nursing interventions, but also about the reliability and precision of nursing assessment measures, the antecedents or determinants of health and well-being, and the nature of patients' experiences. Confidence in the evidence is enhanced when the research methods are compelling, when there have been multiple confirmatory studies, and when the evidence has been systematically evaluated and synthesized.

Of course, there continue to be clinical practice questions for which there is relatively little research information. In such situations, nursing practice must rely on other sources—for example, bench-marking data, pathophysiologic data, chart review, quality improvement and risk data, and clinical expertise. As Sackett and colleagues (2000) have noted, one benefit of the EBP movement is that a new research agenda can emerge when clinical questions arise for which there is no satisfactory evidence.

EBP Challenges

Nurses have completed many studies about the translation of research into practice, including research on factors that are barriers to EBP. This is an important area of research, because the findings suggest ways in which EBP efforts can be promoted or undermined, and thus raise issues that need to be addressed in advancing evidence-based nursing.

Studies that have explored barriers to EBP have been done in numerous countries and have yielded similar results about constraints on clinical nurses. Most barriers fall into one of three categories: (1) quality and nature of the research, (2) characteristics of nurses, and (3) organizational factors.

With regard to the research, one problem is the limited availability of high-quality research evidence for some practice areas. There remains an ongoing need for research that directly addresses pressing clinical problems, for replication of studies in a range of settings, and for greater collaboration between researchers and clinicians. Another issue is that nurse researchers need to improve their ability to communicate evidence, and the clinical implications of evidence, to practicing nurses.

Nurses' attitudes and education are also potential barriers to EBP. Studies have found that some nurses do not value or know much about research, and others simply resist change. Fortunately, there is growing evidence that many nurses do value research and want to be involved in research-related activities. Nevertheless, many nurses do not know how to access research evidence and do not possess the skills to critically evaluate research findings— and even those who do may not know how to effectively incorporate research evidence into clinical decision making. Among nurses in non–English-speaking countries, another impediment is that most research evidence is reported in English.

Finally, many of the challenges to using research in practice are organizational. "Unit culture" can undermine research use, and administrative and other organizational barriers also play a major role. Although many organizations support the idea of EBP in theory, they do not always provide the necessary supports in terms of staff release time and availability of resources. Nurses' time constraints are a crucial deterrent to the use of evidence at the bedside. Strong leadership in healthcare organizations is essential to making evidence-based practice happen.

RESOURCES FOR EVIDENCE-BASED PRACTICE

The translation of research evidence into nursing practice is an ongoing challenge, but resources to support EBP are now widely available. We urge you to explore other ideas with your health information librarian, because there has been an explosion of EBP resources, and the list is growing as we write.

Preappraised Evidence

Research evidence comes in various forms, the most basic of which is in individual studies. Primary studies published in professional journals are not preappraised for quality and use in practice. Chapter 5 discusses how to access primary studies for a literature review.

Preprocessed (preappraised) evidence is evidence that has been selected from primary studies and evaluated for use by clinicians. DiCenso and colleagues (2005) have described a hierarchy of preprocessed evidence. On the first rung above primary studies are synopses of single studies, followed by systematic reviews, and then synopses of systematic reviews. Clinical practice guidelines are at the top of the hierarchy. A somewhat different hierarchy is offered by Guyatt et al. (2008), who placed a category they called "Systems" (textbook-like resources) at the top. At each successive step in the hierarchy, there is greater ease in applying the evidence to clinical practice. We describe several types of preappraised evidence sources in this section.

Systematic Reviews

Evidence-based practice relies on meticulous integration of research evidence on a topic. The emphasis on *best evidence* in EBP implies that evidence about a clinical problem has been gathered, evaluated, and synthesized so that conclusions can be drawn about the most effective practices. Systematic reviews are a pivotal component of EBP: their "bottom line" is a summary of what the best evidence is at the time the review was written.

A systematic review is not just a literature review, such as ones we describe in Chapter 5. A systematic review is in itself a methodical, scholarly inquiry that follows many of the same steps as those for primary studies. Chapter 27 offers guidelines on conducting and critiquing systematic reviews.

Systematic reviews can take various forms. Until recently, the most common type of systematic review was a traditional narrative integration of research findings. Narrative reviews of quantitative studies are still common, but a type of systematic review called a meta-analysis has emerged as an important EBP tool.

Meta-analysis is a method of integrating quantitative findings statistically. In essence, meta-analysis treats the findings from a study as one piece of information. The findings from multiple studies on the same topic are combined and analyzed statistically. Instead of people being the **unit of analysis** (the basic entity of the analysi), individual studies are the unit of analysis in a meta-analysis. Meta-analysis provides a convenient, objective method of integrating a large body of findings and of observing patterns that might otherwise have gone undetected.

Example of a meta-analysis: Jung and colleagues (2009) conducted a meta-analysis on the effectiveness of fear of falling treatment programs for the elderly. The researchers integrated results from 6 studies. The aggregated evidence indicated that such interventions are effective in decreasing elders' fear of falling.

Integrative reviews of qualitative studies often take the form of metasyntheses, which are rich resources for EBP (Beck, 2009). A **metasynthesis** involves integrating qualitative research findings on a specific topic that are themselves interpretive syntheses of narrative information. A metasynthesis is distinct from a quantitative meta-analysis: A metasynthesis is less about reducing information and more about amplifying and interpreting it. Strategies are also being developed in the area of **mixed methods synthesis**, which are efforts to integrate and synthesize both quantitative and qualitative evidence (Thorne, 2009).

Example of a meta-synthesis: Meeker and Jezewski (2009) did a metasynthesis of 13 studies of the experiences of family members confronted with decisions about withdrawing life-sustaining treatments from seriously ill patients. The analysis suggested that family members engage in a process of decision making that encompasses reframing reality, relating to others, and integrating (reconciling and going on).

Some systematic reviews are published in professional journals that can be accessed using standard literature search procedures; others are available in dedicated databases. In particular, the Cochrane Database of Systematic Reviews contains thousands of systematic reviews (mostly meta-analyses) relating to health care interventions. Cochrane reviews are done with great rigor, and have the advantage of being checked and updated regularly. For interventions that are socially or behaviorally oriented, systematic reviews are available in another resource called the Campbell Collaboration, *www.campbellcollaboration.org*.

Example of Cochrane review: Dobbins and a team of Canadian nurse researchers (2009) summarized evidence on the effectiveness of school-based interventions for promoting physical fitness in children and adolescents. The evidence from 104 studies supported the conclusion that such interventions have positive benefits on some outcomes (e.g., television viewing, blood cholesterol), but little effect on others (e.g., leisure time physical activity, blood pressure).

Many other resources are available for locating systematic reviews, as well as synopses of such reviews. Some of the more prominent ones include the following:

- The Agency for Healthcare Research and Quality (AHRQ) awarded contracts to establish Evidence-Based Practice Centers that issue *evidence reports* (*www.ahrq.gov*).
- The Centre for Reviews and Dissemination at the University of York (England) produces useful systematic reviews (*http://www.york.ac.uk/inst/crd/index.htm*).
- The Joanna Briggs Institute in Australia is another useful source for systematic reviews in nursing and other health fields (*www.joannabriggs.edu.au*).
- In Canada, the Ontario Ministry of Health and Long-Term Care sponsors the Effective Public Health Practice Project (EPHPP), which undertakes and disseminates systematic reviews on health topics (*www.hamilton.ca/phcs/ephpp*).
- The University of Texas Health Science Center offers a search website called SUMSearch that allows you to type in queries for evidence (*http://sumsearch.uthscsa.edu/*).

➲ TIP: Websites cited in this chapter, plus additional websites with useful content relating to EBP, are listed in the Toolkit with the accompanying *Resource Manual*. This will allow you to simply use the "Control/Click" feature to go directly to the website, without having to type in the URL and risk a typographical error.

Clinical Practice Guidelines and Care Bundles

Evidence-based **clinical practice guidelines**, like systematic reviews, represent an effort to distill a large body of evidence into a manageable form, but guidelines are different in a number of respects. First, clinical practice guidelines, which are usually based on systematic reviews, give specific recommendations for evidence-based decision making. Their intent is to influence what clinicians do. Second, guidelines attempt to address all of the issues relevant to a clinical decision, including the balancing of benefits and risks. Third, systematic reviews are evidence-driven—that is, they are undertaken when a body of evidence has been produced and needs to be synthesized. Guidelines, by contrast, are "necessity-driven" (Sackett et al., 2000), meaning that guidelines are developed to guide clinical practice—even when available evidence is limited or of unexceptional quality. Fourth, systematic reviews are done by researchers, but guideline development typically involves the consensus of a group of researchers, experts, and clinicians. For this reason, guidelines based on the same evidence may result in different recommendations that take into account contextual factors—for example, guidelines appropriate in the United States may be unsuitable in Taiwan or Sweden.

Also, organizations are developing and adopting **care bundles**—a concept developed by the Institute for Healthcare Initiatives—that encompass a set of interventions to treat or prevent a specific cluster of symptoms (*www.ihi.org*). There is growing evidence that a combination or bundle of strategies produces better outcomes than a single intervention.

Example of a review of care bundle effects: In a review conducted for an EBP project, O'Keefe-McCarthy and colleagues (2008) found evidence that implementation of a care bundle for ventilator-associated pneumonia is associated with decreased ventilator days, ICU length of stay, and mortality rates.

Guidelines and bundles are available for many diagnostic and therapeutic decisions. Typically, they define a minimum set of services and actions appropriate for certain clinical conditions. Most guidelines allow for a flexible approach in their application to individual patients who fall outside the scope of their guideline (e.g., those with significant comorbidities).

It can be challenging to find clinical practice guidelines because they have proliferated and there is no one single guideline repository. One useful approach is to search for guidelines in comprehensive guideline databases, or through specialty organizations that have sponsored guideline development. It would be impossible to list all possible sources, but a few deserve special mention.

- In the United States, nursing and other health care guidelines are maintained by the National Guideline Clearinghouse (*www.guideline.gov*).
- In Canada, information about clinical practice guidelines can be found through the Registered Nurses Association of Ontario (RNAO) (*www.rnao.org/bestpractices*) and the Canadian Medical Association (*http://mdm.ca/cpgsnew/cpgs/index.asp*).
- In the United Kingdom, two sources for clinical guidelines are the Translating Research into Practice (TRIP) database (*http://www.tripdatabase.com*) and the National Institute for Clinical Excellence (*www.nice.org.uk*).
- Another resource is the EBM-Guidelines, which offer recommendations relative to primary care in several languages (*www.ebm-guidelines.com*).
- The Guidelines International Network makes available guidelines from around the world (*www.g-i-n.net*).

Professional societies and organizations also maintain collections of guidelines of relevance to their area of specialization. In nursing, the Association of Women's Health, Obstetric and Neonatal Nurses (AWHONN) has provided extraordinary leadership in advocating EBP and has developed a host of clinical practice guidelines (*www.awhonn.org*).

In addition to looking for guidelines in national clearinghouses and in the websites of professional organizations, you can search bibliographic databases such as MEDLINE or EMBASE. Search terms such as the following can be used: *practice guideline, clinical practice guideline, best practice guideline, evidence-based guideline, standards,* and *consensus statement.* Be aware, though, that a standard search for guidelines in bibliographic databases will yield many references—but often a frustrating mixture of citations to not only the actual guidelines, but also to commentaries, anecdotes, case studies, and so on.

Example of a nursing clinical practice guideline: In 2008, the RNAO updated a 2005 best practice guideline called "Care and Maintenance to Reduce Vascular Access Complications."

Developed by a panel under the leadership of Susanne Nelson, the guideline "incorporates best practices related to the care and maintenance of vascular access devices applicable to all adult clients requiring this kind of care." (*www.rnao.org*). The guideline offers a repertoire of evidence-based recommendations and indicates the strength of evidence supporting each one.

There are many topics for which practice guidelines have not yet been developed, but the opposite problem is also true: The dramatic increase in the number of guidelines means that there are sometimes multiple guidelines on the same topic. Worse yet, because of variation in the rigor of guideline development and in interpreting the evidence, different guidelines sometimes offer different and even conflicting recommendations. Thus, those who wish to adopt clinical practice guidelines are urged to critically appraise them to identify ones that are based on the strongest and most up-to-date evidence, have been meticulously developed, are user-friendly, and are appropriate for local use. We offer some assistance with these tasks later in this chapter.

Clinical Decision Support Tools

Clinical decision support tools are designed to help nurses and other health care professionals to organize information, guide their assessments, and apply appropriate interventions. Among such decision support tools are **clinical decision rules**, which synthesize the best available evidence into convenient guides for practice (Shapiro & Driever, 2004; Shapiro, 2005). Such decision rules, by standardizing aspects of patient assessments and prescribing specific evidence-based actions, can minimize clinical uncertainty and reduce variations in practice at the bedside.

It has been argued that, to be useful, decision support tools must offer speedy guidance in real time. Technological advances are making such point-of-care decision-making assistance possible. Computerized decisional support (both on computers and personal digital assistants or PDAs) is now available for various clinical settings and specific clinical problems (e.g., Doran, 2009; Doran et al., 2007).

Other Preappraised Evidence

Several other types of preprocessed evidence are useful for EBP. These include the following:

- Synopses of systematic reviews and of single studies are available in evidence-based abstract journals such as *Clinical Evidence* (*www.clinicalevidence.com*) and *Evidence-Based Nursing* (*www.evidencebasednursing.com*). *Evidence-Based Nursing* presents critical summaries of studies and systematic reviews from more than 150 journals.
- An "evidence digest" feature appears in each issue of *Worldviews on Evidence-Based Nursing*. These digests offer concise summaries of clinically important studies, along with practice implications.
- The website Bandolier in the United Kingdom provides abstracts and critical summaries of systematic reviews of health interventions (*www.medicine.ox.ac.uk/bandolier/index.html*).
- AHRQ launched its Healthcare Innovations Exchange program in 2008, which offers a repository of hundreds of effective healthcare innovations (*www.innovations.ahrq.gov*).
- The American Association of Critical-Care Nurses regularly publishes "practice alerts," which

are evidence-based recommendations for practice changes (*www.aacn.org*).
- The Nursing Reference Center™ is a comprehensive reference resource that provides an array of clinical information for nurses, including evidence-based care sheets, best practice guidelines, and point-of-care drug information (*www.ebcohost.com*).

Models for EBP

Several models of EBP have been developed. These models offer frameworks for designing and implementing EBP projects in practice settings. Some models focus on the use of research from the perspective of individual clinicians (e.g., the Stetler Model), but most focus on institutional EBP efforts (e.g., the Iowa Model). Another way to categorize existing models is to distinguish models that are process-oriented models (e.g., the Iowa Model) and models that are explicitly mentor models, such as the Clinical Nurse Scholar Model and the ARCC Model.

The many worthy EBP models are too numerous to list comprehensively, but a few are shown in Box 2.1. For those wishing to follow a formal EBP model, the cited references should be consulted.

BOX 2.1 Selected Models for Evidence-Based Practice

- ACE Star Model of Knowledge Transformation (Academic Center for Education-Based Practice, 2009)
- Advancing Research and Clinical Practice Through Close Collaboration (ARCC) Model (Melnyk & Fineout-Overholt, 2011)
- Clinical Nurse Scholar Model (Schultz, 2005)
- Diffusion of Innovations Theory (Rogers, 1995)
- Framework for Adopting an Evidence-Based Innovation (DiCenso et al., 2005)
- Iowa Model of Evidence-Based Practice to Promote Quality Care (Titler et al., 2001)
- Johns Hopkins Nursing EBP Model (Newhouse et al., 2005)
- Model for Change to Evidence-Based Practice (Rosswurm & Larabee, 1999)
- Ottawa Model of Research Use (Logan & Graham, 1998)
- Pipeline Model (Wimpenny et al., 2008)
- Promoting Action on Research Implementation in Health Services (PARiHS) Model, (Rycroft-Malone et al., 2002)
- Stetler Model of Research Utilization (Stetler, 2001)

Gawlinski and Rutledge (2008) offer suggestions for selecting an EBP model.

Although each model offers different perspectives on how to translate research findings into practice, several of the steps and procedures are similar across the models. The most prominent of these models have been the **Diffusion of Innovations Theory**, the **Stetler Model**, and the **Iowa Model**. The latter two, developed by nurses, were originally crafted with an emphasis on research utilization, but they have been updated to incorporate EBP processes.

We provide an overview of key activities and issues in EBP initiatives, based on a distillation of common elements from EBP models, in a subsequent section of this chapter. We rely especially heavily on the Iowa Model, a diagram for which is shown in Figure 2.2.

Example of the application of an EBP model: Boyer and colleagues (2009) described how Russworm and Larrabee's 6-step model for EBP was used as a guiding framework for an EBP project. The model, which focuses on *planned change*, guided a medical–surgical team in the implementation and evaluation of an evidence-based bladder scanner protocol.

EVIDENCE-BASED PRACTICE IN INDIVIDUAL NURSING PRACTICE

This section and the following one, which are based on the various models of EBP, provide an overview of how research can be used in clinical settings. More extensive guidance is available in textbooks devoted to evidence-based nursing (e.g., Brown, 2009; Craig & Smyth, 2007; DiCenso et al., 2005; Houser & Bokovoy, 2006; Melnyk & Fineout-Overholt, 2011). We first discuss strategies and steps for individual clinicians and then describe activities used by teams of nurses.

Clinical Scenarios and the Need for Evidence

Individual nurses make many decisions and are called upon to provide health care advice, and so

they have ample opportunity to put research into practice. Here are four clinical scenarios that provide examples of such opportunities:

- *Clinical Scenario 1*. You work on an intensive care unit and notice that *Clostridium difficile* infection has become more prevalent among surgical patients in your hospital. You want to know if there is a reliable screening tool for assessing the risk of infection so that preventive measures could be initiated in a more timely and effective manner.
- *Clinical Scenario 2*. You work in a rehabilitation hospital and one of your elderly patients, who had total hip replacement, tells you she is planning a long airplane trip to visit her daughter after rehabilitation treatments are completed. You know that a long plane ride will increase her risk of deep vein thrombosis and wonder if compression stockings are an effective in-flight treatment. You decide to look for the best possible evidence to answer this question.
- *Clinical Scenario 3*. You work in an allergy clinic and notice how difficult it is for many children to undergo allergy scratch tests. You wonder if there is an intervention to help allay children's fears about skin tests when they are being tested for allergens.
- *Clinical Scenario 4*. You are caring for a hospitalized cardiac patient who tells you that he has sleep apnea. He confides in you that he is reluctant to undergo continuous positive airway pressure (CPAP) treatment because he worries it will hinder intimacy with his wife. You wonder if there is any evidence about what it is like to undergo CPAP treatment so that you can better understand how to address your patient's concerns.

In these and thousands of other clinical situations, research evidence can be put to good use to improve the quality of nursing care. Some situations might lead to unit-wide or institution-wide scrutiny of current practices, but in other situations, individual nurses can personally investigate the evidence to help them address specific problems.

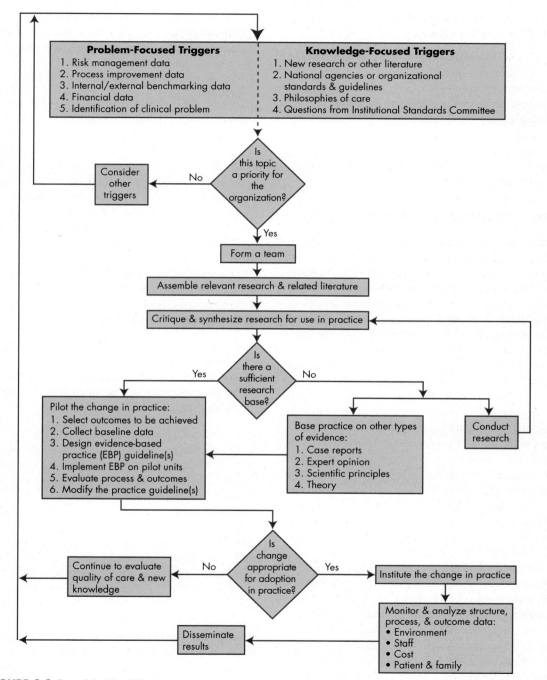

FIGURE 2.2 Iowa Model of Evidence-Based Practice to Promote Quality Care. (Adapted from Titler, et al. [2001]. The Iowa Model of Evidence-Based Practice to Promote Quality Care. *Critical Care Nursing Clinics of North America, 13*, 497–509. Reprinted with permission.)

For individual-level EBP efforts, the major steps in EBP include the following:

1. Asking clinical questions that can be answered with research evidence
2. Searching for and retrieving relevant evidence
3. Appraising and synthesizing the evidence
4. Integrating the evidence with your own clinical expertise, patient preferences, and local context
5. Assessing the effectiveness of the decision, intervention, or advice

Asking Well-Worded Clinical Questions

Converting information needs into well-worded clinical questions that can be answered with research evidence is a crucial first step in EBP. Some EBP writers distinguish between background and foreground questions. *Background questions* are general, foundational questions about a clinical issue, for example: What is cancer cachexia (progressive body wasting)? What is its pathophysiology? Answers to such background questions are typically found in textbooks. *Foreground questions*, by contrast, are those that can be answered based on current best research evidence on diagnosing, assessing, or treating patients, or on understanding the meaning or prognosis of their health problems. For example, we may wonder, is a fish oil–enhanced nutritional supplement effective in stabilizing weight in patients with advanced cancer? The answer to such a question may provide guidance on how best to address the needs of patients with cachexia—that is, the answer provides an opportunity for EBP.

Textbooks on EBP provide guidance on how to phrase clinical foreground questions in a manner that makes it easier to search for an answer. For example, DiCenso and colleagues (2005) and Guyatt and colleagues (2008) advise that, for questions that call for quantitative information (e.g., about the effectiveness of a treatment), three components should be identified:

1. the *population* (What are the characteristics of the patients or clients?);

2. the *intervention or exposure* (What is the intervention of interest? or, What is the potentially harmful exposure about which we are concerned?); and
3. the *outcome* (What is the outcome in which we are interested?).

Dissecting our question about cachexia according to this scheme, our population is cancer patients with advanced cancer or cachexia; the intervention is fish oil–enhanced nutritional supplements; and the outcome is weight stabilization. As another example, in the first clinical scenario about *Clostridium difficile* cited earlier, the population is surgical patients in the ICU, the intervention is a risk assessment tool, and the outcome is early detection of risk for infection.

For questions that can best be answered with qualitative information (e.g., about the meaning of an experience or health problem) DiCenso et al. (2005) suggest two components:

1. the *population* (What are the characteristics of the patients or clients?),
2. the *situation* (What conditions, experiences, or circumstances are we interested in understanding?).

For example, suppose our question was, What is it like to suffer from cachexia? In this case, the question calls for rich qualitative information. The population is patients with advanced cancer, and the situation is the experience of cachexia.

Fineout-Overholt and Johnston (2005) recommended a 5-component scheme for formulating EBP questions, using the acronym PICOT as a guide: population (P), intervention or issue (I), comparison of interest (C), outcome (O), and time (T). Their scheme contrasts an intervention (or issue) with a specific comparison. For example, we might want to learn whether fish oil–enhanced supplements are better than melatonin in stabilizing weight in cancer patients. In some cases, it is important to designate a specific comparison, while in others we might not have a specific comparison in mind. For example, in searching for evidence about the effectiveness of fish oil supplements, we might want to search for studies that compared such supplements to melatonin, placebos, other treatments, or no treatments. The final component in the Fineout-Overholt and Johnston scheme is a time frame, that is, the time frame in which an intervention might be appropriate. Like the "C" component, the "T" is not always needed.

Table 2.1 offers question templates for asking well-framed clinical questions in selected circumstances. The right hand panel includes questions with an explicit comparison (PICO questions), while the left panel does not.

> **TIP:** The Toolkit section of Chapter 2 in the accompanying *Resource Manual* includes Table 2.1 in a Word file that can be adapted for your use, so that the template questions can be readily "filled in." Additional EBP resources from this chapter are also in the Toolkit.

Finding Research Evidence

By asking clinical questions in the forms suggested, you should be able to more effectively search the research literature for the information you need. By using the templates in Table 2.1, the information you insert into the blanks constitute the *keywords* for undertaking an electronic search.

For an individual EBP endeavor, the best place to begin is to search for evidence in a systematic review or other preappraised source because this leads to a quicker answer—and potentially a superior answer as well if your methodologic skills are limited. Researchers who prepare reviews and clinical guidelines usually have strong research skills and use exemplary standards in evaluating the evidence. Moreover, preappraised evidence is usually developed by teams of researchers, which means that the conclusions are cross-validated. Thus, when preprocessed evidence is available to answer a clinical question, you may not need to look any farther, unless the review is not recent. When preprocessed evidence cannot be located or is old, you will need to look for best evidence in primary studies, using strategies we describe in Chapter 5.

> **TIP:** In Chapter 5, we provide guidance on using the free internet resource, PubMed, for searching the bibliographic database MEDLINE®. Of special interest to those engaged in an EBP search, PubMed offers a special resource for those seeking evidence for clinical decisions. The "Clinical Queries" link appears under the heading PubMed Tools on the PubMed Home Page. In another important database, CINAHL®, it is now also possible to delimit a search with a "Clinical Queries" or "Evidence-Based Practice" limiter.

Appraising the Evidence

After locating relevant evidence, it should be appraised before taking clinical action. Critical appraisal for EBP may involve several types of assessments (Box 2.2).

The thoroughness of your appraisal depends on several factors, the most important of which is the nature of the clinical action for which evidence is being sought. Some actions have implications for patient safety, while others are more relevant to patients' satisfaction. Using best evidence to guide nursing practice is important for a wide range of outcomes, but appraisal standards would be especially strict for evidence that could affect patient safety and morbidity.

Evidence Quality

The first appraisal issue is the extent to which the findings are valid. That is, were the study methods sufficiently rigorous that the evidence is credible? We offer guidance on critiquing studies and evaluating the strength of evidence from primary studies throughout this book. If there are several primary studies and no existing systematic review, you would need to draw conclusions about the body of evidence taken as a whole. There are several systems for "grading" the quality of a body of evidence, such as the one developed by AHRQ (*http://www.ahrq.gov/clinic/uspstf/grades.htm#post*), and we discuss integration in Chapter 27. Clearly, you would need to put most weight on the most rigorous studies. Preappraised evidence is already screened and evaluated, but you may still need to judge its integrity.

TABLE 2.1	Question Templates for Selected Clinical Foreground Questions

TYPE OF QUESTION	QUESTION TEMPLATE FOR QUESTIONS *WITHOUT* AN EXPLICIT COMPARISON	QUESTION TEMPLATE FOR QUESTIONS *WITH* AN EXPLICIT COMPARISON (PICO)
Treatment/ Intervention	In _____ (population), what is the effect of _____ (intervention) on _____ (outcome)?	In _____ (population), what is the effect of _____ (intervention), in comparison to _____ (comparative/ alternative intervention), on _____ (outcome)?
Diagnosis/ assessment	For _____ (population), does _____ (tool/procedure) yield accurate and appropriate diagnostic/assessment information about _____ (outcome)?	For _____ (population), does _____ (tool/procedure) yield more accurate or more appropriate diagnostic/assessment information than _____ (comparative tool/procedure) about _____ (outcome)?
Prognosis	For _____ (population), does _____ (disease or condition) increase the risk of or influence _____ (outcome)?	For _____ (population), does _____ (disease or condition), relative to _____ (comparative disease or condition) increase the risk of or influence _____ (outcome)?
Causation/ Etiology/ Harm	Does _____ (exposure or characteristic) increase the risk of _____ (outcome) in _____ (population)?	Does _____ (exposure or characteristic) increase the risk of _____ (outcome) compared to _____ (comparative exposure or condition) in _____ (population)?
Meaning or Process	What is it like for _____ (population) to experience _____ (condition, illness, circumstance)? OR What is the process by which _____ (population) cope with, adapt to, or live with _____ (condition, illness, circumstance)?	(Explicit comparisons not typical in these types of question)

BOX 2.2 Questions for Appraising the Evidence

What is the quality of the evidence—that is, how rigorous and reliable is it?
What *is* the evidence—what is the magnitude of effects?
How precise is the estimate of effects?
What evidence is there of any side effect or side benefits?
What is the financial cost of applying (and not applying) the evidence?
Is the evidence relevant to my particular clinical situation?

Magnitude of Effects

You also need to assess what the results actually *are*, and whether they are clinically important. This criterion considers not whether the results are valid, but what they are and how powerful are the effects. For example, consider clinical scenario number 2 cited earlier, which leads to the following clinical question: Does the use of compression stockings lower the risk of flight-related deep vein thrombosis for high-risk patients? In our search, we find a relevant systematic review in the nursing literature—a meta-analysis of nine randomized controlled trials (Hsieh & Lee, 2005)—and another in the Cochrane database (Clarke et al., 2006). The conclusion of these reviews, based on reliable evidence, is that compression stockings are effective and the magnitude of the effect, in terms of risk reduction, is fairly substantial. Thus, advice about the use of compression stockings may be appropriate, pending an appraisal of other factors.

Determining the magnitude of the effect for quantitative findings is especially important when an intervention is costly or when there are potentially negative side effects. If, for example, there is good evidence that an intervention is only marginally effective in improving a health problem, it is important to consider other factors (e.g., evidence of effects on quality of life).

There are various ways to quantify the magnitude of effects, many of which are described later in this book. An index known as the *effect size*, for example, can provide estimates of the magnitude of effects for outcomes for which average values can be computed (e.g., average body temperature). When outcomes can be dichotomized (e.g., occurrence versus nonoccurrence of a health problem), estimates of magnitude of the effect can be calculated as *absolute risk reduction (ARR)* or *relative risk reduction (RRR)*. For example, if the RRR for the use of compression stockings was 50%, this would mean that this intervention reduced the risk of deep vein thrombosis by 50%, relative to what would occur in its absence. We describe methods of calculating these and other related indexes in Chapter 16.

Precision of Estimates

Another consideration, relevant with quantitative evidence, is how precise the estimate of effect is. This level of appraisal requires some statistical sophistication, and so we postpone our discussion of *confidence intervals* to Chapter 17. Suffice it to say that research results provide only an estimate of effects and it is useful to understand not only the exact estimate, but also the range within which the actual effect probably lies.

Peripheral Effects

If the evidence is judged to be valid and the magnitude of effects supports further consideration, supplementary information may still be important in guiding decisions. One issue concerns peripheral benefits and costs, evidence for which would typically have emerged during your search. In framing your clinical question, you would have identified the key outcomes in which you were interested—for example, weight stabilization or weight gain for interventions to address cancer cachexia. Primary research on this topic, however, would likely have examined other outcomes that would need to be taken into account—for example, quality of life, side effects, satisfaction, and so on.

Financial Issues

Another issue concerns the financial cost of using the evidence. In some cases, costs may be small or nonexistent. For example, in clinical scenario 4, where the question concerned the experience of CPAP treatment, nursing action would be cost-neutral because the evidence would be used to provide information and reassurance to the patient. Some interventions, however, are costly and so the amount of resources needed to put best evidence into practice would need to be factored into any decision. Of course, while the cost of a clinical decision needs to be considered, the cost of *not* taking action is equally important.

Clinical Relevance

Finally, it is important to appraise the evidence in terms of its relevance for the clinical situation at hand—that is, for *your* patient in a specific clinical setting. Best practice evidence can most readily be applied to an individual patient in your care if he or she is similar to people in the study or studies under review. Would your patient have qualified for participation in the study—or is there some factor such as age, illness severity, or comorbidity that would have excluded him or her? DiCenso and colleagues (2005), who advised clinicians to ask whether there is some compelling reason to conclude that the results may *not* be applicable in their clinical situation, have written some useful tips on applying research results to individual patients.

Actions Based on Evidence Appraisals

Appraisals of the evidence may lead you to different courses of action. You may reach this point and conclude that the evidence is not sufficiently sound, or that the likely effect is too small, or that the cost of applying the evidence is too high. The integration of appraisal information may suggest that "usual care" is the best strategy—or it may suggest the need for a new EBP inquiry. For instance, in the example about cachexia, you likely would have learned that recent best evidence suggests that fish oil–enhanced nutritional supplements may be an ineffective treatment (Dewey et al., 2007). However, during your search you may have come across a Cochrane review that concluded that megestrol acetate improves appetite and weight gain in patients with cancer (Berenstein & Ortiz, 2005). This may lead to a new evidence inquiry and to discussions with other members of your health care team about nutrition protocols for your clinical setting. If, however, the initial appraisal of evidence suggests a promising clinical action, then you can proceed to the next step.

Integrating Evidence

As the definition for EBP implies, research evidence needs to be integrated with other types of information, including your own clinical expertise and knowledge of your clinical setting. You may be aware of factors that would make implementation of the evidence, no matter how sound or promising, inadvisable.

Patient preferences and values are also important. A discussion with the patient may reveal negative attitudes toward a potentially beneficial course of action, contraindications (e.g., comorbidities), or possible impediments (e.g., lack of health insurance).

One final issue is the importance of integrating evidence from qualitative research, which can provide rich insights about how patients experience a problem, or about barriers to complying with a treatment. A new intervention with strong potential benefits may fail to achieve desired outcomes if it is not implemented with sensitivity and understanding of the patients' perspectives. As Morse (2005) has so aptly noted, evidence from an RCT may tell you whether a pill is effective, but qualitative research can help you understand why patients may not swallow the pill.

Implementing the Evidence and Evaluating Outcomes

After the first four steps of the EBP process have been completed, you can use the resulting information to make an evidence-based decision or to provide research-informed advice. Although the steps in the process, as just described, may seem complicated, in reality the process can be efficient—*if* there is an adequate evidence base, and especially if it has been skillfully preprocessed. EBP is most challenging when findings from research are contradictory, inconclusive, or "thin"—that is to say, when better quality evidence is needed.

One last step in an individual EBP effort concerns evaluation. Part of the evaluation involves determining if your action achieved the desired outcome. Another part concerns an evaluation of how well you are performing EBP. Sackett and colleagues (2000) offer self-evaluation questions that relate to the five EBP steps, such as asking answerable questions (Am I asking any clinical questions at all? Am I asking well-formulated questions?) and finding external evidence (Do I know the best sources of current evidence? Am I becoming more efficient in my searching?). A self-appraisal may lead you to conclude that at least some of the clinical questions in which you are interested are best addressed as a group effort.

EVIDENCE-BASED PRACTICE IN AN ORGANIZATIONAL CONTEXT

Most nurses practice in organizations, such as hospitals or long-term care settings. For some clinical scenarios that trigger an EBP effort, individual nurses may have sufficient autonomy that they can implement research-informed actions on their own (e.g., answering questions about experiences with CPAP). In many situations, however, decisions are best made among a team of nurses working together to solve a common clinical problem. This section describes some additional considerations that are relevant to institutional efforts at EBP—efforts designed to result in a formal policy or protocol affecting the practice of many nurses.

Many of the steps in organizational EBP projects are similar to the ones described in the previous section. For example, asking questions and gathering and appraising evidence are key activities in both. However, there are additional issues of relevance at the organizational level.

Selecting a Problem for an Organizational EBP Project

An institutional EBP effort can emerge in response to clinical scenarios such as those presented earlier, but can also arise in other contexts such as quality improvement efforts. Some EBP projects are "bottoms-up" efforts that originate in discussions among clinicians who propose problem-solving innovations with their supervisors. Others are "top-down" efforts in which administrators take steps to stimulate creative thought and the use of research evidence among clinicians. This latter approach often occurs as part of the Magnet recognition process.

Several EBP models distinguish two types of "triggers" for an EBP project—(1) *problem-focused triggers*—a clinical practice problem in need of solution, or (2) *knowledge-focused triggers*—readings in the research literature. Problem-focused triggers may arise in the normal course of clinical practice, as in the clinical scenarios described earlier. A problem-focused approach is likely to have staff support if the problem is widespread.

A second catalyst, knowledge-focused triggers, is research evidence itself. Sometimes this catalyst is a new clinical guideline, and in other cases, the impetus emerges from discussions in a journal club. For EBP projects with knowledge-focused triggers, an assessment of clinical relevance might be needed—that is, will a problem of significance to nurses in that setting be solved by introducing an innovation? Titler and Everett (2001) offered suggestions for selecting interventions, using concepts from Rogers' Diffusion of Innovations Model.

With both types of triggers, consensus about the problem's importance and the need for improving practice is crucial. In the Iowa Model (see Figure 2.2), the first decision point involves determining whether the topic is a priority for the organization considering practice changes. Titler and colleagues (2001) advised that, when finalizing a topic, the following issues be taken into account: the topic's fit with the organization's strategic plan, the magnitude of the problem, the number of people invested in the problem, support of nurse leaders and of those in other disciplines, costs, and possible barriers to change.

Addressing Practical Issues in Organizational EBP Efforts

The most pervasive barriers to EBP are organizational, and so one upfront issue is that nurse administrators need to create structures and processes that facilitate research translation. Nursing leaders can support EBP as an approach to clinical decision making in many ways, including providing nurses with sufficient time away from their daily clinical responsibilities to undertake EBP activities, making available financial and material resources, and developing collaborations with mentors who can provide guidance and direction in the search for and appraisal of evidence.

In an organizational EBP project, some practical matters should be resolved even before a search for evidence begins. One issue concerns the team itself. A motivated and inspiring team leader is essential. The recruitment and development of EBP team members often requires an interdisciplinary perspective. Identifying tasks to be undertaken, developing a realistic timetable and budget, assigning members to tasks, and scheduling meetings are necessary to ensure that the effort will progress. Finally, it is wise for the team to solicit the support of stakeholders who might affect project activities and the eventual implementation of EBP changes.

Finding and Appraising Evidence for Organizational EBP

For an organizational EBP effort, the best possible scenario involves identifying an appropriate clinical practice guideline, care bundle, or other decision support tool that has been based on rigorous research evidence. For some problem areas, however, clinical guidelines will need to be *developed* based on the evidence and not just implemented or adapted for use.

If a relevant guideline is identified, it should be carefully appraised. Several guideline appraisal instruments are available, but the one that has gained the broadest support is the Appraisal of Guidelines

Research and Evaluation (AGREE) Instrument (AGREE Collaboration, 2001). This tool has been translated into over a dozen languages and has been endorsed by the World Health Organization. The AGREE instrument consists of ratings of quality on a 4-point scale (strongly agree, agree, disagree, and strongly disagree) for 23 quality dimensions organized in six domains: scope and purpose, stakeholder involvement, rigor of development, clarity and presentation, application, and editorial independence. As examples, one of the statements in the Scope and Purpose domain is: "The patients to whom the guideline is meant to apply are specifically described"; one of the statements in the Rigor of Development domain is: "The guideline has been externally reviewed by experts prior to its publication." The AGREE instrument should be applied to the guideline under consideration by a team of 2 to 4 appraisers. The instrument and instructions for its use are available at *www.agreecollaboration.org*.

One final issue is that guidelines change more slowly than the evidence. If a high-quality guideline is not recent, it is advisable to determine whether more up-to-date evidence would alter (or strengthen) the guideline's recommendations. It has been recommended that, to avoid obsolescence, guidelines should be reassessed for validity every 3 years.

Making Decisions Based on Evidence Appraisals

In the Iowa Model, the synthesis and appraisal of research evidence provides the basis for a second major decision. The crux of the decision concerns whether the evidence is sufficient to justify an EBP change—for example, whether an existing clinical practice guideline is of sufficient quality that it can be used or adapted locally, or whether (in the absence of a guideline) research evidence is sufficiently rigorous to recommend a practice innovation.

Coming to conclusions about the adequacy of research evidence can result in several possible outcomes leading to different paths. If the research base is weak, the team could either abandon the EBP project, or they could assemble other types of evidence (e.g., through consultation with experts or surveys of clients) and assess whether these sources suggests a practice change. Another possibility is to pursue an original clinical study to address the question directly. This course of action may be impractical and would result in years of delay before conclusions could be drawn. If, on the other hand, there is a solid evidence base or a high-quality clinical practice guideline, then the team could develop plans for moving forward with implementing a practice innovation.

Assessing Implementation Potential

In some EBP models, the next step is the development and testing of the innovation, followed by an assessment of organizational "fit." Other models recommend early steps to assess the appropriateness of the innovation within the organizational context. In some cases, such an assessment may be warranted even before searching for and appraising evidence. We think an early assessment of the *implementation potential* (or *environmental readiness*) of a clinical innovation is often sensible, although there are situations with little need for a formal assessment.

In determining the implementation potential of an innovation in a particular setting, several issues should be considered, particularly the transferability of the innovation, the feasibility of implementing it, and its cost–benefit ratio.

- *Transferability*. The main transferability issue is whether it makes sense to implement the innovation in your practice setting. If some aspects of the setting are fundamentally incongruent with the innovation—in terms of its philosophy, type of clients served, staff, or administrative structure—then it might not make sense to try to adopt the innovation, even if there is evidence of clinical effectiveness in other contexts. One possibility, however, is that some organizational changes could be made to make the "fit" better.
- *Feasibility*. Feasibility questions address practical concerns about the availability of staff and resources, the organizational climate, the need

for and availability of external assistance, and the potential for clinical evaluation. An important issue is whether nurses will have, or share, control over the innovation. If nurses will not have control over a new procedure, the interdependent nature of the project should be identified early so that the EBP team will have needed interdisciplinary representatives.
- *Cost–benefit ratio*. A critical part of a decision to proceed with an EBP project is a careful assessment of costs and benefits of the change. The cost–benefit assessment should encompass likely costs and benefits to various groups (e.g., clients, nurses, and the overall organization). If the degree of risk in introducing an innovation is high, then potential benefits must be great and the evidence must be very sound. A cost–benefit assessment should consider the opposite side of the coin as well: the costs and benefits of *not* instituting an innovation. The status quo bears its own risks and failure to change—especially when such change is based on firm evidence—can be costly to clients, to organizations, and to the entire nursing community.

➔ **T I P :** The Toolkit for Chapter 2 in the *Resource Manual* has a worksheet with a series of questions for assessing the implementation potential of a potential innovation.

If the implementation assessment suggests that there might be problems in testing the innovation in that particular practice setting, then the team can either begin the process anew with a different innovation, or pursue a plan to improve the implementation potential (e.g., seeking external resources if costs were the inhibiting factor).

➔ **T I P :** Documentation of all steps in the EBP process, including the implementation potential of an innovation, is highly recommended. Committing ideas to writing is useful because it can help to resolve ambiguities, serve as a problem-solving tool if problems emerge, and be used to persuade others of the value of the project. All aspects of the EBP project should be transparent.

Developing Evidence-Based Protocols

If the implementation criteria are met and the evidence is adequate, the team can prepare an action plan to move the effort forward, which includes laying out strategies for designing and piloting the new clinical practice. In most cases, a key activity will involve developing a local evidence-based clinical practice protocol or guideline, or adapting an existing one.

If a relevant clinical practice guideline has been judged to be of sufficiently high quality, the EBP team needs to decide whether to (1) adopt it in its entirety, (2) adopt only certain recommendations, while disregarding others (e.g., recommendations for which the evidence is less sound), or (3) make adaptations deemed necessary based on local circumstances. The risk in modifying guidelines is that the adaptation will not adequately incorporate the research evidence.

If there is no existing clinical practice guideline, or if existing guidelines are weak, the team will need to develop its own protocol or guideline reflecting the accumulated research evidence. Strategies for developing clinical practice guidelines are suggested in most textbooks on EBP and in several handbooks (e.g., Turner et al., 2008). Whether a guideline is developed "from scratch" or adapted from an existing one, independent peer review is advisable to ensure that the guidelines are clear, comprehensive, and congruent with best existing evidence.

> **TIP:** Guidelines should be user-friendly. Visual devices such as flow charts and decision trees are often useful.

Implementing and Evaluating the Innovation

Once an EBP protocol has been developed, the next step is to **pilot test** it (give it a trial run) in a clinical setting and to evaluate the outcome. Building on the Iowa Model, this phase of the project likely would involve the following activities:

1. Developing an evaluation plan (e.g., identifying outcomes to be achieved, deciding how many clients to involve, settling on when and how often to collect outcome information)
2. Collecting information on the outcomes prior to implementing the innovation, to develop a comparison against which the outcomes of the innovation can be assessed
3. Training staff in the use of the new protocol and, if necessary, "marketing" the innovation to users so that it is given a fair test
4. Trying the protocol out on one or more units or with a group of clients
5. Evaluating the pilot project, in terms of both process (e.g., how was the innovation received, what implementation problems were encountered?) and outcomes (e.g., how were outcomes affected, what were the costs?)

> **TIP:** DiCenso and her colleagues (2002) have developed a toolkit designed to facilitate the implementation of clinical practice guidelines. The toolkit is available at *www.rnao.org.*

A variety of research strategies and designs can be used to evaluate the innovation (see Chapter 11). In most cases, an informal evaluation will be adequate, for example, comparing outcome information from hospital records before and after the innovation and gathering information about patient and staff satisfaction. Qualitative information can also contribute to the evaluation: qualitative data can uncover subtleties about the implementation process and help to explain findings.

Evaluation information should be gathered over a sufficiently long period (6 to 12 months) to allow for a true test of a "mature" innovation. An even longer timeframe is useful for learning about the *sustainability* of an innovation. The end result is a decision about whether to adopt the innovation, to modify it for ongoing use, or to revert to prior practices. Another advisable step is to disseminate the results so that other nurses and nursing administrators can benefit. Finally, the EBP team should develop a plan for when the new protocol will be reviewed and, if necessary, updated based on new research evidence or ongoing feedback about outcomes.

TIP: Every nurse can play a role in using research evidence. Here are some strategies:

- *Read widely and critically.* Professionally accountable nurses keep abreast of important developments and read journals relating to their specialty, including research reports in them.
- *Attend professional conferences.* Nursing conferences include presentations of studies with clinical relevance. Conference attendees have opportunities to meet researchers and to explore practice implications.
- *Insist on evidence that a procedure is effective.* Every time nurses or nursing students are told about a standard nursing procedure, they have a right to ask: Why? Nurses need to develop expectations that the clinical decisions they make are based on sound, evidence-based rationales.
- *Become involved in a journal club.* Many organizations that employ nurses sponsor journal clubs that review studies with potential relevance to practice. The traditional approach for a journal club (nurses coming together as a group to discuss and critique an article) is in some settings being replaced with online journal clubs that acknowledge time constraints and the inability of nurses from all shifts to come together at one time.
- *Pursue and participate in EBP projects.* Several studies have found that nurses who are involved in research activities (e.g., an EBP project or data collection activities) develop more positive attitudes toward research and better research skills.

RESEARCH EXAMPLE

Thousands of EBP projects are underway in practice settings. Many that have been described in the nursing literature offer useful information about planning and implementing such an endeavor. One is described here, and another full article is included in the *Resource Manual*.

Study: Care of the patient with enteral tube feeding: An evidence-based protocol (Kenny & Goodman, 2010)

Purpose: The TriService Nursing Research Program sought to create a culture of incorporating best evidence into nursing practices in military hospitals throughout the United States. Kenny and Goodman's article described a protocol development and testing project that was implemented at a large military medical center under that initiative. The purpose of this project was to understand the evidence for managing enteral tube feedings in adult patients, to develop and implement an evidence-based protocol, and to evaluate its effects. A secondary aim was to educate the nursing staff about the EBP process.

Framework: The project used the Iowa Model as its guiding framework. The decision to select enteral feedings was based on a serious patient sentinel event, and so had a problem-focused trigger.

Protocol Development: When the project began, nursing practice relating to enteral feedings in the medical center was based on tradition, and varied from nurse to nurse. The topic had support from clinical nursing staff and administrators, and fit with organizational priorities. A project team was formed of nurses, a physician, a clinical nurse specialist, and a nutrition care specialist. The team met regularly for about 6 months to review evidence and develop a protocol. The work began with a thorough review and "grading" of existing evidence on managing enteral tube feedings. The evidence base was not especially strong, but the team identified many practices with sufficient research support to craft a set of recommendations. The team developed relevant educational materials (e.g., one-page *Nursing Cliff Notes*, tabletop education in a tripanel acrylic sign holder), and offered inservice sessions on each ward to explain the new protocol and its evidence base.

Evaluation: The outcomes of the project were assessed at three levels: patient, nursing, and organization. At the patient level, outcomes were assessed using anecdotal reports of tube clogging incidents. Nursing outcomes included knowledge of evidence-based intervention (measured before and after the protocol implementation), and process measures to examine compliance with the new protocol, as measured on a documentation checklist. The organizational outcome was actions performed by executives demonstrating support of the EBP model.

Findings and Conclusions: Anecdotal data supported a tentative conclusion of better patient outcomes (e.g., a decrease in clogged tubes). There was a significant increase in staff knowledge and implementation of evidence-based processes. The authors concluded that "the project has infused the creation of a culture of value for EBP from the level of the clinical staff nurse to the nursing executive level" (p. S29).

⬤⬤⬤⬤⬤⬤⬤⬤⬤⬤⬤⬤⬤⬤⬤⬤⬤⬤⬤⬤

SUMMARY POINTS

- **Evidence-based practice (EBP)** is the conscientious integration of current best evidence with clinical expertise and patient preferences in making clinical decisions; it is a clinical problem-solving strategy that de-emphasizes decision making based on custom.
- **Research utilization (RU)** and EBP are overlapping concepts that concern efforts to use research as a basis for clinical decisions, but RU *starts* with a research-based innovation that gets evaluated for possible use in practice.
- Two underpinnings of the EBP movement are the Cochrane Collaboration (which is based on the work of British epidemiologist Archie Cochrane), and the clinical learning strategy called *evidence-based medicine* developed at the McMaster Medical School.
- EBP typically involves weighing various types of evidence in an effort to determine *best evidence*; an **evidence hierarchy** may be used to rank study findings according to the strength of evidence provided. Hierarchies for evaluating evidence about health care interventions typically put systematic reviews of *randomized controlled trials* (RCTs) at the pinnacle.
- Resources to support EBP are growing at a phenomenal pace. Among the resources are systematic reviews (and electronic databases that make them easy to locate); evidence-based clinical practice guidelines, care bundles, and other decision support tools; a wealth of other preappraised evidence that makes it possible to practice EBP efficiently; and models of EBP that provide a framework for undertaking EBP efforts.
- **Systematic reviews** are rigorous integrations of research evidence from multiple studies on a topic. Systematic reviews can involve either qualitative, narrative approaches to integration (including **metasynthesis** of qualitative studies), or quantitative methods (**meta-analysis**) that integrate findings statistically.

- Evidence-based **clinical practice guidelines** combine a synthesis and appraisal of research evidence with specific recommendations for clinical decision making. Clinical practice guidelines should be carefully and systematically appraised, for example using the Appraisal of Guidelines Research and Evaluation (AGREE) instrument.
- **Care bundles**, which encompass a set of interventions to treat or prevent a cluster of symptoms, are another research-based strategy that can be used in EBP.
- Many models of EBP have been developed, including models that provide a framework for individual clinicians (e.g., the **Stetler Model**) and others for organizations or teams of clinicians (e.g., the **Iowa Model** of Evidence-Based Practice to Promote Quality Care). Another widely used model is Rogers' **Diffusion of Innovations Theory**.
- Individual nurses can put research into practice, using 5 basic steps: (1) framing an answerable clinical question, (2) searching for relevant research evidence, (3) appraising and synthesizing the evidence, (4) integrating evidence with other factors, and (5) assessing effectiveness.
- An appraisal of the evidence involves such considerations as the validity of study findings, their clinical importance, the precision of estimates of effects, associated costs and risks, and utility in a particular clinical situation.
- EBP in an organizational context involves many of the same steps as an individual EBP effort, but tends to be more formalized and must take organizational and interpersonal factors into account. "Triggers" for an organizational project include both pressing clinical problems and existing knowledge.
- Team-based or organizational EBP projects typically involve the development or adaptation of clinical protocols. Before these products can be tested, there should be an assessment of the *implementation potential* of the innovation, which includes the dimensions of transferability of findings, feasibility of using the findings in the new setting, and the cost–benefit ratio of a new practice.

- Once an evidence-based protocol or guideline has been developed and deemed worthy of implementation, the team can move forward with a **pilot test** of the innovation and an assessment of the outcomes prior to widespread adoption.

STUDY ACTIVITIES

Chapter 2 of the *Resource Manual for Nursing Research: Generating and Assessing Evidence for Nursing Practice, 9th ed.*, offers study suggestions for reinforcing concepts presented in this chapter. In addition, the following questions can be addressed in classroom or online discussions:

1. Think about your own clinical situation and identify a problem area. Now, pose a well-worded clinical question using the templates in Table 2.1. Identify the various components of the question—that is, population, intervention or issue, comparison, and outcome.
2. Discuss the overall approach used in the example featured at the end of this chapter (Kenny & Goodman, 2010).

STUDIES CITED IN CHAPTER 2

Berenstein, E. G., & Ortiz, Z. (2005). Megestrol acetate for the treatment of anorexia-cachexia syndrome. *Cochrane Database of Systematic Reviews,* No. CD004310.

Boyer, D., Steltzer, N., & Larrabee, J. (2009). Implementation of an evidence-based bladder scanner protocol. *Journal of Nursing Care Quality, 24,* 10–16.

Clarke, M., Hopewell, S., Juszczak, E., Eisinga, A., & Kjeldstrom, M. (2006). Compression stockings for preventing deep vein thrombosis in airline passengers. *Cochrane Database of Systematic Reviews,* No. CD004002.

Dewey, A., Baughan, C., Dean, T., Higgins, B., & Johnson, I. (2007). Eicosapentaenoic acid (EPA, an omega-3 fatty acid from fish oils) for the treatment of cancer cachexia. *Cochrane Database of Systematic Reviews,* No. CD004597.

Dobbins, M., DeCorby, K., Robeson, P., Husson, H., Trillis, D. (2009). School-based physical activity programs for promoting physical activity and fitness in children and adolescents aged 6-18. *Cochrane Database of Systematic Reviews, 21,* No. CD007651.

Doran, D. (2009). The emerging role of PDAs in information use and clinical decision making. *Evidence Based Nursing, 12,* 35–38.

Doran, D., Mylopoulos, J., Kushniruk, A., Nagle, L., Laurie-Shaw, Sidani, S., Tourangeau, A. E., Lefebre, N., Reid-Haughian, C., Carryer, J. R., Cranley, L. A., & McArthur, G. (2007). Evidence in the palm of your hand: Development of an outcomes-focused knowledge translation intervention. *Worldviews of Evidence-Based Nursing, 4,* 69–77.

Estabrooks, C. A. (1999). The conceptual structure of research utilization. *Research in Nursing & Health, 22,* 203–216.

Hsieh, H. F., & Lee, F. P. (2005). Graduated compression stockings as prophylaxis for flight-related venous thrombosis: Systematic literature review. *Journal of Advanced Nursing, 51,* 83–98.

Jung, D., Lee, J., & Lee, S. (2009). A meta-analysis of fear of falling treatment programs for the elderly. *Western Journal of Nursing Research, 31,* 6–16.

Kenny, D. J., & Goodman, P. (2010). Care of the patient with enteral tube feeding: An evidence-based practice protocol. *Nursing Research, 59,* S22–S31.

Meeker, M., & Jezewski, M. (2009). Metasynthesis: Withdrawing life-sustaining treatments—the experience of family decision makers. *Journal of Clinical Nursing, 18,* 163–173.

O'Keefe-McCarthy, S., Santiago, C., & Lau, G. (2008). Ventilator-associated pneumonia bundled strategies: An evidence-based practice. *Worldview of Evidence-Based Nursing, 5,* 193–204.

Methodologic and nonresearch references cited in this chapter can be found in a separate section at the end of the book.

3 | Key Concepts and Steps in Qualitative and Quantitative Research

This chapter covers a lot of ground—but, for many of you, it is familiar ground. For those who have taken an earlier research course, this chapter provides a review of key terms and steps in the research process. For those without previous exposure to research methods, this is an important chapter that offers basic grounding in research terminology.

Research, like any discipline, has its own language—its own *jargon*. Some terms are used by both qualitative and quantitative researchers, but others are used predominantly by one or the other group. To make matters more complex, much of the jargon used in nursing research has its roots in the social sciences, but sometimes different terms for the same concepts are used in medical research; we cover both but acknowledge that social science jargon predominates.

FUNDAMENTAL RESEARCH TERMS AND CONCEPTS

When researchers address a problem through research—regardless of the underlying paradigm—they undertake a **study** (or an **investigation**). Studies involve various people working together in different roles.

The Faces and Places of Research

Studies with humans involve two sets of people: those who do the research and those who provide the information. In a quantitative study, the people being studied are called **subjects** or **study participants** (Table 3.1). In a qualitative study, the individuals cooperating in the study are called **informants**, **key informants**, or study participants. Collectively, both in qualitative and quantitative studies, study participants comprise the **sample**.

The person who conducts a study is the **researcher** or **investigator**. Studies are often undertaken by several people. When a study is done by a team, the person directing the study is the **principal investigator (PI)**. Two or three researchers collaborating equally are **co-investigators**. **Reviewers** are sometimes called on to critique a study and offer feedback. If these people are at a similar level of experience to the researchers, they are **peer reviewers**.

In large-scale projects, dozens of individuals may be involved in planning, managing, and conducting the study. The examples of staffing configurations that follow span the continuum from an extremely large project to a more modest one.

Examples of staffing on a quantitative study: The first author of this book was involved in a multicomponent, interdisciplinary study of poor

	TABLE 3.1	Key Terms in Quantitative and Qualitative Research

CONCEPT	QUANTITATIVE TERM	QUALITATIVE TERM
Person Contributing Information	Subject Study participant —	— Study participant Informant, key informant
Person Undertaking the Study	Researcher Investigator	Researcher Investigator
That Which Is Being Investigated	— Concepts Constructs Variables	Phenomena Concepts — —
System of Organizing Concepts	Theory, theoretical framework Conceptual framework, conceptual model	Theory Conceptual framework, sensitizing framework
Information Gathered	Data (numerical values)	Data (narrative descriptions)
Connections Between Concepts	Relationships (cause-and- effect, functional)	Patterns of association
Logical reasoning processes	Deductive reasoning	Inductive reasoning

women living in four major cities (Cleveland, Los Angeles, Miami, and Philadelphia). As part of the study, she and two colleagues prepared a report documenting the health problems of about 4,000 welfare mothers who were interviewed in 1998 and again in 2001 (Polit et al., 2001). The project staff included over 100 people, including 2 co-PIs; lead investigators (Polit was one) of 6 project components; over 50 interviewers and supervisors; and dozens of other researchers, research assistants, computer programmers, and other support staff. Several health consultants, including a prominent nurse researcher (Linda Aiken), were reviewers.

Examples of staffing on a qualitative study:
Beck (2009) conducted a qualitative study focusing on the experiences of mothers caring for their children with a brachial plexus injury. The team consisted of Beck as the PI (who gathered and analyzed all the data), members of the United Brachial Plexus

Executive Board (who helped to recruit mothers for the study), a transcriber (who listened to the tape-recorded interviews and typed them up verbatim), and an undergraduate nursing student (who checked the accuracy of the interview transcripts against the tape-recorded interviews). (Beck's study appears in its entirety in the accompanying *Resource Manual*).

Research can be undertaken in a variety of *settings* (the specific places where information is gathered), and in one or more *sites*. Some studies take place in **naturalistic settings** in the field, such as in people's homes, but some studies are done in controlled **laboratory settings**. Researchers make decisions about where to conduct a study based on the nature of the research question and type of information needed. Qualitative researchers are especially likely to engage in **fieldwork** in natural settings because they are interested in the contexts of people's experiences. The *site* is the overall location for the research—it could be an entire community (e.g., a Haitian neighborhood in Miami) or an institution (e.g., a hospital in Toronto). Researchers sometimes engage in **multisite studies** because the use of multiple sites offers a larger or more diverse sample of study participants.

The Building Blocks of Research

Phenomena, Concepts, and Constructs

Research involves abstractions. For example, *pain, quality of life*, and *resilience* are abstractions of particular aspects of human behavior and characteristics. These abstractions are called **concepts** or, in qualitative studies, **phenomena**.

Researchers may also use the term **construct**. Like a concept, a construct is an abstraction inferred from situations or behaviors. Kerlinger and Lee (2000) distinguish concepts from constructs by noting that constructs are abstractions that are deliberately and systematically invented (constructed) by researchers. For example, *self-care* in Orem's model of health maintenance is a construct. The terms *construct* and *concept* are sometimes used interchangeably but, by convention, a construct refers to a more complex abstraction than a concept.

Theories and Conceptual Models

A **theory** is a systematic, abstract explanation of some aspect of reality. Theories, which knit concepts together into a coherent system, play a role in both qualitative and quantitative research.

Quantitative researchers may start with a theory, *framework*, or *conceptual model* (distinctions are discussed in Chapter 6). Based on theory, they make predictions about how phenomena will behave in the real world *if the theory is true*. Specific predictions deduced from theory are tested through research; results are used to support, reject, or modify the theory.

In qualitative research, theories may be used in various ways. Sometimes conceptual or **sensitizing frameworks**, derived from qualitative research traditions we describe later in this chapter, provide an impetus for a study or offer an orienting world view. In such studies, the framework helps to guide the inquiry and to interpret gathered information. In other qualitative studies, theory is the *product* of the research: The investigators use information from participants inductively to develop a theory rooted in the participants' experiences. The goal is to develop a theory that explains phenomena *as they exist*, not as they are preconceived.

Variables

In quantitative studies, concepts are usually called **variables**. A variable, as the name implies, is something that varies. Weight, anxiety, and blood pressure are variables—each varies from one person to another. In fact, most aspects of humans are variables. If everyone weighed 150 pounds, weight would not be a variable, it would be a *constant*. It is precisely because people and conditions *do* vary that most research is conducted. Quantitative researchers seek to understand how or why things vary, and to learn if differences in one variable are related to differences in another. For example, lung cancer research is concerned with the variable of lung cancer, which is a variable because not everyone has this disease. Researchers have studied factors that might be linked to lung cancer, such as cigarette smoking. Smoking is also a variable because not everyone smokes. A variable, then, is any quality of a person, group, or situation that varies or takes on different values. Variables are the building blocks of quantitative studies.

When an attribute is extremely varied in the group under study, the group is **heterogeneous** with respect to that variable. If the amount of variability is limited, the group is **homogeneous**. For example, for the variable height, a group of 2-year-old children is likely to be more homogeneous than a group of 18-year-olds. Degree of **variability** or **heterogeneity** of a group of people has implications for study design.

Variables may be inherent characteristics of people, such as their age, blood type, or weight. Sometimes, however, researchers *create* a variable. For example, if a researcher tests the effectiveness of patient-controlled analgesia as opposed to intramuscular analgesia in relieving pain after surgery, some patients would be given patient-controlled analgesia and others would receive intramuscular analgesia. In the context of this study, method of pain management is a variable because different patients get different analgesic methods.

Continuous, Discrete, and Categorical Variables. Some variables take on a wide range of values. A person's age, for instance, can take on values from zero to more than 100, and the values are not restricted to whole numbers. **Continuous variables** have values along a continuum and, in theory, can assume an infinite number of values between two points. Consider the continuous variable *weight*: between 1 and 2 pounds, the number of values is limitless: 1.05, 1.8, 1.333, and so on.

By contrast, a **discrete variable** has a finite number of values between any two points, representing discrete quantities. For example, if people were asked how many children they had, they might answer 0, 1, 2, 3, or more. The value for number of children is discrete, because a number such as 1.5 is not meaningful. Between 1 and 3, the only possible value is 2.

Other variables take on a small range of values that do not represent a *quantity*. Blood type, for example, has four values—A, B, AB, and O. Variables that take on a handful of discrete nonquantitative values are **categorical variables**. When categorical variables take on only two values, they are **dichotomous variables**. Gender, for example, is dichotomous: male and female.

Dependent and Independent Variables. Many studies seek to unravel and understand causes of phenomena. Does a nursing intervention *cause* improvements in patient outcomes? Does smoking *cause* lung cancer? The presumed cause is the **independent variable**, and the presumed effect is the **dependent variable**. Some researchers use the term **outcome variable**—the variable capturing the outcome of interest—in lieu of dependent variable.

Variability in the dependent variable is presumed to *depend on* variability in the independent variable. For example, researchers study the extent to which lung cancer (the dependent variable) depends on smoking (the independent variable). Or, investigators may study the extent to which patients' pain (the dependent variable) depends on different nursing actions (the independent variable).

Frequently, the terms *independent variable* and *dependent variable* are used to indicate *direction of influence* rather than a causal mechanism. For example, suppose a researcher studied the mental health of caregivers caring for spouses with Alzheimer's disease and found better mental health outcomes for wives than for husbands. The researcher might be unwilling to conclude that caregivers' mental health was *caused* by gender. Yet the direction of influence clearly runs from gender to mental health: It makes *no* sense to suggest that caregivers' mental health influenced their gender! Although the researcher cannot infer a cause-and-effect connection, it is appropriate to conceptualize mental health as the dependent variable and gender as the independent variable, because it is the caregivers' mental health that the researcher is interested in understanding, explaining, or predicting.

Most dependent variables have multiple causes or antecedents. If we were studying factors that influence people's weight, we might consider their height, physical activity, and diet as independent variables. Two or more *dependent* variables also may be of interest. For example, a researcher may compare the effects of two methods of nursing care for children with cystic fibrosis. Several dependent variables could be used to assess treatment effectiveness, such as length of hospital stay, number of recurrent respiratory infections, and so on. It is common to design studies with multiple independent and dependent variables.

Variables are not *inherently* dependent or independent. A dependent variable in one study could be an independent variable in another. For example, a study might examine the effect of a nurse-initiated exercise intervention (the independent variable) on osteoporosis (the dependent variable). Another study might investigate the effect of osteoporosis (the independent variable) on bone fracture incidence (the dependent variable). In short, whether a variable is independent or dependent is a function of the role that it plays in a particular study.

> **Example of independent and dependent variables:** *Research question:* Do women with diabetes differ from those without diabetes in terms of cancer screening behaviors? (Marshall et al., 2010)
> *Independent variable:* Status of having or not having diabetes
> *Dependent variable:* Cancer screening behaviors

Conceptual and Operational Definitions

Study concepts need to be defined and explicated, and dictionary definitions are seldom adequate. Two types of definitions are of particular relevance—conceptual and operational.

Concepts are abstractions of observable phenomena, and researchers' world views shapes how those concepts are defined. A **conceptual definition** presents the abstract or theoretical meaning of the concepts being studied. Even seemingly straightforward terms need to be conceptually defined. The classic example is the concept of *caring*. Morse and colleagues (1990) scrutinized the works of numerous writers to determine how *caring* was defined, and identified five different classes of conceptual definition: as a human trait, a moral imperative, an affect, an interpersonal relationship, and a therapeutic intervention. Researchers undertaking studies concerned with caring need to make clear which conceptual definition they have adopted—both to themselves and to their readers. In qualitative studies, conceptual definitions of key phenomena may be the major end product of the endeavor, reflecting the intent to have the meaning of concepts defined by those being studied.

In quantitative studies, however, researchers clarify and define concepts at the outset. This is necessary because quantitative researchers must indicate how the variables will be observed and measured. An **operational definition** of a concept specifies the operations that researchers must perform to measure it. Operational definitions should be congruent with conceptual definitions.

Variables differ in the ease with which they can be operationalized. The variable *weight*, for example, is easy to define and measure. We might operationally define weight as the amount that an object weighs, to the nearest full pound. This definition designates that weight will be measured using one system (pounds) rather than another (grams). We could also specify that weight will be measured using a spring scale with participants fully undressed after 10 hours of fasting. This operational definition clearly indicates what we mean by the variable *weight*.

Few variables are operationalized as easily as weight. Most variables can be measured in different ways, and researchers must choose the one that best captures the variables as they conceptualize them. Take, for example, *anxiety*, which can be defined in terms of both physiologic and psychological functioning. For researchers choosing to emphasize physiologic aspects, the operational definition might involve a physiologic measure such as the Palmar Sweat Index. If researchers conceptualize anxiety as a psychological state, the operational definition might involve a paper-and-pencil measure such as the State Anxiety Scale. Readers of research articles may not agree with how variables were conceptualized and measured, but definitional precision has the advantage of communicating exactly what terms mean within the study.

> **Example of conceptual and operational definitions:** Schim, Doorenbos, and Borse (2006) tested an intervention to expand cultural competence among hospice workers. Cultural competence encompassed several aspects, such as cultural awareness, which was conceptually defined as a care provider's knowledge about areas of cultural expression in which cultural groups may differ. The researchers measured their constructs with the Cultural Competence Assessment (CCA) instrument. The CCA operationalizes cultural awareness by having healthcare staff indicate their level of agreement with such statements as, "I understand that people from different cultural groups may define the concept of 'healthcare' in different ways."

Data

Research **data** (singular, datum) are the pieces of information obtained in a study. In quantitative

---

BOX 3.1 Example of Quantitative Data

Question: Thinking about the past week, how depressed would you say you have been on a scale from 0 to 10, where 0 means "not at all" and 10 means "the most possible"?

Data:
9 (Subject 1)
0 (Subject 2)
4 (Subject 3)

---

studies, researchers identify variables, develop conceptual and operational definitions, and then collect relevant data. Quantitative researchers collect primarily **quantitative data**—data in numeric form. For example, suppose we conducted a quantitative study in which a key variable was depression. We might ask, "Thinking about the past week, how depressed would you say you have been on a scale from 0 to 10, where 0 means 'not at all' and 10 means 'the most possible'?" Box 3.1 presents quantitative data for three fictitious people. Subjects provided a number along the 0 to 10 continuum representing their degree of depression—*9* for subject 1 (a high level of depression), *0* for subject 2 (no depression), and *4* for subject 3 (little depression). The numeric values for all people, collectively, would comprise the data on depression.

In qualitative studies, researchers collect **qualitative data**, that is, narrative descriptions. Narrative information can be obtained by having conversations with participants, by making detailed notes about how people behave in naturalistic settings, or by obtaining narrative records, such as diaries. Suppose we were studying depression qualitatively. Box 3.2 presents qualitative data for three people responding conversationally to the question, "Tell me about how you've been feeling lately—have you felt sad or depressed at all, or have you generally been in good spirits?" The data consist of rich descriptions of each participant's emotional state.

Relationships

Researchers are rarely interested in isolated concepts, except in descriptive studies. For example, a researcher might describe the percentage of patients receiving intravenous (IV) therapy who experience IV infiltration. In this example, the variable is IV

BOX 3.2 Example of Qualitative Data

Question: Tell me about how you've been feeling lately—have you felt sad or depressed at all, or have you generally been in good spirits?

Data: "Well, actually, I've been pretty depressed lately, to tell you the truth. I wake up each morning and I can't seem to think of anything to look forward to. I mope around the house all day, kind of in despair. I just can't seem to shake the blues, and I've begun to think I need to go see a shrink." (Participant 1)

"I can't remember ever feeling better in my life. I just got promoted to a new job that makes me feel like I can really get ahead in my company. And I've just gotten engaged to a really great guy who is very special." (Participant 2)

"I've had a few ups and downs the past week, but basically things are on a pretty even keel. I don't have too many complaints." (Participant 3)

infiltration versus no infiltration. Usually, however, researchers study phenomena in relation to other phenomena—that is, they focus on relationships. A **relationship** is a bond or a connection between phenomena. For example, researchers repeatedly have found a *relationship* between cigarette smoking and lung cancer. Both qualitative and quantitative studies examine relationships, but in different ways.

In quantitative studies, researchers examine the relationship between the independent and dependent variables. The research question asks whether variation in the dependent variable is systematically related to variation in the independent variable. Relationships are usually expressed in quantitative terms, such as *more than*, *less than*, and so on. For example, let us consider as our dependent variable a person's weight. What variables are related to (associated with) body weight? Some possibilities are height, caloric intake, and exercise. For each independent variable, we can make a prediction about its relationship to the dependent variable:

Height: Taller people will weigh more than shorter people.
Caloric intake: People with higher caloric intake will be heavier than those with lower caloric intake.
Exercise: The lower the amount of exercise, the greater will be the person's weight.

Each statement expresses a predicted relationship between weight (the dependent variable) and a measurable independent variable. Terms such as *more than* and *heavier than* imply that as we observe a change in one variable, we are likely to observe a change in weight. If Nate were taller than Tom, we would predict (in the absence of any other information) that Nate is also heavier than Tom.

Quantitative studies can address one or more of the following questions about relationships:

- Does a relationship between variables *exist*? (e.g., is cigarette smoking related to lung cancer?)
- What is the *direction* of the relationship between variables? (e.g., are people who smoke *more* likely or *less* likely to get lung cancer than those who do not?)

- How *strong* is the relationship between the variables? (e.g., how powerful is the link between smoking and lung cancer? How much higher is the risk that smokers will develop lung cancer?)
- What is the *nature* of the relationship between variables? (e.g., does smoking *cause* lung cancer? Does some other factor *cause* both smoking and lung cancer?)

As the last question suggests, variables can be related to one another in different ways. One type of relationship is called a **cause-and-effect** (or **causal**) **relationship**. Within the positivist paradigm, natural phenomena are assumed not to be haphazard; they have antecedent causes that are presumably discoverable. In our example about a person's weight, we might speculate that there is a causal relationship between caloric intake and weight: consuming more calories causes weight gain. As noted in Chapter 1, many quantitative studies are *cause-probing*—they seek to illuminate the causes of phenomena.

Example of a study of causal relationships:
Lin and colleagues (2010) studied whether a therapeutic lifestyle program caused reductions in cardiac risk factors following coronary artery bypass graft surgery.

Not all relationships between variables can be interpreted as cause-and-effect relationships. There is a relationship, for example, between a person's pulmonary artery and tympanic temperatures: people with high readings on one tend to have high readings on the other. We cannot say, however, that pulmonary artery temperature *caused* tympanic temperature, nor that tympanic temperature *caused* pulmonary artery temperature. This type of relationship is called a **functional** (or an **associative**) **relationship** rather than a causal relationship.

Example of a study of functional relationships:
Al-Akour and co-researchers (2010) examined the relationship between quality of life among Jordanian adolescents with type 1 diabetes on the one hand, and gender and age on the other.

Qualitative researchers are not concerned with quantifying relationships, nor in testing causal relationships. Qualitative researchers seek patterns of association as a way to illuminate the underlying meaning and dimensionality of phenomena. Patterns of interconnected themes and processes are identified as a means of understanding the whole.

Example of a qualitative study of patterns: Gaudine and colleagues (2010) studied HIV-related stigma in a Vietnamese community. In-depth interviews were conducted with people living with HIV, family members, community members, and healthcare professionals. The researchers identified four dimensions of HIV-related stigma, the manifestation of which differed for each group.

MAJOR CLASSES OF QUANTITATIVE AND QUALITATIVE RESEARCH

Researchers usually work within a paradigm that is consistent with their world view, and that gives rise to questions that excite their curiosity. The maturity of the focal concept also may lead to one or the other paradigm: When little is known about a topic, a qualitative approach is often more fruitful than a quantitative one. In this section, we briefly describe broad categories of quantitative and qualitative research.

Quantitative Research: Experimental and Nonexperimental Studies

A basic distinction in quantitative studies is between experimental and nonexperimental research. In **experimental research**, researchers actively introduce an intervention or treatment. In **nonexperimental research**, researchers are bystanders—they collect data without intervening. For example, if a researcher gave bran flakes to one group of people and prune juice to another to evaluate which method facilitated elimination more effectively, the study would be experimental because the researcher intervened in the normal course of things. If, however, a researcher compared elimination patterns of two groups of people whose regular eating patterns

differed—for example, some normally took foods that stimulated bowel elimination and others did not—there is no intervention, and the study is nonexperimental. In medical and epidemiologic research, an experimental study usually is called a **clinical trial**, and a nonexperimental inquiry is called an **observational study**. As we discuss in Chapter 11, a *randomized controlled trial* or RCT is a particular type of clinical trial.

Experimental studies are explicitly cause-probing—they test whether an intervention *caused* changes in (affected) the dependent variable. Sometimes nonexperimental studies also seek to elucidate or detect causal relationships, but the resulting evidence is usually less conclusive. Experimental studies offer the possibility of greater control over confounding influences than nonexperimental studies, and so, causal inferences are more plausible.

Example of experimental research: Twiss and colleagues (2009) tested the effect of an exercise intervention for breast cancer survivors with bone loss on the women's muscle strength, balance, and fall frequency. Some women received the 24-month intervention, and others did not.

In this example, the researcher intervened by giving some patients the opportunity to participate in the exercise program, while others were not given this opportunity. In other words, the researcher *controlled* the independent variable, which in this case was the exercise intervention.

Example of nonexperimental research: Vallance and co-researchers (2010) studied factors that predicted exercise and physical activity among breast cancer survivors. They examined the association between physical activity on the one hand and demographic, psychosocial, and motivational factors measured 6 months earlier on the other.

This nonexperimental study did not involve an intervention. The researchers were interested in similar variables as in the previously described experimental study (physical activity and exercise) and in a similar population (patients with breast cancer), but their intent was to explore existing relationships rather than to evaluate an intervention.

Qualitative Research: Disciplinary Traditions

The majority of qualitative studies can best be described as **qualitative descriptive research**. Many qualitative studies, however, are rooted in research traditions that originated in anthropology, sociology, and psychology. Three such traditions, prominent in qualitative nursing research, are briefly described here. Chapter 19 provides a fuller discussion of these traditions and the methods associated with them.

The **grounded theory** tradition, with roots in sociology, seeks to describe and understand the key social psychological processes that occur in a social setting. Grounded theory was developed in the 1960s by two sociologists, Glaser and Strauss (1967). The focus of most grounded theory studies is on a developing social experience—the social and psychological stages and phases that characterize a particular event or episode. A major component of grounded theory is the discovery of a *core variable* that is central in explaining what is going on in that social scene. Grounded theory researchers strive to generate explanations of phenomena that are grounded in reality.

Example of a grounded theory study: Propp and colleagues (2010) conducted a grounded theory study to examine critical healthcare team processes. They identified specific nurse–team communication practices that were perceived by team members to enhance patient outcomes.

Phenomenology, rooted in a philosophical tradition developed by Husserl and Heidegger, is concerned with the lived experiences of humans. Phenomenology is an approach to thinking about what life experiences of people are like and what they mean. The phenomenological researcher asks the questions: What is the *essence* of this phenomenon as experienced by these people? Or, what is the meaning of the phenomenon to those who experience it?

Example of a phenomenological study: Schachman (2010) conducted in-depth interviews to explore the lived experience of first-time fatherhood from the perspective of military men deployed to combat regions during birth.

Ethnography is the primary research tradition within anthropology, and provides a framework for studying the lifeways and experiences of a defined cultural group. Ethnographers typically engage in extensive fieldwork, often participating in the life of the culture under study. Ethnographic research is in some cases concerned with broadly defined cultures (e.g., Hmong refugee communities), but sometimes focuses on more narrowly defined cultures (e.g., the culture of an emergency department). Ethnographers strive to learn from members of a cultural group, to understand their world view, and to describe their customs and norms.

Example of an ethnographic study: Hessler (2009) conducted ethnographic fieldwork to investigate physical activity and active play among rural preschool children.

MAJOR STEPS IN A QUANTITATIVE STUDY

In quantitative studies, researchers move from the beginning of a study (posing a question) to the end point (obtaining an answer) in a reasonably linear sequence of steps that are broadly similar across studies. In some studies, the steps overlap; in others, certain steps are unnecessary. Still, a general flow of activities is typical in a quantitative study (See Figure 3.1). This section describes that flow, and the next section describes how qualitative studies differ.

Phase 1: The Conceptual Phase

Early steps in a quantitative study typically have a strong conceptual or intellectual element. These activities include reading, conceptualizing, theorizing, and reviewing ideas with colleagues or advisers. During this phase, researchers call on such skills as creativity, deductive reasoning, and a firm grounding in previous research on the topic of interest.

Step 1: Formulating and Delimiting the Problem

Quantitative researchers begin by identifying an interesting, significant research problem and

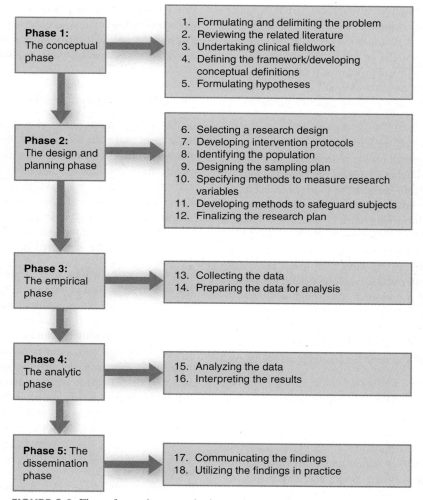

FIGURE 3.1 Flow of steps in a quantitative study.

formulating **research questions**. Good research depends to a great degree on good questions. In developing research questions, nurse researchers must attend to substantive issues (What kind of new evidence is needed?), theoretical issues (Is there a conceptual context for understanding this problem?), clinical issues (How could evidence from this study be used in clinical practice?), methodologic issues (How can this question best be studied to yield high-quality evidence?), and ethical issues (Can this question be rigorously addressed without committing ethical transgressions?).

➲ T I P : A critical ingredient in developing good research questions is personal interest. Begin with topics that fascinate you or about which you have a passionate interest or curiosity.

Step 2: Reviewing the Related Literature
Quantitative research is typically conducted in the context of previous knowledge. To contribute new

evidence, quantitative researchers strive to understand existing evidence. A thorough **literature review** provides a foundation on which to base new evidence and usually is conducted before data are collected. For clinical problems, it may also be necessary to learn the "status quo" of current procedures, and to review existing practice guidelines or protocols.

Step 3: Undertaking Clinical Fieldwork

Unless the research problem originated in a clinical setting, researchers embarking on a clinical nursing study benefit from spending time in clinical settings, discussing the problem with clinicians and administrators, and observing current practices. Clinical fieldwork can provide perspectives on recent clinical trends, current diagnostic procedures, and relevant healthcare-delivery models; it can also help researchers better understand clients and the settings in which care is provided. Such fieldwork can also be valuable in gaining access to an appropriate site or in developing methodologic strategies. For example, in the course of clinical fieldwork researchers might discover the need for research assistants who are bilingual.

Step 4: Defining the Framework and Developing Conceptual Definitions

Theory is the ultimate aim of science: It transcends the specifics of a particular time, place, and group and aims to identify regularities in the relationships among variables. When quantitative research is performed within the context of a theoretical framework, the findings may have broader significance and utility. Researchers should have a conceptual rationale and conceptual definitions of key variables.

Step 5: Formulating Hypotheses

A **hypothesis** is a statement of the researcher's expectations or predictions about relationships among study variables. The research question identifies the study concepts and asks how the concepts might be related; a hypothesis is the predicted answer. For example, the research question might be: Is preeclamptic toxemia related to stress during pregnancy? This might be translated into the following hypothesis: Women with high levels of stress during pregnancy will be more likely than women with lower stress to experience preeclamptic toxemia. Most quantitative studies are designed to test hypotheses through statistical analysis.

Phase 2: The Design and Planning Phase

In the second major phase of a quantitative study, researchers make decisions about the methods they will use to address the research question. Researchers usually have considerable flexibility in designing a study, and they make many decisions. These methodologic decisions have crucial implications for the integrity of the resulting evidence. If the methods used to collect and analyze research data are flawed, then the evidence from the study may have little value.

Step 6: Selecting a Research Design

The **research design** is the overall plan for obtaining answers to the research questions. Many experimental and nonexperimental research designs are available. In designing the study, researchers select a specific design and identify strategies to minimize bias. Research designs indicate how often data will be collected, what types of comparisons will be made, and where the study will take place. The research design is the architectural backbone of the study.

Step 7: Developing Protocols for the Intervention

In experimental research, researchers actively intervene, which means that participants are exposed to different treatment conditions. For example, if we were interested in testing the effect of biofeedback in treating hypertension, the independent variable would be biofeedback compared with either an alternative treatment (e.g., relaxation), or no treatment. An **intervention protocol** for the study must be developed, specifying exactly what the biofeedback treatment would entail (e.g., who would administer it, how frequently, over how long a period the treatment would last, and so on) *and* what the alternative condition would be. The goal of well-articulated protocols is to have all people in each group treated in the same way. (In nonexperimental research, this step is not necessary.)

Step 8: Identifying the Population to be Studied

Quantitative researchers need to clarify the group to whom study results can be generalized—that is, they must identify the population to be studied. A **population** is *all* the individuals or objects with common, defining characteristics. For example, the population of interest might be all patients undergoing chemotherapy in San Diego.

Step 9: Designing the Sampling Plan

Researchers collect data from a sample, which is a subset of the population. Using samples is more practical than collecting data from an entire population, but the risk is that the sample might not reflect the population's traits. In a quantitative study, a sample's adequacy is assessed by its size and **representativeness**. The quality of the sample depends on how typical, or representative, the sample is of the population. The **sampling plan** specifies how the sample will be selected and recruited, and how many subjects there will be.

Step 10: Specifying Methods to Measure Research Variables

Quantitative researchers must develop or borrow methods to measure the research variables accurately. Based on the conceptual definitions, researchers identify appropriate methods to operationalize variables and collect the data. The primary methods of data collection are *self-reports* (e.g., interviews), *observations* (e.g., observing the sleep–wake state of infants), and *biophysiologic measurements*. Measuring research variables and developing a **data collection plan** are challenging activities.

Step 11: Developing Methods to Safeguard Human/Animal Rights

Most nursing research involves humans, and so procedures need to be developed to ensure that the study adheres to ethical principles. Each aspect of the study plan needs to be scrutinized to determine whether the rights of participants have been adequately protected. A formal presentation to an ethics committee is often required.

Step 12: Reviewing and Finalizing the Research Plan

Before collecting their data, researchers often take steps to ensure that plans will work smoothly. For example, they may evaluate the *readability* of written materials to determine if participants with low reading skills can comprehend them, or they may *pretest* their measuring instruments to see if they work well. Normally, researchers also have their research plan critiqued by peers, consultants, or other reviewers before implementing it. Researchers seeking financial support submit a **proposal** to a funding source, and reviewers usually suggest improvements.

Phase 3: The Empirical Phase

The empirical phase of quantitative studies involves collecting data and preparing the data for analysis. Often, the empirical phase is the most time-consuming part of the investigation. Data collection typically requires many weeks, or even months, of work.

Step 13: Collecting the Data

The actual collection of data in quantitative studies often proceeds according to a preestablished plan. The plan specifies where and when the data will be gathered, procedures for describing the study to participants, and methods for recording information. Technological advances have expanded possibilities for automating data collection.

Step 14: Preparing the Data for Analysis

Data collected in a quantitative study are rarely amenable to direct analysis—preliminary steps are needed. One such step is **coding**, which is the process of translating verbal data into numeric form. For example, patients' responses to a question about their gender might be coded "1" for female and "2" for male (or vice versa). Another preliminary step involves entering the data onto computer files for analysis.

Phase 4: The Analytic Phase

Quantitative data are not reported in *raw* form (i.e., as a mass of numbers). They are subjected to analysis and interpretation, which occurs in the fourth major phase of a project.

Step 15: Analyzing the Data

Quantitative researchers analyze their data through **statistical analyses**, which include simple procedures (e.g., computing an average) as well as ones that are complex. Some analytic methods are computationally formidable, but the underlying logic of statistical tests is fairly easy to grasp. Computers have eliminated the need to get bogged down with mathematic operations.

Step 16: Interpreting the Results

Interpretation involves making sense of study results and examining their implications. Researchers attempt to explain the findings in light of prior evidence, theory, and their own clinical experience—and in light of the adequacy of the methods, they used in the study. Interpretation also involves envisioning how the new evidence can best be used in clinical practice, and what further research is needed.

Phase 5: The Dissemination Phase

In the analytic phase, the researcher comes full circle: questions posed at the outset are answered. Researchers' responsibilities are not completed, however, until study results are disseminated.

Step 17: Communicating the Findings

A study cannot contribute evidence to nursing practice if the results are not shared. Another—and often final—task of a study, therefore, is the preparation of a **research report** that summarizes the study. Research reports can take various forms: dissertations, journal articles, conference presentations, and so on. Journal articles—reports appearing in such professional journals as *Nursing Research*—usually are the most useful because they are available to a broad, international audience. We discuss journal articles later in this chapter.

Step 18: Utilizing the Findings in Practice

Ideally, the concluding step of a high-quality study is to plan for the use of the evidence in practice settings. Although nurse researchers may not themselves be able to implement a plan for using the evidence, they can contribute to the process by including in their research reports recommendations regarding how the study evidence could be used in practice, by ensuring that adequate information has been provided for a meta-analysis, and by pursuing opportunities to disseminate the findings to clinicians.

ACTIVITIES IN A QUALITATIVE STUDY

Quantitative research involves a fairly linear progression of tasks—researchers plan the steps to be taken to maximize study integrity and then follow those steps as faithfully as possible. In qualitative studies, by contrast, the progression is closer to a circle than to a straight line—qualitative researchers are continually examining and interpreting data and making decisions about how to proceed based on what has already been discovered (Figure 3.2).

Because qualitative researchers have a flexible approach, it is impossible to define the flow of activities in a study precisely—the flow varies from one study to another, and researchers themselves do not know ahead of time exactly how the study will proceed. We try to provide a sense of how qualitative studies are conducted, however, by describing some major activities and indicating how and when they might be performed.

Conceptualizing and Planning a Qualitative Study

Identifying the Research Problem

Qualitative researchers usually begin with a broad topic area, focusing on an aspect of a topic that is poorly understood and about which little is known. They may not pose refined research questions at the outset. The general topic area may be narrowed and clarified on the basis of self-reflection and discussion with others, but researchers may proceed

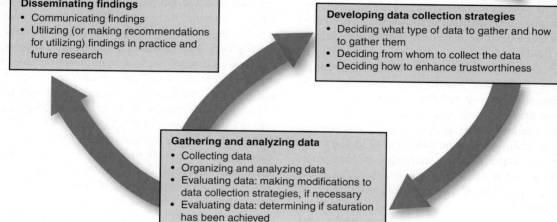

Planning the study
- Identifying the research problem
- Doing a literature review
- Developing an overall approach
- Selecting and gaining entrée into research sites
- Developing methods to safeguard participants

Disseminating findings
- Communicating findings
- Utilizing (or making recommendations for utilizing) findings in practice and future research

Developing data collection strategies
- Deciding what type of data to gather and how to gather them
- Deciding from whom to collect the data
- Deciding how to enhance trustworthiness

Gathering and analyzing data
- Collecting data
- Organizing and analyzing data
- Evaluating data: making modifications to data collection strategies, if necessary
- Evaluating data: determining if saturation has been achieved

FIGURE 3.2 Flow of activities in a qualitative study.

initially with a fairly broad research question that allows the focus to be delineated more clearly, once the study is underway.

Doing a Literature Review

Qualitative researchers do not all agree about the value of an upfront literature review. Some believe that researchers should not consult the literature before collecting data, because prior studies could influence conceptualization of the focal phenomenon. In this view, the phenomena should be explicated based on participants' viewpoints rather than on prior knowledge. Those sharing this opinion often do a literature review at the end of the study. Other researchers conduct a brief preliminary review to get a general grounding. Still others believe that a full early literature review is appropriate. In any case, qualitative researchers typically find a fairly small body of relevant

previous work because of the types of question they ask.

Selecting and Gaining Entrée into Research Sites

Before going into the field, qualitative researchers must identify an appropriate site. For example, if the topic is the health beliefs of the urban poor, an inner-city neighborhood with low-income residents must be identified. Researchers may need to engage in anticipatory fieldwork to identify a suitable and information-rich environment for the study. In some cases, researchers have ready access to the study site, but in others, they need to **gain entrée**. A site may be well suited to the needs of the research, but if researchers cannot "get in," the study cannot proceed. Gaining entrée typically involves negotiations with **gatekeepers** who have the authority to permit entry into their world.

Developing an Overall Approach in Qualitative Studies

Quantitative researchers do not collect data until the research design has been finalized. Qualitative researchers, by contrast, use an **emergent design** that materializes during the course of data collection. Certain design features may be guided by the qualitative research tradition within which the researcher is working, but nevertheless, few qualitative studies adopt rigidly structured designs that prohibit changes while in the field.

Although qualitative researchers do not always know in advance exactly how the study will progress, they nevertheless must have some sense of how much time is available for fieldwork and must also arrange for and test needed equipment, such as tape recorders or laptop computers. Other planning activities include such tasks as hiring and training interviewers to assist in the collection of data, securing interpreters if the informants speak a different language, and hiring appropriate consultants, transcribers, and support staff.

Addressing Ethical Issues

Qualitative researchers, like quantitative researchers, must also develop plans for addressing ethical issues—and, indeed, there are special concerns in qualitative studies because of the more intimate nature of the relationship that typically develops between researchers and study participants. Chapter 7 describes these concerns.

Conducting a Qualitative Study

In qualitative studies, the tasks of sampling, data collection, data analysis, and interpretation typically take place iteratively. Qualitative researchers begin by talking with or observing a few people with first-hand experience with the focal phenomenon. The discussions and observations are loosely structured, allowing for the expression of a full range of beliefs, feelings, and behaviors. Analysis and interpretation are ongoing, concurrent activities that guide choices about the kinds of people to sample next and the types of questions to ask or observations to make.

Data analysis involves clustering together related types of narrative information into a coherent scheme. As analysis and interpretation progress, researchers begin to identify **themes** and categories, which are used to build a rich description or theory of the phenomenon. The kinds of data obtained and the people selected as participants tend to become increasingly purposeful as the conceptualization is developed and refined. Concept development and verification shape the sampling process—as a conceptualization or theory develops, the researcher seeks participants who can confirm and enrich the theoretical understandings, as well as participants who can potentially challenge them and lead to further theoretical development.

Quantitative researchers decide upfront how many people to include in a study, but qualitative researchers' sampling decisions are guided by the data. Qualitative researchers use the principle of **data saturation**, which occurs when themes and categories in the data become repetitive and redundant, such that no new information can be gleaned by further data collection.

Quantitative researchers seek to collect high-quality data by using measuring instruments that have been demonstrated to be accurate and valid. Qualitative researchers, by contrast, must take steps to demonstrate the *trustworthiness* of the data while in the field. The central feature of these efforts is to confirm that the findings accurately reflect the experiences and viewpoints of participants. One confirmatory activity, for example, involves going back to participants and sharing preliminary interpretations with them so that they can evaluate whether the researcher's thematic analysis is consistent with their experiences.

Qualitative researchers sometimes need to develop appropriate strategies for leaving the field. Because qualitative researchers may develop strong relationships with participants and entire communities, they need to be sensitive to the fact that their departure might seem like a form of abandonment. Graceful departures and methods of achieving closure are important.

Disseminating Qualitative Findings

Qualitative nursing researchers also strive to share their findings with others at conferences and in journal articles. Qualitative findings, because of their depth and richness, also lend themselves to book-length manuscripts. Regardless of researchers' positions about *when* a literature review should be conducted, they usually include a summary of prior research in their reports as a means of providing context for the study.

Quantitative reports almost never contain **raw data**—that is, data in the form they were collected, which are numeric values. Qualitative reports, by contrast, are usually filled with rich verbatim passages directly from participants. The excerpts are used in an evidentiary fashion to support or illustrate researchers' interpretations and thematic construction.

Example of raw data in a qualitative report: Langegard and Ahlberg (2009) explored things that patients with incurable cancer had found consoling during the course of the disease. In-depth interviews with 10 hospice patients revealed that a major theme was acceptance, as illustrated by the following quote:

"Talking about it is a way of getting the truth into my head. Through putting my situation into words, it becomes a way of understanding and then I have a possibility to be consoled. If I don't understand the consequences of my disease, I can't possibly be consoled ... It's not about giving up, but it's about realizing that this is the way it is. It's over, it's incurable" (p. 104).

Like quantitative researchers, qualitative nurse researchers want their findings used by others. Qualitative findings often are the basis for formulating hypotheses that are tested by quantitative researchers, for developing measuring instruments for both research and clinical purposes, and for designing effective nursing interventions. Qualitative studies help to shape nurses' perceptions of a problem or situation, their conceptualizations of potential solutions, and their understanding of patients' concerns and experiences.

RESEARCH JOURNAL ARTICLES

Research **journal articles**, which summarize the context, design, and results of a study, are the primary method of disseminating research evidence. This section reviews the content and style of research journal articles to ensure that you will be equipped to delve into the research literature. A more detailed discussion of the structure of journal articles is presented in Chapter 28, which provides guidance on writing research reports.

Content of Journal Articles

Many quantitative and qualitative journal articles follow a conventional organization called the **IMRAD format**. This format, which loosely follows the steps of quantitative studies, involves organizing material into four main sections—**I**ntroduction, **M**ethod, **R**esults, **a**nd **D**iscussion. The main text of the report is usually preceded by an abstract and followed by references.

The Abstract

The **abstract** is a brief description of the study placed at the beginning of the article. The abstract answers, in about 200 words, the following: What were the research questions? What methods did the researcher use to address the questions? What did the researcher find? What are the implications for nursing practice? Readers can review an abstract to assess whether the entire report is of interest. Some journals have moved from traditional abstracts—single paragraphs summarizing the study's main features—to slightly longer, structured abstracts with specific headings. For example, abstracts in *Nursing Research* organize study information under the following headings: Background, Objectives, Method, Results, and Conclusions.

The Introduction

The introduction communicates the research problem and its context. The introduction, which often is not specifically labeled "Introduction," follows immediately after the abstract. This section usually describes:

- The central phenomena, concepts, or variables under study
- The current state of evidence, based on a literature review
- The theoretical or conceptual framework
- The study purpose, research questions, or hypotheses to be tested
- The study's significance

Thus, the introduction sets the stage for a description of what the researcher did and what was learned. The introduction corresponds roughly to the conceptual phase (Phase 1) of a study.

The Method Section

The method section describes the methods used to answer the research questions. This section lays out methodologic decisions made in the design and planning phase (Phase 2), and may offer rationales for those decisions. In a quantitative study, the method section usually describes:

- The research design;
- The sampling plan;
- Methods of data collection and specific instruments used;
- Study procedures (including ethical safeguards); and
- Analytic procedures and methods.

Qualitative researchers discuss many of the same issues, but with different emphases. For example, a qualitative study often provides more information about the research setting and the study context, and less information on sampling. Also, because formal instruments are not used to collect qualitative data, there is less discussion about data collection methods, but there may be more information on data collection procedures. Increasingly, reports of qualitative studies are including descriptions of the researchers' efforts to enhance the rigor of the study.

The Results Section

The results section presents the **findings** (results) obtained in the data analyses. The text summarizes key findings, often accompanied by more detailed tables or figures. Virtually all results sections contain descriptive information, including a description of the participants (e.g., average age, percent male/female).

In quantitative studies, the results section provides information about **statistical tests**, which are used to test hypotheses and evaluate the believability of the findings. For example, if the percentage of smokers who smoke two packs or more daily is computed to be 40%, how *probable* is it that the percentage is accurate? If the researcher finds that the average number of cigarettes smoked weekly is lower for those in an intervention group than for those not getting the intervention, how *probable* is it that the intervention effect is *real*? Is the effect of the intervention on smoking likely to be replicated with a new sample of smokers—or does the result reflect a peculiarity of the sample? Statistical tests help to answer such questions. Researchers typically report:

- *The names of statistical tests used.* Different tests are appropriate for different situations, but they are based on common principles. You do not have to know the names of all statistical tests—there are dozens of them—to comprehend the findings.
- *The value of the calculated statistic.* Computers are used to calculate a numeric value for the particular statistical test used. The value allows researchers to draw conclusions about the meaning of the results. The *actual* numeric value of the statistic, however, is not inherently meaningful and need not concern you.
- *The significance.* A critical piece of information is whether the value of the statistic was significant (not to be confused with important or clinically relevant). When researchers report that results are **statistically significant**, it means the findings are probably reliable and replicable with a new sample. Research reports also indicate the **level of significance**, which is an index of how probable it is that the findings are reliable. For example, if a report says that a finding was significant at the .05 level, this means that

only 5 times out of 100 (5 ÷ 100 = .05) would the result be spurious. In other words, 95 times out of 100, similar results would be obtained with a new sample. Readers can have a high degree of confidence—but not total assurance—that the evidence is reliable.

Example from the results section of a quantitative study: Cook and colleagues (2009) studied degree of agreement between blood glucose values obtained by laboratory analysis versus by a point-of-care device. Their results indicated that, "Laboratory glucose values for blood from a catheter differed significantly from point-of-care values for blood from the catheter ($t = -9.18$, $p < .001$)" (p. 65). The average glucose value was 124 mg/dL for the point-of-care analysis, compared to 114 mg/dL for the laboratory analysis.

In this study, Cook and colleagues found that glucose values from the lab were significantly lower than those obtained from point-of-care devices. The average difference of 10 mg/dL was not likely to have been a haphazard difference, and would probably be replicated with a new sample. This finding is highly reliable: less than one time in 1,000 ($p < 0.001$) would a difference this great have occurred as a fluke. To understand this finding, you do not have to understand what a t statistic is, nor do you need to worry about the actual value of the statistic, -9.18.

Qualitative researchers often organize findings according to the major themes, processes, or categories identified in the data. Results sections of qualitative reports often have several subsections, the headings of which correspond to the themes. Excerpts from the raw data are presented to support and provide a rich description of the thematic analysis. The results section of qualitative studies may also present the researcher's emerging theory about the phenomenon under study.

The Discussion Section

In the discussion section, researchers draw conclusions about what the results mean, and how the evidence can be used in practice. The discussion often reviews study limitations and the implications of the limitations for the integrity of the results. Researchers are in the best position to point out sample deficiencies, design problems, weaknesses in data collection, and so forth. A discussion section that presents these limitations demonstrates to readers that the author was aware of these limitations and probably took them into account in interpreting the findings.

The Style of Research Journal Articles

Research reports tell a story. However, the style in which many research journal articles are written—especially reports of quantitative studies—makes it difficult for many readers to figure out or become interested in the story. To unaccustomed audiences, research reports may seem stuffy, pedantic, and bewildering. Four factors contribute to this impression:

1. *Compactness.* Journal space is limited, so authors compress a lot of information into a short space. Interesting, personalized aspects of the study cannot be reported; in qualitative studies, only a handful of supporting quotes can be included.
2. *Jargon.* The authors of research reports use terms that may seem esoteric.
3. *Objectivity.* Quantitative researchers tell their stories objectively, often in a way that makes them sound impersonal. For example, most quantitative reports are written in the passive voice (i.e., personal pronouns are avoided), which tends to make a report less inviting and lively than use of the active voice. Qualitative reports, by contrast, are more subjective and personal, and written in a more conversational style.
4. *Statistical information.* The majority of nursing studies are quantitative, and thus most reports summarize the results of statistical analyses. Numbers and statistical symbols can intimidate readers who do not have statistical training.

In this textbook, we try to assist you in dealing with these issues and also strive to encourage you to tell *your* research stories in a manner that makes them accessible to practicing nurses.

Tips on Reading Research Reports

As you progress through this textbook, you will acquire skills for evaluating various aspects of research reports critically. Some preliminary hints on digesting research reports follow.

- Grow accustomed to the style of research articles by reading them frequently, even though you may not yet understand all the technical points.
- Read from an article that has been copied (or downloaded and printed) so that you can highlight portions and write marginal notes.
- Read articles slowly. Skim the article first to get major points and then read it more carefully a second time.
- On the second reading of a journal article, train yourself to be an *active* reader. Reading actively means that you constantly monitor yourself to assess your understanding of what you are reading. If you have problems, go back and reread difficult passages or make notes so that you can ask someone for clarification. In most cases, that "someone" will be your research instructor, but also consider contacting researchers themselves via e-mail.
- Keep this textbook with you as a reference while you are reading articles so that you can look up unfamiliar terms in the glossary or index.

- Try not to get bogged down in (or scared away by) statistical information. Try to grasp the gist of the story without letting numbers frustrate you.
- Until you become accustomed to research journal articles, you may want to "translate" them by expanding compact paragraphs into looser constructions, by translating jargon into familiar terms, by recasting the report into an active voice, and by summarizing findings with words rather than numbers. (Chapter 3 in the accompanying *Resource Manual* has an example of such a translation).

GENERAL QUESTIONS IN REVIEWING A RESEARCH STUDY

Most chapters of this book contain guidelines to help you evaluate different aspects of a research report critically, focusing primarily on the researchers' methodologic decisions. Box 3.3 ⊗ presents some further suggestions for performing a preliminary overview of a research report, drawing on concepts explained in this chapter. These guidelines supplement those presented in Box 1.1, Chapter 1.

BOX 3.3 Additional Questions for a Preliminary Review of a Study

1. What is the study all about? What are the main phenomena, concepts, or constructs under investigation?
2. If the study is quantitative, what are the independent and dependent variables?
3. Do the researchers examine relationships or patterns of association among variables or concepts? Does the report imply the possibility of a causal relationship?
4. Are key concepts clearly defined, both conceptually and operationally?
5. What type of study does it appear to be, in terms of types described in this chapter: Quantitative—experimental? nonexperimental? Qualitative—descriptive? grounded theory? phenomenology? ethnography?
6. Does the report provide any information to suggest how long the study took to complete?
7. Does the format of the report conform to the traditional IMRAD format? If not, in what ways does it differ?

RESEARCH EXAMPLES

In this section, we illustrate the progression of activities and discuss the time schedule of two studies (one quantitative and the other qualitative) conducted by the second author of this book.

Project Schedule for a Quantitative Study

Beck and Gable (2001) undertook a study to evaluate a scale they developed, the Postpartum Depression Screening Scale (PDSS).

Phase 1. Conceptual Phase:
1 Month

This phase was short, because much of the conceptual work had been done in an earlier study, in which Beck and Gable developed the PDSS. The literature had already been reviewed and Beck had done extensive fieldwork. The same framework and conceptual definitions that had been used in the first study were used in the new study.

Phase 2. Design and Planning Phase:
6 Months

The second phase included fine tuning the research design, gaining entrée into the hospital where subjects were recruited, and obtaining approval of the hospital's human subjects review committee. During this period, Beck met with statistical consultants and with Gable, an instrument development specialist, numerous times.

Phase 3. Empirical Phase:
11 Months

Data collection took almost a year to complete. The design called for administering the PDSS to 150 mothers at 6 weeks postpartum, and scheduling them for a psychiatric diagnostic interview to determine if they were suffering from postpartum depression. Recruitment of the women, which occurred in prepared childbirth classes, began 4 months before data collection. The researchers then waited until 6 weeks after delivery to gather data. The nurse psychotherapist, who had her own clinical practice, was able to come to the hospital only 1 day a week to conduct the diagnostic interviews; this contributed to the time required to achieve the desired sample size.

Phase 4. Analytic Phase:
3 Months

Statistical tests were performed to determine a cutoff score on the PDSS above which mothers would be identified as having screened positive for postpartum depression. Data analysis also was undertaken to determine the accuracy of the PDSS in predicting diagnosed postpartum depression. During this phase, Beck met with Gable and statisticians to interpret results.

Phase 5. Dissemination Phase:
18 Months

The researchers prepared and submitted their report to the journal *Nursing Research* for possible publication. It was accepted within 4 months, but it was "in press" (awaiting publication) for 14 months before being published. During this period, the authors presented their findings at regional and international conferences.

Project Schedule for a Qualitative Study

Beck (2004) conducted a phenomenological study on women's experiences of birth trauma. Total time from start to finish was approximately 3 years.

Phase 1. Conceptual Phase:
3 Months

Beck, who is renowned for her program of research on postpartum depression, became interested in birth trauma when she delivered the keynote address at a conference in New Zealand. She was asked to speak on perinatal anxiety disorders. In preparing for her address, Beck located only a handful of articles on birth trauma and its resulting post-traumatic stress disorder (PTSD). Following her keynote speech, a mother made a riveting presentation about her experience of

PTSD due to a traumatic childbirth. The mother, Sue Watson, was one of the founders of Trauma and Birth Stress (TABS), a charitable trust in New Zealand. Watson and Beck discussed the possibility of Beck conducting a qualitative study with the mothers who were members of TABS. Gaining entrée into TABS was facilitated by Watson and four other founders of TABS.

Phase 2. Design and Planning Phase: 3 Months

Beck selected a phenomenological design to describe the experience of a traumatic birth. Beck and Watson decided that Beck would write an introductory letter explaining the study, and Watson would write a letter endorsing the study. Both letters were to be sent to mothers who were members of TABS, asking for their cooperation. Once the basic design was developed, the research proposal was submitted to and approved by the ethics committee at Beck's university.

Phase 3. Empirical/Analytic Phases: 24 months

Data for the study were collected over an 18-month period, during which 40 mothers sent their stories of birth trauma to Beck via e-mail attachments. For the next 6 months, Beck analyzed the mothers' stories. Four themes emerged from data analysis: To care for me: Was that too much to ask? To communicate with me: Why was this neglected? To provide safe care: You betrayed my trust and I felt powerless, and The end justifies the means: At whose expense, at what price?

Phase 4 Dissemination Phase: 9 Months

A manuscript describing this study was submitted for publication to *Nursing Research* in April 2003. In June, Beck received a letter indicating that the reviewers' recommended she revise and resubmit the paper. Six weeks later, Beck resubmitted her revised manuscript, and in September, she was notified that her revised manuscript had been accepted for publication. The article was published in the January/February 2004 issue. Beck also has presented the findings at numerous national and international research conferences.

SUMMARY POINTS

- The people who provide information to the **researchers** (investigators) in a study are called **subjects** or **study participants** (in quantitative research) or study participants or **informants** in qualitative research; collectively they comprise the **sample**.
- The *site* is the overall location for the research; researchers sometimes engage in **multisite studies**. *Settings* are the more specific places where data collection occurs. Settings can range from totally naturalistic environments to formal laboratories.
- Researchers investigate **concepts** and **phenomena** (or **constructs**), which are abstractions or mental representations inferred from behavior or characteristics.
- Concepts are the building blocks of **theories**, which are systematic explanations of some aspect of the real world.
- In quantitative studies, concepts are called *variables*. A **variable** is a characteristic or quality that takes on different values (i.e., varies from one person to another). Groups that are varied with respect to an attribute are **heterogeneous**; groups with limited variability are **homogeneous**.
- **Continuous variables** can take on an infinite range of values along a continuum (e.g., weight). **Discrete variables** have a finite number of values between two points (e.g., number of children). **Categorical variables** have distinct categories that do not represent a quantity (e.g., gender).
- The **dependent** (or **outcome**) variable is the behavior or characteristic the researcher is interested in explaining, predicting, or affecting. The **independent variable** is the presumed cause of, antecedent to, or influence on the dependent variable.

- A **conceptual definition** describes the abstract or theoretical meaning of a concept being studied. An **operational definition** specifies procedures required to measure a variable.
- **Data**—information collected during a study—may take the form of narrative information (**qualitative data**) or numeric values (**quantitative data**).
- A **relationship** is a bond or connection between two variables. Quantitative researchers examine the relationship between the independent variable and dependent variable.
- When the independent variable causes or affects the dependent variable, the relationship is a **cause-and-effect** (or **causal**) **relationship**. In a **functional (associative) relationship**, variables are related in a noncausal way.
- A basic distinction in quantitative studies is between **experimental research**, in which researchers actively intervene, and **nonexperimental** (or **observational**) **research**, in which researchers make observations of existing phenomena without intervening.
- Qualitative research sometimes is rooted in research traditions that originate in other disciplines. Three such traditions are grounded theory, phenomenology, and ethnography.
- **Grounded theory** seeks to describe and understand key social psychological processes that occur in a social setting.
- **Phenomenology** focuses on the lived experiences of humans and is an approach to learning what the life experiences of people are like and what they mean.
- **Ethnography** provides a framework for studying the meanings and lifeways of a culture in a holistic fashion.
- Quantitative researchers usually progress in a fairly linear fashion from asking research questions to answering them. The main phases in a quantitative study are the conceptual, planning, empirical, analytic, and dissemination phases.
- The *conceptual phase* involves (1) defining the problem to be studied, (2) doing a **literature review**, (3) engaging in **clinical fieldwork** for

clinical studies, (4) developing a framework and conceptual definitions, and (5) formulating **hypotheses** to be tested.
- The *planning phase* entails (6) selecting a **research design**, (7) developing **intervention protocols** if the study is experimental, (8) specifying the **population**, (9) developing a **sampling plan**, (10) specifying methods to measure the research variables, (11) developing strategies to safeguard the rights of participants, and (12) finalizing the research plan (e.g., *pretesting* instruments).
- The *empirical phase* involves (13) collecting data and (14) preparing data for analysis.
- The *analytic phase* involves (15) analyzing data through **statistical analysis** and (16) interpreting the results.
- The *dissemination phase* entails (17) communicating the findings in a **research report** and (18) promoting the use of the study evidence in nursing practice.
- The flow of activities in a qualitative study is more flexible and less linear. Qualitative studies typically involve an **emergent design** that evolves during **fieldwork**.
- Qualitative researchers begin with a broad question regarding a phenomenon, often focusing on a little-studied aspect. In the early phase of a qualitative study, researchers select a site and seek to **gain entrée** into it, which typically involves enlisting the cooperation of **gatekeepers**.
- Once in the field, researchers select informants, collect data, and then analyze and interpret them in an iterative fashion; field experiences help in an ongoing fashion to shape the design of the study.
- Early analysis in qualitative research leads to refinements in sampling and data collection, until **saturation** (redundancy of information) is achieved.
- Both qualitative and quantitative researchers disseminate their findings, most often in **journal articles** that concisely communicate what the researchers did and what they found.

- Journal articles often consist of an **abstract** (a brief synopsis) and four major sections in an **IMRAD format**: an **I**ntroduction (explanation of the study problem and its context), **M**ethod section (the strategies used to address the problem), **R**esults section (study findings), **and D**iscussion (interpretation of the findings).
- Research reports are often difficult to read because they are dense and contain a lot of jargon. Quantitative research reports may be intimidating at first because, compared to qualitative reports, they are more impersonal and report on statistical tests.
- **Statistical tests** are procedures for testing research hypotheses and evaluating the believability of the findings. Findings that are **statistically significant** are ones that have a high probability of being "real."

STUDY ACTIVITIES

Chapter 3 of the *Resource Manual for Nursing Research: Generating and Assessing Evidence for Nursing Practice, 9th ed.*, offers study suggestions for reinforcing concepts presented in this chapter. In addition, the following questions can be addressed in classroom or online discussions:

1. Suggest ways of conceptually and operationally defining the following concepts: nursing competency, aggressive behavior, pain, postsurgical recovery, and body image.
2. Name five continuous, five discrete, and five categorical variables and identify which, if any, are dichotomous.
3. In the following research problems, identify the independent and dependent variables:
   a. Does screening for intimate partner violence among pregnant women improve birth and delivery outcomes?
   b. Do elderly patients have lower pain thresholds than younger patients?
   c. Are the sleeping patterns of infants affected by different forms of stimulation?
   d. Can home visits by nurses to released psychiatric patients reduce readmission rates?

STUDIES CITED IN CHAPTER 3

Al-Akour, N., Khader, Y., & Shatnawi, N. (2010). Quality of life and associated factors among *Jordanian* adolescents with type 1 diabetes mellitus. *Journal of Diabetes and its Complications, 24*, 43–47.

Beck, C. T. (2004). Birth trauma: In the eye of the beholder. *Nursing Research, 53*, 28–35.

Beck, C. T. (2009). The arm: There is no escaping the reality for mothers of children with obstetric brachial plexus injuries. *Nursing Research, 58*, 237–245.

Beck, C. T., & Gable, R. K. (2001). Further validation of the Postpartum Depression Screening Scale. *Nursing Research, 50*, 155–164.

Cook, S., Laughlin, D., Moore, M., North, D., Wilkins, K., Wong, G., Wallace-Scroggs, A., & Halvorson, L. (2009). Differences in glucose values obtained from point-of-care glucose meters and laboratory analysis in critically ill patients. *American Journal of Critical Care, 18*, 65–71.

Gaudine, A., Gien, L., Thuan, T., & Dung-do, V. (2010). Perspectives of HIV-related stigma in a community in Vietnam. *International Journal of Nursing Studies, 47*, 38–48.

Hessler, K. (2009). Physical activity behaviors of rural preschoolers. *Pediatric Nursing, 35*, 246–253.

Langegard, U., & Ahlberg, K. (2009). Consolation in conjunction with incurable cancer. *Oncology Nursing Forum, 36*, 99–107.

Lin, H., Tsai, Y., Lin, P., & Tsay, P. (2010). Effects of a therapeutic lifestyle change programme on cardiac risk factors after coronary artery bypass graft. *Journal of Clinical Nursing, 19*, 60–68.

Marshall, J., Cowell, J., Campbell, E., & McNaughton, D. (2010). Regional variations in cancer screening rates found in women with diabetes. *Nursing Research, 59*, 34–41.

Polit, D. F., London, A., & Martinez, J. (2001). *The health of poor urban women.* New York: Manpower Demonstration Research Corporation. (Report available online at: www.mdrc.org)

Propp, K., Apker, J., Ford, W., Wallace, N., Serbenski, M., & Hofmeister, N. (2010). Meeting the complex needs of the health care team: Identification of nurse-team communication practices perceived to enhance patient outcomes. *Qualitative Health Research, 20*, 15–28.

Schachman, K. (2010). Online fatherhood: The experience of first-time fatherhood in combat-deployed troops. *Nursing Research, 59*, 11–17.

Schim, S., Doorenbos, A., & Borse, N. (2006) Enhancing cultural competence among hospice staff. *The American Journal of Hospice & Palliative Care, 23*, 404–411.

Twiss, J., Waltman, N., Berg, K., Ott, C., Gross, G., & Lindsey, A. (2009). An exercise intervention for breast cancer survivors with bone loss. *Journal of Nursing Scholarship, 41*, 20–27.

Vallance, J., Plotnikoff, R., Karvinen, K., Mackey, J., & Courneya, K. (2010). Understanding physical activity maintenance in breast cancer survivors. *American Journal of Health Behavior, 34*, 225–236.

Methodologic and nonresearch references cited in this chapter can be found in a separate section at the end of the book.

PART 2

CONCEPTUALIZING AND PLANNING A STUDY TO GENERATE EVIDENCE FOR NURSING

4 | Research Problems, Research Questions, and Hypotheses

OVERVIEW OF RESEARCH PROBLEMS

Studies begin much like an EBP effort—as problems that need to be solved, or as questions that need to be answered. This chapter discusses the development of research problems. We begin by clarifying some relevant terms.

Basic Terminology

At a general level, a researcher selects a **topic** or a phenomenon on which to focus. Examples of research topics are claustrophobia during MRI tests, pain management for sickle cell disease, and nutrition during pregnancy. Within these broad topic areas are many potential research problems. In this section, we illustrate various terms using the topic *side effects of chemotherapy.*

A **research problem** is an enigmatic or troubling condition. Researchers identify a research problem within a broad topic area of interest. The purpose of research is to "solve" the problem—or to contribute to its solution—by generating relevant evidence. A **problem statement** articulates the problem and describes the need for a study through the development of an *argument.* Table 4.1 presents a simplified problem statement related to the topic of side effects of chemotherapy.

Research questions are the specific queries researchers want to answer in addressing the problem. Research questions guide the types of data to collect in a study. Researchers who make specific predictions about answers to research questions pose **hypotheses** that are then tested.

Many reports include a **statement of purpose** (or purpose statement), which summarizes the study goals. Researchers might also identify several **research aims** or **objectives**—the specific accomplishments they hope to achieve by conducting the study. The objectives include answering research questions or testing research hypotheses, but may also encompass broader aims (e.g., developing an effective intervention).

These terms are not always consistently defined in research methods textbooks, and differences among them are often subtle. Table 4.1 illustrates the interrelationships among terms as we define them.

Research Problems and Paradigms

Some research problems are better suited to qualitative versus quantitative methods. Quantitative studies usually focus on concepts that are fairly well developed, about which there is an existing body of evidence, and for which there are reliable methods of measurement. For example, a quantitative study might be undertaken to explore whether

TABLE 4.1	Example of Terms Relating to Research Problems
TERM	**EXAMPLE**
Topic/focus	Side effects of chemotherapy
Research problem (Problem statement)	Nausea and vomiting are common side effects among patients on chemotherapy, and interventions to date have been only moderately successful in reducing these effects. New interventions that can reduce or prevent these side effects need to be identified.
Statement of purpose	The purpose of the study is to test an intervention to reduce chemotherapy-induced side effects—specifically, to compare the effectiveness of patient-controlled and nurse-administered antiemetic therapy for controlling nausea and vomiting in patients on chemotherapy.
Research question	What is the relative effectiveness of patient-controlled antiemetic therapy versus nurse-controlled antiemetic therapy with regard to (a) medication consumption and (b) control of nausea and vomiting in patients on chemotherapy?
Hypotheses	Subjects receiving antiemetic therapy by a patient-controlled pump will (1) be less nauseous, (2) vomit less, and (3) consume less medication than subjects receiving the therapy by nurse administration.
Aims/objectives	This study has as its aim the following objectives: (1) to develop and implement two alternative procedures for administering antiemetic therapy for patients receiving moderate emetogenic chemotherapy (patient controlled versus nurse controlled), (2) to test three hypotheses concerning the relative effectiveness of the alternative procedures on medication consumption and control of side effects, and (3) to use the findings to develop recommendations for possible changes to clinical procedures.

older people with chronic illness who continue working are less (or more) depressed than those who retire. There are relatively accurate measures of depression that would yield quantitative information about the level of depression in a sample of employed and retired chronically ill older people.

Qualitative studies are often undertaken because some aspect of a phenomenon is poorly understood, and the researcher wants to develop a rich and context-bound understanding of it. Qualitative studies are often initiated to heighten awareness and create a dialogue about a phenomenon. Qualitative methods would not be well suited to comparing levels of depression among employed and retired seniors, but they would be ideal for exploring, for example, the *meaning* of depression among chronically ill retirees. Thus, the nature of the research question is closely allied to paradigms and to research traditions within paradigms.

Sources of Research Problems

Where do ideas for research problems come from? At a basic level, research topics originate with researchers' interests. Because research is a time-consuming enterprise, inquisitiveness about and interest in a topic are essential. Research reports rarely indicate the source of researchers' inspiration, but a variety of explicit sources can fuel their curiosity, including the following:

- *Clinical experience.* Nurses' everyday clinical experience is a rich source of ideas for research topics. Immediate problems that need a solution—analogous to problem-focused triggers discussed in Chapter 2—may generate more enthusiasm than abstract problems inferred from a theory, and they have high potential for clinical significance.
- *Quality improvement efforts.* Important clinical questions sometimes emerge in the context of findings from quality improvement studies. Personal involvement on a quality improvement team can sometimes generate ideas for a study.
- *Nursing literature.* Ideas for studies often come from reading the nursing literature. Research articles may suggest problems indirectly by stimulating the reader's curiosity and directly by identifying needed research. Familiarity with existing research or with emerging clinical issues is an important route to developing a research topic.
- *Social issues.* Topics are sometimes suggested by global social or political issues of relevance to the healthcare community. For example, the feminist movement raised questions about such topics as gender equity in healthcare. Public awareness about health disparities has led to research on healthcare access and culturally sensitive interventions.
- *Theories.* Theories from nursing and related disciplines are another source of research problems. Researchers ask, If this theory is correct, what would I predict about people's behaviors, states, or feelings? The predictions can then be tested through research.
- *Ideas from external sources.* External sources and direct suggestions can sometimes provide the impetus for a research idea. For example, ideas for studies may emerge by reviewing a funding agency's research priorities or from brainstorming with other nurses.

Additionally, researchers who have developed a *program of research* on a topic area may get inspiration for "next steps" from their own findings or from a discussion of those findings with others.

Example of a problem source for a quantitative study: Beck, one of this book's authors, has developed a strong research program on postpartum depression (PPD). Beck was approached by Dr. Carol Lammi-Keefe, a professor in nutritional sciences, who had been researching the effect of DHA (docosahexaemoic acid, a fat found in cold-water fish) on fetal brain development. The literature suggested that DHA might play a role in reducing the severity of PPD and so the two researchers are collaborating in a project to test the effectiveness of dietary supplements of DHA on the incidence and severity of PPD. Their clinical trial, funded by the Donaghue Medical Research Foundation, is currently underway.

➲ TIP: Personal experiences in clinical settings are a provocative source of research ideas. Here are some hints on how to proceed:

- Watch for a recurring problem and see if you can discern a pattern in situations that lead to the problem.

Example: Why do many patients complain of being tired after being transferred from a coronary care unit to a progressive care unit?

- Think about aspects of your work that are frustrating or do not result in the intended outcome—then try to identify factors contributing to the problem that could be changed.

Example: Why is suppertime so frustrating in a nursing home?

- Critically examine your own clinical decisions. Are they based on tradition, or are they based on systematic evidence that supports their efficacy?

Example: What would happen if you used the return of flatus to assess the return of GI motility after abdominal surgery, rather than listening to bowel sounds?

DEVELOPING AND REFINING RESEARCH PROBLEMS

Unless a research problem is based on an explicit suggestion, actual procedures for developing one are difficult to describe. The process is rarely a smooth and orderly one; there are likely to be false starts, inspirations, and setbacks. The few suggestions offered here are not intended to imply that there are techniques for making this first step easy but rather to encourage you to persevere in the absence of instant success.

Selecting a Topic

Developing a research problem is a creative process. In the early stages of generating research ideas, it is unwise to be too self-critical. It is better to relax and jot down areas of interest as they come to mind. It matters little if the terms you use to remind you of the ideas are abstract or concrete, broad or specific, technical or colloquial—the important point is to put ideas on paper.

After this first step, the ideas can be sorted in terms of interest, knowledge about the topics, and the perceived feasibility of turning the topics into a study. When the most fruitful idea has been selected, the list should not be discarded; it may be necessary to return to it.

➲ **TIP:** The process of selecting and refining a research problem usually takes longer than you might think. The process involves starting with some preliminary ideas, having discussions with colleagues and advisers, persuing the research literature, looking at what is happening in clinical settings, and a lot of reflection.

Narrowing the Topic

Once you have identified a topic of interest, you can begin to ask some broad questions that can lead you to a researchable problem. Examples of question stems that may help to focus an inquiry include the following:

- What is going on with . . . ?
- What is the process by which . . . ?
- What is the meaning of . . . ?
- What is the extent of . . . ?
- What influences or causes . . . ?
- What differences exist between . . . ?

- What are the consequences of . . . ?
- What factors contribute to . . . ?

Again, early criticism of ideas can be counterproductive. Try not to jump to the conclusion that an idea sounds trivial or uninspired without giving it more careful consideration or exploring it with others.

Beginning researchers often develop problems that are too broad in scope or too complex for their level of methodologic expertise. The transformation of the general topic into a workable problem is typically accomplished in uneven steps. Each step should result in progress toward the goals of narrowing the scope of the problem and sharpening and defining the concepts.

As researchers move from general topics to more specific researchable problems, multiple potential problems can emerge. Consider the following example. Suppose you were working on a medical unit and were puzzled by the fact that some patients always complained about having to wait for pain medication when certain nurses were assigned to them. The general problem area is discrepancy in patient complaints regarding pain medications administered by different nurses. You might ask: What accounts for the discrepancy? How can I improve the situation? These queries are not research questions, but they may lead you to ask such questions as the following: How do the two groups of nurses differ? What characteristics do the complaining patients share? At this point, you may observe that the ethnic background of the patients and nurses could be relevant. This may lead you to search the literature for studies about ethnicity in relation to nursing care, or it may provoke you to discuss the observations with others. These efforts may result in several research questions, such as the following:

- What is the essence of patient complaints among patients of different ethnic backgrounds?
- Is the ethnic background of nurses related to the frequency with which they dispense pain medication?
- Does the number of patient complaints increase when patients are of dissimilar ethnic backgrounds as opposed to when they are of the same ethnic background as nurses?

- Do nurses' dispensing behaviors change as a function of the similarity between their own ethnic background and that of patients?

These questions stem from the same problem, yet each would be studied differently; for example, some suggest a qualitative approach and others suggest a quantitative one. A quantitative researcher might become curious about ethnic differences in nurses' dispensing behaviors. Both ethnicity and nurses' dispensing behaviors are variables that can be measured reliably. A qualitative researcher who noticed differences in patient complaints would likely be more interested in understanding the *essence* of the complaints, the patients' *experience* of frustration, or the *process* by which the problem got resolved. These are aspects of the research problem that would be difficult to quantify.

Researchers choose a problem to study based on several factors, including its inherent interest and its compatibility with a paradigm of preference. In addition, tentative problems vary in their feasibility and worth. A critical evaluation of ideas is appropriate at this point.

Evaluating Research Problems

There are no rules for making a final selection of a research problem, but some criteria should be kept in mind. Four important considerations are the problem's significance, researchability, feasibility, and interest to you.

Significance of the Problem

A crucial factor in selecting a problem is its significance to nursing. Evidence from the study should have potential to contribute meaningfully to nursing practice. Within the existing body of evidence, the new study should be the right "next step." The right next step could involve an original inquiry, but it could also be a replication to answer previously asked questions with greater rigor or with different types of people.

In evaluating the significance of an idea, the following kinds of questions are relevant: Is the problem important to nursing and its clients? Will patient care

benefit from the evidence? Will the findings challenge (or lend support to) untested assumptions? If the answer to all these questions is "no," then the problem should be abandoned.

Researchability of the Problem

Not all problems are amenable to research inquiry. Questions of a moral or ethical nature, although provocative, cannot be researched. For example, should assisted suicide be legalized? There are no *right* or *wrong* answers to this question, only points of view. To be sure, it is possible to ask related questions that could be researched, such as the following:

- What are nurses' attitudes toward assisted suicide?
- What moral dilemmas are perceived by nurses who might be involved in assisted suicide?
- Do terminally ill patients living with high levels of pain hold more favorable attitudes toward assisted suicide than those with less pain?

The findings from studies addressing such questions would have no bearing on whether assisted suicide should be legalized, but the information could be useful in developing a better understanding of the issues.

Feasibility of Addressing the Problem

A third consideration concerns feasibility, which encompasses several issues. Not all of the following factors are universally relevant, but they should be kept in mind in making a decision.

Time. Most studies have deadlines or goals for completion, so the problem must be one that can be studied in the given time. The scope of the problem should be sufficiently restricted so that there will be enough time for the various steps reviewed in Chapter 3. It is prudent to be conservative in estimating time for various tasks because research activities often require more time than anticipated.

Availability of Study Participants. In any study involving humans, researchers need to consider whether people with the desired characteristics will be available and willing to cooperate. Securing people's cooperation is sometimes easy (e.g., getting nursing students to complete a questionnaire), but other situations pose more difficulties. Some people may not have the time or interest, and others may not feel well enough to participate. If the research is time-consuming or demanding, researchers may need to exert extra effort in recruiting participants, or may have to offer a monetary incentive.

Cooperation of Others. It may be insufficient to get the cooperation of prospective participants alone. As noted in Chapter 3, it may be necessary to gain entrée into an appropriate community or setting, and to develop the trust of gatekeepers. In institutional settings (e.g., hospitals), access to clients, personnel, or records requires authorization. Most healthcare organizations require approval of proposed studies.

Facilities and Equipment. All studies have resource requirements, although needs are sometimes modest. It is prudent to consider what facilities and equipment will be needed and whether they will be available before embarking on a study. For example, if technical equipment is needed, can it be secured, and is it functioning properly? Availability of space, office equipment, and research support staff may also need to be considered.

Money. Monetary needs for studies vary widely, ranging from $100 to $200 for small student projects to hundreds of thousands of dollars for large-scale research. If you are on a limited budget, you should think carefully about projected expenses before selecting a problem. Major categories of research-related expenditures include:

- Personnel costs—payments to individuals hired to help with the study (e.g., for conducting interviews, coding, data entry, transcribing, word processing)
- Participant costs—payments to participants as an incentive for their cooperation or to offset their expenses (e.g., transportation or baby-sitting costs)
- Supplies—paper, envelopes, computer disks, postage, audiotapes, and so on
- Printing and duplication costs—expenses for reproducing forms, questionnaires, and so forth
- Equipment—laboratory apparatus, computers and software, audio or video recorders, calculators, and the like

- Laboratory fees for the analysis of biophysiologic data
- Transportation costs (e.g., travel to participants' homes)

Researcher Experience. The problem should be chosen from a field about which you have some prior knowledge or experience. Researchers may struggle with a topic that is new and unfamiliar—although upfront clinical fieldwork may make up for certain deficiencies. The issue of technical expertise also should be considered. Beginning researchers with limited methodologic skills should avoid research problems that might require the development of sophisticated measuring instruments or that involve complex analyses.

Ethical Considerations. A research problem may be unfeasible if an investigation of the problem would pose unfair or unethical demands on participants. An overview of major ethical considerations in research is presented in Chapter 7 and should be reviewed when considering the study's feasibility.

Researcher Interest

Even if a tentative problem is researchable, significant, and feasible, there is one more criterion: your own interest in the problem. Genuine fascination with the chosen research problem is an important prerequisite to a successful study. A lot of time and energy are expended in a study; there is little sense devoting these resources to a project about which you are not enthusiastic.

➲ **TIP:** Beginning researchers often seek suggestions about a topic area, and such assistance may be helpful in getting started. Nevertheless, it is rarely wise to be talked into a topic toward which you are not personally inclined. If you do not find a problem attractive or stimulating during the beginning phases of a study, then you are bound to regret your choice later.

COMMUNICATING RESEARCH PROBLEMS

Every study needs a problem statement—an articulation of what it is that is problematic and that is the impetus for the research. Most research reports also present either a statement of purpose, research questions, or hypotheses, and often combinations of these elements are included.

Many beginning researchers do not really understand problem statements and may even have trouble identifying them in a research article—not to mention developing one. A problem statement is presented early, and often begins with the very first sentence after the abstract. Specific research questions, purposes, or hypotheses appear later in the introduction. Typically, however, researchers *begin* their inquiry with a research question or a purpose, and *then* develop an argument in a problem statement to present the rationale for the new research. This section describes the wording of statements of purpose and research questions, followed by a discussion of problem statements.

Statements of Purpose

Many researchers articulate their goals as a statement of purpose, worded declaratively. The purpose statement establishes the study's general direction and captures its essence. It is usually easy to identify a purpose statement because the word *purpose* is explicitly stated: "The purpose of this study was . . ."—although sometimes the words *aim, goal, intent,* or *objective* are used instead, as in "The aim of this study was. . . ."

In a quantitative study, a statement of purpose identifies the key study variables and their possible interrelationships, as well as the population of interest.

Example of a statement of purpose from a quantitative study: "The primary purpose of this study was to determine the incidence of and associated risk for falls and fractures among adults 12 to 60 months after they underwent RYGB (Roux-en-Y gastric bypass) for morbid obesity" (Berarducci et al., 2009, p. 35).

This purpose statement identifies the population—individuals who have undergone RYGB surgery—and indicates two goals. The first is descriptive, that is, to describe the incidence of falls and fractures

within the population. The second is to examine the effect of risk factors, such as use of analgesics, diuretics, and sedatives (the independent variables) on fall and fracture incidence (the dependent variables).

In qualitative studies, the statement of purpose indicates the key concept or phenomenon, and the group, community, or setting under study.

Example of a statement of purpose from a qualitative study: "The purpose of this study was to explore the characteristics of and the contexts related to sexual behaviors among institutionalized residents with dementia" (Tzeng et al., 2009, p. 991).

This statement indicates that the central phenomenon was the characteristics and contexts of sexual behavior, and that the group under study was institutionalized residents with dementia.

The statement of purpose communicates more than just the nature of the problem. Researchers' selection of verbs in a purpose statement suggests how they sought to solve the problem, or the state of knowledge on the topic. A study whose purpose is to *explore* or *describe* a phenomenon is likely an investigation of a little-researched topic, sometimes involving a qualitative approach such as a phenomenology or ethnography. A statement of purpose for a qualitative study—especially a grounded theory study—may also use verbs such as *understand, discover, develop,* or *generate.* Statements of purpose in qualitative studies may "encode" the tradition of inquiry, not only through the researcher's choice of verbs, but also through the use of "buzz words" associated with those traditions, as follows:

- *Grounded theory*: Processes, social structures, social interactions
- *Phenomenological studies*: experience, lived experience, meaning, essence
- *Ethnographic studies*: culture, roles, lifeways, cultural behavior

Quantitative researchers also suggest the nature of the inquiry through their selection of verbs. A statement indicating that the purpose of the study is to *test* or *evaluate* something (e.g., an intervention) suggests an experimental design, for example. A study whose purpose is to *examine* or *explore* the relationship between two variables is more likely to involve a nonexperimental design. In some cases, the verb is ambiguous: a purpose statement indicating that the researcher's intent is to *compare* could be referring to a comparison of alternative treatments (using an experimental approach) or a comparison of two pre-existing groups (using a nonexperimental approach). In any event, verbs such as *test*, *evaluate*, and *compare* suggest an existing knowledge base and quantifiable variables.

Note that the choice of verbs in a statement of purpose should connote objectivity. A statement of purpose indicating that the intent of the study was to *prove*, *demonstrate*, or *show* something suggests a bias.

⮞ **T I P :** In wording your statement of purpose, it may be useful to look at published research articles for models. Unfortunately, some reports fail to state unambiguously the study purpose, leaving readers to infer the purpose from such sources as the title of the report. In other reports, the purpose is clearly stated but may be difficult to find. Researchers most often state their purpose toward the end of the report's introduction.

Research Questions

Research questions are, in some cases, direct rewordings of statements of purpose, phrased interrogatively rather than declaratively, as in the following example:

- The purpose of this study is to assess the relationship between the dependency level of renal transplant recipients and their rate of recovery.
- What is the relationship between the dependency level of renal transplant recipients and their rate of recovery?

The question form has the advantage of simplicity and directness. Questions invite an answer and help to focus attention on the kinds of data that would have to be collected to provide that answer. Some research reports thus omit a statement of purpose and state only research questions. Other researchers use a set of research questions

to clarify or lend greater specificity to a global purpose statement.

Research Questions in Quantitative Studies

In Chapter 2, we discussed the framing of clinical foreground questions to guide an EBP inquiry. Many of the EBP question templates in Table 2.1 could yield questions to guide a study as well, but *researchers* tend to conceptualize their questions in terms of their *variables*. Take, for example, the first question in Table 2.1, which states, "In (population), what is the effect of (intervention) on (outcome)? A researcher would likely think of the question in these terms: "In (population), what is the effect of (independent variable) on (dependent variable)? The advantage of thinking in terms of variables is that researchers must consciously decide how to operationalize their variables and how to guide an analysis strategy with their variables. Thus, we can say that in quantitative studies, research questions identify key study variables, the relationships among them, and the population under study. The variables are all measurable, quantifiable concepts.

Most research questions concern relationships among variables, and so many quantitative research questions could be articulated using a general question template: "In (population), what is the relationship between (independent variable or IV) and (dependent variable or DV)?" Examples of minor variations include the following:

- *Treatment, intervention*: In (population), what is the effect of (IV: intervention) on (DV)?
- *Prognosis*: In (population), does (IV: disease, condition) affect or increase the risk of (DV: adverse consequences)?
- *Causation, etiology*: In (population), does (IV: exposure, characteristic) cause or increase the risk of (DV: disease, health problem)?

There is one important distinction between the clinical foreground questions for an EBP-focused evidence search as described in Chapter 2 and a research question for an original study. As shown in Table 2.1, sometimes clinicians ask questions about explicit comparisons (e.g., they want to compare intervention A to intervention B) and sometimes they do not (e.g., they want to learn the effects of intervention A, compared to any other intervention or to the absence of an intervention). In a research question, there must *always* be a designated comparison, because the independent variable must be operationally defined; this definition would articulate exactly what is being studied.

Another distinction between EBP and research questions is that research questions sometimes are more complex than clinical foreground questions for EBP. As an example, suppose that we began with an interest in nurses' use of humor with cancer patients, and the effects that humor has on these patients. One research question might be, "What is the effect of nurses' use of humor (versus absence of humor, the IV) on stress (the DV) in hospitalized cancer patients (the population)? But we might also be interested in whether the relationship between the IV and the DV is influenced by or *moderated* by a third variable. For example: Does nurses' use of humor have a different effect on stress in male versus female patients? In this example, gender is a **moderator variable**—a variable that affects the strength or direction of an association between the independent and dependent variable. Identifying moderators may be important in understanding *when* to expect a relationship between the IV and DV, and often has clinical relevance. Moderator (or *moderating*) variables can be characteristics of the population (e.g., male versus female patients) or of the circumstances (e.g., rural versus urban settings). Here are examples of question templates that involve a moderator variable (MV):

- *Treatment, intervention*: In (population), does the effect of (IV: intervention) on (DV) vary by (MV)?
- *Prognosis*: In (population), does the effect of (IV: disease, condition) on (DV) vary by (MV)?
- *Causation, etiology*: In (population), does (IV: exposure, characteristic) cause or increase risk of (DV) differentially by (MV)?

When a study purpose is to understand *causal pathways*, research questions may involve a **mediating variable**—a variable that intervenes between

the IV and the DV and helps to explain why the relationship exists. In our example, we might ask the following: Does nurses' use of humor have a direct effect on the stress of hospitalized patients with cancer, or is the effect *mediated by* humor's effect on natural killer cell activity?

Some research questions are primarily descriptive. As examples, here are some descriptive questions that could be answered in a study on nurses' use of humor:

- What is the frequency with which nurses use humor as a complementary therapy with hospitalized cancer patients?
- What are the attitudes of hospitalized cancer patients to nurses' use of humor?
- What are the characteristics of nurses who use humor as a complementary therapy with hospitalized cancer patients?

Answers to such questions might, if addressed in a methodologically sound study, be useful in developing strategies for reducing stress in patients with cancer.

Example of a research question from a quantitative study: Robbins and colleagues (2009) studied gender differences in middle school children's attitudes toward physical activity. One of their key research questions was: *Do middle school boys and girls differ in their perceived benefits of and barriers to physical activity?*

➔ TIP: The toolkit section of Chapter 4 of the accompanying *Resource Manual* includes a Word document that can be "filled in" to generate many types of research questions for both qualitative and quantitative studies.

Research Questions in Qualitative Studies

Research questions for qualitative studies state the phenomenon of interest and the group or population of interest. Researchers in the various qualitative traditions vary in their conceptualization of what types of questions are important. Grounded theory researchers are likely to ask *process* questions, phenomenologists tend to ask *meaning* questions, and ethnographers generally ask *descriptive* questions about cultures. The terms associated with the various traditions, discussed previously in connection with purpose statements, are likely to be incorporated into the research questions.

Example of a research question from a phenomenological study: What is women's lived experience of fear of childbirth? (Nilsson & Lundgren, 2009).

Not all qualitative studies are rooted in a specific research tradition. Many researchers use qualitative methods to describe or explore phenomena without focusing on cultures, meaning, or social processes.

Example of a research question from a descriptive qualitative study: Horne and colleagues (2010) conducted a descriptive qualitative study that asked, *What do young older adults perceive to be the influence of primary healthcare professionals in encouraging exercise and physical activity?*

In qualitative studies, research questions may evolve over the course of the study. Researchers begin with a *focus* that defines the broad boundaries of the study, but the boundaries are not cast in stone. The boundaries "can be altered and, in the typical naturalistic inquiry, will be" (Lincoln & Guba, 1985, p. 228). The naturalist begins with a research question that provides a general starting point but does not prohibit discovery; qualitative researchers are sufficiently flexible that questions can be modified as new information makes it relevant to do so.

Problem Statements

Problem statements express the dilemma or troubling situation that needs investigation and that provides a rationale for a new inquiry. A problem statement identifies the nature of the problem that is being addressed and its context and significance. A problem statement is *not* merely a statement of the purpose of the study, it is a well-structured formulation of what it is that is problematic, what it is that

"needs fixing," or what it is that is poorly understood. Problem statements, especially for quantitative studies, often have most of the following six components:

1. *Problem identification*: What is wrong with the current situation?
2. *Background*: What is the context of the problem that readers need to understand?
3. *Scope of the problem*: How big a problem is it, how many people are affected?
4. *Consequences of the problem*: What is the cost of not fixing the problem?
5. *Knowledge gaps*: What information about the problem is lacking?
6. *Proposed solution*: What is the basis for believing that the proposed study would contribute to the solution of the problem?

TIP: The toolkit section of Chapter 4 of the accompanying *Resource Manual* includes these questions in a Word document that can be "filled in" and reorganized as needed, as an aid to developing a problem statement.

Suppose our topic was humor as a complimentary therapy for reducing stress in hospitalized patients with cancer. Our research question is, "What is the effect of nurses' use of humor on stress and natural killer cell activity in hospitalized cancer patients?" Box 4.1 presents a rough draft of a problem statement for such a study. This problem statement is a reasonable first draft. The draft has several, but not all, of the six components.

Box 4.2 illustrates how the problem statement could be strengthened by adding information about scope (component 3), long-term consequences (component 4), and possible solutions (component 6). This second draft builds a more compelling argument for new research: millions of people are affected by cancer, and the disease has adverse consequences not only for those diagnosed and their families, but also for society. The revised problem statement also describes preliminary findings on which the new study might build.

As this example suggests, the problem statement is usually interwoven with supportive evidence from the research literature. In many research articles, it

---

BOX 4.1 Draft Problem Statement on Humor and Stress

A diagnosis of cancer is associated with high levels of stress. Sizeable numbers of patients who receive a cancer diagnosis describe feelings of uncertainty, fear, anger, and loss of control. Interpersonal relationships, psychological functioning, and role performance have all been found to suffer following cancer diagnosis and treatment.

A variety of alternative/complementary therapies have been developed in an effort to decrease the harmful effects of stress on psychological and physiological functioning, and resources devoted to these therapies (money and staff) have increased in recent years. However, many of these therapies have not been carefully evaluated to determine their efficacy, safety, or cost effectiveness. For example, the use of humor has been recommended as a therapeutic device to improve quality of life, decrease stress, and perhaps improve immune functioning, but the evidence to justify its popularity is scant.

---

is difficult to disentangle the problem statement from the literature review, unless there is a subsection specifically labeled "Literature Review."

Problem statements for a qualitative study similarly express the nature of the problem, its context, its scope, and information needed to address it, as in this example with bracketed citations:

Example of a problem statement from a qualitative study: "An unhealthy diet and lack of activity are two of the major risk factors responsible for increases in non-communicable diseases in modern societies. Problems such as cardiovascular and coronary heart disease, obesity, diabetes, and cancer account for more than half of deaths (60%) and nearly half (47%) of the burden of disease worldwide [1] . . . As prevention is a priority, the impact that children's activity levels and diet could have on their current and future health is of special concern [3] . . . Parents have a great influence on food [5] and activity [6,7] choices and behaviours of their offspring . . . This study used a qualitative design . . . to investigate how mothers and fathers contributed to food and activity choices and maintenance of a healthy lifestyle in children" (Lopez-Dicastillo et al., 2010).

BOX 4.2 Some Possible Improvements to Problem Statement on Humor and Stress

Each year, more than 1 million people are diagnosed with cancer, which remains one of the top causes of death among both men and women (citations). Numerous studies have documented that a diagnosis of cancer is associated with high levels of stress. Sizeable numbers of patients who receive a cancer diagnosis describe feelings of uncertainty, fear, anger, and loss of control (citations). Interpersonal relationships, psychological functioning, and role performance have all been found to suffer following cancer diagnosis and treatment (citations). These stressful outcomes can, in turn, adversely affect health, long-term prognosis, and medical costs among cancer survivors (citations).

A variety of alternative/complementary therapies have been developed in an effort to decrease the harmful effects of stress on psychological and physiological functioning, and resources devoted to these therapies (money and staff) have increased in recent years (citations). However, many of these therapies have not been carefully evaluated to determine their efficacy, safety, or cost effectiveness. For example, the use of humor has been recommended as a therapeutic device to improve quality of life, decrease stress, and perhaps improve immune functioning (citations), but the evidence to justify its popularity is scant. Preliminary findings from a recent small-scale endocrinology study with a healthy sample exposed to a humorous intervention (citation), however, holds promise for further inquiry with immunocompromised populations.

Qualitative studies that are embedded in a particular research tradition usually incorporate terms and concepts in their problem statements that foreshadow their tradition of inquiry (Creswell, 2006). For example, the problem statement in a grounded theory study might refer to the need to generate a theory relating to social processes. A problem statement for a phenomenological study might note the need to gain insight into people's experiences or the meanings they attribute to those experiences. And an ethnographer might indicate the need to understand how cultural forces affect people's behavior.

RESEARCH HYPOTHESES

A hypothesis is a prediction, almost always a prediction about the relationship between variables. In qualitative studies, researchers do not have an *a priori* hypothesis, in part because there is too little known to justify a prediction, and in part, because qualitative researchers want the inquiry to be guided by participants' viewpoints rather than by their own hunches. Thus, our discussion here focuses on hypotheses in quantitative research.

Function of Hypotheses in Quantitative Research

Research questions, as we have seen, are usually queries about relationships between variables. Hypotheses are predicted answers to these queries. For instance, the research question might ask: Does sexual abuse in childhood affect the development of irritable bowel syndrome in women? The researcher might predict the following: Women who were sexually abused in childhood have a higher incidence of irritable bowel syndrome than women who were not.

Hypotheses sometimes follow from a theoretical framework. Scientists reason from theories to hypotheses and test those hypotheses in the real world. The validity of a theory is evaluated through hypothesis testing. Take, as an example, the theory of reinforcement, which maintains that behavior that is positively reinforced (rewarded) tends to be learned or repeated. If the theory is valid, it should be possible to make predictions about human behavior. For example, the following hypothesis is deduced from reinforcement theory: Pediatric patients who are given a reward (e.g., a balloon or permission to watch television) when they cooperate during nursing procedures tend to be more cooperative during those procedures than nonrewarded peers. The theory gains support if the hypothesis is confirmed.

Not all hypotheses are derived from theory. Even in the absence of a theory, well-conceived hypotheses offer direction and suggest explanations. For example, suppose we hypothesized that the incidence of bradycardia in extremely low-birth-weight infants undergoing intubation and ventilation would be lower using the closed tracheal suction system (CTSS) than using the partially ventilated endotracheal suction method (PVETS). We could justify our speculation based on earlier studies or clinical observations, or both. *The development of predictions in and of itself forces researchers to think logically, to exercise critical judgment, and to tie together earlier research findings.*

Now, let us suppose the preceding hypothesis is not confirmed: We find that rates of bradycardia are similar for both the PVETS and CTSS methods. *The failure of data to support a prediction forces researchers to analyze theory or previous research critically, to carefully review the limitations of the study's methods, and to explore alternative explanations for the findings.* The use of hypotheses in quantitative studies tends to induce critical thinking and to facilitate understanding and interpretation of the data.

To illustrate further the utility of hypotheses, suppose we conducted the study guided only by the research question, Is there a relationship between suction method and rates of bradycardia? The investigator without a hypothesis is apparently prepared to accept any results. The problem is that it is almost always possible to explain something superficially after the fact, no matter what the findings are. Hypotheses guard against superficiality and minimize the risk that spurious results will be misconstrued.

Characteristics of Testable Hypotheses

Testable hypotheses state the expected relationship between the independent variable (the presumed cause or antecedent) and the dependent variable (the presumed effect or outcome) within a population.[1]

Example of a research hypothesis: Moore and co-researchers (2009) tested patency time in long-term indwelling urethral catheters among patients in three groups: those receiving standard care, a normal saline washout, or an acidic washout solution. The researchers hypothesized that time to first catheter change would be longest among patients who had the acidic washout solution.

In this example, the population is patients with long-term indwelling urethral catheters, the independent variable is method of managing blockages, and the dependent variable is the length of time elapsed until first catheter change. The hypothesis predicts that these two variables are related within the population—longer catheter life was expected for those receiving the acidic washout solution.

When researchers' hypotheses do not make a relational statement, the hypothesis is difficult to test. Take the following example: *Pregnant women who receive prenatal instruction regarding postpartum experiences are not likely to experience postpartum depression.* This statement expresses no anticipated relationship. There is only one variable (postpartum depression), and a relationship by definition requires at least two variables.

The problem is that without a prediction about an anticipated relationship, the hypothesis is difficult to test using standard procedures. In our example, how would we know whether the hypothesis was supported—what standard could be used to decide whether to accept or reject it? To illustrate this concretely, suppose we asked a group of mothers who had been given instruction on postpartum experiences the following question 1 month after delivery: On the whole, how depressed have you been since you gave birth? Would you say (1) extremely depressed, (2) moderately depressed, (3) a little depressed, or (4) not at all depressed?

Based on responses to this question, how could we compare the actual outcome with the predicted outcome? Would *all* the women have to say they were "not at all depressed?" Would the prediction be supported if 51% of the women said they were "not at all depressed" *or* "a little depressed?" It is difficult to test the accuracy of the prediction.

A test is simple, however, if we modify the prediction to the following: Pregnant women who receive prenatal instruction are less likely to experience postpartum depression than those with no prenatal instruction. Here, the dependent variable is the women's depression, and the independent variable is receipt versus nonreceipt of prenatal instruction. The relational aspect of the prediction is embodied in the phrase *less than*. If a hypothesis lacks a phrase such as *more than, less than, greater than, different from, related to, associated with,* or something similar, it is probably not amenable to testing in a quantitative study. To test this revised hypothesis, we could ask two groups of women with different prenatal instruction experiences to respond to the question on depression and then compare the groups' responses. The absolute degree of depression of either group would not be at issue.

Hypotheses should be based on justifiable rationales. Hypotheses often follow from previous research findings or are deduced from a theory. When a relatively new area is being investigated, the researcher may have to turn to logical reasoning or clinical experience to justify predictions.

The Derivation of Hypotheses

Many students ask, How do I go about developing hypotheses? Two basic processes—induction and deduction—are the intellectual machinery involved in deriving hypotheses.

An **inductive hypothesis** is a generalization inferred from observed relationships. Researchers observe certain patterns or associations among phenomena and then make predictions based on the observations. Related literature should be examined to learn what is known on a topic, but an

---

[1]It is possible to test hypotheses about the value of a single variable, but this happens rarely. See Chapter 17 for an example.

important source for inductive hypotheses is clinical experiences, combined with critical analysis. For example, a nurse might notice that presurgical patients who ask a lot of questions about pain or who express pain-related fears have a more difficult time than other patients in learning appropriate postoperative procedures. The nurse could formulate a testable hypothesis, such as: Patients who are stressed by fear of pain will have more difficulty in deep breathing and coughing after their surgery than patients who are not stressed. Qualitative studies are an important source of inspiration for inductive hypotheses.

Example of deriving an inductive hypothesis: In Beck and Watson's (2008) qualitative study on the impact of birth trauma on breastfeeding, one of their findings was that many mothers who had experienced birth trauma experienced intrusive, unwelcome flashbacks that caused them great distress. A hypothesis that can be derived from this qualitative finding might be as follows: Women who experience a traumatic childbirth have more flashbacks of their labor and delivery during breastfeeding than women who do not experience birth trauma.

Deduction is the other mechanism for deriving hypotheses. Theories of how phenomena interrelate cannot be tested directly but researchers can, through deductive reasoning, develop hypotheses based on theoretical principles. Inductive hypotheses begin with specific observations and move toward generalizations. **Deductive hypotheses** have theories as a starting point. Researchers ask: If this theory is valid, what are the implications for the variables of interest? Researchers deduce that if the general theory is true, then certain outcomes can be expected. Specific predictions derived from general principles must then be subjected to testing through data collection and analysis. If hypotheses are supported, then the theory is strengthened.

The advancement of nursing knowledge depends on both inductive and deductive hypotheses. Ideally, an iterative process is set in motion wherein observations are made (e.g., in a qualitative study), inductive hypotheses are formulated, systematic observations are made to test the hypotheses, theories are developed on the basis of the results,

deductive hypotheses are formulated from the theory, new data are gathered, theories are modified, and so forth. Researchers need to be organizers of concepts (think inductively), logicians (think deductively), and critics and skeptics of resulting formulations, constantly demanding evidence.

Wording of Hypotheses

A good hypothesis is worded clearly and concisely, and in the present tense. Researchers make predictions about relationships that exist in the population, and not just about a relationship that will be revealed in a particular sample. There are various types of hypotheses.

Simple versus Complex Hypotheses

In this book, we define a **simple hypothesis** as a hypothesis that states an expected relationship between *one* independent and *one* dependent variable. A **complex hypothesis** is a prediction of a relationship between two or more independent variables and/or two or more dependent variables.

Simple hypotheses state a relationship between one independent variable, which we will call X, and one dependent variable, which we will call Y. Y is the predicted effect, outcome, or consequence of X, which is the presumed cause or antecedent. This relationship is shown graphically in Figure 4.1A. The circles represent variables X and Y, and the hatched area designates the strength of the relationship between them. If there were a one-to-one correspondence between X and Y, the two circles would overlap completely. If the variables were unrelated, the circles would not overlap at all. The previously cited study of catheter patency time in three catheter management groups (Moore et al., 2009) illustrates a simple hypothesis.

Most phenomena are affected by a multiplicity of factors. A person's weight, for example, is affected simultaneously by such factors as height, diet, bone structure, activity level, and metabolism. If Y in Figure 4.1A was weight, and X was a person's caloric intake, we would not be able to explain or understand individual variation in weight very well. For example, knowing that Nate

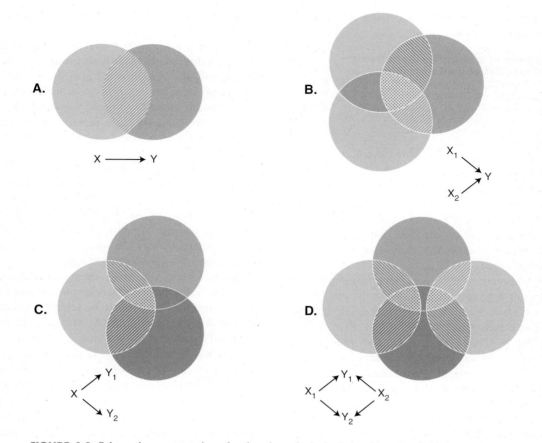

FIGURE 4.1 Schematic representation of various hypothetical relationships. (X = Independent variable; Y = Dependent variable.)

O'Hara's daily caloric intake averages 2,500 calories would not permit a good prediction of his weight. Knowledge of other factors, such as his height, would improve the accuracy with which his weight could be predicted.

Figure 4.1B presents a schematic representation of the effect of two independent variables (X_1 and X_2) on one dependent variable (Y). To pursue the preceding example, the hypothesis might be: Taller people (X_1) and people with higher caloric intake (X_2) weigh more (Y) than shorter people and those with lower caloric intake. As the figure shows, a larger proportion of the area of Y is hatched when there are two independent variables than when

there is only one. This means that caloric intake *and* height do a better job in helping us explain variation in weight (Y) than caloric intake alone. Complex hypotheses have the advantage of allowing researchers to capture some of the complexity of the real world.

Just as a phenomenon can result from more than one independent variable, so a single independent variable can influence more than one phenomenon, as illustrated in Figure 4.1C. A number of studies have found, for example, that cigarette smoking (the independent variable, X), can lead to both lung cancer (Y_1) and coronary disorders (Y_2). Complex hypotheses are common in studies that try to assess the impact of a nursing intervention on multiple outcomes.

> **Example of a complex hypothesis—multiple dependent variables:** Lundberg and colleagues (2009) hypothesized that mental health patients who experienced stigmatizing rejection experiences [X] would, compared to those without such experiences, have lower self-esteem [Y_1], lower sense of empowerment [Y_2], and lower sense of coherence [Y_3].

A more complex type of hypothesis, which links two or more independent variables to two or more dependent variables, is shown in Figure 4.1D. An example might be a hypothesis that smoking *and* the consumption of alcohol during pregnancy might lead to lower birth weights *and* lower Apgar scores in infants.

Hypotheses are also complex if mediating or moderator variables are included in the prediction. For example, it might be hypothesized that the effect of caloric intake (X) on weight (Y) is moderated by gender (Z)—that is, the relationship between height and weight is different for men and women. Or, we might predict that the effect of ephedra (X) on weight (Y) is indirect, mediated by ephedra's effect on metabolism (Z).

Directional versus Nondirectional Hypotheses

Hypotheses can be stated in a number of ways, as in the following examples:

1. Older patients are more at risk of experiencing a fall than younger patients.
2. There is a relationship between the age of a patient and the risk of falling.
3. The older the patient, the greater the risk that he or she will fall.
4. Older patients differ from younger ones with respect to their risk of falling.
5. Younger patients tend to be less at risk of a fall than older patients.
6. The risk of falling increases with the age of the patient.

In each example, the hypothesis indicates the population (patients), the independent variable (patients'

age), the dependent variable (a fall), and the anticipated relationship between them.

Hypotheses can be either directional or nondirectional. A **directional hypothesis** is one that specifies not only the existence but also the expected direction of the relationship between variables. In the six versions of the hypothesis, versions 1, 3, 5, and 6 are directional because there is an explicit prediction that older patients are at greater risk of falling than younger ones.

A **nondirectional hypothesis**, by contrast, does not state the direction of the relationship. Versions 2 and 4 in the example illustrate nondirectional hypotheses. These hypotheses state the prediction that a patient's age and risk of falling are related, but they do not stipulate whether the researcher thinks that *older* patients or *younger* ones are at greater risk.

Hypotheses derived from theory are almost always directional because theories provide a rationale for expecting variables to be related in a certain way. Existing studies also offer a basis for directional hypotheses. When there is no theory or related research, when findings of prior studies are contradictory, or when researchers' own experience leads to ambivalence, nondirectional hypotheses may be appropriate. Some people argue, in fact, that nondirectional hypotheses are preferable because they connote impartiality. Directional hypotheses, it is said, imply that researchers are intellectually committed to certain outcomes, and such a commitment might lead to bias. This argument fails to recognize that researchers typically *do* have hunches about outcomes, whether they state those expectations explicitly or not. We prefer directional hypotheses—when there is a reasonable basis for them—because they clarify the study's framework and demonstrate that researchers have thought critically about the phenomena under study. Directional hypotheses may also permit a more sensitive statistical test through the use of a *one-tailed test*—a rather fine point we discuss in Chapter 17.

Research versus Null Hypotheses

Hypotheses can be described as either research hypotheses or null hypotheses. **Research hypotheses** (also called *substantive* or *scientific* hypotheses) are statements of expected relationships between variables. All hypotheses presented thus far are research hypotheses that indicate actual expectations.

Statistical inference uses a logic that may be confusing. This logic requires that hypotheses be expressed as an expected *absence* of a relationship. **Null hypotheses** (or *statistical hypotheses*) state that there is no relationship between the independent and dependent variables. The null form of the hypothesis used in our example might be: "Patients' age is unrelated to their risk of falling" or "Older patients are just as likely as younger patients to fall." The null hypothesis might be compared with the assumption of innocence of an accused criminal in English-based systems of justice: The variables are assumed to be "innocent" of any relationship until they can be shown "guilty" through appropriate statistical procedures. The null hypothesis represents the formal statement of this assumption of innocence.

➲ **TIP:** Avoid stating hypotheses in null form in a proposal or a report, because this gives an amateurish impression. When statistical tests are performed, the underlying null hypothesis is assumed without being explicitly stated.

Hypothesis Testing

Researchers seek evidence through statistical analysis that their research hypotheses have a high probability of being correct. However, hypotheses are never *proved* through hypothesis testing; rather, they are *accepted* or *supported*. Findings are always tentative. Certainly, if the same results are replicated in numerous studies, then greater confidence can be placed in the conclusions. Hypotheses come to be increasingly supported with mounting evidence.

Let us look at why this is so. Suppose we hypothesized that height and weight are related. We predict that, on average, tall people weigh more than short people. We then obtain height and weight measurements from a sample and analyze the data. Now, suppose we happened by chance to get a sample that consisted of short, heavy people, and tall,

thin people. Our results might indicate that there is no relationship between height and weight. Would we be justified in stating that this study *proved* that height and weight are unrelated?

As another example, suppose we hypothesized that tall nurses are more effective than short ones. In reality, we would expect no relationship between height and a nurse's job performance. Now, suppose that, by chance again, we drew a sample in which tall nurses received better job evaluations than short ones. Could we conclude that height is related to a nurse's performance? These two examples illustrate the difficulty of using observations from a sample to generalize to a population. Other issues, such as the accuracy of the measures and the effects of uncontrolled variables prevent researchers from concluding with finality that hypotheses are proved.

➲ **TIP:** If a researcher uses any statistical tests (as is true in most quantitative studies), it means that there are underlying hypotheses—regardless of whether the researcher explicitly stated them—because statistical tests are designed to test hypotheses. In planning a quantitative study of your own, do not be afraid to make predictions, that is, to state hypotheses.

CRITIQUING RESEARCH PROBLEMS, RESEARCH QUESTIONS, AND HYPOTHESES

In critiquing research articles, you need to evaluate whether researchers have adequately communicated their problem. The delineation of the problem, purpose statement, research questions, and hypotheses sets the stage for the description of what was done and what was learned. Ideally, you should not have to dig too deeply to decipher the research problem or to discover the questions.

A critique of the research problem is multidimensional. Substantively, you need to consider whether the problem is significant and has the potential to produce evidence to improve nursing practice. Studies that build in a meaningful way on existing knowledge are well-poised to contribute to

BOX 4.3 Guidelines for Critiquing Research Problems, Research Questions, and Hypotheses

1. What is the research problem? Is the problem statement easy to locate and is it clearly stated? Does the problem statement build a cogent and persuasive argument for the new study?
2. Does the problem have significance for nursing? How might the research contribute to nursing practice, administration, education, or policy?
3. Is there a good fit between the research problem and the paradigm within which the research was conducted? Is there a good fit between the problem and the qualitative research tradition (if applicable)?
4. Does the report formally present a statement of purpose, research question, and/or hypotheses? Is this information communicated clearly and concisely, and is it placed in a logical and useful location?
5. Are purpose statements or questions worded appropriately? For example, are key concepts/variables identified and is the population of interest specified? Are verbs used appropriately to suggest the nature of the inquiry and/or the research tradition?
6. If there are no formal hypotheses, is their absence justified? Are statistical tests used in analyzing the data despite the absence of stated hypotheses?
7. Do hypotheses (if any) flow from a theory or previous research? Is there a justifiable basis for the predictions?
8. Are hypotheses (if any) properly worded—do they state a predicted relationship between two or more variables? Are they directional or nondirectional, and is there a rationale for how they were stated? Are they presented as research or as null hypotheses?

evidence-based nursing practice. Researchers who develop a systematic *program of research*, building on their own earlier findings, are especially likely to make important contributions (Conn, 2004). For example, Beck's series of studies relating to postpartum depression have influenced women's healthcare worldwide. Also, research problems stemming from established research priorities (Chapter 1) have a high likelihood of yielding important new evidence for nurses because they reflect expert opinion about areas of needed research.

Another dimension in critiquing the research problem is methodologic—in particular, whether the research problem is compatible with the chosen research paradigm and its associated methods. You should also evaluate whether the statement of purpose or research questions have been properly worded and lend themselves to empirical inquiry.

In a quantitative study, if the research article does not contain explicit hypotheses, you need to consider whether their absence is justified. If there are hypotheses, you should evaluate whether they are

logically connected to the problem and are consistent with existing evidence or relevant theory. The wording of hypotheses should also be assessed. To be testable, the hypothesis should contain a prediction about the relationship between two or more measurable variables. Specific guidelines for critiquing research problems, research questions, and hypotheses are presented in Box 4.3.

RESEARCH EXAMPLES

This section describes how the research problem and research questions were communicated in two nursing studies, one quantitative and one qualitative.

Research Example of a Quantitative Study

Study: The relationship among self-esteem, stress, coping, eating behavior, and depressive mood in adolescents (Martyn-Nemeth et al., 2009).

Problem Statement: "The prevalence of adolescent overweight has increased from 5% to 17% over the past 30 years in the United States . . . There are serious long-term health consequences for adolescents who are overweight . . . In addition, all overweight adolescents are at increased risk for depressive mood and clinical depression. Overweight adolescents tend to remain overweight as adults, with an increased risk of diabetes, cardiovascular disease, and cancer . . . The overall estimated economic burden of obesity in the nation for the year 2002 was 93 billion dollars . . . Self-esteem is associated with overeating and weight gain in adolescents, and stress-induced eating and inadequate coping skills have been related to overeating and obesity in adults . . . Important questions remain about the relationship of self-esteem, stress, social support, and coping to eating patterns in racially/ethnically diverse male and female adolescents" (p. 98).

Statement of Purpose: The purpose of this study "was to examine relationships among self-esteem, stress, social support, and coping, and to test a model of their effects on eating behavior and depressive mood in a sample of high school students" (p. 96).

Research Questions: The authors posed three research questions about relationships among the study variables (e.g., "Does the use of food as a coping mechanism relate to being overweight?" p. 99) One question focused on a mediating variable: "Does coping mediate the relationship of low self-esteem, increased stress, and decreased social support with the outcomes of unhealthy eating behavior and depressive mood" (p. 99).

Hypotheses: It was hypothesized that adolescents with low self-esteem, increased stress, and decreased social support would predominantly use avoidance mechanisms of coping, which would in turn mediate the negative outcomes of unhealthy eating and depressive mood.

Study Methods: The study was conducted with a multiracial sample of 102 students from two public high schools in Midwestern United States. Data were collected through self-administered questionnaires.

Key Findings: The results indicated that low self-esteem and stress were related to avoidant coping and depressive mood. Also, low self-esteem and avoidant coping were related to unhealthy eating, thus offering partial support for the researchers' hypotheses.

Research Example of a Qualitative Study

Study: Sustaining self: The lived experience of transition to long-term ventilation (Briscoe & Woodgate, 2010).

Problem Statement: "Chronic respiratory failure (CRF) occurs as a result of irreversible and/or progressive deterioration in ventilation and gas exchange, and is a common end point of a number of conditions that affect the lung, chest wall, and/or neurologic system . . . The only treatment for CRF is mechanical ventilation (MV), which can be delivered invasively via a tracheotomy tube, or noninvasively via a tightly sealed nasal or face mask, mouthpiece, or negative-chest-pressure device . . . A consensus of measuring incidence of CRF and prevalence of ventilator utilization is reflected in the literature . . . Care for individuals requiring long-term mechanical ventilation (LTMV) is evolving, and there is growing impetus to comprehensively address operational, financial, ethical, and client-centered concerns . . . Gaining a comprehensive understanding of both the burdens and benefits of ventilator treatment is vital for health professionals, ventilator users, and families . . . Especially lacking is an understanding of their transition, or journey, from spontaneous breathing to the stable reliance on LTMV" (pp. 57–58) (Citations were omitted to streamline the presentation).

Statement of Purpose: "The purpose of this phenomenological study was to acquire a detailed description of the experience of transition to LTMV from individuals requiring ventilation" (p. 58). (No specific research questions were articulated in this article).

Method: Study participants were 11 ventilated individuals recruited from two respiratory care facilities in western Canada. All participants were interviewed on one or more occasions, and all interviews were audiorecorded. Participants shared pictures and other memorabilia, which assisted them in telling their stories of transition to LTMV. Conversational questions were posed, such as "Can you please tell me about the time when the ventilator was first introduced to you? Analysis began with the first interview and continued with ongoing interviews over a 4-month period.

Key Findings: The transition journey was found to be a time of psychological, physical, and spiritual challenge. "Sustaining self" was identified as the essence of ventilator users' transition experience.

SUMMARY POINTS

- A **research problem** is a perplexing or enigmatic situation that a researcher wants to address through disciplined inquiry. Researchers usually identify a broad **topic,** narrow the problem scope, and identify questions consistent with a paradigm of choice.

- Common sources of ideas for nursing research problems are clinical experience, relevant literature, quality improvement initiatives, social issues, theory, and external suggestions.
- Key criteria in assessing a research problem are that the problem should be clinically significant; researchable; feasible; and of personal interest.
- Feasibility involves the issues of time, cooperation of participants and other people, availability of facilities and equipment, researcher experience, and ethical considerations.
- Researchers communicate their aims as problem statements, statements of purpose, research questions, or hypotheses.
- A **statement of purpose**, which summarizes the overall study goal, identifies key concepts (variables) and the population. Purpose statements often communicate, through the use of verbs and other key terms, the underlying research tradition of qualitative studies, or whether study is experimental or nonexperimental in quantitative ones.
- A **research question** is the specific query researchers want to answer in addressing the research problem. In quantitative studies, research questions usually concern the existence, nature, strength, and direction of relationships.
- Some research questions are about **moderator variables** that affect the strength or direction of a relationship between the independent and dependent variables; others are about **mediating variables** that intervene between the independent and dependent variable and help to explain why the relationship exists.
- **Problem statements,** which articulate the nature, context, and significance of a problem, include several components: problem identification; the background, scope, and consequences of the problem; knowledge gaps; and possible solutions to the problem.
- In quantitative studies, a **hypothesis** is a statement of predicted relationships between two or more variables.

- **Simple hypotheses** express a predicted relationship between one independent variable and one dependent variable, whereas **complex hypotheses** state an anticipated relationship between two or more independent variables and two or more dependent variables (or state predictions about mediating or moderator variables).
- **Directional hypotheses** predict the direction of a relationship; **nondirectional hypotheses** predict the existence of relationships, not their direction.
- **Research hypotheses** predict the existence of relationships; **null hypotheses,** which express the absence of a relationship, are the hypotheses subjected to statistical testing.
- Hypotheses are never proved or disproved in an ultimate sense—they are accepted or rejected, supported or not supported by the data.

STUDY ACTIVITIES

Chapter 4 of the *Resource Manual for Nursing Research: Generating and Assessing Evidence for Nursing Practice, 9th ed.*, offers study suggestions for reinforcing concepts presented in this chapter. In addition, the following questions can be addressed in classroom or online discussions:

1. Think of a frustrating experience you have had as a nursing student or as a practicing nurse. Identify the problem area. Ask yourself a series of questions until you have one that you think is researchable. Evaluate the problem in terms of the evaluation criteria discussed in this chapter.
2. To the extent possible, use the critiquing questions in Box 4.3 to appraise the research problems for the two studies used as research examples at the end of this chapter.

STUDIES CITED IN CHAPTER 4

Beck, C. T., & Watson, S. (2008). The impact of birth trauma on breastfeeding: A tale of two pathways. *Nursing Research, 57,* 228–236.

Berarducci, A., Haines, K., & Murr, M. (2009). Incidence of bone loss, falls, and fractures after Roux-en-Y gastric bybass for morbid obesity. *Applied Nursing Research, 22*, 35–41.

Briscoe, W., & Woodgate, R. (2010). Sustaining self: The lived experience of transition to long-term ventilation. *Qualitative Health Research, 20*, 57–67.

Horne, M., Skelton, D., Speed, S., & Todd, C. (2010). The influence of primary health care professionals in encouraging exercise and physical activity uptake among white and South Asian older adults. *Patient Education & Counseling, 78*, 97–103.

Lopez-Dicastillo, O., Grande, G., & Callery, P. (2010). Parents' contrasting views on diet versus activity of children. *Patient Education and Counseling, 78*, 117–123.

Lundberg, B., Hansson, L., Wentz, E., & Bjorkman, T. (2009). Are stigmatizing experiences among persons with mental illness related to perceptions of self-esteem, empowerment, and sense of coherence? *Journal of Psychiatric & Mental Health Nursing, 16*, 516–522.

Martyn-Nemeth, P., Penckofer, S., Gulanick, M., Velsor-Friedrich, B., & Bryant, F. (2009). The relationship among self-esteem, stress, coping, eating behavior, and depressive mood in adolescents. *Research in Nursing & Health, 32*, 96–109.

Moore, K., Hunter, H., McGinnis, R., Bascu, C., Fader, M., Gray, M., Getliffe, K., Chobanuk, J., Puttagunta, L., & Voaklander, D. C. (2009). Do catheter washouts extend patency time in long-term indwelling urethral catheters? *Journal of Wound, Ostomy, and Continence Nursing, 36*, 82–90.

Nilsson, C., & Lundgren, I. (2009). Women's lived experience of fear of childbirth. *Midwifery, 25*, 1–9.

Robbins, L., Sikorski, A., Hamel, L., Wu, T., & Wilbur, J. (2009). Gender comparisons of perceived benefits of and barriers to physical activity in middle school youth. *Research in Nursing & Health, 32*, 163–176.

Tzeng, Y. L., Lin, L., Shyr, Y., & Wen, J. (2009). Sexual behavior of institutionalized residents with dementia. *Journal of Clinical Nursing, 18*, 991–1001.

Methodologic and nonresearch references cited in this chapter can be found in a separate section at the end of the book.

5 | Literature Reviews: Finding and Critiquing Evidence

Researchers typically conduct research within the context of existing knowledge by undertaking a thorough **literature review**. This chapter describes activities associated with literature reviews, including locating and critiquing studies. Many of these activities overlap with early steps in an EBP project, as described in Chapter 2.

GETTING STARTED ON A LITERATURE REVIEW

Before discussing the steps involved in doing a research-based literature review, we briefly discuss some general issues. The first concerns the viewpoint of qualitative researchers.

Literature Reviews in Qualitative Research Traditions

As noted in Chapter 3, qualitative researchers have varying opinions about reviewing the literature before doing a new study. Some of the differences reflect viewpoints associated with qualitative research traditions.

Grounded theory researchers often collect their data before reviewing the literature. The grounded theory takes shape as data are analyzed. Researchers then turn to the literature when the theory is sufficiently developed, seeking to relate prior findings to the theory. Glaser (1978) warned that, "It's hard enough to generate one's own ideas without the 'rich' detailment provided by literature in the same field" (p. 31). Thus, grounded theory researchers may defer a literature review, but then consider how previous research fits with or extends the emerging theory. McGhee and colleagues (2007), however, have noted how researchers can use reflexivity (a concept discussed at length later in this book) to prevent prior knowledge from distorting grounded theory analysis.

Phenomenologists often undertake a search for relevant materials at the outset of a study. In reviewing the literature, phenomenological researchers look for experiential descriptions of the phenomenon being studied (Munhall, 2012). The purpose is to expand the researcher's understanding of the phenomenon from multiple perspectives, and this may include an examination of artistic sources in which the phenomenon is described (e.g., in novels or poetry).

Even though "ethnography starts with a conscious attitude of almost complete ignorance" (Spradley, 1979, p. 4), literature that led to the choice of the cultural problem to be studied is often reviewed before data collection. A second, more thorough literature review is often done during data analysis and interpretation so that findings can be compared with previous findings.

Regardless of tradition, if funding is sought for a qualitative project, an upfront literature review is usually necessary. Reviewers need to understand the context for the proposed study, and must be persuaded that it should be funded.

Purposes and Scope of Research Literature Reviews

Written literature reviews are undertaken for many different purposes. The length of the product depends on its purpose. Regardless of length, a good review requires thorough familiarity with available evidence. As Garrard (2006) advised, you must strive to *own* the literature on a topic to be confident of preparing a state-of-the-art review. The major types of written research review include the following:

- *A review in a research report.* Literature reviews in the introduction to a report provide readers with an overview of existing evidence, and contribute to the argument for the new study. These reviews are usually only 2 to 4 double-spaced pages, and so, only key studies can be cited. The emphasis is on summarizing and evaluating an overall body of evidence.
- *A review in a proposal.* A literature review in a proposal provides context, confirms the need for new research, and demonstrates the writer's "ownership" of the literature. The length of such reviews is established in proposal guidelines, but is often just a few pages. This means that the review must reflect expertise on the topic in a very succinct fashion.
- *A review in a thesis or dissertation.* Dissertations in the traditional format (see Chapter 28) often include a thorough, critical literature review. An entire chapter may be devoted to the review, and such chapters are often 15 to 25 pages long. These reviews typically include an evaluation of the overall body of literature as well as critiques of key individual studies.
- *Free-standing literature reviews.* Nurses also prepare reviews that critically appraise and summarize a body of research, sometimes for a course or for an EBP project. Researchers who are experts

in a field also may do systematic reviews that are published in journals (Chapter 27). Free-standing reviews are usually 15 to 25 pages long.

This chapter focuses on the preparation of a review as a component of an original study, but most activities are similar for other types of review. By doing a thorough review, researchers can determine how best to make a contribution to existing evidence—for example, whether there are gaps or inconsistencies in a body of research, or whether a replication with a new population is the right next step. A literature review also plays a role at the end of the study when researchers try to make sense of their findings.

Types of Information for a Research Review

Written materials vary in their quality and the kind of information they contain. In performing a literature review, you will have to decide what to read and what to include in a written review. We offer some suggestions that may help in making such decisions.

The most important type of information for a research review is findings from prior studies. You should rely mostly on **primary source** research reports, which are descriptions of studies written by the researchers who conducted them.

Secondary source research documents are descriptions of studies prepared by someone other than the original researcher. Literature reviews, for example, are secondary sources. If reviews are recent, they are a good place to start because they provide an overview of the topic and a valuable bibliography. Secondary sources are not substitutes for primary sources because they typically fail to provide much detail about studies, and are seldom completely objective.

> **➲ TIP:** For an EBP project, a recent, high-quality review may be sufficient to provide needed information about existing evidence, although it is wise to search for recent studies not covered by the review.

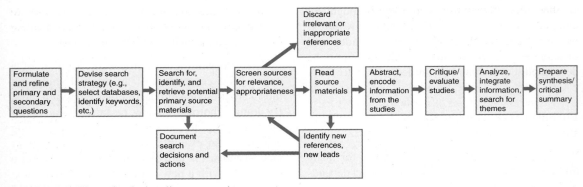

FIGURE 5.1 Flow of tasks in a literature review.

Examples of primary and secondary sources:

- Primary source, an original study of palliative patients and family caregivers regarding preferences for location of death: Stajduhar, K., Allan, D., Cohen, S., & Heyland, D. (2008). Preferences for location of death of seriously ill hospitalized patients. *Palliative Medicine, 22,* 85–88.
- Secondary source, a review of factors affecting place of end-of-life care for patients with cancer: Murray, M., Fiset, V., Young, S., & Kryworuchko, J. (2009). Where the dying live: Review of determinants of place of end-of-life cancer care. *Oncology Nursing Forum, 36,* 69–77.

In addition to research reports, your search may yield nonresearch references, such as case reports, anecdotes, or clinical descriptions. Nonresearch materials may broaden understanding of a problem, demonstrate a need for research, or describe aspects of clinical practice. These writings may help in formulating research ideas, but they usually have limited utility in written research reviews because they do not address the central question: What is the current state of *evidence* on this research problem?

Major Steps and Strategies in Doing a Literature Review

Conducting a literature review is a little like doing a full study, in the sense that reviewers start with a question, formulate and implement a plan for gathering information, and then analyze and interpret information. The "findings" must then be summarized in a written product.

Figure 5.1 outlines the literature review process. As the figure shows, there are several potential feedback loops, with opportunities to retrace earlier steps in search of more information. This chapter discusses each step, but some steps are elaborated in Chapter 27 in our discussion of systematic reviews.

Conducting a high-quality literature review is more than a mechanical exercise—it is an art and a science. Several qualities characterize a high-quality review. First, the review must be comprehensive, thorough, and up-to-date. To "own" the literature (Garrard, 2006), you must be determined to become an expert on your topic, which means that you need to be creative and diligent in hunting down leads for possible sources of information.

> **TIP:** Locating all relevant information on a research question is a bit like being a detective. The literature retrieval tools we discuss in this chapter are a tremendous aid, but there inevitably needs to be some digging for the clues to evidence on a topic. Be prepared for sleuthing!

Second, a high-quality review is systematic. Decision rules should be clear, and criteria for including or excluding a study need to be explicit. This is because a third characteristic of a good review is that it is reproducible, which means that another diligent reviewer would be able to apply the same decision rules and criteria and come to similar conclusions about the evidence.

Another desirable attribute of a literature review is the absence of bias. This is more easily achieved when systematic rules for evaluating information are followed—although reviewers cannot totally elude personal opinions. For this reason, systematic reviews are often conducted by teams of researchers who can evaluate each other's conclusions. Finally, reviewers should strive for a review that is insightful and that is more than "the sum of its parts." Reviewers have an opportunity to contribute to knowledge through an astute and incisive synthesis of the evidence.

We recommend thinking of doing a literature review as similar to doing a qualitative study. This means having a flexible approach to "data collection" and thinking creatively about ideas for new sources of information. It means pursuing leads until "saturation" is achieved—that is, until your search strategies yield redundant information about studies to include. And it also means that the analysis of your "data" will typically involve a search for important themes.

Primary and Secondary Questions for a Review

For free-standing literature reviews and EBP projects, the reviewer may seek to summarize research evidence about a single focused question, such as those described in Chapter 2 (see Table 2.1 for question templates). For those who are undertaking a literature review as part of a new study, the *primary question* for the literature review is the same as the actual research question for the new study. The researcher wants to know: What is the current state of knowledge on the question that I will be addressing in *my* study?

If you are doing a review for a new study, you inevitably will need to search for existing evidence on several *secondary questions* as well because you will need to develop an argument (a rationale) for the new study in the problem statement. An example (which we will use throughout this chapter) will clarify this point.

Suppose that we were conducting a study to address the following question: What characteristics of nurses are associated with effective pain management for hospitalized children? In other words, our primary question is whether there are characteristics of nurses that are associated with appropriate responses to children's pain. Such a question would arise within the context of a perceived problem, such as a concern that nurses' treatment of children's pain is not always optimal. A basic statement of the problem might be as follows:

• • •

Many children are hospitalized annually and many hospitalized children experience high levels of pain. There are long-lasting harmful effects to the nervous system when severe or persistent pain in children is untreated. Although effective analgesic and nonpharmacologic methods of controlling children's pain exist, and although there are reliable methods of assessing children's pain, nurses do not always manage children's pain effectively. *What characteristics distinguish nurses who are effective and those who are not?*

• • •

This rudimentary problem statement suggests a number of *secondary questions* for which evidence from the literature will need to be located and evaluated. Examples of such secondary questions include the following:

- How many children are hospitalized annually?
- What types and levels of pain do hospitalized children experience?
- What are the consequences of untreated pain in children?
- How can pain in hospitalized children be reliably assessed and effectively treated?
- How adequately do nurses manage pain in hospitalized pediatric patients?

Thus, conducting a literature review tends to be a multipronged endeavor when it is done as part of a new study. While most of the "detective work" in searching the literature that we describe in this chapter applies principally to the primary question, it is important to keep in mind other questions for which information from the research literature needs to be retrieved.

LOCATING RELEVANT LITERATURE FOR A RESEARCH REVIEW

As shown in Figure 5.1, an early step in a literature review is devising a strategy to locate relevant studies. The ability to locate research documents on a topic is an important skill that requires adaptability. Rapid technological changes have made manual methods of finding information obsolete, and sophisticated methods of searching the literature are being introduced continuously. We urge you to consult with librarians, colleagues, or faculty for suggestions.

Formulating a Search Strategy

There are many ways to search for research evidence, and it is wise to begin a search with some strategies in mind. Cooper (2010) has identified several approaches, one of which we describe in some detail in this chapter: searching for references in bibliographic databases. Another approach, called the *ancestry approach*, involves using citations from relevant studies to track down earlier research on the same topic (the "ancestors"). A third method, the *descendancy approach*, is to find a pivotal early study and to search forward in citation indexes to find more recent studies ("descendants") that cited the key study. Other strategies exist for tracking down what is called the *grey literature*, which refers to studies with more limited distribution, such as conference papers, unpublished reports, and so on. We describe these strategies in Chapter 27 on systematic reviews. If your intent is to "own" the literature, then you will likely want to adopt all of these strategies, but in many cases, the first two or three might suffice.

> **TIP:** You may be tempted to begin a literature search through an Internet search engine, such as Yahoo, Google, or Google Scholar. Such a search is likely to yield a lot of "hits" on your topic, but is not likely to give you full bibliographic information on *research* literature on your topic—and you might become frustrated with searching through vast numbers of website links.

Search plans also involve decisions about delimiting the search. These decisions need to be explicit to ensure reproducibility. If you are not multilingual, you may need to constrain your search to studies written in your own language. You may also want to limit your search to studies conducted within a certain time frame (e.g., within the past 15 years). You may want to exclude studies with certain types of participants. For instance, in our example of a literature search about nurses' characteristics and treatment of children's pain, we might want to exclude studies in which the children were neonates. Finally, you may choose to limit your search based on how your key variables are defined. For instance, in our example, you may (or may not) wish to exclude studies in which the focus was on nurses' *attitudes* toward children's pain.

> **TIP:** Constraining your search might help you to avoid irrelevant material, but be cautious about putting too many restrictions on your search, especially initially. You can always make decisions to exclude studies at a later point, provided you have clear criteria and a rationale. Be sure not to limit your search to very recent studies or to studies exclusively in the nursing literature.

Searching Bibliographic Databases

Reviewers typically begin by searching bibliographic databases that can be accessed by computer. The databases contain entries for thousands of journal articles, each of which has been coded to facilitate retrieval. For example, articles may be coded for language used (e.g., English), subject matter (e.g., pain), type of journal (e.g., nursing), and so on. Several commercial vendors (e.g., Aries Knowledge Finder, Ovid, EBSCOhost, ProQuest) offer software for retrieving information from these databases. Most programs are user-friendly, offering menu-driven systems with on-screen support so that retrieval can proceed with minimal instruction. Some providers offer discount rates for students and trial services that allow you to test them before subscribing. In most cases, however, your university or hospital library has a subscription.

Getting Started with a Bibliographic Database

Before searching an electronic database, you should become familiar with the features of the software you are using to access the database. The software gives you options for limiting your search, for combining the results of two searches, for saving your search, and so on. Most programs have tutorials that can improve the efficiency and effectiveness of your search. In many cases, a "Help" button will provide you with a lot of information.

You will also need to learn how to get from "point A" (the constructs in which you are interested) to "point B" (the way that the program stores and organizes information about the constructs). Most software you are likely to use has mapping capabilities. *Mapping* is a feature that allows you to search for topics using your own **keywords**, rather than needing to enter a term that is exactly the same as a **subject heading** (subject codes) in the database. The software translates ("maps") the keywords you enter into the most plausible subject heading. In addition to mapping your term onto a database-specific subject heading, most programs will also search in the *text fields* of records (usually the title and abstract) for the keyword entered.

⬤ TIP: The keywords you begin with are usually your key independent or dependent variables, and perhaps your population. If you have used the question templates in Table 2.1 or in the Toolkit for Chapter 4, the words you entered in the blanks would be keywords.

Even when there are mapping capabilities, you should learn the relevant subject headings of the database you are using because keyword searches and subject heading searches yield overlapping but nonidentical results. Subject headings for databases can be located in the database's thesaurus or other reference tools.

⬤ TIP: To identify all major research reports on a topic, you need to be flexible and to think broadly about the keywords that could be related to your topic. For example, if you are interested in anorexia nervosa, you might look under *anorexia, eating disorder,* and *weight loss,* and perhaps under *appetite, eating behavior, food habits, bulimia,* and *body weight change.*

General Database Search Features

Some features of an electronic search are similar across databases. One feature is that you usually can use **Boolean operators** to expand or delimit a search. Three widely used Boolean operators are AND, OR, and NOT (usually in all caps). The operator *AND* delimits a search. If we searched for *pain AND children,* the software would retrieve only records that have both terms. The operator *OR* expands the search: *pain OR children* could be used in a search to retrieve records with either term. Finally, *NOT* narrows a search: *pain NOT children* would retrieve all records with pain that did not include the term children.

Wildcard and truncation symbols are other useful tools for searching databases. These symbols vary from one database to another, but their function is to expand the search. A **truncation symbol** (often an asterisk, *) expands a search term to include all forms of a root word. For example, a search for *child** would instruct the computer to search for any word that begins with "child" such as children, childhood, or childrearing. **Wildcard symbols** (often a question mark or asterisk) inserted into the middle of a search term permits a search for alternative spellings. For example, a search for *behavio?r* would retrieve records with either *behavior* or *behaviour.* Also, a search for *wom?n* would retrieve records with either *woman* or *women.* For each database, it is important to learn what these special symbols are and how they work. For example, many databases require at least three letters at the beginning of a search term before a wildcard or truncation symbol can be used (e.g., ca* would not be allowed). Moreover, not every database (including PubMed) allows wildcard codes in the middle of a search term.

Another important thing to know is that use of special symbols usually turns off a software's mapping feature. For example, a search for *child** would retrieve records in which any form of "child" appeared in text fields, but it would not map any of these concepts onto the database's subject headings (e.g., pediatric).

Sometimes it is important to keep words together in a search, as in a search for records with *blood pressure.* Some bibliometric software would treat this as *blood AND pressure,* and would search for records with both terms somewhere in text fields, even if they are not contiguous. Quotation marks often can be used to ensure that the words are searched only in combination, as in *"blood pressure."*

Key Electronic Databases for Nurse Researchers

Two especially useful electronic databases for nurse researchers are CINAHL (**C**umulative **I**ndex to **N**ursing and **A**llied **H**ealth **L**iterature) and MEDLINE (**Med**ical Literature On-**Line**), which we discuss in the next sections. Other potentially useful bibliographic databases for nurses include:

- British Nursing Index
- Cochrane Database of Systematic Reviews
- Dissertation Abstracts online
- EMBASE (the **E**xcerpta **M**edica data**base**)
- HaPI (**H**ealth **a**nd **P**sychosocial **I**nstruments database)
- Health Source: Nursing/Academic Edition
- ISI Web of Knowledge
- Nursing and Allied Health Source (ProQuest)
- PsycINFO (**Psyc**hology **Info**rmation)
- Scopus

Note that a search strategy that works well in one database does not always produce good results in another. Thus, it is important to explore strategies in each database and to understand how each database is structured—for example, what subject headings are used and how they are organized in a hierarchy. Each database and software program also has certain peculiarities. For example, using PubMed (to be discussed later) to search the MEDLINE database, you might restrict your search to nursing journals. However, if you did this you would be excluding studies in several journals in which nurses often publish, such as *Birth* and *Qualitative Health Research* because these journals are not coded for the nursing subset of PubMed.

➲ **TIP:** In the next two sections, we provide specific information about using CINAHL and MEDLINE via PubMed. Note, however, that databases and the software through which they are accessed change from time to time, and our instructions may not be precisely accurate. For example, a redesigned interface was implemented in PubMed in late 2009 and was later revised in February 2010, requiring us to rewrite parts of the MEDLINE section.

Cumulative Index to Nursing and Allied Health Literature

CINAHL is an important electronic database: It covers references to virtually all English-language nursing and allied health journals, as well as to books, dissertations, and selected conference proceedings in nursing and allied health fields. There are several versions of the CINAHL database (e.g., CINAHL, CINAHL Plus), each with somewhat different features relating to full text availability and journal coverage. All are offered through EBSCOhost.

The basic CINAHL database indexes material from nearly 3,000 journals dating from 1981, and contains more than 1 million records. In addition to providing information for locating references (i.e., author, title, journal, year of publication, volume, and page numbers), CINAHL provides abstracts of most citations. Supplementary information, such as names of data collection instruments, is available for many records. CINAHL can be accessed through CINAHL (*www.ebscohost.com/cinahl/*) or through institutional libraries. We illustrate features of CINAHL, but note that some may be labeled differently at your institution.

At the outset, you might begin with a "basic search" by simply entering keywords or phrases relevant to your primary question. In the basic search screen, you could limit your search in a number of ways, for example, by limiting the records retrieved to those with certain features (e.g., only ones with abstracts or only those in journals with peer review), to specific publication dates (e.g., only those from 2005 to the present), or to those coded as being in a particular subset (e.g., nursing). The basic search screen also allows you to expand your search by clicking an option labeled "Apply related words."

As an example, suppose we were interested in recent research on nurses' pain management for children. If we searched for *pain*, we would get nearly 20,000 records. Searching for *pain AND child* AND nurs** would bring the number down to about 2,000. (In CINAHL, an asterisk is the truncation symbol and a question mark is the wildcard). We could pare the number down to about 300 in a basic search by limiting the search to articles with abstracts published in nursing journals after 2004.

The advanced search mode in CINAHL permits even more fine-tuning. For example, we could stipulate that we wanted only research articles published in English. These restrictions, which take only seconds to execute, would get us down to a more manageable number of records (130) that could be searched more carefully for relevance. The advanced search mode offers many additional search options that should be more fully explored.

The full records for the 130 references would then be displayed on the monitor in a Results List. The Results List has sidebar options that allow you to narrow your search even farther, if desired. From the Results List, we could place promising references into a folder for later scrutiny, or we could immediately retrieve and print full bibliographic information for records of interest. An example of an abridged CINAHL record entry for a study identified through the search on children's pain is presented in Figure 5.2. The record begins with the article title, the authors' names and affiliation, and source. The source indicates the following:

- Name of the journal (*Pediatric Nursing*)
- Year and month of publication (2008 Jul–Aug)
- Volume (34)
- Issue (4)
- Page numbers (297–397)
- Number of cited references (40)

The record also shows the major and minor CINAHL subject headings that were coded for this study. Any of these headings could have been used to retrieve this reference. Note that the subject headings include substantive codes such as *Pain – Nursing*, and also methodologic codes (e.g., *Questionnaires*) and sample characteristic codes (e.g., *Child*). Next, the abstract for the study is shown. Based on the abstract, we would decide whether this reference was pertinent. Additional information on the record includes the journal subset, special interest category, instrumentation, and (if relevant) funding for the study. Each entry shows an accession number that is the unique identifier for each record in the database, as well as other identifying numbers.

An important feature of CINAHL and other databases is that it allows you to easily find other relevant references once a good one has been found. For example, in Figure 5.2 you can see that the record offers many embedded links on which you can click. For example, you could click on any of the authors' names to see if they have published other related articles. You could also click on any of the subject headings to track down other leads. There is also a link in each record called *Cited References*. By clicking this link, the entire reference list for the record (i.e., all the references cited in the article) would be retrieved, and you could then examine any of the citations. Finally, there is a sidebar link in each record called "*Find similar results*," which would retrieve additional records for articles with a similar focus.

In CINAHL, you can also explore the structure of the database's thesaurus to get additional leads for searching. The tool bar at the top of the screen has a tab called *CINAHL Headings*. When you click on this tab and enter a term in the "Browse" field, you can enter a term of interest and select one of three options: Term Begins With, Term Contains, or Relevance Ranked (which is the default). For example, if we entered *pain* and then clicked on Browse, we would be shown the 52 relevant subject headings relating to pain. We could then search the database for any of the listed subject headings. Also, many terms have an "Explode" option, which allows you to create a search query in which headings are exploded to retrieve all references indexed to that term.

Title:	Nurse characteristics and inferences about children's pain
Authors:	Griffin RA; Polit DF; Byrne MW
Affiliation:	Boston College, School of Nursing, Chestnut Hill, MA
Source:	Pediatric Nursing (PEDIATR **NURS**), 2008 Jul–Aug; 34(4): 297–307 (40 ref)
Publication Type:	journal article – CEU, exam questions, **research**, tables/charts
Language:	English
Major Subjects:	Child, Hospitalized Nurse Attitudes – Evaluation Pain – Nursing Pain – Therapy – In Infancy and Childhood Pediatric Nursing
Minor Subjects:	Analysis of Variance; Child; Cross Sectional Studies; Demography; Descriptive Statistics; Female; Mail; Male; Multiple Regression; Post Hoc Analysis; Questionnaires; Random Sample; Scales; Survey Research; T-Tests; United States; Vignettes; Visual Analog Scaling
Abstract:	The purpose of this study was to describe pediatric **nurses'** projected responses to **children's pain** as described in vignettes of hospitalized **children** and to explore **nurse** characteristics that might influence those responses. A survey was mailed to a national random sample of 700 RNs, and 334 **nurses** responded. The survey included case reports of three hospitalized school-aged **children** experiencing **pain.** **Nurses** were asked to rate their perceptions of the **children's pain** levels and to indicate how much analgesia they would recommend. Contrary to earlier studies, in response to the scenarios, **nurses** in this sample perceived high levels of **pain**, said they would administer doses of analgesia close to the maximum prescribed by physicians, and recommended an array of non-pharmacologic methods to treat **pain**. Variation in **pain** perceptions and decisions was not related to key personal and professional characteristics of the **nurses**, including their education level, race/ethnicity, age, years of clinical experience, and receipt of continuing education about **pain**. Findings from this large national study suggest that most **nurses** would make appropriate decisions relating to the treatment of **children's pain**, perhaps reflecting changes in the emphasis on **pain** management.
Journal Subset:	Core nursing; Nursing; Peer reviewed; USA
Special Interest:	Pain and Pain Management; Pediatric Care
Instrumentation:	FACES pain scale (FPS)
Accession No.	2010006653

FIGURE 5.2 Example of a record from a CINAHL search.

CINAHL can also be used to pursue descendancy searches. In the Results List, there is a notation for each record entry for the number of times the article was cited in the CINAHL database. Clicking on the link would show the full list of articles that had cited this study.

⊃ TIP: The Institute for Scientific Information (ISI) maintains a multidisciplinary resource called the Web of Knowledge, which offers searching opportunities in several bibliographic databases. The Web of Knowledge is widely used for its citation feature, which can be helpful in applying a descendancy strategy, using a link labeled "Cited Reference."

The MEDLINE Database

The MEDLINE database was developed by the U.S. National Library of Medicine (NLM), and is widely recognized as the premier source for bibliographic coverage of the biomedical literature. MEDLINE covers about 5,000 medical, nursing, and health journals published in about 70 countries and contains more than 15 million records dating back to the mid 1960s. In 1999, abstracts of reviews from the Cochrane Collaboration became available through MEDLINE.

The MEDLINE database can be accessed online through a commercial vendor such as Ovid, but this database can be accessed for free through the PubMed website (*http://www.ncbi.nlm.nih.gov/PubMed*). This means that anyone, anywhere in the world, with Internet access can search for journal articles, and thus, PubMed is a lifelong resource regardless of your institutional affiliation. PubMed has an excellent tutorial.

On the Home page of PubMed, you can launch a basic search that looks for your keyword in text fields of the record. As you begin to enter your keyword (or a key phrase) in the search box, automatic suggestions will display, and you can click on the one that is the best match.

MEDLINE uses a controlled vocabulary called MeSH (Medical Subject Headings) to index articles. MeSH provides a consistent way to retrieve information that may use different terms for the same concepts. You can learn about relevant MeSH terms by clicking on the "MeSH database" link on the home page (under "More Resources"). If, for example, we searched the MeSH database for "pain," we would find that Pain is a MeSH subject heading (a definition is provided) and there are 39 additional related categories—for example, "pain measurement" and "somatoform disorders." MeSH subject headings may overlap with, but are not identical to, subject headings used in CINAHL.

If you begin using your own keyword in a basic search, you can see how your term mapped onto MeSH terms by scrolling down and looking in the right-hand panel for a section labeled "Search Details." For example, if we entered the keyword "children" in the search field of the initial screen, Search Details would show us that PubMed searched for all references that have "child" or "children" in text fields of the database record, *and* it also searched for all references that had been coded "child" as a subject heading, because "child" is a MeSH subject heading. When you initiate a search, PubMed offers an "Also Try" feature (also in the right panel) that suggests other terms to enter in the search field (e.g., pain children).

If we did a PubMed search of MEDLINE similar to the one we described earlier for CINAHL, we would find that a simple search for *pain* would yield about 420,000 records, and *pain AND child* AND nurs** would yield nearly 2,500. We can place restrictions on the search by clicking the blue "Limits" link

right above the search box. Limits include date (e.g., published in the last 2 years), language (e.g., English), journal subset (e.g., Nursing journals), and text options (e.g., only those with abstracts). If we limited our search to entries with abstracts, written in English, published within the past 5 years, and coded in the Nursing subset, the search would yield about 300 citations. This PubMed search yielded more references than the CINAHL search, but we were not able to limit the search to research reports: PubMed does not have a generic category that distinguishes all research articles from nonresearch articles. Further options for building the search are available by clicking the "Advanced Search" link, which is directly to the right of the "Limits" link.

Figure 5.3 shows the full citation for the same study we located earlier in CINAHL (Figure 5.2). Beneath the abstract, when you click on "MeSH Terms" the display presents all of the MeSH terms that were used for this particular study, and also any "Substances." As you can see, the MeSH terms are quite different from the subject headings for the same reference in CINAHL. As with CINAHL, you can click on highlighted record entries (author names and MeSH terms) for possible leads. You can also click on a link labeled "LinkOut," which provides more resources for the article. In this example, the link tells us that there are three full text sources for this study: EBSCO, Ovid, and ProQuest (not shown in Figure 5.3).

In the right panel of the screen for PubMed records there is a list of "Related Articles," which is a useful feature once you have found a study that is a good exemplar of the evidence for which you are looking. Further down in the right panel, PubMed provides a list of any articles in the MEDLINE database that had cited this study, which is useful for a descendancy search.

➲ **TIP:** Searching for qualitative studies can pose special challenges. Walters and colleagues (2006) described how they developed optimal search strategies for qualitative studies in the EMBASE database, and Wilczynski and colleagues (2007) offered advice for searching in CINAHL. Flemming and Briggs (2006) compared three alternative strategies for finding qualitative research.

Pediatr Nurs. 2008 Jul–Aug;34(4):297–305.

Nurse characteristics and inferences about children's pain.

Griffin RA, Polit DF, Byrne MW.

Boston College, School of Nursing, Chestnut Hill, MA, USA.

The purpose of this study was to describe pediatric nurses' projected responses to children's pain as described in vignettes of hospitalized children and to explore nurse characteristics that might influence those responses. A survey was mailed to a national random sample of 700 RNs, and 334 nurses responded. The survey included case reports of three hospitalized school-aged children experiencing pain. Nurses were asked to rate their perceptions of the children's pain levels and to indicate how much analgesia they would recommend. Contrary to earlier studies, in response to the scenarios, nurses in this sample perceived high levels of pain, said they would administer doses of analgesia close to the maximum prescribed by physicians, and recommended an array of non-pharmacologic methods to treat pain. Variation in pain perceptions and decisions was not related to key personal and professional characteristics of the nurses, including their education level, race/ethnicity, age, years of clinical experience, and receipt of continuing education about pain. Findings from this large national study suggest that most nurses would make appropriate decisions relating to the treatment of children's pain, perhaps reflecting changes in the emphasis on pain management.

PMID: 18814563 [PubMed - indexed for MEDLINE]

MeSH Terms:

Analgesics, Opioid/administration & dosage	Male
Child	Middle Aged
Cross-Sectional Studies	Pain/drug therapy
Female	Pain/nursing*
Health Care Surveys	Pain Measurement*
Health Knowledge, Attitudes, Practice*	United States
Humans	

Substances: Analgesics, Opioid

FIGURE 5.3 Example of a record from a PubMed search.

Screening and Gathering References

References that have been identified through a literature search need to be screened. One screen is a practical one: Is the reference accessible? For example, some references may be written in a language you do not read, or published in a journal that you cannot retrieve. A second screen is relevance, which you can usually infer by reading the abstract. If an abstract is unavailable, you will need to guess about relevance based on the title. When screening an article, keep in mind that some of the articles judged to be not relevant for your primary question may be appropriate for a secondary question. A third screening criterion may be the study's methodologic quality—i.e., the quality of evidence the study yields, a topic discussed in a later section.

We strongly urge you to obtain full copies of relevant studies rather than taking notes. It is often necessary to reread an article or to get further details about a study, which can easily be done if you have a copy. Online retrieval of full text articles has increasingly become possible. An article that is not directly available online through your institution can be retrieved through a commercial vendor, by photocopying it from a hardcopy journal, or by requesting a copy from the lead author via e-mail communication.

Each obtained article should be filed in a manner that permits easy access. Some authors (Garrard, 2006) advocate a chronological filing method (e.g., by date of publication), but we think that alphabetical filing (using last name of the first author) is easier.

Documentation in Literature Retrieval

If your goal is to "own" the literature, you will be using a variety of databases, keywords, subject headings, and strategies in your effort to pursue all possible leads. As you meander through the complex world of research information, you will likely lose track of your efforts if you do not document your actions from the outset.

It is highly advisable to maintain a notebook (or computer database program) to record your search strategies and search results. You should make note of information such as databases searched; limits put on your search; specific keywords, subject headings, or authors used to direct the search; combining strategies adopted; studies used to inaugurate a "Related Articles" or "descendancy" search; websites visited; links pursued; authors contacted to request further information or copies of articles not readily available; and any other information that would help you keep track of what you have done. Part of your strategy usually can be documented by printing your search history from electronic databases.

By documenting your actions, you will be able to conduct a more efficient search—that is, you will not inadvertently duplicate a strategy you have already pursued. Documentation will also help you to assess what else needs to be tried—where to go next in your search. Finally, documenting your efforts is a step in ensuring that your literature review is reproducible.

➥ **TIP:** The Toolkit section of the accompanying *Resource Manual* offers a template for documenting certain types of information during a literature search. The template, as a Word document, can easily be augmented and adapted.

ABSTRACTING AND RECORDING INFORMATION

Tracking down relevant research on a topic is only the beginning of doing a literature review. Once you have a stack of useful articles, you need to develop a strategy for making sense of the information in them. If a literature review is fairly simple, it may be sufficient to jot down notes about key features of the studies under review and to use these notes as the basis for your analysis. However, literature reviews are often complex—for example, there may be dozens of studies, or study findings may vary. In such situations, it is useful to adopt a formal system of recording key information about each study. We describe two mechanisms for doing this, formal protocols and matrices. First, though, we discuss the advantages of developing a coding scheme.

Coding the Studies

Reviewers who undertake systematic reviews often develop extensive coding systems to support statistical analyses. Coding may not be necessary in less formal reviews, but we do think that coding can be useful, so we offer some simple suggestions and an example.

To develop a coding scheme, you will need to read at least a subset of studies and look for opportunities to categorize information. One approach is to code for key variables or themes. Let us take the example we have used in this chapter, the relationship between nurses' characteristics (the independent variable) on the one hand and nurses' responses to children's pain (the dependent variable) on the other. By perusing the articles we retrieved, we find that several nurse characteristics have been studied—for example, their age, gender, clinical experience, and so on. We can assign codes to each characteristic. Now let us consider the dependent variable, nurses' responses to children's pain. We find that some studies have focused on nurses' perceptions of children's pain, others have examined nurses' use of analgesia, and so on. These different outcomes can also be coded. An

---

BOX 5.1 Codes for Results Matrix/Coding in Margins

CODES FOR NURSE CHARACTERISTICS (INDEPENDENT VARIABLES)

1. Age
2. Gender
3. Education
4. Years of clinical experience
5. Race/ethnicity
6. Personal experience with pain
7. Nurse practitioner status

CODES FOR RESPONSES TO CHILDREN'S PAIN (DEPENDENT VARIABLES)

a. Perceptions of children's pain
b. Pain treatment (use of analgesia)
c. Pain treatment (use of nonpharmacologic methods)
d. Other (e.g., perceived barriers to optimal pain management)

---

example of a simple coding scheme is presented in Box 5.1.

The codes can then be applied to the studies. You can record these codes in a protocol or matrices (which we discuss next), but you should also note the codes in the margins of the articles themselves, so you can easily find the information. Figure 5.4, which presents an excerpt from the results of a study by Vincent and Denyes (2004), shows marginal coding of key variables.

Coding can be a useful organizational tool even when a review is focused. For example, if our research question was about nurses' use of non-

pharmacologic methods of pain treatment (i.e., not about use of analgesics or about pain perceptions), the outcome categories could be specific nonpharmacologic approaches, such as distraction, guided imagery, massage, and so on. The point is to organize information in a way that facilitates retrieval and analysis.

Literature Review Protocols

One method of organizing information from research articles is to use a formal protocol. Protocols are a means of recording various aspects of a study

---

For research question 2, the only significant relationship found between nurse characteristics (basic conditioning factors) and either the two nursing agency variables of knowledge and attitude, and ability to overcome barriers, or the nursing action/system variable of analgesic administration was a positive correlation between nurses' years of practice and nurses' abilities to overcome barriers to optimal pain management, $r = .41$, $p = .001$. Nurses who had longer practice experience with children also reported greater ability to overcome barriers to optimal pain management.

1b 1d
3b 3d
4b 4d
5b 5d
6b 6d

FIGURE 5.4 Coded excerpt from Results section. From Vincent, C. V., & Denyes, M. J. [2004]. Relieving children's pain: Nurses' abilities and analgesic administration practices. *Journal of Pediatric Nursing, 19*[1], 40–50.

systematically, including the full citation, theoretical foundations, methodologic features, findings, and conclusions. Evaluative information (e.g., your assessment of the study's strengths and weaknesses) can also be noted.

There is no fixed format for such a protocol—you must decide what elements are important to record *consistently* across studies to help you organize and analyze information. The example in Figure 5.5 ✪ can be adapted to fit your needs. (Although many

Citation:	Authors: _____
	Title: _____
	Journal: _____
	Year: _____ Volume: _____ Issue: _____ Pages: _____
Type of Study:	☐ Quantitative ☐ Qualitative ☐ Mixed Method
Location/Setting:	_____
Key concepts/ Variables:	Concepts: _____
	Intervention/Independent Variable: _____
	Dependent Variable: _____
	Controlled Variable: _____
Framework/Theory:	_____
Design Type:	☐ Experimental ☐ Quasi-experimental ☐ Nonexperimental
	Specific Design: _____
	Blinding? ☐ None ☐ Single: _____ ☐ Double _____
	Descrip. of Intervention: _____
	_____
	_____
	Comparison group(s): _____
	☐ Cross-sectional ☐ Longitudinal/Prospective No. of data collection points: ___
Qual. Tradition:	☐ Grounded theory ☐ Phenomenology ☐ Ethnography ☐ Other: _____
Sample:	Size: _____ Sampling method: _____
	Sample characteristics: _____
Data Sources:	Type: ☐ Self-report ☐ Observational ☐ Biophysiologic ☐ Other _____
	Description of measures: _____
	_____
	_____
	Data Quality: _____
Statistical Tests:	Bivariate: ☐ *t*-test ☐ ANOVA ☐ Chi-square ☐ Pearson's *r* ☐ Other: _____
	Multivar: ☐ Multiple Regression ☐ MANOVA ☐ Logistic Regression ☐ Other: ____
Findings/ Effect Sizes/ Themes	_____
	_____
	_____
	_____
	_____
	_____
Recommendations:	_____
Strengths:	_____
Weaknesses:	_____

FIGURE 5.5 ✪ Example of a literature review protocol.

terms on this protocol may not be familiar to you yet, you will learn their meaning in later chapters.) If you developed a coding scheme, you can use the codes to record information about study variables rather than writing out their names. Once you have developed a draft protocol, you should pilot test it with several studies to make sure it is sufficiently comprehensive.

Literature Review Matrices

For traditional narrative reviews of the literature, we prefer using two-dimensional matrices to organize information, because matrices directly support a thematic analysis. The content of the matrices, and number of matrices, can vary. A matrix can be constructed in hand-written form, in a word processing table, or in a spreadsheet. One advantage of computer files is that the information in the matrices can then be manipulated and sorted (e.g., the matrix entries can be sorted chronologically, or by authors' last name). We present some basic ideas, but there is room for creativity in designing matrices to organize information.

We think three types of matrix are useful:

- A Methodologic Matrix, which organizes information to answer: How have researchers studied this research question?
- Results Matrices, which address: What have researchers *found*?
- An Evaluation Matrix, to answer: How much confidence do we have in the evidence?

A Methodologic Matrix is used to record key features of study methods. Each row is for a study, and columns are for the kinds of methodologic information you want to capture across studies. An abbreviated example of such a matrix for the question about nurses' characteristics in relation to response to children's pain is presented in Figure 5.6 (available in the Toolkit). ⊗ This matrix only has six entries (other relevant studies were omitted to save space), yet it is clear that information arrayed in this fashion allows us to see patterns that might otherwise have gone unnoticed. For example, by looking down the columns, we can readily discern that the broad research question has attracted international interest,

samples of convenience have predominated, and self-report methods of data collection are most often used. When such a matrix is completed for all studies, it is easy to draw conclusions about how research questions have been addressed.

To discern themes in the pattern of *results*, we recommend developing multiple Results Matrices. It is useful to have as many Results Matrices as there are codes for either the independent or dependent variables, whichever is greater. In our coding scheme in Box 5.1, there are 7 independent variables and 4 dependent variables, so we would have 7 Results Matrices, one for each independent variable. The matrix in Figure 5.7 ⊗, for example, is for recording information for studies that examined *nurses' education* in relation to responses to children's pain. Other matrices would focus on nurses' age, years of experience, and so on. In each matrix, columns are used for dependent variables, and rows represent separate studies. Findings about the relationship between a particular independent variable and a particular dependent variable are noted in the cells. The cell entries can indicate more precisely how dependent variables were operationalized, the direction of any relationships, level of significance, or other types of statistical information. Although there are only four studies in this Results Matrix, we can detect some patterns: the evidence, although not consistent, mostly suggests that nurses' level of education is unrelated to their responses to children's pain. Older studies were more likely than recent ones to find that more education was associated with better pain management.

Care should be taken in abstracting results information. Researchers sometimes point out only the findings that are statistically significant. Take, for example, the coded paragraph in Figure 5.4. The researchers (Vincent & Denyes, 2004) only elaborated results about the relationship between the nurses' years of experience and their ability to overcome barriers to optimal pain management. However, as indicated in the entry in the Methodologic Matrix (see Figure 5.6), this study gathered and analyzed data about 5 nurse characteristics in relation to 2 pain management outcomes, and so

Authors	Pub Yr	Country	Dependent Variables	Independent Variables	Study Design	Sample Size	Sampling Method	Data Collection	Age of Children
Griffin et al.	2008	U.S.A.	Perception of child's pain, Use of analgesics, Use of nonpharmacologic methods	Nurses' age, clinical experience, education, nurse practitioner status	Cross-sectional, correlational	332 nurses, national sample	Random	Self-report questionnaire	8–10
Twycross	2007	U.K.	Pain management practices	Knowledge of pain management.	Cross-sectional, correlational	13 nurses, 1 surgical ward	Convenience	Observation, self-report	0–16
Vincent & Denyes	2004	U.S.A.	Use of analgesics, Perceived barriers to optimal pain management	Nurses' age, race, clinical experience, education, pain experience	Cross-sectional, correlational	67 nurses from 7 hospital units	Convenience	Observation, self-report questionnaire	3–17
Polkki et al.	2001	Finland	Nurses' use of nonpharmacologic methods	Nurses' age, education, clinical experience, # own kids	Cross-sectional, correlational	162 nurses from 5 hospitals	Convenience	Self-report questionnaire	8–12
Hamers et al.	1997	Netherlands	Assessments of child's pain, Confidence in assessment, Use of analgesics	Level of experience in pediatric nursing	Cross-sectional, correlational	695 nurses	Convenience	Video, vignette, self-reports	5–10
Margolius et al.	1995	U.S.A.	Perceptions of child's pain, Perceived adequacy of pain management	Nurses' education, age, years of nursing experience	Cross-sectional, correlational	228 nurses, 1 pediatric setting	Convenience	Self-report questionnaire	NA

FIGURE 5.6 Example of a methodologic matrix for recording key methodologic features of studies for a literature review: nurse characteristics and management of children's pain.

Independent Variable: *Nurses' Education* (Code 3)

Authors	Pub Year	DV.a Pain Perceptions	DV.b Use of Analgesics	DV.c Use of Nonpharmacologics	DV.d Other
Griffin et al.	2008	Rating of child's pain: no significant relationship	Amount used within PRN: no significant relationship	Number of nonpharmacologic strategies used: no significant relationship	—
Vincent & Denyes	2004	—	Percent of prescribed medications administered: no significant relation	—	Perceived barriers to optimal pain management: no significant relationship
Polkki et al.	2001	—	—	Use of nonpharmacologic methods higher in those with more education ($p < .05$)	—
Margolius et al.	1995	Perception of children's pain: higher with more education ($p < .05$)	—	—	—

FIGURE 5.7 ⊗ Example of a results matrix for recording key findings for a literature review: nurses' education and management of children's pain.

there are 10 codes in the margin of Figure 5.4. Thus, although nothing in the paragraph mentions nurses' education, we have entered "no significant relationship" in two cells of the Results Matrix in Figure 5.7 because the paragraph implies that all relationships, except one, were nonsignificant.

⮕ **TIP:** Results matrices can also be used for qualitative studies. Instead of columns for independent or dependent variables, columns can be used to record themes, concepts, or categories.

CRITIQUING STUDIES AND EVALUATING THE EVIDENCE

In drawing conclusions about a body of research, reviewers must record not only factual information about studies—methodologic features and findings—but must also make judgments about the worth of the evidence. This section discusses issues relating to research critiques.

Research Critiques of Individual Studies

A research **critique** is a careful appraisal of the strengths and weaknesses of a study. A good critique objectively identifies areas of adequacy and inadequacy. Although our emphasis in this chapter is on the evaluation of a body of research evidence for a literature review, we pause to offer advice about other types of critiques.

Many critiques focus on a single study rather than on aggregated evidence. For example, most journals that publish research articles have a policy of soliciting critiques by two or more peer reviewers who prepare written critiques and make a recommendation about whether or not to publish the report. Peer reviewers' critiques typically are brief and focus on key substantive and methodologic issues.

Students taking a research course may be asked to critique a study, to document their mastery of methodologic concepts. Such critiques usually are expected to be comprehensive, encompassing various dimensions of a report. This might include

substantive and theoretical aspects, ethical issues, methodologic decisions, interpretation, and the report's organization and presentation. The purpose of such thorough critique is to cultivate critical thinking, to induce students to use and document newly acquired research skills, and to prepare students for a professional nursing career in which evaluating research will almost surely play a role. Writing research critiques is an important first step on the path to developing an evidence-based practice.

⮕ **TIP:** When doing a research critique, you should read the article you are critiquing at least twice because the first step in preparing a critique is to understand what the report is saying. We encourage you to write in the margins of the article and to circle keywords.

We provide support for such comprehensive critiques of individual studies in several ways. First, detailed critiquing suggestions corresponding to chapter content are included in most chapters. Second, we offer an abbreviated set of key critiquing guidelines for quantitative and qualitative reports here in this chapter, in Boxes 5.2 ✖ and 5.3 ✖, respectively. Finally, it is always illuminating to have a good model, and so Appendices H and I of the accompanying *Resource Manual* include completed comprehensive research critiques of a quantitative and qualitative study (the studies themselves are printed in their entirety as well).

⮕ **TIP:** The guidelines in Boxes 5.2 and 5.3, which are available in the Toolkit of the accompanying *Resource Manual*, can be used to critique the quantitative and qualitative components of mixed methods studies that combine the two approaches (see Chapter 25). In addition, the questions in Box 25.1 should be addressed for a comprehensive critique of mixed methods studies.

The guidelines in Boxes 5.2 and 5.3 are organized according to the structure of most research articles—Abstract, Introduction, Method, Results, and Discussion. The second column lists key critiquing questions that have broad applicability to

BOX 5.2 Guide to an Overall Critique of a Quantitative Research Report

Aspect of the Report	Critiquing Questions	Detailed Critiquing Guidelines
Title	• Is the title a good one, succinctly suggesting key variables and the study population?	
Abstract	• Does the abstract clearly and concisely summarize the main features of the report (problem, methods, results, conclusions)?	
Introduction Statement of the problem	• Is the problem stated unambiguously, and is it easy to identify? • Does the problem statement build a cogent, persuasive argument for the new study? • Does the problem have significance for nursing? • Is there a good match between the research problem and the paradigm and methods used? Is a quantitative approach appropriate?	Box 4.3, page 90
Hypotheses or research questions	• Are research questions and/or hypotheses explicitly stated? If not, is their absence justified? • Are questions and hypotheses appropriately worded, with clear specification of key variables and the study population? • Are the questions/hypotheses consistent with the literature review and the conceptual framework?	Box 4.3, page 90
Literature review	• Is the literature review up to date and based mainly on primary sources? • Does the review provide a state-of-the-art synthesis of evidence on the problem? • Does the literature review provide a sound basis for the new study?	Box 5.4, page 122
Conceptual/ theoretical framework	• Are key concepts adequately defined conceptually? • Is there a conceptual/theoretical framework, rationale, and/or map, and (if so) is it appropriate? If not, is the absence of one justified?	Box 6.3, page 145
Method Protection of human rights	• Were appropriate procedures used to safeguard the rights of study participants? Was the study externally reviewed by an IRB/ethics review board? • Was the study designed to minimize risks and maximize benefits to participants?	Box 7.3, page 170

BOX 5.2 Guide to an Overall Critique of a Quantitative Research Report (continued) ✖

Aspect of the Report	Critiquing Questions	Detailed Critiquing Guidelines
Research design	• Was the most rigorous possible design used, given the study purpose? • Were appropriate comparisons made to enhance interpretability of the findings? • Was the number of data collection points appropriate? • Did the design minimize biases and threats to the internal, construct, and external validity of the study (e.g., was blinding used, was attrition minimized)?	Box 9.1, page 230; Box 10.1, page 254
Population and sample	• Is the population described? Is the sample described in sufficient detail? • Was the best possible sampling design used to enhance the sample's representativeness? Were sampling biases minimized? • Was the sample size adequate? Was a power analysis used to estimate sample size needs?	Box 12.1, page 289
Data collection and measurement	• Are the operational and conceptual definitions congruent? • Were key variables operationalized using the best possible method (e.g., interviews, observations, and so on) and with adequate justification? • Are specific instruments adequately described and were they good choices, given the study purpose, variables being studied, and the study population? • Does the report provide evidence that the data collection methods yielded data that were reliable and valid?	Box 13.1, page 309; Box 14.1, page 347
Procedures	• If there was an intervention, is it adequately described, and was it rigorously developed and implemented? Did most participants allocated to the intervention group actually receive it? Is there evidence of intervention fidelity? • Were data collected in a manner that minimized bias? Were the staff who collected data appropriately trained?	Box 9.1, page 230; Box 10.1, page 254
Results Data analysis	• Were analyses undertaken to address each research question or test each hypothesis? • Were appropriate statistical methods used, given the level of measurement of the variables, number of groups being compared, and assumptions of the tests? • Was the most powerful analytic method used (e.g., did the analysis help to control for confounding variables)? • Were Type I and Type II errors avoided or minimized? • In intervention studies, was an intention-to-treat analysis performed? • Were problems of missing values evaluated and adequately addressed?	Box 16.1, page 400; Box 17.1, page 429

(box continues on page 114)

BOX 5.2 Guide to an Overall Critique of a Quantitative Research Report (continued)

Aspect of the Report	Critiquing Questions	Detailed Critiquing Guidelines
Findings	• Is information about statistical significance presented? Is information about effect size and precision of estimates (confidence intervals) presented? • Are the findings adequately summarized, with good use of tables and figures? • Are findings reported in a manner that facilitates a meta-analysis, and with sufficient information needed for EBP?	Box 17.1, page 429; Box 28.1, page 687
Discussion Interpretation of the findings	• Are all major findings interpreted and discussed within the context of prior research and/or the study's conceptual framework? • Are causal inferences, if any, justified? • Are interpretations well-founded and consistent with the study's limitations? • Does the report address the issue of the generalizability of the findings?	Box 19.1, page 482
Implications/ recommendations	• Do the researchers discuss the implications of the study for clinical practice or further research—and are those implications reasonable and complete?	Box 19.1, page 482
Global Issues Presentation	• Is the report well-written, organized, and sufficiently detailed for critical analysis? • In intervention studies, is a CONSORT flow chart provided to show the flow of participants in the study? • Is the report written in a manner that makes the findings accessible to practicing nurses?	Box 28.2, page 698
Researcher credibility	• Do the researchers' clinical, substantive, or methodologic qualifications and experience enhance confidence in the findings and their interpretation?	
Summary assessment	• Despite any limitations, do the study findings appear to be valid—do you have confidence in the *truth* value of the results? • Does the study contribute any meaningful evidence that can be used in nursing practice or that is useful to the nursing discipline?	

quantitative and qualitative studies, and the third column has cross-references to the detailed guidelines in the various chapters of the book. Many critiquing questions are likely too difficult for you to answer at this point, but your methodologic and critiquing skills will develop as you progress through this book. We developed these guidelines based on our years of experience as researchers and research methodologists, but they do not represent a formal, rigorously developed set of questions that

BOX 5.3 Guide to an Overall Critique of a Qualitative Research Report

Aspect of the Report	Critiquing Questions	Detailed Critiquing Guidelines
Title	● Is the title a good one, suggesting the key phenomenon and the group or community under study?	
Abstract	● Does the abstract clearly and concisely summarize the main features of the report?	
Introduction Statement of the problem	● Is the problem stated unambiguously and is it easy to identify? ● Does the problem statement build a cogent and persuasive argument for the new study? ● Does the problem have significance for nursing? ● Is there a good match between the research problem on the one hand and the paradigm, tradition, and methods on the other?	Box 4.3, page 90
Research questions	● Are research questions explicitly stated? If not, is their absence justified? ● Are the questions consistent with the study's philosophical basis, underlying tradition, or ideological orientation?	Box 4.3, page 90
Literature review	● Does the report adequately summarize the existing body of knowledge related to the problem or phenomenon of interest? ● Does the literature review provide a sound basis for the new study?	Box 5.4, page 122
Conceptual underpinnings	● Are key concepts adequately defined conceptually? ● Is the philosophical basis, underlying tradition, conceptual framework, or ideological orientation made explicit and is it appropriate for the problem?	Box 6.3, page 145
Method Protection of participants' rights	● Were appropriate procedures used to safeguard the rights of study participants? Was the study subject to external review by an IRB/ethics review board? ● Was the study designed to minimize risks and maximize benefits to participants?	Box 7.3, page 170
Research design and research tradition	● Is the identified research tradition (if any) congruent with the methods used to collect and analyze data? ● Was an adequate amount of time spent in the field or with study participants? ● Did the design unfold in the field, giving researchers opportunities to capitalize on early understandings? ● Was there an adequate number of contacts with study participants?	Box 20.1, page 510

(box continues on page 116)

BOX 5.3 Guide to an Overall Critique of a Qualitative Research Report (continued) ⊗

Aspect of the Report	Critiquing Questions	Detailed Critiquing Guidelines
Sample and setting	• Was the group or population of interest adequately described? Were the setting and sample described in sufficient detail? • Was the approach used to recruit participants or gain access to the site productive and appropriate? • Was the best possible method of sampling used to enhance information richness and address the needs of the study? • Was the sample size adequate? Was saturation achieved?	Box 21.1, page 528
Data collection	• Were the methods of gathering data appropriate? Were data gathered through two or more methods to achieve triangulation? • Did the researcher ask the right questions or make the right observations, and were they recorded in an appropriate fashion? • Was a sufficient amount of data gathered? Were the data of sufficient depth and richness?	Box 22.1, page 548
Procedures	• Are data collection and recording procedures adequately described and do they appear appropriate? • Were data collected in a manner that minimized bias? Were the staff who collected data appropriately trained?	Box 22.1, page 548
Enhancement of trustworthiness	• Did the researchers use effective strategies to enhance the trustworthiness/integrity of the study, and was the description of those strategies adequate? • Were the methods used to enhance trustworthiness appropriate and sufficient? • Did the researcher document research procedures and decision processes sufficiently that findings are auditable and confirmable? • Is there evidence of researcher reflexivity? • Is there "thick description" of the context, participants, and findings, and was it at a sufficient level to support transferability?	Box 24.1, page 598; Table 24.1, page 587
Results Data analysis	• Are the data management and data analysis methods sufficiently described? • Was the data analysis strategy compatible with the research tradition and with the nature and type of data gathered? • Did the analysis yield an appropriate "product" (e.g., a theory, taxonomy, thematic pattern)? • Do the analytic procedures suggest the possibility of biases?	Box 23.1, page 559

BOX 5.3 Guide to an Overall Critique of a Qualitative Research Report (continued)

Aspect of the Report	Critiquing Questions	Detailed Critiquing Guidelines
Findings	• Are the findings effectively summarized, with good use of excerpts and supporting arguments? • Do the themes adequately capture the meaning of the data? Does it appear that the researcher satisfactorily conceptualized the themes or patterns in the data? • Does the analysis yield an insightful, provocative, authentic, and meaningful picture of the phenomenon under investigation?	Box 23.1, page 559
Theoretical integration	• Are the themes or patterns logically connected to each other to form a convincing and integrated whole? • Are figures, maps, or models used effectively to summarize conceptualizations? • If a conceptual framework or ideological orientation guided the study, are the themes or patterns linked to it in a cogent manner?	Box 23.1, page 559; Box 6.3, page 145
Discussion		
Interpretation of the findings	• Are the findings interpreted within an appropriate social or cultural context? • Are major findings interpreted and discussed within the context of prior studies? • Are the interpretations consistent with the study's limitations?	Box 23.1, page 559
Implications/ recommendations	• Do the researchers discuss the implications of the study for clinical practice or further inquiry—and are those implications reasonable and complete?	
Global Issues		
Presentation	• Is the report well written, organized, and sufficiently detailed for critical analysis? • Is the description of the methods, findings, and interpretations sufficiently rich and vivid?	Box 28.2, page 698
Researcher credibility	• Do the researchers' clinical, substantive, or methodologic qualifications and experience enhance confidence in the findings and their interpretation?	
Summary assessment	• Do the study findings appear to be trustworthy—do you have confidence in the *truth* value of the results? • Does the study contribute any meaningful evidence that can be used in nursing practice or that is useful to the nursing discipline?	

are appropriate for a formal systematic review. They should, however, facilitate beginning efforts to critically appraise nursing studies. (Some formal guidelines are referenced in Chapter 27).

A few comments about these guidelines are in order. First, the questions call for a yes or no answer (although for some, the answer may be "Yes, *but* . . ."). In all cases, the desirable answer is "yes." That is, a "no" suggests a possible limitation and a "yes" suggests a strength. Therefore, the more "yeses" a study gets, the stronger it is likely to be. These guidelines can thus cumulatively suggest a global assessment: a report with 25 "yeses" is likely to be superior to one with only 10. Not all "yeses" are equal, however. Some elements are more important in drawing conclusions about study rigor than others. For example, the inadequacy of the article's literature review is less damaging to the worth of the study's *evidence* than the use of a faulty design. In general, questions about methodologic decisions (i.e., the questions under "Method") and about the analysis are especially important in evaluating the study's evidence.

Although the questions in these boxes elicit yes or no responses, a comprehensive critique would need to do more than point out what the researchers did and did not do. Each relevant issue would need to be discussed and your criticism justified. For example, if you answered "no" to the question about whether the problem was easy to identify, you would need to describe your concerns and perhaps offer suggestions for improvement.

Our simplified critiquing guidelines have a number of shortcomings. In particular, they are generic despite the fact that critiquing cannot use a one-size-fits-all list of questions. Some critiquing questions that are relevant to, say, clinical trials do not fit into a set of general questions for all quantitative studies. Thus, you would need to use some judgment about whether the guidelines are sufficiently comprehensive for the type of study you are critiquing, and perhaps supplement them with the more detailed critiquing questions in each chapter of this book.

Finally, there are questions in these guidelines for which there are no objective answers. Even experts sometimes disagree about what are the best method-

ologic strategies for a study. Thus, you should not be afraid to express an evaluative opinion—but be sure that your comments have some basis in methodologic principles discussed in this book.

⊃ TIP: It is appropriate to assume the posture of a skeptic when you are critiquing a research article. Just as a careful clinician seeks evidence from research findings that certain practices are or are not effective, you as a reviewer should demand evidence from the article that the researchers' decisions and their conclusions were sound.

Evaluating a Body of Research

In reviewing the literature, you typically would not undertake a *comprehensive* critique of each study—but you would need to assess the quality of evidence in each study so that you could draw conclusions about the overall body of evidence. Critiques for a literature review tend to focus on methodologic aspects.

In systematic reviews, methodologic quality often plays a role in selecting studies because investigations judged to be of low quality are sometimes screened out from further consideration. Using methodologic quality as a screening criterion is controversial, however. Systematic reviews sometimes involve the use of a formal evaluation instrument that gives quantitative ratings to aspects of the study, so that appraisals across studies ("scores") can be compared. Methodologic screening and formal scoring instruments are described in Chapter 27.

In literature reviews for a new primary study, methodologic features of studies under review need to be assessed with an eye to answering a broad question: To what extent do the findings reflect the *truth* or, conversely, to what extent do biases undermine the believability of the findings? The "truth" is most likely to be revealed when researchers use powerful designs, good sampling plans, strong data collection instruments and procedures, and appropriate analyses.

Judgments about the rigor of studies under review can be entered in an Evaluation Matrix.

Authors	Year of Publication	Major Strengths	Major Weaknesses	Quality Score*
Vincent & Denyes	2004	• Measured actual use of analgesics, not self-report • Linkage to Orem's theory • Good descriptive info on knowledge, attitudes, and use of analgesics	• Small and unrepresentative sample ($N = 67$), strong likelihood of Type II error (questionable power analysis) • Weak design for studying Q1 (effect of knowledge on analgesic use, effect of analgesic use on actual pain); several internal validity threats • Possibility that nurses' behavior in administering analgesics was affected by knowing they were in a study	12
Study 2				
Study 3				

*The quality score is fictitious and is shown here to indicate that information of this type could be recorded in the evaluation matrix.

FIGURE 5.8 Example of an evaluation matrix for recording strengths and weaknesses of studies for a literature review: nurse characteristics and management of children's pain.

Alternatively, additional columns for evaluative information can be added to the Methodologic Matrix. The advantage of combining information in one matrix is that methodologic features and assessments about those features are in a single table. The disadvantage is that the matrix would have so many columns that it might be cumbersome. A simple Evaluation Matrix is presented in Figure 5.8 , which provides space in the columns for noting major strengths and weaknesses for each study (the rows). If a "score" for overall quality is derived from a formal scoring instrument (e.g., by counting all the "yeses" from Boxes 5.2 or 5.3), this information can be added to the Evaluation Matrix.

ANALYZING AND SYNTHESIZING INFORMATION

Once all the relevant studies have been retrieved, read, abstracted, and critiqued, the information has to be analyzed and synthesized. As previously noted, doing a literature review is similar to doing a qualitative study, particularly with respect to the analysis of the "data" (i.e., information from the retrieved studies). In both, the focus is on identifying important *themes*.

A thematic analysis essentially involves detecting patterns and regularities, as well as inconsistencies. Several different types of themes can be identified, as described in Table 5.1. The reason we have recommended using various matrices should be clear from reading this list of possible themes: it is easier to discern patterns by reading down the columns of the matrices than by flipping through a stack of review protocols.

Clearly, it is not possible—even in lengthy free-standing reviews—to analyze all the themes we have identified. Reviewers have to make decisions about which patterns to pursue. In preparing a review as part of a new study, you would need to determine which pattern is of greatest relevance for developing an argument and providing a context for the new research.

TABLE 5.1	Thematic Possibilities for a Literature Review
TYPE OF THEME	**QUESTIONS FOR THEMATIC ANALYSIS**
Substantive	What is the pattern of evidence? How much evidence is there? How consistent is the body of evidence? How powerful are the observed effects? How persuasive is the evidence? What gaps are there in the body of evidence?
Theoretical	What theoretical or conceptual frameworks have been used to address the primary question—or has most research been atheoretical? How congruent are the theoretical frameworks? Do findings vary in relation to differences in frameworks?
Generalizability/ Transferability	To what types of people or settings do the findings apply? Do the findings vary for different types of people (e.g., men versus women) or setting (e.g., urban versus rural)?
Historical	Have there been substantive, theoretical, or methodologic trends over time? Is the evidence getting better? When was most of the research conducted?
Researcher	Who has been doing the research, in terms of discipline, specialty area, nationality, prominence, and so on? Has the research been developed within a systematic program of research?

PREPARING A WRITTEN LITERATURE REVIEW

Writing literature reviews can be challenging, especially when voluminous information must be condensed into a small number of pages, as is typical for a journal article or proposal. We offer a few suggestions, but acknowledge that skills in writing literature reviews develop over time.

Organizing the Review

Organization is crucial in a written review. Having an outline helps to structure the flow of presentation. If the review is complex, a written outline is recommended; a mental outline may suffice for simpler reviews. The outline should list the main topics or themes to be discussed, and indicate the order of presentation. The important point is to have a plan before starting to write so that the review has a coherent flow. The goal is to structure the review in such a way that the presentation is logical, demonstrates meaningful thematic integration, and leads to a conclusion about the state of evidence on the topic.

Writing a Literature Review

Although it is beyond the scope of this textbook to offer detailed guidance on writing research reviews, we offer a few comments on their content and style. Additional assistance is provided in books such as those by Fink (2009) and Galvan (2009).

Content of the Written Literature Review

A written research review should provide readers with an objective, organized synthesis of evidence on a topic. A review should be neither a series of quotes nor a series of abstracts. The central tasks are to summarize and critically evaluate the overall evidence so as to reveal the current state of knowledge—not simply to describe what researchers have done.

Although key studies may be described in some detail, it is not necessary to provide particulars for every reference, especially when there are page constraints. Studies with comparable findings often can be summarized together.

> **Example of grouped studies:** Considine and McGillivray (2010) summarized several studies as follows in their introduction to a study of emergency nursing care for acute stroke: "Although the use of thrombolysis as a treatment option for acute stroke is discussed in most stroke guidelines..., most current evidence does not support the use of thrombolysis in acute ischaemic stroke beyond three hours (Hacke et al., 1995; Clarke et al., 1999, 2000; Kothari et al., 2001; National Stroke Foundation, 2003) to 4–5 hours after symptom onset (Haack et al., 2008, Wahlgren et al., 2008)."

The literature should be summarized in your own words. The review should demonstrate that you have considered the cumulative worth of the body of research. Stringing together quotes from various documents fails to show that previous research has been assimilated and understood.

The review should be objective, to the extent possible. Studies that are at odds with your hypotheses should not be omitted, and the review should not ignore a study because its findings contradict other studies. Inconsistent results should be analyzed and the supporting evidence evaluated objectively.

A literature review typically concludes with a concise summary of current evidence on the topic and gaps in the evidence. If the review is conducted for a new study, this critical summary should demonstrate the need for the research and should clarify the basis for any hypotheses.

➡ **T I P :** As you progress through this book, you will acquire proficiency in critically evaluating studies. We hope you will understand the *mechanics* of doing a review after reading this chapter, but we do not expect you to be able to write a state-of-the-art review until you have gained more skills in research methods.

Style of a Research Review

Students preparing their first written research review often face stylistic challenges. In particular, students sometimes accept research findings uncritically, perhaps reflecting a common misunderstanding about the conclusiveness of research. You should keep in mind that hypotheses cannot be proved or disproved by empirical testing, and no research question can be definitely answered in a single study. This does not mean that research evidence should be ignored. The problem is partly semantic: hypotheses are not proved, they are *supported* by research findings. Research reviews should be written in a style that suggests tentativeness.

➡ **T I P :** When describing study findings, you can use phrases indicating tentativeness of the results, such as the following:

- Several studies have *found* . . .
- Findings thus far *suggest* . . .
- Results from a landmark study *indicated* . . .
- The data *supported* the hypothesis . . .
- There *appears* to be strong evidence that . . .

A related stylistic problem is the interjection of opinions into the review. The review should include opinions sparingly, if at all, and should be explicit about their source. Reviewers' own opinions do not belong in a review, except for assessments of study quality.

The left-hand column of Table 5.2 presents several examples of stylistic flaws for a review. The right-hand column offers suggestions for rewordings that are more acceptable for a research literature review. Many alternative wordings are possible.

TABLE 5.2	Examples of Stylistic Difficulties for Research Literature Reviews
PROBLEMATIC STYLE OR WORDING	**IMPROVED STYLE OR WORDING**
Women who do not participate in childbirth preparation classes manifest a high degree of anxiety during labor.	*Studies have found that* women who participate in childbirth preparation classes *tend to* manifest less anxiety than those who do not (Franck, 2011; Kim, 2010; Yepsen, 2011).
Studies have proved that doctors and nurses do not fully understand the psychobiologic dynamics of recovery from a myocardial infarction.	Studies by Fortune (2010) and Crampton (2011) *suggest that many* doctors and nurses do not fully understand the psychobiologic dynamics of recovery from a myocardial infarction.
Attitudes cannot be changed quickly.	Attitudes *have been found to be* relatively stable, enduring attributes that do not change quickly (Nicolet, 2010; Brusser & Lace, 2011)
It is known that uncertainty engenders stress.	*According to* Dr. A. Cassard (2011), an expert on stress and anxiety, uncertainty is a stressor.

Note: Italicized words in the improved version indicate key alternations.

CRITIQUING RESEARCH LITERATURE REVIEWS

It is often difficult to critique a research review because the author is almost invariably more knowledgeable about the topic than the readers. It is thus not usually possible to judge whether the author has included all relevant literature and has adequately summarized evidence on that topic. Many aspects of a review, however, are amenable to evaluation by readers who are not experts on the topic. Some suggestions for critiquing written research reviews are presented in Box 5.4. When a review is published as

BOX 5.4 Guidelines for Critiquing Literature Reviews

1. Is the review thorough—does it include all of the major studies on the topic? Does it include recent research? Are studies from other related disciplines included, if appropriate?
2. Does the review rely on appropriate materials (e.g., mainly on primary source research articles)?
3. Is the review merely a summary of existing work, or does it critically appraise and compare key studies? Does the review identify important gaps in the literature?
4. Is the review well organized? Is the development of ideas clear?
5. Does the review use appropriate language, suggesting the tentativeness of prior findings? Is the review objective? Does the author paraphrase, or is there an over reliance on quotes from original sources?
6. If the review is part of a research report for a new study, does the review support the need for the study?
7. If it is a review designed to summarize evidence for clinical practice, does the review draw reasonable conclusions about practice implications?

a stand-alone article, it should include information to help readers evaluate the reviewer's search strategies, as discussed in Chapter 27.

In assessing a literature review, the key question is whether it summarizes the current state of research evidence adequately. If the review is written as part of an original research report, an equally important question is whether the review lays a solid foundation for the new study.

RESEARCH EXAMPLES OF LITERATURE REVIEWS

The best way to learn about the style, content, and organization of a research literature review is to read reviews in nursing journals. We present excerpts from two reviews here and urge you to read others on a topic of interest to you.*

Literature Review from a Quantitative Research Report

Study: Accuracy of vaginal symptom self-diagnosis algorithms for deployed military women (Ryan-Wenger et al, 2010)

Statement of Purpose: The major purpose of this study was to evaluate the accuracy of a prototype of the Women in the Military Self-Diagnosis (WMSD) kit for the diagnosis of vaginal symptoms. Another aim was to predict potential self-medication omission and commission error rates.

Literature Review (Excerpt): "Deployment settings are typically austere, characterized by extreme temperatures, primitive sanitary conditions, and limited hygiene and laundry facilities. These factors increase military women's risk for vaginitis. . . . Ryan-Wenger and Lowe (2000) surveyed 1,537 military women about their symptoms of genitourinary infections and healthcare experiences in their home duty stations and during deployment. Of the 841 women who had been deployed, 87% ($n = 732$) reported that they experienced vaginal symptoms such as itching, discharge, or foul odor at some time during deployment. Because of these symptoms, nearly half the women (48%) noted a decrease in the quality of their work performance and 24% lost from

a few hours to more than a day of work time. . . . In focus groups conducted by DACOWITS [Defense Department Advisory Committee on Women in the Services], in our survey, and in a phenomenological study of soldier care, women evaluated deployment healthcare services for women as inadequate, citing lack of confidence in the knowledge and skills of the provider, lack of privacy, and lack of confidentiality (DACOWITS, 2007; Jennings, 2005; Ryan-Wenger & Lowe, 2000). . . . We proposed that a viable solution to the problem is a field-expedient kit for self-diagnosis and self-treatment of common genitourinary symptoms. . . .

Despite . . . diagnostic standards, studies show that clinicians often misdiagnose vaginal infections. For example, in one study, 197 vaginal samples were analyzed by culture, Gram stain, microscopy, and DNA hybridization with Affirm TM VPIII to derive a diagnosis of BV [bacterial vaginosis], TV [trichomonas vaginitis], and/or CV [candida vaginitis] (Schweiertz et al., 2006). Compared with laboratory diagnoses, physicians misdiagnosed CV in 77.1% of 109 cases, BV in 61.3% of 80 cases, and 87.5% of eight mixed infections. One reason for such high levels of inaccuracy is that many providers do not use the common office-based tests that are recommended to achieve a diagnosis. This point is illustrated by a study of diagnostic procedures used by physicians with 52 women who made 150 visits to a vaginitis clinic (Wiesenfeld & Macio, 1999). Microscopic assessment was done in 63% of the visits, and whiff and pH tests were conducted in only 3% of visits. In another study, 556 nurse practitioners and 608 physicians reported their diagnostic practices on a Web-based survey (Anderson & Karasz, 2005). An average of 79% of these providers indicated that they 'often or always' examined women with vaginal symptoms, 47% conducted whiff tests, and only 33.5% conducted pH tests on vaginal fluid" (pp. 2–4).

Literature Review from a Qualitative Research Report

Study: Young people's experience of living with ulcerative colitis and an ostomy (Savard & Woodgate, 2009)

Statement of Purpose: The purpose of this study was to understand the lived experiences of young adults with inflammatory bowel disease and an ostomy.

Literature Review (Excerpt): "Ulcerative colitis (UC) and Crohn's disease are collectively referred to as inflammatory bowel disease (IBD). . . . Approximately 25% of all new Crohn's disease cases and between 15% and 40% of all new UC cases are diagnosed in individuals younger

---

*Consult the full research reports for references cited in these excerpted literature reviews.

than 20 years of age (Kim & Ferry, 2004; Rayhorn, 2001). Individuals with IBD experience a range of symptoms including abdominal pain, cramping, and loose stools (Listrom & Holt, 2004; Pearson, 2004; Rayhorn, 2001; Veronesi, 2003). Some individuals may at some point during their illness require surgery, resulting in an ostomy (Reynaud & Meeker, 2002).

Although there has been discussion in the literature about what it is like to have IBD with or without an ostomy, young people (i.e., adolescents and young adults) have rarely been asked about their experiences (Daniel, 2001; Decker, 2000). Of the research done on young people, a lack of consensus remains as to how IBD affects this population socially and psychologically. Some studies reveal that IBD has negative psychological effects such as alienation, reduced living space, feelings of helplessness, self-blame, depression, and anxiety (Brydolf & Segesten, 1996; Daniel, 2001; Dudley-Brown, 1996; Mackner & Crandall, 2006; Wood et al., 1987), whereas others reveal that people with IBD cope well and are psychologically healthy (Joachim & Milne, 1987; Mackner & Crandall, 2005).

Studies carried out on individuals living with ostomies reveal that they face many lifestyle challenges that include physical and psychological adjustments (Manderson, 2005; Reynaud & Meeker, 2002; Rheaume & Gooding, 1991; Slater, 1992). Others have found that individuals with a temporary or permanent stoma perceive negative body image feelings and express difficulties in coming to terms with having the stoma (Black, 2004; Casati et al., 2000; Junkin & Beitz, 2005; . . .), especially the young population (O'Brien, 1999; Willis, 1998). . . .

A limitation of the work to date is that it has mainly been approached from a quantitative paradigm, and hence is not focused on capturing the meanings that young people ascribe to their experience. The literature review revealed four qualitative studies, two Swedish and two Canadian, that focus on the lived experienced of young individuals with IBD (Brydoff & Segeston, 1996; Daniel, 2001; Nicholas et al., 2007; Reichenberg et al., 2007). Although involving young people from different countries, common findings included the young people experiencing a reduced living space because of their dependency on needing to be near a toilet, feelings of embarrassment, a loss of control, and alienation from oneself and from others. . . . In summary, there is a need for more qualitative research that is directed at gaining understanding about the lived experiences of young people living with IBD and an ostomy" (pp. 33–34).

SUMMARY POINTS

- A research **literature review** is a written summary of evidence on a research problem.
- The major steps in preparing a written research review include formulating a question, devising a search strategy, conducting a search, retrieving relevant sources, abstracting information, critiquing studies, analyzing aggregated information, and preparing a written synthesis.
- Study findings are the major focus of research reviews. Information in nonresearch references—for example, opinion articles, case reports—may broaden understanding of a research problem, but has limited utility in research reviews.
- A **primary source** is the original description of a study prepared by the researcher who conducted it; a **secondary source** is a description of the study by a person unconnected with it. Literature reviews should be based on primary source material.
- Strategies for finding studies on a topic include the use of bibliographic tools, but also include the **ancestry approach** (tracking down earlier studies cited in a reference list of a report) and the **descendancy approach** (using a pivotal study to search forward to subsequent studies that cited it.)
- An important method for locating references is an electronic search of bibliographic databases. For nurses, the CINAHL and MEDLINE databases are especially useful.
- In searching a database, users can perform a **keyword search** that looks for searcher-specified terms in text fields of a database record (or that maps keywords onto the database's subject codes) or can search according to **subject heading** codes themselves.
- References must be screened for relevance, and then pertinent information must be abstracted for analysis. Formal review protocols and matrices facilitate abstraction.
- Matrices (two-dimensional arrays) are a convenient means of abstracting and organizing information for a literature review. A reviewer

might use a Methodologic Matrix to record methodologic features of a set of studies, a set of Results Matrices to record research findings, and an Evaluation Matrix to record quality assessment information. The use of such matrices facilitates thematic analysis of the retrieved information.

- A research **critique** is a careful appraisal of a study's strengths and weaknesses. Critiques for a research review tend to focus on the methodologic aspects of a set of studies. Critiques of individual studies tend to be more comprehensive.

- The analysis of information from a literature search involves the identification of important themes—regularities (and inconsistencies) in the information. Themes can take many forms, including substantive, methodologic, and theoretical themes.

- In preparing a written review, it is important to organize materials logically, preferably using an outline. The written review should not be a succession of quotes or abstracts. The reviewers' role is to describe study findings, the dependability of the evidence, evidence gaps, and (in the context of a new study) contributions that the new study would make.

STUDY ACTIVITIES

Chapter 5 of the *Resource Manual for Nursing Research: Generating and Assessing Evidence for Nursing Practice, 9th ed.*, offers study suggestions for reinforcing concepts presented in this chapter. In addition, the following questions can be addressed in classroom or online discussions:

1. Suppose you were planning to study the relationship between chronic transfusion therapy and quality of life in adolescents with sickle cell disease. Identify 5 to 10 keywords that could be used to search for relevant studies, and compare them with those found by other students.

2. Suppose you were studying factors affecting the discharge of chronic psychiatric patients. Obtain references for 5 studies for this topic, and compare them with those of other students.

3. Carefully examine Figures 5.6 and 5.7 and see how many themes you can identify. Also, see how many incongruities there are among studies in the matrixes (i.e., the absence of consistent themes).

STUDIES CITED IN CHAPTER 5

Considine, J., & McGillivray, B. (2010). An evidence-based practice approach to improving nursing care of acute stroke in an Australian Emergency Department. *Journal of Clinical Nursing, 19,* 138–144.

Griffin, R. A., Polit, D. F., & Byrne, M. W. (2008). Nurse characteristics and inferences about children's pain. *Pediatric Nursing, 34,* 297–307.

Hamers, J. P., van den Hout, M. A., Halfens, R. J., Abu-Saad, H. H., & Heijltes, A. E. (1997). Differences in pain assessment and decisions regarding the administration of analgesics between novices, intermediates and experts in pediatric nursing. *International Journal of Nursing Studies, 34,* 325–334.

Margolius, F. R., Hudson, K. A., & Miche, Y. (1995). Beliefs and perceptions about children in pain: A survey. *Pediatric Nursing, 21,* 111–115.

Murray, M., Fiset, V., Young, S., & Kryworuchko, J. (2009). Where the dying live: Review of determinants of place of end-of-life cancer care. *Oncology Nursing Forum, 36,* 69–77.

Polkki T., Vehvilainen-Julkunen K., & Pietila, A. M. (2001). Nonpharmacological methods in relieving children's postoperative pain: A survey on hospital nurses in Finland. *Journal of Advanced Nursing, 34,* 483–492.

Ryan-Wenger, N., Neal, J., Jones, A., & Lower, N. (2010). Accuracy of vaginal symptom self-diagnosis algorithms for deployed military women. *Nursing Research, 59,* 2–10.

Savard, J., & Woodgate, R. (2009). Young people's experience of living with ulcerative colitis and an ostomy. *Gastroenterology Nursing, 32,* 33–41.

Stajduhar, K., Allan, D., Cohen, S., & Heyland, D. (2008). Preferences for location of death of seriously ill hospitalized patients. *Palliative Medicine, 22,* 85–88.

Twycross, A. (2007). What is the impact of theoretical knowledge of children's nurses' post-operative pain management practices? *Nurse Education Today, 27,* 697–707.

Vincent, C. V., & Denyes, M. J. (2004). Relieving children's pain: Nurses' abilities and analgesic administration practices. *Journal of Pediatric Nursing, 19,* 40–50.

Methodologic and nonresearch references cited in this chapter can be found in a separate section at the end of the book.

6

Theoretical Frameworks

High-quality studies achieve a high level of *conceptual integration*. This means that the methods are appropriate for the research questions, the questions are consistent with existing research evidence, and there is a plausible conceptual rationale for the way things are expected to unfold—including a rationale for hypotheses to be tested or for the design of an intervention.

For example, suppose we hypothesized that a smoking cessation intervention would reduce rates of smoking among patients with cardiovascular disease. Why would we make this prediction? That is, what is our "theory" (our theoretical rationale) about how the intervention might bring about behavior change—do we predict that the intervention will change patients' knowledge, attitudes, motivation, social supports, or sense of control over their decision making? Our view of how the intervention would "work" should guide the design of the intervention and the study. To use a nonexperimental example, suppose we hypothesized gender differences in coping with the loss of a child. What is our "theory" for why men and women would differ—do we suspect biological differences, role socialization differences, social expectation differences, or differences in social capital?

In designing research, there needs to be a well-deliberated conceptualization of people's behaviors or characteristics, and how these affect or are affected by interpersonal, environmental, or biologic forces. In high-quality research, a clear, defensible conceptualization is made explicit. This chapter discusses theoretical and conceptual contexts for nursing research problems.

THEORIES, MODELS, AND FRAMEWORKS

Many terms are used in connection with conceptual contexts for research, including theories, models, frameworks, schemes, and maps. We offer guidance in distinguishing these terms, but note that our definitions are far from universal—indeed a confusing aspect of theory-related writings is that there is no consensus about terminology.

Theories

The term *theory* is used in many ways. For example, nursing instructors and students often use the term to refer to classroom content, as opposed to the actual practice of performing nursing actions. In both lay and scientific usage, the term theory connotes an abstraction.

In research circles, the term theory is used differently by different authors. Classically, scientists have used **theory** to refer to an abstract generalization that offers a systematic explanation about how phenomena are interrelated. In this traditional definition, a theory embodies at least two concepts that are related in a manner that the theory purports to explain. Thus, traditional theories typically have explanation or prediction as their purpose.

Others, however, use the term *theory* less restrictively to refer to a broad characterization that can thoroughly describe a single phenomenon. Some authors refer to this type of theory as *descriptive theory,* while others have used the term *factor isolating theory*. Broadly speaking, descriptive theories are ones that describe or categorize characteristics of individuals, groups, or situations by abstracting common features observed across multiple manifestations. Descriptive theory plays an important role in qualitative studies. Qualitative researchers often strive to develop conceptualizations of phenomena that are grounded in actual observations. Descriptive theory is often a precursor to predictive and explanatory theories.

Components of a Traditional Theory

Writings on scientific theory include such terms as *proposition*, *premise*, *axiom*, *principle*, and so forth. Here, we present a simplified analysis of the components of a theory.

Concepts are the basic building blocks of a theory. Classical theories comprise a set of propositions that indicate relationships among the concepts. Relationships are denoted by such terms as "is associated with," "varies directly with," or "is contingent on." The propositions form a logically interrelated deductive system. This means that the theory provides a mechanism for logically deriving new statements from the original propositions.

Let us illustrate with the **Theory of Planned Behavior** (TPB) (Ajzen, 2005), which is an extension of another theory called the *Theory of Reasoned Action* or TRA (Fishbein & Ajzen, 2009). TPB provides a framework for understanding people's behavior and its psychological determinants. A greatly simplified construction of the TPB consists of the following propositions:

1. Behavior that is volitional is determined by people's intention to perform that behavior.

2. Intention to perform or not perform a behavior is determined by three factors:
   - Attitudes toward the behavior (i.e., the overall evaluation of performing the behavior)
   - Subjective norms (i.e., perceived social pressure to perform or not perform the behavior)
   - Perceived behavioral control (i.e., self-efficacy beliefs—the anticipated ease or difficulty of engaging in the behavior)
3. The relative importance of the three factors in influencing intention varies across behaviors and situations.

TIP: There are websites devoted to many of the theories and conceptual models mentioned in this chapter, including the TPB. Several specific websites are listed in the "Useful Websites for Chapter 6" table in the Toolkit of the accompanying *Resource Manual,* for you to click on directly. An excellent Internet resource that describes theories of relevance to nursing is: *http://www.nursingtheory.net/*. Another useful website provides links to many key nursing theories: *http://nursing.clayton.edu/eichelberger/nursing.htm*.

The concepts that form the basis of the TPB include behaviors, intentions, attitudes, subjective norms, and perceived self-control. The theory, which specifies the nature of the relationship among these concepts, provides a framework for generating hypotheses relating to health behaviors. We might hypothesize on the basis of the TPB, for example, that compliance with a medical regimen (the behavior) could be enhanced by influencing people's attitudes toward compliance, or by increasing their sense of control. The TPB has been used as the underlying theory in studying a wide range of health decision-making behaviors (e.g., contraceptive choice, condom use, preventive health screening) as well as in developing health-promoting interventions.

Example using the TPB: Peddle and colleagues (2009) used the Theory of Planned Behavior to predict adherence to a presurgical exercise training intervention in patients awaiting surgery for suspected malignant lung lesions. Perceived behavioral control and subjective norms were found to predict adherence.

Levels of Theories

Theories differ in their level of generality and abstraction. The most common labels used in nursing for levels or scope of theory are *grand*, *middle-range*, and *micro* or *practice*.

Grand theories or *macrotheories* purport to describe and explain large segments of the human experience. In nursing, there are several grand theories that offer explanations of the whole of nursing and that address the nature, goals, and mission of nursing practice as distinct from the discipline of medicine. An example of a nursing theory that has been described as a grand theory is Parse's Theory of Human Becoming (Parse, 1999).

Theories of relevance to researchers are often less abstract than grand theories. **Middle-range theories** attempt to explain such phenomena as decision making, stress, comfort, health promotion, and unpleasant symptoms. In comparison with grand theories, middle-range theories tend to involve fewer concepts or propositions, are more specific, and are more amenable to empirical testing (Peterson & Bredow, 2009). Nurse researchers are increasingly turning to middle-range theories for their conceptual inspiration. There are literally dozens of middle-range theories developed by or used by nurses, several of which will be briefly described in this chapter.

The least abstract level of theory is *practice theory* (sometimes called *micro theory* or *situation-specific theory*). Such theories are highly specific, narrow in scope, and have an action orientation. They are seldom associated with research, and there is ongoing debate about whether they should be called "theory" (Peterson & Bredow, 2009).

Models

Conceptual models, **conceptual frameworks**, or **conceptual schemes** (we use the terms interchangeably) are a less formal means of organizing phenomena than theories. Like theories, conceptual models deal with abstractions (concepts) that are assembled by virtue of their relevance to a common theme. What is absent from conceptual models is the deductive system of propositions that assert and explain relationships among concepts. Conceptual models provide a perspective regarding interrelated phenomena, but are more loosely structured and more abstract than theories. A conceptual model broadly presents an understanding of the phenomenon of interest and reflects the assumptions and philosophical views of the model's designer. Conceptual models can serve as springboards for generating hypotheses, but conceptual models are not formally "tested."

The term *model* is often used in connection with symbolic representations of a conceptualization. **Schematic models** (or *conceptual maps*) are visual representations of some aspect of reality; like conceptual models and theories, they use concepts as building blocks, but with a minimal use of words. A visual or symbolic representation of a theory or conceptual framework often helps to express abstract ideas in a concise and convenient form.

Schematic models, which are common in both qualitative and quantitative research, represent phenomena graphically. Concepts and the linkages between them are represented through the use of boxes, arrows, or other symbols. As an example, Figure 6.1 shows **Pender's Health Promotion Model**, which is a model for explaining and predicting the health-promotion component of lifestyle (Pender et al., 2006). Such schematic models can be useful in clarifying and succinctly communicating linkages among concepts.

Frameworks

A **framework** is the overall conceptual underpinnings of a study. Not every study is based on a formal theory or conceptual model, but every study has a framework—that is, a conceptual rationale. In a study based on a theory, the framework is a **theoretical framework**; in a study that has its roots in a specified conceptual model, the framework is a **conceptual framework** (although the terms conceptual framework and theoretical framework are frequently used interchangeably).

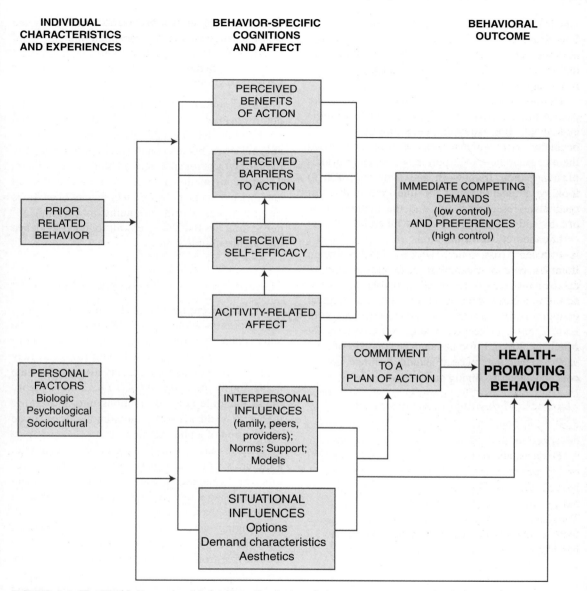

| INDIVIDUAL CHARACTERISTICS AND EXPERIENCES | BEHAVIOR-SPECIFIC COGNITIONS AND AFFECT | BEHAVIORAL OUTCOME |

FIGURE 6.1 The Health Promotion Model (from Pender's website, *www.nursing.umich.edu/faculty/pender/chart.gif*; retrieved July 10, 2010).

In most nursing studies, the framework is not an explicit theory or conceptual model, and often, the underlying conceptual rationale for the inquiry is not explained. Frameworks are often implicit, without being formally acknowledged or described. In studies that fail to articulate a conceptual frame-work, it may be difficult to figure out what the researchers thought was "going on."

Sometimes researchers fail even to adequately describe key constructs at the conceptual level. The concepts in which researchers are interested are by definition abstractions of observable phenomena, and our world view, and views on nursing, shape how those concepts are defined and operationalized. Researchers should make clear the conceptual definition of their key variables, thereby providing information about the study's framework.

In most qualitative studies, the frameworks are part of the research tradition in which the study is embedded. For example, ethnographers usually begin their work within a theory of culture. Grounded theory researchers incorporate sociological principles into their framework and their approach to looking at phenomena. The questions that most qualitative researchers ask and the methods they use to address those questions inherently reflect certain theoretical formulations.

In recent years, *concept analysis* has become an important enterprise among students and nurse scholars. Several methods have been proposed for undertaking a concept analysis and clarifying conceptual definitions (Morse et al., 1996; Schwartz-Barcott & Kim, 2000; Walker & Avant, 2005; Weaver & Mitcham, 2008). Efforts to analyze concepts of relevance to nursing practice should facilitate greater conceptual clarity among nurse researchers.

Example of developing a conceptual definition: Hodges (2009) examined a variety of writings in her analysis of the concept of *life purpose*. She considered philosophical underpinnings, relevant theoretical frameworks, and empirical support for the construct's attributes. She proposed the following conceptual definition of *life purpose* as it applies to older adults in critical care settings:

"The degree to which a person realizes his/her own interpersonal, intrapersonal, and psychological uniqueness on the basis of life experiences that correspond with spiritual values and goals at a specific time in life" (p. 169).

THE NATURE OF THEORIES AND CONCEPTUAL MODELS

Theories and conceptual models have much in common, including their origin, general nature, purposes, and role in research. In this section, we examine some general characteristics of theories

and conceptual models. We use the term *theory* in a broad sense, inclusive of conceptual models.

Origin of Theories and Models

Theories, conceptual frameworks, and models are not *discovered*; they are created and invented. Theory building depends not only on facts and observable evidence, but also on the originator's ingenuity in pulling facts together and making sense of them. Theory construction is a creative and intellectual enterprise that can be undertaken by anyone who is insightful, has a firm grounding in existing evidence, and has the ability to knit together evidence into an intelligible pattern.

Tentative Nature of Theories and Models

Theories and conceptual models cannot be proved—they represent a theorist's best effort to describe and explain phenomena. Today's flourishing theory may be discredited or revised tomorrow. This may happen if new evidence or observations undermine a previously accepted theory. Or, a new theory might integrate new observations into an existing theory to yield a more parsimonious or accurate explanation of a phenomenon.

Theories and models that are not congruent with a culture's values also may fall into disfavor over time. For example, certain psychoanalytical and structural social theories, which had broad support for decades, have come to be challenged as a result of changing views about women's roles. Theories are deliberately invented by humans, and so they are not free from human values, which can change over time.

Thus, theories and models are never considered final and verified. We have no way of knowing the ultimate accuracy and utility of any theory and so should treat all theories as tentative.

The Role of Theories and Models

Theoretical and conceptual frameworks play several interrelated roles in the progress of a science.

Theories allow researchers to integrate observations and facts into an orderly scheme. They are efficient mechanisms for drawing together accumulated facts, often from separate and isolated investigations. The linkage of findings into a coherent structure can make a body of evidence more accessible and, thus, more useful.

In addition to summarizing, theories and models can guide a researcher's understanding of not only the *what* of natural phenomena but also the *why* of their occurrence. Theories often provide a basis for predicting phenomena. Prediction, in turn, has implications for the control of those phenomena. A utilitarian theory has potential to bring about desirable changes in people's behavior or health. Thus, theories are an important resource for the development of nursing interventions.

Theories and conceptual models help to stimulate research and the extension of knowledge by providing both direction and impetus. Thus, theories may serve as a springboard for advances in knowledge and the accumulation of evidence for practice.

Relationship between Theory and Research

The relationship between theory and research is reciprocal and mutually beneficial. Theories and models are built inductively from observations, and an excellent source for those observations is prior research, including in-depth qualitative studies. Concepts and relationships that are validated through research become the foundation for theory development. The theory, in turn, must be evaluated by testing deductions from it (i.e., hypotheses). Thus, research plays a dual and continuing role in theory building and testing. Theory guides and generates ideas for research; research assesses the worth of the theory and provides a foundation for new theories.

> **Example of theory development:** Jean Johnson (1999) developed a middle-range theory called Self-Regulation Theory that explicates relationships between healthcare experiences, coping, and health outcomes. Here is how she described theory development:

> "The theory was developed in a cyclic process. Research was conducted using the self-regulation theory of coping with illness. Propositions supported by data were retained, other propositions were altered when they were not supported, and new theoretical propositions were added when research produced unexpected findings. This cycle has been repeated many times over three decades leading to the present stage of development of the theory" (pp. 435–436). Many nurse researchers have grounded their studies in Self-Regulation Theory, including Kirchhoff and colleagues (2008), who used the theory to structure messages for an intervention to prepare families of intensive care patients for withdrawal of life support.

CONCEPTUAL MODELS AND THEORIES USED IN NURSING RESEARCH

Nurse researchers have used both nursing and nonnursing frameworks to provide a conceptual context for their studies. This section briefly discusses several frameworks that have been found useful.

Conceptual Models and Theories of Nursing

In the past few decades, several nurses have formulated theories and models of nursing practice. These models constitute formal explanations of what nursing is and what the nursing process entails, according to the model developer's point of view. As Fawcett (2005) has noted, four concepts are central to models of nursing: *human beings*, *environment*, *health*, and *nursing*. The various conceptual models, however, define these concepts differently, link them in diverse ways, and emphasize different relationships among them. Moreover, different models view different processes as being central to nursing. For example, Sister Calista Roy's Adaptation Model identifies adaptation of patients as a critical phenomenon (Roy & Andrews, 1999). Martha Rogers (1994), by contrast, emphasized the centrality of the individual as a unified whole, and her model views nursing as a process in which clients are aided in achieving maximum well-being within their potential.

The conceptual models were not developed primarily as a base for nursing research. Indeed, most models have had more impact on nursing education and clinical practice than on research. Nevertheless, nurse researchers have been inspired by these conceptual frameworks in formulating research questions and hypotheses. Table 6.1 lists 10 conceptual models in nursing that have been used by researchers. The table briefly describes the model's key feature and identifies a study that has claimed the model as its framework. Two nursing models that have generated particular interest as a basis for research are described in greater detail.

Roy's Adaptation Model

In **Roy's Adaptation Model**, humans are viewed as biopsychosocial adaptive systems who cope with environmental change through the process of adaptation (Roy & Andrews, 2009). Within the human system, there are four subsystems: physiological/physical, self-concept/group identity, role function, and interdependence. These subsystems constitute adaptive modes that provide mechanisms for coping with environmental stimuli and change. Health is viewed as both a state and a process of being and becoming integrated and whole that reflects the mutuality of persons and environment. The goal of nursing, according to this model, is to promote client adaptation. Nursing also regulates stimuli affecting adaptation. Nursing interventions usually take the form of increasing, decreasing, modifying, removing, or maintaining internal and external stimuli that affect adaptation. Like several other broad conceptual models of nursing, Roy's Adaptation Model has been the basis for several middle-range theories.

Example using Roy's Adaptation Model:
DeSanto-Madeya (2009) studied adaptation to spinal cord injury for family members and individuals, using concepts from Roy's Adaptation Model. The physical, emotional, functional, and social components of adaptation were studied for those 1 year and 3 years post-injury.

Rogers' Science of Unitary Human Beings

The building blocks of **Rogers' Science of Unitary Human Beings** (Rogers, 1990, 1994) are five assumptions relating to human life processes: wholeness (a human as a unified whole, more than the sum of the parts), openness (humans and the environment continuously exchanging matter and energy), unidirectionality (life processes existing along an irreversible space/time continuum), pattern and organization (which identify humans and reflect their wholeness), and sentience and thought (a human as capable of abstraction, imagery, language, and sensation). Four critical elements are basic to Rogers' proposed system. First, *energy fields* are the fundamental unit of the living (human energy fields) and the nonliving (environmental energy field). Second, *open systems* describe the open nature of the fields, which allow for an interchange of energy. Third, *pattern* is the distinguishing characteristic of energy fields, and human behavior can be regarded as manifestations of changing pattern. And fourth, *pandimensionality* describes a nonlinear domain without temporal or spatial attributes. The key to Rogers' conceptual framework are her principles of homeodynamics, which represent a way of viewing unitary human beings and provide guidance to nursing practice. The principles include integrality, helicy, and resonancy. *Integrality* concerns the continuous and mutual processes between human and environmental fields—changes in one field will bring about changes in the other. *Helicy* refers to the continuous and innovative diversity of human and environmental field patterns. Finally, *resonancy* describes the continuous change from lower to higher frequency wave patterns in human and environmental energy fields. Rogerian science continues to be developed by theorists and researchers, and specific research methods have been developed based on Rogerian principles (e.g., Cowling, 2004).

Example using a Rogerian framework:
Farren (2010) examined the relationships among power, uncertainty, self-transcendence, and quality of life in breast cancer survivors from the perspective of Rogers' Science of Unitary Human Beings.

TABLE 6.1	Conceptual Models and Theories of Nursing Used by Nurse Researchers		
THEORIST AND REFERENCE	**NAME OF MODEL/THEORY**	**KEY THESIS OF THE MODEL**	**RESEARCH EXAMPLE**
F. Moyra Allen, 2002	McGill Model of Nursing	Nursing is the science of health-promoting interactions. Health promotion is a process of helping people cope and develop; the goal of nursing is to actively promote patient and family strengths and the achievement of life goals.	Cossette et al. (2002) included elements of the McGill Model in their study to document the types of nursing approaches that were associated with reductions in psychological distress among patients with postmyocardial infarction.
Madeline Leininger, 2006	Theory of Culture Care Diversity and Universality	Caring is a universal phenomenon but varies transculturally. Fundamental belief that people in different cultures can inform and are capable of guiding healthcare professionals to receive the kind of care they need and desire.	Guided by Leininger's theory, Schumacher (2010) explored the meanings, beliefs, and practices of care for rural residents in the Dominican Republic.
Myra Levine, 1996	Conservation Model	Conservation of energy, structural integrity, personal integrity, and social integrity by nurses contributes to maintenance of a person's wholeness.	Mock et al. (2007) used concepts from Levine's model to examine the effects of exercise on fatigue and physical functioning in cancer patients.
Betty Neuman, 2001	Health Care Systems Model	Each person is a complete system; the goal of nursing is to assist in maintaining client system stability.	Yarcheski et al. (2010) used Neuman's model as the framework for their study of stress and wellness in early adolescents.
Margaret Newman, 1994, 1997	Health as Expanding Consciousness	Health is viewed as an expansion of consciousness with health and disease parts of the same whole; health is seen in an evolving pattern of the whole in time, space, and movement.	Ness (2009) used Newman's theory to study pain expression in the perioperative period among Somali women.

(Table continues on page 134)

| TABLE 6.1 | Conceptual Models and Theories of Nursing Used by Nurse Researchers (continued) |

THEORIST AND REFERENCE	NAME OF MODEL/THEORY	KEY THESIS OF THE MODEL	RESEARCH EXAMPLE
Dorothea Orem, 2003	Self-Care Deficit Nursing Theory	Self-care activities are what people do on their own behalf to maintain health and well-being; the goal of nursing is to help people meet their own therapeutic self-care demands.	Moore et al. (2009) tested the effect of a community-based nutrition education program on nutrition outcomes in Nicaraguan adolescent girls, using concepts from Orem's model.
Rosemarie Rizzo Parse, 1999	Theory of Human Becoming	Health and meaning are co-created by indivisible humans and their environment; nursing involves having clients share views about meanings.	Doucet (2009) studied the lived experience of trusting another person, interpreted within the human becoming school of thought.
Martha Rogers, 1990, 1994	Science of Unitary Human Beings	The individual is a unified whole in constant interaction with the environment; nursing helps individuals achieve maximum well-being within their potential.	Shearer et al. (2009) studied the rhythm of health in 51 older women with chronic illness, using a Rogerian perspective.
Sr. Callista Roy, 1999, 2006	Adaptation Model	Humans are adaptive systems that cope with change through adaptation; nursing helps to promote client adaptation during health and illness.	Weiss et al. (2009) used Roy's model in their study of women's physical, emotional, functional, and social adaptation during the first 2 weeks following caesarean birth.
Jean Watson, 2005	Theory of Caring	Caring is the moral ideal, and entails mind–body–soul engagement with one another.	Watson's conceptual theory of caring underpinned a study of patients' perceptions of being cared for within a multicultural context in Saudi Arabia (Suliman et al., 2009)

Other Models and Middle-Range Theories Developed by Nurses

In addition to conceptual models that are designed to describe and characterize the nursing process, nurses have developed middle-range theories and models that focus on more specific phenomena of interest to nurses. Examples of middle-range theories that have been used in research include:

- Beck's (2012) Theory of Postpartum Depression
- Kolcaba's (2003) Comfort Theory
- Reed's (1991) Self-Transcendence Theory
- Symptom Management Model (Dodd et al., 2001)
- Theory of Transitions (Meleis et al., 2000)
- Theory of Unpleasant Symptoms (Lenz et al., 1997)
- Peplau's (1997) Theory of Interpersonal Relations
- Pender's Health Promotion Model (Pender et al., 2006)
- Mishel's Uncertainty in Illness Theory (1990)

The latter two are briefly described here.

The Health Promotion Model

Nola Pender's (2006) Health Promotion Model (HPM) focuses on explaining health-promoting behaviors, using a wellness orientation. According to the revised model (see Figure 6.1), *health promotion* entails activities directed toward developing resources that maintain or enhance a person's well-being. The model embodies a number of theoretical propositions that can be used in developing interventions and understanding health behaviors. For example, one HPM proposition is that people commit to engaging in behaviors from which they anticipate deriving valued benefits, and another is that perceived competence or self-efficacy relating to a given behavior increases the likelihood of actual performance of the behavior. Greater perceived self-efficacy is viewed as resulting in fewer perceived barriers to a specific health behavior. The model also incorporates interpersonal and situational influences on a person's commitment to health-promoting actions.

Example using the HPM: McElligott and colleagues (2009) tested the HPM to explain health-promoting lifestyle behaviors of acute care nurses.

Uncertainty in Illness Theory

Mishel's Uncertainty in Illness Theory (Mishel, 1990) focuses on the concept of uncertainty—the inability of a person to determine the meaning of illness-related events. According to this theory, people develop subjective appraisals to assist them in interpreting the experience of illness and treatment. Uncertainty occurs when people are unable to recognize and categorize stimuli. Uncertainty results in the inability to obtain a clear conception of the situation, but a situation appraised as uncertain will mobilize individuals to use their resources to adapt to the situation. Mishel's theory, as originally conceptualized, was most relevant to patients in an acute phase of illness or in a downward illness trajectory, but it has been reconceptualized to include constant uncertainty in chronic or recurrent illness. Mishel's conceptualization of uncertainty (and her Uncertainty in Illness Scale) have been used in many nursing studies.

Example using Uncertainty in Illness Theory: Bailey and colleagues (2009) examined the constructs of the Uncertainty in Illness Theory in a study of the relationship between uncertainty, symptoms, and quality of life in persons with chronic hepatitis C.

Other Models and Theories Used by Nurse Researchers

Many concepts in which nurse researchers are interested are not unique to nursing; therefore, their studies are sometimes linked to frameworks that are not models from the nursing profession. Several of these alternative models have gained special prominence in the development of nursing interventions to promote health-enhancing behaviors. In addition to the previously described Theory of Planned Behavior, four nonnursing models or theories have often been used in nursing studies: Bandura's Social Cognitive Theory, Prochaska's Transtheoretical (Stages of Change) Model, the Health Belief Model, and Lazarus and Folkman's Theory of Stress and Coping.

Bandura's Social Cognitive Theory

Social Cognitive Theory (Bandura, 1985, 1997, 2001), which is sometimes called **self-efficacy theory**, offers an explanation of human behavior using the concepts of self-efficacy and outcome expectations. Self-efficacy expectations are focused on people's belief in their own capacity to carry out particular behaviors (e.g., smoking cessation). Self-efficacy expectations, which are context-specific, determine the behaviors a person chooses to perform, their degree of perseverance, and the quality of the performance. Bandura identified four factors that influence a person's cognitive appraisal of self-efficacy: (1) their own mastery experience; (2) verbal persuasion; (3) vicarious experience; and (4) physiological and affective cues, such as pain and anxiety. The role of self-efficacy has been studied in relation to numerous health behaviors such as weight control, self-management of chronic illness, and smoking.

TIP: Bandura's self-efficacy construct is a key mediating variable in several theories discussed in this chapter. Self-efficacy has repeatedly been found to explain a significant amount of variation in people's behaviors and to be amenable to change, and so self-efficacy enhancement is often a goal in interventions designed to change people's health-related behaviors (Conn et al., 2001).

Example using Social Cognitive Theory: Nahm and colleagues (2009) explored the effect of a theory-based website designed to prevent hip fractures on health behaviors among older adults. The theoretical basis of the website was Social Cognitive Theory.

The Transtheoretical (Stages of Change) Model

There are several dimensions in the **Transtheoretical Model** (Prochaska & Velicer, 1997, Prochaska et al., 2002), a model that has been the basis of numerous interventions designed to change people's behavior such as smoking. The core construct around which the other dimensions are organized are the *stages of change*, which conceptualizes a continuum of *motivational readiness* to change problem behavior. The five stages of change are precontemplation, contemplation, preparation, action, and maintenance. Transitions from one stage to the next are affected by processes of change. Studies have shown that successful self-

changers use different processes at each particular stage, thus suggesting the desirability of interventions that are individualized to the person's stage of readiness for change. The model also incorporates a series of intervening variables, one of which is self-efficacy.

Example using the Transtheoretical Model: Daley and colleagues (2009) developed and tested a 5-week stage-specific education and counseling intervention aimed at improving exercise-related outcomes for women with elevated blood pressure.

The Health Belief Model

The **Health Belief Model** (HBM) (Becker, 1976, 1978) has become a popular framework in nursing studies focused on patient compliance and preventive healthcare practices. The model postulates that health-seeking behavior is influenced by a person's perception of a threat posed by a health problem and the value associated with actions aimed at reducing the threat. The major components of the HBM include perceived susceptibility, perceived severity, perceived benefits and costs, motivation, and enabling or modifying factors. Perceived susceptibility is a person's perception that a health problem is personally relevant or that a diagnosis is accurate. Even when one recognizes personal susceptibility, action will not occur unless the individual perceives the severity to be high enough to have serious implications. Perceived benefits are the patients' beliefs that a given treatment will cure the illness or help prevent it, and perceived barriers include the complexity, duration, and accessibility of the treatment. Motivation is the desire to comply with a treatment. Among the modifying factors that have been identified are personality variables, patient satisfaction, and sociodemographic factors.

Example using the HBM: Kara and Acikel (2009) used the HBM as a guiding framework in their study of breast self-examination (BSE) in a sample of Turkish nursing students and their mothers. Consistent with the model, mothers—who practiced self-examination less frequently than their daughters—reported higher barriers, lower motivation, and lower perceived benefits of BSE.

Lazarus and Folkman's Theory of Stress and Coping

The **Theory of Stress and Coping** (Lazarus, 2006; Lazarus & Folkman, 1984) is an effort to explain people's methods of dealing with stress, that is, environmental and internal demands that tax or exceed a person's resources and endanger his or her well-being. The model posits that coping strategies are learned, deliberate responses used to adapt to or change stressors. According to this model, a person's perception of mental and physical health is related to the ways he or she evaluates and copes with the stresses of living.

> **Example using the Theory of Stress and Coping:** Using Lazarus and Folkman's Theory of Stress and Coping as a framework, Burton and colleagues (2009) compared the level of perceived stress and somatization of spouses of deployed versus nondeployed American servicemen, and examined the relationship between stress and somatization.

➲ **TIP:** Several controversies surround the issue of theoretical frameworks in nursing. One concerns whether there should be a single, unified model of nursing or multiple, competing models. Another controversy involves the source of theories for nursing research. Some commentators advocate the development of unique nursing theories, claiming that only through such development can knowledge to guide nursing practice be produced. Others argue that well-respected theories from other disciplines, such as physiology or psychology (so-called *borrowed theories*), can and should be applied to nursing problems. (When the appropriateness of borrowed theories for nursing inquiry are confirmed, the theories are sometimes called *shared theories*). Nurse researchers are likely to continue on their current path of conducting studies within a multidisciplinary, multitheoretical perspective, and we are inclined to see the use of multiple frameworks as a healthy part of the development of nursing science.

Selecting a Theory or Model for Nursing Research

As we discuss in the next section, theory can be used by qualitative and quantitative researchers in various ways. A task common to many efforts to develop a study with a conceptual context, however, is the identification of an appropriate model or theory—a task made especially daunting because of the burgeoning number available. There are no rules for how this can be done, but there are two places to start—with the theory or model, or with the phenomenon being studied.

Readings in the theoretical literature often give rise to research ideas, so it is useful to become familiar with a variety of grand and middle-range theories. Table 6.1 provides references to the writings of a few major nurse theorists, and several nursing theory textbooks provide good overviews (e.g., Fawcett, 2005; McEwen & Wills, 2006; Alligood & Tomey, 2010). Resources for learning more about middle-range theories include Smith and Liehr (2003), Alligood and Tomey (2010), and Peterson and Bredow (2009). Additionally, the Toolkit in the *Resource Manual* for this textbook offers a list of references for about 100 middle-range theories and models that have been used in nursing research, organized in broad domains (e.g., aging, mental health, and pain). ✪

If you begin with a particular research problem or topic and are looking for a theory, a good strategy is to examine the conceptual contexts of existing studies on a similar topic. You may find that several different models or theories have been used, and so the next step is to learn as much as possible about the most promising ones so that you can select an appropriate one for your own study.

➲ **TIP:** Although it may be tempting to read about the features of a theory in a secondary source, it is best to consult a primary source, and to rely on the most up-to-date reference because models are often revised as research accumulates. However, it is also a good idea to review studies that have used the theory, including studies that focused on a research problem that is *not* similar to your own. By reading other studies, you will be better able to judge how much empirical support the theory has received, how key variables were measured, and perhaps how the theory should be adapted.

Many writers have offered advice on how to do an analysis and evaluation of a theory for use in nursing practice and nursing research (e.g., Barnum,

BOX 6.1 Some Questions for a Preliminary Assessment of a Model or Theory

Issue	Questions
Theoretical clarity	• Are key concepts defined and are definitions sufficiently clear? • Do all concepts "fit" within the theory? Are concepts used in the theory in a manner compatible with conceptual definitions? • Are basic assumptions consistent with one another? • Are schematic models compatible with the text? Are schematic models needed but not presented? • Can the theory be followed—is it adequately explained? Are there ambiguities?
Theoretical complexity	• Is the theory sufficiently rich and detailed? • Is the theory overly complex? • Can the theory be used to explain or predict, or only to describe phenomena?
Theoretical grounding	• Are the concepts identifiable in reality? • Is there a research basis for the theory, and is the basis solid?
Appropriateness of the theory	• Are the tenets of the theory compatible with nursing's philosophy? • Are key concepts within the domain of nursing?
Importance of the theory	• Could research based on this theory answer critical questions? • How will testing the theory contribute to nursing's evidence base?
General issue	• Are there other theories or models that do a better job of explaining phenomena of interest?

1998; Chinn & Kramer, 2004; Fawcett, 2005; Parker, 2006). Box 6.1 ⊗ presents some basic questions that can be asked in a preliminary assessment of a theory or model.

In addition to evaluating the general integrity of the model or theory, it is important to make sure that there is a proper "fit" between the theory and the research question to be studied. A critical issue is whether the theory has done a good job of explaining, predicting, or describing constructs that are key to your research problem. A few additional questions include the following:

• Has the theory been applied to similar research questions, and do the findings from prior research lend credibility to the theory's utility for research?
• Are the theoretical constructs in the model or theory readily operationalized? Are there existing instruments of adequate quality?

• Is the theory compatible with your world view, and with the world view implicit in the research question?

⊃ **TIP:** If you begin with a research problem and need to identify a suitable framework, it is wise to confer with people who may be familiar with a broad range of theoretical perspectives. By having an open discussion, you are more likely to identify an appropriate framework.

TESTING, USING, AND DEVELOPING A THEORY OR FRAMEWORK

The manner in which theory and conceptual frameworks are used by qualitative and quantitative researchers is elaborated on in the following section.

In the discussion, we use the term *theory* broadly to include conceptual models, formal theories, and frameworks.

Theories and Qualitative Research

Theory is almost always present in studies that are embedded in a qualitative research tradition such as ethnography, phenomenology, or grounded theory. These research traditions inherently provide an overarching framework that gives qualitative studies a theoretical grounding. However, different traditions involve theory in different ways.

Sandelowski (1993b) made a useful distinction between **substantive theory** (conceptualizations of the target phenomenon that is being studied) and theory that reflects a conceptualization of human inquiry. Some qualitative researchers insist on an atheoretical stance vis-à-vis the phenomenon of interest, with the goal of suspending *a priori* conceptualizations (substantive theories) that might bias their collection and analysis of data. For example, phenomenologists are in general committed to theoretical naiveté, and explicitly try to hold preconceived views of the phenomenon in check. Nevertheless, they are guided in their inquiries by a framework or philosophy that focuses their analysis on certain aspects of a person's life. That framework is based on the premise that human experience is an inherent property of the experience itself, not constructed by an outside observer.

Ethnographers typically bring a strong cultural perspective to their studies, and this perspective shapes their initial fieldwork. Fetterman (2010) has observed that most ethnographers adopt one of two cultural theories: **ideational theories**, which suggest that cultural conditions and adaptation stem from mental activity and ideas, or **materialistic theories**, which view material conditions (e.g., resources, money, and production) as the source of cultural developments.

The theoretical underpinning of grounded theory is a melding of sociological formulations (Glaser, 2003). The most prominent theoretical system in grounded theory is **symbolic interaction** (or *interactionism*), which has three underlying premises (Blumer, 1986). First, humans act toward things based on the meanings that the things have for them. Second, the meaning of things arises out of the interaction humans have with other fellow humans. Last, meanings are handled in, and modified through, an interpretive process in dealing with the things humans encounter. Despite having a theoretical umbrella, grounded theory researchers, like phenomenologists, attempt to hold prior substantive theory (existing knowledge and conceptualizations about the phenomenon) in abeyance until their own substantive theory begins to emerge.

Example of a grounded theory study:
Edwards and Sines (2008) conducted a study based on a symbolic interactionist framework to develop a substantive grounded theory of the process of initial assessment by nurses at triage—a process they described as "passing the audition" of credibility.

Grounded theory methods are designed to facilitate the generation of theory that is *conceptually dense*, that is, with many conceptual patterns and relationships. Grounded theory researchers seek to develop a conceptualization of a phenomenon that is *grounded* in actual observations—that is, to explicate an empirically based conceptualization for integrating and making sense of a process or phenomenon. During the ongoing analysis of data, the researchers move from specific pieces of data to abstract generalizations that synthesize and give structure to the observed phenomenon. The goal is to use the data to provide a description or an explanation of events as they occur—not as they have been conceptualized in existing theories. Once the grounded theory begins to take shape, however, previous literature is used for comparison with the emerging and developing categories of the theory. Sandelowski (1993b) has noted that previous substantive theories or conceptualizations, when used in this manner, are essentially data themselves, and can be taken into consideration, along with study data, as part of an inductively driven new conceptualization.

TIP: The use of theory in qualitative studies has been the topic of some debate. Morse (2002a) called for qualitative researchers to not be "theory ignorant but theory smart" (p. 296) and to "get over" their theory phobia. Morse elaborated (2004a) by noting that qualitative research does not necessarily begin with holding in check all prior knowledge of the phenomenon under study. She suggested that if the boundaries of the concept of interest can be identified, a qualitative researcher can use these boundaries as a scaffold to inductively explore the attributes of the concept.

In recent years, some qualitative nurse researchers have adopted a perspective known as critical theory as their framework. **Critical theory** is a paradigm that involves a critique of society and societal processes and structures, as we discuss in greater detail in Chapter 20.

Qualitative researchers sometimes use conceptual models of nursing as an interpretive framework. For example, some qualitative nurse researchers acknowledge that the philosophic roots of their studies lie in conceptual models of nursing developed by Newman, Parse, and Rogers.

Example of using nursing theory in a qualitative study: Yang and colleagues (2009) conducted a phenomenological inquiry, using Newman's Theory of Expanding Consciousness as a guiding framework, to identify meaningful patterns of health among Hmong American women living with diabetes.

One final note is that a systematic review of qualitative studies on a specific topic is another strategy leading to theory development. In metasyntheses, qualitative studies on a topic are scrutinized to identify their essential elements. The findings from different sources are then used for theory building. Paterson (2001), for example, used the results of 292 qualitative studies that described the experiences of adults with chronic illness to develop the shifting perspectives model of chronic illness. This model depicts living with chronic illness as an ongoing, constantly shifting process in which individuals' perspectives change in the degree to which illness is in the foreground or background in their lives.

Theories and Models in Quantitative Research

Quantitative researchers, like qualitative researchers, link research to theory or models in several ways. The classic approach is to test hypotheses deduced from an existing theory.

Testing an Existing Theory

Theories sometimes stimulate new studies. For example, a nurse might read about Pender's Health Promotion Model (see Figure 6.1) and, as reading progresses, reasoning such as the following might occur: "If the HPM is valid, then I would expect that patients with osteoporosis who perceived the benefit of a calcium-enriched diet would be more likely to alter their eating patterns than those who perceived no benefits." Such a conjecture can serve as a starting point for testing the model.

In testing a theory or model, quantitative researchers deduce implications (as in the preceding example) and develop hypotheses, which are predictions about the manner in which variables would be interrelated if the theory were valid. The hypotheses are then subjected to testing through systematic data collection and analysis.

The testing process involves a comparison between observed outcomes with those predicted in the hypotheses. Through this process, a theory is continually subjected to potential disconfirmation. If studies repeatedly fail to disconfirm a theory, it gains support and acceptance. Testing continues until pieces of evidence cannot be interpreted within the context of the theory but *can* be explained by a new theory that also accounts for previous findings. Theory-testing studies are most useful when researchers devise logically sound deductions from the theory, design a study that reduces the plausibility of alternative explanations for observed relationships, and use methods that assess the theory's validity under maximally heterogeneous situations so that potentially competing theories can be ruled out.

Researchers sometimes base a new study on a theory in an effort to explain earlier descriptive findings. For example, suppose several researchers had found that nursing home residents demonstrate greater levels of anxiety and noncompliance with nursing staff around bedtime than at other times. These findings shed no light on underlying causes of the problem, and so suggest no way to improve it. Several explanations, rooted in models such as Transition Theory or Lazarus and Folkman's Theory of Stress and Coping, may be relevant in explaining the residents' behavior. By directly testing the theory in a new study (i.e., deducing hypotheses derived from the theory), a researcher might learn *why* bedtime is a vulnerable period for the elderly in nursing homes.

Researchers sometimes combine elements from more than one theory as a basis for generating hypotheses. In doing this, researchers need to be thoroughly knowledgeable about *both* theories to see if there is an adequate conceptual basis for conjoining them. If underlying assumptions or conceptual definitions of key concepts are not compatible, the theories should not be combined (although perhaps elements of the two can be used to create a new conceptual framework with its own assumptions and definitions).

Another strategy sometimes used in theory-testing research is to test two competing theories directly— that is, to test alternative explanations of a phenomenon. There are competing theories for such phenomena as stress, behavior change, quality of life, and so on, and each competing theory suggests alternative approaches to facilitating positive outcomes or minimizing negative ones. Researchers who deliberately test multiple theories with a single sample of participants may be able to make powerful comparisons about the utility of competing explanations. Such a study requires considerable advance planning and the measurement of a wider array of constructs than would otherwise be the case, but may yield important results.

Example of a test of competing theories: Mahon and Yarcheski (2002) tested two alternative models of happiness in early adolescents: a theory linking happiness to enabling mechanisms and a theory of happiness based on adolescents' personality traits. The findings suggested that enabling mechanisms had more explanatory power than personality characteristics in predicting happiness.

Tests of a theory increasingly are taking the form of testing theory-based interventions. If a theory is correct, it has implications for strategies to influence people's health-related attitudes or behavior, and hence their health outcomes. And, if an intervention is developed on the basis of an explicit conceptualization of human behavior and thought, then it likely has a greater chance of being effective than if it is developed in a conceptual vacuum. The role of theory in the development of interventions is discussed at greater length in Chapter 26.

Example of theory testing in an intervention study: Mishel and co-researchers (2009) tested the effects of a theory-based decision-making uncertainty management intervention for newly diagnosed prostate cancer patients.

Using a Model or Theory as an Organizing Structure

Many researchers who cite a theory or model as their framework are not directly testing it. Silva (1986), in her analysis of 62 studies that claimed their roots in 5 nursing models, found that only 9 were direct and explicit tests of the models cited. The most common use of the models was to provide an organizing structure for the studies. In such an approach, researchers begin with a broad conceptualization of nursing (or stress, health beliefs, and so on) that is consistent with that of the model developers. The researchers *assume* that the models they espouse are valid, and then use the model's constructs or schemas to provide an organizational or interpretive context. Using models in this fashion can serve a valuable organizing purpose, but such studies do not address the issue of whether the theory itself is sound.

To our knowledge, Silva's study has not been replicated with a recent sample of studies, but we suspect that, even today, most quantitative studies that cite models and theories as their frameworks are using them primarily as organizational or interpretive tools. Silva (1986) offered seven evaluation criteria for assessing whether a study is actually testing a theory. Box 6.2 ⊗ presents a set of

BOX 6.2 Criteria to Determine if a Theory or Model is Being Tested in a Study

1. Is the purpose of the study to assess the validity of a theory's assumptions or propositions?
2. Does the report explicitly note that the theory is the framework for the research?
3. Is the theory discussed in sufficient detail that the relationship between the theory on the one hand and study hypotheses or research questions on the other is clear?
4. Are study hypotheses directly deduced from the theory?
5. Are study hypotheses empirically tested in an appropriate manner, so as to shed light on the validity of the theory?
6. Is the validity of the theory's assumptions or propositions supported (or challenged) based on evidence from the empirical tests?
7. Does the report discuss how evidence from empirical tests supports or refutes the theory, or how the theory explains relevant aspects of the findings?

Adapted from Silva, M. C. (1986). Research testing nursing theory: State of the art. *Advances in Nursing Science, 9,* 1–11.

evaluative questions broadly adapted from Silva's criteria. More recently, Keller and colleagues (2009) offered some guidelines for assessing fidelity to theory in intervention studies.

We should note that the framework for a quantitative study need not be a formal theory such as those described in the previous section. Sometimes quantitative studies are undertaken to further explicate constructs developed in grounded theory or other qualitative research.

Example of using qualitatively derived constructs as organizing structure: Hobdell and colleagues (2007) studied correlates of *chronic sorrow*, a construct that was developed and refined into a middle-range theory based on numerous qualitative studies, in families of children with epilepsy.

Fitting a Problem to a Theory

Researchers sometimes develop a set of research questions or hypotheses, and then subsequently try to devise a theoretical context in which to frame them. Such an approach may in some cases be worthwhile, but we caution that an after-the-fact linkage of theory to a problem does not always enhance a study. An important exception is when the researcher is struggling to make sense of findings and calls on an existing theory to help explain or interpret them.

If it is necessary to find a relevant theory or model after a research problem is selected, the search for such a theory must begin by first conceptualizing the problem on an abstract level. For example, take the research question: "Do daily telephone conversations between a psychiatric nurse and a patient for 2 weeks after hospital discharge reduce rates of readmission by short-term psychiatric patients?" This is a relatively concrete research problem, but it might profitably be viewed within the context of Orem's Self-Care Deficit Theory, reinforcement theory, a theory of social support, or a theory of crisis resolution. Part of the difficulty in finding a theory is that a single phenomenon of interest can be conceptualized in a number of ways.

Fitting a problem to a theory after the fact should be done with circumspection. Although having a theoretical context can enhance the meaningfulness of a study, artificially linking a problem to a theory is not the route to scientific utility, nor to enhancing nursing's evidence base. There are many published studies that purport to have a conceptual framework when, in fact, the tenuous *post hoc* linkage is all too evident. In Silva's (1986) analysis of 62 studies that claimed roots in a nursing model, about one third essentially paid only lip service to a model. If a conceptual model is really linked to a problem, then the design of the study, decisions about what to measure and how to measure it, and the interpretation of the findings *flow* from that conceptualization.

⊃ **TIP :** If you begin with a research question and then subsequently identify a theory or model, be willing to adapt or augment your original research problem as you gain greater understanding of the theory. The linking of theory and research question may involve an iterative approach.

Developing a Framework in a Quantitative Study

Novice researchers may think of themselves as unqualified to develop a conceptual scheme of their own. But theory development depends less on research experience than on powers of observation, grasp of a problem, and knowledge of prior research. There is nothing to prevent a creative and astute person from formulating an original conceptual framework for a study. The conceptual scheme may not be a full-fledged formal theory, but it should place the issues of the study into some broader perspective.

The basic intellectual process underlying theory development is induction—that is, reasoning from particular observations and facts to broader generalizations. The inductive process involves integrating what one has experienced or learned into an organized scheme. For quantitative research, the observations used in the inductive process usually are findings from other studies. When patterns of relationships among variables are derived in this fashion, one has the makings of a theory that can be put to a more rigorous test. The first step in the development of a framework, then, is to formulate a generalized scheme of relevant concepts that is firmly grounded in the research literature.

Let us use as an example a hypothetical study question that we described in Chapter 4, namely,

What is the effect of humor on stress in patients with cancer? (See the problem statement in Box 4.2, page 83). In undertaking a literature review, we find that researchers and reviewers have suggested a myriad of complex relationships among such concepts as humor, social support, stress, coping, appraisal, immune function, and neuroendocrine function on the one hand and various health outcomes (pain tolerance, mood, depression, health status, and eating and sleeping disturbances) on the other (e.g., Christie and Moore, 2005). While there is a fair amount of research evidence for the existence of these relationships, it is not clear how they all fit together. Without some kind of "map" or conceptualization of what might be going on, it would be difficult to design a strong study—we might, for example, not measure all the key variables or we might not undertake an appropriate analysis. And, if our goal is to design a humor therapy, we might struggle in developing a strong intervention in the absence of a framework.

The conceptual map in Figure 6.2 represents an attempt to put the pieces of the puzzle together for a study involving a test of a humor intervention to improve health outcomes for patients with cancer. According to this map, stress is affected by a cancer diagnosis and treatment both directly and indirectly, through the person's appraisal of the situation. That appraisal, in turn, is affected by the patient's coping skills, personality factors, and available social supports (factors which themselves are interrelated). Stress and physiological function (neuroendocrine and immunologic) have reciprocal relationships.

Note that we have not yet put in a "box" for humor in Figure 6.2. How do we think humor might operate? If we see humor as having primarily a direct effect on physiologic response, we would place humor near the bottom and draw an arrow from the box to immune and neuroendocrine function. But perhaps humor reduces stress because it helps a person cope (i.e., its effects are primarily psychological). Or maybe humor will affect the person's appraisal of the situation. Alternatively, a nurse-initiated humor therapy might have its effect primarily because it is a form of social support.

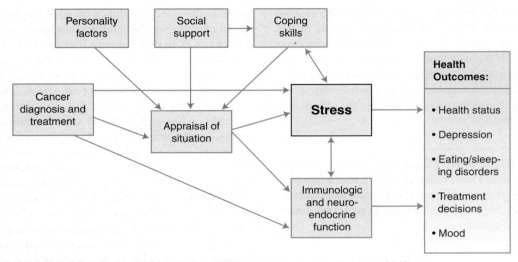

FIGURE 6.2 Conceptual Model of Stress and Health Outcomes in Patients with Cancer.

Each conceptualization has a different implication for study design. To give but one example, if the humor therapy is viewed primarily as a form of social support, then we might want to compare our intervention to an alternative intervention that involves the presence of a comforting nurse (another form of social support), without any special effort at including humor.

This type of inductive conceptualization based on existing research is a useful means of providing theoretical grounding for a study. Of course, our research question in this example could have been addressed within the context of an existing conceptualization, such as Lazarus and Folkman's Theory of Stress and Coping or the psychoneuroimmunology (PNI) framework (McCain et al., 2005), but hopefully our example illustrates how developing an original framework can inform researchers' decisions and strengthen the study.

Example of model development: Hoffman and colleagues (2009) studied the role of perceived self-efficacy for fatigue self-management on physical function status in patients with cancer, based on their own conceptual model. The model represented a synthesis of findings from the literature and from two existing theories—the Theory of Unpleasant Symptoms and Self-Efficacy Theory.

CRITIQUING FRAMEWORKS IN RESEARCH REPORTS

It is often challenging to critique the theoretical context of a published research report—or its absence—but we offer a few suggestions.

In a qualitative study in which a grounded theory is developed and presented, you probably will not be given enough information to refute the proposed theory because only evidence supporting it is presented. You can, however, assess whether the theory seems logical, whether the conceptualization is insightful, and whether the evidence in support of it is persuasive. In a phenomenological study, you should look to see if the researcher addresses the philosophical underpinnings of the

⊖ **TIP:** We strongly encourage you to draw a conceptual map before launching an investigation based on either a formal theory or your own inductive conceptualization—even if you do not plan to formally test the entire model or present the model in a report. Such maps are valuable heuristic devices in planning a study.

study. The researcher should briefly discuss the philosophy of phenomenology upon which the study was based.

Critiquing a theoretical framework in a quantitative report is also difficult, especially because you are not likely to be familiar with a range of relevant theories and models. Some suggestions for evaluating the conceptual basis of a quantitative study are offered in the following discussion and in Box 6.3. ⊗

The first task is to determine whether the study does, in fact, have a theoretical or conceptual framework. If there is no mention of a theory, model, or framework, you should consider whether the study's contribution is weakened by the absence of a conceptual context. Nursing has been criticized for producing pieces of isolated research that are difficult to integrate because of the absence of a theoretical foundation, but in some cases, the research may be so pragmatic that it does not really need a theory to enhance its usefulness. For exam-

ple, research designed to determine the optimal frequency of turning patients has a utilitarian goal; a theory might not enhance the value of the findings. If, however, the study involves the test of an intervention, the absence of a formally stated theoretical framework or rationale suggests conceptual fuzziness.

If the study does have an explicit framework, you must then ask whether the particular framework is appropriate. You may not be in a position to challenge the researcher's use of a particular theory or to recommend an alternative, but you can evaluate the logic of using that framework and assess whether the link between the problem and the theory is genuine. Does the researcher present a convincing rationale for the framework used? Do the hypotheses flow from the theory? Will the findings contribute to the validation of the theory? Does the researcher interpret the findings within the context of the framework? If the answer to such questions is no, you may have grounds for criticizing the

---

BOX 6.3 Guidelines for Critiquing Theoretical and Conceptual Frameworks

1. Does the report describe an explicit theoretical or conceptual framework for the study? If not, does the absence of a framework detract from the usefulness or significance of the research?
2. Does the report adequately describe the major features of the theory or model so that readers can understand the conceptual basis of the study?
3. Is the theory or model appropriate for the research problem? Would a different framework have been more fitting?
4. If there is an intervention, was there a cogent theoretical basis or rationale for the intervention?
5. Was the theory or model used as the basis for generating hypotheses, or was it used as an organizational or interpretive framework? Was this appropriate?
6. Do the research problem and hypotheses (if any) naturally flow from the framework, or does the purported link between the problem and the framework seem contrived? Are deductions from the theory logical?
7. Are the concepts adequately defined in a way that is consistent with the theory? If there is an intervention, are intervention components consistent with the theory?
8. Is the framework based on a conceptual model of nursing or on a model developed by nurses? If it is borrowed from another discipline, is there adequate justification for its use?
9. Did the framework guide the study methods? For example, was the appropriate research tradition used if the study was qualitative? If quantitative, do the operational definitions correspond to the conceptual definitions?
10. Does the researcher tie the study findings back to the framework in the Discussion section? Do the findings support or challenge the framework? Are the findings interpreted within the context of the framework?

study's framework, even though you may not be able to articulate how the conceptual basis of the study could be improved.

RESEARCH EXAMPLES

Throughout this chapter, we have mentioned studies that were based on various conceptual and theoretical models. This section presents more detailed examples of the linkages between theory and research from the nursing research literature—one from a quantitative study and the other from a qualitative study.

Research Example from a Quantitative Study: Health Promotion Model

Study: Clinical trial of tailored activity and eating newsletters with older rural women (Walker et al., 2009)

Statement of Purpose: The purpose of the study was to evaluate the effects of a tailored intervention, based on Pender's Health Promotion Model (HPM), on such health outcomes as physical activity and healthy eating among older rural women. The intervention involved a series of newletters.

Theoretical Framework: The HPM (see Figure 6.1) was used as the framework for the intervention "because midlife and older women may be more interested in enhancing health to maintain independence than in avoiding specific disease as they age" (p. 75). In designing the tailored intervention, the researchers selected four behavior-specific cognitions from the HPM—perceived benefits, barriers, self-efficacy, and interpersonal influences. These cognitions are viewed in the model as determinants of behavior, and have been found to be modifiable. The intervention targeted change on health behaviors themselves, and also on these known influences on the behaviors.

Method: In this community-based study, two similar rural sites were assigned, at random, to either the tailored intervention protocol or to a generic intervention. A sample of 225 women aged 50 to 69 years were recruited to participate. Over a 12-month period, the women received by mail either 18 generic newsletters or 18 newsletters tailored on the four HPM behavior-specific cognitions, as well as

on the behaviors of interest—activity and diet. Tailored newsletters included content relevant to individual recipients, as suggested in their assessment responses. Newsletters also included information about HPM determinants—that is, the benefits of healthy eating and activity, overcoming barriers to change, building confidence in the ability to change, and obtaining social support from friends and family. Outcome data were collected at 6 and 12 months after the start of the intervention. Assessments of the HPM behavioral determinants for tailoring purposes were completed at the outset and at 3, 6, and 9 months later. Outcomes focused on physical activity and eating, and included both behavioral markers (e.g., self-reported daily servings of fruits and vegetables, time engaged daily in moderate or high intensity activity) and biomarkers (e.g., serum lipid levels, percentage of body fat).

Key Findings: Women in both groups showed improvement in certain outcomes over the course of the study, such as increased fruit and vegetable servings and decreased percentage of calories from fat. Improvements in other outcomes, however, were only observed in the tailored intervention group, including increased moderate or high intensity activity and decreased blood pressure. The researchers concluded that the theory-based tailored newsletters were more effective than generic newsletters in facilitating behavior change over the 12-month period.

Research Example from a Qualitative Study: A Grounded Theory

Study: Getting "to the point": The experience of mothers getting assistance for their adult children who are violent and mentally ill (Copeland & Heileman, 2008).

Statement of Purpose: The purposes of the study were to describe how mothers understand violent behavior directed at them by their adult children with mental illness, and to explain the process mothers used to get assistance and access mental health treatment when violence occurred.

Method: Grounded theory methods were used. Data were collected by means of in-depth interviews with 8 mothers of mentally ill adult children. Every woman was asked, "Can you tell me about a time when your son/daughter has been violent in your family." Additional questions probed what the mother then did, how and by whom decisions were made, whether decisions led to desired results, and whether the mother wished another course had been taken. Interviews, which were conducted in the participants' homes or in another private location of their choice, were audiotaped and later transcribed for analysis. Interviews lasted between 1.5 and 2 hours.

Theoretical Framework: A grounded theory method was adopted, with symbolic interactionism used as a theoretical foundation. As noted by the authors, this theory proposes that people derive meaning through social interaction and through their interpretation of those interactions. "It was therefore assumed that mothers interpret their children's mental illness and violent behavior in a way that makes sense to them in the context of their daily lives and that the meaning of both affects their responses to the violence they experience" (p. 137).

Key Findings: The grounded theory methods led to the development of a theoretical map of the process mothers used to get assistance when their children became violent. As shown in Figure 6.3, the process of getting assistance ("getting to the point") involved a period of hypervigilance in which the mothers felt on high alert—although they felt there was little they could do. While their children decompensated, the mothers waited for the inevitable point at which their children would meet criteria for involuntary hospitalization. Fear and uncertainty eventually outweighed their ability to manage their children's behavior, at which time they called psychiatric evaluation teams (PET) who were the gatekeepers to mental health treatment.

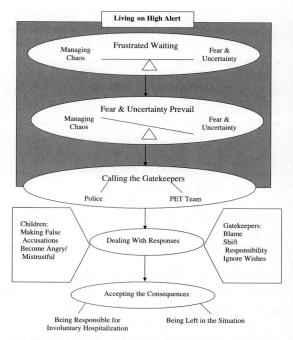

FIGURE 6.3 A grounded theory of mothers' process of getting assistance when their adult children with mental illness become violent toward them. From Copeland, D. A., & Heileman, M. (2008). Getting "to the point": The experience of mothers getting assistance for their adult children who are violent and mentally ill. *Nursing Research, 57*, p. 139.

SUMMARY POINTS

- High-quality research requires *conceptual integration*, one aspect of which is having a defensible theoretical rationale for undertaking the study in a given manner or for testing specific hypotheses. Researchers demonstrate their conceptual clarity through the delineation of a theory, model, or framework on which the study is based.

- A **theory** is a broad abstract characterization of phenomena. As classically defined, a theory is an abstract generalization that systematically explains relationships among phenomena. **Descriptive theory** thoroughly describes a phenomenon.

- The basic components of a theory are concepts; classically defined theories consist of a set of propositions about the interrelationships among concepts, arranged in a logically interrelated system that permits new statements to be derived from them.

- **Grand theories** (or *macrotheories*) attempt to describe large segments of the human experience. **Middle-range theories** are more specific to certain phenomena and are increasingly important in nursing research.

- Concepts are also the basic elements of **conceptual models**, but concepts are not linked in a logically ordered, deductive system. Conceptual models, like theories, provide context for nursing studies.

- The goal of theories and models in research is to make findings meaningful, to integrate knowledge into coherent systems, to stimulate new research, and to explain phenomena and relationships among them.

- **Schematic models** (or **conceptual maps**) are graphic, theory-driven representations of phenomena and their interrelationships using symbols or diagrams and a minimal use of words.

- A **framework** is the conceptual underpinning of a study, including an overall rationale and conceptual definitions of key concepts. In qualitative studies, the framework often springs from distinct research traditions.

- Several conceptual models and grand theories of nursing have been developed. The concepts central to models of nursing are human beings, environment, health, and nursing. Two major conceptual models of nursing used by researchers are Roy's Adaptation Model and Rogers' Science of Unitary Human Beings.

- Non-nursing models used by nurse researchers (e.g., Bandura's Social Cognitive Theory) are **borrowed theories**; when the appropriateness of borrowed theories for nursing inquiry is confirmed, the theories become **shared theories**.

- In some qualitative research traditions (e.g., phenomenology), the researcher strives to suspend previously held **substantive theories** of the phenomena under study, but nevertheless there is a rich theoretical underpinning associated with the tradition itself.

- Some qualitative researchers specifically seek to develop *grounded theories*, data-driven explanations to account for phenomena under study through inductive processes.

- In the classical use of theory, researchers test hypotheses deduced from an existing theory. An emerging trend is the testing of theory-based interventions.

- In both qualitative and quantitative studies, researchers sometimes use a theory or model as an organizing framework, or as an interpretive tool.

- Researchers sometimes develop a problem, design a study, and *then* look for a conceptual framework; such an after-the-fact selection of a framework usually is less compelling than a more systematic application of a particular theory.

- Even in the absence of a formal theory, quantitative researchers can inductively weave together the findings from prior studies into a conceptual scheme that provides methodologic and conceptual direction to the inquiry.

STUDY ACTIVITIES

Chapter 6 of the *Resource Manual for Nursing Research: Generating and Assessing Evidence for Nursing Practice, 9th ed.*, offers study suggestions for reinforcing concepts presented in this chapter. In addition, the following questions can be addressed in classroom or online discussions:

1. Select one of the conceptual models or theories described in this chapter. Formulate a research question and one or two hypotheses that could be used empirically to test the utility of the conceptual framework or model in nursing practice.

2. Answer appropriate questions from Box 6.3 regarding the Walker and colleagues (2009) intervention study for rural older women described at the end of the chapter. Also, consider what the implications of the study are in terms of the utility of the HPM.

3. Answer appropriate questions from Box 6.3 regarding Copeland and Heileman's grounded theory study of mothers dealing with their violent mentally ill adult children: (a) In what way was the use of theory different in this study than in the previous study by Walker and colleagues? (b) Comment on the utility of the schematic model shown in Figure 6.3.

STUDIES CITED IN CHAPTER 6

Bailey, D., Landerman, L., Barroso, J., Bixby, P. Mishel, M., Muir, A., Strickland, L., & Clipp, E. (2009). Uncertainty, symptoms, and quality of life in persons with chronic hepatitis C. *Psychosomatics, 50,* 138–146.

Burton, T., Farley, D., & Rhea, A. (2009). Stress-induced somatization in spouses of deployed and nondeployed servicemen. *Journal of the American Academy of Nurse Practitioners, 21*, 332–329.

Christie, W., & Moore, C. (2005). The impact of humor on patients with cancer. *Clinical Journal of Oncology Nursing, 9*, 211–218.

Copeland, D. A., & Heileman, M. (2008). Getting "to the point": The experience of mothers getting assistance for their adult children who are violent and mentally ill. *Nursing Research, 57*, 136–143.

Cossette, S., Frasure-Smith, N., & Lespérance, F. (2002). Nursing approaches to reducing psychological distress in men and women recovering from myocardial infarction. *International Journal of Nursing Studies, 39*, 479–494.

Daley, L., Fish, A., Frid, D., & Mitchell, G. (2009). Stage-specific education/counseling intervention in women with elevated blood pressure. *Progress in Cardiovascular Nursing, 24*, 45–52.

DeSanto-Madeya, S. (2009). Adaptation to spinal cord injury for families post-injury. *Nursing Science Quarterly, 22*, 57–66.

Doucet, T. J. (2009). Trusting another: A Parse research method study. *Nursing Science Quarterly, 22*, 259–266.

Edwards, B., & Sines, D. (2008). Passing the audition—the appraisal of client credibility and assessment by nurses at triage. *Journal of Clinical Nursing, 17*, 2444–2451.

Farren, A. T. (2010). Power, uncertainty, self-transcendence, and quality of life in breast cancer survivors. *Nursing Science Quarterly, 23*, 63–71.

Hobdell, E., Grant, M., Valencia, I., Mare, J., Kothare, S., Legido, A., & Kurana, D. (2007). Chronic sorrow and coping in families of children with epilepsy. *Journal of Neuroscience Nursing, 39*, 76–82.

Hodges, P. J. (2009). The essence of life purpose. *Critical Care Nursing Quarterly, 32*, 163–170.

Hoffman, A., von Eye, A., Gift, A., Given, B., Given, C., & Rothert, M. (2009). Testing a theoretical model of perceived self-efficacy for cancer-related fatigue self-management and optimal physical functioning status. *Nursing Research, 58*, 32–41.

Kara, B., & Acikel, C. (2009). Health beliefs and breast self-examination in a sample of Turkish nursing students and their mothers. *Journal of Clinical Nursing, 18*, 1412–1421.

Kirchhoff, K., Palzkill, J., Kowalkowski, J., Mork, A., & Gretarsdottir, E. (2008). Preparing families of intensive care patients for withdrawal of life support. *American Journal of Critical Care, 17*, 113–121.

Mahon, N. E., & Yarcheski, A. (2002). Alternative theories of happiness in early adolescents. *Clinical Nursing Research, 11*, 306–323.

McElligott, D., Siemers, S., Thomas, L., & Kohn, N. (2009). Health promotion in nurses: Is there a healthy nurse in the house? *Applied Nursing Research, 22*, 211–215.

Mishel, M., Germino, B., Lin, L., Pruthi, R., Wallen, E., Crandell, J., & Bivler, D. (2009). Managing uncertainty about treatment decision making in early prostate cancer. *Patient Education & Counseling, 77*, 349–359.

Mock, V., St. Ours, C., Hall, S., Bositis, A., Tillery, M., Belcher, A., Krumm, S., McCorkle, R., & Wald, F. (2007). Using a conceptual model in nursing research—mitigating fatigue in cancer patients. *Journal of Advanced Nursing, 58*, 503–512.

Moore, J., Pawloski, L., Rodriguez, C., Lubi, L., & Ailinger, R. (2009). The effect of a nutrition education program on the nutritional knowledge, hemoglobin levels, and nutritional status of Nicaraguan adolescent girls. *Public Health Nursing, 26*, 144–152.

Nahm, E., Resnick, B., DeGrezia, M., & Brotemarkle, R. (2009). Use of discussion boards in a theory-based health website for older adults. *Nursing Research, 58*, 419–426.

Ness, S. M. (2009). Pain expression in the perioperative period: Insights from a focus group of Somali women. *Pain Management Nursing, 10*, 65–75.

Paterson, B. L. (2001). The shifting perspectives model of chronic illness. *Journal of Nursing Scholarship, 33*, 21–26.

Peddle, C., Jones, L., Eves, N., Reiman, T., Sellar, C., Winton, T., Courneya, K. (2009). Correlates of adherence to supervised exercise in patients awaiting surgical removal of malignant tumor lesions. *Oncology Nursing Forum, 36*, 287–295.

Schumacher, G. (2010). Culture care meanings, beliefs, and practices in rural Dominican Republic. *Journal of Transcultural Nursing, 21*, 93–103.

Shearer, N., Fleury, J., & Reed, P. (2009). The rhythm of health in older women with chronic illness. *Research and Theory for Nursing Practice, 23*, 148–160.

Suliman, W., Welmann, E., Omer, T., & Thomas, L. (2009). Applying Watson's nursing theory to assess patient perceptions of being cared for in a multicultural environment. *Journal of Nursing Research, 17*, 293–297.

Walker, S. N., Pullen, C., Boeckner, L., Hageman, P., Hertzog, M., Oberdorfer, M., Rutledge, M. J. (2009). Clinical trial of tailored activity and eating newsletters with older rural women. *Nursing Research, 58*, 74–85.

Weiss, M., Fawcett, J., & Aber, C. (2009). Adaptation, postpartum concerns, and learning needs in the first two weeks after caesarean birth. *Journal of Clinical Nursing, 18*, 2938–2948.

Yang, A., Xiong, D., Vang, E., & Pharris, M. (2009). Hmong American women living with diabetes. *Journal of Nursing Scholarship, 41*, 139–148.

Yarcheski, T., Mahon, N., Yarcheski, A., & Hanks, M. (2010). Perceived stress and wellness in early adolescents using the Neuman Systems Model. *Journal of School Nursing, 26*, 230–237.

Methodologic and nonresearch references cited in this chapter can be found in a separate section at the end of the book.

7

Ethics in Nursing Research

In studies involving human beings or animals, researchers must deal with ethical issues. Ethics can be challenging because ethical requirements sometimes conflict with the desire to produce rigorous evidence. This chapter discusses major ethical principles that must be considered in designing research.

ETHICS AND RESEARCH

When humans are used as study participants, care must be exercised to ensure that their rights are protected. Ethical research conduct may strike you as self-evident, but ethical considerations have not always been given adequate attention.

Historical Background

The Nazi medical experiments of the 1940s are a famous example of disregard for ethical conduct. Nazi research involved the use of prisoners of war and racial "enemies" in experiments testing human endurance and reaction to untested drugs. The studies were unethical not only because they exposed people to harm and even death, but also because people could not refuse participation. Similar wartime experiments that raised ethical concerns were conducted in Japan and Australia (McNeill, 1993).

More recently, researchers investigated the effects of syphilis among poor African American men between 1932 and 1972 in the Tuskegee Syphilis Study, sponsored by the U.S. Public Health Service. Medical treatment was deliberately withheld to study the course of the untreated disease. A public health nurse recruited many participants (Vessey and Gennarao, 1994). Similarly, Dr. Herbert Green studied women with cervical cancer in Auckland, New Zealand in the 1980s; patients with carcinoma were not given treatment so that the natural progression of the disease could be studied.

In the Willowbrook Study, Dr. Saul Krugman conducted research on hepatitis during the 1960s. At Willowbrook, an institution for the mentally retarded on Staten Island, children were deliberately infected with the hepatitis virus. Even more recently, it was revealed in 1993 that U.S. federal agencies had sponsored radiation experiments since the 1940s on hundreds of people, many of them prisoners or elderly hospital patients. And in 2010, it was revealed that a U.S. doctor who worked on the Tuskegee Study inoculated prisoners in Guatemala with syphilis in the 1940s (Reverby, in press). Many other examples of studies with ethical transgressions—often more subtle than these examples—have emerged to give ethical concerns the high visibility they have today.

Codes of Ethics

In response to human rights violations, various **codes of ethics** have been developed. The *Nuremberg Code*, developed after Nazi atrocities were made public in the Nuremberg trials, was an international effort to establish ethical standards. The *Declaration of Helsinki*, another international set of standards, was adopted in 1964 by the World Medical Association and was most recently revised in 2008.

Most disciplines (e.g., psychology, sociology, medicine) have established their own ethical codes. In nursing, the American Nurses Association (ANA) issued *Ethical Guidelines in the Conduct, Dissemination, and Implementation of Nursing Research* (Silva, 1995). ANA also published in 2001 a revised *Code of Ethics for Nurses with Interpretive Statements*, a document that covers primarily ethical issues for practicing nurses but that also includes principles that apply to nurse researchers. In Canada, the Canadian Nurses Association published a document entitled *Ethical Research Guidelines for Registered Nurses* in 2002. In Australia, three nursing organizations collaborated to develop the *Code of Ethics for Nurses in Australia* (2008).

Some nurse ethicists have called for an international ethics code for nursing, but nurses in most countries have developed their own professional codes or follow the codes established by their governments. The International Council of Nurses (ICN), however, has developed the *ICN Code of Ethics for Nurses*, updated in 2006.

➔ **TIP:** In their study of 27 ethical review boards in the United States, Rothstein & Phuong (2007) found nurses to be more sensitive to ethical issues than members from other disciplines.

Government Regulations for Protecting Study Participants

Governments throughout the world fund research and establish rules for adhering to ethical principles. For example, Health Canada specified the *Tri-Council Policy Statement: Ethical Conduct for Research Involving Humans* as the guidelines to protect study participants in all types of research. In Australia, the National Health and Medical Research Council issued the *National Statement on Ethical Conduct in Research Involving Humans* in 2007 and also issued a special statement about incentive payments to study participants in 2009.

In the United States, the National Commission for the Protection of Human Subjects of Biomedical and Behavioral Research adopted a code of ethics in 1978. The commission, established by the National Research Act, issued the **Belmont Report**, which provided a model for many disciplinary guidelines. The Belmont Report also served as the basis for regulations affecting research sponsored by the U.S. government, including studies supported by NINR. The U.S. Department of Health and Human Services (DHHS) has issued ethical regulations that have been codified as Title 45 Part 46 of the Code of Federal Regulations (45 CFR 46). These regulations, revised most recently in 2005, are among the most widely used guidelines in the United States for evaluating the ethical aspects of studies.

➔ **TIP:** There are many useful websites devoted to ethical principles, only some of which are mentioned in this chapter. Several websites are listed in the "Useful Websites for Chapter 7" file in the Toolkit of the accompanying *Resource Manual*, for you to click on directly.

Ethical Dilemmas in Conducting Research

Research that violates ethical principles is rarely done specifically to be cruel, but usually occurs out of a conviction that knowledge is important and potentially beneficial in the long run. There are situations in which participants' rights and study demands are in direct conflict, posing **ethical dilemmas** for researchers. Here are examples of research problems in which the desire for rigor conflicts with ethical considerations:

1. *Research question:* Are nurses equally empathic in their treatment of male and female patients in the ICU?

   Ethical dilemma: Ethics require that participants be aware of their role in a study. Yet if the researcher informs nurse participants that their empathy in treating male and female ICU patients will be scrutinized, will their behavior be "normal?" If the nurses' usual behavior is altered because of the known presence of research observers, then the findings will be inaccurate.

2. *Research question:* What are the coping mechanisms of parents whose children have a terminal illness?

   Ethical dilemma: To answer this question, the researcher may need to probe into the psychological state of parents at a vulnerable time; such probing could be painful or traumatic. Yet knowledge of the parents' coping mechanisms might help to design effective interventions for dealing with parents' grief and stress.

3. *Research question:* Does a new medication prolong life in patients with cancer?

   Ethical dilemma: The best way to test the effectiveness of an intervention is to administer the intervention to some participants but withhold it from others to see if differences between the groups emerge. However, if the intervention is untested (e.g., a new drug), the group receiving the intervention may be exposed to potentially hazardous side effects. On the other hand, the group *not* receiving the drug may be denied a beneficial treatment.

4. *Research question:* What is the process by which adult children adapt to the day-to-day stresses of caring for a parent with Alzheimer's disease?

   Ethical dilemma: Sometimes, especially in qualitative studies, a researcher may get so close to participants that they become willing to share "secrets" and privileged information. Interviews can become confessions—sometimes of unseemly or even illegal behavior. In this example, suppose a woman admitted to physically abusing her mother—how does the researcher respond to that information without undermining a pledge of confidentiality? And, if the researcher divulges the information to authorities, how can a pledge of confidentiality be given in good faith to other participants?

As these examples suggest, researchers are sometimes in a bind. Their goal is to develop high-quality evidence for practice, using the best methods available, but they must also adhere to rules for protecting human rights. Another dilemma can arise if nurse researchers are confronted with conflict-of-interest situations, in which their expected behavior as researchers conflicts with their expected behavior as nurses (e.g., deviating from a research protocol to give assistance to a patient). It is precisely because of such conflicts and dilemmas that codes of ethics have been developed to guide researchers' efforts.

ETHICAL PRINCIPLES FOR PROTECTING STUDY PARTICIPANTS

The *Belmont Report* articulated three broad principles on which standards of ethical conduct in research are based: beneficence, respect for human dignity, and justice. We briefly discuss these principles and then describe procedures researchers adopt to comply with them.

Beneficence

Beneficence imposes a duty on researchers to minimize harm and maximize benefits. Human research should be intended to produce benefits for participants or—a situation that is more common—for others. This principle covers multiple dimensions.

The Right to Freedom from Harm and Discomfort

Researchers have an obligation to avoid, prevent, or minimize harm (*nonmaleficence*) in studies with humans. Participants must not be subjected to unnecessary risks of harm or discomfort, and their participation must be essential to achieving scientifically and societally important aims that could not otherwise be realized. In research with humans, *harm* and *discomfort* can be physical (e.g., injury, fatigue), emotional (e.g., stress, fear), social (e.g., loss of social support), or financial (e.g., loss of wages). Ethical researchers must use strategies to minimize all types of harms and discomforts, even ones that are temporary.

Research should be conducted only by qualified people, especially if potentially dangerous equipment or specialized procedures are used. Ethical researchers must be prepared to terminate a study if they suspect that continuation would result in injury, death, or undue distress to participants. When a new medical procedure or drug is being tested, it is usually advisable to experiment with animals or tissue cultures before proceeding to tests with humans. (Guidelines for the ethical treatment of animals are discussed later in this chapter.)

Protecting human beings from physical harm may be straightforward, but the psychological consequences of study participation are usually subtle and require close attention and sensitivity. For example, participants may be asked questions about their personal views, weaknesses, or fears. Such queries might lead people to reveal sensitive personal information. The point is not that researchers should refrain from asking questions, but that they need to be aware of the nature of the intrusion on people's psyches.

The need for sensitivity may be greater in qualitative studies, which often involve in-depth exploration on highly personal topics. In-depth probing may actually expose deep-seated fears that study participants had previously repressed. Qualitative researchers, regardless of the underlying research tradition, must be especially vigilant in anticipating such problems.

Example of intense self-scrutiny in a qualitative study: Caelli (2001) conducted a phenomenological study to illuminate nurses' understandings of health, and how such understandings translated into nursing practice. One participant, having explored her experience of health with the researcher over several interview sessions, resigned from her city hospital job as a result of gaining a new recognition of the role health played in her life.

The Right to Protection from Exploitation

Involvement in a study should not place participants at a disadvantage or expose them to damages. Participants need to be assured that their participation, or information they might provide, will not be used against them. For example, people describing their finances to a researcher should not be exposed to the risk of losing public healthcare benefits; those divulging illegal drug use should not fear exposure to criminal authorities.

Study participants enter into a special relationship with researchers, and it is crucial that this relationship not be exploited. Exploitation may be overt and malicious (e.g., sexual exploitation, use of donated blood for developing a commercial product), but might also be more subtle. For example, suppose people agreed to participate in a study requiring 30 minutes of their time and then the researcher decided 1 year later to go back to them, to follow their progress. Unless the researcher had previously warned participants that there might be a follow-up study, the researcher might be accused of not adhering to the agreement previously reached and of exploiting the researcher–participant relationship.

Because nurse researchers may have a nurse–patient (in addition to a researcher–participant) relationship, special care may be required to avoid exploiting that bond. Patients' consent to participate in a study may result from their understanding of the researcher's role as *nurse*, not as *researcher*.

In qualitative research, psychological distance between researchers and participants often declines as the study progresses. The emergence of a pseudotherapeutic relationship is not uncommon, which heightens the risk that exploitation could inadvertently occur (Eide & Kahn, 2008). On the other hand, qualitative researchers often are in a better position than quantitative researchers to *do good*, rather than just to avoid doing harm, because of the relationships they often develop with participants. Munhall (2012) has argued that qualitative nurse researchers have the responsibility of ensuring that, if there are any conflicts, the clinical and therapeutic imperative of nursing takes precedence over the research imperative of advancing knowledge.

Example of therapeutic research experiences:
Beck (2005) reported that participants in her studies on birth trauma and post-traumatic stress disorder (PTSD) expressed a range of benefits from their e-mail exchanges with Beck. Here is what one informant voluntarily shared:

"You thanked me for everything in your e-mail, and I want to THANK YOU for caring. For me, it means a lot that you have taken an interest in this subject and are taking the time and effort to find out more about PTSD. For someone to even acknowledge this condition means a lot for someone who has suffered from it" (p. 417).

Respect for Human Dignity

Respect for human dignity is the second ethical principle in the *Belmont Report*. This principle includes the right to self-determination and the right to full disclosure.

The Right to Self-Determination

Humans should be treated as autonomous agents, capable of controlling their actions. **Self-determination** means that prospective participants can voluntarily decide whether to take part in a study, without risk of prejudicial treatment. It also means that people have the right to ask questions, to refuse to give information, and to withdraw from the study.

A person's right to self-determination includes freedom from **coercion**, which involves threats of penalty from failing to participate in a study or excessive rewards from agreeing to participate. Protecting people from coercion requires careful thought when the researcher is in a position of authority or influence over potential participants, as is often the case in a nurse–patient relationship. The issue of coercion may require scrutiny even when there is not a pre-established relationship. For example, a generous monetary incentive (or **stipend**) offered to encourage participation among an economically disadvantaged group (e.g., the homeless) might be considered mildly coercive because such incentives might pressure prospective participants into cooperation.

The Right to Full Disclosure

People's right to make informed, voluntary decisions about study participation requires full disclosure. **Full disclosure** means that the researcher has fully described the nature of the study, the person's right to refuse participation, the researcher's responsibilities, and likely risks and benefits. The right to self-determination and the right to full disclosure are the two major elements on which informed consent—discussed later in this chapter—is based.

Full disclosure is not always straightforward because it can create biases and sample recruitment problems. Suppose we were testing the hypothesis that high school students with a high rate of absenteeism are more likely to be substance abusers than students with good attendance. If we approached potential participants and fully explained the study purpose, some students likely would refuse to participate, and nonparticipation would be selective; those least likely to volunteer might well be substance abusing students—the group of primary interest. Moreover, by knowing the research question, those who *do* participate might not give candid responses. In such a situation, full disclosure could undermine the study.

A technique that is sometimes used in such situations is **covert data collection** (*concealment*), which is the collection of data without participants' knowledge and consent. This might happen, for example, if a researcher wanted to observe people's behavior in real-world settings and worried that doing so openly would affect the behavior of interest. Researchers might choose to obtain the information through concealed methods, such as by videotaping with hidden equipment or observing while pretending to be engaged in other activities. Covert data collection may in some cases be acceptable if risks are negligible and participants' right to privacy has not been violated. Covert data collection is least likely to be ethically tolerable if the study is focused on sensitive aspects of people's behavior, such as drug use or sexual conduct.

A more controversial technique is the use of **deception**, which involves deliberately withholding information about the study or providing participants with false information. For example, in studying high school students' use of drugs, we might describe the research as a study of students' health practices, which is a mild form of misinformation.

Deception and concealment are problematic ethically because they interfere with participants' right to make truly informed decisions about personal costs and benefits of participation. Some people argue that deception is never justified. Others, however, believe that if the study involves minimal risk to participants and if there are anticipated benefits to society, then deception may be justified to enhance the validity of the findings. ANA guidelines offer this advice about deception and concealment:

• • •

The investigator understands that concealment or deception in research is controversial, depending on the type of research. Some investigators believe that concealment or deception in research can never be morally justified. The investigator further understands that before concealment or deception is used, certain criteria must be met: (1) The study must be of such small risk to the research participant and of such great significance to the advancement of the public good that concealment or deception can be morally justified . . . (2) The acceptability of concealment or deception is related to the degree of risks to research participants . . . (3) Concealment or deception are used only as last resorts, when no other approach can ensure the validity of the study's findings . . . (4) The investigator has a moral responsibility to inform research participants of any concealment or deception as soon as possible and to explain the rationale for its use. (Silva, 1995, p. 10, Section 4.2).

• • •

Another issue that has emerged in this era of electronic communication concerns data collection over the Internet. For example, some researchers analyze the content of messages posted to chat rooms, blogs, or listserves. The issue is whether such messages can be treated as research data without permission and informed consent. Some researchers believe that messages posted electronically are in the public domain and can be used without consent for research purposes. Others, however, feel that standard ethical rules should apply in cyberspace research and that electronic researchers must carefully protect the rights of those who are participants in "virtual" communities. Guidance for

the ethical conduct of health research on the Internet has been developed by such writers as Ellett and colleagues (2004), Flicker and colleagues (2004), and Holmes (2009).

Justice

The third broad principle articulated in the *Belmont Report* concerns justice, which includes participants' right to fair treatment and their right to privacy.

The Right to Fair Treatment

One aspect of justice concerns the equitable distribution of benefits and burdens of research. Participant selection should be based on study requirements and not on a group's vulnerability. Participant selection has been a key ethical issue historically, with some researchers selecting groups with lower social standing (e.g., poor people, prisoners) as participants. The principle of justice imposes particular obligations toward individuals who are unable to protect their own interests (e.g., dying patients) to ensure that they are not exploited.

Distributive justice also imposes duties to neither neglect nor discriminate against individuals or groups who may benefit from research. During the 1980s and early 1990s, there was strong evidence that women and minorities were being unfairly excluded from many clinical studies in the United States. This led to the promulgation of regulations requiring that researchers who seek funding from the National Institutes of Health (NIH) include women and minorities as participants. The regulations also require researchers to examine whether clinical interventions have differential effects (e.g., whether benefits are different for men than for women), although this provision has had limited adherence (Polit & Beck, 2009).

The fair treatment principle covers issues other than participant selection. The right to fair treatment means that researchers must treat people who decline to participate (or who withdraw from the study after initial agreement) in a nonprejudicial manner; that they must honor all agreements made with participants (including payment of any promised stipends); that they demonstrate respect for the beliefs, habits, and lifestyles of people from different backgrounds or cultures; that they give participants access to research staff for desired clarification; and that they afford participants courteous and tactful treatment at all times.

The Right to Privacy

Most research with humans involves intrusions into personal lives. Researchers should ensure that their research is not more intrusive than it needs to be and that participants' privacy is maintained continuously. Participants have the right to expect that their data will be kept in strictest confidence.

Privacy issues have become especially salient in the U.S. healthcare community since the passage of the Health Insurance Portability and Accountability Act of 1996 (HIPAA), which articulates federal standards to protect patients' health information. In response to the HIPAA legislation, the U.S. Department of Health and Human Services issued the regulations *Standards for Privacy of Individually Identifiable Health Information*. For most healthcare providers who transmit health information electronically, compliance with these regulations, known as the Privacy Rule, was required as of April 14, 2003.

___

➲ TIP: Some information relevant to HIPAA compliance is presented in this chapter, but you should confer with any organizations that are involved in the research (if they are covered entities) regarding their practices and policies relating to HIPAA provisions. Also, there are websites that provide extensive information about the implications of HIPAA for health research: *http://privacyruleandresearch.nih.gov/* and *www.hhs.gov/ocr/hipaa/guidelines/research.pdf.*

___

PROCEDURES FOR PROTECTING STUDY PARTICIPANTS

Now that you are familiar with fundamental ethical principles in research, you need to understand procedures that researchers use to adhere to them.

Risk/Benefit Assessments

One strategy that researchers can use to protect participants is to conduct a **risk-benefit assessment**. Such an assessment is designed to examine whether the benefits of participating in a study are in line with the costs, be they financial, physical, emotional, or social—that is, whether the *risk/benefit* ratio is acceptable. The assessment of risks and benefits that individual participants might experience should be shared with them so that they can evaluate whether it is in their best interest to participate. Box 7.1 summarizes major costs and benefits of research participation.

___

➲ TIP: The Toolkit in the accompanying *Resource Manual* includes a Word document with the factors in Box 7.1 arranged in worksheet form for you to complete in doing a risk/benefit assessment. By completing the worksheet, it may be easier for you to envision opportunities for "doing good" and to avoid possibilities of doing harm.

___

The risk/benefit ratio should also consider whether risks to participants are on a par with benefits to society and to nursing in terms of the evidence produced. A broad guideline is that the degree of risk by participants should never exceed the potential humanitarian benefits of the knowledge to be gained. Thus, the selection of a significant topic that has the potential to improve patient care is the first step in ensuring that research is ethical.

All research involves some risks, but risk is sometimes minimal. **Minimal risk** is defined as risks no greater than those ordinarily encountered in daily life or during routine tests or procedures. When the risks are not minimal, researchers must proceed with caution, taking every step possible to diminish risks and maximize benefits. If expected risks to participants outweigh the anticipated benefits of the study, the research should be redesigned.

In quantitative studies, most details of the study usually are spelled out in advance, so a reasonably accurate risk/benefit ratio assessment can be developed. Qualitative studies, however, usually evolve as data are gathered, so it may be more difficult to

BOX 7.1 Potential Benefits and Risks of Research to Participants

MAJOR POTENTIAL BENEFITS TO PARTICIPANTS

- Access to a potentially beneficial intervention that might otherwise be unavailable to them
- Comfort in being able to discuss their situation or problem with a friendly, objective person
- Increased knowledge about themselves or their conditions, either through opportunity for introspection and self-reflection or through direct interaction with researchers
- Escape from normal routine, excitement of being part of a study
- Satisfaction that information they provide may help others with similar problems or conditions
- Direct monetary or material gains through stipends or other incentives

MAJOR POTENTIAL RISKS TO PARTICIPANTS

- Physical harm, including unanticipated side effects
- Physical discomfort, fatigue, or boredom
- Psychological or emotional distress resulting from self-disclosure, introspection, fear of the unknown, discomfort with strangers, fear of eventual repercussions, anger or embarrassment at the type of questions being asked
- Social risks, such as the risk of stigma, adverse effects on personal relationships, loss of status
- Loss of privacy
- Loss of time
- Monetary costs (e.g., for transportation, child care, time lost from work)

assess all risks at the outset. Qualitative researchers must remain sensitive to potential risks throughout the study.

Example of ongoing risk/benefit assessment: Carlsson and colleagues (2007) discussed ethical issues relating to the conduct of interviews with people who have brain damage. The researchers noted the need for ongoing vigilance and attention to cues about risks and benefits. For example, one interview had to be interrupted because the participant displayed signs of distress. Afterward, however, the participant expressed gratitude for the opportunity to discuss his experience.

One potential benefit to participants is monetary. Stipends offered to prospective participants are rarely viewed as an opportunity for financial gain, but there is ample evidence that stipends are useful incentives to participant recruitment and retention (Edwards et al., 2009; Robinson et al., 2007). Financial incentives are especially effective when the group under study is difficult to recruit, when the

study is time-consuming or tedious, or when participants incur study-related costs (e.g., for child care or transportation). Stipends range from $1 to hundreds of dollars, but most are in the $20 to $30 range.

TIP: In evaluating the anticipated risk/benefit ratio of a study design, you might want to consider how comfortable *you* would feel about being a study participant.

Informed Consent and Participant Authorization

A particularly important procedure for safeguarding study participants involves obtaining their informed consent. **Informed consent** means that participants have adequate information about the research, comprehend that information, and have the ability to consent to or decline participation voluntarily. This section discusses procedures for obtaining informed consent and for complying with HIPAA rules regarding accessing patients' health information.

The Content of Informed Consent

Fully informed consent involves communicating the following pieces of information to participants:

1. *Participant status.* Prospective participants need to understand the distinction between *research* and *treatment.* They should be told which healthcare activities are routine and which are implemented specifically for the study. They also should be informed that data they provide will be used for research purposes.

2. *Study goals.* The overall goals of the research should be stated, in lay rather than technical terms. The use to which the data will be put should be described.

3. *Type of data.* Prospective participants should be told what type of data will be collected.

4. *Procedures.* Prospective participants should be given a description of the data collection procedures and of procedures to be used in any innovative treatment.

5. *Nature of the commitment.* Participants should be told the expected time commitment at each point of contact and the number of contacts within a given timeframe.

6. *Sponsorship.* Information on who is sponsoring or funding the study should be noted; if the research is part of an academic requirement, this information should be shared.

7. *Participant selection.* Prospective participants should be told how they were selected for recruitment and how many people will be participating.

8. *Potential risks.* Prospective participants should be informed of any foreseeable risks (physical, psychological, social, or economic) or discomforts and efforts that will be taken to minimize risks. The possibility of unforeseeable risks should also be discussed, if appropriate. If injury or damage is possible, treatments that will be made available to participants should be described. When risks are more than minimal,

prospective participants should be encouraged to seek advice before consenting.

9. *Potential benefits.* Specific benefits to participants, if any, should be described, as well as possible benefits to others.

10. *Alternatives.* If appropriate, participants should be told about alternative procedures or treatments that might be advantageous to them.

11. *Compensation.* If stipends or reimbursements are to be paid (or if treatments are offered without fee), these arrangements should be discussed.

12. *Confidentiality pledge.* Prospective participants should be assured that their privacy will at all times be protected. If anonymity can be guaranteed, this should be stated.

13. *Voluntary consent.* Researchers should indicate that participation is strictly voluntary and that failure to volunteer will not result in any penalty or loss of benefits.

14. *Right to withdraw and withhold information.* Prospective participants should be told that, after consenting, they have the right to withdraw from the study or to withhold any specific piece of information. Researchers may need to describe circumstances under which researchers would terminate the study.

15. *Contact information.* The researcher should tell participants whom they could contact in the event of further questions, comments, or complaints.

In qualitative studies, especially those requiring repeated contact with participants, it may be difficult to obtain meaningful informed consent at the outset. Qualitative researchers do not always know in advance how the study will evolve. Because the research design emerges during data collection, researchers may not know the exact nature of the data to be collected, what the risks and benefits to participants will be, or how much of a time commitment they will be expected to make. Thus, in a qualitative study, consent is often viewed as an ongoing, transactional process, sometimes called **process consent**. In process consent, the researcher continually renegotiates the consent, allowing participants to play a collaborative role in the decision-making process regarding ongoing participation.

> **Example of process consent:** Treacy and colleagues (2007) conducted a three-round longitudinal study of children's emerging perspectives and experiences of cigarette smoking. Parents and children consented to the children's participation. At each round, consent to continue participating in the study was reconfirmed.

Comprehension of Informed Consent

Consent information is normally presented to prospective participants while they are being recruited, either orally or in writing. Written notices should not, however, take the place of spoken explanations, which provide opportunities for elaboration and for participants to question and "screen" the researchers.

> **Example of "screening" of researchers:** Speraw (2009) did an in-depth study of adults and children with disabilities. Parental consent was obtained for child participants, and Speraw noted that:
>
> ". . . extensive discussion with parents took place via telephone. Additional conversations took place in the participants' homes prior to the interview. This period of rapport building was deemed essential, allowing parents ample opportunity to screen the researcher and make a determination of the suitability of the study for their child" (p. 736).

Because informed consent is based on a person's evaluation of the potential risks and benefits of participation, critical information must not only be communicated, but also understood. Researchers may have to play a "teacher" role in communicating consent information. They should be careful to use simple language and to avoid jargon and technical terms whenever possible; they should also avoid language that might unduly influence the person's decision to participate. Written statements should be consistent with the participants' reading levels and educational attainment. For participants from a general population (e.g., patients in a hospital), the statement should be written at about the 7th or 8th grade reading level.

> **TIP:** Yates and colleagues (2009) described an innovative visual presentation of informed consent information designed to improve communication and enhance participation rates.

For some studies, especially those involving more than minimal risk, researchers need to make special efforts to ensure that prospective participants understand what participation will entail. In some cases, this might involve testing participants for their comprehension of the informed consent material before deeming them eligible. Such efforts are especially warranted with participants whose native tongue is not English or who have cognitive impairments.

> **Example of confirming comprehension in informed consent:** Horgas and colleagues (2008) studied the relationship between pain and functional disability in older adults. Prospective participants had to demonstrate ability to provide informed consent:
>
> "Ability to consent was ascertained by explaining the study to potential participants, who were then asked to describe the study" (p. 344). All written materials for the study, including consent forms, were at the 8th-grade reading level and printed in 14-point font.

Documentation of Informed Consent

Researchers usually document informed consent by having participants sign a **consent form**. In the United States, federal regulations for studies funded by the government require written consent of participants, except under certain circumstances. When the study does not involve an intervention and data are collected anonymously—or when existing data from records or specimens are used and identifying information is not linked to the data—regulations requiring written informed consent do not apply. HIPAA legislation is explicit about the type of information that must be eliminated from patient records for the data to be considered **de-identified**.

The consent form should contain all the information essential to informed consent. Prospective participants (or a legally authorized representative) should have ample time to review the document before signing it. The consent form should also be signed by the researcher, and a copy should be retained by both parties.

An example of a written consent form used in a study of one of the authors is presented in Figure 7.1. The numbers in the margins of this figure correspond to the types of information for informed consent outlined earlier. (The form does not indicate how people were selected; prospective participants knew they were recruited from a particular support group.)

TIP: In developing a consent form, the following suggestions might prove helpful:

1. Organize the form coherently so that prospective participants can follow the logic of what is being communicated. If the form is complex, use headings as an organizational aid.
2. Use a large enough font so that the form can be easily read, and use spacing that avoids making the document appear too dense. Make the form attractive and inviting.
3. In general, simplify. Use clear, consistent terminology. Avoid technical terms if possible. If technical terms are needed, include definitions. Some suggestions are offered in the Toolkit.
4. Assess the form's reading level by using a **readability formula** to ensure an appropriate level for the group under study. There are several such formulas, the most widely used being the FOG Index (Gunning, 1968), the Flesch Reading Ease score, and Flesch-Kincaid grade level score (Flesch, 1948). Microsoft Word provides Flesch readability statistics.
   - In Word 2003, click Tools → Options → Spelling and Grammar → Show Readability Statistics.
   - In Word 2007, click the Microsoft Office button (upper left corner) → Word Options → Proofing → Check Grammar with Spelling + Show Readability Statistics.
   - In Word 2010, click the blue Office button (upper left corner) → Options → Proofing → Check Grammar with Spelling + Show Readability Statistics.
5. Test the form with people similar to those who will be recruited, and ask for feedback.

In certain circumstances (e.g., with non–English-speaking participants), researchers with NIH funding have the option of presenting the full information orally and then summarizing essential information in a **short form**. If a short form is used, however, the oral presentation must be witnessed by a third party, and the witness's signature must appear on the short consent form. The signature of a third-party witness is also advisable in studies involving more than minimal risk, even when a comprehensive consent form is used.

When the primary means of data collection is through a self-administered questionnaire, some researchers do not obtain written informed consent because they assume **implied consent** (i.e., that the return of the completed questionnaire reflects voluntary consent to participate). This assumption, however, may not always be warranted (e.g., if patients feel that their treatment might be affected by failure to cooperate with the researcher).

TIP: The Toolkit in the accompanying *Resource Manual* includes several informed consent forms as Word documents that can be adapted for your use. (Many universities offer templates for consent forms.) The Toolkit also includes several other resources designed to help you with the ethical aspects of a study.

Authorization to Access Private Health Information

Under HIPAA regulations in the United States, a covered entity such as a hospital can disclose individually identifiable health information (IIHI) from its records if the patient signs an authorization. The authorization can be incorporated into the consent form, or it can be a separate document. Using a separate authorization form may be advantageous to protect the patients' confidentiality because the form does not need to provide detailed information about the purpose of the research. If the research purpose is not sensitive, or if the hospital or entity is already cognizant of the study purpose, an integrated authorization and consent form may suffice.

The authorization, whether obtained separately or as part of the consent form, must include the following: (1) who will receive the information, (2) what type of information will be disclosed, and (3) what further disclosures the researcher

Informed Consent Form

1 2 3,5 4 12 11 8	I understand that I am being asked to participate in a research study at Saint Francis Hospital and Medical Center. This research study will evaluate: What it is like being a mother of multiples during the first year of the infants' lives. If I agree to participate in the study, I will be interviewed for approximately 30 to 60 minutes about my experience as a mother of multiple infants. The interview will be tape-recorded and take place in a private office at Saint Francis Hospital. No identifying information will be included when the interview is transcribed. I understand I will receive $25.00 for participating in the study. There are no known risks associated with this study.
7	I realize that I may not participate in the study if I am younger than 18 years of age or I cannot speak English.
10	I realize that the knowledge gained from this study may help either me or other mothers of multiple infants in the future.
13 14	I realize that my participation in this study is entirely voluntary, and I may withdraw from the study at any time I wish. If I decide to discontinue my participation in this study, I will continue to be treated in the usual and customary fashion.
12	I understand that all study data will be kept confidential. However, this information may be used in nursing publications or presentations.
8	I understand that if I sustain injuries from my participation in this research project, I will not be automatically compensated by Saint Francis Hospital and Medical Center.
15	If I need to, I can contact Dr. Cheryl Beck, University of Connecticut, School of Nursing, any time during the study.
1,2	The study has been explained to me. I have read and understand this consent form, all of my questions have been answered, and I agree to participate. I understand that I will be given a copy of this signed consent form.

_____   _____
Signature of Participant   Date

_____   _____
Signature of Witness   Date

_____   _____
Signature of Investigator   Date

FIGURE 7.1 Example of an informed consent form.

anticipates. The need for patient authorization to access IIHI can be waived only under certain circumstances. Patient authorization usually must be obtained for data that are *created* as part of the research, as well as for information already maintained in institutional records (Olsen, 2003).

Confidentiality Procedures

Study participants have the right to expect that data they provide will be kept in strict confidence. Participants' right to privacy is protected through various confidentiality procedures.

Anonymity

Anonymity, the most secure means of protecting confidentiality, occurs when the researcher cannot link participants to their data. For example, if questionnaires were distributed to a group of nursing home residents and were returned without any identifying information, responses would be anonymous. As another example, if a researcher reviewed hospital records from which all identifying information (e.g., name, social security number, and so on) had been expunged, anonymity would again protect participants' right to privacy. Whenever it is possible to achieve anonymity, researchers should strive to do so. Distributed questionnaires through the mail, to groups of participants, or over the Internet are especially conducive to anonymity.

Example of anonymity: Wagner and colleagues (2009) distributed anonymous questionnaires to members of gerontological nursing organizations in the United States and Canada. The questionnaires elicited nurses' perceptions of workplace safety culture in long-term care settings.

Confidentiality in the Absence of Anonymity

When anonymity is impossible, confidentiality procedures need to be implemented. A promise of **confidentiality** is a pledge that any information participants provide will not be publicly reported in a manner that identifies them, and will not be accessible to others. This means that research information should not be shared with strangers nor with people known to participants (e.g., relatives, doctors, other nurses), unless participants give explicit permission to do so.

Researchers can take a number of steps to ensure that a *breach of confidentiality* does not occur, including the following:

- Obtain identifying information (e.g., name, address) from participants only when essential.
- Assign an **identification** (ID) **number** to each participant and attach the ID number rather than other identifiers to the actual data.
- Maintain identifying information in a locked file.
- Restrict access to identifying information to only a few people on a need-to-know basis.
- Enter no identifying information onto computer files.
- Destroy identifying information as quickly as practical.
- Make research personnel sign confidentiality pledges if they have access to data or identifying information. ✪
- Report research information in the aggregate; if information for an individual is reported, disguise the person's identity, such as through the use of a fictitious name.

⊃ T I P : Researchers who plan to collect data from participants multiple times (or who use multiple forms that need to be linked) do not have to forego anonymity. A technique that has been successful is to have participants themselves generate an ID number. They might be instructed, for example, to use their birth year and the first three letters of their mother's maiden names as their ID code (e.g., 1946CRU). This code would be put on every form so that forms could be linked, but researchers would not know participants' identities.

Qualitative researchers may need to take extra steps to safeguard participants' privacy. Anonymity is almost never possible in qualitative studies because researchers typically become closely involved with participants. Moreover, because of the in-depth nature of qualitative studies, there may be a greater invasion of privacy than is true in quantitative research. Researchers who spend time in the home of a participant may, for example, have difficulty segregating the public behaviors that the participant is willing to share from private behaviors that unfold during data collection. A final issue is adequately disguising participants in reports. Because the number of participants is small, qualitative researchers may need to take extra precautions to safeguard identities. This may mean more than simply using a fictitious name. Qualitative researchers may have to slightly distort identifying information, or provide only general descriptions. For example, a 49-year-old antique dealer with ovarian cancer might be described as "a middle-aged cancer patient who worked in retail sales" to avoid identification that could occur with the more detailed description.

> **Example of confidentiality procedures in a qualitative study:** Graffigna and Olson (2009) studied how young people talk about HIV/AIDS in a group interview. Potential participants were assured of confidentiality and the voluntary nature of participation. Participants signed consent forms in the presence of researchers so that questions could be addressed. Names and identifying information were removed from data and stored separately in the researchers' office. Transcripts of the group discussion were analyzed anonymously.

Certificates of Confidentiality

There are situations in which confidentiality can create tensions between researchers and legal or other authorities, especially if participants are involved in criminal or dangerous activity (e.g., substance abuse, unprotected sexual intercourse). To avoid the possibility of forced, involuntary disclosure of sensitive research information (e.g., through a court order or subpoena), researchers in the United States can apply for a **Certificate of Confidentiality** from the National Institutes of Health (Lutz et al., 2000). Any research that involves the collection of personally identifiable, sensitive information is potentially eligible for a Certificate, even if the study is not federally funded. Information is considered sensitive if its release might damage participants' financial standing, employability, or reputation or might lead to discrimination; information about a person's mental health, as well as genetic information, is also considered sensitive.

A Certificate of Confidentiality protects against the forced disclosure of research data in a wide range of situations. A Certificate allows researchers to refuse to disclose identifying information on study participants in any civil, criminal, administrative, or legislative proceeding at the federal, state, or local level.

A Certificate of Confidentiality helps researchers to achieve their research objectives without threat of involuntary disclosure and can be helpful in recruiting participants. Researchers who obtain a Certificate should alert prospective participants about this valuable protection in the consent form, and should note any planned exceptions to those protections. For example, a researcher might decide to voluntarily comply with state child abuse reporting laws even though the Certificate would prevent authorities from punishing researchers who chose not to comply.

> **Example of obtaining a Certificate of Confidentiality:** Laughon (2007) conducted an in-depth study of the ways in which poor, urban African American women with a history of physical abuse stay healthy. Interviews covered a range of sensitive topics (domestic violence, substance abuse), so the researcher obtained a Certificate of Confidentiality.

Debriefings, Communications, and Referrals

Researchers can often show their respect for participants—and proactively minimize emotional risks—by carefully attending to the nature of the interactions· they have with them. For example, researchers should always be gracious and polite, should phrase questions tactfully, and should be sensitive to cultural and linguistic diversity.

Researchers can also use more formal strategies to communicate respect and concern for participants' well-being. For example, it is sometimes useful to offer **debriefing** sessions after data collection is completed to permit participants to ask questions or air complaints. Debriefing is especially important when the data collection has been stressful or when ethical guidelines had to be "bent" (e.g., if any deception was used in explaining the study).

Example of debriefing: Sandgren and colleagues (2006) studied strategies that palliative cancer nurses used to avoid being emotionally overloaded. After each in-depth interview with 46 nurses,

"... we made sure that the participants were doing well, and we assessed possible needs for emotional support" (p. 81).

It is also thoughtful to communicate with participants after the study is completed to let them know that their participation was appreciated. Researchers sometimes demonstrate their interest in study participants by offering to share study findings with them once the data have been analyzed (e.g., by mailing them a summary or advising them of an appropriate website).

Example of thanking participants: Hsiao and Van Riper (2009) studied individual and family adaptation in Taiwanese families with relatives who had severe and persistent mental illness. At the end of the study, each participant was sent a thank you card to convey gratitude for their time.

Finally, in some situations, researchers may need to assist study participants by making referrals to appropriate health, social, or psychological services.

Example of referrals: Caldwell and Redeker (2009) studied psychological distress in women living in inner cities. All participants were offered the opportunity to obtain counseling at a local health center. Women whose psychological distress scores were moderate were referred to the health center. Those whose scores were severe were escorted to the psychiatric emergency room where they were immediately evaluated by a clinician.

Treatment of Vulnerable Groups

Adherence to ethical standards is often straightforward, but additional procedures and heightened sensitivity may be required to protect the rights of special vulnerable groups. **Vulnerable populations** may be incapable of giving fully informed consent (e.g., mentally retarded people) or may be at risk of unintended side effects because of their circumstances (e.g., pregnant women). Researchers interested in studying high-risk groups should understand guidelines governing informed consent, risk/benefit assessments, and acceptable research

procedures for such groups. In general, research with vulnerable groups should be undertaken only when the risk/benefit ratio is low or when there is no alternative (e.g., studies of childhood development require child participants).

Among the groups that nurse researchers should consider vulnerable are the following:

- *Children.* Legally and ethically, children do not have competence to give informed consent, so the informed consent of children's parents or legal guardians must be obtained. It is appropriate, however—especially if the child is at least 7 years old—to obtain the child's assent as well. **Assent** refers to the child's affirmative agreement to participate. If the child is mature enough (e.g., a 12-year-old) to understand basic informed consent information, it is advisable to obtain written assent from the child as well, as evidence of respect for the child's right to self-determination. Lindeke and colleagues (2000) and Kanner and colleagues (2004) provided guidance on children's assent and consent to participate in research. The U.S. government has issued special regulations (Subpart D of the Code of Federal Regulations, 2005) for the additional protection of children as study participants.
- *Mentally or emotionally disabled people.* Individuals whose disability makes it impossible for them to weigh the risks and benefits of participation (e.g., people affected by cognitive impairment, coma, and so on) also cannot legally or ethically provide informed consent. In such cases, researchers should obtain the written consent of a legal guardian. To the extent possible, informed consent or assent from participants themselves should be sought as a supplement to consent by a guardian. NIH guidelines note that studies involving people whose autonomy is compromised by disability should focus in a direct way on their condition.
- *Severely ill or physically disabled people.* For patients who are very ill or undergoing certain treatments, it might be necessary to assess their ability to make reasoned decisions about study participation. For example, Higgins and Daly

(1999) described a process they used to assess decisional capacity in mechanically ventilated patients. For certain disabilities, special procedures for obtaining consent may be required. For example, with deaf participants, the entire consent process may need to be in writing. For people who have a physical impairment preventing them from writing or for participants who cannot read and write, alternative procedures for documenting informed consent (such as audiotaping or videotaping consent proceedings) should be used.

- *The terminally ill.* Terminally ill people who participate in studies seldom expect to benefit personally from the research, so the risk/benefit ratio needs to be carefully assessed. Researchers must also take steps to ensure that the healthcare and comfort of terminally ill participants are not compromised. Special procedures may be needed to obtain informed consent if they are physically or mentally incapacitated.

- *Institutionalized people.* Particular care is required in recruiting institutionalized people because they depend on healthcare personnel and may feel pressured into participating, or may believe that their treatment would be jeopardized by failure to cooperate. Inmates of prisons and other correctional facilities, who have lost their autonomy in many spheres of activity, may similarly feel constrained in their ability to withhold consent. The U.S. government has issued specific regulations for the protection of prisoners as study participants (see Code of Federal Regulations, 2005, Subpart C). Researchers studying institutionalized groups need to emphasize the voluntary nature of participation.

- *Pregnant women.* The U.S. government has issued additional requirements governing research with pregnant women and fetuses (Code of Federal Regulations, 2005, Subpart B). These requirements reflect a desire to safeguard both the pregnant woman, who may be at heightened physical and psychological risk, and the fetus, who cannot give informed consent. The regulations stipulate that a pregnant woman cannot be involved in a study unless its purpose is to meet the health needs of the pregnant woman, and risks to her and the fetus are minimized or there is only a minimal risk to the fetus.

Example of research with a vulnerable group: Kelly and colleagues (2009) studied dating violence among girls (average age of 15) in the juvenile justice system who were participating in a health promotion program in Bexar County, Texas. The authors noted that because of the high prevalence of violence and neglect in this population, the ethics review committee of Kelly's university waived obtaining parental consent as being a source of potential harm. Girls were assured in person that participation was voluntary and that lack of participation would not affect their detention or probation status.

It should go without saying that researchers need to proceed with great caution in conducting research with people who might fall into two or more vulnerable categories, as was the case in the preceding example.

➲ **TIP:** Jacobson (2005) has astutely pointed out the need to be vigilant on behalf of persons not traditionally identified as vulnerable and, therefore, not covered in standard protocols regarding vulnerable participants. *Anybody* may be vulnerable at any given time due to acute illness or special circumstances that challenge the capacity to provide truly informed consent.

External Reviews and the Protection of Human Rights

Researchers, who often have a strong commitment to their research, may not be objective in their risk/benefit assessments or in their efforts to protect participants' rights. Because of the possibility of a biased self-evaluation, the ethical dimensions of a study should normally be subjected to external review.

Most institutions where research is conducted have formal committees for reviewing proposed research plans. These committees are sometimes called *human subjects committees*, *ethical advisory boards*, or *research ethics committees*. In the United States, the committee likely will be called an **Institutional Review Board (IRB)**, whereas in Canada it is called a **Research Ethics Board (REB)**.

➲ **T I P :** You should find out early what an institution's require-ments are regarding ethics, in terms of its forms, procedures, and review schedules. Also, it is wise to allow a generous amount of time for negotiating with IRBs, which may require procedural modifications and re-review.

Qualitative researchers in various countries have expressed some concerns that standard ethical review procedures are not sensitive to special issues and cir-cumstances faced in qualitative research. There is concern that regulations were " . . . created for quanti-tative work, and can actually impede or interrupt work that is not hypothesis-driven 'hard science'" (Van de Hoonaard, 2002, p. i). Thus, qualitative researchers may need to take extra care to explain their methods, rationales, and approaches to review board members unfamiliar with qualitative research.

Institutional Review Boards

In the United States, federally sponsored studies are subject to strict guidelines for evaluating the treatment of human participants. (Guidance on human subjects issues in grant applications is pro-vided in Chapter 29.) Before undertaking such a study, researchers must submit research plans to the IRB, and must also go through formal training on ethical conduct and a certification process that can be completed online.

The duty of the IRB is to ensure that the pro-posed plans meet federal requirements for ethical research. An IRB can approve the proposed plans, require modifications, or disapprove the plans. The main requirements governing IRB decisions may be summarized as follows (Code of Federal Regu-lations, 2005, §46.111):

- Risks to participants are minimized.
- Risks to participants are reasonable in relation to anticipated benefits, if any, and the impor-tance of the knowledge that may reasonably be expected to result.
- Selection of participants is equitable.
- Informed consent will be sought, as required, and appropriately documented.
- Adequate provision is made for monitoring the research to ensure participants' safety.

- Appropriate provisions are made to protect par-ticipants' privacy and confidentiality of the data.
- When vulnerable groups are involved, appro-priate additional safeguards are included to pro-tect their rights and welfare.

Example of IRB approval: Jones and her colleagues (2010) studied the meaning of surviving cancer among Latino adolescents and young adults. The procedures and protocols for the study were approved by the IRBs of two cancer clinics where the study was conducted.

Many studies require a full IRB review involv-ing a meeting at which a majority of IRB members are present. An IRB must have five or more mem-bers, at least one of whom is not a researcher (e.g., a member of the clergy or a lawyer may be appro-priate). One IRB member must be a person who is not affiliated with the institution and is not a family member of an affiliated person. To protect against potential biases, the IRB cannot comprise entirely men, women, or members from a single profession.

For certain research involving no more than minimal risk, the IRB can use expedited review procedures, which do not require a meeting. In an **expedited review**, a single IRB member (usually the IRB chairperson) carries out the review. An example of research that qualifies for an expedited IRB review is minimal-risk research ". . . employ-ing survey, interview, focus group, program evalua-tion, human factors evaluation, or quality assurance methodologies" (Code of Federal Regulations, 2005, §46.110).

Federal regulations also allow certain types of research in which there are no apparent risk to par-ticipants to be exempt from IRB review. The web-site of the Office of Human Research Protections, in its policy guidance section, includes decision charts designed to clarify whether a study is exempt.

➲ **T I P :** Researchers seeking a Certificate of Confidentiality must first obtain IRB approval because such approval is a prerequisite for the Certificate. Applications for the Certificate should be submitted at least 3 months before participants are expected to enroll in the study.

Data and Safety Monitoring Boards

In addition to IRBs, researchers in the United States may have to communicate information about ethical aspects of their studies to other groups. For example, some institutions have established separate **Privacy Boards** to review researchers' compliance with provisions in HIPAA, including review of authorization forms and requests for waivers.

For researchers evaluating interventions in clinical trials, NIH also requires review by a **data and safety monitoring board** (DSMB). The purpose of a DSMB is to oversee the safety of participants, to promote data integrity, and to review accumulated outcome data on a regular basis to determine whether study protocols should be altered, or the study stopped altogether. Members of a DSMB are selected based on their clinical, statistical, and methodologic expertise. The degree of monitoring by the DSMB should be proportionate to the degree of risk involved.

Example of a Data and Safety Monitoring Board: Artinian and colleagues (2007) tested the effectiveness of a nurse-managed telemonitoring intervention for lowering blood pressure among hypertensive African Americans. In a separate article, the researchers presented a good description of their data and safety monitoring plan and discussed how IRBs and DSMBs differ (Artinian et al., 2004).

Building Ethics into the Design of the Study

Researchers need to give careful thought to ethical requirements while planning a study, and should ask themselves whether intended safeguards for protecting humans are sufficient. They must continue their vigilance throughout the course of the study as well, because unforeseen ethical dilemmas may arise. Of course, first steps in doing ethical research include scrutinizing the research question to determine if it is clinically significant and designing the study in a manner that yields sound evidence—it can be construed as unethical to do poorly conceived or weakly designed research because it would be a poor use of people's time.

The remaining chapters of the book offer advice on how to design studies that yield high-quality

evidence for practice. Methodologic decisions about rigor, however, must be made within the context of ethical requirements. Box 7.2 presents some examples of the kinds of questions that might be posed in thinking about ethical aspects of study design.

➔ **TIP:** After study procedures have been developed, researchers should undertake a self-evaluation of those procedures to determine if they meet ethical requirements. Box 7.3, later in this chapter, provides some guidelines that can be used for such a self-evaluation.

OTHER ETHICAL ISSUES

In discussing ethical issues relating to the conduct of nursing research, we have given primary consideration to the protection of human participants. Two other ethical issues also deserve mention: the treatment of animals in research and research misconduct.

Ethical Issues in Using Animals in Research

Some nurse researchers use animals rather than human beings as their subjects, typically focusing on biophysiologic phenomena. Despite some opposition to such research by animal rights activists, researchers in health fields likely will continue to use animals to explore physiologic mechanisms and to test interventions that could pose risks to humans.

Ethical considerations are clearly different for animals and humans; for example, the concept of *informed consent* is not relevant for animal subjects. Guidelines have been developed governing treatment of animals in research. In the United States, the Public Health Service issued a policy statement on the humane care and use of animals, most recently amended in 2002. The guidelines articulate nine principles for the proper treatment of animals used in

BOX 7.2 Examples of Questions for Building Ethics into a Study Design

RESEARCH DESIGN

- Will participants get allocated fairly to different treatment groups?
- Will steps to reduce bias or enhance integrity add to the risks participants will incur?
- Will the setting for the study protect against participant discomfort?

INTERVENTION

- Is the intervention designed to maximize good and minimize harm?
- Under what conditions might a treatment be withdrawn or altered?

SAMPLE

- Is the population defined so as to unwittingly and unnecessarily exclude important segments of people (e.g., women or minorities)?
- Will potential participants be recruited into the study equitably?

DATA COLLECTION

- Will data be collected in such a way as to minimize respondent burden?
- Will procedures for ensuring confidentiality of data be adequate?
- Will data collection staff be appropriately trained to be sensitive and courteous?

REPORTING

- Will participants' identities be adequately protected?

biomedical and behavioral research. These principles cover such issues as the transport of research animals, alternatives to using animals, pain and distress in animal subjects, researcher qualifications, the use of appropriate anesthesia, and euthanizing animals under certain conditions. In Canada, researchers who use animals in their studies must adhere to the policies and guidelines of the Canadian Council on Animal Care (CCAC) as articulated in the two-volume *Guide to the Care and Use of Experimental Animals.*

Holtzclaw and Hanneman (2002) noted several important considerations in the use of animals in nursing research. First, there must be a compelling reason to use an animal model—not simply convenience or novelty. Second, study procedures should be humane, well planned, and well funded. Animal studies are not necessarily less costly than those with human participants, and they require serious ethical and scientific consideration to justify their use.

Example of research with animals: Raines and other nurse anesthetists (2009) studied the anxiolytic effects of luteolin, a lemon balm flavenoid, in male Sprague-Dawley rats. In all, 55 rats were used in the study. Protocols for the use of the rats were in accordance with NIH's Guide for the Care and Use of Laboratory Animals and they received approval from an Institutional Animal Care and Use Committee.

Research Misconduct

Ethics in research involves not only the protection of human and animal subjects, but also protection of the public trust. The issue of **research misconduct** (or *scientific misconduct*) has received greater attention in recent years as incidents of researcher fraud and misrepresentation have come to light. Currently, the U.S. agency responsible for overseeing efforts to improve research integrity and for handling allegations of research misconduct is the Office of Research Integrity (ORI) within DHHS. Researchers seeking funding from NIH must demonstrate that they have received training on research integrity and the responsible conduct of research.

Research misconduct, as defined by a 2005 U.S. Public Health Service regulation (42 CFR Part 93), is "fabrication, falsification, or plagiarism in proposing, performing, or reviewing research, or in reporting research results." To be construed as misconduct, there must be a significant departure from accepted practices in the research community, and the misconduct must have been committed intentionally, knowingly, or recklessly. *Fabrication* involves making up data or study results. *Falsification* involves manipulating research materials, equipment, or processes; it also involves changing or omitting data, or distorting results such that the research is not accurately represented in reports. *Plagiarism* involves the appropriation of someone's ideas, results, or words without giving due credit, including information obtained through the confidential review of research proposals or manuscripts.

Although the official definition focuses on only three types of misconduct, there is widespread agreement that research misconduct covers many other issues including improprieties of authorship, poor data management, conflicts of interest, inappropriate financial arrangements, failure to comply with governmental regulations, and unauthorized use of confidential information. Conflicts of interest may be a particularly salient issue in health-related research funded by for-profit organizations.

Example of research misconduct: In 2008, the U.S. Office of Research Integrity ruled that a nurse in Missouri engaged in scientific misconduct in research supported by the National Cancer Institute. The nurse falsified and fabricated data that were reported to the National Surgical Adjuvant Breast and Bowel Project (NIH Notice Number NOT-OD-08-096).

Research integrity is an important concern in nursing. Jeffers and Whittemore (2005), for example, engaged in work to identify and describe research environments that promote integrity. In a study that focused on ethical issues faced by editors of nursing journals, Freda and Kearney (2005) found that 64% of the 88 editors reported some type of ethical dilemma, such as duplicate publication, plagiarism, or conflicts of interest. Editors in several major nursing journals subsequently wrote editorials about this topic (e.g., Baggs, 2008; Broome, 2008). Habermann and colleagues (2010) studied 1,645 research coordinators' experiences with research misconduct in their clinical environments. More than 250 coordinators, most of them nurses, said they had first-hand knowledge of scientific misconduct that included protocol violations, consent violations, fabrication, falsification, and financial conflicts of interest.

Example of research on research integrity: In 2005, Gwen Anderson was awarded a grant through NINR under its Research on Research Integrity initiative. Her study explored common daily practices and systems in gene therapy clinical research, and sought to describe institutional cultures that promote or protect research integrity—as well as those that do not. In another study, Dr. Anderson (2008) examined the ethical preparedness and performance of gene therapy study coordinators.

CRITIQUING THE ETHICS OF RESEARCH STUDIES

Guidelines for critiquing ethical aspects of a study are presented in Box 7.3. Members of an ethics committee should be provided with sufficient information to answer all these questions. Research journal articles, however, do not always include detailed information about ethics because of space constraints. Thus, it is not always possible to critique researchers' adherence to ethical guidelines, but we offer a few suggestions for considering a study's ethical aspects.

Many research reports acknowledge that study procedures were reviewed by an IRB or ethics committee. When a report specifically mentions a formal review, it is usually safe to assume that a group of concerned people did a conscientious review of the study's ethical issues.

BOX 7.3 Guidelines for Critiquing the Ethical Aspects of a Study

1. Was the study approved and monitored by an Institutional Review Board, Research Ethics Board, or other similar ethics review committee?
2. Were participants subjected to any physical harm, discomfort, or psychological distress? Did the researchers take appropriate steps to remove, prevent, or minimize harm?
3. Did the benefits to participants outweigh any potential risks or actual discomfort they experienced? Did the benefits to society outweigh the costs to participants?
4. Was any type of coercion or undue influence used to recruit participants? Did they have the right to refuse to participate or to withdraw without penalty?
5. Were participants deceived in any way? Were they fully aware of participating in a study and did they understand the purpose and nature of the research?
6. Were appropriate informed consent procedures used? If not, were there valid and justifiable reasons?
7. Were adequate steps taken to safeguard participants' privacy? How was confidentiality maintained? Were Privacy Rule procedures followed (if applicable)? Was a Certificate of Confidentiality obtained? If not, *should* one have been obtained?
8. Were vulnerable groups involved in the research? If yes, were special precautions used because of their vulnerable status?
9. Were groups omitted from the inquiry without a justifiable rationale, such as women (or men), minorities, or older people?

You can also come to some conclusions based on a description of the study methods. There may be sufficient information to judge, for example, whether study participants were subjected to physical or psychological harm or discomfort. Reports do not always specifically state whether informed consent was secured, but you should be alert to situations in which the data could not have been gathered as described if participation were purely voluntary (e.g., if data were gathered unobtrusively).

In thinking about ethical issues, you should also consider who the study participants were. For example, if a study involved vulnerable groups, there should be more information about protective procedures. You might also need to attend to who the study participants were *not*. For example, there has been considerable concern about the omission of certain groups (e.g., minorities) from clinical research.

It is often difficult to determine whether the participants' privacy was safeguarded unless the researcher mentions pledges of confidentiality or anonymity. A situation requiring special scrutiny arises when data are collected from two people simultaneously (e.g., a husband and wife who are jointly interviewed); in

such situations, the absence of privacy raises not only ethical concerns, but also questions regarding participants' candor. As noted by Forbat and Henderson (2003), ethical issues arise when two people in an intimate relationship are interviewed about a common issue, even when they are interviewed privately. They described the potential for being "stuck in the middle" when trying to get two sides of a story, and facing the dilemma of how to ask one person probing questions after having been given confidential information about the topic by the other.

RESEARCH EXAMPLES

Two research examples that highlight ethical issues are presented in the following sections.

Research Example from a Quantitative Study

Study: Health status in an invisible population: Carnival and migrant worker children (Kilanowski & Ryan-Wenger, 2007).

Study Purpose: The purpose of the study was to examine the health status of children of itinerant carnival workers and migrant farm workers in the United States.

Research Methods: A total of 97 boys and girls younger than 13 years were recruited into the study. All children received an oral health screening and were measured for height and weight. Parents completed questionnaires about their children's health and healthcare, and most brought health records from which information about immunizations was obtained.

Ethics-Related Procedures: The families were recruited through the cooperation of gatekeepers at farms and carnival communities in 7 states. Parents were asked to complete informed consent forms, which were available in both English and Spanish. Children who were older than 9 were also asked whether they would like to participate, and gave verbal assent. Confidentiality was a concern to both the families and the gatekeepers. The researchers needed to assure all parties that the data would be confidential and not used against families or facilities. Data were gathered in locations and time periods that had been suggested by the carnival managers and farm owners so that parents did not need to forfeit work hours to participate in the study. Migrant farm workers were often eager to participate, and often waited in line to sign the consent forms. At the conclusion of the encounter, the researchers gave the parents a written report of the children's growth parameters and recommendations for follow-up. In appreciation of the parents' time, $10 was given to the parents, and the child was given an age-appropriate nonviolent toy (worth about $10) of their choice. Children were also given a new toothbrush. The IRB of the Ohio State University approved this study.

Key Findings: Carnival children were less likely than migrant children to have regularly scheduled well-child examinations and to have seen a dentist in the previous year. Among children ages 6 to 11, the itinerant children in both groups were substantially more likely to be overweight than same-aged children nationally.

Research Example from a Qualitative Study

Study: Storying childhood sexual abuse (Draucker & Martsolf, 2008).

Study Purpose: The purpose of the study was to describe and explain how individuals disclose their experience of childhood sexual abuse.

Study Methods: Drauker and Martsolf used grounded theory methods to develop a framework explaining how survivors of childhood sexual abuse tell others about their abuse experiences. The study data were from open-ended interviews with 74 individuals (40 women and 34 men) who had experienced ongoing sexual abuse by a family member or close acquaintance. The interviews were audiotaped for subsequent analysis.

Ethics-Related Procedures: Prospective participants were screened before enrollment in the study to ensure that they were not experiencing psychiatric distress or current abuse that would make participation risky. Informed consent was obtained from individuals who passed the screening. Participants were paid $35 for their time and travel expenses. Emergency mental health referral procedures were developed in case a participant experienced acute distress during the interview. No one required an emergency referral, but several people requested information about counseling resources. The researchers obtained IRB approval from their university prior to data collection. A Certificate of Confidentiality was obtained to ensure participants' privacy.

Key Findings: The psychological problem faced by participants was that childhood sexual abuse both demands and defies explanation. The core psychological process used in response to this problem was called "storying childhood sexual abuse." Processes included: (1) starting the story: the story-not-yet-told; (2) coming out with the story: the story-first-told; (3) shielding the story: the story-as-secret; (4) revising the story: the story-as-account; and (5) sharing the story: the story-as-message.

SUMMARY POINTS

- Because research has not always been conducted ethically and because researchers face **ethical dilemmas** in designing studies that are both ethical and rigorous, **codes of ethics** have been developed to guide researchers.
- Three major ethical principles from the *Belmont Report* are incorporated into most guidelines: beneficence, respect for human dignity, and justice.
- **Beneficence** involves the performance of some good and the protection of participants from

physical and psychological harm and exploitation (*nonmaleficence*).

- **Respect for human dignity** involves participants' **right to self-determination,** which means they have the freedom to control their own actions, including voluntary participation.

- **Full disclosure** means that researchers have fully divulged participants' rights and the risks and benefits of the study. When full disclosure could yield biased results, researchers sometimes use **covert data collection** or **concealment** (the collection of information without the participants' knowledge or consent) or **deception** (either withholding information from participants or providing false information).

- **Justice** includes the **right to fair treatment** and the **right to privacy.** In the United States, privacy has become a major issue because of the Privacy Rule regulations that resulted from the Health Insurance Portability and Accountability Act (HIPAA).

- Various procedures have been developed to safeguard study participants rights, including risk/benefit assessments, informed consent procedures, and confidentiality procedures.

- In a **risk/benefit assessment,** the potential benefits of the study to participants and to society are weighed against the costs to individuals.

- **Informed consent** procedures, which provide prospective participants with information needed to make a reasoned decision about participation, normally involve signing a **consent form** to document voluntary and informed participation.

- In qualitative studies, consent may need to be continually renegotiated with participants as the study evolves, through **process consent** procedures.

- Privacy can be maintained through **anonymity** (wherein not even researchers know participants' identities) or through formal **confidentiality procedures** that safeguard the information participants provide.

- U.S. researchers can seek a **Certificate of Confidentiality** that protects them against the forced disclosure of confidential information through a court order or other legal or administrative process.

- Researchers sometimes offer **debriefing** sessions after data collection to provide participants with more information or an opportunity to air complaints.

- **Vulnerable groups** require additional protection. These people may be vulnerable because they are unable to make a truly informed decision about study participation (e.g., children), because of diminished autonomy (e.g., prisoners), or because circumstances heighten the risk of physical or psychological harm (e.g., pregnant women).

- External review of the ethical aspects of a study by an ethics committee, Research Ethics Board (REB), or **Institutional Review Board (IRB)** is highly desirable and may be required by either the agency funding the research or the organization from which participants are recruited.

- In studies in which risks to participants are minimal, an **expedited review** (review by a single member of the IRB) may be substituted for a full board review; in cases in which there are no anticipated risks, the research may be exempted from review.

- Researchers need to give careful thought to ethical requirements throughout the study's planning and implementation and to ask themselves continually whether safeguards for protecting humans are sufficient.

- Ethical conduct in research involves not only protection of the rights of human and animal subjects, but also efforts to maintain high standards of integrity and avoid such forms of **research misconduct** as *plagiarism, fabrication* of results, or *falsification* of data.

STUDY ACTIVITIES

Chapter 7 of the *Resource Manual for Nursing Research: Generating and Assessing Evidence for Nursing Practice, 9th ed.,* offers study suggestions for reinforcing concepts presented in this chapter. In addition, the following questions can be addressed in classroom or online discussions:

1. For one of the two studies described in the research example section (Kilanowski and Ryan-Wegner, 2007, or Draucker and Martsolf, 2008), draft a consent form that includes required information, as described in the section on informed consent.

2. Answer the relevant questions in Box 7.3 regarding the Kilanowski and Ryan-Wenger (2007) study. Also consider the following questions: (a) Could the data for this study have been collected anonymously? Why or why not? (b) Might a Certificate of Confidentiality have been helpful in this study?

3. Answer the relevant questions in Box 7.3 regarding the Draucker and Martsolf (2008) study. Also consider the following questions: (a) The researchers paid participants a $35 stipend—was this ethically appropriate? (b) Why do you think the researchers obtained a Certificate of Confidentiality for this research?

STUDIES CITED IN CHAPTER 7

Anderson, G. (2008). Ethical preparedness and performance of gene therapy study coordinators. *Nursing Ethics, 15*, 208–221.

Artinian, N., Flack, J., Nordstrom, C., Hockman, E., Washington, O., Jen, K., & Fathy, M. (2007). Effects of nurse-managed telemonitoring on blood pressure at 12-month follow-up among urban African Americans. *Nursing Research, 56*, 312–322.

Caelli, K. (2001). Engaging with phenomenology: Is it more of a challenge than it needs to be? *Qualitative Health Research, 11*, 273–281.

Caldwell, B., & Redeker, N. (2009). Sleep patterns and psychological distress in women living in the inner city. *Research in Nursing & Health, 32*, 177–190.

Carlsson, E., Paterson, B., Scott-Findley, S., Ehnfors, M., & Ehrenberg, A. (2007). Methodological issues in interviews involving people with communication impairments after acquired brain damage. *Qualitative Health Research, 17*, 1361–1371.

Draucker, C. B., & Martsolf, D. (2008). Storying childhood sexual abuse. *Qualitative Health Research, 18*, 1034–1048.

Freda, M. C., & Kearney, M. (2005). Ethical issues faced by nursing editors. *Western Journal of Nursing Research, 27*(4), 487–499.

Graffigna, G., & Olson, K. (2009). The ineffable disease: Exploring young people's discourses about HIV/AIDS in Alberta, Canada. *Qualitative Health Research, 19*, 790–801.

Habermann, B., Broome, M., Pryor, E., & Ziner, K. W. (2010). Research coordinators' experiences with scientific misconduct and research integrity. *Nursing Research, 59*, 51–57.

Horgas, A., Yoon, S., Nichols, A., & Marsiske, M (2008). The relationship between pain and functional disability in black and white older adults. *Research in Nursing & Health, 31*, 341–354.

Hsiao, C. Y., & Van Riper, M. (2009). Individual and family adaptation in Taiwanese families of individuals with severe and persistent mental illness. *Research in Nursing & Health, 32*, 307–320.

Jones, B., Volker, D., Vinajeras, Y., Butros, L., Fitchpatrick, C., & Rossetto, K. (2010). The meaning of surviving cancer for Latino adolescents and emerging young adults. *Cancer Nursing, 33*, 74–81.

Kelly, P., Cheng, A., Peralez-Dieckmann, E., & Martinez, E. (2009). Dating violence and girls in the juvenile justice system. *Journal of Interpersonal Violence, 24*, 1536–1551.

Kilanowski, J., & Ryan-Wenger, N. (2007). Health status in an invisible population: Carnival and migrant worker children. *Western Journal of Nursing Research, 29*, 100–120.

Laughon, K. (2007). Abused African American women's processes of staying healthy. *Western Journal of Nursing Research, 29*, 365–384.

Polit, D. F., & Beck, C. T. (2009). International gender bias in nursing research, 2005–2006: A quantitative content analysis. *International Journal of Nursing Studies, 46*, 1102–1110.

Raines, T., Jones, P., Moe, N., Duncan, R., McCall, S., & Caremuga, T. (2009). Investigation of the anxiolytic effects of luteolin, a lemon balm flavonoid in the male Sprague-Dawley rat. *AANA Journal, 77*, 33–36.

Rothstein, W., & Phuong, L. (2007). Ethical attitudes of nurse, physician, and unaffiliated members of Institutional Review Boards. *Journal of Nursing Scholarship, 39*, 75–81.

Sandgren, A., Thulesius, H., Fridlund, B., & Petersson, K. (2006). Striving for emotional survival in palliative cancer nursing. *Qualitative Health Research, 16*, 79–96.

Speraw, S. (2009). "Talk to me—I'm human": The story of a girl, her personhood, and the failures of health care. *Qualitative Health Research, 19*, 732–743.

Treacy, M., Hyde, A., Boland, J., Whitaker, T., Abaunza, P. S., & Stewart-Knox, B. (2007). Children talking: Emerging perspectives and experiences of cigarette smoking. *Qualitative Health Research, 17*, 238–249.

Wagner, L., Capezuti, E., & Rice, J. (2009). Nurses' perceptions of safety culture in long-term care settings. *Journal of Nursing Scholarship, 41*, 184–192.

Methodologic and nonresearch references cited in this chapter can be found in a separate section at the end of the book.

8

Planning a Nursing Study

A dvance planning is required for all research, and is especially important for quantitative studies because the study design is typically finalized before the study proceeds. This chapter provides advice for planning qualitative and quantitative studies.

Researchers face numerous challenges in conducting a study, including financial challenges (Will I have enough money?), administrative challenges (Can I obtain institutional approval?), practical challenges (Will I meet my deadlines?), ethical challenges (Can the study be designed to be both rigorous and ethical?), clinical challenges (Will research goals conflict with clinical goals?), and methodologic challenges (Will the methods used to address the research question yield accurate and valid results?). This book provides guidance primarily on methodologic challenges. Yet, other challenges impinge on a researcher's ability to design methodologically sound studies and need to be considered at the planning stage.

TOOLS AND CONCEPTS FOR PLANNING RIGOROUS RESEARCH

In planning a study, it is important to keep in mind not only the challenges of doing rigorous research, but also options for addressing them. This section discusses key methodologic concepts and tools in meeting those challenges.

Inference

Inference is an integral part of doing and evaluating research. An **inference** is a conclusion drawn from the study evidence, taking into account the methods used to generate that evidence. Inference is the attempt to come to conclusions based on limited information, using logical reasoning processes.

Inference is necessary because researchers use proxies that "stand in" for the things that are fundamentally of interest. A sample of participants is a proxy for an entire population. A study site is a proxy for all relevant sites in which the phenomena of interest could unfold. A measuring tool yields proxy information about constructs that are captured through fallible approximations. A control group that does not receive an intervention is a proxy for what would happen to the *same* people if they simultaneously received *and* did not receive the intervention.

Researchers face the challenge of using methods that yield good and persuasive evidence in support of inferences that they wish to make.

Reliability, Validity, and Trustworthiness

Researchers want their findings to reflect the *truth*. Research cannot contribute evidence to guide clinical practice if the findings are inaccurate, biased, fail to represent the experiences of the target group, or result in misinterpretations. Consumers of research need to assess the quality of a study's evidence by evaluating the conceptual and methodologic decisions the researchers made, and those who do research must strive to make decisions that result in evidence of the highest possible quality.

Quantitative researchers use several criteria to assess the quality of a study, sometimes referred to as its **scientific merit**. Two especially important criteria are reliability and validity. **Reliability** refers to the accuracy and consistency of information obtained in a study. The term is most often associated with the methods used to measure variables. For example, if a thermometer measured Alan's temperature as 98.1°F one minute and as 102.5°F the next minute, the reliability of the thermometer would be highly suspect. The concept of reliability is also important in interpreting statistical results. *Statistical reliability* refers to the probability that the results would hold with a wider group than the people who participated in the study—that is, the results support an inference about what is true in a population.

Validity is a more complex concept that broadly concerns the *soundness* of the study's evidence—that is, whether the findings are unbiased and well grounded. Like reliability, validity is an important criterion for evaluating methods to measure variables. In this context, the validity question is whether the methods are really measuring the concepts that they purport to measure. Is a paper-and-pencil measure of depression *really* measuring depression? Or, is it measuring something else, such as loneliness or low self-esteem? Researchers strive for solid conceptual definitions of research variables and valid methods to operationalize them.

Validity is also relevant with regard to inferences about the effect of the independent variable on the dependent variable. Did a nursing intervention *really* bring about improvements in patients' outcomes—or were other factors responsible for patients' progress? Researchers make numerous

methodologic decisions that influence this type of study validity.

Qualitative researchers use somewhat different criteria (and different terminology) in evaluating a study's quality. Qualitative researchers discuss methods of enhancing the **trustworthiness** of the study's data (Lincoln & Guba, 1985). Trustworthiness encompasses several dimensions—credibility, transferability (discussed later in the chapter), confirmability, and dependability. **Dependability** refers to evidence that is consistent and stable. **Confirmability**, similar to objectivity, is the degree to which study results are derived from characteristics of participants and the study context, not from researchers' biases.

Credibility is achieved to the extent that the research methods engender confidence in the truth of the data and researchers' interpretations. Credibility in a qualitative study can be enhanced through various approaches (Chapter 24), but one strategy merits early discussion because it has implications for the design of all studies, including quantitative ones. **Triangulation** is the use of multiple sources or referents to draw conclusions about what constitutes the truth. In a quantitative study, this might mean having multiple measures of a dependent variable to determine if predicted effects are consistent. In a qualitative study, triangulation might involve trying to reveal the complexity of a phenomenon by using multiple means of data collection to converge on the truth (e.g., having in-depth discussions with study participants, as well as watching their behavior in natural settings). Or, it might involve triangulating the ideas and interpretations of multiple researchers working together as a team. Nurse researchers are increasingly triangulating across paradigms—that is, integrating both qualitative and quantitative data in a single study to enhance the validity of the conclusions.

Example of triangulation: Martinsen and colleagues (2009) described the phenomenon of *sensitive cooperation* as a basis for assisted feeding in people with high cervical spinal cord injury (hcSCI). Sixteen people with hcSCI were interviewed on two occasions, and the second interview included direct observation.

Nurse researchers need to design their studies in such a way that the reliability, validity, and trustworthiness of their studies are maximized. This book offers advice on how to do this.

Bias

Bias can threaten the study's ability to reveal the truth and so is a major concern in designing a study. A **bias** is an influence that produces a distortion or error in the study results. Biases can affect evidence quality in both qualitative and quantitative studies.

Bias can result from a number of factors that need to be considered in planning a study. These include the following:

- *Participants' lack of candor*. Sometimes people distort their behavior or statements—consciously or subconsciously—so as to present themselves in the best light.
- *Researcher subjectivity*. Investigators may distort inferences in the direction of their expectations, or in line with their own experiences—or they may unintentionally communicate their expectations to participants and thereby induce biased behavior or disclosures.
- *Sample imbalances*. The sample itself may be biased; for example, if a researcher studying abortion attitudes included only members of right-to-life (or pro-choice) groups in the sample, the results would be distorted.
- *Faulty methods of data collection*. An inadequate method of capturing key concepts can lead to biases; for example, a flawed measure of patient satisfaction with nursing care may exaggerate or underestimate patients' concerns.
- *Inadequate study design*. A researcher may structure the study in such a way that an unbiased answer to the research question cannot be achieved.
- *Flawed implementation*. Even a well-designed study can sustain biases if the design (or the intervention, if any) is not carefully implemented. Monitoring for bias throughout the study is important.

Example of respondent bias: Collins and colleagues (2005) studied 316 pages of interview transcripts from three phenomenological studies and searched for instances in which participants may have distorted their responses in a manner that would make them "look good," or that would flatter the interviewers. They identified only six potential instances of what they called "problematic interviewee behavior." Yet they concluded, based on these instances, that "it is probably not a good idea for nurses to interview patients to whom they have personally delivered (or will deliver) care" (p. 197).

A researcher's job is to reduce or eliminate bias to the extent possible, to establish mechanisms to detect or measure it when it exists, and to take known biases into account in interpreting study findings. And, it is the job of consumers to carefully scrutinize methodologic decisions to draw conclusions about whether biases undermined the study evidence.

Unfortunately, bias can seldom be avoided totally because the potential for its occurrence is pervasive. Some bias is haphazard and affects only small data segments. As an example of such **random bias** (or *random error*), a handful of participants might provide inaccurate information because of extreme fatigue. When error is random, distortions are as likely to bias results in one direction as the other. **Systematic bias**, on the other hand, is consistent and distorts results in a single direction. For example, if a spring scale consistently measured people's weight as being 2 pounds heavier than their true weight, there would be systematic bias in the data on weight.

Researchers adopt a variety of strategies to eliminate or minimize bias and strengthen study rigor. Triangulation is one such approach, the idea being that multiple sources of information or points of view can help counterbalance biases and offer avenues to identify them. Methods that quantitative researchers use to combat bias often involve research control.

Research Control

A central feature of quantitative studies is that they usually involve efforts to control aspects of the research. **Research control** most typically involves holding constant other influences on the dependent variable so that the true relationship between the independent and dependent variables can be understood. In other words, research control attempts to eliminate contaminating factors that might obscure the relationship between the variables of central interest.

The issue of contaminating factors—called **confounding** (or **extraneous**) **variables**—can best be illustrated with an example. Suppose we wanted to study whether teenage women are at higher risk of having low-birth-weight infants than older mothers *because of their age*. In other words, we want to test whether there is something about women's maturational development that causes differences in birth weight. Studies have shown that, in fact, teenagers have a higher rate of low-birth-weight babies than women in their 20s. The question here is whether maternal age itself (the independent variable) causes differences in birth weight (the dependent variable), or whether there are other mechanisms that account for the relationship between age and birth weight. We need to design a study so as to control other potential determinants of the dependent variable that are also related to the independent variable.

Two confounding variables in this study are women's nutritional habits and prenatal care. Teenagers tend to be less careful than older women about nutrition, and are also less likely to obtain adequate prenatal care. Both nutrition and the amount of care could, in turn, affect the baby's birth weight. Thus, if these two factors are not controlled, then any observed relationship between a mother's age and her infant's birth weight could be caused by the mother's age itself, her diet, or her prenatal care.

These three possible explanations might be portrayed schematically as follows:

1. Mother's age → infant birth weight
2. Mother's age → prenatal care → infant birth weight
3. Mother's age → nutrition → infant birth weight

The arrows here symbolize a causal mechanism or an influence. In models 2 and 3, the effect of maternal age on infant birth weight is *mediated* by prenatal care and nutrition, respectively. Some research is specifically designed to test paths of mediation, but in the present example, these variables are extraneous to the research question. Our task is to design a study so that the first explanation can be tested. Both nutrition and prenatal care must be controlled if the goal is to shed light on the validity of explanation 1.

How can we impose such control? There are a number of ways, as discussed in Chapter 10, but the general principle underlying each alternative is that the confounding variables must be **held constant**. The confounding variables must somehow be handled so that, *in the context of the study*, they are not related to the independent or dependent variable. As an example, let us say we want to compare the birth weights of infants born to two groups of women: those aged 15 to 19 years and those aged 25 to 29 years. We must design a study in such a way that the nutritional and prenatal healthcare practices of the two groups are comparable, even though, in general, the two groups are not comparable in these respects.

To illustrate, consider a control method called **matching**, which involves deliberately selecting participants in such a way that both older and younger mothers have similar eating habits and amounts of prenatal attention. Each teenage pregnant woman would be matched to a pregnant woman in the older group in terms of the two confounding variables. For example, if a 16-year-old had 1 prenatal visit and a poor score on a measure of nutrition, a woman in her late 20s with the same characteristics would be sought for the older group. Then, if the two groups differ in terms of their infants' birth weight, we might infer that age (and not diet or prenatal care) influenced birth weight. If the groups did not differ, however, we might tentatively conclude that it is not mother's age *per se* that causes young women to have a higher percentage of low-birth-weight babies, but rather some other factor, such as nutrition or prenatal care. Of course, although we have designated prenatal care and nutrition as extraneous variables in this study, they are not at all extraneous to a full understanding of factors that influence birth weight; in other studies, nutritional practices and prenatal care would be key independent variables.

By exercising control in this example, we have taken a step toward explaining the relationship between variables. The world is complex, and many variables are interrelated in complicated ways. When studying a particular problem in a quantitative study, it is difficult to examine this complexity directly; researchers must usually analyze a couple of relationships at a time and put pieces together like a jigsaw puzzle. That is why even modest studies can make contributions to knowledge. The extent of the contribution in a quantitative study, however, is often directly related to how well researchers control confounding influences.

In the present example, we identified three variables that could affect birth weight, but dozens of others might be relevant, such as maternal stress, mothers' use of alcohol during pregnancy, and so on. Researchers need to isolate the independent and dependent variables in which they are interested and then identify confounding variables that need to be controlled.

Example of control through matching: King and colleagues (2009) compared risk for coronary heart disease in nondiabetic women either with or without a history of gestational diabetes. To control confounding variables, the two groups were matched in terms of age, body mass index, and time since the pregnancy.

It is often unnecessary to control all variables that affect the dependent variable. Confounding variables need to be controlled only if they simultaneously are related to both the dependent and independent variables. This is illustrated in Figure 8.1, which has the following elements:

- Each circle represents all the variability associated with a particular variable.
- The large circle in the center stands for the dependent variable, birth weight.
- Smaller circles stand for factors affecting birth weight.
- Overlapping circles indicate the degree to which the variables are related to each other.

In this hypothetical example, four variables are related to birth weight: mother's age, amount of prenatal care, nutritional practices, and smoking

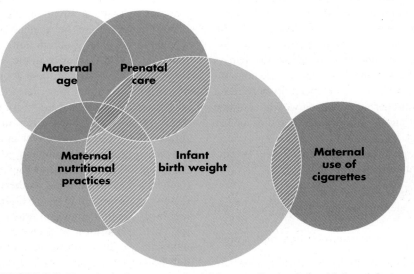

FIGURE 8.1 Hypothetical representation of factors affecting infant birth weight.

during pregnancy. The first three variables are also interrelated; this is shown by the fact that these three circles overlap not only with birth weight, but also with each other. Younger mothers tend to have different patterns of prenatal care and nutrition than older mothers. Mothers' smoking, however, is unrelated to these three variables. In other words, women who smoke during their pregnancies (according to this fictitious representation) are as likely to be young as old, to eat properly as not, and to get adequate prenatal care as not. If this representation were accurate, then maternal smoking would not need to be controlled to study the effect of maternal age on infant birth weight. If this scheme is incorrect—if teenage mothers smoke more or less than older mothers—then maternal smoking practices should be controlled.

Figure 8.1 does not show birth weight as being totally explained by the four other variables. The middle area of the birth weight circle shows "unexplained" variability in birth weight. Other determinants cause babies to be born weighing different amounts. Genetic traits, events occurring during pregnancy, and medical treatments administered prenatally are examples of other factors that can affect an infant's birth weight. In designing a study, quantitative researchers should attempt to control variables that overlap with both independent and dependent variables to understand fully the relationship between the main variables of interest.

Research control is a critical tool for managing bias and for enhancing validity in quantitative studies. There are situations, however, in which too much control can introduce bias. For example, if researchers tightly control the ways in which key study variables are manifested, it is possible that the true nature of those variables will be obscured. In studying phenomena that are poorly understood or whose dimensions have not been clarified, then an approach that allows flexibility and exploration is more appropriate. Research rooted in the constructivist paradigm does not impose controls. Qualitative researchers typically adopt the view that imposing controls on a research setting removes some of the meaning of reality.

Randomness

For quantitative researchers, a powerful tool for eliminating bias involves **randomness**—having certain features of the study established by chance rather than by design or researcher preference. When people are selected at random to participate in the study, for example, each person in the initial pool has an equal probability of being selected. This in turn means that there are no systematic biases in the make-up of the sample. Men and women have an equal chance of being selected, for example. Similarly, if participants are allocated randomly to groups that will be compared (e.g., an intervention and "usual care" group), then there can be no systematic biases in the composition of the groups. Randomness is a compelling method of controlling confounding variables and reducing bias.

Qualitative researchers almost never consider randomness a desirable tool. Qualitative researchers tend to use information obtained early in the study in a purposeful (nonrandom) fashion to guide their inquiry and to pursue information-rich sources that can help them expand or refine their conceptualizations. Researchers' judgments are viewed as indispensable vehicles for uncovering the complexities of phenomena of interest.

Reflexivity

Qualitative researchers do not use methods such as research control or randomness, but they are as interested as quantitative researchers in discovering the true state of human experience. Qualitative researchers often rely on reflexivity to guard against personal bias in making judgments. **Reflexivity** is the process of reflecting critically on the self and of analyzing and making note of personal values that could affect data collection and interpretation.

Schwandt (2007) has described reflexivity as having two aspects. The first concerns the acknowledgment that the researcher is part of the setting, context, or social phenomenon under study. The second involves the process of self-reflection about one's own biases, preferences, stakes in, and fears about the research and theoretical inclinations.

Qualitative researchers are encouraged to explore these issues, to be reflexive about every decision made during the inquiry, and to note their reflexive thoughts in personal journals and memos.

Reflexivity can be a useful tool in quantitative as well as qualitative research. Self-awareness and introspection can enhance the quality of any study.

Example of reflexivity: Ray (2009) studied the experience of peacekeepers deployed in Somalia, Rwanda, and the former Yugoslavia with regard to their healing from trauma. Ray, who worked as a clinical nurse specialist with veterans and enlisted personnel, made efforts to recognize her own biases and assumptions about the phenomenon by maintaining a reflective journal.

Generalizability and Transferability

Nurses increasingly rely on evidence from research in their clinical practice. Evidence-based practice is based on the assumption that study findings are not unique to the people, places, or circumstances of the original research (Polit & Beck, 2010).

Generalizability is a criterion used in quantitative studies to assess the extent to which findings can be applied to other groups and settings. How do researchers enhance the generalizability of a study? First and foremost, they must design studies strong in reliability and validity. There is no point in wondering whether results are generalizable if they are not accurate or valid. In selecting participants, researchers must also give thought to the types of people to whom the results might be generalized—and then select participants in such a way that the sample reflects the population of interest. If a study is intended to have implications for male and female patients, then men and women should be included as participants. Chapters 10 and 12 describe issues to consider to enhance generalizability.

Qualitative researchers do not specifically seek to make their findings generalizable. Nevertheless, they usually want to generate evidence that could be useful in other situations. Lincoln and Guba (1985), in their influential book on naturalistic inquiry, discussed the concept of **transferability**, the extent to which qualitative findings can be transferred to other settings, as an aspect of a study's trustworthiness. One mechanism for promoting transferability is the amount of information qualitative researchers provide about study contexts. The issue of generalizability and transferability in qualitative research is discussed in Chapter 21.

> **TIP:** When planning a study, it is wise to keep a sharp focus on the potential your study could have for evidence-based nursing practice—it may play a role in some of the methodologic decisions you make. Make an effort to think about generalizability and transferability throughout the study.

OVERVIEW OF RESEARCH DESIGN FEATURES

The research design of a study spells out the basic strategies that researchers adopt to develop evidence that is accurate and interpretable. The research design incorporates some of the most important methodologic decisions that researchers make, particularly in quantitative studies. Thus, it is important to understand design options when planning a research project.

Table 8.1 describes seven design features that typically need to be considered in planning a quantitative study, and several are also pertinent in qualitative studies. These features include the following:

- Whether or not there will be an *intervention*
- How confounding variables will be *controlled*
- Whether *blinding* will be used to avoid biases
- What the relative timing of collecting data on dependent and independent variables will be
- What types of *comparisons* will be made to enhance interpretability
- What the *location* of the study will be
- What *timeframes* will be adopted

This section discusses the last three features because they are relevant in planning both qualitative and quantitative studies. Chapters 9 and 10 elaborate on the first four.

TABLE 8.1	Key Research Design Features in Quantitative Studies	
FEATURE	**KEY QUESTIONS**	**DESIGN OPTIONS**
Intervention	Will there be an intervention? What will the intervention entail? What specific design will be used?	Experimental (RCT)*, quasi-experimental (controlled trial), nonexperimental (observational) design
Control over confounding variables	How will confounding variables be controlled? Which confounding variables will be controlled?	Matching, homogeneity, blocking, crossover, randomization, statistical control
Blinding (masking)	From whom will critical information be withheld to avoid bias?	Open versus closed study; single-blind, double-blind, triple-blind
Relative timing	When will information on independent and dependent variables be collected— looking backward or forward?	Retrospective, prospective design
Comparisons	What type of comparisons will be made to illuminate key processes or relationships? What is the nature of the comparison?	Within-subject design, between-subject design, mixed design, external comparisons
Location	Where will the study take place?	Single site versus multisite; in the field versus controlled setting
Timeframes	How often will data be collected? When, relative to other events, will data be collected?	Cross-sectional, longitudinal design; repeated measures design

*RCT: Randomized controlled trial

Note: Several terms in this table are explained in subsequent chapters

➲ T I P : You will make many important design decisions that will affect the believability of your findings during the planning stage. In some cases, the decisions will influence whether you receive funding (if you seek financial support) or are able to publish your findings (if you submit to a journal). Therefore, a great deal of care and thought should go into these decisions.

Comparisons

In most quantitative (and some qualitative) studies, researchers incorporate comparisons into their design to provide a context for interpreting results. As noted in Chapter 4, most quantitative research questions are phrased in terms of a comparison because the comparison typically embodies the independent variable. For example, if our research question asks, what is the effect of massage on anxiety in hospitalized children, the implied comparison is massage versus no massage—that is, the independent variable.

Researchers can structure their studies to examine various types of comparison, the most common of which are as follows:

1. *Comparison between two or more groups.* For example, if we were studying the emotional consequences of having an abortion, we might compare the emotional status of women who had an abortion with that of women with an unintended pregnancy who delivered the baby. Or, we might compare those receiving a special intervention with those receiving "usual care." In a qualitative study, we might compare mothers and fathers with respect to their experience of having a child diagnosed with schizophrenia.

2. *Comparison of one group's status at two or more points in time.* For example, we might want to compare patients' levels of stress before and after introducing a new procedure to reduce preoperative stress. Or, we might want to compare coping processes among caregivers of patients with AIDS early and later in the caregiving experience.

3. *Comparison of one group's status under different circumstances.* For example, we might compare people's heart rates during two different types of exercise.

4. *Comparison based on relative rankings.* If, for example, we hypothesized a relationship between the pain level and degree of hopefulness in patients with cancer, we would be asking whether those with high levels of pain felt less hopeful than those with low levels of pain. This research question involves a comparison of those with different rankings—higher versus lower—on both variables.

5. *Comparison with external data.* Researchers may directly compare their results with results from other studies or with *norms* (standards from a large and representative sample), sometimes using statistical procedures. This type of comparison often supplements rather than replaces other comparisons. In quantitative studies, this approach is useful primarily when the dependent variable is measured with a widely accepted method (e.g., blood pressure readings or scores on a standard measure of depression).

> **Example of using comparative data from external sources:** White and Groh (2007) studied depression and quality of life among women after a myocardial infarction. They used a measure of health and well-being for which national comparison data were available (the Short-Form 36), which enabled them to compare their sample's outcomes to national norms for healthy women aged 55 to 64.

Research designs for quantitative studies can be categorized based on the type of comparisons that are made. Studies that compare groups of different people (as in examples 1 and 4) are **between-subjects designs**. Sometimes, however, it is preferable to make comparisons for the *same* participants at different times or under difference circumstances, as in examples 2 and 3. Such designs are **within-subjects designs**. When two or more groups of people are followed over time, the design is sometimes called a **mixed design** because comparisons can be both within groups over time, or between groups.

Comparisons are often the central focus of a quantitative study, but even when they are not, they provide a context for interpreting the findings. In the example of studying the emotional status of women who had an abortion, it would be difficult to know whether their emotional state was worrisome without comparing it to that of others—or without comparing it to their state at an earlier time (e.g., prior to pregnancy).

Sometimes a natural comparison group suggests itself. For example, if we were testing the effectiveness of a new nursing procedure for burn patients, an obvious comparison group would be burn patients receiving usual care rather than the innovation. In other cases, however, the choice of a comparison group is less clear-cut, and decisions about a comparison group can affect the interpretability of the findings. In the example about the emotional consequences of an abortion, we proposed women who had delivered a baby as a comparison group. This comparison focuses on pregnancy *outcome* (i.e., pregnancy termination versus live birth). An alternative comparison group might be women who had a miscarriage. In this case, the comparison focuses not on the outcome (in both groups, the outcome is pregnancy loss) but rather on the *determinant* of the outcome. Thus, in designing a study, quantitative researchers choose comparisons that will best illuminate the central issue under investigation.

Qualitative researchers sometimes plan to make comparisons when they undertake an in-depth study, but comparisons are rarely their primary focus. Nevertheless, patterns emerging in the data often suggest that certain comparisons have strong descriptive and explanatory value.

> ➲ **TIP:** Try not to make design decisions single-handedly. Seek the advice of faculty, colleagues, or consultants. Once you have made design decisions, it may be useful to write out a rationale for your choices, and share it with others to see if they can find flaws in your reasoning or if they can suggest improvements. A worksheet for documenting design decisions and rationales is available as a Word document in the Toolkit section of the accompanying *Resource Manual.*

Research Location

An important planning task is to identify sites for the study. There are some situations in which a site for the study is a "given," as might be the case for a clinical study conducted in a hospital or institution with which researchers are affiliated, but in other studies, the identification of an appropriate site involves considerable effort.

Planning for this aspect of the study involves two types of activities—selecting the site or sites, and gaining access to them. While some of the issues we discuss here are of particular relevance to qualitative researchers working in the field, many quantitative studies also need to attend to these matters in planning a project, especially in intervention studies.

Site Selection

The primary consideration in site selection is whether the site is appropriate—that is, whether it has people with the behaviors, experiences, or characteristics of interest. The site must also have a sufficient *number* of these kinds of people and adequate *diversity* or mix of people to achieve research

goals. In addition, the site must be one in which access to study participants can be granted. The site should also be one that matches other requirements, such as space needs, personnel, laboratory facilities, and so forth. In a good site, both methodologic goals (e.g., ability to exert needed controls) and ethical requirements (e.g., ability to ensure privacy and confidentiality) can be achieved. Finally, the site should be one in which the researcher will be allowed to maintain an appropriate role vis-à-vis study participants and clinical staff for the duration of the study.

> ➲ **TIP:** Before searching for a suitable site, it might be helpful to jot down the site characteristics that you would ideally like to have so that you can more clearly assess the degree to which the reality matches the ideal. Once you have compiled a list, it might be profitable to brainstorm with colleagues, advisors, or other professionals about your needs to see if they can help you to identify potential sites.

In some cases, researchers may have to decide *how many* sites to include. Having multiple sites is advantageous in terms of enhancing the generalizability of the study findings, but multisite studies are complex and pose management, financial, and logistic challenges. Multiple sites are a good strategy when several co-investigators from different institutions are working together on a project.

Site visits to potential sites and clinical fieldwork are usually required to assess the "fit" between what the researcher needs and what the site has to offer. In essence, site visits involve "prior ethnography" (Erlandson et al., 1993) in which the researcher must make and record observations and converse with key gatekeepers or stakeholders in the site to better understand its characteristics and constraints. Buckwalter and colleagues (2009) have noted particular issues of concern when working in sites that are "unstable" research environments, such as critical care units or long-term care facilities.

Gaining Access

Researchers must gain entrée into those sites deemed suitable for the inquiry. If the site is an entire community, a multitiered effort of gaining acceptance from gatekeepers may be needed. For example, it may be necessary to enlist the cooperation first of community leaders and subsequently of administrators and staff in specific institutions (e.g., domestic violence organizations) or leaders of specific groups (e.g., support groups).

Because establishing *trust* is a central issue, gaining entrée requires strong interpersonal skills, as well as familiarity with the site's customs and language. Researchers' ability to gain the gatekeepers' trust can occur only if researchers are congenial, are candid about research requirements, and—especially—express genuine interest in and concern for the people in the site. Gatekeepers might be especially cooperative if they are persuaded that there will be direct benefits to them or their constituents.

Information to help gatekeepers make a decision about granting access usually should be put in writing, even if the negotiation takes place in person. An information sheet should cover the following points: (1) the purpose of the research and who the beneficiaries would be; (2) why the site was chosen; (3) what the research would entail, including when the study would start, how long research staff would be at the site, how much disruption there likely would be, and what the resource requirements are; (4) how ethical guidelines would be maintained, including how results would be reported; and (5) what the gatekeeper or others at the site have to gain from cooperating in the study. Figure 8.2 ⊗ presents an example of a letter of inquiry for gaining entrée into a facility.

Gaining entrée may be an ongoing process of establishing relationships and rapport with gatekeepers and others at the site, including prospective informants. The process might involve *progressive entry*, in which certain privileges are negotiated at first and then are subsequently expanded (Erlandson et al., 1993). Morse and Field (1995) advised ongoing communication with gatekeepers between the time that access is granted and the start-up of the study, which may be a lengthy period if funding decisions or study preparations (e.g., instrument development) are time-consuming. It is not only courteous to keep people informed, but it may also prove critical to the success of the project because circumstances (and leadership) at the site can change.

Bernard (2006) offered five guidelines for entering the field: (1) If you have a choice, select a field site that gives you the easiest access to data; (2) bring along multiple copies of written documentation about yourself and your study; (3) if you have personal contacts, use them to help you enter the field site; (4) be prepared to address questions about yourself and your study; and (5) take time to become familiar with the physical and social layout of your field site.

Timeframes

Research designs designate when, and how often, data will be collected. In many studies, data are collected at one point in time. For example, patients might be asked on a single occasion to describe their health-promoting behaviors. Some designs, however, call for multiple contacts with participants, often to assess changes over time. Thus, in planning a study, researchers must decide on the number of data collection points needed to address the research question properly. The research design also designates *when*, relative to other events, data will be collected. For example, the design might call for measurement of cholesterol levels 4 weeks and 8 weeks after an exercise intervention.

Designs can be categorized in terms of study timeframes. The major distinction, for both qualitative and quantitative researchers, is between cross-sectional and longitudinal designs.

Cross-Sectional Designs

Cross-sectional designs involve the collection of data once the phenomena under study are captured during a single period of data collection. Cross-sectional studies are appropriate for describing the status of phenomena or for describing relationships among phenomena at a fixed point in time. For example, we might be interested in determining whether psychological symptoms in menopausal women are correlated contemporaneously with physiologic symptoms.

Ms. Wendy Smith, R.N.
Family Birth Place
General Hospital
Hartford, CT

Dear Ms. Smith:

I am the Principal Investigator of a study whose primary goal is to improve the detection of postpartum depression in Hispanic mothers. The study will involve testing a standard Spanish version of the Postpartum Depression Screening Sale (PDSS). Postpartum depression is a cross-cultural mental illness that can have devastating effects for 10%–15% of new mothers and their families. It has been estimated that up to 50% of all cases go undetected. Non–English-speaking women in this country may be even more disadvantaged and isolated in their environments and may thus be at even higher risk for depression than English-speaking women, and thus effective screening with a valid instrument may be especially important.

Your hospital would be a desirable site for this research because of the high percentage of Hispanic women who deliver at your Family Birth Place. The research would require a sample of 75 Hispanic mothers 18 years of age or older who have given birth within the past 3 months. Each mother would complete the PDSS-Spanish Version and would participate in a diagnostic interview for *DSM-IV* depressive disorders, conducted by a female Hispanic psychologist. If a woman is diagnosed with postpartum depression, she would be referred for psychiatric follow-up. Each mother would be given a gift certificate for $25.00 for participating in the study.

If feasible, I would like to approach the 75 Hispanic women to invite them to participate in the study soon after delivery, while they are on the postpartum unit. The mothers would be recruited by a Hispanic research assistant who is an RN. Prospective participants will be asked to sign an informed consent form, which will be available in both English and Spanish (whichever language version participants prefer). Confidentiality will be strictly maintained. No name or identifying information will be written on any of the data collection forms. All data will be kept in a locked file cabinet in my office at the University of Connecticut.

Results of the study will be presented at research conferences and in a nursing research journal. The study findings will provide you with a more complete picture of your own Hispanic population and the percentage suffering from postpartum depression. A Spanish version of the PDSS will be made available for your use for screening Hispanic mothers at your hospital.

If it is possible, I would like to schedule an appointment with you so that we can discuss the possibility of my conducting this research on your unit.

Sincerely,
Cheryl Tatano Beck, DNSc, CNM, FAAN
Professor

FIGURE 8.2 ⊗ Sample letter of inquiry for gaining entrée into a research site (fictitious).

Example of a cross-sectional qualitative study: Woodgate (2009) studied the experience of dyspnea in school-aged children with asthma. Thirty children diagnosed with asthma were interviewed at a single point in time.

Cross-sectional designs are sometimes used for time-related purposes, but the results may be misleading or ambiguous. For example, we might test the hypothesis, using cross-sectional data, that a determinant of excessive alcohol consumption is low impulse control, as measured by a psychological test. When both alcohol consumption and impulse control are measured concurrently, how-ever, it is difficult to know which variable influenced the other, if either. Cross-sectional data can most appropriately be used to infer time sequence under two circumstances: (1) when a cogent theoretical rationale guides the analysis or (2) when there is evidence or logical reasoning indicating that one variable preceded the other—for example, in a study of the effects of low birth weight on morbidity in school-aged children, it is clear that birth weight came first.

Cross-sectional studies can be designed to permit inferences about processes evolving over time, but such designs are usually less persuasive than longitudinal ones. Suppose, for example, we were studying changes in children's health promotion activities between ages 10 and 13. One way to study this would be to interview children at age 10 and then 3 years later at age 13—a longitudinal design. On the other hand, we could use a cross-sectional design by interviewing *different* children ages 10 and 13 and then comparing their responses. If 13-year-olds engaged in more health-promoting activities than 10-year-olds, it might be inferred that children improve in making healthy choices as they age. To make this kind of inference, we would have to assume that the older children would have responded as the younger ones did had they been questioned 3 years earlier, or, conversely, that 10-year-olds would report more health promoting activities if they were questioned again 3 years later. Such a design, which involves a comparison of multiple age cohorts, is sometimes called a **cohort comparison design**.

Cross-sectional studies are economical, but inferring changes over time with such designs is problematic. In our example, 10- and 13-year old children may have different attitudes toward health promotion, independent of maturation. Rapid social and technological changes may make it risky to assume that differences in the behaviors or traits of different age groups are the result of time passing rather than of cohort or generational differences. In cross-sectional studies designed to explore change, there are often alternative explanations for the findings—and that is precisely what good research design tries to avoid.

Example of a cross-sectional study with inference of change over time: DiIorio and colleagues (2007) examined the relationship between adolescents' age on the one hand and their intimate behaviors and discussions about sex on the other in a cross-sectional study of African American youth aged 12, 13, 14, and 15. Intimate behavior and peer discussions increased with age, but discussions with mothers did not.

Longitudinal Designs

A study in which researchers collect data at more than one point in time *over an extended period* is a **longitudinal design**. There are four situations in which a longitudinal design is appropriate:

1. *Studying time-related processes.* Some research problems specifically concern phenomena that evolve over time (e.g., healing, physical growth).
2. *Determining time sequences.* It is sometimes important to determine the sequencing of phenomena. For example, if it is hypothesized that infertility results in depression, then it would be important to ascertain that the depression did not precede the fertility problem.
3. *Assessing changes over time.* Some studies examine whether changes have occurred over time. For example, an experimental study might examine whether an intervention had both short-term and long-term benefits. A qualitative study might explore the evolution of grieving in the spouses of palliative care patients.
4. *Enhancing research control.* Quantitative researchers sometimes collect data at multiple points to enhance the interpretability of the results. For example, when two groups are being compared with regard to the effects of alternative interventions, the collection of data before any intervention occurs allows the researcher to detect—and control—any initial differences between groups.

There are several types of longitudinal designs. Most involve collecting data from one group of study participants multiple times, but others involve different samples. **Trend studies**, for example, are investigations in which samples from a population are studied over time with respect to some phenomenon. Trend studies permit researchers to examine patterns and rates of change and to predict future developments. Many trend studies document trends in public health issues, such as smoking, obesity, child abuse, and so on.

Example of a trend study: Small and colleagues (2009) conducted a trend study to assess changes over time in pediatric nurse practitioners' ability to assess and manage childhood obesity. Data were obtained in both 1999 and 2005.

In a more typical longitudinal study, the *same* people provide data at two or more points in time. Longitudinal studies of general (nonclinical) populations are sometimes called **panel studies**. The term *panel* refers to the sample of people providing data. Because the same people are studied over time, researchers can examine different patterns of change (e.g., those whose health improved or deteriorated). Panel studies are intuitively appealing as an approach to studying change, but they are expensive.

Example of a panel study: The U.S. government sponsors numerous large-scale panel studies, and many nurse researchers have analyzed data from these studies. For example, Atkins and Hart (2008) studied the effect of childhood personality, as assessed at age 5 or 6, on the initiation of sexual activity before age 16. The researchers used three waves of data from a panel study of men and women who, together with their children, were studied for decades.

Follow-up studies are similar to panel studies, but are undertaken to determine the subsequent development of individuals who have a specified condition or who have received a specific intervention. For example, patients who have received a particular nursing intervention or clinical treatment may be followed to ascertain long-term effects. Or, in a qualitative study, patients initially interviewed shortly after a diagnosis of prostate cancer may be followed to assess their experiences during or after treatment decisions have been made.

Example of a qualitative follow-up study: Roe and colleagues (2009) followed up a sample of older patients who had fallen. In-depth data were collected at two points in time to examine how the fall affected their health status, lifestyle, service use, and fall prevention efforts.

Some longitudinal studies are called **cohort studies**, in which a group of people (the cohort) is tracked over time to see if subsets with exposure to different factors differ in terms of subsequent outcomes or risks. For example, in a cohort of women, those with or without a history of childbearing could be tracked to examine differences in rates of ovarian cancer. This type of study, often called a *prospective study*, is discussed in Chapter 9.

Longitudinal studies are appropriate for studying the dynamics of a phenomenon over time, but a major problem is **attrition**—the loss of participants over time. Attrition is problematic because those who drop out of the study often differ in important ways from those who continue to participate, resulting in potential biases and difficulty with generalizing to the original population.

In longitudinal studies, researchers must make decisions about the number of data collection points and the intervals between them based on the nature of the study and available resources. When change or development is rapid, numerous time points at short intervals may be needed to document it. Researchers interested in outcomes that may occur years after the original data collection must use longer-term follow-up. However, the longer the interval, the greater the risk of attrition and resulting biases.

Repeated Measures Designs

Studies with multiple points of data collection are sometimes described as having a **repeated measures design**, which usually signifies a study in which data are collected three or more times. Longitudinal studies, such as follow-up and cohort studies, sometimes use a repeated measures design.

Repeated measures designs, however, can also be used in studies that are essentially cross-sectional. For example, a study involving the collection of postoperative patient data on vital signs hourly over an 8-hour period would not be described as longitudinal because the study does not involve an extended time perspective. Yet, the design could be characterized as repeated measures. Researchers are especially likely to use the term *repeated measures design* when they use a repeated measures approach to statistical analysis (see Chapter 17).

Example of a repeated measures follow-up study: King and colleagues (2009) studied changes in level of depression among men recovering from coronary artery bypass surgery. Depression was measured in a sample of cardiac patients at hospital discharge and at 6, 12, and 36 weeks postoperatively.

➲ **T I P :** In making design decisions, you will often need to balance various considerations, such as time, cost, ethical issues, and study integrity. Try to get a firm understanding of your "upper limits" before finalizing your design. That is, what is the *most* money that can be spent on the project? What is the *maximal amount* of time available for conducting the study? What is the limit of acceptability with regard to attrition? These limits often eliminate some design options. With these constraints in mind, the central focus should be on designing a study that maximizes the validity or trustworthiness of the study.

PLANNING DATA COLLECTION

In planning a study, researchers must select methods to gather their research data. This section provides an overview of various methods of data collection for qualitative and quantitative studies.

Overview of Data Collection and Data Sources

As in the case of research designs, there is an array of alternative data collection methods and approaches from which to choose. Most often, researchers collect new data, and one key planning decision concerns the basic types of data to gather. Three approaches have been used most frequently by nurse researchers: self-reports, observation, and biophysiologic measures. In some cases, researchers may be able to use data from existing sources, such as records.

Self-Reports

A good deal of information can be gathered by questioning people, a method known as **self-report**. If, for example, we were interested in learning about patients' perceptions of hospital care or about preoperative fears, we would likely gather data by asking them relevant questions. The unique ability of humans to communicate verbally on a sophisticated level makes direct questioning a particularly important part of nurse researchers' data collection repertoire. The vast majority of nursing studies involve data collected by self-report.

The self-report method is strong in directness and versatility. If we want to know what people think, feel, or believe, the most efficient means of gathering information is to ask them about it. The strongest argument that can be made for the self-report method is that it can yield information that would be impossible to gather by any other means. Behaviors can be observed, but only if participants engage in them publicly. Furthermore, observers can observe only those behaviors occurring at the time of the study. Through self-reports, researchers can gather *retrospective data* about events occurring in the past, or information about behaviors in which people plan to engage in the future. Information about feelings, values, or opinions can sometimes be inferred through observation, but behaviors and feelings do not always correspond exactly. Self-report methods can capture psychological characteristics through direct communication with participants.

Despite these advantages, verbal report methods have some weaknesses. The most serious issue concerns the validity and accuracy of self-reports: Can we be sure that respondents feel or act the way they say they do? Can we trust the information that they provide, particularly if true answers would reveal embarrassing behavior? Investigators often have no alternative but to assume that participants have been frank. Yet, we all have a tendency to want to present ourselves positively, and this may conflict with the truth. Researchers who gather self-report data should recognize these limitations and take them into consideration when interpreting the results.

Example of a study using self-reports:
Ahlström and colleagues (2010) studied the meaning of major depression in family life from the perspective of the ill parent. The data came from in-depth interviews with 8 respondents.

Self-report methods normally depend on respondents' willingness to share personal information, but **projective techniques** are sometimes used to obtain data indirectly about people's ways of thinking. Projective techniques present participants with a stimulus of low structure, permitting them to "read in" and then describe their own interpretations. The Rorschach test is one example of a projective technique. Other projective methods encourage self-expression through the construction of some product (e.g., drawings). The assumption is that people express their needs, motives, and emotions by working with or manipulating materials. Projective methods are used infrequently by nurse researchers, the major exception being studies using expressive methods to explore sensitive topics with children.

Example of a study using projective methods: In an ethnographic study, Lindsay-Waters (2008) explored the experience of having a long-term renal illness among children in a hospital renal unit. An understanding of their experiences was obtained through in-depth interviews, observations, and an analysis of their drawings.

Observation

For certain research problems, an alternative to self-reports is **observation** of people's behaviors or characteristics. Observation can be done directly through the human senses or with the aid of technical apparatus, such as video equipment. Observational methods are versatile and can be used to gather information about a wide range of phenomena, including the following:

- Characteristics and conditions of individuals (e.g., patients' sleep–wake state)
- Verbal communication (e.g., nurse–patient dialogue)
- Nonverbal communication (e.g., facial expressions)
- Activities and behavior (e.g., geriatric patients' self-grooming)
- Skill attainment (e.g., diabetic patients' skill in testing their urine)
- Environmental conditions (e.g., architectural barriers in nursing homes).

Observation in healthcare environments is an important data-gathering strategy. Nurses are in an advantageous position to observe, relatively unobtrusively, the behaviors of patients, their families, and hospital staff. Moreover, nurses may, by training, be especially sensitive observers.

Observational methods may yield better data than self-reports when people are unaware of

their own behavior (e.g., manifesting preoperative symptoms of anxiety), when people are embarrassed to report activities (e.g., displays of aggression), when behaviors are emotionally laden (e.g., grieving), or when people are not capable of describing their actions (e.g., young children). Observation is intrinsically appealing in its ability to capture a record of behaviors and events. Furthermore, with an observational approach, humans—the observers—are used as measuring instruments and provide a uniquely sensitive and intelligent tool.

Shortcomings of observation include behavior distortions when participants are aware of being observed—a problem called **reactivity**. Reactivity can be eliminated if observations are made without people's knowledge, through some type of concealment—but this poses ethical concerns because of the inability to obtain truly informed consent. Another problem is **observer biases**. A number of factors interfere with objective observations, including the following:

- Emotions, prejudices, and values of observers may result in faulty inference.
- Personal commitment may color what is seen in the direction of what observers want to see.
- Anticipation of what is to be observed may affect what *is* observed.
- Hasty decisions before adequate information is collected may result in erroneous classifications or conclusions.

Observational biases probably cannot be eliminated completely, but they can be minimized through careful training.

Example of a study using observation: Holliday-Welsh and colleagues (2009) studied the effect of a massage on the agitated behavior of cognitively impaired nursing home residents. Various aspects of agitation were observed and recorded.

Biophysiologic Measures

Many clinical studies rely on the use of quantitative **biophysiologic measures**. Physiologic and physical variables typically require specialized technical instruments and equipment for their measurement.

Because such equipment is generally available in healthcare settings, the costs of these measures to nurse researchers may be small or nonexistent.

A major strength of biophysiologic measures is their objectivity. Nurse A and nurse B, reading from the same spirometer output, are likely· to record the same tidal volume measurements. Furthermore, barring the possibility of equipment malfunctioning, two different spirometers are likely to produce identical tidal volume readouts. Another advantage of physiologic measurements is the relative precision and sensitivity they normally offer. By *relative*, we are implicitly comparing physiologic instruments with measures of psychological phenomena, such as self-report measures of anxiety or pain. Biophysiologic measures usually yield data of exceptionally high quality.

Example of a study using biophysiologic measures: Tang and colleagues (2010) studied factors related to fatigue in patients with chronic heart failure. They studied several biophysiologic measures (e.g., ejection fraction, hemoglobin) in relation to fatigue.

Records

Most researchers create original data for their studies, but they sometimes take advantage of available information, such as in **records**. Hospital records, patient charts, physicians' order sheets, care plan statements, and the like all constitute rich data sources to which nurse researchers may have access.

Research data obtained from records and other documents are advantageous because they are economical: the collection of original data is often time-consuming and costly. Also, records avoid problems stemming from people's awareness of and reaction to study participation. Furthermore, investigators do not have to rely on participants' cooperation.

On the other hand, when researchers are not responsible for collecting data, they may be unaware of the records' limitations and biases. Two major types of bias in records are **selective deposit** and **selective survival**. If the available records are not the entire set of all possible such records, researchers must question how representative existing records are. Many record keepers *intend* to

maintain an entire universe of records but may not succeed. Lapses may be the result of systematic biases, and careful researchers should attempt to learn what those biases may be. Eder and colleagues (2005) have suggested some strategies for enhancing the reliability of data extracted from medical records.

Other difficulties also may be relevant. Sometimes records have to be verified for their authenticity or accuracy, a task that may be difficult if the records are old. Researchers using records must be prepared to deal with systems they do not understand. Codes and symbols that had meaning to the record keeper may have to be translated. In using records to study trends, researchers should be alert to possible changes in record-keeping procedures.

Another problem is the increasing difficulty of gaining access to institutional records. As mentioned in Chapter 7, federal legislation in the United States (HIPAA) has created some obstacles to accessing records for research purposes. Thus, although records may be plentiful, inexpensive, and accessible, they should not be used without paying attention to potential problems. Moreover, it is often difficult to find existing data that are ideally suited to answering a research question.

Example of a study using records: Graham and co-researchers (2010) investigated nurses' compliance with discharge risk screening policies, the accuracy of the screening, and factors associated with screening completion by auditing the medical records of 99 acute care patients.

⊃ **TIP:** Researchers' decisions about data collection methods are independent of decisions about research design. Researchers using an experimental design can rely on self-report data—as can a researcher doing an ethnography, for example. The research *question* may dictate which specific data collection method to use, but researchers often have great latitude in designing a data collection plan.

Dimensions of Data Collection Approaches

Data collection methods vary along three key dimensions: structure, researcher obtrusiveness, and objectivity. In planning a study, researchers make decisions about where on these dimensions the data collection methods should fall.

Structure

In structured data collection, information is gathered from participants in a comparable, prespecified way. For example, most self-administered questionnaires are highly structured: They include a fixed set of questions to be answered in a specified sequence and with predesignated response options (e.g., agree or disagree). Structured methods give participants limited opportunities to qualify their answers or to explain the meaning of their responses. By contrast, qualitative studies rely mainly on loosely structured methods of data collection.

There are advantages and disadvantages to both approaches. Structured methods often take considerable effort to develop and refine, but they yield data that are relatively easy to analyze because the data can be readily quantified. Structured methods are seldom appropriate for an in-depth examination of a phenomenon, however. Consider the following two methods of asking people about their levels of stress:

Structured: During the past week, would you say you felt stressed:

1. rarely or none of the time,
2. some or a little of the time,
3. occasionally or a moderate amount of the time, or
4. most or all of the time?

Unstructured: How stressed or anxious have you been this past week? Tell me about the kinds of tensions and stresses you have been experiencing.

Structured questioning would allow researchers to compute what percentage of respondents felt stressed most of the time, but would provide no information about the cause or circumstances of the stress. The unstructured question allows for deeper and more thoughtful responses, but may pose difficulties for people who are not good at expressing themselves. Moreover, the unstructured question yields data that are much more difficult to analyze.

When data are collected in a structured fashion, researchers must develop (or borrow) a data collection **instrument**, which is the formal written document used to collect and record information, such as a questionnaire. When unstructured methods are used, there is typically no formal instrument, although there may be a list of the types of information needed.

Researcher Obtrusiveness

Data collection methods differ in the degree to which people are aware of the data gathering process. If people know they are under scrutiny, their behavior and responses may not be "normal," and distortions can undermine the value of the research. When data are collected unobtrusively, however, ethical problems may emerge, as discussed in Chapter 7.

Study participants are most likely to distort their behavior and their responses to questions under certain circumstances. Researcher obtrusiveness is likely to be most problematic when: (1) a program is being evaluated and participants have a vested interest in the evaluation outcome, (2) participants are engaged in socially unacceptable or unusual behavior, (3) participants have not complied with medical and nursing instructions, and (4) participants are the type of people who have a strong need to "look good." When researcher obtrusiveness is unavoidable under these circumstances, researchers should make an effort to put participants at ease, to stress the importance of candor and naturalistic behavior, and to adopt a neutral and nonjudgmental demeanor.

Objectivity

Objectivity refers to the degree to which two independent researchers can arrive at similar "scores" or make similar observations regarding concepts of interest, that is, make judgments regarding participants' attributes or behavior that are not biased by personal feelings or beliefs. Some data collection approaches require more subjective judgment than others, and some research problems require a higher degree of objectivity than others.

Researchers with a positivist orientation usually strive for a high degree of objectivity. In research based on the constructivist paradigm, however, the subjective judgment of investigators is considered an asset because subjectivity is viewed as essential for understanding human experiences.

Developing a Data Collection Plan

In planning a study, researchers make many decisions about the type and amount of data to collect. The task involves weighing several factors, but the key is to identify the kinds of data that will yield the most accurate, valid, meaningful, and trustworthy information for addressing the research question.

Most researchers face the issue of balancing the need for rich, extensive information against the risk of overburdening participants. In many studies, more data are collected than are needed or analyzed. Although it is better to have adequate data than to have unwanted omissions, minimizing *participant burden* should be an important goal. Careful advance planning is essential to ensure good data coverage without placing undue demands on participants.

In developing a data collection plan, researchers need to give thought to the kind of evidence they want to provide to their colleagues in practice settings. Some concepts are especially well suited to the development of an evidence-based nursing practice. For example, Ingersoll (2005) has identified a number of evidence-based, nurse-sensitive outcome indicators that should be given consideration in designing studies, especially for studies that test the effects of nursing interventions. Examples include health-related quality of life, functional status, risk-reduction behaviors, compliance, and health-promoting behaviors.

Specific guidance on developing a data collection plan is offered later in this book for quantitative studies (Chapter 13) and qualitative studies (Chapter 22).

ORGANIZATION OF A RESEARCH PROJECT

Studies typically take many months to complete and longitudinal studies require years of work. During the planning phase, it is important to make preliminary estimates of how long various tasks will require. This may be easier to accomplish for quantitative studies than for qualitative ones because the former tend to have a more linear progression of pre-specified activities and strategies, but even qualitative studies profit from a tentative schedule.

Almost all studies are conducted under time constraints. Students in research courses have end-of-term deadlines; government-sponsored research involves funds granted for a specified time. Those who do not have formal time limits (e.g., graduate students working on dissertations) have their own goals for project completion. Setting up a timetable in advance may help in meeting such goals. Having deadlines helps to delimit tasks that might otherwise continue indefinitely, such as problem selection and literature reviews.

Chapter 3 presented a sequence of steps that quantitative researchers follow in a study. The steps represented an idealized conception: the research process rarely follows a neatly prescribed sequence of procedures, even in quantitative studies. Developments in one step, for example, may require alterations in a previous activity. Iteration and backtracking are the norm. For example, sample size decisions may require rethinking how many sites are needed. Selection of data collection methods might require changes to how the population is defined, and so on. Nevertheless, preliminary time estimates are valuable. In particular, it is important to have a sense of how much total time the study will require and when it will begin.

◗ TIP: It is not possible to give even approximate figures for the relative percentage of time that should be spent on each task. Some projects need many months to develop and test new instruments, whereas other studies use previously existing ones, for example. Clearly, not all steps are equally time-consuming. It would not make sense simply to divide the available time by the number of tasks.

Researchers sometimes develop visual timelines to help them organize a study. These devices are especially useful if funding is sought because the schedule helps researchers to understand when and for how long staff support (e.g., for transcribing interviews) is needed. This can best be illustrated with an example, in this case of a hypothetical quantitative study.

Suppose a researcher was studying the following problem: Is a woman's decision to have an annual mammogram related to her perceived susceptibility to breast cancer? Using the organization of steps outlined in Chapter 3, here are some of the tasks that might be undertaken:*

1. The researcher is concerned that many older women do not get mammograms regularly. Her specific *research question* is whether mammogram practices are different for women who have different views about their susceptibility to breast cancer.

2. The researcher *reviews the research literature* on breast cancer, mammography use, and factors affecting mammography decisions.

3. The researcher does *clinical fieldwork* by discussing the problem with nurses and other healthcare professionals in various clinical settings (health clinics, private obstetrics and gynecology practices) and by informally discussing the problem with women in a support group for breast cancer patients.

4. The researcher seeks theories and models for her problem. She finds that the Health Belief Model is relevant, and this helps her to develop a *theoretical framework* and a conceptual definition of susceptibility to breast cancer.

5. Based on the framework, the following *hypothesis is developed*: Women who perceive themselves as not susceptible to breast cancer are less likely than other women to get an annual mammogram.

6. The researcher adopts a nonexperimental, cross-sectional, between-subjects *research design*. Her comparison strategy will be to compare women with different rankings on susceptibility to breast cancer. She designs the study to control the confounding variables of age, marital status, and health insurance status. Her research site will be Los Angeles.

7. There is no *intervention* in this study (the design is nonexperimental) and so this step is unnecessary.

8. The researcher designates that the *population* of interest is women between the ages of 50 and 65 years living in Los Angeles who have not been previously diagnosed as having any form of cancer.

9. The researcher will recruit 250 women living in Los Angeles as her *research sample*; they are identified at random using a telephone procedure known as random-digit dialing, so she does not need to gain entrée into any institution or organization.

10. *Research variables will be measured* by self-report; that is, the independent variable (perceived susceptibility), dependent variable (mammogram history), and confounding variables will be measured by asking participants a series of questions. The researcher will use existing measuring instruments, rather than developing new ones.

11. The IRB at the researcher's institution is asked to review the plans to ensure that the study *adheres to ethical standards*.

12. *Plans for the study are finalized*: The methods are reviewed and refined by colleagues with clinical and methodologic expertise and by the IRB, the data collection instruments are pretested, and interviewers who will collect the data are trained.

13. *Data are collected* by conducting telephone interviews with the research sample.

14. *Data are prepared for analysis* by coding them and entering them onto a computer file.

15. *Data are analyzed* using a statistical software package.

16. The results indicate that the hypothesis is supported; however, the researcher's *interpretation* must take into consideration that many women who were asked to participate declined to do so.

---

*This is only a partial list of tasks and is designed to illustrate the flow of activities; the flow in this example is more orderly than would ordinarily be true.

17. The researcher presents an early report on her findings and interpretations at a conference of Sigma Theta Tau International. She subsequently publishes the report in the *Western Journal of Nursing Research.*

18. The researcher seeks out clinicians to discuss how the study findings can be *utilized in practice.*

The researcher plans to conduct this study over a 2-year period, and Figure 8.3 presents a hypothetical schedule. Many steps overlap or are undertaken concurrently; some steps are projected to involve little time, whereas others require months of work. (The Toolkit section of the accompanying *Resource Manual* includes the timeline in Figure 8.3 as a Word document for you to adapt for your study). ✖

In developing a time schedule, several considerations should be kept in mind, including researchers' level of knowledge and methodologic competence. Resources available to researchers, in terms of research funds and personnel, greatly influence time estimates. In the present example, if the researcher needed funding to help pay for the cost of hiring interviewers, the timeline would need to be expanded to accommodate the period required to prepare a proposal and await the funding decision.

It is also important to consider the practical aspects of performing the study, which were not enumerated in the preceding section. Obtaining supplies, securing permissions, getting approval for using forms or instruments, hiring staff, and holding meetings are all time-consuming, but necessary, activities.

Calendar Months:	1	2	3	4	5	6	7	8	9	10	11	12	13	14	15	16	17	18	19	20	21	22	23	24
Conceptual Phase																								
1. Problem identification	→																							
2. Literature review	→	→																						
3. Clinical fieldwork	→																							
4. Theoretical framework	→	→																						
5. Hypothesis formulation			→																					
Design/Planning Phase																								
6. Research design				→	→																			
7. Intervention protocols (NA)																								
8. Population specification				→	→																			
9. Sampling plan					→	→																		
10. Data collection plan					→	→																		
11. Ethics procedures						→	→																	
12. Finalization of plans					→	→	→																	
Empirical Phase																								
13. Collection of data										→	→	→	→	→										
14. Data preparation										→	→	→	→											
Analytic Phase																								
15. Data analysis															→	→	→							
16. Interpretation of results															→	→	→							
Dissemination Phase																								
17. Presentations/reports																			→	→	→	→	→	→
18. Utilization of findings																			→	→	→	→	→	→
Calendar Months:	1	2	3	4	5	6	7	8	9	10	11	12	13	14	15	16	17	18	19	20	21	22	23	24

FIGURE 8.3 ✖ Project timeline (in months) for a hypothetical study of women's mammography decisions.

Individuals differ in the kinds of tasks that appeal to them. Some people enjoy the preliminary phase, which has a strong intellectual component, whereas others are more eager to collect the data, a task that is more interpersonal. Researchers should, however, allocate a reasonable amount of time to do justice to each activity.

⊃ **TIP:** Getting organized for a study has many dimensions beyond having a timeline. One especially important issue concerns having the right team and mix of skills for a research project, and developing plans for hiring and monitoring research staff (Kang et al., 2005; Nelson & Morrison-Beedy, 2008). We discuss research teams in connection with proposal development (Chapter 29).

PILOT STUDIES

A consistent conclusion in systematic reviews is that the quality of evidence on problems of relevance to nursing and healthcare is less than optimal. This means that "best evidence" available for nursing practice is seldom the best evidence possible. There is a growing recognition that it takes a lot of skill and effort to do research that has strong evidentiary value.

Researchers sometimes incorporate a pilot study into their plans. A **pilot study** is a small-scale version or trial run designed to test the methods to be used in a larger, more rigorous study. Pilot studies are not just studies with a small number of participants, nor are they small, exploratory studies. The focus of pilot studies is not substantive in that their primary purpose is not to answer research questions. The purpose of a pilot study is to prevent an expensive fiasco—that is, a costly but flawed large-scale study. For this reason, pilot studies are sometimes called **feasibility studies**.

⊃ **TIP:** Many studies in the nursing research literature are called pilots when, in fact, they appear to be small-scale exploratory efforts, often with numerous methodologic flaws. Avoid using the term *pilot study* unless you truly plan to use lessons from the pilot to assess the feasibility of developing a stronger, larger investigation on the same topic.

Pilot studies can serve a number of important functions in planning a rigorous larger study, including evaluation of the following:

- Adequacy of study methods and procedures
- Likely success of a participant recruitment strategy
- Appropriateness and quality of instruments
- Strength of relationships between key variables so that the number of needed study participants can be estimated
- Identification of confounding variables that need to be controlled
- Adequacy of training materials for research staff
- Potential problems, such as loss of participants during the course of the study
- Extent to which the preliminary evidence justifies more rigorous research
- Project costs for budgeting purposes

Pilot studies play an especially important role in research involving new interventions—a topic we discuss in greater detail in Chapter 26. In intervention research, the pilot is a test of not only the research methods, but also of the intervention itself, providing opportunities for refining and improving it. The pilot can also offer insights into the feasibility of implementing the intervention in real-world settings. Data from pilot testing an intervention can shed light on a number of things, including the following:

- The acceptability of the intervention to intended beneficiaries (e.g., patients), intervention agents (e.g., nurses), and administrators
- The adequacy, comprehensiveness, and clarity of intervention protocols
- The appropriateness of the "dose" of the intervention
- The extent to which *intervention fidelity* can be maintained (i.e., the faithfulness with which the protocols are actually adhered to)
- The rate of retention in the intervention
- The safety of the intervention, and any unforeseen side effects it might yield

In summary, the outcomes of a pilot study are *lessons* that can inform subsequent efforts to generate valid evidence for nursing practice. Thus, in planning a study, it is wise to consider the many possible benefits of undertaking a pilot.

➲ **TIP:** Researchers usually should not seek funding for a full-fledged intervention study until they have completed pilot work and can describe the lessons learned.

CRITIQUING PLANNING ASPECTS OF A STUDY

Researchers typically do not reveal much about the planning process or about problems that arose during the course of a study. Thus, there is typically little that a reader can do to critique the researcher's planning efforts. What *can* be critiqued, of course, are the outcomes of the planning—that is, the actual methodologic decisions themselves. Guidelines for critiquing those decisions are provided in subsequent chapters of this book.

There are, however, a few things that readers can be alert to relating to the planning of a study. First, evidence of careful conceptualization provides a clue that the project was well planned. If a conceptual map is presented (or implied) in the report, it means that the researcher had a "road map" that facilitated planning.

Second, readers can consider whether the researcher's plans reflect adequate attention to concerns about EBP. For example, was the comparison group strategy designed to reflect a realistic practice concern? Was the setting one that maximizes potential for the generalizability of the findings? Did the timeframes for data collection correspond to clinically important milestones? Was the intervention sensitive to the constraints of a typical practice environment?

Finally, confidence in the efficacy of study planning can be strengthened by evidence that the researcher devoted sufficient time and resources in preparing for the study. For example, if the report indicates that the study was preceded by a pilot test, this suggests that some "bugs" were probably worked out. If the report indicates that the study grew out of earlier research on a similar topic, or

that the researcher had previously used the same instruments, or had completed other studies in the same setting, this also suggests that the researcher was not plunging into unfamiliar waters. Unrealistic planning can sometimes be inferred from a discussion of sample recruitment. If the report indicates that the researcher was unable to recruit the originally hoped-for number of participants, or if recruitment took months longer than anticipated, this suggests that the researcher may not have done adequate homework during the planning phase.

RESEARCH EXAMPLE

In this section, we describe the outcomes of a pilot study for a larger intervention study.

Study: Tales from the field: What the nursing research textbooks will not tell you (Smith et al., 2008)

Purpose: The purpose of the article was to describe some of the setbacks and lessons learned in a pilot for an intervention study designed to test a multiphase management strategy for persons with dementia.

Pilot Study Methods: The researchers undertook a 1-year pilot study in the first phase of a multiyear project. The purpose of the pilot was to assess and refine data collection methods and procedures, review recruitment strategies and criteria used to select participants, evaluate the acceptability of the screening and outcome measures, and gather information for improving the intervention. The plan was to recruit and assess 20 people with probable or possible Alzheimer's disease living in assisted living facilities (ALF).

Pilot Study Findings: The researchers were faced with numerous challenges and setbacks in their pilot effort. Passive methods of recruiting family members, who were needed for signing consent (placing posters and informational handouts in ALFs) yielded no participants, so other strategies had to be developed. Eventually, 17 participants were enrolled, but not a single one met the stringent criteria for inclusion in the study that the researchers had originally developed. Data collection took longer than anticipated. Staff at the ALF facilities were not always cooperative. Problems with obtaining IRB approval resulted in months of delay.

Conclusions: The researchers found that "the information learned was quite valuable and was used to shape changes in subsequent research" (p. 235). They noted the value of undertaking pilot work and of doing a systematic analysis about midway through the pilot. Other recommendations included doing good upfront assessments of study sites, allowing plenty of time for revisions for the IRB, and having a "Plan B" when things go awry.

SUMMARY POINTS

- Researchers face numerous conceptual, practical, ethical, and methodologic challenges in planning a study. The major methodologic challenge is designing a study that is reliable and valid (quantitative studies) or trustworthy (qualitative studies).
- **Reliability** refers to the accuracy and consistency of information obtained in a study. **Validity** is a more complex concept that broadly concerns the *soundness* of the study's evidence—that is, whether the findings are cogent, convincing, and well grounded.
- **Trustworthiness** in qualitative research encompasses several different dimensions. **Dependability** refers to evidence that is believable, consistent, and stable over time. **Confirmability** refers to evidence of the researcher's objectivity. **Credibility** is achieved to the extent that the research methods engender confidence in the truth of the data and in the researchers' interpretations.
- **Triangulation**, the use of multiple sources or referents to draw conclusions about what constitutes the truth, is one approach to establishing credibility.
- A **bias** is an influence that distorts study results. **Systematic bias** results when a bias is consistent across particular subgroups of participants or in particular situations and operates in a consistent direction.
- In quantitative studies, **research control** is used to **hold constant** outside influences on the dependent variable so that its relationship to the independent variable can be better understood. Researchers use various strategies to control **confounding** (or **extraneous**) **variables**, which are extraneous to the study purpose and can obscure understanding.

- In quantitative studies, a powerful tool to eliminate bias is **randomness**—having certain features of the study established by chance rather than by design or personal preference.
- **Reflexivity**, the process of reflecting critically on the self and of scrutinizing personal values that could affect interpretation, is an important tool in qualitative research.
- **Generalizability** in a quantitative study concerns the extent to which findings can be generalized and applied to other groups and settings. **Transferability** is the extent to which qualitative findings are meaningful and can be transferred to other settings.
- In planning a study, researchers make many design decisions, including whether to have an intervention, how to control confounding variables, what type of comparisons will be made, where the study will take place, and what the timeframes of the study will be.
- Quantitative researchers often incorporate comparisons into their designs to enhance interpretability. In **between-subjects designs**, different groups of people are compared. **Within-subjects designs** involve comparisons of the same people at different times or in different circumstances. In **mixed designs** researchers can compare two or more groups at fixed points in time, and can also compare people within groups across time.
- Site selection for a study often requires **site visits** to evaluate suitability and feasibility. Gaining entrée into a site involves developing and maintaining trust with gatekeepers.
- **Cross-sectional designs** involve collecting data at one point in time, whereas **longitudinal designs** involve data collection two or more times over an extended period.
- **Trend studies** have multiple points of data collection with different samples from the same population. **Panel studies** gather data from the same people, usually from a general population, more than once. In a **follow-up study**, data are gathered two or more times from a more well-defined group (e.g., those with a particular health problem). In a **cohort study**, a cohort of people is tracked over time to see if subsets with

different exposures to risk factors differ in terms of subsequent outcomes.

- A **repeated measures design** typically involves collecting data three or more times, either in a longitudinal fashion or in rapid succession over a shorter timeframe.
- Longitudinal studies are typically expensive, time-consuming, and at risk of **attrition** (loss of participants over time), but are essential for illuminating time-related phenomena.
- Researchers also develop a **data collection plan**. In nursing, the most widely used methods are self-report, observation, biophysiologic measures, and existing records.
- **Self-report** data are obtained by directly questioning people about phenomena of interest. Self-reports are versatile and powerful but a drawback is the potential for respondents' deliberate or inadvertent misrepresentations.
- A wide variety of human activity and traits is amenable to **direct observation**. However, observation is subject to **observer biases** and distorted participant behavior (**reactivity**).
- **Biophysiologic measures** tend to yield high-quality data that are objective and valid, and often cost-efficient for nurse researchers.
- Existing **records** and documents are an economical source of research data, but two potential biases in records are **selective deposit** and **selective survival**.
- Data collection methods vary in terms of structure, researcher obtrusiveness, and objectivity, and researchers must make decisions about these dimensions in their plan.
- A **pilot** (or **feasibility**) **study** is a small-scale trial run designed to test methods to be used in a larger, more rigorous study. Pilot studies provide invaluable *lessons* that can enhance the quality of evidence the larger study can yield.

●◉●◉●◉●◉●◉●◉●◉●◉●◉●◉●◉●◉●

STUDY ACTIVITIES

Chapter 8 of the *Resource Manual for Nursing Research: Generating and Assessing Evidence for Nursing Practice, 9th ed.*, offers study suggestions for reinforcing concepts presented in this chapter. In addition, the following questions can be addressed in classroom or online discussions:

1. Find a study published in a nursing journal in 2000 or earlier that is described as a pilot study. Do you think the study really is a pilot study, or do you think this label was used inappropriately? Search forward for a larger subsequent study to evaluate your response.
2. Suppose you wanted to study how children's attitudes toward smoking change over time. Design a cross-sectional study to research this question, specifying the samples that you would want to include. Now, design a longitudinal study to research the same problem. Identify the strengths and weaknesses of each approach.

●◉●◉●◉●◉●◉●◉●◉●◉●◉●◉●◉●◉●

STUDIES CITED IN CHAPTER 8

Ahlström, B., Skärsäter, I., & Danielson, E. (2010). The meaning of major depression in family life: The viewpoint of the ill parent. *Journal of Clinical Nursing, 19*, 284–293.

Atkins, R., & Hart, D. (2008). The under-controlled do it first: Childhood personality and sexual debut. *Research in Nursing & Health, 31*, 626–639.

Collins, M., Shattell, M., & Thomas, S. P. (2005). Problematic interviewee behaviors in qualitative research. *Western Journal of Nursing Research, 27*, 188–199.

DiIorio, C., McCarty, F., Denzmore, P., & Landis, A. (2007). The moderating influence of mother-adolescent discussion on early and middle African American adolescent sexual behavior. *Research in Nursing & Health, 30*, 193–202.

Graham, J., Gallagher, R., & Bothe, J. (2010). Early completion of the discharge risk screen by nurses in acute care wards. *Journal of Nursing Care Quality, 25*, 80–86.

Holliday-Welsh, D., Gessert, C., & Renier, C. (2009). Massage in the management of agitation in nursing home residents with cognitive impairment. *Geriatric Nursing, 30*, 108–117.

King, K., Colella, T., Faris, P., & Thompson, D. (2009). Using the cardiac depression scale in men recovering from coronary artery bypass surgery. *Journal of Clinical Nursing, 18*, 1617–1624.

King, K., Gerich, J., Guzick, D., King, K., & McDermott, M. (2009). Is a history of gestational diabetes related to risk factors for coronary heart disease? *Research in Nursing & Health, 32*, 298–306.

Lindsay-Waters, A. (2008). An ethnography of a children's renal unit: Experiences of children and young people with long-term renal illness. *Journal of Clinical Nursing, 17*, 3103–3114.

Martinsen, B., Harder, I., & Biering-Sorensen, F. (2009). Sensitive cooperation: A basis for assisted feeding. *Journal of Clinical Nursing, 18*, 708–715.

Mishel, M., Germino, B., Lin, L., Pruthi, R., Wallen, E., Crandell, J., & Blyler, D. (2009). Managing uncertainty about treatment decision-making in early stage prostate cancer: A randomized clinical trial. *Patient Education & Counseling, 77*, 349–359.

Ray, S. L. (2009). The experience of contemporary peacekeepers healing from trauma. *Nursing Inquiry, 16*, 53–63.

Roe, B., Howell, F., Riniotis, K., Beech, R., Crome, P., & Ong, B. (2009). Older people and falls: Health status, quality of life, lifestyle, care networks, prevention and views on service use following a recent fall. *Journal of Clinical Nursing, 18*, 2261–2272.

Small, L., Anderson, D., Sidora-Arcoleo, K., & Gance-Cleveland, B. (2009). Pediatric nurse-practitioners' assessment and management of childhood overweight/obesity: Results from 1999 and 2005 cohort surveys. *Journal of Pediatric Health Care, 23*, 231–241.

Smith, M., Buckwalter, K., Kang, H., Schultz, S., & Ellingrod, V. (2008). Tales from the field: What the nursing research textbooks will not tell you. *Applied Nursing Research, 21*, 232–236.

Tang, W., Yu, C., & Yeh, S. (2010). Fatigue and its related factors in patients with chronic heart failure. *Journal of Clinical Nursing, 19*, 69–78.

White, M., & Groh, C. (2007). Depression and quality of life in women after a myocardial infarction. *Journal of Cardiovascular Nursing, 22*, 138–144.

Woodgate, R. (2009). The experience of dyspnea in school-age children with asthma. *MCN: The American Journal of Maternal Child Nursing, 34*, 154–161.

Methodologic and nonresearch references cited in this chapter can be found in a separate section at the end of the book.

PART 3

DESIGNING AND CONDUCTING QUANTITATIVE STUDIES TO GENERATE EVIDENCE FOR NURSING

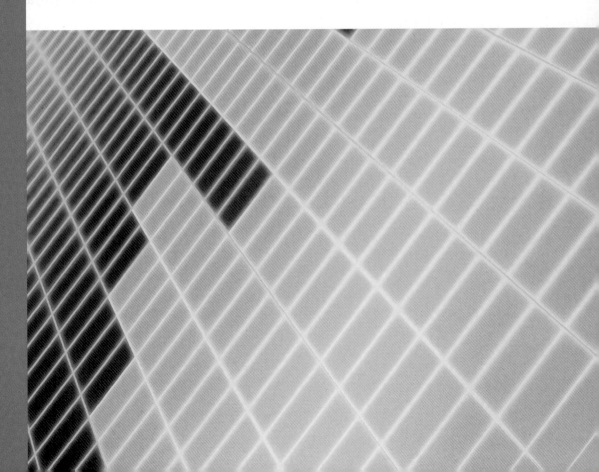

9

Quantitative Research Design

GENERAL DESIGN ISSUES

Part 3 of this book (Chapters 9 through 19) focuses on methods of doing quantitative research.

This chapter describes options for designing quantitative studies. We begin by discussing several broad issues.

Causality

As noted in Chapter 2, several broad categories of research questions are relevant to evidence-based nursing practice—questions about interventions, diagnosis and assessment, prognosis, etiology and harm, and meaning or process (Table 2.1). Questions about meaning or process call for a qualitative approach, which we describe in Chapter 20. Questions about diagnosis or assessment, as well as questions about the status quo of health-related situations, are typically descriptive. Many research questions, however, are about *causes* and *effects*:

- Does a telephone therapy intervention for patients diagnosed with prostate cancer *cause* improvements in their decision-making skills? (intervention question)

- Do birthweights under 1,500 grams *cause* developmental delays in children? (prognosis question)
- Does cigarette smoking *cause* lung cancer? (etiology/harm question)

Although causality is a hotly debated philosophical issue, we all understand the general concept of a **cause**. For example, we understand that failure to sleep *causes* fatigue and that high-caloric intake *causes* weight gain.

Most phenomena have multiple causes. Weight gain, for example, can be the effect of high-caloric consumption, but other factors also cause weight gain. Causes of health-related phenomena usually are not *deterministic*, but rather *probabilistic*—that is, the causes increase the probability that an effect will occur. For example, there is ample evidence that smoking is a cause of lung cancer, but not everyone who smokes develops lung cancer, and not everyone with lung cancer was a smoker.

The Counterfactual Model

While it might be easy to grasp what researchers have in mind when they talk about a *cause,* what exactly is an **effect**? Shadish and colleagues (2002), who wrote a widely acclaimed book on research design and causal inference, explained that a good way to grasp the meaning of an effect is by conceptualizing a counterfactual. In a research context, a **counterfactual** is what would have happened *to the same people* exposed to a causal factor if they *simultaneously* were *not* exposed to the causal factor. An effect represents the difference between what actually did happen with the exposure and what would have happened without it. This counterfactual model is an idealized conception that can never be realized, but it is a good model to keep in mind in designing a study to provide cause-and-effect evidence. As Shadish and colleagues (2002) noted, "A central task for all cause-probing research is to create reasonable approximations to this physically impossible counterfactual" (p. 5).

Criteria for Causality

Several writers have proposed criteria for establishing a cause-and-effect relationship. Lazarsfeld (1955), reflecting ideas of John Stuart Mill, identified three criteria for causality. The first is *temporal*: A cause must precede an effect in time. If we were testing the hypothesis that aspertame causes fetal abnormalities, it would be necessary to demonstrate that the abnormalities did not develop before the mothers' exposure to aspertame. The second requirement is that there be an *empirical relationship* between the presumed cause and the presumed effect. In the aspertame example, we would have to find an association between aspertame consumption and fetal abnormalities, that is, that a higher percentage of aspertame users than nonusers had infants with fetal abnormalities. The final criterion for inferring causality is that the relationship cannot be explained as being *caused by a third variable*. Suppose, for instance, that people who used aspertame tended also to drink more coffee than nonusers of aspertame. There would then be a possibility that any relationship between maternal aspertame use and fetal abnormalities reflects an underlying causal relationship between a substance in coffee and the abnormalities.

Additional criteria were proposed by Bradford-Hill (1971) as part of the discussion about the causal link between smoking and lung cancer. Two of Bradford-Hill's criteria foreshadow the importance of meta-analyses, techniques for which had not been fully developed when the criteria were

proposed. The criterion of *coherence* involves having similar evidence from multiple sources, and the criterion of *consistency* involves having similar levels of statistical relationship in several studies. Another important criterion is *biologic plausibility*, that is, evidence from laboratory or basic physiologic studies that a causal pathway is credible.

Researchers investigating causal relationships must provide persuasive evidence about these criteria through their study design. Some designs are better at revealing cause-and-effect relationships than others, but not all research questions can be answered using the strongest designs because of ethical or practical constraints. Much of this chapter concerns designs for illuminating causal relationships.

Design Terminology

It is easy to get confused about terms used for research designs because there is inconsistency among writers. Moreover, design terms used by medical and epidemiologic researchers are usually different from those used by social scientists. Many early nurse researchers got their research training in social science fields such as psychology or sociology before doctoral-level training became available in schools of nursing, and so social scientific design terms have predominated in the nursing research literature.

Nurses interested in establishing an evidence-based practice must to be able to understand studies from many disciplines. We use both medical and social science terms in this book, although the latter predominate. Table 9.1 provides a list of several design terms used by social scientists and the corresponding terms used by medical researchers.

EXPERIMENTAL DESIGN

A basic distinction in quantitative research design is between experimental and nonexperimental research. In an **experiment** (or **randomized controlled trial, RCT**), researchers are active agents,

TABLE 9.1	Research Design Terminology in the Social Scientific and Medical Literature
SOCIAL SCIENTIFIC TERM	**MEDICAL RESEARCH TERM**
Experiment, true experiment, experimental study	Randomized controlled trial, randomized clinical trial, RCT
Quasi-experiment, quasi-experimental study	Controlled trial, controlled trial without randomization
Nonexperimental study, correlational study	Observational study
Retrospective study	Case-control study
Prospective nonexperimental study	Cohort study
Group or condition (e.g., experimental or control group/condition)	Group or arm (e.g., intervention or control arm)
Experimental group	Treatment or intervention group

not passive observers. Early physical scientists learned that although pure observation of phenomena is valuable, complexities occurring in nature often made it difficult to understand relationships. This problem was addressed by isolating phenomena in a laboratory and controlling the conditions under which they occurred. Procedures developed by physical scientists were profitably adopted by biologists during the 19th century, resulting in many achievements in physiology and medicine. The 20th century witnessed the increased use of experimental methods by researchers interested in human behavior.

The controlled experiment is considered to be the gold standard for yielding reliable evidence about causes and effects. Experimenters can be relatively confident in the genuineness of causal relationships because they are observed under controlled conditions and typically meet the criteria for establishing causality. As we pointed out in Chapter 4, hypotheses are never proved or disproved by scientific methods, but true experiments offer the most convincing evidence about the effect one variable has on another.

A true experimental or RCT design is characterized by the following properties:

- *Manipulation:* The researcher *does* something to at least some participants—that is, there is some type of intervention.
- *Control:* The researcher introduces controls over the experimental situation, including devising an approximation of a counterfactual—usually, a control group that does not receive the intervention.
- *Randomization*: The researcher assigns participants to a control or experimental condition on a random basis.

Design Features of True Experiments

Researchers have many options in designing an experiment. We begin by discussing several features of experimental designs.

Manipulation: The Experimental Intervention

Manipulation involves *doing* something to study participants. Experimenters manipulate the independent variable by administering a **treatment** (**intervention**) to some people and withholding it from others, or administering a different treatment. Experimenters deliberately *vary* the independent variable (the presumed cause) and observe the effect on the outcome.

For example, suppose we hypothesized that gentle massage is an effective pain relief strategy for nursing home residents. The independent variable, receipt of gentle massage, can be manipulated by giving some patients the massage intervention and withholding it from others. We would then compare pain levels (the dependent variable) in the two groups to see if differences in receipt of the intervention resulted in differences in average pain levels.

In designing RCTs, researchers make many decisions about what the experimental condition entails, and these decisions can affect the conclusions. To get a fair test, the intervention should be appropriate to the problem, consistent with a theoretical rationale, and of sufficient intensity and duration that effects might reasonably be expected. The full nature of the intervention must be delineated in formal protocols that spell out exactly what the treatment is. Among the questions researchers need to address are the following:

- What *is* the intervention, and how does it differ from usual methods of care?
- What specific procedures are to be used with those receiving the intervention?
- What is the dosage or intensity of the intervention?
- Over how long a period will the intervention be administered, how frequently will it be administered, and when will the treatment begin (e.g., 2 hours after surgery)?
- Who will administer the intervention? What are their credentials, and what type of special training will they receive?
- Under what conditions will the intervention be withdrawn or altered?

The goal in most RCTs is to have an identical intervention for all people in the treatment group. For example, in most drug studies, those in the experimental group are given the exact same ingredient, in the same dose, administered in exactly the same manner—all according to well-articulated protocols. There is, however, growing interest in **patient-centered interventions** or **PCIs** (Lauver et al.,

2002). The purpose of PCIs is to enhance treatment efficacy by taking people's characteristics or needs into account. In tailored interventions, each person receives an intervention customized to certain characteristics, such as demographic characteristics (e.g., gender), cognitive factors (e.g., reading level), or affective factors (e.g., motivation). Interventions based on the Transtheoretical (stages of change) Model (Chapter 6) usually are PCIs, because the intervention is tailored to fit people's readiness to change their behavior. There is some evidence that tailored interventions are more effective than standardized interventions (e.g., Lauver et al., 2003). More research in this area is needed, however, and such research is likely to play an important role in our current evidence-based practice environment in which there is a strong interest in understanding not only *what* works, but what works for *whom*.

➲ TIP: Although PCIs are not universally standardized, they are typically administered according to well-defined procedures and guidelines, and the intervention agents are carefully trained in making decisions about who should get what type of treatment.

Manipulation: The Control Condition

Evidence about relationships requires making at least one comparison. If we were to supplement the diet of premature infants with a special nutrient for 2 weeks, their weight at the end of 2 weeks would tell us nothing about treatment effectiveness. At a bare minimum, we would need to compare posttreatment weight with pretreatment weight to determine if, at least, their weight had increased. But, let us assume that we find an average weight gain of 1 pound. Does this gain support the conclusion that the nutrition supplement (the independent variable) caused weight gain (the dependent variable)? No, it does not. Babies normally gain weight as they mature. Without a control group—a group that does *not* receive the supplement—it is impossible to separate the effects of maturation from those of the treatment.

The term **control group** refers to a group of participants whose performance on an outcome is used to evaluate that of the treatment group on the same outcome. As noted in Table 9.1, researchers with training from a social science tradition use the term "group" or "condition" (e.g., the experimental group or the control condition), but medical researchers often use the term "arm," as in the intervention arm or the control arm of the study.

The control condition is a proxy for an ideal counterfactual. Researchers have choices about what to use as the counterfactual. Their decision is sometimes based on theoretical or substantive grounds, but may be driven by practical or ethical concerns. In some research, control group members receive no treatment at all—they are merely observed with respect to performance on the outcome. This type of control condition is not usually feasible in nursing research. For example, if we wanted to evaluate the effectiveness of a nursing intervention for hospital patients, we would not devise an RCT in which patients in the control group received no nursing care at all. Among the possibilities for the counterfactual are the following:

1. An alternative intervention; for example, participants could receive two different types of distraction as alternative therapies for pain.
2. A **placebo** or pseudointervention presumed to have no therapeutic value; for example, in studies of the effectiveness of drugs, some patients get the experimental drug and others get an innocuous substance. Placebos are used to control for the nonpharmaceutical effects of drugs, such as the attention being paid to participants. (There can, however, be **placebo effects**—changes in the dependent variable attributable to the placebo condition—because of participants' expectations of benefits or harms).

Example of a placebo control group: In a study of the effect of sucrose on infant pain responses during routine immunizations, Hatfield (2008) randomly assigned infants to groups administered either a sucrose solution or sterile water.

3. Standard methods of care—the usual procedures used to care for patients. This is the most typical control condition in nursing studies.
4. Different doses or intensities of treatment wherein all participants get some type of intervention, but the experimental group gets

an intervention that is richer, more intense, or longer. This approach is attractive when there is a desire to analyze **dose-response effects**, that is, to test whether larger doses are associated with larger benefits, or whether a smaller (and perhaps less costly or burdensome) dose would suffice.

Example of different dose groups: Martinez and colleagues (2009) used an experimental design to test the relative effect of three "doses" of a walking intervention for patients with peripheral arterial disease. Participants were randomly assigned to a walking program lasting 2 to 9 weeks, 10 to 14 weeks, or 15 to 94 weeks.

5. **Wait-list control group**, with delayed treatment; the control group eventually receives the full experimental intervention, after all research outcomes are assessed.

Example of a wait-list control group: Heidrich and colleagues (2009) assessed the efficacy of an individualized intervention to improve symptom management in older breast cancer survivors. In one of their pilot studies, participants were assigned at random to the treatment condition or to a wait-list control group.

Methodologically, the best test is between two conditions that are as different as possible, as when the experimental group gets a strong treatment and the control group gets no treatment. Ethically, the most appealing counterfactual is probably the delay of treatment approach (number 5), which may be hard to do pragmatically. Testing two competing interventions (number 1) also has ethical appeal, but the risk is that the results will be inconclusive because it is difficult to detect differential effects if both interventions are at least moderately effective.

Some researchers combine two or more comparison strategies. For example, they might test two alternative treatments (option 1) against a placebo (option 3). Another option is to compare an intervention, a placebo, and no treatment. The use of multiple comparison groups is often attractive but, of course, adds to the cost and complexity of the study.

Example of a three-group design: Nikolajsen and colleagues (2009) randomly assigned patients undergoing placement of a femoral nerve block to one of three groups: two alternative intervention groups (audiovisual stimulation versus audio stimulation) or a "usual care" control group. Differences in pain were then assessed.

Sometimes researchers include an **attention control group** when they want to rule out the possibility that intervention effects are caused by the special attention given to those receiving the intervention, rather than by the actual treatment content. The idea is to separate the "active ingredients" of the treatment from the "inactive ingredients" of special attention.

Example of an attention control group: Seers and colleagues (2008) studied the effectiveness of relaxation for reducing postoperative pain and anxiety in orthopedic surgery patients. The design involved four groups—total body relaxation, jaw relaxation, attention control, and usual care control. Those in the attention control group received usual care, plus extra attention by being asked to describe what they do, feel, and think when they are in pain.

The control group decision should be based on an underlying conceptualization of how the intervention might "cause" the intended effect, and should also reflect consideration of what it is that needs to be controlled. For example, if attention control groups are being considered, there should be an underlying conceptualization of the construct of "attention" (Gross, 2005).

Whatever decision is made about a control group strategy, researchers need to be as careful in spelling out the counterfactual as in delineating the intervention. In research reports, researchers sometimes say that the control group got "usual methods of care" without explaining what that condition was and how different it was from the intervention being tested. In drawing on an evidence base for practice, nurses need to understand exactly what happened to study participants in different conditions. Barkauskas and colleagues (2005) and Shadish and colleagues (2002) offer useful advice about developing a control group strategy.

Randomization

Randomization (also called **random assignment** or **random allocation**) involves assigning participants to treatment conditions at random. *Random* means that everyone has an equal chance of being assigned to any group. If people are placed in groups randomly, there is no systematic bias in the groups with respect to preintervention attributes that could affect outcome variables.

Randomization Principles. The overall purpose of random assignment is to approximate the ideal—but impossible—counterfactual of having the same people in multiple treatment groups simultaneously. For example, suppose we wanted to study the effectiveness of a contraceptive counseling program for multiparous women who have just given birth. Two groups of women are included—one will be counseled and the other will not. Women in the sample are likely to differ from one another in many ways, such as age, marital status, financial situation, and the like. Any of these characteristics could affect a woman's diligence in practicing contraception, independent of whether she receives counseling. We need to have the "counsel" and "no counsel" groups equal with respect to these confounding characteristics to assess the impact of counseling on subsequent pregnancies. A counterfactual group needs to be equivalent, to the fullest extent possible, to the intervention group. Random assignment of people to one group or the other is designed to perform this equalization function. One method might be to flip a coin (more elaborate procedures are discussed later). If the coin comes up "heads," a participant would be assigned to one group; if it comes up "tails," she would be assigned to the other group.

Although randomization is the preferred method for equalizing groups, there is no *guarantee* that the groups will be equal. As an example, suppose the study sample involves 10 women who have given birth to 4 or more children. Five of the 10 women are aged 35 years or older, and the remaining 5 are younger than age 35. We would expect random assignment to result in two or three women from the two age ranges in each group. But suppose that, by chance, the older five women all ended up in the counseling group.

These women, who are nearing the end of childbearing years, have a lower likelihood of conceiving. Thus, follow-up of their subsequent childbearing might suggest that the counseling program was effective in reducing subsequent pregnancies; yet, a higher birth rate in the control group may reflect age and fecundity differences, not lack of exposure to counseling.

Despite this possibility, randomization is the most trustworthy method of equalizing groups. Unusual or deviant assignments such as this one are rare, and the likelihood of getting markedly unequal groups is reduced as the sample size increases.

You may wonder why we do not consciously control characteristics that are likely to affect the outcome through matching (Chapter 8). For example, if matching were used in the contraceptive counseling study, we could ensure that if there were a married, 38-year-old woman with six children in the experimental group, there would be a married, 38-year-old woman with six children in the control group. There are two problems with matching, however. First, to match effectively, we must know the characteristics that are likely to affect the outcome, but this knowledge is not always available. Second, even if we knew the relevant traits, the complications of matching on more than two or three characteristics simultaneously are prohibitive. With random assignment, *all* personal characteristics—age, income, intelligence, religiosity, and so on—are likely to be equally distributed in all groups. Over the long run, the groups tend to be counterbalanced with respect to an infinite number of biologic, psychological, economic, and social traits.

Basic Randomization. To demonstrate how random assignment is performed, we turn to another example. Suppose we were testing two alternative interventions to lower the anxiety of children who are about to undergo tonsillectomy. One intervention involves giving structured information about the surgical team's activities (procedural information); the other involves structured information about what the child will feel (sensation information). A third control group receives no special intervention. With a sample of 15 children, five will be randomly assigned to each group.

Researchers can use a **table of random numbers** to randomize. A small portion of such a table is shown in Table 9.2. In a table of random numbers, any digit from 0 to 9 is equally likely to follow any other digit. Going in any direction from any point in the table produces a random sequence.

In our example, we would number the 15 children from 1 to 15, as shown in column 2 of Table 9.3, and then draw numbers between 01 and 15 from the random number table. To find a random starting point, you can close your eyes and let your finger fall at some point on the table. For this example, assume that our starting point is at number 52, bolded in Table 9.2. We can move in any direction from that point, selecting numbers that fall between 01 and 15. Let us move to the right, looking at two-digit combinations. The number to the right of 52 is 06. The person whose number is 06, Nathan O., is assigned to group I. Moving along, the next number within our range is 11. (To find numbers in the desired range, we bypass numbers between 16 and 99.) Alaine J., whose number is 11, is also assigned to group I. The next three numbers are 01, 15, and 14. Thus, Kristina N., Chris L., and Paul M. are assigned to group I. The next five numbers between 01 and 15 in the table are used to assign five children to group II, and the remaining five are put into group III. Note that numbers that have already been used often reappear in the table before the task is completed. For example, the number 15 appeared four times during this randomization. This is normal because the numbers are random.

We can look at the three groups to see if they are equal for one readily discernible trait, gender. We started out with eight girls and seven boys. As Table 9.4 shows, randomization did a good job of allocating boys and girls about equally across the three groups. We must accept on faith the probability that other characteristics (e.g., race, age, initial anxiety) are also well distributed in the randomized groups. The larger the sample, the stronger the likelihood that the groups will be comparable across all factors that could affect the outcomes.

Researchers usually assign participants proportionately to groups being compared. For example, a sample of 300 participants in a 2-group design would generally be allocated 150 to the experimental

TABLE 9.2	Small Table of Random Digits

46 85 05 23 26	34 67 75 83 00	74 91 06 43 45
69 24 89 34 60	45 30 50 75 21	61 31 83 18 55
14 01 33 17 92	59 74 76 72 77	76 50 33 45 13
56 30 38 73 15	16 **52** 06 96 76	11 65 49 98 93
81 30 44 85 85	68 65 22 73 76	92 85 25 58 66
70 28 42 43 26	79 37 59 52 20	01 15 96 32 67
90 41 59 36 14	33 52 12 66 65	55 82 34 76 41
39 90 40 21 15	59 58 94 90 67	66 82 14 15 75
88 15 20 00 80	20 55 49 14 09	96 27 74 82 57
45 13 46 35 45	59 40 47 20 59	43 94 75 16 80
70 01 41 50 21	41 29 06 73 12	71 85 71 59 57
37 23 93 32 95	05 87 00 11 19	92 78 42 63 40
18 63 73 75 09	82 44 49 90 05	04 92 17 37 01
05 32 78 21 62	20 24 78 17 59	45 19 72 53 32
95 09 66 79 46	48 46 08 55 58	15 19 02 87 82
43 25 38 41 45	60 83 32 59 83	01 29 14 13 49
80 85 40 92 79	43 52 90 63 18	38 38 47 47 61
81 08 87 70 74	88 72 25 67 36	66 16 44 94 31
84 89 07 80 02	94 81 03 19 00	54 10 58 34 36

group and 150 to the control group. If there were 3 groups, there would be 100 per group. It is also possible (and sometimes desirable ethically) to have a different allocation. For example, if an especially promising treatment were developed, we could assign 200 to the treatment group and 100 to the control group. Such an allocation does, however, make it more difficult to detect treatment effects at statistically significant levels—or, to put it another way, the overall sample size must be larger to attain the same level of statistical reliability.

Computerized resources are available for free on the Internet to help with randomization. One such website is *www.randomizer.org*, which has a useful tutorial. Standard statistical software packages (e.g., SPSS or SAS) can also be used (see Shadish et al., 2002, p. 311). We also offer 2-digit and 3-digit ran-

dom number tables in the Toolkit included with the accompanying *Resource Manual*. ⊗

➲ TIP: There is considerable confusion—even in research methods textbooks—about random assignment versus random sampling. Randomization (random assignment) is a *signature* of an experimental design. If there is no random allocation of participants to conditions, then the design is not a true experiment. Random *sampling*, by contrast, is a method of selecting people for a study (see Chapter 12). Random sampling is *not* a signature of an experimental design. In fact, most RCTs do *not* involve random sampling.

Randomization Procedures. The success of randomization depends on two factors. First, the allocation process should be truly random. Second, there must be strict adherence to the randomization schedule. The latter can be achieved if the alloca-

TABLE 9.3	Example of Random Assignment Procedure

CHILD'S NAME	NUMBER	GROUP ASSIGNMENT
Kristina N.	01	I
Derek A.	02	III
Trinity A.	03	III
Lauren J.	04	II
Grace S.	05	II
Nathan O.	06	I
Norah J.	07	III
Thomas N.	08	III
Daniel B.	09	II
Rita T.	10	III
Alaine J.	11	I
Maren B.	12	II
Vadim B.	13	II
Paul M.	14	I
Chris L.	15	I

tion is unpredictable (for both participants and those enrolling them) and tamperproof. Random assignment should involve **allocation concealment** that prevents those who enroll participants from knowing upcoming assignments. Allocation concealment is intended to prevent biases that could stem from knowledge of allocations before assignments actually occur. To use an exaggerated example, if the person doing the enrollment knew that the next person enrolled would be assigned to a promising intervention, he or she might defer enrollment until a particularly needy patient came

TABLE 9.4	Breakdown of the Gender Composition of the Three Groups

GENDER	GROUP I	GROUP II	GROUP III
Boys	3	2	2
Girls	2	3	3

along. Allocation concealment can always be implemented, regardless of the intervention.

Several methods have been devised to ensure allocation concealment, many of which involve developing a randomization schedule before the study begins. This is advantageous when people do not enter a study simultaneously, but rather on a *rolling enrollment* basis. In such situations, the sequence of allocation can be predetermined before enrollment. One widely used method is to have sequentially numbered, opaque sealed envelopes (SNOSE) containing assignment information. As each participant enters the study, he or she receives the next envelope in the sequence (for procedural suggestions, see Vickers, 2006, or Doig & Simpson, 2005). Envelope systems, however, can be subject to tampering (Vickers, 2006). A preferred method is to have treatment allocation information communicated to interventionists by a person unconnected with enrollment or treatment, by telephone or email. This person is trained to strictly follow the randomization schedule. In multisite trials, centralized randomization is strongly recommended.

TIP: Padhye and colleagues (2009) have described an easy-to-use spreadsheet method for randomization in small studies.

The timing of randomization is also important. Study eligibility—whether a person meets the criteria for inclusion—should be ascertained before randomization. If **baseline data** (preintervention data) are collected to measure key outcomes, this should occur before randomization to rule out any possibility that group assignment in itself might affect outcomes prior to treatment. Randomization should occur as closely as possible to the start of the intervention to maximize the likelihood that all randomized people will actually receive the condition to which they have been assigned. Figure 9.1 illustrates the sequence of steps that occurs in most RCTs, including the timing for obtaining informed consent.

Randomization Variants. In most cases, randomization involves the random assignment of individuals to different conditions. An alternative is **cluster randomization**, which involves randomly assigning *clusters* of people to different treatment groups (Christie et al.,

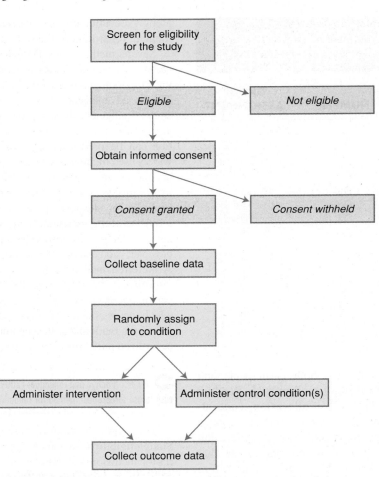

FIGURE 9.1 Sequence of steps in a conventional randomization design.

2009). Cluster randomization may enhance the feasibility of conducting an experiment. Groups of patients who enter a hospital unit at the same time, or patients at different sites, can be randomly assigned to a treatment condition as a unit—thus ruling out, in some situations, practical impediments to randomization. This approach also reduces the risk of **contamination of treatments**, that is, the co-mingling of people in the groups, which could cloud the results if they exchange information. The main disadvantages of cluster randomization are that the statistical analysis of data obtained through this approach is more complex, and sample size requirements are usually greater for a given level of accuracy. Moreover, the number of

units being randomized must be fairly large for the randomization to be successful in equalizing across units. Cluster randomization can also complicate efforts at research synthesis using meta-analysis. Donner and Klar (2004) and Christie and colleagues (2009) offer useful discussions about planning a study with cluster randomization.

Example of cluster randomization: Huizing and colleagues (2009) tested an educational intervention to reduce the use of restraints in psychogeriatric nursing home wards. Fourteen wards were randomly assigned to receive the intervention or not. In all, 105 nursing home residents were included in the analyses.

Simple randomization is usually adequate for creating groups with comparable characteristics, but researchers sometimes take steps to ensure that subgroups of participants are allocated equally to conditions through **stratification**. For example, if a researcher stratified on the basis of gender, men and women would be randomly assigned to conditions separately, thus ensuring that both men and women received the intervention in the right proportions.

⬤ **T I P :** Sometimes stratification is called *blocking*, and the resulting design is called a **randomized block design**. This should not be confused with the design described next. When a cluster randomized design is used, it is almost always a good idea to first stratify units along a dimension of importance before randomizing.

Sometimes people are randomly assigned in blocks through **permuted block randomization**. Rather than having a randomization schedule for the entire sample, randomization occurs for blocks of participants—for example, 6 or 8 at a time. If the entire sample is randomly allocated to conditions, the first 5 or 6 people could be allocated to one or another condition, by chance alone. If allocation is done in randomly permuted blocks in randomly selected sizes, randomization within the small blocks would guarantee a balanced distribution across conditions while maintaing allocation concealment. Such a system is especially appropriate when enrollment occurs over a long period of time because the type of people enrolling might change—or the intervention itself might change due to improved proficiency in implementing it. The Toolkit in the *Resource Manual* offers guidance on block randomization. ✲

Example of stratified, permuted block randomization: Lai and colleagues (2006) studied the effect of music during kangaroo care on maternal anxiety and infant response. Mother–infant dyads were randomly assigned to the treatment or control group using permuted block randomization, stratified on infant gender.

A controversial randomization variant is called **randomized consent** or a **Zelen design** after its originator (Zelen, 1979). Study participants some-

times have a preference about which condition they want. If randomization occurs *after* informed consent (as in Figure 9.1), people who are not assigned to their preferred condition may opt out of the study. Zelen proposed a simple solution: randomize first and *then* obtain consent, thus eliminating the possibility that the consent process will generate preferences. Those in the intervention group are then approached and offered the intervention, which they can accept or decline. If the control group condition is standard care, control group members may not even be asked for their consent, as they would not be getting anything different. The ethical controversies surrounding this form of randomization, as well as its merits and other limitations, have been described by Homer (2002).

Example of the Zelen design: Steiner and colleagues (2001) compared postacute intermediate care in a nurse-led unit versus conventional care on general medical wards in terms of such outcomes as patients' length of stay and mortality. The investigators, who used the Zelen design to randomize patients, argued that conventional randomization was distressful and confusing to many older patients.

Another method of addressing preferences is **partially randomized patient preference (PRPP)**, wherein all participants are asked preferences about treatment conditions. Only those without a strong preference are randomized, but all participants are followed up. Lambert and Wood (2000) outlined the benefits and problems of this approach.

Blinding or Masking

A rather charming (but problematic) quality of people is that they usually want things to turn out well. Researchers want their ideas to work, and they want their hypotheses supported. Participants often want to be helpful and also want to present themselves in a positive light. These tendencies can lead to biases because they can affect what participants do and say (and what researchers ask and perceive) in ways that distort the truth.

A procedure called **blinding** (or **masking**) is used in some RCTs to prevent biases stemming from *awareness*. Blinding involves concealing information from participants, data collectors, care providers, intervention agents, or data analysts to enhance objectivity and minimize **expectation bias**. For example, if participants are not aware of whether they are getting an experimental drug or a placebo, then their outcomes cannot be influenced by their expectations of its efficacy. Blinding typically involves disguising or withholding information about participants' status in the study (e.g., whether they are in the experimental or control group), but can also involve withholding information about study hypotheses, baseline performance on outcomes, or preliminary study results.

The absence of blinding can result in different biases. **Performance bias** refers to systematic differences in the care provided to members of different groups of participants, apart from an intervention that is the focus of the inquiry. For example, participants in a "usual care" group may seek to obtain an innovative intervention elsewhere. Those delivering an intervention might treat participants in groups differently, apart from the intervention itself. Blinding of participants, and blinding agents delivering treatments, is used to avoid performance bias. **Detection** (or **ascertainment**) bias, which concerns systematic differences between groups in how outcome variables are measured, verified, or recorded, is addressed by blinding those who collect the outcome data or, in some cases, those who analyze them.

Unlike allocation concealment, blinding is not always possible. Drug studies often lend themselves to blinding, but many nursing interventions do not. For example, if the intervention were a smoking cessation program, participants would know that they were receiving the intervention, and the interventionist would be aware of who was in the program. However, it is usually possible, and desirable, to at least mask participants' treatment status from people collecting outcome data and from other clinicians providing normal care.

⟳ TIP: Although blinding is useful for minimizing bias, it may not be necessary if subjectivity and error risk are low. For example, participants' ratings of pain are subjective and susceptible to biases stemming from their own or data collectors' awareness of group

status or study hypotheses. Hospital readmission and length of hospital stay, on the other hand, are variables less likely to be affected by people's awareness.

When blinding is not used, the study is an **open study**, in contrast to a **closed study** that results from masking. When blinding is used with only one group of people (e.g., study participants), it is sometimes described as a **single-blind study**. When it is possible to mask with two groups (e.g., those delivering an intervention and those receiving it), it is sometimes called **double-blind**, and when three groups are masked, it may be called **triple-blind**. However, recent guidelines have recommended that researchers not use these terms without explicitly stating which groups were blinded to avoid any ambiguity (Moher et al., 2010).

The term *blinding*, though widely used, has fallen into some disfavor because of possible pejorative connotations, and some organizations (e.g., the American Psychological Association) have recommended using masking instead. Medical researchers, however, appear to prefer *blinding* unless the people in the study have vision impairments (Schulz et al., 2002). Similarly, the vast majority of nurse researchers use the term *blinding* rather than *masking* (Polit et al., 2010).

Example of a single-blind experiment: Pölkki and colleagues (2008) tested an imagery-induced relaxation intervention to reduce postoperative pain in 8- to 12-year-old children. The nurse who collected the data did not know whether children were in the intervention group or the usual care control group.

Specific Experimental Designs

There are numerous experimental designs, including many that are not discussed in this book, such as *nested designs* and the *Solomon four-group design*. Some popular designs described in this section are summarized in Table 9.5. The second column (schematic diagram) depicts design notation from a classic monograph (Campbell & Stanley, 1963). In this notation, R means random assignment, O represents an observation (i.e., data collection on

TABLE 9.5 — Design Alternatives: Selected Experimental (Randomized) Designs

TYPE OF DESIGN	SCHEMATIC DIAGRAM	SITUATIONS THAT ARE BEST SUITED TO THIS DESIGN	DRAWBACKS OF THIS DESIGN
1. Basic posttest-only design	R X O_1 / R O_1 or R X_A O_1 / R X_B O_1	When the outcome is not relevant until after the intervention is complete (e.g., length of stay in hospital)	Does not permit an evaluation of whether the two groups were comparable at the outset on the outcome of interest
2. Basic pretest-posttest design (with optional repeated follow-ups)	R O_1 X O_2 / R O_1 O_2 R O_1 X O_2 O_3 O_4 / R O_1 O_2 O_3 O_4	a. When the focus of the intervention is on change (e.g., behaviors, attitudes) b. When the researcher wants to assess both group differences (experimental comparison), and change within groups (quasi-experimental)	Sometimes the pretest itself can affect the outcomes of interest
3. Multiple intervention design	R O_1 X_A O_2 / R O_1 X_B O_2 / R O_1 O_2	Can be used to disentangle effects of different components of a complex intervention, or to test competing interventions	a. Requires larger sample than basic designs b. May be at risk to threats to statistical conclusion validity* if A and B are not very different (small effects)
4. Wait-list (delay of treatment) design	R O_1 X O_2 O_3 / R O_1 O_2 X O_3	a. Attractive when there is patient preference for the innovative treatment b. Can strengthen inferences by virtue of replication aspect for the second group	a. Controls may drop out of study before they get deferred treatment b. Not suitable if key outcomes are measured long after treatment (e.g., mortality) or if there is an interest in assessing long-term effects (waitlist period is then too long)
5. Crossover design—participants serve as their own controls	R O_1 X_A O_2 X_B O_3 / R O_1 X_B O_2 X_A O_3	a. Appropriate only if there is no expectation of carryover effects from one period to the next (effects should have rapid onset, short halflife) b. Useful when recruitment is difficult—smaller sample is needed; excellent for controlling confounding variables	a. Often cannot be assumed that there are no carryover effects b. If the first treatment received "fixes" a problem for participants, they may not remain in the study for the second one c. History threat* to validity a possibility
6. Factorial design	R O_1 X_{A1B1} O_2 / R O_1 X_{A1B2} O_2 / R O_1 X_{A2B1} O_2 / R O_1 X_{A2B2} O_2	a. Efficient for testing two interventions simultaneously b. Can be useful in illuminating interaction effects, but most useful when strong synergistic/additive effects (or no interaction effects) are expected	Power needed to detect interactions could require larger sample size than when testing each intervention separately

KEY: R = Randomization
X = Intervention (X_A = one treatment, X_B = alternative treatment, dose, etc.)
O = Observation or measurement of the dependent variable/outcome

*Validity threats are discussed in Chapter 10.

the outcome variable), and X stands for exposure to the intervention. Each row designates a different group, and time is portrayed moving from left to right. Thus, in Row 2 (a basic pretest–posttest design), the top line represents the group that was randomly assigned (R) to an intervention (X) and from which data were collected prior to (O_1) and after (O_2) the intervention. The second row is the control group, which differs from the experimental group only by absence of the treatment (no X). (Note that some information in the "drawbacks" column of Table 9.5 is not discussed until Chapter 10.)

Basic Experimental Designs

Earlier in this chapter, we described a study that tested the effect of gentle massage on pain in nursing home residents. This example illustrates a simple design that is sometimes called a **posttest-only design** (or **after-only design**) because data on the dependent variable are collected only once—after randomization and completion of the intervention.

A second basic design involves the collection of baseline data, as shown in the flow chart (Figure 9.1). Suppose we hypothesized that convective airflow blankets are more effective than conductive water-flow blankets in cooling critically ill febrile patients. Our design involves assigning patients to the two types of blankets (the independent variable) and measuring the dependent variable (body temperature) twice, before and after the intervention. This design allows us to examine whether one blanket type is more effective than the other in *reducing* fever—that is, with this design researchers can examine *change*. This design is a **pretest–posttest design** or a **before–after design**. Many pretest–posttest designs include data collection at multiple postintervention points (sometimes called *repeated measures designs*, as noted in Chapter 8). Designs that involve collected data multiple times from two groups can be described as mixed designs: analyses can examine both differences *between* groups and changes *within* groups over time.

These basic designs can be "tweaked" in various ways—for example, the design could involve comparison of three or more groups or could have

a wait-listed control group. These designs are included in Table 9.5.

Example of a pretest–posttest experimental design: Wentworth and colleagues (2009) tested the efficacy of a 20-minute massage on tension, anxiety, and pain in patients awaiting invasive cardiovascular procedures. Outcomes were measured before and after the massage.

Factorial Design

Most experimental designs involve manipulating only one independent variable, but it is possible to manipulate two or more variables simultaneously. Suppose we were interested in comparing two therapies for premature infants: tactile stimulation versus auditory stimulation. We also want to learn if the daily *amount* of stimulation (15, 30, or 45 minutes) affects infants' progress. The outcomes are measures of infant development (e.g., weight gain, cardiac responsiveness). Figure 9.2 illustrates the structure of this RCT.

This **factorial design** allows us to address three research questions:

1. Does auditory stimulation have a more beneficial effect on premature infants' development than tactile stimulation, or vice versa?
2. Is the duration of stimulation (independent of type) related to infant development?
3. Is auditory stimulation most effective when linked to a certain dose and tactile stimulation most effective when coupled with a different dose?

The third question shows the strength of factorial designs: they permit us to test not only **main effects**

Type of stimulation

		Auditory A1		Tactile A2	
Daily dose	15 Min. B1	A1	B1	A2	B1
	30 Min. B2	A1	B2	A2	B2
	45 Min. B3	A1	B3	A2	B3

FIGURE 9.2 Example of a 2 × 3 factorial design.

(effects from experimentally manipulated variables, as in questions 1 and 2), but also **interaction effects** (effects from combining treatments). It may be insufficient to say that auditory stimulation is better than tactile stimulation (or vice versa) and that 45 minutes of daily stimulation is more effective than 15 or 30 minutes. How these two variables interact (how they behave in combination) is also of interest. Our results may indicate that 45 minutes of auditory stimulation is the most beneficial treatment. We could not have learned this by conducting two separate studies that manipulated one independent variable and held the second one constant.

In factorial experiments, people are randomly assigned to a specific combination of conditions. In our example in Figure 9.2, infants would be assigned randomly to one of six **cells**—that is, six treatment conditions or boxes in the diagram. The two independent variables in a factorial design are the **factors**. Type of stimulation is factor A and amount of daily exposure is factor B. Level 1 of factor A is auditory and level 2 of factor A is tactile. When describing the dimensions of the design, researchers refer to the number of **levels**. The design in Figure 9.2 is a 2 × 3 design: two levels in factor A times three levels in factor B. Factorial experiments can be performed with multiple independent variables (factors), but designs with more than three factors are rare.

> **Example of a factorial design:** Munro and colleagues (2009) used a 2 × 2 factorial design to test treatments to prevent ventilator-associated pneumonia in critically ill adults. Patients were randomly assigned to 1 of 4 conditions: 0.12% solution chlorhexidine oral swab twice daily, toothbrushing three times daily, both treatments, or neither treatment.

Crossover Design

Thus far, we have described RCTs in which different people are randomly assigned to different treatments. For instance, in the previous example, infants exposed to auditory stimulation were not the same infants as those exposed to tactile stimulation. A **crossover design** involves exposing the same people to more than one condition. This type of within-subjects design has the advantage of ensuring the highest possible equivalence among participants exposed to different conditions—the groups being compared are equal with respect to age, weight, health, and so on because they are composed of the same people.

Because randomization is a signature characteristic of an experiment, participants in a crossover design must be randomly assigned to different orderings of treatments. For example, if a crossover design were used to compare the effects of auditory and tactile stimulation on infant development, some infants would be randomly assigned to receive auditory stimulation first, and others would be assigned to receive tactile stimulation first. When there are three or more conditions to which participants will be exposed, the procedure of **counterbalancing** can be used to rule out ordering effects. For example, if there were three conditions (A, B, C), participants would be randomly assigned to one of six counterbalanced orderings:

A, B, C	A, C, B
B, C, A	B, A, C
C, A, B	C, B, A

Although crossover designs are extremely powerful, they are inappropriate for certain research questions because of the problem of **carry-over effects**. When people are exposed to two different treatments or conditions, they may be influenced in the second condition by their experience in the first condition. As one example, drug studies rarely use a crossover design because drug B administered *after* drug A is not necessarily the same treatment as drug B administered *before* drug A. When carry-over effects are a potential concern, researchers often have a **washout period** in between the treatments (i.e., a period of no treatment exposure).

Crossover designs usually involve treatments administered in a time sequence. Crossover designs can, however, involve simultaneous tests on two sides of a person's body.

> **Example of a crossover design:** Pinar and colleagues (2009) tested two leg bag products (with and without latex) on a sample of men postradical prostatectomy. Each product was tested, in a randomized order, for 4 to 5 days.

Strengths and Limitations of Experiments

In this section, we explore the reasons why experimental designs are held in high esteem and examine some limitations.

Experimental Strengths

An experimental design is the gold standard for testing interventions because it yields strong evidence about intervention effects. Through randomization and the use of a comparison condition, experimenters come as close as possible to attaining the "ideal" counterfactual. Experiments offer greater corroboration than any other approach that, *if* the independent variable (e.g., diet, drug, teaching approach) is manipulated, *then* certain consequences in the dependent variable (e.g., weight loss, recovery, learning) may be expected to ensue. The great strength of RCTs, then, lies in the confidence with which causal relationships can be inferred. Through the controls imposed by manipulation, comparison, and—especially—randomization, alternative explanations can often be ruled out or discredited. It is because of these strengths that meta-analyses of RCTs, which integrate evidence from multiple studies using an experimental design, are at the pinnacle of evidence hierarchies for questions about treatment (Figure 2.1, p. 28).

Experimental Limitations

Despite the benefits of experimental research, this type of design also has limitations. First, there are often constraints that make an experimental approach impractical or impossible. These constraints are discussed later in this chapter.

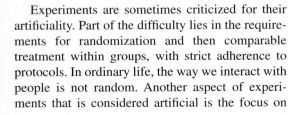

TIP: Shadish and colleagues (2002) described 10 situations that are especially conducive to randomized experiments; these are summarized in a table in the Toolkit.

Experiments are sometimes criticized for their artificiality. Part of the difficulty lies in the requirements for randomization and then comparable treatment within groups, with strict adherence to protocols. In ordinary life, the way we interact with people is not random. Another aspect of experiments that is considered artificial is the focus on only a handful of variables while holding all else constant. This requirement has been criticized as being reductionist and as artificially constraining human experience. Experiments that are undertaken without a guiding theoretical framework are sometimes criticized for suggesting causal connections without any explanation for *why* the intervention affected observed outcomes.

A problem with RCTs conducted in clinical settings is that it is often clinical staff, rather than researchers, who administer an intervention; therefore, it can sometimes be difficult to determine if those in the intervention group actually received the treatment and if those in the control group did not. It may be especially difficult to maintain the integrity of the intervention and control conditions if the study period extends over time. Moreover, clinical studies are conducted in environments over which researchers may have little control—and control is a critical factor in RCTs. McGuire and colleagues (2000) have described some issues relating to the challenges of testing interventions in clinical settings.

Sometimes a problem emerges if participants have discretion about participation in the treatment. Suppose, for example, that we randomly assigned patients with HIV infection to a special support group intervention or to a control group. Experimental subjects who elect not to participate in the support groups, or who participate infrequently, actually are in a "condition" that looks more like the control condition than the experimental one. The treatment is diluted through nonparticipation, and it may become difficult to detect any treatment effects, no matter how effective it might otherwise have been. We discuss this at greater length in the next chapter.

Another potential problem is the **Hawthorne effect**, a placebo-type effect caused by people's expectations. The term is derived from a set of experiments conducted at the Hawthorne plant of the Western Electric Corporation in which various environmental conditions, such as light and working hours, were varied to test their effects on worker productivity. Regardless of what change was introduced, that is, whether the light was made better or worse, productivity increased. Knowledge of being included in the study (not just knowledge of being in a particular group) appears to have affected people's behavior, thus obscuring the effect of the treatment.

In sum, despite the superiority of RCTs for testing causal hypotheses, they are subject to a number of limitations, some of which may make them difficult to apply to real-world problems. Nevertheless, with the growing demand for evidence-based practice, true experimental designs are increasingly being used to test the effects of nursing interventions.

QUASI-EXPERIMENTS

Quasi-experiments, called *controlled trials without randomization* in the medical literature, involve an intervention but they lack randomization, the signature of a true experiment. Some quasi-experiments even lack a control group. The signature of a quasi-experimental design, then, is an intervention in the absence of randomization.

Quasi-Experimental Designs

The most widely used quasi-experimental designs are summarized in Table 9.6, which depicts designs using the schematic notation we introduced earlier.

Nonequivalent Control Group Designs

The **nonequivalent control group pretest–posttest design** involves two groups of participants, from whom outcome data are collected before and after implementing an intervention. For example, suppose we wished to study the effect of a new hospital-wide model of care that involved having a patient care facilitator (PCF) be the primary point person for all patients during their stay. Our main outcome is patient satisfaction. The new system is being implemented throughout the hospital, and so, randomization is not possible. For comparative purposes, we decide to collect data in a similar hospital that is not instituting the PCF model. Data on patient satisfaction is collected in both hospitals

at baseline, before the change is made, and again after its implementation.

The first row of Table 9.6 depicts this study symbolically. The top line represents the experimental (PCF) hospital, and the second row is the comparison hospital. This diagram is identical to the experimental pretest–posttest design (see Table 9.5), *except* there is no "R"—participants have not been randomized to groups. The design in Table 9.6 is weaker because *it cannot be assumed that the experimental and comparison groups are equivalent at the outset*. Because there is no randomization, quasi-experimental comparisons are farther from an ideal counterfactual than experimental comparisons. The design is nevertheless strong, because baseline data allow us to assess whether patients in the two hospitals had similar satisfaction initially. If the comparison and experimental groups are similar at baseline, we could be relatively confident inferring that any posttest difference in satisfaction was the result of the new care model. If patient satisfaction is different initially, however, it will be difficult to interpret posttest differences. Note that in quasi-experiments, the term **comparison group** is often used in lieu of *control group* to refer to the group against which treatment group outcomes are evaluated.

Now, suppose we had been unable to collect baseline data. This design, diagrammed in Row 2 of Table 9.6, has a major flaw. We no longer have information about the initial equivalence of the two hospitals. If we find that patient satisfaction in the experimental hospital is higher than that in the control hospital at posttest, can we conclude that the new care delivery method *caused* improved satisfaction? An alternative explanation for posttest differences is that patient satisfaction in the two hospitals differed initially. Campbell and Stanley (1963) called this *nonequivalent control group posttest-only design* preexperimental rather than quasi-experimental because of its fundamental weakness—although Shadish, and colleagues (2002), in their more recent book on causal inference, simply called this a weaker quasi-experimental design.

TABLE 9.6 Design Alternatives: Selected Quasi-Experimental Designs

TYPE OF DESIGN	SCHEMATIC DIAGRAM	SITUATIONS THAT ARE BEST SUITED	DRAWBACKS
1. Nonequivalent control group, pretest–posttest design	O_1 X O_2 O_1 O_2	Attractive when an entire unit must get the intervention and a similar unit not getting the intervention is available	a. Selection threat* remains a nearly intractable problem, but less so than when there is no pretest b. History threat* also a possibility
2. Nonequivalent control group, posttest only design	X O_1 O_1	A reasonable choice only when there is some a priori knowledge about comparability of groups with regard to key outcomes	Extremely vulnerable to selection threat,* possibility of other threats as well, especially history threat*
3. One-group pretest–posttest design	O_1 X O_2	A reasonable choice only when intervention impact is expected to be dramatic and other potential causes have little credibility	Typically provides very weak support for causal inference—vulnerable to many internal validity threats (maturation, history, etc.)*
4. Time series design	O_1 O_2 O_3 O_4 X O_5 O_6 O_7 O_8	a. Good option when there are abundant data on key outcome in existing records b. Addresses maturation threat and change from secular trends & random fluctuation	a. Complex statistical analysis that is most appropriate with very large number of data points (100+) b. History threat* remains, and (sometimes) selection threat* if the population changes over time
5. Time series nonequivalent control group design	O_1 O_2 O_3 O_4 X O_5 O_6 O_7 O_8 O_1 O_2 O_3 O_4 O_5 O_6 O_7 O_8	Attractive when an entire unit/institution adopts the intervention and a similar unit not adopting it is available, *and* if comparable data are readily available in records of both	a. Selection threat* remains, as two units or institutions are rarely identical b. Analyses may be very complex
6. Time series with withdrawn and reinstituted treatment	O_1 O_2 X O_3 O_4 –X O_5 O_6 X O_7 O_8	*Attractive if effects of an intervention are short-term	a. May be untenable to assume that there are no carryover effects b. May be difficult ethically to withdraw treatment if it is efficacious

KEY: X = Intervention
O = Observation or measurement of the dependent variable/outcome

*Validity threats are discussed in Chapter 10.

Example of a nonequivalent control group pretest–posttest design: Yuan and colleagues (2009) tested the effectiveness of an exercise intervention on nurses' physical fitness. The researchers used nurses from different units of a medical center in Taiwan to be in either an intervention group or a comparison group.

Example of a historical comparison group: Swadener-Culpepper and colleagues (2008) studied the effect of continuous lateral rotation therapy on patients at high risk for pulmonary complications. Length of stay for those receiving the therapy was compared to that for a high-risk historical comparison group.

Sometimes researchers use *matching* within a pretest–posttest nonequivalent control group design to ensure that the groups are, in fact, equivalent on at least some key variables related to the outcomes. For example, if an intervention was designed to reduce patient anxiety, then it might be desirable to not only *measure* preintervention anxiety in the intervention and comparison group, but to take steps to ensure that the groups' anxiety levels were comparable by matching participants' initial anxiety. Because matching on more than a couple variables is unwieldy, a more sophisticated method of matching, called **propensity matching**, can be used by researchers with statistical sophistication. This method involves the creation of a single **propensity score** that captures the conditional probability of exposure to a treatment given various preintervention characteristics. Experimental and comparison group members can then be matched on this score (Qin et al., 2008). Both conventional and propensity matching are most easily implemented when there is a large pool of potential comparison group participants from which good matches to treatment group members can be selected.

In lieu of using a contemporaneous nonrandomized comparison group, researchers sometimes use a **historical comparison group**. That is, comparison data are gathered about a group of people before implementing the intervention. Even when the people are from the same institutional setting, however, it is risky to assume that the two groups are comparable, or that the environments are comparable in all respects except for the new intervention. There remains the possibility that something other than the intervention could account for any observed differences in outcomes.

Time Series Designs

In the designs just described, a control group was used but randomization was not, but some quasi-experiments have neither. Suppose that a hospital implemented rapid response teams (RRTs) in its acute care units. Administrators want to examine the effects on patient outcomes (e.g., unplanned admissions to the ICU, mortality rate) and nurse outcomes (e.g., stress). For the purposes of this example, assume no other hospital could serve as a good comparison. The only kind of comparison that can be made is a before—after contrast. If RRTs were implemented in January, one could compare the mortality rate (for example) during the 3 months before RRTs with the mortality rate during the subsequent 3-month period. The schematic representation of such a study is shown in the third row of Table 9.6.

This one-group pretest–posttest design seems straightforward, but it has weaknesses. What if either of the 3-month periods is atypical, apart from the innovation? What about the effects of any other policy changes inaugurated during the same period? What about the effects of external factors that influence mortality, such as a flu outbreak or seasonal migration? This design (also called preexperimental by Campbell and Stanley) cannot control these factors.

> **TIP:** One-group pretest–posttest designs are not always unproductive. For example, if a study tested a brief teaching intervention, with baseline knowledge data obtained immediately before the intervention and posttest knowledge data collected immediately after it, it may be reasonable to infer that the intervention is the most plausible explanation for knowledge gains.

In our RRT example, the design could be modified so that some alternative explanations for changes in mortality could be ruled out. One such design is the **time series design** (sometimes called an *interrupted time series design*), diagramed in Row 4 of Table 9.6. In a time series design, data are collected over an extended period and an intervention is introduced during that period. In the diagram, O_1 through O_4 represent four separate instances of data collection on an outcome before treatment, X is the introduction of the intervention, and O_5 through O_8 represent four posttreatment observations. In our example, O_1 might be the number of deaths in January through March in the year before the new RRT system, O_2 the number of deaths in April through June, and so forth. After RRTs are implemented, data on mortality are similarly collected for four consecutive 3-month periods, giving us observations O_5 through O_8.

Even though the time series design does not eliminate all problems of interpreting changes in mortality, the extended time period strengthens the ability to attribute change to the intervention. Figure 9.3 demonstrates why this is so. The two line graphs (*A* and *B*) in the figure show two possible outcome patterns for eight mortality observations. The vertical dotted line in the center represents the timing of

the RRT system. Patterns *A* and *B* both reflect a feature common to most time series studies—fluctuation from one data point to another. These fluctuations are normal. One would not expect that, if 480 patients died in a hospital in 1 year, the deaths would be spaced evenly with 40 per month. It is precisely because of these fluctuations that the one-group pretest–posttest design, with only one observation before and after the intervention, is so weak.

Let us compare the interpretations that can be made for the outcomes shown in Figure 9.3. In both patterns *A* and *B*, mortality decreased between O_4 and O_5, immediately after RRTs were implemented. In *B*, however, mortality rose at O_6 and continued to rise at O_7. The decrease at O_5 looks similar to other apparently haphazard fluctuations in mortality. In *A*, by contrast, the number of deaths decreases at O_5 and remains relatively low for subsequent observations. There may be other explanations for a change in the mortality rate, but the time series design does permit us to rule out the possibility that the data reflect unstable measurements at only two points in time. If we had used a simple pretest–posttest design, it would have been analogous to obtaining the measurements at O_4 and

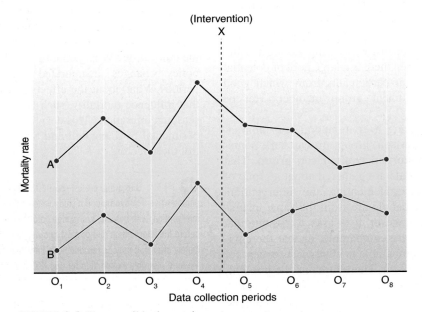

FIGURE 9.3 Two possible time series outcome patterns.

O_5 of Figure 9.3 only. The outcomes in both *A* and *B* are the same at these two time points. The broader time perspective leads us to draw different conclusions about the effects of RRTs. Nevertheless, the absence of a comparison group means that the design is far from yielding an ideal counterfactual.

Time series designs are often especially important in *quality improvement studies*, because in such efforts randomization is rarely possible, and only one institution is involved in the inquiry.

> **Example of a time series design:** Kratz (2008) used a time series design to test the effects of implementing research-based protocols to decrease negative outcomes associated with delirium and acute confusion. Kratz used 3 years of hospital records data prior to and 4 years of records data after implementing the new protocols, for such outcomes as patient falls and use of restraints.

One drawback of a time series design is that a large number of data points—100 or more—is recommended for a traditional analysis (Shadish et al., 2002), and the analyses are complex. Nurse researchers are, however, beginning to use a little-known but versatile and compelling approach called *statistical process control* to assess effects when they have collected data sequentially over a period of time before and after implementing an intervention or practice change (Polit & Chaboyer, in review).

A powerful quasi-experimental design results when time series and nonequivalent control group designs are combined (Row 5 of Table 9.6). In the example just described, a time series nonequivalent control group design would involve collecting data over an extended period from both the hospital introducing the RRTs and another similar hospital not implementing RRTs. Information from another hospital with similar characteristics would make inferences regarding the effects of RRTs more convincing because other factors influencing the trends would likely be comparable in both groups.

Numerous variations on the time series design are possible. For example, additional evidence regarding the effects of a treatment can be achieved by instituting the treatment at several different points in time, strengthening the treatment over time, or instituting the treatment at one point and then withdrawing it at a later point, sometimes with reinstitution (Row 6 of Table 9.6). Clinical nurse researchers may be in a good position to use such time series designs because many measures of patient functioning are routinely made at multiple points over an extended period.

> **Example of a time series design with withdrawal and reinstitution:** Hicks-Moore (2005) studied the effect of relaxing music at mealtime on agitated behaviors of nursing home residents with dementia. Music was introduced in week 2, removed in week 3, and then reinstituted in week 4. The pattern of agitated behaviors was consistent with the hypothesis that relaxing music has a calming effect.

A particular application of a time series approach is called **single-subject experiments** (*N-of-1 studies*). Single-subject studies use time series designs to gather information about intervention effects based on a single patient (or a small number of patients) under controlled conditions. The most basic single-subject design involves a baseline phase of data gathering (A) and an intervention phase (B), yielding an **AB design**. If the treatment is withdrawn, it would be an **ABA design**; if a withdrawn treatment is reinstituted, it would be an **ABAB design**. Portney and Watkins (2000) offer valuable guidance about single-subject studies in clinical settings.

> **Example of a single-subject ABAB design:** Elliott and Horgas (2009) used an ABAB design in which the intervention (a scheduled dose of acetaminophen) was administered, withdrawn, and then reinstituted in three people with dementia. Data on pain-related behaviors were collected daily for 24 days.

Other Quasi-Experimental Designs

Several other quasi-experimental designs offer alternatives to RCTs. One such design, the **regression discontinuity design**, will not be elaborated on here because it is rarely used in nursing studies. This design, which involves *systematic* assignment of people to groups based on cut-off scores on a preintervention measure (e.g., giving an intervention to the most severely ill patients), is considered attractive from an ethical standpoint and merits consideration. Its features have been described in the nursing literature by Atwood and Taylor (1991).

Earlier in this chapter, we described partially randomized patient preference or PRPP. This design has advantages in terms of participant recruitment to participate in a study, because those with a strong preference get to choose their treatment condition. Those without a strong preference are randomized, but those *with* a preference are given the condition they prefer and are followed up as part of the study. The two randomized groups are part of a true experiment, but the two groups who get their preference are in a quasi-experiment. This design can yield valuable information about the kind of people who prefer one condition over another. The evidence of treatment effectiveness is weak in the quasi-experimental segment because the people who elected a certain treatment likely differ from those who opted for the alternative—and these preintervention differences, rather than the alternative treatments, could account for any observed differences in outcomes. Yet, evidence from the quasi-experiment could usefully support or qualify evidence from the experimental portion of the study.

Example of a PRPP design: Coward (2002) used a PRPP design in a pilot study of a support group intervention for women with breast cancer. She found that the majority of women did *not* want to be randomized, but rather had a strong preference for either being in or not being in the support group. Her article describes the challenges she faced.

Another quasi-experimental approach—often embedded within a true experiment—is a **dose-response** design in which the outcomes of those receiving different doses of a treatment—not as a result of randomization—are compared. For example, in complex and lengthy interventions, some people attend more sessions or get more intensive treatment than others. The rationale for a quasi-experimental dose-response analysis is that if a larger dose corresponds to better outcomes, this provides supporting evidence for inferring that the treatment caused the outcome. The difficulty, however, is that people tend to get different doses of the treatment because of differences in motivation,

physical function, or other characteristics that could be driving outcome differences—and not the different doses themselves. Nevertheless, when a dose-response analyses may yield useful information.

Example of a dose-response analysis within a true experiment: Lai and Good (2005) randomly assigned community dwelling elders who had difficulty sleeping to a control group or to an intervention group that listened to 45-minute sedative music tapes at bedtime. Those in the intervention group experienced significantly better sleep quality than those in the control group. Moreover, over the 3-week study period, sleep improved weekly, which suggested a cumulative dose effect.

Experimental and Comparison Conditions

Researchers using a quasi-experimental approach, like those adopting an experimental design, should strive to develop strong interventions that provide an opportunity for a fair test, and should develop protocols documenting what the interventions entail. Researchers need to be especially careful in understanding and documenting the counterfactual in quasi-experiments. In the case of nonequivalent control group designs, this means understanding the conditions to which the comparison group is exposed. In our example of using a hospital with traditional nursing systems as a comparison for the new primary nursing system, the nature of that traditional system should be fully understood. In time series designs, the counterfactual is the condition existing before implementing the intervention. Blinding should be used, to the extent possible—indeed, this is often more feasible in a quasi-experiment than in an RCT.

Strengths and Limitations of Quasi-Experiments

A major strength of quasi-experiments is that they are practical. In clinical settings, it is often impossible to conduct true experimental tests of nursing interventions. Quasi-experimental designs introduce some research control when full experimental rigor is not possible.

Another advantage of quasi-experiments is that patients are not always willing to relinquish control over their treatment condition. Indeed, there is some evidence that people are increasingly unwilling to volunteer to be randomized in clinical trials (Gross & Fogg, 2001). Quasi-experimental designs, because they do not involve random assignment, are likely to be acceptable to a broader group of people. This, in turn, has implications for the generalizability of the results—but the problem is that the results may be less conclusive.

Thus, researchers using quasi-experimental designs need to be cognizant of their weaknesses and need to take steps to counteract those weaknesses or at least take them into account in interpreting results. When a quasi-experimental design is used, there may be several **rival hypotheses** competing with the experimental manipulation as explanations for the results. (This issue relates to *internal validity* and is discussed further in Chapter 10.) Take as an example the case in which we administer a special diet to frail nursing home residents to assess its effects on weight gain. If we use no comparison group or if we use a nonequivalent control group and then observe a weight gain, we must ask the questions: Is it *plausible* that some other factor caused the gain? Is it *plausible* that pretreatment differences between the experimental and comparison groups resulted in differential gain? Is it *plausible* that the elders, on average, gained weight simply because the most frail died or were transferred to a hospital? If the answer is "yes" to any of these questions, then inferences about the causal effect of the intervention are weakened. The plausibility of any particular rival explanation cannot be answered unequivocally. Usually, judgment must be exercised. Because the conclusions from quasi-experiments ultimately depend in part on human judgment, rather than on more objective criteria, cause-and-effect inferences are less compelling.

NONEXPERIMENTAL RESEARCH

Many research questions—including ones seeking to establish causal relationships—cannot be addressed with an experimental or quasi-experimental design. For example, at the beginning of this chapter, we posed this prognosis question: Do birth weights under 1,500 grams *cause* developmental delays in children? Clearly, we cannot manipulate birth weight, the independent variable. Babies are born with weights that are neither random nor subject to research control. One way to answer this question is to compare two groups of infants—babies with birth weights above and below 1,500 grams at birth—in terms of their subsequent development. When researchers do not intervene by manipulating the independent variable, the study is **nonexperimental**, or, in the medical literature, **observational**.

Most nursing studies are nonexperimental, mainly because most human characteristics (e.g., birth weight, ethnicity, lactose intolerance) cannot be experimentally manipulated. Also, many variables that could *technically* be manipulated cannot be manipulated ethically. For example, if we were studying the effect of prenatal care on infant mortality, it would be unethical to provide such care to one group of pregnant women while deliberately depriving a randomly assigned second group. We would need to locate a naturally occurring group of pregnant women who had not received prenatal care. Their birth outcomes could then be compared with those of women who had received appropriate care. The problem, however, is that the two groups of women are likely to differ in terms of many other characteristics, such as age, education, and income, any of which individually or in combination could affect infant mortality, independent of prenatal care. This is precisely why experimental designs are so strong in demonstrating cause-and-effect relationships. Many nonexperimental studies are designed to explore causal relationships when experimental work is not possible—although, some studies have primarily a descriptive intent.

Correlational Cause-Probing Research

When researchers study the effect of a potential *cause* that they cannot manipulate, they use **correlational designs** to examine relationships between variables. A **correlation** is a relationship or association between two variables, that is, a tendency for variation in one variable to be related to variation in another. For example, in human adults, height and weight are correlated because there is a tendency for taller people to weigh more than shorter people.

As mentioned early in this chapter, one criterion for causality is that an empirical relationship (correlation) between variables must be demonstrated. It is risky, however, to infer causal relationships in correlational research. In experiments, researchers have direct control over the independent variable; the experimental treatment can be administered to some and withheld from others, and the two groups can be equalized with respect to everything except the independent variable through randomization. In correlational research, on the other hand, investigators do not control the independent variable, which often has already occurred. Groups being compared could differ in many respects that could affect outcomes of interest. Although correlational studies are inherently weaker than experimental studies in elucidating cause-and-effect relationships, different designs offer different degrees of supportive evidence.

Retrospective Designs

Studies with a **retrospective design** are ones in which a phenomenon existing in the present is linked to phenomena that occurred in the past. The signature of a retrospective study is that the researcher begins with the dependent variable (the effect) and then examines whether it is correlated with one or more previously occurring independent variables (potential causes).

Most early studies of the smoking–lung cancer link used a retrospective **case-control design**, in which researchers began with a group of people who had lung cancer (*cases*) and another group who did not (*controls*). The researchers then looked for differences between the two groups in antecedent behaviors or conditions, such as smoking.

In designing a case-control study, researchers try to identify controls without the disease or condition who are as similar as possible to the cases with regard to key confounding variables (e.g., age, gender). Researchers sometimes use matching or other techniques to control for confounding variables. (Sometimes they opt to match two or more controls for each case). To the degree that researchers can demonstrate comparability between cases and controls with regard to confounding traits, inferences regarding the presumed cause of the disease are enhanced. The difficulty, however, is that the two groups are almost never totally comparable with respect to all potential factors influencing the dependent variable.

Example of a case-control design: Swenson and colleagues (2009) used a case-control design to assess risk factors for lymphedema following breast cancer surgery. Women with and without lymphedema were matched on type of axillary surgery and surgery date, and then compared to such antecedent risk factors as weight, number of positive nodes, and treatments received.

Not all retrospective studies can be described as using a case-control design. Sometimes researchers use a retrospective approach to identify risk factors for different *amounts* of a problem or condition. That is, the outcome is not "caseness" but rather *degree* of some condition. For example, a retrospective design might be used to identify factors predictive of the length of time new mothers breastfed their infants. Essentially, such a design is intended to understand factors that *cause* women to make different breastfeeding decisions.

Retrospective studies are often cross-sectional, with data on both the dependent and independent variables collected at a single point in time. In such studies, data for the independent variable are based on recollection (retrospection). One problem, however, is that recollection is often less accurate than contemporary measurement. Asking people if they had a headache at any time in the previous 12 months might not be difficult to answer, but asking them to report how many times they had a headache, or what it felt like to have a headache 6 months ago, is likely to result in unreliable answers.

Example of a retrospective design: Musil and colleagues (2009) used cross-sectional data in their retrospective study designed to identify antecedent factors to predict depressive symptoms in grandmothers raising their grandchildren. The independent variables included family stresses and strains, social support, and demographic variables such as age and employment status.

Prospective Nonexperimental Designs

In correlational studies with a **prospective design** (called a **cohort design** in medical circles), researchers start with a presumed cause and then go forward in time to the presumed effect. For example, we might want to test the hypothesis that rubella during pregnancy (the independent variable) is related to birth defects (the dependent variable). To test this hypothesis prospectively, we would begin with a sample of pregnant women, including some who contracted rubella during pregnancy and others who did not. The subsequent occurrence of congenital anomalies would be assessed for all participants, and we would examine whether women with rubella were more likely than other women to bear infants with birth defects.

Prospective studies are more costly than retrospective studies, in part because prospective studies require at least two rounds of data collection. A substantial follow-up period may be needed before the outcome of interest occurs, as is the case in prospective studies of cigarette smoking and lung cancer. Also, prospective designs require large samples if the outcome of interest is rare, as in the example of malformations associated with maternal rubella. Another issue is that in a good prospective study, researchers take steps to confirm that all participants are free from the effect (e.g., the disease) at the time the independent variable is measured, and this may be difficult or expensive to do. For example, in prospective smoking–lung cancer studies, lung cancer may be present initially but not yet diagnosed.

Despite these issues, prospective studies are considerably stronger than retrospective studies. In particular, any ambiguity about whether the presumed cause occurred before the effect is resolved in prospective research if the researcher has confirmed the initial absence of the effect. In addition, samples are more likely to be representative, and investigators may be in a position to impose controls to rule out competing explanations for the results.

➡ **TIP:** The term "prospective" is not synonymous with "longitudinal." Although most nonexperimental prospective studies *are* longitudinal, prospective studies are not *necessarily* longitudinal. Prospective means that information about a possible cause is obtained prior to information about an effect. RCTs are inherently prospective because the researcher introduces the intervention and then determines its effect. An RCT that collected data 1 hour after an intervention would be prospective, but not longitudinal.

Some prospective studies are exploratory. Researchers sometimes measure a wide range of possible "causes" at one point in time, and then examine an outcome of interest at a later point (e.g., length of stay in hospital). Such studies are usually stronger than retrospective studies if it can be determined that the outcome was not present initially because time sequences are clear. They are not, however, as powerful as prospective studies that involve specific *a priori* hypotheses and the comparison of cohorts known to differ on a presumed cause. Researchers doing exploratory retrospective or prospective studies are sometimes accused of going on "fishing expeditions" that can lead to erroneous conclusions because of spurious or idiosyncratic relationships in a particular sample of participants.

Example of a prospective nonexperimental study: Wiklund and colleagues (2009) conducted a prospective cohort study of first-time mothers to examine the effect of mode of delivery (vaginal versus cesarean) on changes in the mothers' personality from predelivery to 9 months after delivery.

Natural Experiments

Researchers are sometimes able to study the outcomes of a "**natural experiment**" in which a group exposed to a phenomenon with potential health consequences is compared with a nonexposed group. Natural experiments are nonexperimental because the researcher does not intervene, but they are called "natural *experiments*" if people are affected essentially at random. For example, the psychological well-being of people living in a community struck with a natural disaster (e.g., a volcanic eruption) could be compared with the well-being of people living in a similar but unaffected community to determine the toll exacted by the disaster (the independent variable). Note that the independent variable or "cause" does not need to be a "natural" phenomenon. It could, for example, be a fire or winning the lottery. Moreover, the groups being compared do not need to be different people; if pre-event measures have been obtained, before–after comparisons might be profitable.

Example of a natural experiment: Liehr and colleagues (2004) were in the midst of collecting data from healthy students over a 3-day period (September 10 to 12, 2001) when the events of September 11 unfolded. The researchers seized the opportunity to examine what people go through in the midst of stressful upheaval. Both pre- and post-tragedy data were available for the students' blood pressure, heart rate, and television viewing.

Path Analytic Studies

Researchers interested in testing theories of causation based on nonexperimental data are increasingly using a technique known as **path analysis** (or similar techniques). Using sophisticated statistical procedures, researchers test a hypothesized causal chain among a set of independent variables, mediating variables, and a dependent variable. Path analytic procedures, described briefly in Chapter 18, allow researchers to test whether nonexperimental data conform sufficiently to the underlying model to justify causal inferences. Path analytic studies can be done within the context of both cross-sectional and longitudinal designs, the latter providing a stronger basis for causal inferences because of the ability to sort out time sequences.

Example of a path analytic study: Chen and Tzeng (2009) tested a model to explain adherence to pelvic floor muscle exercise among women with urinary incontinence. Their path analysis tested hypothesized causal pathways between adherence on the one hand and self-efficacy, exercise knowledge and attitudes, and severity of urine loss on the other.

Descriptive Research

A second broad class of nonexperimental studies is **descriptive research**. The purpose of descriptive studies is to observe, describe, and document aspects of a situation as it naturally occurs and sometimes to serve as a starting point for hypothesis generation or theory development.

Descriptive Correlational Studies

Sometimes researchers are better able to simply describe relationships than to comprehend causal pathways. Many research problems are cast in noncausal terms. We ask, for example, whether men are less likely than women to bond with their newborn infants, not whether a particular configuration of sex chromosomes *caused* differences in parental attachment. Unlike other types of correlational research—such as the cigarette smoking and lung cancer investigations—the aim of **descriptive correlational research** is to describe relationships among variables rather than to support inferences of causality.

Example of a descriptive correlational study: Jacob and colleagues (2010) conducted a descriptive correlational study to examine the relationship between respiratory symptoms and pain experiences in children and adolescents with sickle cell disease.

Studies designed to address diagnosis/assessment questions—that is, whether a tool or procedure yields accurate assessment or diagnostic information about a condition or outcome—typically involve descriptive correlational designs. Procedures are discussed in Chapter 15.

Univariate Descriptive Studies

The aim of some descriptive studies is to describe the frequency of occurrence of a behavior or condition, rather than to study relationships. **Univariate descriptive studies** are not necessarily focused on only one variable. For example, a researcher might be interested in women's experiences during menopause. The study might describe the frequency of various symptoms, the average age at menopause, and the percentage of women using medications to alleviate symptoms. The study involves multiple variables, but the primary purpose is to describe the status of each and not to relate them to one another.

Two types of descriptive study come from the field of epidemiology. **Prevalence studies** are done to estimate the prevalence rate of some condition (e.g., a disease or a behavior, such as smoking) at a particular point in time. Prevalence studies rely on cross-sectional designs in which data are obtained from the population at risk of the condition. The researcher takes a "snapshot" of the population at risk to determine the extent to which the condition of interest is present. The formula for a **prevalence rate** (PR) is:

$$\frac{\text{Number of cases with the condition}}{\text{Number in the population at risk}} \times K$$
$$\text{or disease at a given point in time} \quad of being a case$$

K is the number of people for whom we want to have the rate established (e.g., per 100 or per 1,000 population). When data are obtained from a sample (as would usually be the case), the denominator is the size of the sample, and the numerator is the number of cases with the condition, as identified in the study. If we sampled 500 adults aged 21 years and older living in a community, administered a measure of depression, and found that 80 people met the criteria for clinical depression, then the estimated prevalence rate of clinical depression would be 16 per 100 adults in that community.

Incidence studies estimate the frequency of developing *new* cases. Longitudinal designs are needed to estimate incidence because the researcher must first establish who is at risk of becoming a new case—that is, who is free of the condition at the outset. The formula for an **incidence rate** (IR) is:

$$\frac{\text{Number of new cases with the condition}}{\text{Number in the population at risk of being}} \times K$$
$$\text{or disease over a given time period} \quad a case (free of the condition at the outset)}$$

Continuing with our previous example, suppose in October 2010, we found that 80 in a sample of 500 people were clinically depressed (PR = 16 per 100). To determine the 1-year incidence rate, we would reassess the sample in October 2011. Suppose that, of the 420 previously deemed *not* to be clinically depressed in 2010, 21 were now found to meet the criteria for depression. In this case, the estimated 1-year incidence rate would be 5 per 100 $((21 \div 420) \times 100 = 5)$.

Prevalence and incidence rates can be calculated for subgroups of the population (e.g., for men versus women). When this is done, it is possible to calculate another important descriptive index. **Relative risk** is an estimated risk of "caseness" in one group compared with another. Relative risk is computed by dividing the rate for one group by the rate for another. Suppose we found that the 1-year incidence rate for depression was 6 per 100 women and 4 per 100 men. Women's relative risk for developing depression over the 1-year period would be 1.5, that is, women would be estimated to be 1.5 times more likely to develop depression than men. Relative risk is an important index in assessing the contribution of risk factors to a disease or condition (e.g., by comparing the relative risk for lung cancer for smokers versus nonsmokers).

Example of an incidence and prevalence study: Johansson and colleagues (2009) collected cross-sectional data to estimate the prevalence of malnutrition risk among community-dwelling older people in a Swedish municipality (14.5%). Longitudinal data were also collected to estimate the 1-year incidence rate (7.6%).

⟶ **TIP:** The quality of correlational studies that test hypothesized causal relationships is heavily dependent on design decisions— that is, how researchers design their studies to rule out competing causal explanations for the outcomes. Methods of enhancing the rigor of such studies are described in the next chapter. The quality of descriptive studies, by contrast, is more heavily dependent on having a good (representative) sample (Chapter 12) and high-quality measuring instruments (Chapter 14) than on design.

Strengths and Limitations of Correlational Research

The quality of a study is not necessarily related to its approach; there are many excellent nonexperimental studies as well as flawed experiments. Nevertheless, nonexperimental correlational studies have several drawbacks.

Limitations of Correlational Research
Relative to experimental and quasi-experimental research, nonexperimental studies are weak in their

ability to support causal inferences. In correlational studies, researchers work with preexisting groups that were not formed at random, but rather through **self-selection** (also known as *selection bias*). A researcher doing a correlational study cannot assume that groups being compared are similar before the occurrence of the independent variable—the hypothesized cause. Preexisting differences may be a plausible alternative explanation for any group differences on the outcome variable.

The difficulty of interpreting correlational findings stems from the fact that, in the real world, behaviors, attitudes, and characteristics are interrelated (correlated) in complex ways. An example may help to clarify the problem. Suppose we conducted a cross-sectional study that examined the relationship between level of depression in cancer patients and their social support (i.e., assistance and emotional support from others). We hypothesize that social support (the independent variable) affects levels of depression (the dependent variable). Suppose we find that the patients with weak social support are significantly more depressed than patients with strong support. We could interpret this finding to mean that patients' emotional state is influenced by the adequacy of their social supports. This relationship is diagrammed in Figure 9.4A. Yet, there are alternative explanations. Perhaps a third variable influences *both* social support and depression, such as the patients' marital status. It may be that having a spouse is a powerful

influence on how depressed cancer patients feel *and* on the quality of their social support. This set of relationships is diagramed in Figure 9.4B. In this scenario, social support and depression are correlated simply because marital status affects both. A third possibility is reversed causality (Figure 9.4C). Depressed cancer patients may find it more difficult to elicit needed support from others than patients who are more cheerful or amiable. In this interpretation, the person's depression causes the amount of received social support and not the other way around. Thus, interpretations of most correlational results should be considered tentative, particularly if the research has no theoretical basis and if the design is cross-sectional.

Strengths of Correlational Research

Earlier, we discussed constraints that limit the possibility of applying experimental designs to many research problems. Correlational research will continue to play a crucial role in nursing research precisely because many interesting problems are not amenable to experimentation.

Despite our emphasis on causal inferences, it has already been noted that descriptive correlational research does not focus on understanding causal relationships. Furthermore, if the study is testing a causal hypothesis that has been deduced from an established theory, causal inferences may be possible, especially if strong designs (e.g., a prospective design) are used.

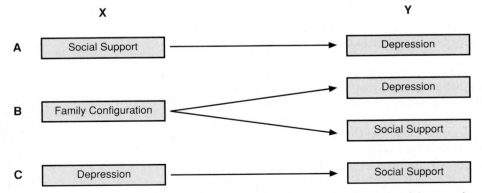

FIGURE 9.4 Alternative explanations for relationship between depression and social support in cancer patients.

Correlational research is often efficient in collecting a large amount of data about a problem. For example, it would be possible to collect extensive information about the health histories and eating habits of a large number of individuals. Researchers could then examine which health problems were associated with which diets, and could thus discover a large number of interrelationships in a relatively short amount of time. By contrast, an experimenter looks at only a few variables at a time. One experiment might manipulate foods high in cholesterol, whereas another might manipulate protein, for example.

Finally, correlational research is often strong in realism. Unlike many experimental studies, correlational research is seldom criticized for its artificiality.

➲ TIP: It is often a good idea to design a study with as many relevant comparisons as possible. Two-group nonequivalent control group posttest-only designs are weak in part because the comparative information they yield is limited. In nonexperimental studies, multiple comparison groups can be effective in dealing with self-selection, especially if comparison groups are chosen to address competing biases. For example, in case–control studies of potential causes of lung cancer, cases would be people with lung cancer, one comparison group could comprise people with a different lung disease and a second could comprise those with no lung disorder.

DESIGNS AND RESEARCH EVIDENCE

Evidence for nursing practice depends on descriptive, correlational, and experimental research. There is often a logical progression to knowledge expansion that begins with rich description, including description from qualitative research. Descriptive studies are valuable in documenting the prevalence, nature, and intensity of health-related conditions and behaviors and are critical in the development of effective interventions. Moreover, in-depth qualitative research may suggest causal links that could be the focus of controlled quantitative research. For example, Colón-Emeric and colleagues (2006) did case studies in two nursing homes. They looked at site differences in communication patterns among the medical and nurs-

ing staff in relation to differences in information flow. Their findings suggested that a "chain of command" type communication style may limit healthcare providers' ability to provide high-quality care. The study suggests a causal hypothesis that merits greater scrutiny with a larger number of nursing homes under more controlled conditions—and also suggests possibilities for interventions. Thus, although qualitative studies are low on the standard evidence hierarchy for *confirming* causal connections (Figure 2.1), they nevertheless serve an important function.

Correlational studies also play a role in developing an evidence base for causal inferences. Retrospective case-control studies may pave the way for more rigorous (but more expensive) prospective studies. As the evidence base builds, conceptual models may be developed and tested using path analytic designs and other theory-testing strategies. These studies can provide hints about how to structure an intervention, who can most profit from it, and when it can best be instituted. Thus, nonexperimental studies can sometimes lead to innovative interventions that can be tested using experimental and quasi-experimental designs.

Many important research questions will never be answered using information from Level I (meta-analyses of RCTs) or Level II studies (RCTs) on the standard evidence hierarchy. An important example is the question of whether smoking causes lung cancer. Despite the inability to randomize people to smoking and nonsmoking groups, few people doubt that this causal connection exists. Thinking about the criteria for causality discussed early in this chapter, there is ample evidence that smoking cigarettes is correlated with lung cancer and, through prospective studies, that smoking precedes lung cancer. The large number of studies conducted has allowed researchers to control for, and thus rule out, other possible "causes" of lung cancer. There has been a great deal of consistency and coherence in the findings. And, the criterion of biologic plausibility has been met through basic physiologic research.

Thus, it may be best to think of alternative evidence hierarchies for questions relating to causality. For "therapy" questions (Table 2.1), experimental designs are the "gold standard." On the next rung of the hierarchy for therapy questions are strong quasi-experimental designs, such as nonequivalent control group pretest–posttest designs. Further down the hierarchy are weaker quasi-experimental designs and then correlational studies.

➲ **T I P :** Studies have shown that evidence from RCTs, quasi-experimental, and observational studies often do not yield the same results. Often the relationship between "causes" and "effects" appears to be stronger in nonexperimental and quasi-experimental studies than in studies in which competing explanations are ruled out through randomization to different conditions.

For questions about prognosis or about etiology and harm (Table 2.1), both of which concern causal relationships, strong prospective (cohort) studies are usually the best design (although there are some situations in which etiology questions can involve randomization). Path analytic studies with longitudinal data and a strong theoretical basis can also be powerful. Retrospective case-control studies are relatively weak, by contrast. Systematic reviews of multiple prospective studies, together with support from theories or biophysiologic research, represent the strongest evidence for these types of question.

CRITIQUING GUIDELINES FOR STUDY DESIGN

The research design used in a quantitative study strongly influences the quality of its evidence and so should be carefully scrutinized. Researchers' design

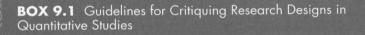

BOX 9.1 Guidelines for Critiquing Research Designs in Quantitative Studies

1. What type of question (therapy, prognosis, etc.) is being addressed? Does the research question concern a possible causal relationship between the independent and dependent variables?
2. What would be the strongest design for the research question? How does this compare with the design actually used?
3. Is there an intervention or treatment? Was the intervention adequately described? Was the control or comparison condition adequately described? Was an experimental or quasi-experimental design used?
4. If the study was an RCT, what specific experimental design was used? Were randomization procedures adequately explained? Does the report provide evidence that randomization was successful—that is, resulted in groups that were comparable prior to the intervention? If cluster randomization was used, was there an adequate number of units?
5. If the design is quasi-experimental, what specific quasi-experimental design was used? Is there justification for deciding not to randomize participants to treatment conditions? Does the report provide evidence that any groups being compared were equivalent prior to the intervention?
6. If the design was nonexperimental, was the study inherently nonexperimental? If not, is there justification for not manipulating the independent variable? What specific nonexperimental design was used? If a retrospective design was used, is there justification for not using a prospective design? What evidence does the report provide that any groups being compared were similar with regard to important confounding characteristics?
7. What types of comparisons are specified in the design (e.g., before–after, between groups)? Do these comparisons adequately illuminate the relationship between the independent and dependent variables? If there are no comparisons, or faulty comparisons, how does this affect the study's integrity and the interpretability of the results?
8. Was the study longitudinal? Was the timing of the collection of data appropriate? Was the number of data collection points reasonable?
9. Was blinding/masking used? If yes, who was blinded—and was this adequate? If not, is there an adequate rationale for failure to mask? Is the intervention a type that could raise expectations that in and of themselves could alter the outcomes?

decisions have more of an impact on study quality than perhaps any other methodologic decision when the research question is about causal relationships.

Actual designs and some controlling techniques (randomization, blinding, allocation concealment) were described in this chapter, and the next chapter explains in greater detail specific strategies for enhancing research control. The guidelines in Box 9.1 ⊗ are the first of two sets of questions to help you in critiquing quantitative research designs.

RESEARCH EXAMPLES

In this section, we present descriptions of an experimental, quasi-experimental, and nonexperimental study.

Research Example of an Experimental Study

Study: The Well Woman Program: A community-based randomized trial to prevent sexually transmitted infections in low-income African American women" (Marion et al., 2009).

Statement of Purpose: The purpose of the study was to determine the effectiveness of an intensive, culturally specific intervention designed to reduce sexually transmitted infections (STIs) among low-income African American women living in high-risk communities.

Treatment Groups: Nurse practitioners and trained peer educators delivered the Well Woman Program (WWP) in two phases. In the 2-month intensive phase, participants in the experimental group had a physical exam, received individual counseling, and attended group sessions led by peer educators. In the maintenance phase (months 3 through 12), they had ongoing tailored counseling and education. Participants in the "minimal intervention" control group received a 10-minute presentation on STIs, STI testing, and care as usual with community providers.

Method: A sample of 342 women from Chicago with a prior history of STIs was randomly assigned to the experimental or control group, using sealed envelopes with randomly generated numbers. Women were randomized in blocks of 10 to ensure comparable numbers in the two groups. Although study participants and those administering the intervention could not be blinded to the women's group status, data collectors were blinded. Data were collected from all women prior to random assignment and then at three follow-up points over the course of 15-months. The primary outcome was biologically confirmed sexually transmitted infection, using nucleic acid amplification tests on vaginal swabs. Participants also completed questionnaires with questions relating to STI risk behavior and other psychological variables.

Key Findings: Randomization appeared to be successful: the two groups were similar in terms of background characteristics that could affect STIs (e.g., age, number of lifetime partners), and in terms of baseline rate of having a positive test for an STI. At month 15, the estimated probability of WWP participants having an STI was 20% less than control group participants, leading the investigators to conclude that "better STI outcomes were due to the intensive individualized intervention" (p. 274).

Research Example of a Quasi-Experimental Study

Study: The impact of a multimedia informational intervention on healthcare service use among women and men newly diagnosed with cancer (Loiselle & Dubois, 2009).

Statement of Purpose: The purpose of the study was to test the effect of a comprehensive cancer informational intervention using information technology on patient satisfaction and the use of healthcare services by men and women newly diagnosed with cancer.

Treatment Groups: The intervention group received a 1-hour training session on the use of information technology, a CD-ROM with information on cancer, and a list of reputable cancer-related web sites. A research assistant was available by telephone or email to answer questions. Intervention materials (including laptop computers for those without a home computer) were available for an 8-week period. The control group received usual care.

Method: Patients from four cancer clinics within large teaching hospitals in Montreal were involved in this study. Eligible patients in three clinics were recruited into the intervention group, while those in the fourth clinic were recruited as the controls. To be eligible, patients had to be newly diagnosed with either breast or prostate cancer and had to plan cancer treatment in one of the study sites. Altogether, 250 patients agreed to participate, 148 in the intervention group and 102 in the comparison group. Data relating to healthcare service use, patient satisfaction, perceptions of information support, and other variables were collected prior to the intervention, 9 weeks later, and then again 3 months later.

Key Findings: The intervention and comparison group members were similar demographically in some respects (e.g., marital status), but several preintervention group differences were found. For example, patients in the intervention group were younger and better educated than those in the comparison group. To address this selection bias problem, these characteristics were controlled statistically, an approach discussed in the next chapter. Patients in the two groups did not differ in their reliance on healthcare services following the intervention. However, patients in the experimental group were significantly more satisfied than those in the comparison group with the cancer information they received.

Research Example of a Correlational Study

Study: Placental position and late stillbirth: A case-control study (Warland, et al., 2009)

Statement of Purpose: The purpose of the study was to examine whether placental position in pregnancy contributes to the risk of having a stillbirth. Earlier research had suggested that some implantation sites may not provide adequate supply of nutrients and oxygen to the fetus.

Method: Pregnant women from two Australian obstetric hospitals were included in the sample. The cases were women with a discharge diagnosis of stillbirth who were at 27 or more weeks gestation. The control group comprised women who gave birth to a live baby at the same hospital during the same period. Controls were matched to cases on maternal age, infant gender, and gestational age. The researchers attempted to match two controls for every case, and were successful for all but five cases. Another nine cases could not be matched to any live-birth mother, and these were removed from the sample. The final sample consisted of 124 cases and 243 controls. The researchers retrospectively reviewed clinical records for all women and recorded the placental position that had been noted during a routine second trimester ultrasound.

Key Finding: Women who had a posterior located placenta were significantly more likely to suffer a still-

birth than women who had a placenta in any other position.

SUMMARY POINTS

- Many quantitative nursing studies aim to elucidate *cause-and-effect relationships*. The challenge of research design is to facilitate inferences about causality.
- Various criteria are used to establish causality. One criterion is that an observed relationship between a presumed cause (independent variable) and an effect (dependent variable) cannot be explained as being caused by other (confounding) variables.
- In an idealized model, a **counterfactual** is what would have happened to the same people simultaneously exposed *and* not exposed to the causal factor. The *effect* represents the difference between the two. The goal of research design is to find a good approximation to the idealized counterfactual.
- **Experiments** (or **randomized controlled trials [RCTs]**) involve **manipulation** (the researcher manipulates the independent variable by introducing a **treatment** or **intervention**); control (including use of a **control group** that is not given the intervention and represents the comparative counterfactual); and **randomization** or **random assignment** (with people allocated to experimental and control groups at random to form groups that are comparable at the outset).
- Everyone in the experimental group usually gets the same intervention as delineated in formal protocols, but some studies involve **patient-centered interventions (PCIs)** that are tailored to meet individual needs or characteristics.
- Researchers can expose the control group to various conditions, including no treatment, an alternative treatment, a **placebo** or pseudointervention, standard treatment ("usual care"), different doses of the treatment, or a **wait-list** (*delayed treatment*) group.
- Random assignment is done by methods that give every participant an equal chance of being in any group, such as by flipping a coin or using

a **table of random numbers**. Randomization is the most reliable method for equating groups on all characteristics that could affect study outcomes. Randomization should involve **allocation concealment** that prevents foreknowledge of upcoming assignments.

- Randomization sometimes involves **stratification** in which participations are first divided into groups (e.g., men and women) before being randomized. In **permuted block randomization**, randomization is done for blocks of people—for example, 6 or 8 at a time in randomly selected block sizes—to ensure a balanced allocation to groups within cohorts of participants.

- **Blinding** (or **masking**) is sometimes used to avoid biases stemming from participants' or research agents' awareness of group status or study hypotheses. **Single-blind studies** involve masking of one group (e.g., participants) and **double-blind studies** involve masking of two groups (e.g., participants, investigators).

- The standard process is to randomize *individuals* to conditions after informed consent and the collection of **baseline data**, but there are variations. **Cluster randomization** involves randomizing larger units (e.g., hospitals) to treatment conditions. **Partially randomized patient preference (PRPP) designs** involve randomizing only patients without a treatment preference. **Randomized consent** (or **Zelen**) **designs** randomize prior to informed consent.

- A **posttest-only** (or **after-only**) **design** involves collecting data only after an intervention. In a **pretest–posttest** (or **before–after**) **design**, data are collected both before and after the intervention, permitting an analysis of change.

- **Factorial designs**, in which two or more independent variables are manipulated simultaneously, allow researchers to test both **main effects** (effects from manipulated independent variables) and **interaction effects** (effects from combining treatments).

- In a **crossover design**, people are exposed to more than one experimental condition, administered in a randomized order, and thus serve as their own controls.

- Experimental designs are the "gold standard" because they come closer than any other design in meeting criteria for inferring causal relationships.

- **Quasi-experimental designs** (*controlled trials without randomization*) involve an intervention but lack randomization. Strong quasi-experimental designs include features in support of causal inferences.

- The **nonequivalent control group pretest–posttest design** involves using a nonrandomized **comparison group** and the collection of pretreatment data so that initial group equivalence can be assessed. Comparability of groups can be sometimes be enhanced through *matching* on individual characteristics or by **propensity matching** that involves matching on a **propensity score** for each participant.

- In a **time series design**, there is no comparison group; information on the dependent variable is collected over a period of time before and after the intervention. Time series designs are often used in **single-subject (*N*-of-1) experiments**.

- Other quasi-experimental designs include the **regression discontinuity design**, quasi-experimental **dose-response analyses**, and the quasi-experimental (nonrandomized) **arms** of a PRPP randomization design (i.e., groups with strong preferences).

- In evaluating the results of quasi-experiments, it is important to ask whether it is plausible that factors other than the intervention caused or affected the outcomes (i.e., whether there are **rival hypotheses** for explaining the results).

- **Nonexperimental** (or **observational**) **research** includes **descriptive research**—studies that summarize the status of phenomena—and **correlational** studies that examine relationships among variables but involve no manipulation of the independent variable (often because it *cannot* be manipulated).

- Designs for correlational studies include **retrospective (case-control) designs** (which begin with the outcome and look back in time for antecedent causes of "caseness" by comparing **cases** that have a disease or condition with controls who do not); **prospective (cohort) designs** (studies that begin with a presumed cause and look forward in time for its effect); **natural experiments** (in which a group is affected by a seemingly random event, such as a disaster); and **path analytic studies** (which test causal models developed on the basis of theory).

- **Descriptive correlational studies** describe how phenomena are interrelated without invoking a causal explanations. **Univariate descriptive studies** examine the frequency or average value of variables.

- Descriptive studies include **prevalence studies** that document the prevalence rate of a condition at one point in time and **incidence studies** that document the frequency of *new* cases, over a given time period. When the incidence rates for two groups are determined, it is possible to compute the **relative risk** of "caseness" for the two.

- The primary weakness of correlational studies for cause-probing questions is that they can harbor biases due to **self-selection** into groups being compared.

STUDY ACTIVITIES

Chapter 9 of the *Resource Manual for Nursing Research: Generating and Assessing Evidence for Nursing Practice, 9th ed.*, offers study suggestions for reinforcing concepts presented in this chapter. In addition, the following questions can be addressed in classroom or online discussions:

1. Assume that you have 10 people—Z, Y, X, W, V, U, T, S, R, and Q—who are going to participate in an RCT you are conducting. Using a table of random numbers, assign five individuals to group 1 and five to group 2.
2. Insofar as possible, use the questions in Box 9.1 to critique the three research examples described at the end of the chapter.
3. Discuss how you would design a prospective study to address the question posed in the Warland and colleagues (2009) case-control study summarized at the end of the chapter.

STUDIES CITED IN CHAPTER 9

Chen, S. Y., & Tzeng, Y. (2009). Path analysis for adherence to pelvic floor exercise among women with urinary incontinence. *Journal of Nursing Research, 17*, 83–92.

Colón-Emeric, C., Ammarell, N, Bailey, D., Corazzini, K., Lekan-Rutledge, D., Piven, M., Utley-Smith, Q., & Anderson, R. A. (2006). Patterns of medical and nursing staff communication in nursing homes. *Qualitative Health Research, 16*, 173–188.

Coward, D. (2002). Partial randomization design in a support group intervention study. *Western Journal of Nursing Research, 24*, 406–421.

Elliott, A., & Horgas, A. (2009). Effects of an analgesic trial in reducing pain behaviors in community-dwelling older adults with dementia. *Nursing Research, 58*, 140–145.

Hatfield, L. A. (2008). Sucrose decreases infant biobehavioral pain response to immunizations: A randomized controlled trial. *Journal of Nursing Scholarship, 40*, 219–225.

Heidrich, S., Brown, R., Egan, J., Perez, O., Phelan, C., Yeom, H., & Ward, S. (2009). An individualized representational intervention to improve symptom management (IRIS) in older breast cancer survivors. *Oncology Nursing Forum, 36*, E133–E143.

Hicks-Moore, S. (2005). Relaxing music at mealtime in nursing homes: Effects on agitated patients with dementia. *Journal of Gerontological Nursing, 31*, 26–32.

Huizing, A., Hamers, J., Gulpers, M., & Berger, M. (2009). Preventing the use of physical restraints on residents newly admitted to psycho-geriatric nursing home wards: A cluster-randomized trial. *International Journal of Nursing Studies, 46*, 459–469.

Jacob, E., Sockrider, M., Dinu, M., Acosta, M., & Mueller, B. (2010). Respiratory symptoms and acute painful episodes in sickle cell disease. *Journal of Pediatric Oncology Nursing, 27*, 33–39.

Johansson, Y., Bachrach-Lindstrom, M., Carstensen, J., & Ek, A. (2009). Malnutrition in a home-living older population: Prevalence, incidence and risk factors. *Journal of Clinical Nursing, 18*, 1354–1364.

Kratz, A. (2008). Use of the acute confusion protocol: A research utilization project. *Journal of Nursing Care Quality, 23*, 331–337.

Lai, H., & Good, M. (2005). Music improves sleep quality in older adults. *Journal of Advanced Nursing, 49*, 234–244.

Lai, H., Chen, C., Peng, T., Chang, F., Hsieh, M., Huang, H., & Chang, S. (2006). Randomized controlled trial of music during kangaroo care on maternal state anxiety and preterm infants' responses. *International Journal of Nursing Studies, 43*, 139–146.

Lauver, D., Settersten, L., Kane, J., & Henriques, J. (2003). Tailored messages, external barriers, and women's utilization of professional breast cancer screening over time. *Cancer, 97*, 2724–2735.

Liehr, P., Mehl, M., Summers, L., & Pennebaker, J. (2004). Connecting with others in the midst of stressful upheaval on September 11, 2001. *Applied Nursing Research, 17*, 2–9.

Loiselle, C., & Dubois, S. (2009). The impact of a multimedia informational intervention on healthcare service use among women and men newly diagnosed with cancer. *Cancer Nursing, 32*, 37–44.

Marion, L. N., Finnegan, L., Campbell, R., & Szalacha, L. (2009). The Well Woman Program: A community-based randomized trial to prevent sexually transmitted infections in low-income African American women. *Research in Nursing & Health, 32*, 274–285.

Martinez, C., Carmelli, E., Barak, S., & Stopka, C. (2009). Changes in pain-free walking based on time in accommodating pain-free exercise therapy for peripheral artery disease. *Journal of Vascular Nursing, 27*, 2–7.

Munro, C., Grap, M., Jones, D., McClish, D., & Sessler, C. (2009). Chlorhexidine, toothbrushing, and preventing ventilator-assisted pneumonia in critically ill adults. *American Journal of Critical Care, 18*, 428–437.

Musil, C., Warner, C., Zauszniewski, J., Wykle, M., & Standing, T. (2009). Grandmother caregiving, family stress and strain, and depressive symptoms. *Western Journal of Nursing Research, 31*, 389–408.

Nikolajsen, L., Lyndgaard, K., Schriver, N., & Mollet, J. (2009). Does audiovisual stimulation with music and nature sights reduce pain and discomfort during placement of a femoral nerve block? *Journal of Perianesthesia Nursing, 24*, 14–18.

Pinar, K., Moore, K., Smits, E., Murphy, K., & Schopflocher, D. (2009). Leg bag comparison: Reported skin health, comfort, and satisfaction. *Journal of Wound, Ostomy, & Continence Nursing, 36*, 319–326.

Pölkki, T., Pietilä, A., Vehviläinen-Julkunen, K., Laukkala, H., & Kiviluoma, K. (2008). Imagery-induced relaxation in children's postoperative pain relief. *Journal of Pediatric Nursing, 23*, 217–224.

Seers, K., Crichton, N., Tutton, L., Smith, L., & Saunders, T. (2008). Effectiveness of relaxation for postoperative pain and anxiety: randomized controlled trial. *Journal of Advanced Nursing, 62*, 681–688.

Steiner, A., Walsh, B., Pickering, R., Wiles, R., Ward, J., Brooking, J., & Southampton NLU Evaluation Team. (2001). Therapeutic nursing or unblocking beds? A randomized controlled trial of a post-acute intermediate care unit. *British Medical Journal, 322*(7284), 453–460.

Swadener-Culpepper, L., Skaggs, R., & Vangilder, C. (2008). The impact of continuous lateral rotation therapy in overall clinical and financial outcomes of critically ill patients. *Critical Care Nursing Quarterly, 31*, 270–279.

Swenson, K., Nissen, M., Leach, J., & Post-White, J. (2009). Case-control study to evaluate predictors of lymphedema after breast cancer surgery. *Oncology Nursing Forum, 36*, 185–193.

Warland, J., McCutcheon, H., & Baghurst, P. (2009). Placental position and late stillbirth: A case control study. *Journal of Clinical Nursing, 18*, 1602–1606.

Wentworth, L., Briese, L., Timimi, F., Bartel, D., Cutshall, S., Tilbury, R., Lennon, R., & Bauer, B. A. (2009). Massage therapy reduces tension, anxiety, and pain in patients awaiting invasive cardiovascular procedures. *Progress in Cardiovascular Nursing, 24*, 155–161.

Wiklund, I., Edman, G., Larsson, C., & Andolf, E. (2009). First-time mothers and changes in personality in relation to mode of delivery. *Journal of Advanced Nursing, 65*, 1636–1644.

Yuan, S., Chou, M., Hwu, L., Chang, Y., Hsu, W., & Kuo, H. (2009). An intervention program to promote health-related physical fitness in nurses. *Journal of Clinical Nursing, 18*, 1404–1411.

Methodologic and nonresearch references cited in this chapter can be found in a separate section at the end of the book.

10

Rigor and Validity in Quantitative Research

VALIDITY AND INFERENCE

This chapter describes strategies for enhancing the rigor of quantitative studies, including ways to minimize biases and control confounding variables. Most of these strategies help to strengthen the inferences that can be made about cause-and-effect relationships.

Validity and Validity Threats

In designing a study, a constructive approach is to anticipate the possible factors that could undermine the **validity** of inferences. Shadish and colleagues (2002) define validity in the context of research design as "the approximate truth of an inference" (p. 34). For example, inferences that an *effect* results from a hypothesized *cause* are valid to the extent that researchers can marshal supporting evidence. Validity is always a matter of degree, not an absolute.

Validity is a property of an inference, not of a research design, but design elements profoundly affect the inferences that can be made. **Threats to validity** are reasons that an inference could be wrong. When researchers introduce design features to minimize potential threats, the validity of the inference is strengthened, and thus evidence is

more persuasive. We identify important validity threats to encourage you to think about ways to address them during the design phase of a study and to evaluate them in interpreting study results.

Types of Validity

Shadish and colleagues (2002) proposed a validity taxonomy that identified four aspects of a good research design, and catalogued dozens of threats to validity. This chapter describes the taxonomy and briefly summarizes major threats, but we urge researchers to consult this seminal work for further guidance on strengthening study validity.

The first type of validity, **statistical conclusion validity**, concerns the validity of inferences that there truly is an empirical relationship, or correlation, between the presumed cause and the effect. The researcher's job is to provide the strongest possible evidence that the relationship is *real* and that the intervention (if any) was given a fair test.

Internal validity concerns the validity of inferences that, given that an empirical relationship exists, it is the independent variable, rather than something else, that caused the outcome. The researcher's job is to develop strategies to rule out the plausibility that something other than the independent variable accounts for the observed relationship.

Construct validity involves the validity of inferences "from the observed persons, settings, and cause-and-effect operations included in the study to the constructs that these instances might represent" (p. 38). One aspect of construct validity concerns the degree to which an intervention is a good representation of the underlying construct that was theorized as having the potential to cause beneficial outcomes. Another concerns whether the measures of the dependent variable are good operationalizations of the constructs for which they are intended.

External validity concerns whether inferences about observed relationships will hold over variations in persons, setting, time, or measures of the outcomes. External validity, then, is about the generalizability of causal inferences, and this is a critical concern for research that aims to yield evidence for evidence-based nursing practice.

These four types of validity and their associated threats are discussed in this chapter. Many validity threats concern inadequate control over confounding variables, so we briefly review methods of controlling variation associated with characteristics of study participants.

Controlling Intrinsic Source of Confounding Variability

This section describes six ways of controlling confounding participant characteristics to rule out rival explanations for cause-and-effect relationships.

Randomization

Randomization is the most effective method of controlling individual characteristics. The primary function of randomization is to secure comparable groups—that is, to equalize groups with respect to confounding variables. A distinct advantage of random assignment, compared with other control methods, is that it controls *all* possible sources of extraneous variation, *without any conscious decision about which variables need to be controlled.*

Crossover

Randomization within a crossover design is an especially powerful method of ensuring equivalence between groups being compared—participants serve

as their own controls. Moreover, fewer participants usually are needed in such a design. Fifty people exposed to two treatments in random order yield 100 pieces of data (50 × 2); 50 people randomly assigned to two different groups yield only 50 pieces of data (25 × 2). Crossover designs are not appropriate for all studies, however, because of the possible carry-over effects: People exposed to two different conditions may be influenced in the second condition by their experience in the first.

Homogeneity

When randomization and crossover are not feasible, alternative methods of controlling confounding characteristics are needed. One method is to use only people who are homogeneous with respect to confounding variables—that is, confounding traits are not allowed to vary. Suppose we were testing the effectiveness of a physical fitness program on the cardiovascular functioning of elders. Our quasi-experimental design involves elders from two different nursing homes, with elders in one of them receiving the physical fitness program. If gender were an important confounding variable (and if the two nursing homes had different proportions of men and women), we could control gender by using only men (or only women) as participants.

Using a homogeneous sample is easy as a control mechanism, but the price is that research findings can be generalized only to the type of people who participated in the study. If the physical fitness program were found to have beneficial effects on the cardiovascular status of a sample of women 65 to 75 years of age, its usefulness for improving the cardiovascular status of men in their 80s would require a separate study. Indeed, one noteworthy criticism of this approach is that researchers sometimes exclude people who are extremely ill, which means that the findings cannot be generalized to those who perhaps are most in need of interventions.

Example of control through homogeneity:
Ngai and colleagues (2010) studied factors that predicted maternal role competence and satisfaction among mothers in Hong Kong. Several variables were controlled through homogeneity, including ethnicity (all were Chinese), parity (all primiparous), and marital status (all were married).

⟳ **T I P :** The principle of homogeneity is often used to control (hold constant) external factors as well as participant characteristics. For example, it may be important to collect outcome data at the same time of the day for all participants if time could affect the outcome (e.g., fatigue). As another example, it may be desirable to maintain **constancy of conditions** in terms of locale of data collection — for example, interviewing all respondents in their own homes, rather than some in their places of work. In each setting, participants assume different roles (e.g., spouse and parent versus employee), and responses may be influenced to some degree by those roles.

Stratification/Blocking

Another approach to controlling confounding variables is to include them in the research design through stratification, as discussed in Chapter 9. To pursue our example of the physical fitness program with gender as the confounding variable, we could build it into the study in a randomized block design in which elderly men and women would be randomly assigned separately to treatment groups. This approach can enhance the likelihood of detecting differences between our experimental and control groups because we can eliminate the effect of the blocking variable (gender) on the dependent variable. In addition, if the blocking variable is of interest substantively, this approach gives researchers the opportunity to study differences in groups created by the stratifying variable (e.g., men versus women). Stratification is appropriate in experiments, and is used in quasi-experimental and correlational studies as well.

Matching

Matching (also called **pair matching**) involves using information about people's characteristics to create comparable groups. If matching were used in our physical fitness example, and age and gender were the confounding variables, we would match a person in the program group with one in the comparison group with respect to age and gender. As noted in the previous chapter, there are reasons why matching is problematic. First, to use matching, researchers must know the relevant confounding variables in advance. Second, it is often difficult to match on more than two or three variables, unless propensity score matching is used—but this method requires technical sophistica-

tion. Yet there are usually many confounding variables that could affect outcomes of interest. For these reasons, matching as the primary control technique should be used only when other, more powerful procedures are not feasible, as might be the case in some nonexperimental studies (e.g., case-control designs).

Sometimes, as an alternative to pair matching, researchers use a *balanced design* with regard to key confounders. In such situations, researchers attempt only to ensure that the groups being compared have similar proportional representation on confounding variables, rather than matching on a one-to-one basis. For example, if gender and age were the two variables of concern, we would strive to ensure that the same percentage of men and women were in the two groups and that the average age was comparable. Such an approach is less cumbersome than pair matching, but has similar limitations. Nevertheless, both pair matching and balancing are preferable to failing to control participant characteristics at all.

Example of control through matching: Luttik and colleagues (2009) studied quality of life in partners of people with congestive heart failure, in comparison to those living with a healthy partner. The two groups of partners were matched in terms of gender and age.

Statistical Control

Another method of controlling confounding variables is through statistical analysis rather than research design. A detailed description of powerful **statistical control** mechanisms will be postponed until Chapter 18, but we will explain underlying principles with a simple illustration of a procedure called **analysis of covariance (ANCOVA)**.

In our physical fitness example, suppose we used a nonequivalent control group design with residents from two nursing homes, and resting heart rate was an outcome. We would expect individual differences in heart rate within the sample—that is, it would vary from one person to the next. The research question is, Can some of the individual differences in heart rate be attributed to a person's participation in physical fitness? We know that differences in heart rate are also related to other characteristics, such as age. In Figure 10.1, the large circles represent the

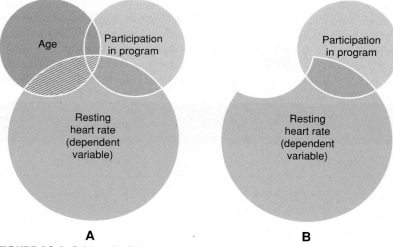

FIGURE 10.1 Schematic diagram illustrating the principle of analysis of covariance.

total extent of individual differences for resting heart rate. A certain amount of variability can be explained by a person's age, which is the small circle on the left in Figure 10.1A. Another part of the variability can perhaps be explained by participation or nonparticipation in the program, represented as the small circle on the right. The two small circles (age and program participation) overlap, indicating a relationship between the two. In other words, people in the physical fitness group are, on average, either older or younger than those in the comparison group, and so age should be controlled. Otherwise, it will be impossible to determine whether postintervention differences in resting heart rate are attributable to differences in age or program participation.

Analysis of covariance controls by statistically removing the effect of confounding variables on the outcome. In the illustration, the portion of heart rate variability attributable to age (the hatched area of the large circle in A) is removed through ANCOVA. Figure 10.1B shows that the final analysis assesses the effect of program participation on heart rate *after removing the effect of age.* By controlling heart rate variability resulting from age, we get a more accurate estimate of the effect of the program on heart rate. Note that even after removing variability due to age, there is still individual variation not associated with the program treatment—the

bottom half of the large circle in B. This means that the study can probably be further enhanced by controlling additional confounders that might account for heart rate differences in the two nursing homes, such as gender, smoking history, and so on. Analysis of covariance and other sophisticated procedures can control multiple confounding variables.

Example of statistical control: Lee and colleagues (2009) tested the effectiveness of a 26-week Tai Chi intervention on health-related quality of life (QOL) in residents from six nursing homes, two of which got the intervention and the other four of which did not. Changes in QOL for residents receiving and not receiving the intervention were compared, while controlling statistically for resident satisfaction.

⊃ **TIP:** Confounding participant characteristics that need to be controlled vary from one study to another, but we can offer some guidance. The best variable is the dependent variable itself, measured before the independent variable occurs. In our physical fitness example, controlling preprogram measures of cardiovascular functioning through ANCOVA would be especially powerful because this would remove the effect of individual variation stemming from many other extraneous factors. Major demographic variables (e.g., age, race/ethnicity, education) and health status indicators are usually good candidates to measure and control. Confounding variables that need to be controlled — variables that correlate with the outcomes — should be identified through a literature review.

Evaluation of Control Methods

Table 10.1 summarizes benefits and drawbacks of the six control mechanisms. Randomization is the most effective method of managing confounding variables—that is, of approximating the ideal but unattainable counterfactual discussed in Chapter 9—because it tends to cancel out individual differences on all possible confounders. Crossover designs are a useful supplement to randomization, but are not always appropriate. The remaining alternatives have a common disadvantage: Researchers must know in advance the relevant confounding variables. To

TABLE 10.1	**Methods of Control over Participant Characteristics**	
METHOD	**BENEFITS**	**LIMITATIONS**
Randomization	• Controls all preintervention confounding variables • Does not require advance knowledge of which variables to control	• Ethical and practical constraints on variables that can be manipulated • Possible artificiality of conditions
Crossover	• If done with randomization, strongest possible approach	• Cannot be used if there are possible carry-over effect from one condition to the next • History threat may be relevant if external factors change over time
Homogeneity	• Easy to achieve in all types of research • Could enhance interpretability of relationships	• Limits generalizability • Requires knowledge of which variables to control • Range restriction could lower statistical conclusion validity
Stratification	• Enhances the ability to detect and interpret relationships • Offers opportunity to examine blocking variable as an independent variable	• Usually restricted to a few stratifying variables • Requires knowledge of which variables to control
Matching	• Enhances ability to detect and interpret relationships • May be easy if there is a large "pool" of potential available controls	• Usually restricted to a few matching variables (except with propensity matching) • Requires knowledge of which variables to match • May be difficult to find comparison group matches, especially if there are more than two matching variables
Statistical control	• Enhances ability to detect and interpret relationships • Relatively economical means of controlling several confounding variables	• Requires knowledge of which variables to control, as well as measurement of those variables • Requires some statistical sophistication

select homogeneous samples, stratify, match, or perform ANCOVA, researchers must know which variables need to be measured and controlled. Yet, when randomization is impossible, the use of any of these strategies is better than no control strategy at all.

STATISTICAL CONCLUSION VALIDITY

As noted in Chapter 9, one criterion for establishing causality is demonstrating that there is a relationship between the independent and dependent variable. Statistical methods are used to support inferences about whether relationships exist. Design decisions can influence whether statistical tests will detect true relationships, so researchers need to make decisions that protect against reaching false statistical conclusions. Even for research that is not cause probing, researchers need to attend to statistical conclusion validity: The issue is whether relationships that exist in reality can be reliably detected in a study. Shadish and colleagues (2002) discussed nine threats to statistical conclusion validity. We focus here on three especially important threats.

Low Statistical Power

Statistical power refers to the ability to detect true relationships among variables. Adequate statistical power can be achieved in various ways, the most straightforward of which is to use a sufficiently large sample. When small samples are used, statistical power tends to be low, and the analyses may fail to show that the independent and dependent variables are related—*even when they are*. Power and sample size are discussed in Chapters 12 and 17.

Another aspect of a powerful design concerns how the independent variable is defined. Both statistically and substantively, results are clearer when differences between groups being compared are large. Researchers should aim to maximize group differences on the dependent variables by maxi-

mizing differences on the independent variable. Conn and colleagues (2001) offer good suggestions for enhancing the power and effectiveness of nursing interventions. Strengthening group differences is usually easier in experimental than in nonexperimental research. In experiments, investigators can devise treatment conditions that are as distinct as money, ethics, and practicality permit. Even in nonexperimental research, however, there may be opportunities to operationalize independent variables in such a way that power to detect differences is enhanced.

Another aspect of statistical power concerns maximizing **precision**, which is achieved through accurate measuring tools, controls over confounding variables, and powerful statistical methods. Precision can best be explained through an example. Suppose we were studying the effect of admission into a nursing home on depression by comparing elders who were or were not admitted. Depression varies from one elderly person to another for various reasons. We want to isolate—as precisely as possible—the portion of variation in depression attributable to nursing home admission. Mechanisms of research control that reduce variability attributable to confounding factors can be built into the research design, thereby enhancing precision. The following ratio expresses what we wish to assess in this example:

$$\frac{\text{Variability in depression}}{\text{Variability in depression due to other factors}}$$
$$\text{(e.g., age, pain, medical condition)}$$

This ratio, greatly simplified here, captures the essence of many statistical tests. We want to make variability in the numerator (the upper half) as large as possible relative to variability in the denominator (the lower half), to evaluate precisely the relationship between nursing home admission and depression. The smaller the variability in depression due to confounding variables (e.g., age, pain), the easier it will be to detect differences in depression between elders who were or were not admitted to a nursing home. Designs that enable researchers to reduce variability caused by confounders can increase statistical conclusion validity. As a purely hypothetical illustration, we will attach some numeric values* to the ratio as follows:

$$\frac{\text{Variability due to nursing home admission}}{\text{Variability due to all confounding variables}} = \frac{10}{4}$$

If we can make the bottom number smaller, say by changing it from 4 to 2, we will have a more precise estimate of the effect of nursing home admission on depression, relative to other influences. Control mechanisms such as those described earlier help to reduce variability caused by extraneous variables and should be considered as design options in planning a study. We illustrate this by continuing our example, singling out age as a key confounding variable. Total variability in levels of depression can be conceptualized as having the following components:

Total variability in depression = Variability
due to nursing home admission + Variability
due to age + Variability due to other
confounding variables

This equation can be taken to mean that part of the reason why some elders are depressed and others are not is that some were admitted to a nursing home and others were not; some were older and some were younger; other factors, such as level of pain and medical condition, also had an effect on depression.

One way to increase precision in this study would be to control age, thereby removing the variability in depression that results from age differences. We could do this, for example, by restricting age to elders younger than 80, thereby reducing the variability in depression due to age. As a result, the

effect of nursing home admission on depression becomes greater, relative to the remaining variability. Thus, this design decision (homogeneity) enabled us to get a more precise estimate of the effect of nursing home admission on level of depression (although, of course, this limits generalizability). Research designs differ considerably in the sensitivity with which effects under study can be detected statistically. Lipsey (1990) has prepared an excellent guide to assist researchers in enhancing the sensitivity of research designs.

Restriction of Range

Although the control of extraneous variation through homogeneity is easy to use and can help to clarify the relationship between key research variables, it can be risky. Not only does this approach limit the generalizability of study findings, but it can also sometimes undermine statistical conclusion validity. When the use of homogeneity restricts the range of values on the outcome variable, relationships between the outcome and the independent variable will be *attenuated*, and may, therefore, lead to an erroneous inference that the variables are unrelated.

In the example just used, we suggested limiting the sample of nursing home residents to elders younger than 80 to reduce variability in the denominator. Our aim was to enhance the variability in depression scores attributable to nursing home admission, relative to depression variability due to other factors. What if, however, few elders under 80 were depressed? With limited variability, relationships cannot be detected—the values in both the numerator and denominator are deflated. For example, if *everyone* had a depression score of 50, depression scores would be totally unrelated to age, pain levels, nursing home admission, and so on. Thus, in designing a study, it is important to consider whether there will be sufficient variability to support the statistical analyses envisioned. The issue of *floor effects* and *ceiling effects*, which involve range restrictions at the lower and upper end of a measure, respectively, are discussed later in this book.

---

*You should not be concerned with how these numbers can be obtained. Analytic procedures are explained in Chapter 17.

TIP: In designing a study, try to anticipate nonsignificant findings, and consider design adjustments that might affect the results. For example, suppose our study hypothesis is that environmental factors such as light and noise affect acute confusion in the hospitalized elderly. With a preliminary design in mind, imagine findings that *fail* to support the hypothesis. Then ask yourself what could be done to decrease the likelihood of getting such negative results, under the assumption that such results do not reflect the truth. Could power be increased by making differences in environmental conditions sharper? Could precision be increased by controlling additional confounding variables? Could bias be eliminated by better training of research staff?

Unreliable Implementation of a Treatment

The strength of an intervention (and hence statistical conclusion validity) can be undermined if an intervention is not as powerful in reality as it is "on paper." **Intervention fidelity** (or **treatment fidelity**) concerns the extent to which the implementation of an intervention is faithful to its plan. There is growing interest in intervention fidelity in the nursing literature and considerable advice on how to achieve it (e.g., Spillane et al., 2007; Stein et al., 2007; Whitmer et al., 2005).

Interventions can be weakened by various factors, which researchers can often influence. One issue concerns the extent to which the intervention is similar from one person to the next. Usually, researchers strive for constancy of conditions in implementing a treatment because lack of standardization adds extraneous variation and can diminish the intervention's full force. Even in tailored, patient-centered interventions there are usually protocols, though different protocols are used with different people. Using the notions just described, when standard protocols are not followed, variability due to the intervention (i.e., in the numerator) can be suppressed, and variability due to other factors (i.e., in the denominator) can be inflated, possibly leading to the erroneous conclusion that the intervention was ineffective. This suggests the need for a certain degree of standardization, the development of procedures manuals, thorough training of personnel, and vigilant monitoring (e.g., through

observations of the delivery of the intervention) to ensure that the intervention is being implemented as planned—and that control group members have not gained access to the intervention.

Determining that the intervention was delivered as intended may need to be supplemented with efforts to ensure that the intervention was *received* as intended. This may involve a **manipulation check** to assess whether the treatment was in place, was understood, or was perceived in an intended manner. For example, if we were testing the effect of soothing versus jarring music on anxiety, we might want to determine whether participants themselves perceived the music as soothing and jarring. Another aspect of treatment fidelity for interventions designed to promote behavioral changes concerns the concept of *enactment* (Bellg et al., 2004). Enactment refers to participants' performance of the treatment-related skills, behaviors, and cognitive strategies in relevant real-life settings.

Example of attention to treatment fidelity: Radziewicz and colleagues (2009) described their efforts to establish treatment fidelity in a telephone intervention to provide support to aging patients with cancer and their family caregivers. Their treatment fidelity plan included monitoring adherence to standards of a protocol, carefully training staff using a standardized manual, monitoring the success of training, and monitoring consistency in delivering the intervention.

Another issue is that participants often fail to receive the desired intervention due to lack of **treatment adherence**. It is not unusual for those in the experimental group to elect not to participate fully in the treatment—for example, they may stop going to treatment sessions. To the extent possible, researchers should take steps to encourage participation among those in the treatment group. This might mean making the intervention as enjoyable as possible, offering incentives, and reducing burden in terms of the intervention and data collection (Polit & Gillespie, 2010). Nonparticipation in an intervention is rarely random, so researchers should document which people got what amount of treatment so that individual differences in "dose" can be taken into account in the analysis or interpretation of results.

➲ **TIP:** Except for small-scale studies, every study should have a **procedures manual** that delineates the protocols and procedures for its implementation. The Toolkit section of the accompanying *Resource Manual* provides a model table of contents for such a procedures manual. The Toolkit also includes a model checklist to monitor delivery of an intervention through direct observation of intervention sessions.

INTERNAL VALIDITY

Internal validity refers to the extent to which it is possible to make an inference that the independent variable, rather than another factor, is truly causing variation in the dependent variable. We infer from an effect to a cause by eliminating (controlling) other potential causes. The control mechanisms reviewed earlier are strategies for improving internal validity. If researchers do not carefully manage extraneous variation, the conclusion that participants' performance on the outcome was caused by the independent variable is open to challenge.

Threats to Internal Validity

True experiments possess a high degree of internal validity because manipulation and random assignment allows researchers to rule out most alternative explanations for the results. Researchers who use quasi-experimental or correlational designs must contend with competing explanations of what caused the outcomes. Major competing explanations, or threats to internal validity, are examined in this section.

Temporal Ambiguity

As noted in Chapter 9, a criterion for inferring a causal relationship is that the cause must precede the effect. In RCTs, researchers themselves create the independent variable and then observe subsequent performance on an outcome variable, so establishing temporal sequencing is never a problem. In correlational studies, however, it may be unclear whether the independent variable preceded the dependent variable, or vice versa.

Selection

Selection (self-selection) encompasses biases resulting from pre-existing differences between groups. When individuals are not assigned to groups randomly, the groups being compared could be nonequivalent. Differences on outcomes could then reflect group differences rather than the effect of the independent variable. For example, if we found that women with an infertility problem were more likely to be depressed than women who were mothers, it would be impossible to conclude that the two groups differed in depression *because* of childbearing differences; women in the two groups might have been different in psychological well-being from the start. The problem of selection is reduced if researchers can collect data on participants' characteristics before the occurrence of the independent variable. In our example, the best design would be to collect data on women's depression before they attempted to become pregnant, and then design the study to control early levels of depression. Selection bias is one of the most problematic and frequently encountered threats to the internal validity of studies not using an experimental design.

History

The threat of **history** refers to the occurrence of external events that take place concurrently with the independent variable, and that can affect the outcomes. For example, suppose we were studying the effectiveness of a nurse-led outreach program to encourage pregnant women in rural areas to improve health practices (e.g., cessation of smoking, earlier prenatal care). The program might be evaluated by comparing the average birth weight of infants born in the 12 months before the outreach program with the average birth weight of those born in the 12 months after the program was introduced, using a time series design. However, suppose that 1 month after the new program was launched, a well-publicized docudrama about the inadequacies of prenatal care for poor women was aired on television. Infants' birth weight might now be affected by both the intervention and the messages in the docudrama, and it becomes impossible to disentangle the two effects.

In a true experiment, history usually is not a threat to a study's internal validity because we can often assume that external events are as likely to affect the experimental as the control group. When this is the case, group differences on the dependent variables represent effects over and above those created by outside factors. There are, however, exceptions. For example, when a crossover design is used, an event external to the study may occur during the first half (or second half) of the experiment, so treatments would be contaminated by the effect of that event. That is, some people would receive treatment A with the event and others would receive treatment A without it, and the same would be true for treatment B.

Selection biases sometimes interact with history to compound the threat to internal validity. For example, if the comparison group is different from the treatment group, then the characteristics of the members of the comparison group could lead them to have different intervening experiences, thereby introducing both history and selection biases into the design.

Maturation

In a research context, **maturation** refers to processes occurring within participants during the course of the study as a result of the passage of time rather than as a result of the independent variable. Examples of such processes include physical growth, emotional maturity, and fatigue. For instance, if we wanted to evaluate the effects of a sensorimotor program for developmentally delayed children, we would have to consider that progress occurs in these children even without special assistance. A one-group pretest—posttest design, for example, is highly susceptible to this threat.

Maturation is often a relevant consideration in nursing research. Remember that maturation here does not refer just to aging, but rather to any change that occurs as a function of time. Thus, maturation in the form of wound healing, postoperative recovery, and other bodily changes could be a rival explanation for the independent variable's effect on outcomes.

Mortality/Attrition

Mortality is the threat that arises from attrition in groups being compared. If different kinds of people remain in the study in one group versus another, then these differences, rather than the independent variable, could account for observed differences on the dependent variables at the end of the study. The most severely ill patients might drop out of an experimental condition because it is too demanding, or they might drop out of the comparison group because they see no advantage to remaining in the study. In a prospective cohort study, there may be differential attrition between groups being compared because of death, illness, or geographic relocation. Attrition bias essentially is a type of selection bias that occurs after the unfolding of the study: Groups initially equivalent can lose comparability because of attrition, and it could be that the differential composition, rather than the independent variable, is the "cause" of any group differences on the dependent variables. Attrition bias can also occur in single-group quasi-experiments if those dropping out of the study are a biased subset that make it look like a change in average values resulted from a treatment.

The risk of attrition is especially great when the length of time between points of data collection is long. A 12-month follow-up of participants, for example, tends to produce higher rates of attrition than a 1-month follow-up (Polit & Gillespie, 2009). In clinical studies, the problem of attrition may be especially acute because of patient death or disability.

If attrition is random (i.e., those dropping out of a study are comparable to those remaining in it), then there would not be bias. However, attrition is rarely random. In general, the higher the rate of attrition, the greater the likelihood of bias.

TIP: In longitudinal studies, attrition may occur because researchers cannot find participants, rather than because they refused to stay in the study. One effective strategy to help **tracing** people is to obtain **contact information** from participants at each point of data collection. Contact information should include the names, addresses, and telephone numbers of two or three people with whom the participant is close (e.g., parents, close friends) — people who would be likely to know how to contact participants if they moved. A sample contact information form that can be adapted for your use is provided in the Toolkit of the accompanying Resource Manual.

Testing and Instrumentation

Testing refers to the effects of taking a pretest on people's performance on a posttest. It has been found, particularly in studies dealing with attitudes, that the mere act of collecting data from people changes them. Suppose a sample of nursing students completed a questionnaire about attitudes toward assisted suicide. We then teach them about various arguments for and against assisted suicide, outcomes of court cases, and the like. At the end of instruction, we give them the same attitude measure and observe whether their attitudes have changed. The problem is that the first questionnaire might sensitize students, resulting in attitude changes regardless of whether instruction follows. If a comparison group is not used, it becomes impossible to segregate the effects of the instruction from the effects of the pretest. Sensitization, or testing, problems are more likely to occur when pretest data are gathered via self-reports (e.g., in a questionnaire), especially if people are exposed to controversial or novel material in the pretest.

Another related threat is **instrumentation**. This bias reflects changes in measuring instruments or methods of measurement between two points of data collection. For example, if we used one measure of stress at baseline and a revised measure at follow-up, any differences might reflect changes in the measuring tool rather than the effect of an independent variable. Instrumentation effects can occur even if the same measure is used. For example, if the measuring tool yields more accurate measures on a second administration (e.g., if data collectors are more experienced) or less accurate measures the second time (e.g., if participants become bored and answer haphazardly), then these differences could bias the results.

Internal Validity and Research Design

Quasi-experimental and correlational studies are especially susceptible to threats to internal validity. Table 10.2 lists specific designs that are *most* vulnerable to the threats just described—although it should not be assumed that threats are irrelevant in

TABLE 10.2	Research Designs and Threats to Internal Validity
THREAT	**DESIGNS MOST SUSCEPTIBLE**
Temporal Ambiguity	Case-control Other retrospective/cross-sectional
Selection	Nonequivalent control group (especially, posttest-only) Case-control "Natural" experiments with two groups Time series, if the population changes over time
History	One-group pretest–posttest Time series Prospective cohort Crossover
Maturation	One-group pretest–posttest
Mortality/ Attrition	Prospective cohort Longitudinal experiments and quasi-experiments One-group pretest–posttest
Testing	All pretest–posttest designs
Instrumentation	All pretest–posttest designs

designs not listed. Each threat represents an alternative explanation that competes with the independent variable as a cause of the dependent variable. The aim of a strong research design is to rule out competing explanations. (Tables 9.5 and 9.6 in Chapter 9 also include information about internal validity threats for specific designs.)

An experimental design normally rules out most rival hypotheses, but even in RCTs, researchers must exercise caution. For example, if there is treatment infidelity or contamination between treatments, then history might be a rival explanation for any group differences (or lack of differences). Mortality can be a salient threat in true experiments. Because the experimenter does things differently with the experimental and control groups, people in the groups may drop out of the study differentially. This is particularly apt to happen if the experimental treatment is painful, inconvenient, or time-consuming or if the control condition is boring or bothersome. When this happens, participants remaining in the study may differ from those who left in important ways, thereby nullifying the initial equivalence of the groups.

In short, researchers should consider how best to guard against and detect all possible threats to internal validity, no matter what design is used.

Internal Validity and Data Analysis

The best strategy for enhancing internal validity is to use a strong research design that includes control mechanisms and design features discussed in this chapter. Even when this is possible (and, certainly, when this is *not* possible), it is advisable to conduct analyses to assess the nature and extent of biases. When biases are detected, the information can be used to interpret substantive results. And, in some cases, biases can be statistically controlled.

Researchers need to be self-critics. They need to consider fully and objectively the types of biases that could have arisen—and then systematically search for evidence of their existence (while hoping, of course, that no evidence can be found). To the extent that biases can be ruled out or controlled, the quality of evidence the study yields will be strengthened.

Selection biases should always be examined. Typically, this involves comparing groups on pretest measures, when pretest data have been collected. For example, if we were studying depression in women who delivered a baby by cesarean delivery versus those who delivered vaginally, selection bias could be assessed by comparing depression in these two groups during or before the pregnancy. If there are significant predelivery differences, then any postdelivery differences would have to be interpreted with initial differences in mind (or with differences controlled). In designs with no pretest measure of the outcome, researchers should assess selection biases by comparing groups with respect to key background vari-

ables such as age, health status, and so on. Selection biases should be analyzed even in RCTs because there is no guarantee that randomization will yield perfectly equivalent groups.

Whenever the research design involves multiple points of data collection, researchers should analyze attrition biases. This is typically achieved through a comparison of those who did and did not complete the study with regard to baseline measures of the dependent variable or other characteristics measured at the first point of data collection.

> **Example of assessing attrition and selection bias:** Resnick and colleagues (2008) used a cluster-randomized design to study the effectiveness of an intervention to enhance the self-efficacy of minority urban-dwelling elders. At the 15-week follow-up, only 62% of the initial participants provided outcome data. Dropouts did not differ from those who completed the study in terms of baseline characteristics (attrition bias), and those in the experimental and control group were also similar at baseline (selection bias).

When people withdraw from an intervention study, researchers are in a dilemma about whom to "count" as being "in" a condition. A procedure that is often used is a **per-protocol analysis**, which includes members in a treatment group only if they actually received the treatment. Such an analysis is problematic, however, because self-selection into a nonintervention condition could undo the initial comparability of groups. This type of analysis will almost always be biased toward finding positive treatment effects. The "gold standard" approach is to use an **intention-to-treat analysis**, which involves keeping participants who were randomized in the groups to which they were assigned (Polit & Gillespie, 2009, 2010). An intention-to-treat analysis may yield an underestimate of the effects of a treatment if many participants did not actually get the assigned treatment—but may be a better reflection of what would happen in the real world. Of course, one difficulty with an intention-to-treat analysis is that it is often difficult to obtain outcome data for people who have dropped out of a treatment, but there are many strategies for estimating outcomes for those with missing data (Polit, 2010).

Example of intention-to-treat analysis:
Skrutkowski and colleagues (2008) used an RCT design to test the impact of a pivot nurse in oncology on symptom relief in patients with lung or breast cancer. They used an intention-to-treat analysis, even though participant loss over the course of the study was fairly high (31%). They stated that, "All participants' data were included, whether or not they provided survey data at each assessment period or died before completing the study" (p. 952).

In a crossover design, history is a potential threat both because an external event could differentially affect people in different treatment orderings and because the different orderings are in themselves a kind of differential history. *Substantive* analyses of the data involve comparing outcomes under treatment A versus treatment B. The analysis of bias, by contrast, involves comparing participants in the different orderings (e.g., A then B versus B then A). Significant differences between the two orderings is evidence of an **ordering bias**.

In summary, efforts to enhance the internal validity of a study should not end once the design strategy has been put in place. Researchers should seek additional opportunities to understand (and possibly to correct) the various threats to internal validity that can arise.

CONSTRUCT VALIDITY

Researchers conduct a study with specific exemplars of treatments, outcomes, settings, and people, which are stand-ins for broad constructs. Construct validity involves inferences from study particulars to the higher-order constructs that they are intended to represent. Construct validity is important because constructs are the means for linking the operations used in a study to a relevant conceptualization and to mechanisms for translating the resulting evidence into practice. If studies contain construct errors, there is a risk that the evidence will be misleading.

Enhancing Construct Validity

The first step in fostering construct validity is a careful explication of the treatment, outcomes, setting, and population constructs of interest; the next step is to carefully select instances that match those constructs as closely as possible. Construct validity is further cultivated when researchers assess the match between the exemplars and the constructs and the degree to which any "slippage" occurred.

Construct validity has most often been a concern to researchers in connection with the measurement of outcomes, an issue we discuss in Chapter 14. There is a growing interest, however, in the careful conceptualization and development of theory-based interventions in which the treatment itself has strong construct validity (see Chapter 26). It is just as important for the independent variable (whether it be an intervention or something not amenable to experimental manipulation) to be a strong instance of the construct of interest as it is for the measurement of the dependent variable to have strong correspondence to the outcome construct. In nonexperimental research, researchers do not create and manipulate the hypothesized cause, so ensuring construct validity of the independent variable is often more difficult.

Shadish and colleagues (2002) broadened the concept of construct validity to cover persons and settings as well as outcomes and treatments. For example, some nursing interventions specifically target groups that are characterized as "disadvantaged," but there is not always agreement on how this term is defined and operationalized. Researchers select specific people to represent the construct of a disadvantaged group about which inferences will be made, so it is important that the specific people are good exemplars of the underlying construct. The construct "disadvantaged" must be carefully delineated before a sample is selected. Similarly, if a researcher is interested in such settings as "immigrant neighborhoods" or "school-based clinics," these are constructs that require careful description—and the selection of exemplars that match those setting constructs. Qualitative description is often a powerful means of enhancing the construct validity of settings.

Threats to Construct Validity

Threats to construct validity are reasons that inferences from a particular study exemplar to an abstract construct could be erroneous. Such a threat could occur if the operationalization of the construct fails to incorporate all the relevant characteristics of the underlying construct, or it could occur if it includes extraneous content—both of which are instances of a mismatch. Shadish and colleagues (2002) identified 14 threats to construct validity (their Table 3.1) and several additional threats specific to case-control designs (their Table 4.3). Among the most noteworthy threats are the following:

1. *Reactivity to the study situation*. As discussed in Chapter 9, participants may behave in a particular manner because they are aware of their role in a study (the Hawthorne effect). When people's responses reflect, in part, their perceptions of participation in research, those perceptions become part of the treatment construct under study. There are several ways to reduce this problem, including blinding, using outcome measures not susceptible to reactivity (e.g., data from hospital records), and using preintervention strategies to satisfy participants' desire to look competent or please the researcher.

Example of a possible Hawthorne effect:
Yap and colleagues (2009) evaluated the effect of tailored email messages on physical activity in manufacturing workers, using a two-group quasi-experimental design. Participants in *both* groups increased their activity, although increases were greater in the intervention group. The researchers speculated that the comparison group's improvement was probably a Hawthorne effect.

2. *Researcher expectancies*. A similar threat stems from the researcher's influence on participant responses through subtle (or not-so-subtle) communication about desired outcomes. When this happens, the researcher's expectations become part of the treatment (or nonmanipulated independent variable) construct that is being tested. Blinding is a strategy to reduce this threat, but another strategy is to use observations during the course of the study to detect verbal or behavioral signals of expectations and correct them.

3. *Novelty effects*. When a treatment is new, participants and research agents alike might alter their behavior. People may be either enthusiastic or skeptical about new methods of doing things. Results may reflect reactions to the novelty rather than to the intrinsic nature of an intervention, so the intervention construct is clouded by novelty content.

4. *Compensatory effects*. In intervention studies, *compensatory equalization* can occur if healthcare staff or family members try to compensate for the control group members' failure to receive a perceived beneficial treatment. The compensatory goods or services must then be part of the construct description of the treatment conditions. *Compensatory rivalry* is a related threat arising from the control group members' desire to demonstrate that they can do as well as those receiving a special treatment.

5. *Treatment diffusion or contamination*. Sometimes alternative treatment conditions can get blurred, which can impede good construct descriptions of the independent variable. This may occur when participants in a control group condition receive services similar to those available in the treatment condition. More often, however, blurring occurs when those in a treatment condition essentially put themselves into the control group by dropping out of the intervention. This threat can also occur in nonexperimental studies. For example, in case-control comparisons of smokers and nonsmokers, care must be taken during screening to ensure that study participants are, in fact, appropriately categorized (e.g., some people may consider themselves nonsmokers even though they smoke regularly, but only on weekends).

Construct validity requires careful attention to what we *call* things (i.e., construct labels) so that appropriate construct inferences can be made. Enhancing construct validity in a study requires careful thought before a study is undertaken, in terms of a well-considered explication of constructs, and also requires poststudy scrutiny to assess the degree to which a match between operations and constructs was achieved.

EXTERNAL VALIDITY

External validity concerns the extent to which it can be inferred that relationships observed in a study hold true over variations in people, conditions, and settings, as well as over variations in treatments and outcomes. External validity has emerged as a very major concern in an EBP world in which there is an interest in generalizing evidence from tightly controlled research settings to real-world clinical practice settings.

External validity questions may take on several different forms (Shadish et al., 2002). We may wish to ask whether relationships observed with a study sample can be generalized to a larger population—for example, whether results from a smoking cessation program found effective with pregnant teenagers in Boston can be generalized to pregnant teenagers throughout the United States. Many EBP questions, however, are about going from a broad study group to a *particular* client—for example, whether the pelvic muscle exercises found to be effective in alleviating urinary incontinence in one study are an effective strategy for Linda Smith. Other external validity questions are about generalizing to types of people, settings, situations, or treatments unlike those in the research (Polit & Beck, 2010). For example, can findings about a pain-reduction treatment in a study of Australian women be generalized to men and women in Canada? Or, would a 6-week intervention to promote dietary changes in patients with diabetes be equally effective if the content were condensed into a 3-week program? Sometimes new studies are needed to answer questions about external validity, but sometimes external validity can be enhanced by decisions that the researcher makes in designing a study.

Enhancements to External Validity

One aspect of external validity concerns the *representativeness* of the exemplars used in the study.

For example, if the sample is selected to be representative of a population to which the researcher wishes to generalize the results, then the findings can more readily be applied to that population (see Chapter 12 for sampling designs). Similarly, if the settings in which the study occurs are representative of the clinical settings in which the findings might be applied, then inferences about relevance in those other settings can be strengthened.

An important concept for external validity is *replication*. Multisite studies are powerful because more confidence in the generalizability of the results can be attained if results have been replicated in several sites—particularly if the sites are different on dimensions considered important (e.g., size, nursing skill mix, and so on). Studies with a varied sample of participants can test whether study results are replicated for subgroups of the sample—for example, whether benefits from an intervention apply to men *and* women, or older *and* younger patients. Systematic reviews are a crucial aid to external validity precisely because they assess relationships in replicated studies across time, space, people, and settings.

Another issue concerns attempts to use or create study situations as similar as possible to real-world circumstances. The real world is a "messy" place, lacking the standardization imposed in studies. Yet, external validity can be jeopardized if study conditions are too artificial. For example, if nurses require 5 days of training to implement a promising intervention, we might ask how realistic it would be for administrators to devote resources to such an intervention.

Threats to External Validity

In the previous chapter, we discussed *interaction effects* that can occur in a factorial design when two treatments are simultaneously manipulated. The interaction question is whether the effects of treatment A hold (are comparable) for all levels of treatment B. Conceptually, questions regarding external validity are similar to this interaction question. Threats to external validity concern ways in which relationships between variables might interact with or be moderated by variations in people, settings, time, and conditions. Shadish and colleagues (2002) described several threats to external validity, such as the following two:

1. *Interaction between relationship and people.* An effect observed with certain types of people might not be observed with other types of people. A common complaint about some RCTs is that many people are excluded not because they would not benefit from the treatment, but rather because they cannot provide needed research data (e.g., cognitively impaired patients, non-English speakers). During the 1980s, the widely held perception that many clinical trials were conducted primarily with white males led to policy changes to ensure that treatment by gender and ethnicity subgroup interactions were explored.

2. *Interaction between causal effects and treatment variation.* An innovative treatment might be effective because it is paired with other elements, and sometimes those elements are intangible—for example, an enthusiastic and dedicated project director. The same "treatment" could never be fully replicated, and thus different results could be obtained in subsequent tests.

Shadish and colleagues (2002) noted that moderators of relationships are the norm, not the exception. With interventions, for example, it is normal for a treatment to "work better" for some people than for others. Thus, in thinking about external validity, the primary issue is whether there is constancy of a relationship (or constancy of causation), and not whether the *magnitude* of the effect is constant.

TRADE-OFFS AND PRIORITIES IN STUDY VALIDITY

Quantitative researchers strive to design studies that are strong with respect to all four types of study validity. Sometimes, efforts to increase one type of validity will also benefit another type. In some instances, however, the requirements for ensuring one type of validity interfere with the possibility of achieving others.

For example, suppose we went to great lengths to ensure intervention fidelity in an RCT. Our efforts might include strong training of staff, careful monitoring of intervention delivery, manipulation checks, and steps to maximize participants' adherence to treatment. Such efforts would have positive effects on statistical conclusion validity because the treatment was made as powerful as possible. Internal validity would be enhanced if attrition biases were minimized as a result of high adherence. Intervention fidelity would also improve the construct validity of the treatment because the content delivered and received would better match the underlying construct. But what about external validity? All of the actions undertaken to ensure that the intervention is strong, construct-valid, and administered according to plan are not consistent with the realities of clinical settings. People are not normally paid to adhere to treatments, nurses are not monitored and corrected to ensure that they are following a script, training in the use of new protocols is usually brief, and so on.

This example illustrates that researchers need to give careful thought to how design decisions may affect various aspects of study validity. Of particular concern are trade-offs between internal and external validity.

Internal Validity and External Validity

Tension between the goals of achieving internal validity and external validity is pervasive. Many control mechanisms that are designed to rule out competing explanations for hypothesized cause-and-effect relationships make it difficult to infer that the relationship holds true in uncontrolled real-life settings.

Internal validity was long considered the "*sine qua non*" of experimental research (Campbell & Stanley, 1963). The rationale was this: If there is insufficient evidence that an intervention really caused an effect, why worry about generalizing the results? This high priority given to internal validity, however, is somewhat at odds with the current emphasis on evidence-based practice. A question that some are now posing is this: If study results can't be generalized to real-world clinical settings, who *cares* if the study has strong internal validity? Clearly, both internal and external validity are important to building an evidence base for nursing practice.

There are several "solutions" to the conflict between internal and external validity. The first (and perhaps most prevalent) approach is to emphasize one and sacrifice the other. Following a long tradition of field experimentation based on Campbell and Stanley's advice, it is often external validity that is sacrificed.

A second approach in some medical trials is to use a phased series of studies. In the earlier phase, there are tight controls, strict intervention protocols, and stringent criteria for including people in the RCT. Such studies are **efficacy studies**. Once the intervention has been deemed to be effective under tightly controlled conditions in which internal validity was the priority, it is tested with larger samples in multiple sites under less restrictive conditions, in **effectiveness studies** that emphasize external validity.

A third approach is to compromise. There has been recent interest in promoting designs that aim to achieve a balance between internal and external validity in a single intervention study. We discuss such *practical* (or *pragmatic*) *clinical trials* in Chapter 11.

Efforts to improve the generalizability of health-care research evidence have given rise to a framework for designing and evaluating intervention research called the **RE-AIM framework** (Glasgow, 2006). The framework involves a scrutiny of five aspects of a study: its **R**each, **E**fficacy, **A**doption, **I**mplementation, and **M**aintenance. *Reach* means reaching the intended population of potential beneficiaries, which concerns the extent to which study participants have characteristics that reflect those of that population. *Efficacy* concerns intervention impacts on critical outcomes. *Adoption* concerns the number and representativeness of settings and staff who are willing to implement the intervention.

Implementation concerns the consistency of delivering the intervention as intended, and also intervention costs. The last component, *maintenance*, involves a consideration of the extent to which, at the individual level, outcomes are maintained over time and, at the institutional level, the intervention becomes part of routine practices and policies. Table 10.3 summarizes some key planning questions for each of these five components. Detailed information about this new framework and advice on how to enhance and assess the five components is available at *www.re-aim.org*.

> **Example of a study using RE-AIM:** Whittemore and colleagues (2009) used the RE-AIM model as the organizing framework for their pilot study of a diabetes prevention program in primary care settings. The study appears in its entirety in Appendix D of the accompanying *Resource Manual*.

> ⟶ **TIP:** The Toolkit section of the *Resource Manual* includes a table listing a number of strategies that can be used to enhance the external validity of a study. The table identifies the potential consequence of each strategy for other types of study validity.

Prioritization and Design Decisions

Unfortunately, it is impossible to avoid all possible threats to study validity. By understanding the various threats, however, you can come to conclusions about the kinds of trade-offs you are willing to make to achieve study goals. Some threats are more worrisome than others in terms of both likelihood of occurrence and consequences to the inferences you would like to make. And some threats are more costly to avoid than others. Resources available for a study must be allocated so that there is a correspondence between expenditures and the importance of different types of validity. For example, with a fixed budget, you need to decide whether it is better to increase the size of the sample and hence power (statistical conclusion validity), or to use the money on efforts to reduce attrition (internal validity).

TABLE 10.3	Key Planning Questions within the RE-AIM Framework

RE-AIM COMPONENT	PLANNING QUESTIONS
Reach	• How can I reach those who need the intervention? • How can I design the intervention and the research so as to persuade those who need it to try it?
Efficacy	• How can I plan the intervention to maximize its efficacy? • How can I design the research to maximize the potential to detect its effects?
Adoption	• How can I best select study sites to represent environments where the intervention might be implemented? • How can I develop organizational support for the delivery of my intervention?
Implementation	• What can I do to enhance the likelihood that the intervention is delivered properly? • How can I best assess and document the extent to which intervention fidelity occurred?
Maintenance	• How can I design the intervention so as to encourage long-term maintenance of needed behaviors? • What can I do to enhance the likelihood that the intervention is maintained and delivered over the long term?

The point here is that you should make conscious decisions about how to structure a study to address validity concerns. Every design decision has both a "payoff" and a cost in terms of study integrity. Being cognizant of the effects that design decisions have on the quality of research evidence is a responsibility that nurse researchers should attend to so that their evidence can have the largest possible impact on clinical practice.

TIP: A useful strategy is to create a matrix that lists various design decisions in the first column (e.g., randomization, crossover design), and then use the next four columns to identify the potential impact of those options on the four types of study validity. (In some cells, there may be no entry if there are no consequences of a design element for a given type of validity). A sixth column could be added for estimates of the design element's financial implications, if any. The Toolkit section of the accompanying *Resource Manual* includes a model matrix as a Word document for you to use and adapt.

CRITIQUING GUIDELINES FOR STUDY VALIDITY

In critiquing a research report to evaluate its potential to contribute to nursing practice, it is crucial to make judgments about the extent to which threats to validity were minimized—or, at least, assessed and taken into consideration during the interpretation of the results. The guidelines in Box 10.1 focus on validity-related issues to further help you in the critique of quantitative research designs. Together with the critiquing guidelines in the previous chapter, they are likely to be the core of a strong critical evaluation of the evidence that quantitative studies yield. From an EBP perspective, it is important to remember that drawing inferences about causal relationships relies not only on how high up on the evidence hierarchy a study is (Figure 2.1), but also, for any given level of the hierarchy, how successful the researcher was in managing study validity and balancing competing validity demands.

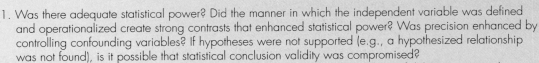

BOX 10.1 Guidelines for Critiquing Design Elements and Study Validity in Quantitative Studies

1. Was there adequate statistical power? Did the manner in which the independent variable was defined and operationalized create strong contrasts that enhanced statistical power? Was precision enhanced by controlling confounding variables? If hypotheses were not supported (e.g., a hypothesized relationship was not found), is it possible that statistical conclusion validity was compromised?
2. In intervention studies, is there evidence that attention was paid to intervention fidelity? For example, were staff adequately trained? Was the implementation of the intervention monitored? Was attention paid to both the delivery and receipt of the intervention?
3. What evidence does the report provide that selection biases were eliminated or minimized? What steps were taken to control confounding participant characteristics that could affect the equivalence of groups being compared? Were these steps adequate?
4. To what extent did the study design rule out the plausibility of other threats to internal validity, such as history, attrition, maturation, and so on? What are your overall conclusions about the internal validity of the study?
5. Were there any major threats to the construct validity of the study? In intervention studies, was there a good match between the underlying conceptualization of the intervention and its operationalization? Was the intervention "pure" or was it confounded with extraneous content, such as researcher expectations? Was the setting or site a good exemplar of the type of setting envisioned in the conceptualization?
6. Was the context of the study sufficiently described to enhance its capacity for external validity? Were the settings or participants representative of the types to which results were designed to be generalized?
7. Overall, did the researcher appropriately balance validity concerns? Was attention paid to certain types of threats (e.g., internal validity) at the expense of others (e.g., external validity)?

RESEARCH EXAMPLE

We conclude this chapter with an example of a study that demonstrated careful attention to many aspects of study validity.

Study: Effects of abdominal massage in management of constipation—A randomized controlled trial (Lämås et al., 2009)

Statement of Purpose: The purpose of the study was to assess the effect of an abdominal massage on gastrointestinal functions and use of laxatives in people with constipation.

Treatment Groups: There were two treatment groups: an intervention group that received an abdominal massage 5 days per week for 8 weeks in addition to previously prescribed laxatives, and a control group that continued with usual laxatives and treatments but no massage.

Method: A sample of 60 people with constipation was recruited from a Swedish community via local newspapers and notices at care centers. Eligible participants were randomly assigned to treatment groups by block randomization, with four patients per block. Gastrointestinal function was assessed with a standardized instrument at baseline, 4 weeks, and 8 weeks. Participants also maintained a daily diary in which they recorded information about bowel movements and use of remedies such as laxatives and fiber.

Additional Study Validity Efforts: The researchers estimated how large a sample was needed to achieve adequate power for statistical conclusion validity, using a procedure called power analysis (Chapter 12). Study protocols and a manual were developed to standardize the massage intervention. Massage interventionists were trained by the lead author. Data were gathered by self-administration (the data collectors were not blinded). Selection bias was assessed by comparing the baseline characteristics of the two groups, who were comparable with regard to demographic characteristics (e.g., age, sex), laxative use, and most indexes of gastrointestinal function. However, those in the intervention group had higher constipation scores, so these baseline scores were statistically adjusted in estimating intervention effects 8 weeks later. Attrition was similar in both groups (10% per group). An intention-to-treat analysis was performed by estimating missing outcome values for those who dropped out of the study.

Key Findings: Those in the intervention group had significantly better outcomes at 8 weeks than those on the control group with regard to constipation and abdominal pain. The massage group also had significantly more bowel movements. The groups had similar usage of laxatives at the end of the study, suggesting massage might be an effective complement to, but not substitute for, laxatives in this population.

SUMMARY POINTS

- Study validity concerns the extent to which appropriate inferences can be made. **Threats to validity** are reasons that an inference could be wrong. A key function of quantitative research design is to rule out validity threats by exercising various types of control.

- Control over confounding participant characteristics is key to managing many validity threats. The best control method is randomization to treatment conditions, which effectively controls all confounding variables—especially within the context of a crossover design.

- When randomization is not possible, other control methods include **homogeneity** (the use of a homogeneous sample to eliminate variability on confounding characteristics); blocking or stratifying, as in the case of a randomized block design; **pair matching** participants on key variables to make groups more comparable (or **balancing** groups to achieve comparability); and **statistical control** to remove the effect of a confounding variable statistically (e.g., through **analysis of covariance**).

- Homogeneity, stratifying, matching, and statistical control share two disadvantages: Researchers must know in advance which variables to control, and they can rarely control all of them.

- Four types of validity affect the rigor of a quantitative study: statistical conclusion validity, internal validity, construct validity, and external validity.

- **Statistical conclusion validity** concerns the validity of inferences that there is an empirical relationship between variables (most often, the presumed cause and the effect).

- Threats to statistical conclusion validity include low **statistical power** (the ability to detect true relationships among variables), low **precision** (the exactness of the relationships revealed after controlling confounding variables), and factors that undermine a strong operationalization of the independent variable (e.g., a treatment).

- **Intervention** (or **treatment) fidelity** concerns the extent to which the implementation of a treatment is faithful to its plan. Intervention fidelity is enhanced through standardized treatment protocols, careful training of intervention agents, monitoring of the delivery and receipt of the intervention, **manipulation checks**, and steps to promote **treatment adherence** and avoid **contamination of treatments**.

- **Internal validity** concerns inferences that outcomes were caused by the independent variable, rather than by factors extraneous to the research. Threats to internal validity include temporal ambiguity (lack of clarity about whether the presumed cause preceded the outcome), **selection** (preexisting group differences), **history** (the occurrence of events external to an independent variable that could affect outcomes), **maturation** (changes resulting from the passage of time), **mortality** (effects attributable to attrition), **testing** (effects of a pretest), and **instrumentation** (changes in the way data are gathered).

- Internal validity can be enhanced through judicious design decisions, but can also be addressed analytically (e.g., through an analysis of selection or attrition biases). When people withdraw from a study, an **intention-to-treat analysis** (analyzing outcomes for all people in their original treatment conditions) is preferred to a **per-protocol analysis** (analyzing outcomes only for those who received the full treatment as assigned) for maintaining the integrity of randomization.

- **Construct validity** concerns inferences from the particular exemplars of a study (e.g., the specific treatments, outcomes, people, and settings) to the higher-order constructs that they are intended to represent. The first step in fostering construct validity is a careful explication of those constructs.

- Threats to construct validity can occur if the operationalization of a construct fails to incorporate all of the relevant characteristics of the construct or if it includes extraneous content. Examples of such threats include *subject reactivity, researcher expectancies, novelty effects, compensatory effects*, and *treatment diffusion*.

- **External validity** concerns inferences about the extent to which study results can be generalized—that is, about whether relationships observed in a study hold true over variations in people, settings, outcome measures, and treatments. External validity can be enhanced by selecting *representative* people, settings, and so on and through replication.

- Researchers need to prioritize and recognize trade-offs among the various types of validity, which sometimes compete with each other. Tensions between internal and external validity are especially prominent. One solution has been to begin with a study that emphasizes internal validity (**efficacy studies**) and then if a causal relationship can be inferred, to undertake **effectiveness studies** that emphasize external validity.

- The **RE-AIM framework** (*Reach, Efficacy, Adoption, Implementation,* and *Maintenance*) is a model for designing and evaluating intervention research that is strong on multiple forms of study validity.

STUDY ACTIVITIES

Chapter 10 of the *Study Guide for Nursing Research: Generating and Assessing Evidence for Nursing Practice*, *9th edition*, offers exercises and study suggestions for reinforcing concepts presented in this chapter. In addition, the following study questions can be addressed:

1. How do you suppose the use of identical twins in a study could enhance control?
2. To the extent possible, apply the questions in Box 10.1 to the massage intervention study described at the end of the chapter (Lämås, et al., 2009).

STUDIES CITED IN CHAPTER 10

Lämås, K., Lindholm, L., Stenlund, H., Engstrom, B., & Jacobsson, C. (2009). Effects of abdominal massage in management of constipation—A randomized controlled trial. *International Journal of Nursing Studies, 46*, 759–767.

Lee, L. Y., Lee, D. T., & Woo, J. (2009). Tai Chi and health-related quality of life in nursing home residents. *Journal of Nursing Scholarship, 41*, 35–43.

Luttik, M., Jaarsma, T., Lesman, I., Sanderman, R., & Hagedoorn, M. (2009). Quality of life in partners of people with congestive heart failure. *Journal of Advanced Nursing, 65*, 1442–1451.

Ngai, F., Chan, S., & Ip, W. (2010). Predictors and correlates of maternal role competence and satisfaction. *Nursing Research, 59*, 185–193.

Radziewicz, R., Rose, J., Bowman, K., Berila, R., O'Toole, E., & Given, B. (2009). Establishing treatment fidelity in a coping and communication support telephone intervention for aging patients with advanced cancer and their family caregivers. *Cancer Nursing, 32*, 193–203.

Resnick, B., Luisi, D., & Vogel, A. (2008). Testing the Senior Exercise Self-efficacy Project (SESEP) for use with urban dwelling minority older adults. *Public Health Nursing, 25*, 221–234.

Skrutkowski, M., Saucier, A., Eades, M., Swidzinski, M., Ritchie, J., Marchionni, C., Ladouceur, M. (2008). Impact of a pivot nurse in oncology on patients with lung or breast cancer. *Oncology Nursing Forum, 35*, 948–954.

Whittemore, R., Melkus, G., Wagner, G., Dziura, J., Northrup, V., & Grey, M. (2009). Translating the diabetes prevention program to primary care. *Nursing Research, 58*, 2–12.

Yap, T., Davis, L., Gates, D., Hemmings, A., & Pan, W. (2009). The effect of tailored emails in the workplace. *AAOHN Journal, 57*, 267–273.

Methodologic and nonresearch references cited in this chapter can be found in a separate section at the end of the book.

11

Specific Types of Quantitative Research

All quantitative studies can be categorized as experimental, quasi-experimental, or non-experimental in design (Chapter 9). This chapter describes types of research that vary in study purpose rather in research design.

The first two types (clinical trials and evaluations) involve interventions, but methods for each have evolved separately because of their disciplinary roots. Clinical trials are associated with medical research, and evaluation research is associated with the fields of education, social work, and public policy. There is overlap in approaches, but to acquaint you with relevant terms, we discuss each separately. Chapter 26 describes the emerging tradition of intervention research that is more clearly aligned with nursing.

CLINICAL TRIALS

Clinical trials are studies designed to assess clinical interventions. The terms associated with clinical trials are used by many nurse researchers.

Phases of a Full Clinical Trial

In medical and pharmaceutical research, clinical trials often adhere to a well-planned sequence of activities. Clinical trials undertaken to test a new drug or an innovative therapy often are designed in a series of four phases, as follows:

Phase I occurs after initial development of the drug or therapy, and is designed primarily to establish safety and tolerance and to determine optimal dose. This phase typically involves small-scale studies using simple designs (e.g., before—after without a control group). The focus is on developing the best possible (and safest) treatment.

Phase II involves seeking preliminary evidence of treatment effectiveness. During this phase, researchers assess the feasibility of launching a rigorous test, seek evidence that the treatment holds promise, look for signs of possible side effects, and identify refinements to improve the intervention. This phase, essentially a pilot test of the treatment, may be designed either as a small-scale experiment or as a quasi-experiment.

Example of an early phase clinical trial:
Chan and colleagues (2007) described the Phase I development of a virtual reality prototype as an approach to reducing pain in pediatric burn patients. In Phase II, the prototype was implemented to assess its usability and to gather preliminary evidence about its effectiveness.

Phase III is a full test of the treatment—an RCT with randomization to an experimental or control group (or to orderings of treatment conditions) under controlled conditions. The goal of this phase is to develop evidence about treatment *efficacy*—that is, whether the treatment is more efficacious than usual care (or an alternative counterfactual). Adverse effects are also monitored. Phase III RCTs often involve a large and heterogeneous sample of participants, sometimes selected from multiple sites to ensure that findings are not unique to a single setting.

Example of a multisite Phase III RCT: Twiss and colleagues (2009) undertook a Phase III randomized controlled trial to test the effectiveness of a 24-month multicomponent exercise intervention for breast cancer survivors with bone loss. Participants, recruited in four research sites, were randomized to either the intervention or a control condition.

Phase IV of clinical trials are studies of the *effectiveness* of an intervention in a general population. As noted in Chapter 10, the emphasis in such studies is on the external validity of an intervention that has shown promise of efficacy under controlled (but often artificial) conditions. Phase IV efforts may also examine the cost-effectiveness of new treatments. In pharmaceutical research, Phase IV trials typically focus on postapproval safety surveillance and on long-term consequences over a larger population and timescale than was possible during earlier phases.

TIP: A typical Phase III clinical trial is a *superiority trial*, designed to assess whether an intervention is *more* effective than standard care or a placebo. Some trials, however, are designed to test whether a new intervention is as good as an established one (an *equivalence trial*) or no worse than the standard of care (a *noninferiority trial*). Such trials face certain challenges, especially with regard to statistical conclusion validity (Christensen, 2007; Lesaffre, 2008).

Sequential Clinical Trials

In a traditional Phase III trial, it may take many months to recruit and randomize a sufficiently large sample. And, in standard trials, it may take years to draw conclusions about efficacy (i.e., until all data have been collected and analyzed). The **sequential clinical trial** is an alternative in which experimental data are continuously analyzed as they become available. Results accumulate, so the experiment can be stopped when the evidence is strong enough to support a conclusion about the intervention's efficacy.

Sequential trials involve a series of "mini-experiments." The first patient is randomly assigned to the experimental (E) or control (C) condition. The next patient is automatically assigned to the alternative condition, creating a series of randomized paired comparisons. Most sequential trials use measures of "preference" for the E or C condition. *Preference*, defined in terms of clinically meaningful outcomes, is measured dichotomously (e.g., improved/did not improve). Using preference measures, each pair is compared, yielding three possibilities: E is preferred, C is preferred, or the two are tied; ties are usually thrown out. All paired comparisons are plotted on graphs for which there are preestablished boundaries with decision rules.

An example is shown in Figure 11.1. The horizontal axis in the middle shows the number of untied pairs (here, 30 pairs). The vertical axis indicates which way the "preference" comparison turned out. When the preference for a given pair favors E, the plotted line goes up; when it favors C, the plotted line goes down. The red butterfly-shaped lines designate decision boundaries. In this example, the first comparison resulted in a preference for the intervention, so the line goes up one unit from the origin. The next comparison favored the control condition, so the plot goes down for pair number two. This procedure continues until the plot crosses a boundary, which designates three **stopping rules**. When the upper boundary (U) is crossed, we would conclude that the intervention is more effective. When the lower boundary (L) is crossed, the conclusion is that the control condition is more effective. When the middle boundary (M) is crossed, the decision is that the two treatments are equally effective. In this example, we tested 18 nontied pairs and were then able to stop, concluding that the E condition was superior to the C condition.

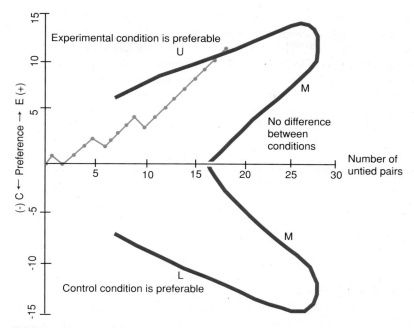

FIGURE 11.1 Example of a sequential clinical trial graph.

Sequential trials are appealing because decisions typically can be reached much earlier than with traditional designs. These trials are not always appropriate, however, (e.g., when three conditions are being compared), or are ambiguous if there are many ties. They may also be complicated if there are multiple outcomes for which preference has to be plotted separately. Portney and Watkins (2000) provide more information about sequential trials.

Practical Clinical Trials

A problem with traditional Phase III RCTs is that, in efforts to enhance internal validity and support causal inference, the designs are so tightly controlled that their relevance to real-life applications can be questioned. Concern about this situation has led to a call for **practical** (or **pragmatic**) **clinical trials**, which strive to maximize external validity with minimal negative effect on internal validity (Glasgow et al., 2005). Tunis and colleagues (2003), in an often-cited paper, defined practical clinical trials (PCTs) as "trials for which the hypotheses and

study design are formulated based on information needed to make a decision" (p. 1626).

Practical clinical trials address practical questions about the benefits and risks of an intervention—as well as its costs—as they would unfold in routine clinical practice. PCTs are thus sensitive to the issues under scrutiny in effectiveness (Phase IV) studies, but there is an increasing interest in developing strategies to bridge the gap between efficacy and effectiveness and to address issues of practicality earlier in the evaluation of promising interventions. As Godwin and colleagues (2003) have noted, achieving a creative tension between generalizability and internal validity is crucial.

Tunis and colleagues (2003) made these recommendations for PCTs: enrollment of diverse populations with fewer exclusions of high-risk patients, recruitment of participants from a variety of practice settings, follow-up over a longer period, inclusion of economic outcomes, and comparisons of clinically viable alternatives. Glasgow and colleagues (2005) have proposed several research designs, including cluster randomization and delayed treatment designs. Carroll and Rounsaville (2003) discussed some options for **hybrid designs** that link efficacy and effectiveness research. Their suggestions combine features of traditional RCTs (e.g., random assignment, assessments of intervention fidelity) with elements of effectiveness research (e.g., assessments of the intervention's cost-effectiveness and of patient satisfaction, few restrictions on eligibility for the study).

Example of a practical clinical trial: Harris and colleagues (2009) conducted a cluster-randomized trial, described as a pragmatic trial, to assess a medication management-training program for community mental health professionals (CMHPs). The intervention was randomly allocated to CMHPs recruited throughout the northwest of England.

➡️ **TIP:** Godwin and colleagues (2003) prepared a useful table that contrasts features of an "explanatory trial" (i.e., a traditional Phase III RCT) and a pragmatic trial. The table can be accessed at *www.biomedcentral.com/content/supplementary/1471-2288-3-28-S1.doc*. This and other websites with material relevant to this chapter are included in the Toolkit of the accompanying *Resource Manual* so that you can "click" on them directly.

EVALUATION RESEARCH

Evaluation research focuses on developing information needed by decision makers about whether to adopt, modify, or abandon a program, practice, procedure, or policy. The term *evaluation research* is most often used when researchers are trying to evaluate a complex program, rather than when they are evaluating a specific entity (e.g., alternative sterilizing solutions).

Evaluations often try to answer broader questions than whether an intervention is effective—for example, they often involve efforts to improve the program (as in Phase II of a clinical trial) or to learn how the program actually "works" in practice. When a program is multidimensional, involving several distinct features or elements, evaluations may address **black box** questions—that is, what is it about the program that is driving observed effects?

Evaluations are often the cornerstone of **policy research**. Nurses have become increasingly aware of the potential contribution their research can make to the formulation of national and local health policies and thus are undertaking evaluations that have implications for policies that affect the allocation of funds for health services (Wood, 2000).

Evaluation researchers often evaluate a program, practice, or intervention that is embedded in a political or organizational context—and so they may confront problems that are organizational or interpersonal. Evaluation research can be threatening. Even when the focus of an evaluation is on a nontangible entity, such as a program, it is *people* who are implementing it. People tend to think that they, or their work, are being evaluated and may feel that their jobs or reputations are at stake. Thus, evaluation researchers need to have more than methodologic skills—they need to be adept in interpersonal relations with people.

Evaluations may involve several project components to answer a variety of questions. Good resources for learning more about evaluation research include the books by Patton (2008) and Rossi and colleagues (2004).

Process or Implementation Analyses

A **process** or **implementation analysis** provides descriptive information about the process by which a program gets implemented and how it actually functions. A process analysis is typically designed to address such questions as the following: Does the program operate the way its designers intended? What are the strongest and weakest aspects of the program? How does the program differ from traditional practices? What were the barriers to its implementation? How do staff and clients feel about the intervention?

A process analysis may be undertaken with the aim of improving a new or ongoing program (a **formative evaluation**). In other situations, the purpose of the process analysis is primarily to describe a program carefully so that it can be replicated by others—or so that people can better understand why the program was or was not effective in meeting its objectives. In either case, a process analysis involves an in-depth examination of the operation of a program, often involving the collection of both qualitative and quantitative data. Process evaluations often overlap with efforts to monitor intervention fidelity.

> **Example of an implementation analysis:** Donaldson and colleagues (2009) did an implementation analysis of a multisite initiative to implement rapid response teams in acute care units. The researchers examined rapid response team composition, the manner in which activation of the team occurred, nurse reactions to the teams, and factors associated with successful implementation.

Outcome Analysis

Evaluations often focus on whether a program or policy is meeting its objectives. Evaluations that assess the worth of a program are sometimes called **summative evaluations**, in contrast to formative evaluations. The intent of such evaluations is to help people decide whether the program should be continued or replicated.

Some evaluation researchers distinguish between an outcome analysis and an impact analysis. An **outcome analysis** (or *outcome evaluation*) does not use a rigorous experimental design. Such an analysis simply documents the extent to which the goals of the program are attained, that is, the extent to which positive outcomes occur. For example, a program may be designed to encourage women in a poor rural community to obtain prenatal care. In an outcome analysis, the researchers might document the percentage of pregnant women who had obtained prenatal care, the average month in which prenatal care was begun, and so on, and perhaps compare this information with existing preintervention community data. Many nursing program evaluations (and quality improvement studies) are outcome analyses, although they are not necessarily labeled as such.

> **Example of an outcome analysis:** Milne and colleagues (2009) undertook an initiative to set up better procedures for managing pressure ulcers in a long-term acute care hospital. Over the course of the project, pressure ulcer prevalence dropped sharply, pressure interventions increased, and documentation improved.

Impact Analysis

An **impact analysis** assesses a program's *net impacts*—impacts that can be attributed to the program, over and above effects of a counterfactual (e.g., standard care). Impact analyses use an experimental or strong quasi-experimental design because their aim is to permit causal inferences about program effects. In the example cited earlier, suppose that the program to encourage prenatal care involved having nurses make home visits to women in rural communities to explain the benefits of early care. If the visits could be made to pregnant women randomly assigned to the intervention, the labor and delivery outcomes of the group of women receiving the home visits and of those not receiving them could be compared to assess the intervention's net impacts, that is, the percentage *increase* in receipt of prenatal care among the experimental group relative to the control group.

> **Example of an impact analysis:** Reynolds (2009) studied the impact of a predischarge patient education program on postdischarge pain management in surgical patients in a rural setting. Patients were randomized either to the intervention or to a usual care control group. The program was found to have beneficial effects on pain scores and interference with activities.

Cost Analysis

New programs or policies are often expensive to implement, but existing programs also may be costly. In our current situation of spiraling healthcare costs, evaluations may include a **cost analysis** (or **economic analysis**) to determine whether the benefits of the program outweigh the monetary costs. Administrators and public policy officials make decisions about resource allocations for health services based not only on whether something "works," but also on whether it is economically viable. Cost analyses are typically done in connection with impact analyses and Phase III clinical trials, that is, when researchers establish strong evidence about program efficacy.

There are several different types of cost analyses (Chang & Henry, 1999), the two most common of which in nursing research are the following:

Cost-benefit analysis, in which monetary estimates are established for both costs and benefits. One difficulty with such an analysis is that it is sometimes difficult to quantify benefits of health services in monetary terms. There is also controversy about methods of assigning dollar amounts to the value of human life.

Cost-effectiveness analysis, which is used to compare health outcomes and resource costs of alternative interventions. Costs are measured in monetary terms, but outcome effectiveness is not. Such analyses estimate what it costs to produce impacts on outcomes that cannot easily be valued in dollars, such as quality of life. Without information on monetary benefits, though, such research faces challenges in persuading decision makers to make changes.

Example of a cost-effectiveness analysis: Olsson and colleagues (2009) compared the hospital costs associated with a new patient-centered integrated care pathway for patients with hip fracture, compared with costs for the usual care system. They found a 40% reduction in the total cost of treatment with the new care system, as well as improved clinical effectiveness.

Cost-utility analyses, although uncommon when Chang and Henry did their analysis in 1999, are now appearing in the nursing literature. This approach is preferred when morbidity and mortality are outcomes of interest, or when quality of life is a major concern. An index called the *quality-adjusted life year* (QALY) is frequently an important outcome indicator in cost-utility analyses.

Example of a cost-utility analysis: Chen and colleagues (2008) undertook a cost-utility analysis in an evaluation of a 12-week walking program for community-dwelling elders in Taiwan. The analysis compared people in the intervention group with those in a control group on such outcomes as healthcare utilization, scores on a health utility index, and estimated quality-adjusted life years.

Researchers doing cost analyses must document what it costs to operate both the new program and its alternative. In doing cost-benefit analyses, researchers must often think about an array of possible short-term costs (e.g., clients' days of work missed within 6 months after the program) and long-term costs (e.g., lost years of productive work life). Often the cost-benefit analyst examines economic gains and losses from several different accounting perspectives—for example, for the target group, hospitals implementing the program, taxpayers, and society as a whole. Distinguishing these different perspectives is crucial if a particular program effect is a loss for one group (e.g., taxpayers) but a gain for another (e.g., the target group).

Nurse researchers are increasingly becoming involved in such cost analyses. Drummond and colleagues (2005) wrote an internationally acclaimed textbook on economic evaluations in healthcare. Duren-Winfield and her colleagues (2000) offer an excellent description of the methods used in a cost-effectiveness analysis of an exercise intervention for patients with chronic obstructive pulmonary disease, and Findorff and colleagues (2005) described how time studies are used to calculate program costs of personnel.

HEALTH SERVICES AND OUTCOMES RESEARCH

Health services research is the broad interdisciplinary field that studies how organizational structures and processes, health technologies, social factors, and personal behaviors affect access to healthcare, the cost and quality of healthcare, and, ultimately, people's health and well-being.

Outcomes research, a subset of health services research, comprises efforts to understand the end results of particular healthcare practices and to assess the effectiveness of healthcare services. Outcomes research overlaps with evaluation research, but evaluation research typically focuses on a specific program or policy, whereas outcomes research is a more global assessment of nursing and healthcare services. The impetus for outcomes research comes from the quality assessment and quality assurance functions that grew out of the professional standards review organizations in the 1970s. Outcomes research represents a response to the increasing demand from policy makers, insurers, and the public to justify care practices and systems in terms of improved patient outcomes and costs. The focus of outcomes research in the 1980s was predominantly on patient health status and costs associated with medical care, but there is a growing interest in studying broader patient outcomes in relation to nursing care—and a greater awareness that evidence-based nursing practice can play a role in quality improvement and healthcare safety, despite the many challenges (Harris et al., 2009).

Although many nursing studies examine patient outcomes, specific efforts to appraise and document the quality of nursing care—as distinct from the care provided by the overall healthcare system—are less common. A major obstacle is attribution—that is, linking patient outcomes to specific nursing actions or interventions, distinct from the actions of other members of the healthcare team. It is also difficult in some cases to attribute a causal link between outcomes and healthcare interventions because other factors (e.g., patient characteristics) affect outcomes in complex ways.

Outcomes research has used a variety of traditional designs and methodologic approaches (primarily quantitative ones), but is also developing a rich array of methods that are not within the traditional research framework. The complex and multidisciplinary nature of outcomes research suggests that this evolving area will offer opportunities for methodologic creativity in the years ahead.

Models of Healthcare Quality

In appraising quality in nursing services, various factors need to be considered. Donabedian (1987), whose pioneering efforts created a framework for outcomes research, emphasized three factors: structure, process, and outcomes. The *structure* of care refers to broad organizational and administrative features. Structure can be appraised in terms of such attributes as size, range of services, technology, organization structure, and organizational climate.

Nursing skill mix and nursing experience are two structural variables that have been found to correlate with patient outcomes. *Processes* involve aspects of clinical management, decision making, and clinical interventions. *Outcomes* refer to the specific clinical end results of patient care. Mitchell and colleagues (1998) noted that "the emphasis on evaluating quality of care has shifted from structures (having the right things) to processes (doing the right things) to outcomes (having the right things happen)" (p. 43).

There have been several suggested modifications to Donabedian's framework for appraising healthcare quality, the most noteworthy of which is the Quality Health Outcomes Model developed by the American Academy of Nursing (Mitchell et al., 1998). This model is less linear and more dynamic than Donabedian's original framework and takes client and system characteristics into account. This model does not link interventions and processes directly to outcomes. Rather, the effects of interventions are seen as mediated by client and system characteristics. This model, and others like it, are increasingly forming the conceptual framework for studies that evaluate quality of care (Mitchell & Lang, 2004).

Outcomes research usually concentrates on various linkages within such models, rather than on testing the overall model. Some studies have examined the effect of healthcare structures on various healthcare processes and outcomes, for example. There are also reliable ways to measure aspects of organizational structures and nurses' practice environments (Aiken & Patrician, 2000; Cummings et al., 2006). Most outcomes research in nursing, however, has focused on the process-patient-outcomes nexus, often using large-scale datasets.

Example of research on structure: Tschanne and Kalisch (2009) studied the effect of variations in nurse staffing (skill mix and hours per patient day) on patient's length of stay in acute care settings. Data were obtained from four medical–surgical units of two midwestern U.S. hospitals.

Nursing Processes and Interventions

To demonstrate nurses' effects on health outcomes, nurses' clinical actions and behaviors must be carefully described and documented, both quantitatively and qualitatively. Examples of nursing process variables include nursing actions such as nurses' problem solving, clinical decision making, clinical competence, nurses' autonomy and intensity, clinical leadership, and specific activities or interventions (e.g., communication, touch).

The work that nurses do is increasingly documented in terms of established classification systems and taxonomies. Indeed, in the United States, the standard use of electronic health records to record all healthcare events, and the submission of the records to national data banks, are imminent. A number of research-based classification systems of nursing interventions are being developed, refined, and tested. Among the most prominent are the Nursing Diagnoses Taxonomy of the North American Nursing Diagnosis Association or NANDA (North American Nursing Diagnosis Association, 2009) and the Nursing Intervention Classification or NIC, developed at the University of Iowa (Bulechek et al., 2008). Many studies have been undertaken to validate classifications internationally.

Patient Risk Adjustment

Patient outcomes vary not only because of the care they receive, but also because of differences in patient conditions and comorbidities. Adverse outcomes can occur no matter what nursing intervention is used. Thus, in evaluating the effects of nursing interventions on outcomes, there needs to be some way of controlling or taking into account patients' risks for poor outcomes, or the mix of risks in a caseload.

Risk adjustments have been used in a number of nursing outcomes studies. These studies typically involve the use of global measures of patient risks or patient acuity, such as the Acute Physiology and Chronic Health Evaluation (APACHE I, II, III, or IV) system. Wheeler (2009) has discussed the pros and cons of the different versions of the system.

Outcomes

Measuring outcomes and linking them to nursing actions is critical in developing an evidence-based

practice and in launching improvement efforts. Outcomes of relevance to nursing can be defined in terms of physical or physiologic function (e.g., heart rate, blood pressure, complications), psychological function (e.g., comfort, life quality, satisfaction), or social function (e.g., relations with family members). Outcomes of interest to nurses may be either short-term and temporary (e.g., postoperative body temperature) or more long-term and permanent (e.g., return to regular employment). Furthermore, outcomes may be defined in terms of the end results to individual patients receiving care, or to broader units such as a community or our entire society, and this would include cost factors.

Just as there have been efforts to develop classifications of nursing interventions, work has progressed on developing nursing-sensitive outcome classification systems. Of particular note is the Nursing-Sensitive Outcomes Classification (NOC), which has been developed by nurses at the University of Iowa College of Nursing to complement the Nursing Intervention Classification (Swanson et al., 2008).

Example of outcomes research: Kutney-Lee and colleagues (2009) defined and operationalized nurse surveillance capacity of hospitals. Using data from nearly 10,000 nurses in 174 hospitals, they found a correlation between a hospital's nurse surveillance capacity (which included measures of education, experience, staffing, and the practice environment) on the one hand and quality of care and adverse events on the other.

SURVEY RESEARCH

A **survey** is designed to obtain information about the prevalence, distribution, and interrelations of phenomena within a population. The decennial census of the U.S. population is an example of a survey, and political opinion polls are another. When a survey uses a sample, as is usually the case, it may be called a **sample survey** (as opposed to a **census**, which covers an entire population). Surveys obtain information from people through **self-report**—that is, participants respond to a series of questions posed by investigators. Surveys, which yield quantitative data primarily, may be cross-sectional or longitudinal (e.g., panel studies).

A great advantage of survey research is its flexibility and broad scope. It can be applied to many populations, it can focus on a wide range of topics, and its information can be used for many purposes. Information obtained in most surveys, however, tends to be relatively superficial: Surveys rarely probe deeply into human complexities. Survey research is better suited to extensive rather than intensive analysis.

The content of a survey is limited only by the extent to which people are able and willing to report on the topic. Any information that can reliably be obtained by direct questioning can be gathered in a survey, although surveys include mostly questions that require brief responses (e.g., yes or no, always/sometimes/never). Surveys often focus on what people do: what they eat, how they care for their health, and so forth. In some instances, the emphasis is on what people plan to do—how they plan to vote, for example.

Survey data can be collected in a number of ways. The most respected method is through **personal interviews** (or *face-to-face interviews*), in which interviewers meet in person with respondents to ask them questions. Personal interviews are often costly because they involve extensive preparation (e.g., interviewer training) and a lot of personnel time. Nevertheless, personal interviews are regarded as the best method of collecting survey data because of the quality of information they yield. A key advantage of personal interviews is that refusal rates tend to be low.

Example of a survey with personal interviews: Voyer and colleagues (2009) conducted face-to-face survey interviews in the homes of nearly 3,000 community-dwelling seniors. The researchers explored factors associated with benzodiazepine dependence.

Telephone interviews are a less costly than in-person interviews, but respondents may be uncooperative on the telephone. Telephoning can be an acceptable method of collecting data if the interview is short, specific, and not too personal or if researchers have had prior personal contact with respondents. Telephone interviews may be difficult for certain groups of respondents, including low-income people (who do not always have a telephone) or the elderly (who may have hearing problems).

Questionnaires, unlike interviews, are self-administered. (They are sometimes called **SAQs**, that is, *self-administered questionnaires*.) Respondents read the questions and give their answers in writing. Because respondents differ in their reading levels and in their ability to communicate in writing, questionnaires are *not* merely a printed form of an interview schedule. Care must be taken in a questionnaire to word questions clearly and simply. Questionnaires are economical but are not appropriate for surveying certain populations (e.g., the elderly, children). In survey research, questionnaires are often distributed through the mail (sometimes called a *postal survey*), but are increasingly being distributed over the Internet.

Example of a mailed survey: Miller and colleagues (2008) mailed a survey to nearly 5,000 randomly selected nurses in 6 states. A major purpose of the survey was to document rates of obesity and overweight in nurses, and to explore whether nurses address obesity issues with patients.

Surveys are relying on new technologies to assist in data collection. Most major telephone surveys now use **computer-assisted telephone interviewing (CATI)**, and growing numbers of in-person surveys use **computer-assisted personal interviewing (CAPI)** with laptop computers. Both procedures involve developing computer programs that present interviewers with the questions to be asked on the monitor; interviewers then enter coded responses directly onto a computer file. CATI and CAPI surveys, although costly, greatly facilitate data collection and improve data quality because there is less opportunity for interviewer error.

Example of CATI: Miller and colleagues (2009) conducted a survey to document the use of dietary supplements in cancer survivors. A sample of over 1,200 adult survivors was interviewed using CATI.

Audio-CASI (computer-assisted self-interview) technology is a state-of-the-art approach for giving respondents more privacy than is possible in an interview (e.g., to collect information about drug use) and is especially useful for populations with literacy problems (Jones, 2003). With audio-CASI, respondents sit at a computer and listen to questions over headphones. Respondents enter their responses (usually simple codes like 1 or 2) directly onto the keyboard, without the interviewer having to see the responses. This approach is also being extended to surveys with personal digital assistants (PDAs).

There are many excellent resources for learning more about survey research, including the books by Fowler (2009) and Dillman and colleagues (2009).

OTHER TYPES OF RESEARCH

Nurse researchers have pursued several other types of research, some of which are briefly described here.

Secondary Analysis

Secondary analysis involves the use of existing data from a previous study to test new hypotheses or answer new questions. In a typical study, researchers collect far more data than are actually analyzed. Secondary analysis of existing data is efficient because data collection is typically the most time-consuming and expensive part of a study. Nurse researchers have undertaken secondary analyses with both large national data sets and smaller, localized sets.

In some cases, a secondary analysis involves examining relationships among variables that were previously unanalyzed (e.g., a dependent variable in the original study could become the independent variable in the secondary analysis). In other cases, a secondary analysis focuses on a particular subgroup of the full original sample (e.g., survey data about health habits from a national sample could be analyzed to study smoking among urban teenagers).

➲ **TIP:** Many graduate students and junior faculty take advantage of existing data sets from mentors or colleagues. In such cases, the secondary analysis might be called a substudy of a larger *parent study*. For example, in an RCT, there is often opportunity for productive exploration of baseline data from participants in both intervention and control conditions.

Researchers interested in performing secondary analyses need to identify, locate, and gain access to suitable databases. They then need to do a thorough assessment of the identified data sets in terms of appropriateness for the research question, adequacy of data quality, and technical usability of the data. Some of these activities may be readily accomplished if the dataset is one made available by a faculty member or colleague.

A number of groups, such as university institutes and federal agencies, have made survey data available to researchers for secondary analysis. Policies regulating public use of data vary, but it is not unusual for a researcher to obtain a dataset at roughly the cost of duplicating data files and documentation. Thus, in some cases in which data collection originally cost hundreds of thousands of dollars, the dataset can be purchased for a fraction of the initial costs. Large-scale datasets on health topics are available from surveys sponsored by the U.S. National Center for Health Statistics. For example, the National Health Interview Survey, the Health Promotion and Disease Prevention Survey, and the National Comorbidity Survey regularly gather health-related information from thousands of people all over the United States. Zeni and Kogan (2007) offered some suggestions about existing health databases. Also, several organizations, such as the Association of Public Data Users, can be helpful in identifying large-scale datasets for secondary analysis. Several useful websites for locating datasets are provided in the Toolkit of the accompanying *Resource Manual*. ✷

The use of available data from large studies makes it possible to bypass time-consuming and costly steps in the research process, but there are some noteworthy disadvantages in working with existing data. In particular, the chances are fairly high that the data set will be deficient in some way, such as in the sample used or the variables measured. Researchers may face many "if only" problems: if only they had asked certain questions or had measured a particular variable differently. Additional issues to consider in doing a secondary analysis of quantitative datasets are described by Bibb (2007) and Magee and colleagues (2006).

Example of a quantitative secondary analysis: Chasens and colleagues (2009) studied the effect of excessive sleepiness on functional outcomes in older adults with diabetes, using data from a subsample of people with a diagnosis of diabetes who participated in a survey of older adults sponsored by the National Sleep Foundation.

➲ **TIP:** Qualitative researchers have also come to recognize the value of secondary analysis of narrative data sets (Manderson et al., 2001). Thorne (1994) identified several types of qualitative secondary analysis, but also warned of potential problems.

Needs Assessments

Researchers conduct **needs assessments** to estimate the needs of a group, community, or organization. The aim of such a study is to assess the need for special services, or to see if a program is meeting the needs of those who are supposed to benefit from it. Because resources are seldom limitless, information that can help in establishing priorities can be valuable.

Various methods can be used in a needs assessment, and the methods are not mutually exclusive. With the **key informant approach**, researchers collect information about a group's needs from people who are in a position to know those needs. The key informants could be community leaders, key healthcare workers, or other knowledgeable people. In-depth interviews are often used to collect the data and they may yield both qualitative and quantitative data.

Needs assessments may rely on a *survey*, which involves collecting data from a sample of the group whose needs are being assessed. In a survey, a representative sample from the group or community would be asked about their needs. Another alternative is to use an **indicators approach**, which relies on facts and statistics available in existing reports or records. This approach is cost-effective because the data are available but need organization and interpretation.

Needs assessments almost always result in recommendations. Researchers conducting a needs assessment typically offer judgments about priorities based on their results (taking costs and feasibility into consideration), and may also offer advice about the means by which the most highly prioritized needs can be addressed.

Example of a needs assessment: Schlairet (2009) used a survey approach to assess the needs for nurses' education relating to end-of-life nursing care. A sample of 567 nurses in one state was surveyed.

Delphi Surveys

Delphi surveys were developed as a tool for short-term forecasting. The technique involves a panel of experts who are asked to complete several rounds of questionnaires focusing on their judgments about a topic of interest. Multiple iterations are used to achieve consensus, without requiring face-to-face discussion. Responses to each round of questionnaires are analyzed, summarized, and returned to the experts with a new questionnaire. The experts can then reformulate their opinions with the panel's viewpoint in mind. The process is usually repeated at least three times until a consensus is obtained.

The Delphi technique is an efficient means of combining the expertise of a geographically dispersed group. The experts are spared the necessity of attending a formal meeting, thus saving time and expense. Another advantage is that a persuasive or prestigious expert cannot have an undue influence on opinions, as could happen in a face-to-face situation. All panel members are on an equal footing. Anonymity probably encourages greater candor than might be expressed in a meeting.

The Delphi technique is, however, time-consuming. Experts must be solicited, questionnaires prepared and distributed, responses analyzed, results summarized, and new questionnaires sent.

Panel members' cooperation may wane in later rounds, so attrition bias is a potential problem. Another concern is how to define consensus (i.e., how many participants have to agree before researchers conclude that consensus has been achieved). Recommendations range from a liberal 51% to a more cautious 70%. Kennedy (2004) and Keeney and colleagues (2006) offer suggestions on using this technique.

Example of a Delphi study: Rauch and colleagues (2009) used a three-round Delphi survey with 57 nurses from 15 countries to obtain feedback about whether the Comprehensive International Classification of Functioning, Disability, and Health Core Set for rheumatoid arthritis captures nursing practice.

Replication Studies

Replication studies are direct attempts to see if findings obtained in a study can be duplicated in another study. A strong evidence-based practice requires replications. Evidence can accumulate through a series of "close-enough-to-compare" studies, but deliberate replications offer special advantages in enhancing the credibility of research findings and extending their generalizability. There are, however, relatively few *published* replication studies, perhaps reflecting a bias for original research on the part of researchers, editors, faculty advisors, and research sponsors.

Various replication strategies exist (Beck, 1994). One strategy is **identical replication** (or *literal* replication), which is an exact duplication of the original methods (e.g., sampling, measurement, analysis). More common is **virtual replication** (or *operational* replication), which involves attempts to approximate the methods used in the reference study as closely as possible, but precise duplication is not sought. A third strategy is **systematic extension replication** (or *constructive* replication), in which methods are not duplicated, but there are deliberate attempts to test the implications of the original research. Many nursing studies that build on earlier research could be described as extension replications, but they are not necessarily conceptualized as systematic extensions.

Reports on replication studies should provide details about what was replicated, and how the replication was similar to or different from the original (Beck, 1994). Researchers should thoroughly critique the original study being replicated, especially if modifications were made on the basis of any shortcoming. Beck also recommended *benchmarking*—comparing the results of the original and replicated study. The comparison should be accompanied by conclusions about both the internal and external validity of the study findings.

Many nurse researchers have called for more deliberate replication studies (e.g., Fahs et al., 2003; Polit & Beck, 2010). The push for an evidence-based practice may strengthen their legitimacy as important scientific endeavors.

Example of a replication study: Duignan and Dunn (2008) replicated a study in Ireland that had been done in the United States. The purpose was to examine the congruence between patients' self-report of pain intensity and emergency nurses' assessments of their pain intensity. In both studies, nurses frequently underestimated patients' pain levels.

Methodologic Studies

Methodologic studies are investigations of the ways of obtaining high-quality data and conducting rigorous research. Methodologic studies address the development and assessment of research tools or methods. The growing demands for sound, reliable outcome measures, and for sophisticated procedures for obtaining data have led to an increased interest in methodologic research.

Many methodologic studies focus on instrument development. Suppose, for example, we developed and tested a new instrument to measure patients' satisfaction with nursing care. In such a study, the purpose is not to describe levels of patient satisfaction or to assess its correlation with staff or patient characteristics. The goal is to develop a high-quality instrument for others to use in clinical or research applications. Instrument development research often involves complex procedures, some of which we describe in Chapter 15.

BOX 11.1 Some Guidelines for Critiquing Studies Described in Chapter 11

1. Does the study purpose match the study design? Was the best possible design used to address the study purpose?
2. If the study was a clinical trial, was adequate attention paid to developing an appropriate intervention? Was the intervention adequately pilot tested?
3. If the study was a clinical trial or evaluation, was there an effort to understand how the intervention was implemented (i.e., a process-type analysis)? Were the financial costs and benefits assessed? If not, should they have been?
4. If the study was an evaluation or needs assessment (or a practical clinical trial), to what extent do the study results serve the practical information needs of key decision makers or intended users?
5. If the study was a survey, was the most appropriate method used to collect the data (i.e., in-person interviews, telephone interviews, mail or Internet questionnaires)?
6. If the study was a secondary analysis, to what extent was the chosen dataset appropriate for addressing the research questions? What were the limitations of the dataset, and were these limitations acknowledged and taken into account in interpreting the results?

Occasionally researchers use an experimental design to test competing methodologic strategies. Suppose we wanted to test whether sending birthday cards to participants reduced rates of attrition in longitudinal studies. Participants could be randomly assigned to a card or no-card condition. The dependent variable would be rates of attrition from the study.

Example of a methodologic study: Hart and colleagues (2009) analyzed the effect of a personalized prenotification (via email or telephone) of a web-based survey on survey response rates. The response rate was 49% among program directors of nurse practitioner programs who were prenotified, compared with 45% among those who were not.

CRITIQUING STUDIES DESCRIBED IN THIS CHAPTER

It is difficult to provide guidance on critiquing the types of studies described in this chapter, because they are so varied and because many of the fundamental methodologic issues that require a critique concern the overall design. Guidelines for critiquing design-related issues were presented in the previous chapters.

Box 11.1 ⊗ offers a few specific questions for critiquing the types of studies included in this chapter. Separate guidelines for critiquing economic evaluations, which are more technically complex, are offered in the Toolkit section of the accompanying *Resource Manual*.

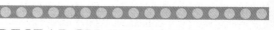

RESEARCH EXAMPLE

This section describes a set of related studies that stemmed from a longitudinal survey. The research example at the end of the next chapter is a good example of an outcomes research project that has generated many secondary analyses.

Studies: Research design and subject characteristics predicting nonparticipation in a panel survey of older families with cancer (Neumark et al., 2001). The influence of end-of-life cancer care on caregivers (Doorenbos et al., 2007).

The Survey: During the mid- to late-1990s, Drs. Barbara and Charles Given conducted a longitudinal survey with over 1,000 older patients who were newly diagnosed with lung, colon, breast, or prostate cancer. The panel study, called the Family Care Study, involved four rounds of telephone interviews as well as self-administered questionnaires with study participants, who were recruited over a 3-year period in multiple hospitals and cancer treatment centers in two states. The purpose of the original parent study was to examine the physical, emotional, and financial outcomes for patients and family members over the first year following cancer diagnosis. Key findings were presented in a report to the funding agency, NINR, and in numerous journal articles (e.g., Given et al., 2000, 2001).

Methodologic Research: The survey data set has been used in several secondary analyses, including one that focused on methodologic issues. Neumark and colleagues (2001) sought to identify factors that could account for loss of participants in the earliest phases of sample accrual. They compared three groups: eligible patients who declined to participate (nonconsenters), patients who originally consented to participate but then later declined (early dropouts), and people who actually took part in the study (participants). The researchers examined two broad types of factors that might explain nonparticipation in the study: participant characteristics and research design characteristics. The aim was to obtain information that would benefit others in designing studies and recruiting participants. They found, for example, that the most powerful design factor was whether a family caregiver was approached to participate. Patients were more likely to give consent and less likely to drop out early when caregivers were also approached.

Substantive Secondary Analysis: Doorenbos, the Givens, and other colleagues (2007) used data from 619 caregivers who completed the year-long study or whose family member died. The analysis focused on whether those caring for family members who ultimately died reported different caregiver depressive symptoms and burden than caregivers whose family survived throughout the study period. The findings suggested that caregiver depressive symptomatology improved over time for both groups, but symptoms were greater among caregivers whose relative died. Among spousal caregivers, those whose spouse died reported greater burden than caregivers whose spouse survived.

SUMMARY POINTS

- **Clinical trials** designed to assess the effectiveness of clinical interventions often involve a series of phases. Features of the intervention are finalized in *Phase I. Phase II* involves seeking

opportunities for refinements and preliminary evidence of efficacy. *Phase III* is a full experimental test of treatment *efficacy*. In *Phase IV*, researchers focus primarily on generalized *effectiveness* and evidence about costs and benefits.

- In a **sequential clinical trial**, data from paired "mini-experiments" are continuously analyzed, using measures of *preference* for the experimental or control condition for pairs of observations. Preferences are plotted on special graphs until the plot crosses one of the boundaries, which designate **stopping rules** for the trial.

- **Practical** (or **pragmatic**) **clinical trials** are designed to provide information to clinical decision makers. They sometimes involve **hybrid designs** that aim to reduce the gap between efficacy and effectiveness studies—that is, between internal and external validity.

- **Evaluation research** assesses the effectiveness of a program, policy, or procedure to assist decision makers. **Process** or **implementation analyses** describe the process by which a program gets implemented and how it functions in practice. **Outcome analyses** describe the status of some condition after the introduction of a program. **Impact analyses** test whether a program caused **net impacts** relative to the counterfactual. **Cost (economic) analyses** assess whether the monetary costs of a program are outweighed by benefits and include **cost-benefit analyses, cost-effectiveness analyses**, and **cost utility analyses**.

- **Outcomes research**, a subset of the broad interdisciplinary field of **health services research**, examines the quality and effectiveness of healthcare and nursing services. A model of healthcare quality encompasses several broad concepts, including: *structure* (factors such as accessibility, range of services, nursing skill mix, and organizational climate), *process* (nursing decisions and actions), client risk factors (e.g., illness severity, comorbidities), and *outcomes* (the specific end results of patient care in terms of patient functioning).

- **Survey research** involves studying people's characteristics, behaviors, and intentions by asking them to answer questions. One survey method is through **personal interviews**, in which interviewers meet respondents face-to-face and question them. **Telephone interviews** are less costly, but are inadvisable if the interview is long or if the questions are sensitive. **Questionnaires** are self-administered (i.e., questions are read by respondents, who then give written responses).

- **Secondary analysis** refers to studies in which researchers analyze previously collected data. Secondary analyses are economical, but it is sometimes difficult to identify an existing dataset that is appropriate.
- **Needs assessments** document the needs of a group or community. The three main needs assessment approaches are the **key informant**, survey, or **indicators approach**.
- The **Delphi technique** is a method of problem solving in which several rounds of questionnaires are sent to a panel of experts. Feedback from previous questionnaires is provided with each new questionnaire so that the experts can converge on a consensus.
- **Replication studies** include *identical replication* (exact duplication of methods of an earlier study), *virtual replication* (close approximation but not exact duplication of methods), and *systematic extension replication* (deliberate attempts to test the implications of the original research).
- In **methodologic studies**, the investigator is concerned with the development, validation, and assessment of methodologic tools or strategies.

STUDY ACTIVITIES

Chapter 11 of the *Study Guide for Nursing Research: Generating and Assessing Evidence for Nursing Practice*, *9th edition*, offers exercises and study suggestions for reinforcing concepts presented in this chapter. In addition, the following study questions can be addressed:

1. Suppose you were interested in doing a survey of nurses' attitudes toward caring for AIDS patients. Would you use a personal interview, telephone

interview, or questionnaire via mail or the Internet to collect your data? Defend your decision.
2. In the research example of the methodologic research by Hart and colleagues (2009), what were the dependent and independent variables? How might other researchers benefit from this research?

STUDIES CITED IN CHAPTER 11

Aiken, L. H., & Patrician, P. A. (2000). Measuring organizational traits of hospitals: The Revised Nursing Work Index. *Nursing Research, 49*, 146–153.

Chan, E. A., Chung, J., Wong, T., Lien, A., & Yang, J. (2007). Application of a virtual reality prototype for pain relief of pediatric burn patients in Taiwan. *Journal of Clinical Nursing, 16*, 786–793.

Chasens, E., Sereika, S., & Burke, L. (2009). Daytime sleepiness and functional outcomes in older adults with diabetes. *The Diabetes Educator, 35*, 455–464.

Chen, I. J., Chou, C., Yu, S., & Cheng, S. (2008). Health services utilization and cost utility analysis of a walking program for residential community elderly. *Nursing Economics, 26*, 263–269.

Cummings, G., Hayduk, L. Estabrooks, C. (2006). Is the Nursing Work Index measuring up? *Nursing Research, 55*, 92–93.

Donaldson, N., Shapiro, S., Scott, M., Foley, M., & Spetz, J. (2009). Leading successful rapid response teams: A multisite implementation evaluation. *Journal of Nursing Administration, 39*, 176–181.

Doorenbos, A., Given, B., Given, C., Wyatt, G., Gift, A., Rahbar, M., & Jeon, S. (2007). The influence of end-of-life cancer care on caregivers. *Research in Nursing & Health, 30*, 270–281.

Duignan, M., & Dunn, V. (2008). Congruence of pain assessment between nurses and emergency department patients: A replication. *International Emergency Nursing, 16*, 23–28.

Given, C., Given, B., Azzouz, F., Stommel, M., & Kozachik, S. (2000). Comparison of changes in physical functioning of elderly patients with new diagnoses of cancer. *Medical Care, 38*, 482–493.

Given, C., Given, B., Azzouz, F., Kozachik, S., & Stommel, M. (2001). Predictors of pain and fatigue in the year following diagnosis among elderly cancer patients. *Journal of Pain and Symptom Management, 21*, 456–466.

Harris, N., Lovell, K., Day, J., & Roberts, C. (2009). An evaluation of a medication management training programme for community mental health professionals. *International Journal of Nursing Studies, 46*, 645–652.

Hart, A., Brennan, C., Sym, D., & Larson, E. (2009). The impact of personalized prenotification on response rates to an electronic survey. *Western Journal of Nursing Research, 31*, 17–23.

Kutney-Lee, A., Lake, E., & Aiken, L. (2009). Development of the hospital nurse surveillance capacity profile. *Research in Nursing & Health, 32*, 217–228.

Miller, P., Vasey, J., Short, P., & Hartman, T. (2009). Dietary supplement use in adult cancer survivors. *Oncology Nursing Forum, 36*, 61–68.

Miller, S., Alpert, P., & Cross, C. (2008). Overweight and obesity in nurses, advanced practice nurses, and nurse educators. *Journal of the American Academy of Nurse Practitioners, 20*, 259–265.

Milne, C., Trigilia, D., Houle, T., Delong, S., & Rosenblum, D. (2009). Reducing pressure ulcer prevalence rates in the long-term acute care setting. *Ostomy Wound Management, 55*, 50–59.

Neumark, D. E., Stommel, M., Given, C. W., & Given, B. A. (2001). Research design and subject characteristics predicting nonparticipation in a panel survey of older families with cancer. *Nursing Research, 50*, 363–368.

Olsson, L., Hansson, E., Ekman, I., & Karlsson, J. (2009). A cost-effectiveness study of a patient-centred integrated care pathway. *Journal of Advanced Nursing, 65*, 1626–1635.

Rauch, A., Kirchberger, I., Boldt, C., Cieza, A., & Stucki, G. (2009). Does the Comprehensive International Classification of Functioning, Disability and Health (ICF) Core Set for rheumatoid arthritis capture nursing practice? A Delphi survey. *International Journal of Nursing Studies, 46*, 1320–1334.

Reynolds, M. A. (2009). Postoperative pain management discharge teaching in a rural population. *Pain Management Nursing, 10*, 76–84.

Schlairet, M. C. (2009). End-of-life nursing care: Statewide survey of nurses' education needs and effects of education. *Journal of Professional Nursing, 25*, 170–177.

Tschannen, D., & Kalisch, B. (2009). The effect of variations in nurse staffing on patient length of stay in the acute care setting. *Western Journal of Nursing Research, 31*, 153–170.

Twiss, J., Waltman, M., Berg, K., Ott, C., Gross, G., & Lindsey, A. (2009). An exercise intervention for breast cancer survivors with bone loss. *Journal of Nursing Scholarship, 41*, 20–27

Voyer, P., Preville, M., Roussel, M., Berbiche, D., & Beland, S. (2009). Factors associated with benzodiazepine dependence among community-dwelling seniors. *Journal of Community Health Nursing, 26*, 101–113.

Methodologic and nonresearch references cited in this chapter can be found in a separate section at the end of the book.

12

Sampling in Quantitative Research

S ampling is familiar to us all. In the course of daily activities, we make decisions and draw conclusions through sampling. A nursing student may select an elective course by sampling two or three classes on the first day of the semester. Patients may generalize about nursing care in a hospital based on the care they received from a sample of nurses. We all come to conclusions about phenomena based on exposure to a limited portion of those phenomena.

Researchers, too, obtain data from samples. In testing the efficacy of a new asthma medication, researchers reach conclusions without giving the drug to all asthmatic patients. Researchers, however, cannot afford to draw conclusions about intervention effects or inter-relationships among variables based on a sample of only three or four people. The consequences of making faulty decisions are more momentous in research than in private decision making.

Quantitative researchers seek to select samples that will allow them to achieve statistical conclusion validity and to generalize their results. They develop a **sampling plan** that specifies in advance how participants are to be selected and how many to include. Qualitative researchers, by contrast, make sampling decisions during the course of data collection, and typically do not have a formal sampling plan. This chapter discusses sampling issues for quantitative studies. Sampling for qualitative research is discussed in Chapter 21.

BASIC SAMPLING CONCEPTS

Let us begin by considering some terms associated with sampling—terms that are used primarily (but not exclusively) in quantitative research.

Populations

A **population** is the entire aggregation of cases in which a researcher is interested. For instance, if we were studying American nurses with doctoral degrees, the population could be defined as all U.S. citizens who are registered nurses (RNs) and who have a PhD, DNSc, DNP, or other doctoral-level degree. Other possible populations might be all male patients who had cardiac surgery in St. Peter's Hospital in 2010, all women with irritable bowel syndrome in Sydney, or all children in Canada with cystic fibrosis. As this list illustrates, a population may be broadly defined to involve thousands of people, or narrowly specified to include only hundreds.

Populations are not restricted to humans. A population might consist of all hospital records in a particular hospital or all blood samples at a particular laboratory. Whatever the basic unit, the population comprises the aggregate of elements in which the researcher is interested.

It is useful to make a distinction between target and accessible populations. The **accessible population** is the aggregate of cases that conform to designated criteria *and* that are accessible for a study. The **target population** is the aggregate of cases about which the researcher would like to generalize. A target population might consist of all diabetic people in the United States, but the accessible population might consist of all diabetic people who attend a particular clinic. Researchers usually sample from an accessible population and hope to generalize to a target population.

➡ **TIP:** A key issue for evidence-based practice is information about the populations on whom research has been conducted. Many quantitative researchers fail to identify their target population, or to discuss the generalizability of the results. The population of interest needs to be carefully considered in planning and reporting a study.

Eligibility Criteria

Researchers must specify criteria that define who is in the population. Consider the population, American nursing students. Does this population include students in all types of nursing programs? How about RNs returning to school for a bachelor's degree? Or students who took a leave of absence for a semester? Do foreign students enrolled in American nursing programs qualify? Insofar as possible, the researcher must consider the exact criteria by which it could be decided whether an individual would or would not be classified as a member of the population. The criteria that specify population characteristics are the **eligibility criteria** or **inclusion criteria**. Sometimes, a population is also defined in terms of characteristics that people must *not* possess (i.e., the **exclusion criteria**). For example, the population may be defined to exclude people who cannot speak English.

Specifications about the population should be driven, to the extent possible, by theoretical consid-erations. In thinking about ways to define the population and delineate eligibility criteria, it is important to consider whether the resulting sample is likely to be a good exemplar of the population construct in which you are interested. A study's construct validity is enhanced when there is a good match between the eligibility criteria and the population construct.

Of course, inclusion or exclusion criteria for a study often reflect considerations other than substantive concerns. Eligibility criteria may reflect one or more of the following:

- *Costs*. Some criteria reflect cost constraints. For example, when non–English-speaking people are excluded, this does not usually mean that researchers are uninterested in non–English speakers, but rather that they cannot afford to hire translators and multilingual data collectors.
- *Practical constraints*. Sometimes, there are other practical constraints, such as difficulty including people from rural areas, people who are hearing impaired, and so on.
- *People's ability to participate in a study*. The health condition of some people may preclude their participation. For example, people with mental impairments, who are in a coma, or who are in an unstable medical condition may need to be excluded.
- *Design considerations*. As noted in Chapter 10, it is sometimes advantageous to a study's internal validity to define a homogeneous population as a means of controlling confounding variables.

The criteria used to define a population for a study have implications for the interpretation of the results and, of course, the external validity of the findings.

Example of inclusion and exclusion criteria: Hafsteindóttir and colleagues (2010) studied malnutrition in hospitalized neurologic patients. Study participants had to be diagnosed with a neurologic or neurosurgical disease and speak Dutch. Patients were excluded if they were bed-bound and if their health condition made participation impossible.

Samples and Sampling

Sampling is the process of selecting cases to represent an entire population so that inferences about the population can be made. A **sample** is a subset of population **elements**, which are the most basic units about which data are collected. In nursing research, elements are usually humans.

Samples and sampling plans vary in quality. *Two key considerations in assessing a sample in a quantitative study are its representativeness and size.* A **representative sample** is one whose key characteristics closely approximate those of the population. If the population in a study of blood donors is 50% male and 50% female, then a representative sample would have a similar gender distribution. If the sample is not representative of the population, the study's external validity (and construct validity) is at risk.

Unfortunately, there is no way to make sure that a sample is representative without obtaining information from the population. Certain sampling procedures are less likely to result in biased samples than others, but a representative sample can never be guaranteed. Researchers operate under conditions in which error is possible. Quantitative researchers strive to minimize errors and, when possible, to estimate their magnitude.

Sampling designs are classified as either probability sampling or nonprobability sampling. **Probability sampling** involves random selection of elements. In probability sampling, researchers can specify the probability that an element of the population will be included in the sample. Greater confidence can be placed in the representativeness of probability samples. In **nonprobability samples**, elements are selected by nonrandom methods. There is no way to estimate the probability that each element has of being included in a nonprobability sample, and every element usually does *not* have a chance for inclusion.

Strata

Sometimes, it is useful to think of populations as consisting of subpopulations, or **strata**. A stratum is a mutually exclusive segment of a population, defined by one or more characteristics. For instance, suppose our population was all RNs in the United States. This population could be divided into two strata based on gender. Or, we could specify three strata of nurses younger than 30 years of age, nurses aged 30 to 45 years, and nurses 46 years or older. Strata are often used in sample selection to enhance the sample's representativeness.

Staged Sampling

Samples are sometimes selected in multiple stages, in what is called **multistage sampling**. In the first stage, large units (such as hospitals or nursing homes) are selected. Then, in a later stage, individual people are sampled. In staged sampling, it is possible to combine probability and nonprobability sampling. For example, the first stage can involve the deliberate (nonrandom) selection of study sites. Then, people within the selected sites can be selected through random procedures.

Sampling Bias

Researchers work with samples rather than with populations because it is cost-effective to do so. Researchers typically do not have the resources to study all members of a population.

It is often possible to obtain reasonably accurate information from a sample, but data from samples *can* lead to erroneous conclusions. Finding 100 people willing to participate in a study is seldom difficult. It is considerably harder to select 100 people who are not a biased subset of the population. **Sampling bias** refers to the systematic over-representation or under-representation of a population segment on a characteristic relevant to the research question.

As an example of consciously biased selection, suppose we were investigating patients' responsiveness to nurses' touch and decide to recruit the first 50 patients meeting eligibility criteria. We decide, however, to omit Mr. Z from the sample because he has been hostile to nursing staff. Mrs. X, who has just lost a spouse, is also bypassed because she is under stress. We have made conscious decisions to exclude certain people, and the decisions do not reflect bona fide eligibility criteria. This can lead to bias because responsiveness to nurses' touch (the dependent variable) may be affected by patients' feelings about nurses or their emotional state.

Sampling bias often occurs unconsciously, however. If we were studying nursing students and systematically interviewed every 10th student who entered the nursing school library, the sample would be biased in favor of library-goers, even if we were conscientious about including every 10th student regardless of his or her age, gender, or other traits.

➡ **TIP:** Internet surveys are attractive because they can be distributed to people all over the world. However, there is an inherent bias in such surveys, unless the population is defined as people who have easy access to, and comfort with, a computer and the Internet.

Sampling bias is partly a function of population homogeneity. If population elements were all identical with respect to key attributes, then any sample would be as good as any other. Indeed, if the population were completely homogeneous, that is, exhibited no variability at all, then a *single* element would be sufficient to draw conclusions about the population. For many physiologic attributes, it may be safe to assume high homogeneity. For example, the blood in a person's veins is relatively homogeneous and so a single blood sample is adequate. For most human attributes, however, homogeneity is the exception rather than the rule. Age, health status, stress, motivation—all these attributes reflect human heterogeneity. When variation occurs in the population, then similar variation should be reflected, to the extent possible, in a sample.

➡ **TIP:** One easy way to increase a study's generalizability is to select participants from multiple sites (e.g., from different hospitals, nursing homes, communities, etc.). Ideally, the different sites would be sufficiently divergent that good representation of the population would be obtained.

NONPROBABILITY SAMPLING

Nonprobability sampling is less likely than probability sampling to produce representative samples. Despite this fact, most studies in nursing and other disciplines rely on nonprobability samples. Four types of nonprobability sampling in quantitative studies are convenience, quota, consecutive, and purposive.

Convenience Sampling

Convenience sampling entails using the most conveniently available people as participants. A faculty member who distributes questionnaires to nursing students in a class is using a convenience sample. The nurse who conducts a study of teenage risk taking at a local high school is also relying on a convenience sample. The problem with convenience sampling is that those who are available might be atypical of the population with regard to critical variables.

Convenience samples do not necessarily comprise individuals known to the researchers. Stopping people at a street corner to conduct an interview is sampling by convenience. Sometimes, researchers seeking people with certain characteristics place an advertisement in a newspaper, put up signs in clinics, or post messages in chat rooms on the Internet. These approaches are subject to bias because people select themselves as pedestrians on certain streets or as volunteers in response to posted notices.

Snowball sampling (also called *network sampling* or *chain sampling*) is a variant of convenience sampling. With this approach, early sample members (called **seeds**) are asked to refer other people who meet the eligibility criteria. This sampling method is often used when the population is people with characteristics who might otherwise be difficult to identify (e.g., people who are afraid of hospitals). Snowballing begins with a few eligible participants and then continues on the basis of participant referrals.

Convenience sampling is the weakest form of sampling. In heterogeneous populations, there is no other sampling approach in which the risk of

TABLE 12.1	Numbers and Percentages of Students in Strata of a Population, Convenience Sample, and Quota Sample		
STRATA	**POPULATION**	**CONVENIENCE SAMPLE**	**QUOTA SAMPLE**
Male	100 (20%)	5 (5%)	20 (20%)
Female	400 (80%)	95 (95%)	80 (80%)
Total	500 (100%)	100 (100%)	100 (100%)

sampling bias is greater. Yet, convenience sampling is the most commonly used method in many disciplines.

Example of a convenience sample: Peddle and colleagues (2009) studied factors that correlated with adherence to supervised exercise in patients awaiting surgery for suspected malignant lung lesions. Their sample of patients was described as a sample of convenience.

⊃ **TIP:** Rigorous methods of sampling *hidden populations*, such as the homeless or injection drug users, are emerging. Because standard probability sampling is inappropriate for such hidden populations, a method called **respondent-driven sampling (RDS)**, a variant of snowball sampling, has been developed. RDS, unlike traditional snowballing, allows the assessment of relative inclusion probabilities based on mathematical models (Magnani et al., 2005).

Quota Sampling

A **quota sample** is one in which the researcher identifies population strata and determines how many participants are needed from each stratum. By using information about population characteristics, researchers can ensure that diverse segments are represented in the sample, preferably in the proportion in which they occur in the population.

Suppose we were interested in studying nursing students' attitude toward working with AIDS patients. The accessible population is a school of nursing with 500 undergraduate students; a sample of 100

students is desired. The easiest procedure would be to distribute questionnaires in classrooms through convenience sampling. We suspect, however, that male and female students have different attitudes, and a convenience sample might result in too many men or women. Table 12.1 presents fictitious data showing the gender distribution for the population and for a convenience sample (second and third columns). In this example, the convenience sample over-represents women and under-represents men. We can, however, establish "quotas" so that the sample includes the appropriate number of cases from both strata. The far-right column of Table 12.1 shows the number of men and women required for a quota sample for this example.

You may better appreciate the dangers of a biased sample with a concrete example. Suppose a key study question was, "Would you be willing to work on a unit that cared exclusively for AIDS patients?" The number and percentage of students in the population who would respond "yes" are shown in the first column of Table 12.2. We would not know these values—they are shown to illustrate a point. Within the population, men are more likely than women to say they would work on a unit with AIDS patients, yet men were under-represented in the convenience sample. As a result, population and sample values on the outcome are discrepant: Nearly twice as many students in the population are favorable toward working with AIDS patients (20%) than we would conclude based on results from the convenience sample (11%). The quota sample does a better

TABLE 12.2	Students Willing to Work on AIDS Unit, in the Population, Convenience Sample, and Quota Sample		
	POPULATION	**CONVENIENCE SAMPLE**	**QUOTA SAMPLE**
Willing males (number)	28	2	6
Willing females (number)	72	9	13
Total number of willing students	100	11	19
Total number of all students	500	100	100
Percentage willing	20%	11%	19%

job of reflecting the views of the population (19%). In actual research situations, the distortions from a convenience sample may be smaller than in this example, but could be larger as well.

Quota sampling does not require sophisticated skills or a lot of effort. Many researchers who use a convenience sample could profitably use quota sampling. Stratification should be based on one or more variables that would reflect important differences in the dependent variable. Such variables as gender, ethnicity, education, and medical diagnosis may be good stratifying variables.

Procedurally, quota sampling is like convenience sampling. The people in any subgroup are a convenience sample from that stratum of the population. For example, the initial sample of 100 students in Table 12.1 constituted a convenience sample from the population of 500. In the quota sample, the 20 men constitute a convenience sample of the 100 men in the population. Because of this fact, quota sampling shares many of the same weaknesses as convenience sampling. For instance, if a researcher is required by a quota-sampling plan to interview 10 men between the ages of 65 and 80 years, a trip to a nursing home might be the most convenient method of obtaining participants. Yet this approach would fail to represent the many older men living independently in the community. Despite its limitations, quota sampling is a major improvement over convenience sampling.

Example of a quota sample: Fox and colleagues (2009) explored perceptions of bed days in patients receiving extended in-patient services for the management of chronic illness. The study used patients from a larger study that used quota sampling to ensure equal representation of people who had different levels of bed days. The strata were defined as people with 0, 2 to 4, and 5 to 7 bed days per week.

Consecutive Sampling

Consecutive sampling involves recruiting *all* of the people from an accessible population who meet the eligibility criteria over a specific time interval, or for a specified sample size. For example, in a study of ventilator-associated pneumonia in ICU patients, if the accessible population were patients in an ICU of a specific hospital, a consecutive sample might consist of all eligible patients admitted to that ICU over a 6-month period. Or it might be the first 250 eligible patients admitted to the ICU, if 250 were the targeted sample size.

Consecutive samples can be selected either for a retrospective or prospective time period. For example, the sample could include every patient who visited a diabetic clinic in the previous 30 days. Or, it could include all of the patients who will enroll in the clinic in the next 30 days.

Consecutive sampling is a far better approach than sampling by convenience, especially if the sampling period is sufficiently long to deal with potential biases that reflect seasonal or other time-related fluctuations. When all members of an accessible population are invited to participate in a study over a fixed time period, the risk of bias is greatly reduced. Consecutive sampling is often the best possible choice when there is "rolling enrollment" into a contained accessible population.

> **Example of a consecutive sample:** O'Meara and colleagues (2008) conducted a study to evaluate factors associated with interruptions in enteral nutrition delivery in mechanically ventilated critically ill patients. A consecutive sample of 59 ICU patients who required mechanical ventilation and were receiving enteral nutrition participated in the study.

Purposive Sampling

Purposive sampling or *judgmental sampling* uses researchers' knowledge about the population to select sample members. Researchers might decide purposely to select people who are judged to be typical of the population or particularly knowledgeable about the issues under study. Sampling in this subjective manner, however, provides no external, objective method for assessing the typicalness of the selected participants. Nevertheless, this method can be used to advantage in certain situations. Newly developed instruments can be effectively pretested and evaluated with a purposive sample of diverse types of people. Purposive sampling is often used when researchers want a sample of experts, as in the case of a needs assessment using the key informant approach or in Delphi surveys.

Purposive sampling is also a good approach in two-staged sampling. That is, sites can first be sampled purposively, and then people can be sampled in some other fashion, as in the following example:

> **Example of purposive sampling:** Dudley-Brown and Freivogel (2009) field tested alternative intake tools for identifying patients at high risk for colorectal cancer in gastroenterology clinics. They began by purposively selecting six sites in four states. Their goal was to select sites so as to "approximate a representative sample for ethnicity and age" (p. 10). In the next stage of sampling, the researchers recruited a consecutive sample of patients over a 2-month period.

Evaluation of Nonprobability Sampling

Except for some consecutive samples, nonprobability samples are rarely representative of the population. When every element in the population does not have a chance of being included in the sample, it is likely that some segment of it will be systematically under-represented. When there is sampling bias, there is a chance that the results could be misleading, and efforts to generalize to a broader population could be misguided.

Nonprobability samples will continue to predominate, however, because of their practicality. Probability sampling requires skill and resources, so there may be no option but to use a nonprobability approach. Strict convenience sampling without explicit efforts to enhance representativeness, however, should be avoided. Indeed, it could be argued that quantitative researchers would do better at achieving representative samples for generalizing to a population if they had an approach that were more purposeful (Polit & Beck, 2010).

Quota sampling is a semi-purposive sampling strategy that is far superior to convenience sampling because it seeks to ensure sufficient representation within key strata of the population. Another purposive strategy for enhancing generalizability is deliberate multisite sampling. For instance, a convenience sample could be obtained from two communities known to differ socioeconomically so that the sample would reflect the experiences and views of both lower- and middle-class participants. In other words, if the population is known to be heterogeneous, you should take steps to capture important variation in the sample.

Even in one-site studies in which convenience sampling is used, researchers can (and should) make an effort to explicitly add cases to correspond more closely to population parameters. Kerlinger and Lee (2000) advised researchers to check their sample for easily verified expectations. For example, if half the population is known to be male, then the researcher can check to see if approximately half the sample is male and use outreach to recruit more males if necessary. Shadish and colleagues (2002) also argued for more purposive sampling, noting that deliberate heterogeneous sampling on presumptively important dimensions is an important strategy for generalization.

Quantitative researchers using nonprobability samples must be cautious about the inferences they make. With efforts to deliberately enhance representativeness, a conservative interpretation of the results with regard to generalizability, and replication of the study with new samples, researchers find that nonprobability samples usually work reasonably well.

PROBABILITY SAMPLING

Probability sampling involves the random selection of elements from a population. **Random sampling** involves a selection process in which each element in the population has an equal, independent chance of being selected. Probability sampling is a complex, technical topic, and books such as those by Levy and Lemeshow (2009) offer further guidance for advanced students.

⬅ **T I P :** Random sampling should not be (but often is) confused with random assignment, which was described in connection with experimental designs in Chapter 9. Random assignment is the process of allocating people to different treatment conditions at random. Random *assignment* has no bearing on how people in an RCT were selected in the first place.

Simple Random Sampling

Simple random sampling is the most basic probability sampling design. In simple random sampling, researchers establish a **sampling frame**, the technical name for the list of elements from which the sample will be chosen. If nursing students at the University of Connecticut were the accessible population, then a roster of those students would be the sampling frame. If the sampling unit were 300-bed or larger hospitals in Taiwan, then a list of all such hospitals would be the sampling frame. In practice, a population may be defined in terms of an existing sampling frame. For example, if we wanted to use a voter registration list as a sampling frame, we would have to define the community population as residents who had registered to vote.

Once a sampling frame has been developed, elements are numbered consecutively. A table of random numbers or computer-generated list of random numbers would then be used to draw a sample of the desired size. An example of a sampling frame for a population of 50 people is shown in Table 12.3. Let us assume we want to randomly sample 20 people. As with random assignment, we could find a starting place in a table of random numbers by blindly placing our finger at some point on the page to

TABLE 12.3	Sampling Frame for Simple Random Sampling Example

(1.)	N. Alexander	(26.)	C. Ball
2.	D. Brady	27.	L. Chodos
3.	D. Carroll	28.	K. DiSanto
4.	M. Dakes	29.	B. Eddy
(5.)	H. Edelman	(30.)	J. Fishon
(6.)	L. Forester	(31.)	R. Griffin
7.	J. Galt	32.	B. Hebert
8.	L. Hall	(33.)	C. Joyce
9.	R. Ivry	(34.)	S. Kane
10.	A. Janosy	35.	C. Lace
11.	J. Kettlewell	36.	M. Montanari
12.	L. Lack	37.	B. Nicolet
(13.)	B. Mastrianni	(38.)	T. Opitz
(14.)	K. Nolte	39.	J. Portnoy
15.	N. O'Hara	40.	G. Queto
16.	T. Piekarz	41.	A. Ryan
(17.)	J. Quint	42.	S. Singleton
(18.)	M. Riggi	(43.)	L. Tower
19.	M. Solomons	44.	V. Vaccaro
20.	S. Thompson	(45.)	B. Wilmot
(21.)	C. VanWagner	(46.)	D. Abraham
22.	R. Walsh	47.	V. Brusser
(23.)	J. Yepsen	48.	O. Crampton
(24.)	M. Zimmerman	49.	R. Davis
25.	A. Arnold	(50.)	C. Eldred

find a two-digit combination between 1 and 50. For this example, suppose that we began with the first number in the random number table of Table 9.2 (p. 208), which is 46. The person corresponding to that number, D. Abraham, is the first person selected to participate in the study. Number 05, H. Edelman, is the second selection, and number 23, J. Yepsen, is the third. This process would continue until 20 participants are chosen. The selected elements are circled in Table 12.3.

Clearly, a sample selected randomly in this fashion is not subject to biases. Although there is no guarantee that a random sample will be representative, random selection ensures that differences in the attributes of the sample and the population are purely a function of chance. The probability of selecting a deviant sample decreases as the size of the sample increases.

Simple random sampling tends to be laborious. Developing a sampling frame, numbering all elements, and selecting elements are time-consuming chores, particularly if the population is large. Imagine enumerating all the telephone subscribers listed in the New York City telephone directory! In actual practice, simple random sampling is not used frequently because it is relatively inefficient. Furthermore, it is not always possible to get a listing of every element in the population, so other methods may be required.

Example of a simple random sample: Lipman and colleagues (2009) documented nurses' practices in an urban children's hospital with regard to whether children's height was measured and plotted on growth charts. Using a random numbers table, a simple random sample of 200 hospital charts was selected for review.

Stratified Random Sampling

In **stratified random sampling**, the population is first divided into two or more strata. As with quota sampling, the aim is to enhance representativeness. Stratified sampling designs subdivide the population into homogeneous subsets (e.g., based on gender or illness severity categories) from which an appropriate number of elements are selected at random.

One difficulty with stratification is that the stratifying attributes must be known in advance and may not be readily discernible. Patient listings, student rosters, or organizational directories may contain information for meaningful stratification, but many lists do not. Quota sampling does not have the same problem because researchers can ask people questions that determine their eligibility for a particular stratum. In stratified sampling, however, a person's status in a stratum must be known before random selection.

The most common procedure for drawing a stratified sample is to group together elements belonging to a stratum and to select randomly the desired number of elements. To illustrate, suppose that the list in Table 12.3 consisted of 25 men (numbers 1 through 25) and 25 women (numbers 26 through 50). Using gender as the stratifying variable, we could guarantee a sample of 10 men and 10 women by randomly sampling 10 numbers from the first half of the list and 10 from the second half. As it turns out, our simple random sampling did result in 10 elements being chosen from each half of the list, but this was purely by chance. It would not have been unusual to draw, say, 8 names from one half and 12 from the other. Stratified sampling can guarantee the appropriate representation of different population segments.

Stratification usually divides the population into unequal subpopulations. For example, if the person's race were used to stratify the population of U.S. citizens, the subpopulation of white people would be larger than that of nonwhite people. We might select participants in proportion to the size of the stratum in the population, using **proportionate stratified sampling**. If the population was students in a nursing school that had 10% African American, 10% Hispanic, 10% Asian, and 70% white students, then a proportionate stratified sample of 100 students, with race/ethnicity as the stratifying variable, would consist of 10, 10, 10, and 70 students from the respective strata.

Proportionate sampling may result in insufficient numbers for making comparisons among strata. In our example, we would not be justified in drawing conclusions about Hispanic nursing students based on only 10 cases. For this reason, researchers may use **disproportionate sampling** when comparisons are sought between strata of greatly unequal size. In the example, the sampling proportions might be altered to select 20 African American, 20 Hispanic, 20 Asian, and 40 white students. This design would ensure a more adequate representation of the three racial/ethnic minorities. When disproportionate sampling is used, however, it is necessary to make an adjustment to arrive at the best estimate of *overall* population values. This adjustment, called **weighting**, is a simple mathematic computation described in textbooks on sampling.

Stratified random sampling enables researchers to sharpen the representativeness of their samples. When it is desirable to obtain reliable information about subpopulations whose memberships are small, stratification provides a means of including a sufficient number of cases in the sample by oversampling for that stratum. Stratified sampling, however, may be impossible if information on the critical variables is unavailable. Furthermore, a stratified sample requires even more labor and effort than simple random sampling because the sample must be drawn from multiple enumerated listings.

Example of stratified random sampling: Ekwall and Hallberg (2007) studied caregiver satisfaction among informal older caregivers who participated in a mail survey in Sweden. The sample was stratified on the basis of age. Questionnaires were mailed to 2,500 elders aged 75 to 79, 2,500 elders aged 80 to 84, 2,000 elders aged 85 to 89, and 1,500 elders aged 90 and over.

Multistage Cluster Sampling

For many populations, it is impossible to get a listing of all elements. For example, the population of full-time nursing students in the United Kingdom would be difficult to list and enumerate for the purpose of drawing a simple or stratified random sample. Large-scale surveys—especially ones involving personal interviews—almost never use simple or stratified random sampling; they usually rely on multistage sampling, beginning with clusters.

Cluster sampling involves selecting broad groups (clusters) rather than selecting individuals, and is typically the first stage of a multistage approach. In drawing a sample of nursing students, we might first draw a random sample of nursing schools and then draw a sample of students from the selected schools. The usual procedure for selecting samples from a general population in the United States is to sample successively such administrative units as census tracts, then households, and then household members. The resulting design can be described in terms of the number of stages (e.g., three-stage sampling). Clusters can be selected either by simple or stratified methods. For instance, in selecting clusters of nursing schools, it may be advisable to stratify on program type.

For a specified number of cases, multistage sampling tends to be less accurate than simple or stratified random sampling. Yet, multistage sampling is more practical than other types of probability sampling, particularly when the population is large and widely dispersed.

Example of multistage sampling: Callaghan and colleagues (2010) studied self-efficacy and exercise behavior in a large sample of Chinese students. High schools were first sampled, with stratification based on geographic location. Students were subsequently sampled from the selected high schools.

Systematic Sampling

Systematic sampling involves selecting every kth case from a list, such as every 10th person on a patient list or every 25th person on a student roster. Systematic sampling is sometimes used to sample every kth person entering a store, or passing down the street, or leaving a hospital, and so forth. In such situations, unless the population is narrowly defined as all those people entering, passing by, or leaving, the sampling is essentially a sample of convenience.

Systematic sampling can, however, be applied so that an essentially random sample is drawn. If we had a list (sampling frame), the following procedure could be adopted. The desired sample size is established at some number (n). The size of the population must be known or estimated (N). By dividing N by n, the sampling interval width (k) is established. The **sampling interval** is the standard distance between sampled elements. For instance, if we wanted a sample of 200 from a population of 40,000, then our sampling interval would be as follows:

$$k = \frac{40,000}{200} = 200$$

In other words, every 200th element on the list would be sampled. The first element should be selected randomly. Suppose that we randomly selected number 73 from a random number table. People corresponding to numbers 73, 273, 473, and so on would be sampled. Alternatively, we could randomly select a number from 1 to the number of elements listed on a page, and then randomly select every kth unit on all pages (e.g., number 38 on every page).

Systematic sampling conducted in this manner yields essentially the same results as simple random sampling, but involves less work. Problems would arise if the list were arranged in such a way that a certain type of element is listed at intervals coinciding with the sampling interval. For instance, if every 10th nurse listed in a nursing staff roster was a head nurse and the sampling interval was 10, then head nurses would either always or never be included in the sample. Problems of this type are rare, fortunately. Systematic sampling may be preferred to simple random sampling because similar results are obtained in a more efficient manner. Systematic sampling can also be applied to lists that have been stratified.

Example of a systematic sample: Houghton and colleagues (2008) surveyed nurse anesthetists about their practices and attitudes regarding smoking intervention. Using the membership list of the American Association of Nurse Anesthetists, every 30th name in the alphabetized list was selected for the sample.

Evaluation of Probability Sampling

Probability sampling is the best method of obtaining representative samples. If all the elements in a popu-

lation have an equal probability of being selected, then the resulting sample is likely to do a good job of representing the population. A further advantage is that probability sampling allows researchers to estimate the magnitude of sampling error. **Sampling error** refers to differences between population values (such as the average age of the population) and sample values (such as the average age of the sample).

The great drawback of probability sampling is its impracticality. It is beyond the scope of most studies to involve a probability sample, unless the population is narrowly defined—and if it *is* narrowly defined, probability sampling may be "overkill." Probability sampling is the preferred and most respected method of obtaining sample elements, but is often unfeasible.

➲ **T I P :** The quality of the sampling plan is of particular importance in survey research, because the purpose of surveys is to obtain information about the prevalence or average values for a population. All national surveys, such as the National Health Interview Survey in the United States, use probability samples (usually multistage cluster samples). Probability samples are rarely used in experimental and quasi-experimental studies, in part because the main focus of such inquiries is on between-group differences rather than absolute values for a population.

SAMPLE SIZE IN QUANTITATIVE STUDIES

Quantitative researchers need to pay attention to the number of participants needed to achieve statistical conclusion validity. A procedure called **power analysis** (Cohen, 1988) can be used to estimate sample size needs, but some statistical knowledge is needed before this procedure can be explained. In this section, we offer guidelines to beginning researchers; advanced students can read about power analysis in Chapter 17 or in a sampling or statistics textbook (e.g., Polit, 2010).

Sample Size Basics

There are no simple formulas that can tell you how large a sample you will need in a given study, but as a general recommendation, you should use the largest sample possible. The larger the sample, the more representative of the population it is likely to be. Every time researchers calculate a percentage or an average based on sample data, they are estimating a population value. Smaller samples tend to produce less precise estimates than larger ones. In other words, the larger the sample, the smaller the sampling error.

Let us illustrate this with an example of monthly aspirin consumption in a nursing home (Table 12.4). The population consists of 15 residents whose aspirin consumption averages 16.0 aspirins per month, as shown in the top row of the table. Eight simple random samples—two each with sample sizes of 2, 3, 5, and 10—have been drawn. Each sample average represents an estimate of the population average (i.e., 16.0). With a sample size of two, our estimate might have been wrong by as many as eight aspirins (sample 1B, average of 24.0), which is 50% greater than the population value. As the sample size increases, the averages get closer to the true population value, *and* the differences in the estimates between samples A and B

get smaller as well. As sample size increases, the probability of getting a markedly deviant sample diminishes. Large samples provide an opportunity to counterbalance atypical values. In the absence of a power analysis, the safest procedure is to obtain data from as large a sample as is feasible.

Large samples are no assurance of accuracy, however. When nonprobability sampling methods are used, even a large sample can harbor extensive bias. The famous example illustrating this point is the 1936 American presidential poll conducted by the magazine *Literary Digest*, which predicted that Alfred M. Landon would defeat Franklin D. Roosevelt by a landslide. About 2.5 million individuals participated in this poll—a substantial sample. Biases resulted from the fact that the sample was drawn from telephone directories and automobile registrations during a depression year when only the well-to-do (who preferred Landon) had a car or telephone. Thus, a large sample cannot correct for a faulty sampling design. Nevertheless, a large nonprobability sample is preferable to a small one.

Because practical constraints such as time, participant cooperation, and resources often limit sample

TABLE 12.4	Comparison of Population and Sample Values and Averages: Nursing Home Aspirin Consumption Example		
NUMBER OF PEOPLE IN GROUP	**GROUP**	**INDIVIDUAL DATA VALUES (NUMBER OF ASPIRINS CONSUMED, PRIOR MONTH)**	**AVERAGE**
15	Population	2, 4, 6, 8, 10, 12, 14, 16, 18, 20, 22, 24, 26, 28, 30	16.0
2	Sample 1A	6, 14	10.0
2	Sample 1B	20, 28	24.0
3	Sample 2A	16, 18, 8	14.0
3	Sample 2B	20, 14, 26	20.0
5	Sample 3A	26, 14, 18, 2, 28	17.6
5	Sample 3B	30, 2, 26, 10, 4	14.4
10	Sample 4A	22, 16, 24, 20, 2, 8, 14, 28, 20, 4	15.8
10	Sample 4B	12, 18, 8, 10, 16, 6, 28, 14, 30, 22	16.4

size, many nursing studies are based on relatively small samples. Most nursing studies use samples of convenience, and many are based on samples that are too small to provide an adequate test of the research hypotheses. Quantitative studies usually are based on samples of fewer than 200 participants, and many have fewer than 100 people (e.g., Polit & Sherman, 1990; Polit & Gillespie, 2009). Power analysis is not done routinely by nurse researchers, and research reports often offer no justification for sample size. When samples are too small, quantitative researchers run the risk of gathering data that will not support their hypotheses, *even when their hypotheses are correct*, thereby undermining statistical conclusion validity.

Factors Affecting Sample Size Requirements in Quantitative Research

Sample size requirements are affected by various factors, some of which we discuss in this section.

Effect Size

Power analysis builds on the concept of an **effect size**, which expresses the strength of relationships among research variables. If there is reason to expect that the independent and dependent variables will be strongly related, then a relatively small sample may be adequate to reveal the relationship statistically. For example, if we were testing a powerful new drug to treat AIDS, it might be possible to demonstrate its effectiveness with a small sample. Typically, however, nursing interventions have modest effects, and variables are usually only moderately correlated with one another. When there is no *a priori* reason for believing that relationships will be strong, then small samples are risky.

Homogeneity of the Population

If the population is relatively homogeneous, a small sample may be adequate. The greater the variability, the greater is the risk that a small sample will not adequately capture the full range of variation. For most nursing studies, it is probably best to assume a fair degree of heterogeneity, unless there is evidence from prior research to the contrary.

Cooperation and Attrition

In most studies, not every one invited to participate in a study agrees to do so. Therefore, in developing a sampling plan, it is good to begin with a realistic, evidence-based estimate of the percentage of people likely to cooperate. Thus, if your targeted sample size is 200 but you expect a 50% refusal rate, you would have to recruit 400 or so eligible people.

In studies with multiple points of data collection, the number of participants usually declines over time. Attrition is most likely to occur if the time lag between data collection points is great, if the population is mobile, or if the population is at risk of death or disability. If the researcher has an ongoing relationship with participants (as might be true in clinical studies), then attrition might be low—but it is rarely 0%. Therefore, in estimating sample size needs, researchers should factor in anticipated loss of participants over time.

Attrition problems are not restricted to longitudinal studies. People who initially agree to cooperate in a study may be subsequently unable or unwilling to participate for various reasons, such as death, deteriorating health, early discharge, discontinued need for an intervention, or simply a change of heart. Researchers should expect a certain amount of participant loss and recruit accordingly.

➔ **TIP:** Polit and Gillespie (2009) found, in a sample of over 100 nursing RCTs, that the average participant loss was 12.5% for studies with follow-up data collection between 31 and 90 days after baseline, and was 18% when the final data collection was more than 6 months after baseline.

Subgroup Analyses

Researchers sometimes wish to test hypotheses not only for an entire population, but also for subgroups. For example, we might be interested in assessing whether a structured exercise program is effective in improving infants' motor skills. After testing the general hypothesis with a sample of infants, we might wish to test whether the intervention is more effective for certain infants (e.g., low-birth-weight versus normal-birth-weight infants). When a sample is divided to test for **subgroup effects**, the sample must be large enough to support analyses with such divisions of the sample.

Sensitivity of the Measures

Instruments vary in their ability to measure key concepts precisely. Biophysiologic measures are usually very sensitive—they measure phenomena accurately, and can make fine discriminations in values. Psychosocial measures often contain some error and lack precision. When measuring tools are imprecise and susceptible to errors, larger samples are needed to test hypotheses adequately.

TIP: Hertzog (2008) has offered guidance on estimating sample size needs for pilot studies.

IMPLEMENTING A SAMPLING PLAN IN QUANTITATIVE STUDIES

This section provides some practical guidance about implementing a sampling plan.

Steps in Sampling in Quantitative Studies

The steps to be undertaken in drawing a sample vary somewhat from one sampling design to the next, but a general outline of procedures can be described.

1. *Identify the population.* You should begin with a clear idea about the target population to which you would like to generalize your results. Unless you have extensive resources, you are unlikely to have access to the entire target population, so you will also need to identify the population that is accessible to you. Researchers sometimes *begin* by identifying an accessible population, and then decide how best to characterize the target population.
2. *Specify the eligibility criteria.* The criteria for eligibility in the sample should then be spelled out. The criteria should be as specific as possible with regard to characteristics that might

exclude potential participants (e.g., extremes of poor health, inability to read English). The criteria might lead you to redefine your target population.

3. *Specify the sampling plan.* Once the accessible population has been identified, you must decide (a) the method of drawing the sample and (b) how large it will be. Sample size specifications should consider the aspects of the study discussed in the previous section. If you can perform a power analysis to estimate the needed number of participants, we highly recommend that you do so. Similarly, if probability sampling is a viable option, that option should be exercised. If you are not in a position to do either, we recommend using as large a sample as possible and taking steps to build representativeness into the design (e.g., by using quota or consecutive sampling).
4. *Recruit the sample.* Once the sampling design has been specified, the next step is to recruit prospective participants according to the plan (after any needed institutional permissions have been obtained) and ask for their cooperation. Issues relating to participant recruitment are discussed next.

Sample Recruitment

Recruiting people to participate in a study involves two major tasks: identifying eligible candidates and persuading them to participate. Researchers may need to spend time early in the project deciding the best sources for recruiting potential participants. Researchers must ask such questions as, Where do large numbers of people matching my population construct live or obtain care? Will I have direct access to people, or will I need to work through gatekeepers? Will there be sufficiently large numbers in one location, or will multiple sites be necessary? During the recruitment phase, it may be necessary to develop a **screening instrument**, which is a brief interview or form that allows researchers to determine whether a prospective participant meets all eligibility criteria for the study.

The next task involves gaining the cooperation of people who have been deemed eligible. It is critical to have an effective recruitment strategy. Many people, given the right circumstances, will agree to cooperate, but—especially in intervention research—some are hesitant. Researchers should ask themselves, What will make this research experience enjoyable, worthwhile, convenient, pleasant, and nonthreatening for people? Researchers have control over such influential factors as the following:

- *Recruitment method.* Face-to-face recruitment is usually more effective than solicitation by a telephone call, letter, or email.
- *Courtesy.* Successful recruitment depends on using recruiters who are pleasant, courteous, and enthusiastic about the study. Cooperation sometimes is enhanced if the recruiters' characteristics are similar to those of prospective participants—particularly with regard to gender, race, and ethnicity.
- *Persistence.* Although high-pressure tactics are never acceptable, persistence may sometimes be needed. When prospective participants are first approached, their initial reaction may be to decline if they are taken off guard. If a person hesitates or gives an equivocal answer at the first attempt, recruiters should ask if they could come back at a later time.
- *Incentives.* Gifts and monetary incentives have been found to have a substantial effect on participation (Edwards et al., 2009).
- *Benefits.* The benefits of participating to the individual and to society should be explained, without exaggeration or misleading information.
- *Sharing results.* Sometimes it is useful to provide people with tangible evidence of their contribution to the study by offering to send them a brief summary of the study results.
- *Convenience.* Every effort should be made to collect data at a time and location that is convenient for participants. In some cases, this may mean making arrangements for transportation or for the care of young children.

- *Endorsements.* It may be valuable to have the study endorsed by a person or organization that has prospective participants' confidence, and to communicate this to them. Endorsements might come from the institution serving as the research setting, a funding agency, or a respected community group or person, such as a church leader. A statement of university sponsorship has positive effects of participation (Edwards et al., 2009). Press releases in advance of recruitment may be advantageous.
- *Assurances.* Prospective subjects should be told who will see the data, what use will be made of the data, and how confidentiality will be maintained.

The issue of participant recruitment—and retention—has received considerable attention in recent years. There are numerous articles on strategies for, and barriers to, recruiting from minority or vulnerable populations (e.g., Russell et al., 2008; Topp et al., 2008; UyBico et al., 2007; Webb et al., 2009), which is a particularly important issue for those interested in health disparities research. Guidance also is available with regard to participant recruitment for RCTs (e.g., Berger et al., 2007; Gul & Ali, 2010; Leathem et al., 2009). In the United States, researchers should be aware of potential recruitment difficulties that have arisen within the context of the Health Insurance Portability and Accountability Act or HIPAA (Wipke-Tevis & Pickett, 2008).

TIP: Participant recruitment often proceeds at a slower pace than researchers anticipate. Once you have determined your sample size needs, it is useful to develop contingency plans for recruiting more people, should the initial plan prove overly optimistic. For example, a contingency plan might involve relaxing the eligibility criteria, identifying another institution through which participants could be recruited, offering incentives to make participation more attractive, or lengthening the recruitment period. When such plans are developed at the outset, it reduces the likelihood that you will have to settle for a less-than-desirable sample size.

Generalizing From Samples

Ideally, the sample is representative of the accessible population, and the accessible population is representative of the target population. By using an appropriate sampling plan, researchers can be reasonably confident that the first part of this ideal has been realized. The second part of the ideal entails greater risk. Are diabetic patients in Atlanta representative of diabetic patients in the United States? Researchers must exercise judgment in assessing the degree of similarity.

The best advice is to be realistic and conservative, and to ask challenging questions: Is it reasonable to assume that the accessible population is representative of the target population? In what ways might they differ? How would such differences affect the conclusions? If differences are great, it would be prudent to specify a more restricted target population to which the findings could be meaningfully generalized.

Interpretations about the generalizability of findings can be enhanced by comparing sample characteristics with population characteristics, when this is possible. Published information about the characteristics of many populations may be available to help in evaluating sampling bias. For example, if you were studying low-income children in Chicago, you could obtain information on the Internet about salient characteristics (e.g., race/ethnicity, age distribution) of low-income American children from the U.S. Bureau of the Census. Population characteristics could then be compared with sample characteristics, and differences taken into account in interpreting the findings. Sousa and colleagues (2004) provide suggestions for drawing conclusions about whether a convenience sample is representative of the population.

Example of comparison of characteristics:
Griffin and colleagues (2008) conducted a survey of over 300 pediatric nurses, whose names had been randomly sampled from a list of 9,000 nurses who subscribed to pediatric nursing journals. Demographic characteristics of the sample (e.g., gender, race/ethnicity, educational background) were compared with characteristics of a nationally representative sample of nurses who participated in a government survey.

CRITIQUING SAMPLING PLANS

In coming to conclusions about the quality of evidence that a study yields, you should carefully scrutinize the sampling plan. If the sample is seriously biased or too small, the findings may be misleading or just plain wrong.

You should consider two issues in your critique of a study's sampling plan. The first is whether the researcher adequately described the sampling strategy. Ideally, research reports should include a description of the following:

- The type of sampling approach used (e.g., convenience, simple random)
- The study population and eligibility criteria for sample selection
- The number of participants and a rationale for the sample size, including whether a power analysis was performed
- A description of the main characteristics of sample members (e.g., age, gender, medical condition, and so forth) and, ideally, of the population
- The number and characteristics of potential participants who declined to participate in the study

If the description of the sample is inadequate, you may not be in a position to deal with the second and principal issue, which is whether the researcher made good sampling decisions. And, if the description is incomplete, it will be difficult to draw conclusions about whether the evidence can be applied in your clinical practice.

Sampling plans should be scrutinized with respect to their effects on the construct, internal, external, and statistical conclusion validity of the study. If a sample is small, statistical conclusion validity will likely be undermined. If the eligibility criteria are restrictive, this could benefit internal validity—but possibly to the detriment of construct and external validity.

We have stressed that a key criterion for assessing the adequacy of a sampling plan in quantitative research is whether the sample is representative of the population. You will never know for sure, but if the sampling strategy is weak or if the sample size

BOX 12.1 Guidelines for Critiquing Quantitative Sampling Designs

1. Is the study population identified and described? Are eligibility criteria specified? Are the sample selection procedures clearly delineated?
2. Do the sample and population specifications support an inference of construct validity with regard to the population construct?
3. What type of sampling plan was used? Would an alternative sampling plan have been preferable? Was the sampling plan one that could be expected to yield a representative sample?
4. If sampling was stratified, was a useful stratification variable selected? If a consecutive sample was used, was the time period long enough to address seasonal or temporal variation?
5. How were people recruited into the sample? Does the method suggest potential biases?
6. Did some factor other than the sampling plan (e.g., a low response rate) affect the representativeness of the sample?
7. Are possible sample biases or weaknesses identified by the researchers themselves?
8. Are key characteristics of the sample described (e.g., mean age, percent female)?
9. Is the sample size sufficiently large to support statistical conclusion validity? Was the sample size justified on the basis of a power analysis or other rationale?
10. Does the sample support inferences about external validity? To whom can the study results reasonably be generalized?

is small, there is reason to suspect some bias. When researchers adopt a sampling plan in which the risk for bias is high, they should take steps to estimate the direction and degree of this bias so that readers can draw some informed conclusions.

Even with a rigorous sampling plan, the sample may be biased if not all people invited to participate in a study agree to do so—which is almost always the case. If certain segments of the population refuse to participate, then a biased sample can result, even when probability sampling is used. Research reports ideally should provide information about **response rates** (i.e., the number of people participating in a study relative to the number of people sampled), and about possible **nonresponse bias**—differences between participants and those who declined to participate (also sometimes referred to as *response bias*). In longitudinal studies, attrition bias should be reported.

Quantitative researchers make decisions about the specification of the population as well as the selection of the sample. If the target population is defined broadly, researchers may have missed opportunities to control confounding variables, and the gap between the accessible and the target population

may be too great. One of your jobs as reviewer is to come to conclusions about the reasonableness of generalizing the findings from the researcher's sample to the accessible population and from the accessible population to a broader target population. If the sampling plan is seriously flawed, it may be risky to generalize the findings at all without replicating the study with another sample.

Box 12.1 ✖ presents some guiding questions for critiquing the sampling plan of a quantitative research report.

RESEARCH EXAMPLE

In this section, we describe in some detail the sampling plan of a quantitative nursing study.

Studies: (1) Quality and strength of patient safety climate on medical–surgical units (Hughes et al., 2009); (2) Organizational effects on patient satisfaction in hospital medical–surgical units (Bacon & Mark, 2009); and (3) Nurse staffing and medication errors: Cross-sectional or longitudinal relationships? (Mark & Belyea, 2009).

Purpose: Barbara Mark, with funding from NINR, launched a large multisite study called the Outcomes Research in Nursing Administration Project-II (ORNA-II). The overall purpose was to investigate relationships of hospital context and structure on the one hand and patient, nurse, and organization outcomes on the other. Data from this project have been used in numerous studies, three of which are cited here.

Design: The project was designed as a prospective correlational study, with data collected in 2003 and 2004.

Sampling Plan: Sampling was multistaged. In the first stage, 146 acute care hospitals were randomly selected from a list of hospitals accredited by the Joint Commission on Accreditation of Health Organizations. To be included, hospitals had to have at least 99 licensed beds. Hospitals were excluded if they were federal, for-profit, or psychiatric facilities. Then, from each selected hospital, two medical, surgical, or medical–surgical units were selected to participate in the study. Units were excluded if they were critical care, pediatric, obstetric, or psychiatric units. Among hospitals with only two eligible units, both participated. Among hospitals with more than two eligible units, an on-site study coordinator selected two to participate. Ultimately, 281 nursing units in 143 hospitals participated in the study. Data from each hospital were gathered in three rounds of data collection over a 6-month period. On each participating unit, all RNs with more than 3 months of experience on that unit were asked to respond to three sets of questionnaires. The response rates were 75% of nurses at Time 1 (4,911 nurses), 58% at Time 2 (3,689 nurses), and 53% at Time 3 (3,272 nurses). Patients were also invited to participate at Time 3. Ten patients on each unit were randomly selected to complete a questionnaire. Patients were included if they were 18 years of age or older, had been hospitalized for at least 48 hours, were able to speak and read English, and were not scheduled for immediate discharge. A total of 2,720 patients participated, and the response rate was 91%.

Key Findings:
- Nurses in Magnet hospitals were more likely to communicate about errors and participate in error-related problem solving (Hughes et al., 2009)
- Greater availability of nursing unit support services was associated with higher levels of patient satisfaction (Bacon & Mark, 2009)
- Nurse staffing was unrelated to medication errors (Mark & Belyea, 2009)

SUMMARY POINTS

- **Sampling** is the process of selecting a portion of the **population**, which is an entire aggregate of cases. An **element** is the basic population unit about which information is collected—usually humans in nursing research.
- **Eligibility criteria** are used to establish population characteristics and to determine who could participate in a study—either who can be included (**inclusion criteria**) or who should be excluded (**exclusion criteria**). Care must be taken to specify eligibility criteria so as to maximize the construct validity of the population construct.
- Researchers usually sample from an **accessible population**, but should identify the **target population** to which they want to generalize their results.
- A sample in a quantitative study is assessed in terms of **representativeness**—the extent to which the sample is similar to the population and avoids bias. **Sampling bias** refers to the systematic over-representation or under-representation of some segment of the population.
- Methods of **nonprobability sampling** (wherein elements are selected by nonrandom methods) include convenience, quota, consecutive, and purposive sampling. Nonprobability sampling designs are practical but usually have strong potential for bias.
- **Convenience sampling** uses the most readily available or convenient group of people for the sample. **Snowball sampling** is a type of convenience sampling in which referrals for potential participants are made by those already in the sample.
- **Quota sampling** divides the population into homogeneous **strata** (subpopulations) to ensure representation of subgroups; within each stratum, people are sampled by convenience.
- **Consecutive sampling** involves taking *all* of the people from an accessible population who meet the eligibility criteria over a specific time interval, or for a specified sample size.

- In **purposive sampling**, elements are handpicked to be included in the sample based on the researcher's knowledge about the population.
- **Probability sampling** designs, which involve the random selection of elements from the population, yield more representative samples than nonprobability designs and permit estimates of the magnitude of **sampling error**.
- **Simple random sampling** involves the random selection of elements from a **sampling frame** that enumerates all the elements; **stratified random sampling** divides the population into homogeneous strata from which elements are selected at random.
- **Cluster sampling** involves sampling of large units. In **multistage sampling**, there is a successive, multistaged selection of random samples from larger units (clusters) to smaller units (individuals) by either simple random or stratified random methods.
- **Systematic sampling** is the selection of every *k*th case from a list. By dividing the population size by the desired sample size, the researcher establishes the **sampling interval**, which is the standard distance between the selected elements.
- In quantitative studies, researchers should use a **power analysis** to estimate **sample size** needs. Large samples are preferable to small ones because larger samples enhance statistical conclusion validity and tend to be more representative, but even large samples do not *guarantee* representativeness.

STUDY ACTIVITIES

Chapter 12 of the *Resource Manual for Nursing Research: Generating and Assessing Evidence for Nursing Practice, 9th edition*, offers exercises and study suggestions for reinforcing concepts presented in this chapter. In addition, the following study questions can be addressed:

1. Answer relevant questions from Box 12.1 with regard to sampling plan for the ORNA studies,

described at the end of the chapter. Also consider the following additional questions: (a) How many stages would you say were involved in the sampling plan? (b) What are some of the likely sources of sampling bias in the final sample of 3,272 nurses?

2. Use the table of random numbers in Table 9.2 to select 10 names from the list of people in Table 12.3. How many names did you draw from the first 25 names and from the second 25 names?

STUDIES CITED IN CHAPTER 12

Bacon, C. T., & Mark, B. (2009). Organizational effects on patient satisfaction in hospital medical-surgical units. *Journal of Nursing Administration, 39*, 220–227.

Callaghan, P., Khalil, E., & Morres, I. (2010). A prospective evaluation of the Transtheoretical Model of Change applied to exercise in young people. *International Journal of Nursing Studies, 47*, 3–12.

Dudley-Brown, S., & Freivogel, M. (2009). Hereditary colorectal cancer in the gastroenterology clinic: How common are at-risk patients and how do we find them? *Gastroenterology Nursing, 32*, 8–16.

Ekwall, A., & Hallberg, I. (2007). The association between caregiving satisfaction, difficulties and coping among older family caregivers. *Journal of Clinical Nursing, 16*, 832–844.

Fox, M., Sidani, S., & Brooks, D. (2009). Perceptions of bed days for individuals with chronic illness in extended care facilities. *Research in Nursing & Health, 32*, 335–344.

Griffin, R., Polit, D., & Byrne, M. (2008). Nurse characteristics and inferences about children's pain. *Pediatric Nursing, 34*, 297–305.

Hafsteindóttir, T., Mosselman, M., Schoneveld, C., Riedstra, Y., & Kruitwagen, C. (2010). Malnutrition is hospitalized neurological patients approximately doubles in 10 days of hospitalisation. *Journal of Clinical Nursing, 19*, 639–645.

Houghton, C., Marcukaitis, A., Marienau, M., Hooten, M., Stevens, S., & Warner, D. (2008). Tobacco intervention attitudes and practices among certified registered nurse anesthetists. *Nursing Research, 57*, 123–129.

Hughes, L., Chang, Y., & Mark, B. (2009). Quality and strength of patient safety climate on medical-surgical units. *Health Care Management Review, 34*, 19–28.

Lipman, T., Euler, D., Markowitz, G., & Ratclifee, S. (2009). Evaluation of linear measurement and growth plotting in an inpatient pediatric setting. *Journal of Pediatric Nursing, 24,* 323–329.

Mark, B., & Belyea, M. (2009). Nurse staffing and medication errors: Cross-sectional or longitudinal relationships? *Research in Nursing & Health, 32,* 18–30.

O'Meara, D., Mireles-Cabodevila, E., Frame, E., Hummell, A., Hammel, J., Dweik, R., & Arroliga, A. C. (2008). Evaluation of delivery of enteral nutrition in critically ill patients receiving mechanical ventilation. *American Journal of Critical Care, 17,* 53–61.

Peddle, C., Jones, L., Eves, N., Reiman, T. Sellar, C., Winton, T., & Courneya, K. S. (2009). Correlates of adherence to supervised exercise in patients awaiting surgical removal of malignant lung lesions. *Oncology Nursing Forum, 36,* 287–295.

Methodologic and nonresearch references cited in this chapter can be found in a separate section at the end of the book.

13

Data Collection in Quantitative Research

Quantitative researchers collect data in a structured manner. Both the people collecting the data and the study participants are constrained during the collection of structured data. Constraints are imposed so that there is consistency in what is asked and how answers are reported, in an effort to enhance objectivity, reduce biases, and facilitate analysis. Major methods of collecting structured data are discussed in this chapter. We begin by discussing broad planning issues.

DEVELOPING A DATA COLLECTION PLAN

Data collection plans for quantitative studies ideally yield accurate, valid, and meaningful data. This is a challenging goal, typically requiring considerable time and effort to achieve. Steps in developing a data collection plan are described in this section. (A flowchart illustrating the sequence of steps is available in the Toolkit of the accompanying *Resource Manual.* ✪)

Identifying Data Needs

Researchers usually begin by identifying the types of data needed for their study. Advance planning may help to avoid "if only" disappointments at the analysis stage. In quantitative studies, researchers may need data for the following purposes:

1. *Testing hypotheses or addressing research questions.* Researchers must include one or more measures of all key variables. Multiple measures of some variables may be needed if a variable is complex or if there is an interest in corroboration and triangulation.

2. *Describing sample characteristics.* Information should be gathered about major demographic and health characteristics of the sample. We advise gathering data about participants' age, gender, race or ethnicity, and education (or income). This information is critical in interpreting results and understanding the population to whom findings can be generalized. If the sample includes participants with a health problem, data on the nature of that problem also should be gathered (e.g., severity, treatments, time since diagnosis).

⤷ **TIP:** Asking demographic questions in the right way is more difficult than you might think. Because the need to collect information about sample characteristics is nearly universal, we have included a demographic form and guidelines in the Toolkit of the accompanying *Resource Manual.* The demographic questionnaire can be adapted as needed.

3. *Controlling confounding variables.* Various approaches can be used to control confounding variables, many of which require measuring those variables. For example, for analysis of covariance, variables that are statistically controlled must be measured.

4. *Analyzing potential biases.* Data that can help the researcher to identify potential biases should be collected. For example, researchers should gather information that would help to identify selection biases in a nonequivalent control group design or attrition biases in RCTs.

5. *Understanding subgroup effects.* It is often desirable to answer research questions for key subgroups of participants. For example, we may wish to know if a special intervention for indigent pregnant women is equally effective for primiparas and multiparas. In such a situation, we would need to collect data about the participants' childbearing history.

6. *Interpreting results.* Researchers should try to anticipate alternative results, and then assess what types of data would best help in interpreting them. For example, if we hypothesized that the presence of school-based clinics in high schools would lower the incidence of sexually transmitted diseases among students but found that the incidence remained constant after the clinic opened, what type of information would help us interpret this result (e.g., information about the students' frequency of intercourse, number of partners, use of condoms, and so on)?

7. *Assessing treatment fidelity.* In intervention studies, it is often useful to monitor treatment fidelity and to assess whether the intended treatment was actually received.

8. *Obtaining administrative information.* It is usually necessary to gather administrative data—for example, dates of data collection and contact information in longitudinal studies.

The list of possible data needs may seem daunting, but many categories overlap. For example, participant characteristics for sample description are often key confounding variables, or useful in creating subgroups. If time or resource constraints make it impossible to collect the full range of variables, then researchers should prioritize data needs.

> **TIP:** In prioritizing data needs, it may be useful to develop a matrix so that decisions about data collection strategies can be made in a systematic way. Such a matrix can help to identify "holes" and redundancies. The matrix might contain such column headings as variable name, purpose (e.g., from the above list), name of instrument to be used, and data quality. A partial example of such a matrix is included in the Toolkit of the *Resource Manual* for you to use and adapt. A conceptual map (Chapter 6) is also a useful tool in identifying data needs.

Selecting Types of Measures

After data needs have been identified, the next step is to select a data collection method (e.g., self-report, records) for each variable. In reviewing data needs, researchers should determine how best to capture each variable in terms of its conceptual or theoretical definition. It is not unusual to combine self-reports, observations, physiologic, or records data in a single study.

Research needs are not the only factors that drive decisions about data collection methods. The decisions must also be guided by ethical considerations (e.g., whether covert data collection is warranted), cost constraints, availability of assistants to help with data collection, and other issues discussed in the next section. Data collection is often the costliest and most time-consuming portion of a study. Because of this, researchers often have to make a number of compromises about the type or amount of data collected.

Selecting and Developing Instruments

Once preliminary decisions have been made about the data collection methods, researchers should determine if there are instruments available for measuring study variables, as will often be the case. Potential data collection instruments should then be assessed. The primary consideration is conceptual relevance: Does the instrument correspond to your conceptual definition of the variable? Another important criterion is whether the instrument will yield high-quality data. Approaches to evaluating data quality are discussed in Chapter 14. Additional factors that may affect your decisions in selecting an instrument are as follows:

1. *Resources.* Resource constraints sometimes prevent the use of the highest-quality measures. There may be some direct costs associated with the measure (e.g., some psychological tests must be purchased), but the biggest cost involves compensation to data collectors if you cannot do it single-handedly—that is, if you have to hire interviewers or observers. In such a situation, the instrument's administration time may determine whether it is a viable option. Also, it may be necessary to pay a participant stipend if data collection procedures are burdensome. Data collection costs should be carefully considered, especially if the use of expensive methods means that you will be forced to cut costs elsewhere (e.g., using a smaller sample).

2. *Availability and familiarity.* You may need to consider how readily available or accessible various instruments are, especially biophysiologic ones. Similarly, data collection strategies with which you have had experience are usually preferable to new ones because administration is usually smoother and more efficient in such cases.

3. *Population appropriateness.* Instruments must be chosen with the characteristics of the target population in mind. Characteristics of special importance include participants' age and literacy levels. If there is concern about participants' reading skills, it may be necessary to calculate the readability of a prospective instrument. If participants include members of minority groups, you should strive to find instruments that are culturally appropriate. If non–English-speaking participants are included in the sample, then the selection of an instrument may be based on the availability of a translated version.

4. *Norms and comparisons.* It may be desirable to select an instrument that has relevant norms.

Norms indicate the "normal" values on the measure for a specified population, and thus offer a built-in comparison. Many standardized scales (e.g., the SF-36 Health Survey from the Medical Outcomes Study) have norms. Similarly, it may be advantageous to select an instrument because it was used in other similar studies, thus providing useful information for interpreting study findings. When a study is an intentional replication, it is often important to use the same instruments as in the original study, even if higher-quality measures are available.

5. *Administration issues.* Some instruments have special requirements that need to be considered. For example, obtaining information about the developmental status of children sometimes requires the skills of a professional psychologist. Another administration issue is that some instruments require or assume stringent conditions with regard to the time of administration, privacy of the setting, and so on. In such a case, requirements for obtaining valid measures must match attributes of the research setting.

6. *Reputation.* Instruments designed to measure the same construct often differ in the reputation they enjoy among specialists in a field, even if they are comparable with regard to documented quality. Thus, it may be useful to seek the advice of knowledgeable people, preferably ones with personal, direct experience using the instruments.

If existing instruments are not suitable for some variables, you may be faced with either adapting an instrument or developing a new one. Creating a new instrument should be a last resort, especially for novice researchers, because it is challenging to develop accurate and valid measuring tools. Chapter 15 provides guidance on developing self-report instruments.

If you are fortunate in identifying a suitable instrument, your next step likely will be to obtain written permission from the author to use it. In general, copyrighted materials always require permission. Instruments that have been developed under a government grant are usually in the public domain, and so may not require permission. When in doubt, it is best to obtain permission. By contacting the instrument's author for permission, you can also request more information about the instrument and its quality. (A sample letter requesting permission to use an instrument is in the Toolkit. ⊗)

➤ **TIP :** In finalizing decisions about instruments, it may be necessary to balance trade-offs between data quality and data quantity (i.e., the number of instruments or questions). If compromises have to be made, it is usually preferable to forego quantity.

Pretesting the Data Collection Package

Researchers who develop a new instrument usually subject it to rigorous **pretesting** so that it can be evaluated and refined. Even when the data collection plan involves existing instruments, however, it is wise to conduct a small pretest.

One purpose of a pretest is to see how much time it takes to administer the entire instrument package. Typically, researchers use multiple instruments and it may be difficult to estimate how long it will take to administer the complete set. Time estimates may be required for informed consent purposes, for developing a budget, or for assessing participant burden.

Pretests can serve many other purposes, including the following:

- Identifying parts of the instrument package that are difficult for participants to read or understand or that may have been misinterpreted
- Identifying questions that participants find objectionable or offensive
- Assessing whether the sequencing of questions or instruments is sensible
- Evaluating training needs for data collectors
- Determining if the measures yield data with sufficient variability

The last purpose requires explanation. For most research questions, the instruments ideally discriminate among participants with different levels of an attribute. If we are asking, for example, whether women experience greater depression than men when they learn of a cancer diagnosis, we need an instrument capable of distinguishing between people with higher and lower levels of depression. If an instrument yields data with limited variability, then it will be impossible to detect a difference in depression between men and women—even when such a difference actually exists. Thus, researchers should look at pretest variation on key research variables. To pursue the example, if the entire pretest sample looks very depressed (or not at all depressed), it would probably be necessary to pretest another instrument.

Example of pretesting: Nyamathi and colleagues (2005) studied the predictors of perceived health status in a sample of 415 homeless adults with tuberculosis. The study involved collecting an extensive array of data via self-reports. All of the instruments had been previously tested with homeless people, and many were pretested in group settings to determine clarity and sensitivity to the population.

Developing Data Collection Forms and Procedures

After the instrument package is finalized, researchers face several administrative tasks, such as the development of various forms (e.g., screening forms to assess eligibility, informed consent forms, records of attempted contacts with participants, logs for recording the receipt of data). It is prudent to design forms that are attractively formatted, legible, and inviting to use, especially if they are to be used by participants themselves. Care should also be taken to design forms to ensure confidentiality. For example, identifying information (e.g., names, addresses) is often recorded on a page that can be detached and kept separate from other data.

➤ **TIP :** Whenever possible, try to avoid reinventing the wheel. It is inefficient and unnecessary to start from scratch — not only in developing instruments but also in creating forms, training materials, and so on. Ask seasoned researchers if they have materials you could borrow or adapt.

In most quantitative studies, researchers develop **data collection protocols** that spell out procedures to be used in data collection. These protocols describe such things as the following:

- Conditions that must be met for collecting the data (e.g., Can others be present at the time of data collection? Where must data collection occur?)
- Specific procedures for collecting the data, including requirements for sequencing multiple instruments and recording information
- Information to provide participants who ask routine questions about the study (i.e., answers to FAQs). Examples include the following: How will the information from this study be used? How did you get my name, and why are you asking me? How long will this take? Who will have access to this information? Can I see the study results? Whom can I contact if I have a complaint? Will I be paid or reimbursed for expenses?
- Procedures to follow in the event that a participant becomes distraught or disoriented, or for any other reason cannot complete the data collection

Researchers also need to decide how to actually gather, record, and manage their data. Technological advances continue to offer new options. As noted in Chapter 11, survey researchers are increasingly using sophisticated computer programs to facilitate collecting, recording, and encoding self-report data (e.g., CATI, CAPI). The Internet is being used to gather data from geographically dispersed populations. Personal digital assistants (PDAs) and audio-enhanced PDAs are also beginning to play a role. Courtney and Craven (2005) and Guadagno and colleagues (2004) offer some suggestions about new technology and data collection.

◗ TIP: Document all major activities and decisions as you develop and implement your data collection plan, and save your documentation. You may need the information later when you write your research report, request funding for a follow-up study, or help other researchers.

STRUCTURED SELF-REPORT INSTRUMENTS

The most widely used data collection method by nurse researchers is structured self-report, which involves a formal, written instrument. The instrument is an **interview schedule** when questions are asked orally in face-to-face or telephone interviews. It is called a **questionnaire** or an **SAQ** (self-administered questionnaire) when respondents complete the instrument themselves, either in a paper-and-pencil format or on a computer. Researchers sometimes embed an SAQ into an interview schedule, with interviewers asking some questions orally but respondents answering others in writing. This section discusses the development and administration of structured self-report instruments.

Types of Structured Questions

Structured instruments consist of a set of questions (often called **items**) in which the wording of both the questions and, in most cases, *response alternatives* is predetermined. When structured instruments are used, people are asked to respond to the same questions, in the same order, and with the same set of response options. In developing structured instruments, much effort must be devoted to the content, form, and wording of questions.

Open and Closed Questions

Structured instruments vary in degree of structure through different combinations of open-ended and closed-ended questions. **Open-ended questions** allow people to respond in their own words, in narrative fashion. The question, "What was your biggest challenge after your surgery?" is an example of an open-ended question. In questionnaires, respondents are asked to give a written reply to open-ended items and so adequate space must be provided to permit a full response. Interviewers are expected to quote oral responses verbatim or as closely as possible.

Closed-ended (or **fixed-alternative**) **questions** offer response options, from which respondents must choose the one that most closely matches the appropriate answer. The alternatives may range from a simple *yes* or *no* ("Have you smoked a cigarette within the past 24 hours?") to complex expressions of opinion or behavior.

Both open- and closed-ended questions have certain strengths and weaknesses. Good closed-ended items are often difficult to construct but easy to administer and, especially, to analyze. With closed-ended questions, researchers need only tabulate the number of responses to each alternative to gain descriptive information. The analysis of open-ended items, by contrast, is more difficult and time-consuming. The usual procedure is to develop categories and code open-ended responses into the categories. That is, researchers essentially transform open-ended responses to fixed categories in a post hoc fashion so that tabulations can be made.

Closed-ended items are more efficient than open-ended questions in that respondents can complete more closed- than open-ended questions in a given amount of time. In questionnaires, participants may be less willing to compose written responses than to check off appropriate alternatives. Closed-ended items are also preferred if respondents are unable to express themselves well verbally. Furthermore, some questions are less objectionable in closed form than in open form. Take the following example:

1. What was your family's total annual income last year?
2. In what range was your family's total annual income last year?
   ❏ 1. Under $25,000,
   ❏ 2. $25,000 to $49,999,
   ❏ 3. $50,000 to $74,999,
   ❏ 4. $75,000 to $99,999, or
   ❏ 5. $100,000 or more

The second question gives respondents a greater measure of privacy than the open-ended question, and is less likely to go unanswered.

A major drawback of closed-ended questions is the possibility of omitting key responses. Such omissions can lead to inadequate understanding of the issues or to outright bias if respondents choose an alternative that misrepresents their position.

Another objection to closed-ended items is that they tend to be superficial. Open-ended questions allow for a richer and fuller perspective on a topic, if respondents are verbally expressive and cooperative. Some of this richness may be lost when researchers tabulate answers they have categorized, but direct excerpts from open-ended responses can be valuable in imparting the flavor of the replies. Finally, some people may object to being forced into choosing from response options that do not reflect their opinions well. Open-ended questions give freedom to respondents and, therefore, offer the possibility of spontaneity and elaboration.

Decisions about the mix of open- and closed-ended questions is based on such considerations as the sensitivity of the questions, respondents' verbal ability, the amount of time available, and the amount of prior research on the topic. Combinations of both types can be used to offset the strengths and weaknesses of each. Questionnaires typically use closed-ended questions primarily, to minimize respondents' writing burden. Interview schedules, on the other hand, tend to be more variable in their mixture of these two question types.

Specific Types of Closed-Ended Questions

The analytic advantages of closed-ended questions are often compelling. Various types of closed-ended questions, illustrated in Table 13.1, are described here. Question types can be intermixed within a structured instrument.

- **Dichotomous questions** require respondents to make a choice between two response alternatives, such as yes/no or male/female. Dichotomous questions are especially appropriate for gathering factual information.
- **Multiple-choice questions** offer three or more response alternatives. Graded alternatives are preferable to dichotomous items for opinion or attitude questions because researchers get more information (intensity as well as direction of opinion) and respondents can express a range of views. Multiple-choice questions typically offer three to seven options.
- **Rank-order questions** ask respondents to rank target concepts along a continuum, such as most to least important. Respondents are asked

TABLE 13.1	Examples of Closed-Ended Questions

QUESTION TYPE	EXAMPLE
1. Dichotomous question	Have you ever been pregnant? 1. Yes 2. No
2. Multiple-choice question	How important is it to you to avoid a pregnancy at this time? 1. Extremely important 2. Very important 3. Somewhat important 4. Not important
3. Rank-order question	People value different things in life. Below is a list of things that many people value. Please indicate their order of importance to you by placing a "1" beside the most important, "2" beside the second-most important, and so on. ____ Career achievement/work ____ Family relationships ____ Friendships, social interactions ____ Health ____ Money ____ Religion
4. Forced-choice question	Which statement most closely represents your point of view? 1. What happens to me is my own doing. 2. Sometimes I feel I don't have enough control over my life.
5. Rating question	On a scale from 0 to 10, where 0 means "extremely dissatisfied" and 10 means "extremely satisfied," how satisfied were you with the nursing care you received during your hospitalization? 0　1　2　3　4　5　6　7　8　9　10 Extremely　　　　　　　　　　　　Extremely dissatisfied　　　　　　　　　　　satisfied

to assign a 1 to the concept that is most important, a 2 to the concept that is second in importance, and so on. Rank-order questions can be useful, but respondents sometimes misunderstand them so good instructions and an example may be needed. Rank-order questions should involve 10 or fewer rankings.

- **Forced-choice questions** require respondents to choose between two statements that represent polar positions or characteristics.
- **Rating questions** ask respondents to evaluate something along an ordered dimension. Rating

questions are typically on a **bipolar scale**, with end points specifying opposite extremes on a continuum. The end points and sometimes intermediary points along the scale are verbally labeled. The number of gradations or points along the scale can vary but often is an odd number, such as 7, 9, or 11, to allow for a neutral midpoint. (In the example in Table 13.1, the rating question has 11 points, numbered 0 to 10.)

- **Checklists** include several questions with the same response format. A checklist is a

The next question is about things that may have happened to you personally. Please indicate how recently, if ever, these things happened to you:

	Yes, within past 12 months	Yes, 2–3 years ago	Yes, more than 3 years ago	No, never
a. Has someone ever yelled at you all the time or put you down on purpose?	1	2	3	4
b. Has someone ever tried to control your every move?	1	2	3	4
c. Has someone ever threatened you with physical harm?	1	2	3	4
d. Has someone ever hit, slapped, kicked, or physically harmed you?	1	2	3	4

FIGURE 13.1 Example of a checklist.

two-dimensional arrangement in which a series of questions is listed along one dimension (usually vertically) and response alternatives are listed along the other. Checklists are relatively efficient and easy to understand, but because they are difficult to read orally, they are used more frequently in SAQs than in interviews. Figure 13.1 presents an example of a checklist.

• **Visual analog scales** (**VAS**) are used to measure subjective experiences, such as pain, fatigue, and dyspnea. The VAS is a straight line, the end anchors of which are labeled as the extreme limits of the sensation or feeling being measured. People are asked to mark a point on the line corresponding to the amount of sensation experienced. Traditionally, the VAS line is 100 mm in length, which facilitates the derivation of a score from 0 to 100 through simple measurement of the distance from one end of the scale to the person's mark on the line. An example of a VAS is shown in Figure 13.2. ⊗

In certain situations, researchers collect information about activities and dates, sometimes using an **event history calendar** (Martyn & Belli, 2002). Such calendars are matrixes that plot time on one dimension (usually the horizontal dimension) and the events or activities on the other. The person recording the data (either the participant or an interviewer) draws lines to indi-

cate the stop and start dates of the specified events or behaviors. Event history calendars are especially useful in collecting information about the occurrence and sequencing of events retrospectively. Data quality about past occurrences is enhanced because the calendar helps participants relate the timing of some events to the timing of others. An example of an event history calendar is included in the Toolkit section of the accompanying *Resource Manual*. ⊗

An alternative to collecting event history data retrospectively is to ask participants to maintain information in an ongoing structured **diary** over a specified time period. This approach is often used to collect quantitative information about sleeping, eating, or exercise behavior.

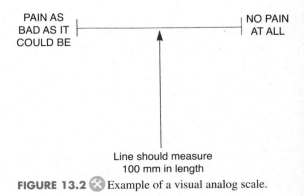

FIGURE 13.2 ⊗ Example of a visual analog scale.

Composite Scales and Other Structured Self-Reports

Several special types of structured self-reports are used by nurse researchers. The most important are composite social-psychological scales that are often included in a questionnaire or interview package. A **scale** provides a numeric score to place respondents on a continuum with respect to an attribute, like a scale for measuring people's weight. Scales are used to discriminate quantitatively among people with different attitudes, fears, and needs. Scales are created by combining several closed-ended items into a composite score. Many sophisticated scaling techniques have been developed, but only two are discussed in this book.* We also briefly describe cognitive and neurologic tests, vignettes, and Q sorts.

Likert Scales

The most widely used scaling technique is the **Likert scale**, named after the psychologist Rensis Likert. A Likert scale consists of several declarative items that express a viewpoint on a topic. Respondents typically are asked to indicate the degree to which they agree or disagree with the opinion expressed by the statement.

Table 13.2 illustrates a six-item Likert-type scale for measuring attitudes toward condom use. Likert scales often include 10 or more statements; the example in Table 13.2 is shown only to illustrate key features. After respondents complete a

Likert scale, their responses are scored. Typically, agreement with positively worded statements and disagreement with negatively worded ones are assigned higher scores. (See Chapter 15, however, for a discussion of problems in including both positive and negative items on a scale). The first statement in Table 13.2 is positively worded; agreement indicates a favorable attitude toward condom use. Thus, a higher score would be assigned to those agreeing with this statement than to those disagreeing with it. With five response alternatives, a score of 5 would be given to those strongly agreeing, 4 to those agreeing, and so forth. The responses of two hypothetical respondents are shown by a check or an X, and their scores are shown in far right columns. Person 1, who agreed with the first statement, has a score of 4, whereas person 2, who strongly disagreed, has a score of 1. The second statement is negatively worded, and so scoring is reversed—a 1 is assigned to those who strongly agree, and so on. This reversal is needed so that a high score consistently reflects positive attitudes toward condoms. A person's total score is computed by adding together individual item scores. Such scales are often called **summated rating scales** because of this feature. The total scores of both respondents are shown at the bottom of Table 13.2. The scores reflect a much more positive attitude toward condoms on the part of person 1 than person 2 does.

The summation feature of such scales makes it possible to make fine discriminations among people with different points of view. A single question allows people to be put into only five categories. A six-item scale, such as the one in Table 13.2, permits finer gradation—from a minimum possible score of 6 (6 × 1) to a maximum possible score of 30 (6 × 5).

Summated rating scales can be used to measure a wide array of attributes. In such cases, the bipolar scale may not be an agree/disagree continuum, but might be always true/never true, very likely/very unlikely, and so on. Constructing a good Likert-type scale requires considerable skill and work. Chapter 15 describes the steps involved in developing and testing such scales.

---

*Other scaling procedures include **ratio scaling, magnitude estimation scaling, multidimensional scaling**, and **multiple scalogram analysis**. Textbooks on psychological scaling and psychometric procedures should be consulted for more information about these scaling strategies.

TABLE 13.2	Example of a Likert Scale							
		RESPONSES†					**SCORE**	
DIRECTION OF SCORING*	**ITEM**	**SA**	**A**	**?**	**D**	**SD**	**Person 1 (✔)**	**Person 2 (✕)**
+	1. Using a condom shows you care about your partner.		✔			✕	4	1
−	2. My partner would be angry if I talked about using condoms.			✕	✔		5	3
−	3. I wouldn't enjoy sex as much if my partner and I used condoms.			✕	✔		4	2
+	4. Condoms are a good protection against AIDS and other sexually transmitted diseases.			✔	✕		3	2
+	5. My partner would respect me if I insisted on using condoms.	✔				✕	5	1
−	6. I would be too embarrassed to ask my partner about using a condom.			✕	✔		5	2
	Total score						26	11

*Researchers would not indicate the direction of scoring on a Likert scale administered to study participants. The scoring direction is indicated in this table for illustrative purposes only.
†SA, strongly agree; A, agree; ?, uncertain; D, disagree; SD, strongly disagree.

Example of a summated rating scale: Lynn and colleagues (2009) developed a Likert-type scale to measure satisfaction in nursing. Examples of statements include the following: "Nurses on my unit enjoy working together" and "I enjoy being responsible for the welfare of my patients." Responses are on a 4-point scale, without a neutral response option.

Semantic Differential Scales

Another technique for measuring attitudes is the **semantic differential** (SD). With the SD, respondents are asked to rate concepts (e.g., dieting, exer-

cise) on a series of *bipolar adjectives*, such as good/bad, effective/ineffective, important/unimportant. Respondents place a check at the appropriate point on a seven-point scale that extends from one extreme of the dimension to the other. Figure 13.3 shows an abbreviated example of the format for an SD for the concept *Assisted Suicide*.

SDs are flexible and easy to construct, and the concept being rated can be virtually anything—a person, concept, controversial issue, and so on. Scoring for SD responses is similar to that for

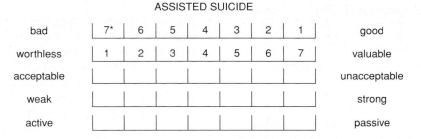

ASSISTED SUICIDE

bad	7*	6	5	4	3	2	1	good
worthless	1	2	3	4	5	6	7	valuable
acceptable								unacceptable
weak								strong
active								passive

*The score values would not be printed on the form administered to actual participants. The numbers are presented here solely for the purpose of illustrating how semantic differentials are scored.

FIGURE 13.3 Example of a semantic differential.

Likert scales. Scores from 1 to 7 are assigned to each bipolar scale response, with higher scores generally associated with the positively worded adjective. Responses are then summed across the bipolar scales to yield a total score.

Researchers can be creative in their choice of bipolar scales, but the adjective pairs should be appropriate for the concepts. The adjective pair large/small for the SD in Figure 13.3 would not make much sense. Another consideration in selecting adjective pairs is the extent to which the adjectives measure the same dimension of the concept. Research with SD scales suggests that adjective pairs tend to cluster along three independent dimensions: evaluation, potency, and activity. Evaluative adjectives, such as effective/ineffective or good/bad are especially important. Potency adjectives include strong/weak and large/small, and examples of activity adjectives are active/passive and fast/slow. These three dimensions need to be scored separately because people's *evaluative* ratings of a concept are independent of their *activity* or *potency* ratings. Researchers must decide how many SD dimensions to include.

Example of a study using an SD: Rempusheski and O'Hara (2005) developed a semantic differential scale, the Grandparent Perceptions of Family Scale (GPFS). Respondents rate stimuli (e.g., "How I view my grandchild") with regard to 22 bipolar adjective pairs. Three adjective pairs were in the action subscale (e.g., active/passive), 11 were in the evaluative subscale (e.g., happy/sad), and 8 were in the potency subscale (e.g., emotionally strong/emotionally weak).

TIP : Most nurse researchers use existing scales rather than developing their own. Resources for locating existing scales include Strickland and DiIorio, 2003; Frank-Stromberg and Olsen, 2004; and Waltz and colleagues, 2010. Also, some helpful websites are included in the Toolkit. Another place to look for existing instruments is in the Health and Psychosocial Instruments (HaPI) database.

Cognitive and Neuropsychological Tests

Nurse researchers sometimes assess study participants' cognitive skills. There are several different types of **cognitive tests**. For example, *intelligence tests* evaluate a person's global ability to perceive relationships and solve problems and *aptitude tests* measure a person's potential for achievement. Some tests have been developed for individual (one-on-one) administration, whereas others have been developed for group use. Individual tests, such as the Stanford-Binet I.Q. test, must be administered by a person with special training. Nurse researchers are especially likely to use ability tests in studies of high-risk groups, such as low-birth-weight children.

Some cognitive tests are specially designed to assess neuropsychological functioning among people with potential cognitive impairments, such as the Mini-Mental Status Examination (MMSE). These tests capture varying types of competence, such as the ability to concentrate and the ability to remember. Nurses have used such tests extensively in studies of elderly patients and patients with Alzheimer's disease. Good sources for learning more about ability tests are the books by Urbina (2004) and the Buros Institute (2007).

Example of a study assessing neuropsychological function: Alpert and colleagues (2009) did a pilot study to evaluate the effect of jazz dance instruction on balance, cognition, and mood in community-dwelling older women. Cognitive outcomes were measured using the MMSE.

Q Sorts

In a **Q sort**, participants are presented with a set of cards on which words or phrases are written. Participants are told to sort the cards along a specified bipolar dimension, such as most important/least important. Typically, there are between 50 and 100 cards to be sorted into 9 or 11 piles, with the number of cards to be placed in each pile predetermined by the researcher (e.g., 2 cards in piles 1 and 9, 4 cards in piles 2 and 8, and so on). It is difficult to achieve reliable results with fewer than 50 cards, but the task becomes tedious and difficult with more than 100.

The sorting instructions and objects to be sorted in a Q sort can vary. For example, attitudes can be studied by writing attitudinal statements on the cards and asking participants to sort them on a continuum from "totally disagree" to "totally agree." Or, patients could be asked to rate nursing behaviors on a continuum from least helpful to most helpful.

Q sorts are versatile and can be applied to a wide variety of problems. Requiring people to place a predetermined number of cards in each pile can reduce biases that are common in Likert scales. On the other hand, it is difficult and time-consuming to administer Q sorts to a large sample of people. Some critics argue that the forced distribution of cards according to researchers' specifications is artificial and excludes information about how participants would ordinarily distribute their responses. Another issue is that Q sorts cannot be incorporated into mailed or Internet questionnaires or administered in telephone interviews. The paper by Akhtar-Danesh and colleagues (2008) provides more information about Q sorts.

Example of a Q sort: Akhtar-Danesh and colleagues (2008) used a 43-card Q sort to examine nurse faculty perceptions of simulation use in nursing education. Statements were sorted into 9 piles on an agree/disagree continuum. An example of a statement in the card sort is: "It's a scheduling nightmare."

Vignettes

Another self-report approach involves the use of **vignettes**, which are brief case reports or descriptions of events to which respondents are asked to react. The descriptions, which can either be fictitious or based on fact, are structured to elicit information about respondents' perceptions of some phenomenon or their projected actions. The vignettes are usually written narrative descriptions, but researchers have also used videotaped vignettes. The questions that follow the vignettes can be open-ended (e.g., How would you describe this patients' level of confusion?) or closed-ended (e.g., Rate how confused you think this patient is on a 7-point scale). Usually 3 to 5 vignettes are included in an instrument.

Sometimes the underlying purpose of vignette studies is not revealed to participants, especially if the technique is used as an indirect measure of prejudices or stereotypes using embedded descriptors, as in the following example.

Example of vignettes: Griffin and colleagues (2007) distributed vignette packets describing three hospitalized children to a national sample of pediatric nurses to explore whether pain management decisions were affected by children's characteristics. Three vignettes described children in pain: one described either a boy or a girl, another described a white or African American child, and the third described a physically attractive or unattractive child. Nurses answered questions about pain treatments they would use without being aware that the child characteristics had been experimentally varied.

Vignettes are an economical means of eliciting information about how people might behave in situations that would be difficult to observe in daily life. Vignettes can be incorporated into questionnaires, and are, therefore, an inexpensive data collection strategy. Also, vignettes often represent an interesting task for participants. The principal problem with vignettes concerns the validity of responses. If respondents describe how they would act in a situation portrayed in the vignette, how accurate is that description of their actual behavior? Thus, although the use of vignettes can be profitable, potential biases should be taken into account in interpreting results.

> **TIP:** Some methods described in this chapter might be appealing because they are unusual and may seem like a creative approach to collecting data. However, the prime considerations in selecting a data collection method should always be the conceptual congruence between the method and the targeted constructs, and the quality of data that the method yields.

Questionnaires Versus Interviews

In developing their data collection plans, researchers need to decide whether to collect data through interviews or questionnaires. Each method has advantages and disadvantages.

Advantages of Questionnaires

Self-administered questionnaires, which can be distributed in person, by mail, or over the Internet, offer some advantages. The strengths of questionnaires include the following:

- *Cost.* Questionnaires, relative to interviews, are much less costly. Distributing questionnaires to groups (e.g., nursing home residents) is inexpensive and expedient. And, with a fixed amount of funds or time, a larger and more geographically diverse sample can be obtained with mailed or Internet questionnaires than with interviews.
- *Anonymity.* Unlike interviews, questionnaires offer the possibility of complete anonymity. A guarantee of anonymity can be crucial in obtaining candid responses, particularly if questions are sensitive. Anonymous questionnaires often result in a higher proportion of socially unacceptable responses (i.e., responses that place respondents in an unfavorable light) than interviews.
- *Interviewer bias.* The absence of an interviewer ensures that there will be no interviewer bias. Interviewers ideally are neutral agents through whom questions and answers are passed. Studies have shown, however, that this ideal is difficult to achieve. Respondents and interviewers interact as humans, and this interaction can affect responses.

Internet surveys are especially economical and can sometimes yield a dataset directly amenable to analysis, without requiring someone to enter data onto a file (the same is also true for CAPI and CATI interviews). Internet surveys also provide opportunities for providing participants with customized feedback and for prompts that can minimize missing responses.

Advantages of Interviews

It is true that interviews are costly, prevent anonymity, and bear the risk of interviewer bias. Nevertheless, interviews are considered superior to questionnaires for most research purposes because of the following advantages:

- *Response rates.* Response rates tend to be high in face-to-face interviews. People are less likely to refuse to talk to an interviewer who directly solicits their cooperation than to ignore a questionnaire or email. A well-designed and properly conducted interview study normally achieves response rates in the vicinity of 80% to 90%, whereas mailed and Internet questionnaires typically achieve response rates of less than 50%. Because nonresponse is not random, low response rates can introduce serious biases. (However, if questionnaires are personally distributed in a particular setting—e.g., patients in a cardiac rehabilitation program—reasonably good response rates often can be achieved.)

> **TIP:** MacDonald and colleagues (2009) have offered useful advice for addressing nonresponse in mailed surveys. Several suggestions are useful for minimizing nonresponse in collecting any type of self-report data. An additional useful resource is a meta-analysis of strategies to increase response to mailed and electronic surveys by Edwards and colleagues (2009).

- *Audience.* Many people cannot fill out a questionnaire. Examples include young children and blind, elderly, illiterate, or uneducated individuals. Interviews, on the other hand, are feasible with most people. For Internet questionnaires, a particularly important drawback is that not everyone has access to computers or uses them regularly.

- *Clarity*. Interviews offer some protection against ambiguous or confusing questions. Interviewers can assess whether questions have been misunderstood and provide clarification. With questionnaires, misinterpreted questions can go undetected.
- *Depth of questioning*. Information obtained from questionnaires tends to be more superficial than from interviews, largely because questionnaires usually contain mostly closed-ended items. Open-ended questions are avoided in questionnaires because most people dislike having to compose a reply. Furthermore, interviewers can enhance the quality of self-report data through *probing*, a topic we discuss later in this chapter.
- *Missing information*. Respondents are less likely to give "don't know" responses or to leave a question unanswered in an interview than on a questionnaire.
- *Order of questions*. In an interview, researchers have control over question ordering. Questionnaire respondents can skip around from one section to another. Sometimes a different ordering of questions from the one intended could bias responses.
- *Sample control*. Interviewers know whether the people being interviewed are the intended respondents. People who receive questionnaires, by contrast, can pass the instrument on to a friend or relative, and this can change the sample composition. Internet surveys are especially vulnerable to the risk that people not targeted by researchers will respond, unless there are password protections.
- *Supplementary data*. Face-to-face interviews can yield additional data through observation. Interviewers can observe and assess respondents' level of understanding, degree of cooperativeness, social class, and so forth. Such information can be useful in interpreting responses.

Many advantages of face-to-face interviews also apply to telephone interviews. Long or detailed interviews or ones with sensitive questions are not well suited to telephone administration, but for relatively brief instruments, telephone interviews are economical and tend to yield a higher response rate than mailed or Internet questionnaires.

Designing Structured Self-Report Instruments

Assembling a high-quality structured self-report instrument is demanding. To design useful, accurate instruments, researchers must carefully analyze the research requirements and attend to minute details. The steps for developing structured self-report instruments follow closely the ones we outlined earlier in the chapter, but a few additional considerations should be mentioned.

Related constructs should be clustered into separate **modules** or areas of questioning. For example, an interview schedule may consist of a module on demographic information, another on health symptoms, a third on stressful life events, and a fourth on health-promoting activities. Thought needs to be given to sequencing modules, and questions within modules, to arrive at an order that is psychologically meaningful and encourages candor. The schedule should begin with questions that are interesting, motivating, and not too sensitive. The instrument also needs to be arranged to minimize bias because early questions sometimes influence responses to subsequent ones. Whenever both general and specific questions about a topic are included, general questions should be placed first to avoid "coaching."

Instruments should be prefaced by introductory comments about the nature and purpose of the study. In interviews, introductory information would be communicated by the interviewer, who would typically follow a script. In questionnaires, the introduction usually takes the form of an accompanying **cover letter**. The introduction should be carefully constructed because it is the first point of contact with potential respondents. An example of a cover letter for a mailed questionnaire is presented in Figure 13.4. ⊗ (This cover letter is included in the Toolkit for you to use and adapt.)

When a first draft of the instrument is in reasonably good order, it should be reviewed by experts in questionnaire construction, by substantive content

Dear Community Resident:

    We are conducting a study to examine how men who are approaching retirement age (55 to 65 years old) feel about various issues relating to their healthcare. This study, which is sponsored by the National Institutes of Health, will enable healthcare providers to better meet the needs of men in your age group. Would you please assist us in this study by completing the enclosed questionnaire? Your opinions and experiences are very important to us and are needed to give an accurate picture of the health-related needs of men in the Capital District.

    Your name was selected at random from a list of residents in your community. The questionnaire is completely anonymous, so you are not asked to put your name on it or identify yourself in any way. We hope, therefore, that you will feel comfortable giving your honest opinions. If you prefer not to answer any particular question, feel free to leave it blank. Please *do* answer questions if you can, though. If you have any comments or concerns about any questions, just write your comments in the margin of the questionnaire or feel free to contact me by email (dfp1@yahoo.com) or by phone (518-587-3994).

    A postage-paid return envelope is enclosed for your convenience. Please take a few minutes to complete and return the questionnaire to us—it should only take about 15 to 20 minutes of your time. **In appreciation for your cooperation, you will be entered into a raffle to win a $250 American Express gift certificate.** Simply return the self-addressed, stamped postcard separately from the questionnaire. To be included in the raffle, your questionnaire must be returned to us by July 10. The raffle winner will be notified by July 17.

    Your participation in the study is completely voluntary. By returning your study booklet, you will be granting your consent to participate in the study. Thank you in advance for your assistance.

FIGURE 13.4 Example of a cover letter.

area specialists, and by someone capable of detecting technical problems, such as spelling mistakes, grammatical errors, and so forth. When these various people have provided feedback, a revised version of the instrument can be pretested. The pretest should be administered to a small sample of individuals (usually 10 to 20) who are similar to actual participants.

In the remainder of this section, we offer some specific suggestions for designing high-quality self-report instruments. Additional guidance is offered in the classic book by Fowler (1995) and by Bradburn and colleagues (2004).

Tips for Wording Questions

We all are accustomed to asking questions, but the proper phrasing of questions for a study is not easy. In wording their questions, researchers should keep four important considerations in mind.

1. *Clarity.* Questions should be worded clearly and unambiguously. This is usually easier said

than done. Respondents do not always have the same mind-set as the researchers.

2. *Ability of respondents to give information.* Researchers need to consider whether respondents can be expected to understand the question or are qualified to provide meaningful information.

3. *Bias.* Questions should be worded in a manner that will minimize the risk of response biases.

4. *Sensitivity.* Researchers should strive to be courteous, considerate, and sensitive to respondents' needs and circumstances, especially when asking questions of a private nature.

Here are some specific suggestions with regard to these four considerations (additional guidance on wording items for composite scales is provided in Chapter 15):

• Clarify in your own mind the information you are seeking. The question, "When do you usually eat your evening meal?" might elicit such responses as "around 6 pm," "when my son gets home from soccer practice," or "when I feel like cooking." The question itself contains no words that are difficult, but the question is unclear because the researcher's intent is not apparent.

- Avoid jargon or technical terms (e.g., parity) if lay terms (e.g., number of children) are equally appropriate. Use words that are simple enough for the *least* educated respondents in the sample. Don't assume that even nurses have extensive knowledge on all aspects of nursing and medical terminology.
- Do not assume that respondents will be aware of, or informed about, issues in which you are interested. Furthermore, avoid giving the impression that they *ought* to be informed. Questions on complex issues sometimes can be worded in such a way that respondents will be comfortable admitting ignorance (e.g., "Many people have not had a chance to learn much about factors that increase the risk of diabetes. Do you happen to know of any contributing factors?") Another approach is to preface a question by a short explanation about terminology or issues.
- Avoid leading questions that suggest a particular answer. A question such as, "Do you agree that nurse-midwives play an indispensable role in the health team?" is not neutral.
- State a range of alternatives within the question itself when possible. For instance, the question, "Do you prefer to get up early in the morning on weekends?" is more suggestive of the "right" answer than "Do you prefer to get up early in the morning or to sleep late on weekends?"
- For questions that deal with controversial topics or socially unacceptable behavior (e.g., excessive drinking, noncompliance with medical regimens), closed-ended questions may be preferred. It is easier to check off having engaged in socially disapproved actions than to verbalize those actions in response to open-ended questions. Moreover, when controversial behaviors are presented as options, respondents are more likely to believe that their behavior is not unique, and admissions of such behavior become less difficult.

- Impersonal wording of questions is sometimes useful in encouraging honesty. To illustrate this point, compare these two statements with which respondents might be asked to agree or disagree: (1) "I am dissatisfied with the nursing care I received during my hospitalization" and (2) "The quality of nursing care in this hospital is unsatisfactory." A respondent might feel more comfortable admitting dissatisfaction with nursing care in the less personally worded second question.

Tips for Preparing Response Alternatives

If closed-ended questions are used, researchers also need to develop response alternatives. Below are some suggestions for preparing them.

- Responses options should cover all significant alternatives. If respondents are forced to choose from options provided by researchers, they should feel comfortable with the available options. As a precaution, researchers often have as a response option a phrase such as "Other— please specify."
- Alternatives should be mutually exclusive. The following categories for a question on a person's age are *not* mutually exclusive: 30 years or younger, 30 to 50 years, or 50 years or older. People who are exactly 30 or 50 would qualify for two categories.
- There should be a rationale for ordering alternatives. Options often can be placed in order of decreasing or increasing favorability, agreement, or intensity. When options have no "natural" order, alphabetic ordering of the alternatives can avoid leading respondents to a particular response (e.g., see the rank order question in Table 13.1).
- Response alternatives should be brief. One sentence or phrase for each option is usually sufficient to express a concept. Response alternatives should be about equal in length.

Tips for Formatting an Instrument

The appearance and layout of an instrument may seem a matter of minor administrative importance. Yet, a poorly designed format can have substantive consequences if respondents (or interviewers) become confused, miss questions, or answer questions they should have omitted. The format is especially important in questionnaires because respondents cannot usually ask for help. The following suggestions may be helpful in laying out an instrument:

- Do not compress too many questions into too small a space. An extra page of questions is better than a form that appears dense and confusing and that provides inadequate space for responses to open-ended questions.
- Set off the response options from the question or stem. Response alternatives are usually aligned vertically (Table 13.1). In questionnaires, respondents can be asked either to circle their answer or to check the appropriate box.
- Give special care to formatting **filter questions**, which are designed to route respondents through different sets of questions depending on their responses. In interview schedules, the typical procedure is to use **skip patterns** that instruct interviewers to skip to a specific question (e.g., SKIP TO Q10). In SAQs, skip instructions may be confusing. It is usually better to put questions appropriate to a subset of respondents apart from the main series of questions, as illustrated in Box 13.1, part B. An important advantage of CAPI, CATI, audio-CASI, and some Internet surveys is that skip patterns are built into the computer program, leaving no room for human error.
- Avoid forcing all respondents to go through inapplicable questions in an SAQ. That is, question 2 in Box 13.1 part B could have been worded as follows: "If you are a member of the American Nurses Association, for how long have you been a member?" Nonmembers may not be sure how to handle this question and may be annoyed at having to read through irrelevant material.

Administering Structured Self-Report Instruments

Administering interview schedules and questionnaires involves different considerations and requires different skills.

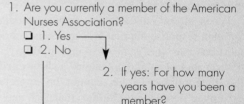

BOX 13.1 Examples of Formats for a Filter Question

A. *Interview Format*

1. Are you currently a member of the American Nurses Association?
   - ❑ 1. Yes
   - ❑ 2. No (SKIP TO Q3)
2. For how many years have you been a member?
   _____ YEARS
3. Do you subscribe to any nursing journals?
   - ❑ 1. Yes
   - ❑ 2. No

B. *Questionnaire Format*

1. Are you currently a member of the American Nurses Association?
   - ❑ 1. Yes
   - ❑ 2. No

   2. If yes: For how many years have you been a member?
   _____ YEARS

3. Do you subscribe to any nursing journals?
   - ❑ 1. Yes
   - ❑ 2. No

Collecting Interview Data

The quality of interview data relies heavily on interviewer proficiency. Interviewers for large survey organizations receive extensive general training in addition to specific training for individual studies. Although we cannot in this introductory book cover all the principles of good interviewing, we can identify some major issues. Additional guidance can be found in the classic handbook by Fowler and Mangione (1990).

A primary task of interviewers is to put respondents at ease so that they will feel comfortable in expressing opinions honestly. Respondents' reactions to interviewers can affect their level of cooperation. Interviewers, therefore, should always be punctual (if an appointment has been made), courteous, and friendly. Interviewers should strive to appear unbiased and to create an atmosphere that encourages candor. All opinions of respondents should be accepted as natural; interviewers should not express surprise, disapproval, or even approval.

With a structured interview schedule, interviewers should follow question wording precisely. Interviewers should not offer spontaneous explanations of what questions mean. Repetition of a question is usually adequate to dispel misunderstandings, especially if the instrument has been pretested. Interviewers should not read questions mechanically. A natural, conversational tone is essential in building rapport, and this tone is impossible to achieve if interviewers are not thoroughly familiar with the questions.

When closed-ended questions have lengthy or complex response alternatives, or when a series of questions has the same response options, interviewers should hand respondents a **show card** that lists the options. People cannot be expected to remember detailed unfamiliar material and may choose the last alternative if they cannot recall earlier ones. (Examples of show cards are included in the Toolkit in the *Resource Manual* ⊗.)

Interviewers record answers to closed-ended items by checking or circling the appropriate alternative, but responses to open-ended questions must be written out in full. Interviewers should not paraphrase or summarize respondents' replies.

Obtaining complete, relevant responses to questions is not always an easy matter. Respondents may reply to seemingly straightforward questions with partial answers. Some may say, "I don't know" to avoid giving their opinions on sensitive topics, or to stall while they think over the question. In such cases, the interviewers' job is to **probe**. The purpose of a probe is to elicit more useful information than respondents volunteered during their initial reply. A probe can take many forms: Sometimes it involves repeating the original question, and sometimes it is a long pause intended to communicate to respondents that they should continue. Frequently, it is necessary to encourage a more complete response to

> **BOX 13.2** Examples of Neutral, Nondirective Probes
>
> - Is there anything else?
> - Go on.
> - Are there any other reasons?
> - How do you mean?
> - Could you please tell me more about that?
> - Would you tell me what you have in mind?
> - There are no right or wrong answers; I'd just like to get your thinking.
> - Could you please explain that?
> - Could you please give me an example?

open-ended questions by a nondirective supplementary question, such as, "How is that?" Interviewers must be careful to use only *neutral* probes that do not influence the content of a response. Box 13.2 gives some examples of neutral, nondirective probes used by professional interviewers to get more complete responses to questions. The ability to probe well is perhaps the greatest test of an interviewer's skill. To know when to probe and how to select the best probes, interviewers must understand the purpose of each question. (The Toolkit for Chapter 14 has material relating to interviewer training that might be useful ⊗.)

Guidelines for telephone interviews are essentially the same as those for face-to-face interviews, but additional effort usually is required to build rapport over the telephone. In both cases, interviewers should strive to make the interview a pleasant and satisfying experience in which respondents are made to understand that the information they are providing is important.

Collecting Questionnaire Data through In-Person Distribution

Questionnaires can be distributed in various ways, including personal distribution, through the mail, and over the Internet. The most convenient procedure is to distribute questionnaires to a group of people who complete the instrument at the same time. This approach has the obvious advantages of maximizing the number of completed questionnaires and allowing respondents to ask questions. Group administrations are often possible in educational settings and in some clinical situations.

Researchers can also hand out questionnaires to individual respondents. Personal contact has a positive effect on response rates, and researchers can answer questions. Individual distribution of questionnaires in clinical settings is often inexpensive and efficient and can yield a relatively high rate of response.

Example of personal distribution of questionnaires: Dirksen and colleagues (2009) explored the relationships between insomnia, depression, and distress in men with prostate cancer. Data were collected by means of questionnaires that were distributed by a research assistant to men receiving treatment in an outpatient ambulatory clinic.

Collecting Questionnaire Data through the Mail

For surveys of a broad population, questionnaires are often mailed. This approach is cost-effective for reaching geographically dispersed respondents, but it tends to yield low response rates. When only a subsample of respondents return their questionnaires, the risk of bias is high. With low response rates, researchers face the possibility that people who did not complete a questionnaire would have answered questions differently from those who did return it.

With response rates greater than 65%, the risk of bias may be relatively small, but lower response rates are the norm. Researchers should attempt to discover how representative respondents are, relative to the selected sample, in terms of basic demographic characteristics, such as age, gender, and race/ethnicity. This comparison may lead researchers to conclude that respondents and nonrespondents are sufficiently similar. When demographic differences are found, investigators can make inferences about the direction of biases.

Response rates can be affected by the manner in which the questionnaires are designed and mailed.

The physical appearance of the questionnaire can influence its appeal, so thought should be given to instrument layout, quality and color of paper, and method of reproduction. The standard procedure for distributing mailed questionnaires is to include a stamped, addressed return envelope—without which, response rates will be seriously jeopardized.

➡ **TIP:** People are more likely to complete a mailed questionnaire if they are encouraged to do so by someone whose name (or position) they recognize. If possible, include a letter of endorsement from someone visible (e.g., a hospital or government official), or write the cover letter on the stationery of a well-respected organization, such as a university.

Follow-up reminders are effective in achieving higher response rates for mailed (and Internet) questionnaires. This procedure involves additional mailings urging nonrespondents to complete and return their forms. Follow-up reminders are typically sent about 10 to 14 days after the initial mailing. Sometimes reminders simply involve a letter or postcard of encouragement to nonrespondents. It is preferable, however, to send a second copy of the questionnaire with the reminder letter because many nonrespondents will have misplaced or discarded the original. Telephone follow-ups can be even more successful, but are costly and time-consuming. With anonymous questionnaires, researchers may be unable to distinguish respondents and nonrespondents for the purpose of sending follow-up letters. In such a situation, the simplest procedure is to send out a follow-up reminder to the entire sample, thanking those who have already answered and asking others to cooperate. ✪ Dillman and colleagues (2009) offer excellent advice for achieving acceptable response rates in mailed and Internet surveys.

Example of mailed questionnaires: Kupferer and colleagues (2009) surveyed women who had discontinued hormone therapy with regard to their use of complementary and alternative medicine for vasomotor symptoms. Questionnaire packets and a postage-paid return envelope were mailed to a random sample of 2,250 women from a purchased mailing list. The response rate was 24%.

Collecting Questionnaire Data via the Internet

The Internet is an economical means of distributing questionnaires. Internet surveys appear to be a promising approach for accessing groups of people interested in specific topics. Internet distribution requires appropriate equipment and some technical skills, but there are a growing number of aids for doing such surveys.

Surveys can be administered through the Internet in several ways. One method is to design a questionnaire in a word processing program, as would be the case for mailed questionnaires. The file with the questionnaire is then attached to an email message and distributed to potential respondents. Respondents can complete the questionnaire and return it as an email attachment or print it and return it by mail or fax. This method may be problematic if respondents have trouble opening attachments or if they use a different word-processing program. Surveys sent via email also run the risk of not getting delivered to the intended party, either because email addresses have changed or because the email messages are blocked by Internet security filters. Blocks are especially common for messages with attachments.

Increasingly, researchers are collecting data through **web-based surveys**. This approach requires researchers to have a website on which the survey is placed or to use a service such as Survey Monkey (*http://www.surveymonkey.com/*). Respondents typically access the website by clicking on a hypertext link. For example, respondents may be invited to participate in the survey through an email message that includes the hyperlink to the survey, or they may be invited to participate when they enter a website related in content to the survey (e.g., the website of a cancer support organization).

Web-based forms are designed for online response, and some can be programmed to include interactive features. By having dynamic features, respondents can receive as well as give information—a feature that can increase motivation to participate. For example, respondents can be given information about their own responses (e.g., how they scored on a scale) or aggregated information about other participants. A major advantage of web-based surveys is that the data are directly amenable to analysis. They can, however, be more expensive than email surveys.

> **Example of a web-based survey:** Sarna and colleagues (2009) conducted a web-based survey to obtain information from nurses in Magnet hospitals about their delivery of smoking cessation interventions. Respondents were solicited through the Chief Nursing Officers (CNOs) at 35 Magnet hospitals meeting inclusion criteria. CNOs were asked to communicate information about the survey web link to their nursing staff. The final response rate was 21%.

Internet surveys will undoubtedly abound in the years ahead. They tend to be economical and can reach a broad audience. However, samples are almost never representative, and response rates tend to be low—often even lower than mailed questionnaires. Several references are available to help researchers who wish to launch an Internet survey. For example, the books by Best and Krueger (2004), Dillman and colleagues (2009), and Fitzpatrick and Montgomery (2004) provide useful information. Weber and colleagues (2005) and Cantrell and Lupinacci (2007) offer guidance on web-based data collection and management.

Evaluation of Structured Self-Reports

Structured self-reports are a powerful data collection method. They are versatile and wide ranging, and yield information that can be readily analyzed statistically. Structured questions can be carefully worded and pretested. In an unstructured interview, by contrast, respondents may answer different questions, and there is no way to know whether question wording affected responses. On the other hand, the questions tend to be much more superficial than questions in unstructured interviews because most structured questions are closed-ended.

Structured self-reports are susceptible to the risk of various **response biases**—many of which are also possible in unstructured self-reports.

Respondents may give biased answers in reaction to the interviewers' behavior or appearance, for example. Perhaps the most pervasive problem is people's tendency to present a favorable image of themselves. **Social desirability response bias** refers to the tendency of some individuals to misrepresent themselves by giving answers that are congruent with prevailing social values. This problem is often difficult to combat. Subtle, indirect, and delicately worded questioning sometimes can help to minimize this response bias. The creation of a permissive atmosphere and provisions for anonymity also encourage frankness. In an interview situation, interviewer training is essential.

Some response biases, called **response sets**, are most commonly observed in composite scales. **Extreme responses** are a bias reflecting consistent selection of extreme alternatives (e.g., "strongly agree"). These extreme responses distort the findings because they do not necessarily signify the most intense feelings about the phenomenon under study, but rather capture a trait of the respondent. There is little a researcher can do to counteract this bias, but there are procedures for detecting it.

Some people have been found to agree with statements regardless of content. Such people are called **yea-sayers**, and the bias is known as the **acquiescence response set**. A less common problem is the opposite tendency for other individuals, called **naysayers**, to disagree with statements independently of question content.

Researchers who construct scales should attempt to eliminate or minimize response set biases. If an instrument or scale is being developed for general use by others, evidence should be gathered to demonstrate that the scale is sufficiently free from response biases to measure the critical variable. Users should consider such evidence in selecting existing scales.

STRUCTURED OBSERVATION

Structured observation is used to document specific behaviors, actions, and events. Structured observation involves using formal instruments and protocols that indicate what to observe, how long to observe it, and how to record information. The challenge of structured observation lies in the formulation of a system for accurately categorizing and recording observations.

In selecting behaviors, conversation, or attributes to be observed, researchers must decide what constitutes a *unit*. A *molar approach* entails observing large units of behavior and treating them as a whole. For example, an entire constellation of verbal and nonverbal behaviors might be construed as signaling confusion in nursing home residents. At the other extreme, a *molecular approach* uses small, specific behaviors or verbal segments as units. Each action, gesture, or phrase is treated as a separate entity. The molar approach is more susceptible to observer errors because of greater ambiguity in what is being observed. On the other hand, in reducing observations to concrete, specific elements, investigators may fail to understand how small elements work in concert in a behavior pattern. The choice of approach depends on the nature of the research problem.

Methods of Recording Structured Observations

Researchers recording structured observations typically use either a checklist or a rating scale. Both types of record-keeping instruments specify the behaviors or events to be observed and are designed to produce numeric information.

⊃ TIP: Compared with the abundance of books designed to provide guidance in developing self-report instruments, there are relatively few resources for researchers who want to design their own observational instruments, except if the focus of the observation is on interpersonal interactions (e.g., Kerig & Lindahl, 2001; Kerig & Baucom, 2004).

Category Systems and Checklists

Structured observation often involves constructing a category system to classify observed phenomena.

A **category system** represents an attempt to designate in a systematic fashion the qualitative behaviors and events transpiring in the observational setting.

Some category systems are constructed so that *all* observed behaviors within a specified domain (e.g., utterances) can be classified into one and only one category. In such an exhaustive system, the categories are mutually exclusive.

Example of exhaustive categories: Foreman and colleagues (2008) analyzed gender differences in the sleep–wake states of 97 preterm infants, who were videotaped in 4-hour segments. The infants' respirations, eye movements, facial expressions, muscle tone, and motor activity were used to classify their sleep–wake state, every 15 seconds, into one of four mutually exclusive categories: awake, drowsy, active sleep, and quiet sleep.

When observers use an exhaustive system—that is, when all behaviors of a certain type, such as verbal interaction, are observed and recorded—researchers must be careful to define categories so that observers know when one behavior ends and a new one begins. Another essential feature is that referent behaviors should be mutually exclusive, as in the previous example. The underlying assumption in using such a category system is that behaviors, events, or attributes that are allocated to a particular category are equivalent to every other behavior, event, or attribute in that same category.

A contrasting technique is to develop a system in which only particular types of behavior (which may or may not be manifested) are categorized. For example, if we were studying autistic children's aggressive behavior, we might develop such categories as "strikes another child," or "kicks or hits walls or floor." In such a category system, many behaviors—all the ones that are nonaggressive—would not be classified. Nonexhaustive systems are adequate for many purposes, but one risk is that resulting data might be difficult to interpret. Problems may arise if a large number of behaviors are not categorized or if long segments of the observation sessions do not involve the target behaviors. In such situations, investigators need to record the amount of time in which the target behaviors occurred, relative to the total time under observation.

Example of nonexhaustive categories: Liaw and colleagues (2006) studied changes in patterns of infants' distress at different phases of a routine tub bath in the NICU. The researchers developed a system to categorize behavioral signs of distress (jerks, tremors, grimaces, arching). Behaviors unrelated to distress were not categorized.

A critical requirement for a good category system is the careful definition of behaviors or characteristics to be observed. Each category must be explained in detail so that observers have relatively clear-cut criteria for identifying the occurrence of a specified phenomenon. Virtually all category systems require observers to make some inferences, to a greater or lesser degree.

Example of low observer inference: Johnston and colleagues (2008) studied the effects of kangaroo mother care on preterm infants' pain from a heel lance. They used the Premature Infant Pain Profile (PIPP) to measure pain. The PIPP includes both physiologic (e.g., heart rate) and behavioral indicators. Three facial actions (brow bulge, eye squeeze, and naso-labial furrow) are scored by observers. The coding system "provides a detailed, anatomically based, and objective description" (p. 4) of newborn behavior.

In this system, assuming that observers were properly trained, relatively little inference would be required to code facial actions. Other category systems, however, require more inference, as in the following example:

Example of moderately high observer inference: Uitterhoeve and colleagues (2008) videotaped oncology nurses interacting with actors playing the role of patients. The videotaped encounters were coded for nurses' responses to patients' cues. Nurses' responses were coded according to both function and form. Function, for example, involved coding whether the patient's cue was *explored*, *acknowledged* but not explored, or elicited a *distancing* response.

In such category systems, even when categories are defined in detail, a moderately heavy inferential burden is placed on observers. The decision concerning degree of observer inference depends on a number of factors, including the research purpose and the observers' skills. Beginning researchers are advised to construct or use category systems that require low to moderate inference.

Category systems are used to construct a **checklist**, which is the instrument observers use to record observed phenomena. The checklist is usually formatted with the list of behaviors or events from the category system on the left and space for tallying the frequency or duration of occurrence of behaviors on the right. With nonexhaustive category systems, categories of behaviors that may or may not be manifested by participants are listed on the checklist. The observer's tasks are to watch for instances of these behaviors and to record their occurrence.

With exhaustive checklists, the observers' task is to place all behaviors in only one category for each element. By **element**, we refer either to a unit of behavior, such as a sentence in a conversation, or to a time interval. To illustrate, suppose we were studying the problem-solving behavior of a group of public health workers discussing a new intervention for the homeless. Our category system involves eight categories: (1) seeks information, (2) gives information, (3) describes problem, (4) offers suggestion, (5) opposes suggestion, (6) supports suggestion, (7) summarizes, and (8) miscellaneous. Observers would be required to classify every group member's contribution—using, for example, each sentence as the element—in terms of one of these eight categories.

Another approach with exhaustive systems is to categorize relevant behaviors at regular time intervals. For example, in a category system for infants' motor activities, the researcher might use 10-second time intervals as the element; observers would categorize infant movements within 10-second periods.

Rating Scales

The major alternative to a checklist for recording structured observations is a **rating scale** that requires observers to rate a phenomenon along a descriptive continuum that is typically bipolar. The ratings are quantified for subsequent analysis.

Observers may be required to rate behaviors or events at specified intervals throughout the observational period (e.g., every 5 minutes). Alternatively, observers may rate entire events or transactions after observations are completed. Postobservation ratings require observers to integrate a number of activities and to judge which point on a scale most closely fits their interpretation of the situation. For example, suppose we were observing children's behavior during a scratch test for allergies. After each session, observers might be asked to rate the children's overall anxiety during the procedure on a graphic rating scale such as the following:

1	2	3	4	5	6	7
Extremely calm			Neither calm nor nervous			Extremely nervous

Rate how calm or nervous the child appeared to be during the procedure.

⮕ TIP: Global observational rating scales are sometimes included at the end of structured interviews. For example, in a study of the health problems of nearly 4,000 low-income mothers, interviewers were asked to observe and rate the safety of the home environment with regard to potential health hazards to the children on a five-point scale, from completely safe to extremely unsafe (Polit et al., 2001).

Rating scales can also be used as an extension of checklists, in which observers not only record the occurrence of a behavior, but also rate some qualitative aspect of it, such as its intensity. A good example is Weiss's (1992) Tactile Interaction Index (TII) for observing patterns of interpersonal touch. The TII comprises four dimensions: location (part of body touched, such as arm, abdomen), action (the specific gesture used, such as grabbing, hitting, patting; duration (temporal length of the touch), and intensity. Observers using the index must both classify the nature and duration of the touch *and* rate intensity on a four-point scale: light, moderate, strong, and deep. When rating scales are coupled with a category scheme, considerable information about a phenomenon can be obtained, but it places an immense burden on observers, particularly if there is extensive activity.

> **Example of observational ratings:** The NEECHAM Confusion Scale, an observational measure to detect the presence and severity of acute confusion, relies on ratings of behavior. For example, one rating concerns alertness/responsiveness, and the ratings are from 0 (responsiveness depressed) to 4 (full attentiveness). The NEECHAM has been used for both clinical and research purposes. For example, McCaffrey (2009) used NEECHAM scores to assess the effects of a music intervention on confusion in older adults after surgery.

> ➲ **TIP:** It is usually useful to spend a period of time with participants before the actual observation and recording of data. Having a warm-up period helps to relax people (especially if audio or video equipment is being used) and can be helpful to observers (e.g., if participants have a linguistic style to which observers must adjust, such as a strong regional accent).

Constructing Versus Borrowing Structured Observational Instruments

As with self-report instruments, we encourage researchers to search for available observational instruments, rather than designing one themselves. The use of an existing instrument not only saves considerable work and time, but also facilitates comparisons among studies.

A few source books describe available observational instruments for certain research applications (e.g., Frank-Stromberg & Olsen, 2004), but the best source for such instruments is recent research literature on the study topic. For example, if you wanted to conduct an observational study of infant pain, a good place to begin would be recent research on this or similar topics to obtain information on how infant pain was operationalized.

Sampling for Structured Observations

Researchers must decide how, when, and for how long structured observational instruments will be used. Observations are usually done for a specific amount of time, and the amount of time is standardized across participants.

Sometimes *sampling* is needed so as to obtain representative examples of behaviors without having to observe for prolonged periods. Observational sampling concerns the selection of *behaviors* (or conversational segments) to be observed, not the selection of participants.

Time sampling involves the selection of time periods during which observations will occur. The time frames may be systematically selected (e.g., 60 seconds at 5-minute intervals) or selected at random. For example, suppose we were studying mothers' interactions with their children in a playground. During a 1-hour observation period, we sample moments to observe, rather than observing the entire session. Let us say that observations are made in 3-minute segments. If we used systematic sampling, we would observe for 3 minutes, then cease observing for a prespecified period, say 3 minutes. With this scheme, a total of ten 3-minute observations would be made. A second approach is to sample randomly 3-minute periods from the total of 20 such periods in an hour; a third is to use all 20 periods. Decisions about the length and number of periods for creating a good sample must be consistent with research aims. In establishing time units, a key consideration is determining a psychologically meaningful time frame. Pretesting and experimentation with different sampling plans is usually necessary.

> **Example of time sampling:** Robb and colleagues (2008) tested the effect of active music engagement on stress and coping behaviors in children with cancer. Participating children received one of three interventions (active music engagement, music listening, or audio storybooks) and were then videotaped. Observers coded selected time segments (10 seconds, followed by 5-second segments) for facial affect, active engagement, and initiation.

Event sampling uses integral behavior sets or events for observation. Event sampling requires that the investigator either have knowledge about the occurrence of events, or be in a position to wait for (or arrange) their occurrence. Examples of integral events suitable for event sampling include shift changes of hospital nurses or cast removals of pediatric patients. This approach is preferable to time sampling when events of interest are infrequent and are at risk of being missed. Still, when behaviors and events are frequent, time sampling has the virtue of enhancing the representativeness of observed behaviors.

Example of event sampling: Bryanton and colleagues (2009) explored whether mothers' perceptions of their childbirth experiences predicted early parenting behaviors. Parenting behaviors were observed during a feeding interaction when the infants were 1 month old.

Technical Aids in Observations

A wide array of technical devices is available for recording behaviors and events, making analysis or categorization at a later time possible. When the target behavior is auditory, recordings can be used to obtain a permanent record. Technological advances have vastly improved the quality, sensitivity, and unobtrusiveness of recording equipment. Auditory recordings can also be subjected to computerized speech software analysis to obtain objective quantitative measures of certain features of the recordings (e.g., volume, pitch).

Videotaping can be used when visual records are desired. In addition to being permanent, videotapes can capture complex behaviors that might elude on-the-spot observers. Visual records are also more capable than the naked eye of capturing fine units of behavior, such as micromomentary facial expressions. Videotapes make it possible to check the accuracy of coders and so are useful as a training aid. Finally, it is easier to conceal a camera than a human observer. Video records also have a few drawbacks, some of which are technical, such as lighting requirements, lens limitations, and so on. Sometimes the camera angle can present a lopsided view of an event. Also, some participants

may be especially self-conscious in front of a video camera. Still, for many applications, permanent visual records offer unparalleled opportunities to expand the scope of observational studies. Haidet and colleagues (2009) offer valuable advice on improving data quality of video-recorded observations.

There is a growing technology for assisting with the encoding and recording of observations. For example, there is equipment that permits observers to enter observational data directly into a computer as the observation occurs, and in some cases, the equipment can record physiologic data concurrently.

Example of using equipment: Brown and colleagues (2009) developed and evaluated an observation system to assess mother–infant feeding interaction relevant to infant neuro-behavior regulation. In developing the system, videotapes of feeding sessions were digitized and stored on the computer so they could be opened for coding. They used a computer-based system (Observer) that offered a means of systematically observing and recording behavior as it occurred in real time. Coding was done by replaying the digitized video recording and entering observational codes into the computer.

Structured Observations by Nonresearch Observers

The observations discussed thus far are made and recorded by research team members. Sometimes, however, researchers ask people not connected with the research to provide structured data, based on their observations of the characteristics or behaviors of others. This method has much in common (in terms of format and scoring) with self-report scales; the primary difference is that the person completing the scale is asked to describe the attributes and behaviors of *another* person, based on observations of that person. For example, a mother might be asked to describe the behavior problems of her preschool child or staff nurses might be asked to evaluate the functional capacity of nursing home residents.

Obtaining observational data from nonresearchers is economical compared with using trained observers. For example, observers might have to watch children for hours or days to describe the nature and intensity of behavior problems, whereas parents or teachers could do this readily. Some behaviors might never lend themselves to outsider observation because of reactivity, occurrence in private situations, or infrequency (e.g., sleepwalking).

On the other hand, such methods may have the same problems as self-report scales (e.g., response-set bias) in addition to observer bias. Observer bias may in some cases be extreme, such as may happen when parents provide information about their children. Nonresearch observers are typically not trained, and interobserver agreement usually cannot be assessed. Thus, this approach has some problems but will continue to be used because, in many cases, there are no alternatives.

Example of observations by nonresearch personnel: Conrad and Altmaier (2009) studied the relationship between social support and levels of adjustment in children with cancer who attended a residential summer camp. Adjustment was measured by having parents complete the Child Behavior Checklist.

Evaluation of Structured Observation

Structured observation is an important data collection method, particularly for recording aspects of people's behaviors when they are not capable of describing them reliably in self-reports. Observational methods are particularly valuable for gathering data about infants and children, older people who are confused or agitated, or people whose communication skills are impaired.

Observations, like self-reports, are vulnerable to biases. One source of bias comes from those being observed. Participants may distort their behaviors in the direction of "looking good." They may also behave atypically because of their awareness of being observed, or their shyness in front of strangers or a camera.

Biases can also reflect human perceptual errors. Observation and interpretation are demanding tasks, requiring attention, perception, and conception. To accomplish these activities in a completely objective fashion is challenging and perhaps impossible. Biases are especially likely to operate when a high degree of observer inference is required.

Several types of observational bias are particularly common. One bias is the **enhancement of contrast effect**, in which observers distort observations in the direction of dividing content into clear-cut entities. The converse effect—a bias toward **central tendency**—occurs when extreme events are distorted toward a middle ground. With **assimilatory biases**, observers distort observations in the direction of identity with previous inputs. This bias would have the effect of miscategorizing information in the direction of regularity and orderliness. Assimilation to the observer's expectations and attitudes also occurs.

Rating scales are also susceptible to bias. The **halo effect** is the tendency of observers to be influenced by one characteristic in judging other, unrelated characteristics. For example, if we formed a positive general impression of a person, we might rate that person as intelligent, loyal, and dependable simply because these traits are positively valued. Ratings may reflect observers' personality. The **error of leniency** is the tendency for observers to rate everything positively, and the **error of severity** is the contrasting tendency to rate too harshly.

The careful construction and pretesting of checklists and rating scales, and the proper training and preparation of observers, play an important role in minimizing biases. To become a good instrument for collecting observational data, observers must be trained to observe in a manner that maximizes accuracy. Even when the lead researcher is the primary observer, self-training and dry runs are essential. The setting during the trial period should resemble as closely as possible the settings that will be the focus of actual observations.

Ideally, training should include practice sessions in which the comparability of observers' recordings is assessed. That is, two or more independent observers should watch a trial situation, and observational coding should then be compared. Procedures for assessing the **interrater reliability** of structured observations are described in the next chapter.

➲ **TIP:** Observations should be made in a neutral, nonjudgmental manner. People being observed are more likely to behave atypically if they think they are being critically appraised. Even positive cues (such as nodding approval) should be withheld because approval may induce repetition of a behavior that might not otherwise have occurred.

BIOPHYSIOLOGIC MEASURES

Settings in which nurses work are typically filled with a wide variety of technical instruments for measuring physiologic functions. It is beyond the scope of this book to describe the many kinds of biophysiologic measures available to nurse researchers. Our goals are to present an overview of biophysiologic measures, to illustrate their use in research, and to note considerations in decisions to use them.

Purposes of Collecting Biophysiologic Data

Clinical nursing studies involve biophysiologic instruments both for creating independent variables (e.g., a biofeedback intervention) and for measuring outcomes. For the most part, our discussion focuses on the use of biophysiologic measures as dependent (outcome) variables. Examples of the purposes of collecting biophysiologic data include the following:

1. *Studies of basic biophysiologic processes that have relevance for nursing care.* These studies involve healthy participants or an animal species. For example, Dorsey and colleagues (2009) studied mechanisms underlying painful peripheral neuropathy in the treatment of HIV using a whole-genome microassay screen with a mouse model.

2. *Descriptions of the physiologic consequences of nursing and healthcare.* These studies do not focus on specific interventions, but rather are designed to learn how standard procedures affect patients' physiologic outcomes. For example, Kang and colleagues (2009) tracked immune recovery (e.g., natural killer cell activity) in the 12 months following cancer treatment among women with early-stage breast cancer.

3. *Evaluations of a specific nursing intervention.* Some studies involve testing the effects of a new intervention, usually in comparison with standard methods of care or alternative interventions. Typically, these studies test the hypothesis that the innovation will result in improved biophysiologic outcomes among patients. As an example, Yeo (2009) tested the effects of a walking versus stretching exercise on preeclampsia risk factors such as heart rate and blood pressure in sedentary pregnant women.

4. *Assessments of products or clinical procedures.* Some studies evaluate products designed to enhance patient health or comfort, or test alternative products and procedures. For example, Mathew and colleagues (2009) collected central catheter blood samples using three alternative methods and compared blood culture results.

5. *Studies of the correlates of physiologic functioning in patients with health problems.* Researchers study possible antecedents and consequences of biophysiologic outcomes to gain insight into potential treatments or modes of care. Nurse researchers have also studied biophysiologic outcomes in relation to social or psychological characteristics. As an example, Neira and colleagues (2009) studied the association between glucose metabolism and cardiometabolic risk factors in Hispanics at risk for metabolic syndrome.

Types of Biophysiologic Measures

Physiologic measurements are either in vivo or in vitro. **In vivo measurements** are performed directly in or on living organisms. Examples include measures of oxygen saturation, blood pressure, and body temperature. An **in vitro measurement**, by contrast, is performed outside the organism's body, as in the case of measuring serum potassium concentration in the blood.

In vivo measures often involve the use of highly complex instrumentation systems, involving (for example) a stimulus, sensing equipment (e.g., transducers), signal-conditioning equipment to reduce interference, display equipment, and recording and data processing equipment. In vivo instruments have been developed to measure all bodily functions, and technological improvements continue to advance our ability to measure biophysiologic phenomena more accurately, more conveniently, and more rapidly than ever before. The uses to which such instruments have been put by nurse researchers are richly diverse.

> **Example of a study with in vivo measures:**
> Ayhan and colleagues (2009) randomly assigned patients undergoing a thyroidectomy to two oxygen-delivery methods (face mask and nasal cannula) and then assessed the effect on peripheral oxygen saturation, measured by pulse oximetry every 5 minutes for 30 minutes.

With in vitro measures, data are gathered by extracting physiologic material from people and submitting it for laboratory analysis. Nurse researchers may or may not be involved in the extraction of the material; however, the analysis is normally done by specialized laboratory technicians. Usually, each laboratory establishes a range of normal values for each measurement, and this information is critical for interpreting the results. Several classes of laboratory analysis have been used by nurse researchers, including chemical measurements (e.g., measures of potassium levels), microbiologic measures (e.g., bacterial counts), and cytologic *or* histologic measures (e.g., tissue biopsies). Laboratory analyses of blood and urine samples are the most frequently used in vitro measures in nursing investigations.

> **Example of a study with in vitro measures:**
> Choi and Rankin (2009) studied factors influencing glucose control in Korean immigrants with type 2 diabetes. A finger stick blood test was used to assess levels of glycosylated hemoglobin (HbA1c).

Selecting a Biophysiologic Measure

The most basic issue in selecting a physiologic measure is whether it will yield good information about research variables. In some cases, researchers need to consider whether the variable should be measured by observation or self-report instead of (or in addition to) using biophysiologic equipment. For example, stress could be measured by asking people questions (e.g., using the State–Trait Anxiety Inventory), by observing their behavior during exposure to stressful stimuli, or by measuring heart rate, blood pressure, or levels of adrenocorticotropic hormone in urine samples.

Several other considerations should be kept in mind in selecting a biophysiologic measure. Some key questions include the following:

- Is the equipment or laboratory analysis you need readily available to you? If not, can it be borrowed, rented, or purchased?
- Can you operate the required equipment and interpret its results, or do you need training? Are resources available to help you with operation and interpretation?
- Will you have difficulty obtaining permission to use the equipment from an Institutional Review Board or other institutional authority?
- Do your activities during data collection permit you to record data simultaneously, or do you need an instrument system with recording equipment (or a research assistant)?
- Is a single measure of the dependent variable sufficient, or are multiple measures needed for a reliable estimate? If the latter, what burden does this place on participants?
- Are your measures likely to be influenced by reactivity (i.e., participants' awareness of their status)? If so, can alternative or supplementary nonreactive measures be identified, or can the extent of reactivity bias be assessed?

- Is the measure you plan to use sufficiently accurate and sensitive to variation?
- Are you thoroughly familiar with rules and safety precautions, such as grounding procedures, especially when using electrical equipment?

Evaluation of Biophysiologic Measures

Biophysiologic measures offer the following advantages to nurse researchers:

- Biophysiologic measures are accurate and precise compared with psychological measures (e.g., self-report measures of anxiety).
- Biophysiologic measures are objective. Two nurses reading from the same sphygmomanometer are likely to obtain the same blood pressure measurements, and two different sphygmomanometers are likely to produce identical readouts. Patients cannot easily distort measurements of biophysiologic functioning deliberately.
- Biophysiologic instruments provide valid measures of targeted variables: thermometers can be depended on to measure temperature and not blood volume, and so forth. For self-report and observational measures, it is often more difficult to be certain that the instrument is really measuring the target concept.

Biophysiologic measures also have a few disadvantages:

- The cost of collecting some types of biophysiologic data may be low or nonexistent, but when laboratory tests are involved, they may be more expensive than other methods (e.g., assessing smoking status by means of cotinine assays versus self-report).
- The measuring tool may affect the variables it is attempting to measure. The presence of a sensing device, such as a transducer, located in a blood vessel partially blocks that vessel and, hence, alters the pressure–flow characteristics being measured.
- Energy must often be applied to the organism when taking the biophysiologic measurements; extreme caution must continually be exercised

to avoid the risk of damaging cells by high-energy concentrations.

The difficulty in choosing biophysiologic measures for nursing studies lies not in their shortage, nor in their questionable utility, nor in their inferiority to other methods. Indeed, they are plentiful, often highly reliable and valid, and extremely useful in clinical nursing studies. Care must be exercised, however, in selecting instruments or laboratory analyses with regard to practical, ethical, medical, and technical considerations.

IMPLEMENTING A DATA COLLECTION PLAN

Data quality in a quantitative study is affected by both the data collection plan and how the plan is implemented.

Selecting Research Personnel

An important decision concerns who will actually collect the research data. In small studies, the lead researcher usually collects the data personally. In larger studies, however, this may not be feasible. When data are collected by others, it is important to select appropriate people. In general, they should be neutral agents through whom data passes—that is, their characteristics or behavior should not affect the substance of the data. Some considerations that should be kept in mind when selecting research personnel are as follows:

- *Experience.* Research staff ideally have had prior experience collecting data (e.g., prior interviewing experience). If this is not feasible, look for people who can readily acquire the necessary skills (e.g., an interviewer should have good verbal and social skills).
- *Congruity with sample characteristics.* If possible, data collectors should match participants with respect to racial or cultural background and gender. The greater the sensitivity of the questions, the greater the desirability of matching characteristics.

- *Unremarkable appearance.* Extremes of appearance should be avoided. For example, data collectors should not dress very casually (e.g., in shorts and tee shirts), nor formally (e.g., in designer clothes). Data collectors should not wear anything that conveys their political, social, or religious views.
- *Personality.* Data collectors should be pleasant (but not effusive), sociable (but not overly talkative), and nonjudgmental (but not unfeeling about participants' lives). The goal is to have nonthreatening data collectors who can put participants at ease.

In some situations, researchers cannot select research personnel. For example, the data collectors may be staff nurses employed at a hospital. Training of the data collection staff is particularly important in such situations. Even if there are no additional data collection staff, researchers should self-monitor their demeanor and prepare for their role with care.

Training Data Collectors

Depending on prior experience, training will need to cover both general procedures (e.g., how to probe in an interview) and ones specific to the study (e.g., how to ask a particular question). Training can often be done in a single day, but complex projects require more time. The lead researcher is usually the best person to conduct the training and to develop training materials.

Data collection protocols usually are a good foundation for a **training manual**. The manual normally includes background materials (e.g., the study aims), general instructions, specific instructions, and copies of all data forms.

➡ **TIP:** A table of contents for a training manual is included in the Toolkit of the accompanying *Resource Manual.* Models for some of the sections in this table of contents (a section on avoiding interviewer bias and another on how to probe) are also available in the Toolkit. If you are collecting the data yourself, you may not need a training manual, but you should learn techniques of professional interviewing.

The agenda for the training should cover the content of the training manual, elaborating on any portion that is especially complex. Training usually includes demonstrations of fictitious data collection sessions, performed either live or on videotape. Finally, training usually involves having trainees do trial runs of data collection (e.g., *mock interviews*) in front of the trainers to demonstrate their understanding of the instructions. Thompson and colleagues (2005) provide some additional tips relating to the training of research personnel.

Example of data collector training: In a two-wave panel study of the health of nearly 4,000 low-income families, Polit and colleagues (2001) trained about 100 interviewers in 4 research sites. Each training session lasted 3 days, including a half day of training on the use of CAPI. At the end of the training, several trainees were not kept on as interviewers because they were not skillful in mastering their assignments.

CRITIQUING STRUCTURED METHODS OF DATA COLLECTION

The goal of a data collection plan is to produce data that are of exceptional quality. Every decision researchers make about data collection methods and procedures is likely to affect data quality, and hence overall study quality. These decisions should be critiqued in evaluating the study's evidence to the extent possible. The critiquing guidelines in Box 13.3 ✖ focus on global decisions about the design and implementation of a data collection plan. Unfortunately, data collection procedures are often not described in detail in research reports, owing to space constraints in journals. A full critique of data collection plans is rarely feasible.

A second set of critiquing guidelines is presented in Box 13.4. ✖ These questions focus on the specific methods of collecting research data in quantitative studies. Further guidance on drawing conclusions about data quality in quantitative studies is provided in the next chapter.

BOX 13.3 Guidelines for Critiquing Data Collection Plans in Quantitative Studies

1. Was the collection of data using structured methods (in contrast with unstructured methods) consistent with study aims?
2. Were the right methods used to collect the data (self-report, observation, etc.)? Was triangulation of methods used appropriately? Should supplementary data collection methods have been used to enrich the data available for analysis?
3. Was the right amount of data collected? Were data collected to address the varied needs of the study? Was *too much* data collected in terms of burdening study participants—and, if so, how might this have affected data quality?
4. Did the researcher select good instruments, in terms of congruence with underlying constructs, data quality, reputation, efficiency, and so on? Were new instruments developed without a justifiable rationale?
5. Were data collection instruments adequately pretested?
6. Did the report provide sufficient information about data collection procedures?
7. Who collected the data? Were data collectors judiciously chosen, with traits that were likely to enhance data quality?
8. Was the training of data collectors described? Was the training adequate? Were steps taken to improve data collectors' ability to elicit or produce high-quality data, or to monitor their performance?
9. Where and under what circumstances were data gathered? Was the setting for data collection appropriate?
10. Were other people present during data collection? Could the presence of others have resulted in any biases?
11. Were data collectors blinded to study hypotheses or to participants' group status?

BOX 13.4 Guidelines for Critiquing Structured Data Collection Methods

1. If self-report methods were used, did the researcher make good decisions about the specific method used to solicit self-report information (e.g., mix of open- and closed-ended questions, use of composite scales, and so on)?
2. Was the instrument package adequately described in terms of reading level of the questions, length of time to complete it, modules included, and so on?
3. Was the mode of obtaining the self-report data appropriate (e.g., in-person interviews, mailed SAQs, Internet questionnaires, and so on)?
4. Were self-report data gathered in a manner that promoted high-quality and unbiased responses (e.g., in terms of privacy, efforts to put respondents at ease, and so on)?
5. If observational methods were used, did the report adequately describe the specific constructs that were observed? What was the unit of observation, and was this appropriate?
6. Was a category system or rating system used to organize and record observations? Was the category system exhaustive? How much inference was required of the observers? Were decisions about exhaustiveness and degree of observer inference appropriate?
7. What methods were used to sample observational units? Was the sampling approach a good one, and did it likely yield a representative sample of behavior?
8. To what degree were observer biases controlled or minimized?
9. Were biophysiologic measures used in the study, and was this appropriate? Did the researcher appear to have the skills necessary for proper interpretation of biophysiologic measures?

●●●●●●●●●●●●●●●●●●●●●●●

RESEARCH EXAMPLE

In the study described next, a variety of data collection approaches was used to measure study variables.

Study: Predicting children's response to distraction from pain (Dr. Ann McCarthy & Dr. Charmaine Kleiber, Principal Investigators, NINR grant 1-R01-NR005269).

Statement of Purpose: Drs. McCarthy and Kleiber developed and tested an intervention to train parents as coaches to distract their children during insertion of an intravenous (IV) catheter. The overall study purpose was to test the effectiveness of the intervention in reducing children's pain and distress, to identify factors that predicted which children benefited from the distraction, and to identify characteristics of parents who were successful in distracting their children.

Design: In this multisite clinical trial, 542 parents were randomly assigned to an intervention group or a usual-care control group. Their children, aged 4 to 10, were scheduled to undergo an IV insertion for a diagnostic medical procedure. Parents in the intervention group received 15 minutes of training regarding effective methods of distraction before the child's IV insertion.

Data Collection Plan: The researchers collected a wide range of data both prior to and following the intervention and IV procedure, using self-report, observational, and biophysiologic measures. Their data collection plan included the use of formal instruments for describing sample characteristics, for assessing key outcomes of children's pain and distress, for measuring parent and child factors they hypothesized would predict the intervention's effectiveness, for capturing characteristics of the IV procedure, and for evaluating treatment fidelity in terms of parental success with distraction coaching. The researchers undertook a thorough literature review to identify factors influencing children's responses to a painful procedure, and developed a model that guided their data collection efforts. Before undertaking the full-scale study, the instruments were pilot tested (Kleiber & McCarthy, 2006). The pilot test was used to assess whether the instruments were understandable, to evaluate the quality of data they would yield, and to explore interrelationships among study variables. The researchers noted "the value of evaluating instruments prior to the initiation of a larger study" (p. 104). Because of the extensiveness of their data collection plan, we describe only a few specific measures here.

Self-Report Instruments: Both parents and children provided self-report data. For example, scores on the Oucher Scale, a self-report measure of children's pain, were used as an outcome variable. Children also reported their level of anxiety on a visual analog scale. Another child self-report instrument (Child Behavioral Style Scale) measured their coping style, using a vignette-type approach with four stressful scenarios. Parents completed self-administered questionnaires that incorporated scales to measure parenting style (Parenting Dimensions Inventory) and anxiety (State-Trait Anxiety Inventory). They also completed instruments that described their children's temperament (Dimensions of Temperament Survey).

Observational Instruments: A research assistant videotaped the parent and the child during the time they were in the treatment room. Videotapes were entered into a computerized video editing program and divided into 10-second intervals for analysis. The authors coded the parents' behavior in terms of the quality and frequency of distraction coaching, using an observational instrument that the researchers carefully developed, the Distraction Coaching Index (Kleiber et al., 2007). The videotapes were also used to code the children's behavioral distress, using the Observation Scale of Behavioral Distress.

Biophysiologic Measures: Children's stress was also measured using salivary cortisol levels. The chew-and-spit technique was used to collect salivary samples. Children chewed a piece of sugarless gum as a salivary stimulant. After discarding the gum, the children spat saliva into a collection tube. Each child provided four salivary cortisol samples: before IV insertion, 20 minutes after IV insertion, and two home samples to assess the child's baseline cortisol levels. Care was taken to ensure the integrity of the samples and to control conditions under which they were obtained (McCarthy et al., 2009).

Key Findings: Results from this extensive study are just appearing in the literature. Early published results have indicated that parents in the intervention group had significantly higher scores than those in the control group for distraction coaching frequency and quality (Kleiber et al., 2007). The researchers also found, using data from control group children, that baseline cortisol levels were lower than levels obtained in the clinics, and that cortisol levels increased following IV insertion, supporting the utility of cortisol levels as a measure of stress response (McCarthy et al., 2009).

SUMMARY POINTS

- Quantitative researchers typically develop a detailed **data collection plan** before they begin to collect their data. For structured data, researchers use formal data collection **instruments** that place constraints on those collecting data and those providing them.

- An early step in developing a data collection plan is the identification and prioritization of data needs. After data needs have been identified, measures of the variables must be located. The selection of existing instruments should be based on such considerations as conceptual suitability, data quality, cost, population appropriateness, and reputation.

- Even when existing instruments are used, the instrument package should be **pretested** to assess its length, clarity, and overall adequacy.

- Structured self-report instruments (**interview schedules** or **questionnaires**) may include open- or closed-ended questions. **Open-ended questions** permit respondents to reply in narrative fashion, whereas **closed-ended** (or **fixed-alternative**) **questions** offer *response alternatives* from which respondents must choose.

- Types of closed-ended questions include (1) **dichotomous questions**, which require a choice between two options (e.g., yes/no); (2) **multiple-choice questions**, which offer a range of alternatives; (3) **rank-order questions**, in which respondents are asked to rank concepts on a continuum; (4) **forced-choice questions**, which require respondents to choose between two competing positions; (5) **rating questions**, which ask respondents to make judgments along a bipolar dimension; (6) **checklists** that have several questions with the same response format; and (7) **visual analog scales** (VASs), which are used to measure subjective experiences such as pain. **Event history calendars** and diaries are used to capture data about the occurrence of events.

- Composite psychosocial **scales** are multiple-item self-report tools for measuring the degree to which individuals possess or are characterized by target attributes.

- **Likert scales** (**summated rating scales**) comprise a series of statements (**items**) about a phenomenon. Respondents typically indicate degree of agreement or disagreement with each statement; a total score is computed by summing item scores, each of which is scored for the intensity and direction of favorability expressed.

- **Semantic differentials** (SDs) consist of a series of bipolar rating scales on which respondents indicate reactions toward a phenomenon; scales can measure an evaluative (e.g., good/bad), activity (e.g., active/passive), or potency (e.g., strong/weak) dimension.

- **Q sorts**, in which people sort a set of card statements into piles according to specified criteria, can be used to measure attitudes, personality, and other psychological traits.

- **Vignettes** are brief descriptions of an event or situation to which respondents are asked to react. They are used to assess respondents' perceptions, hypothetical behaviors, or decisions.

- Questionnaires are less costly and time-consuming than interviews, offer the possibility of anonymity, and run no risk of interviewer bias. Interviews have higher response rates, are suitable for a wider variety of people, and yield richer data than questionnaires.

- Data quality in interviews depends on interviewers' interpersonal skills. Interviewers must put respondents at ease and build rapport, and need to be skillful at *probing* for additional information when respondents give incomplete responses.

- Group administration is the most economical way to distribute questionnaires. Another approach is to mail them, but this method tends to have low **response rates**, which can result in bias. Questionnaires can be distributed via the Internet, most often as a **web-based survey** that is accessed through a hypertext link. Several techniques, such as **follow-up reminders** and good **cover letters**, increase response rates to questionnaires.

- Structured self-reports are vulnerable to the risk of reporting biases. **Response set biases** reflect the tendency of some people to respond to questions in characteristic ways, independently of content. Common response sets include **social desirability, extreme response,** and **acquiescence (yea-saying).**

- Structured observational methods impose constraints on observers, to enhance the accuracy and objectivity of observations and to obtain an adequate representation of phenomena of interest.
- **Checklists** are used in observations to recording the occurrence or frequency of designated behaviors, events, or characteristics. Checklists are based on **category systems** for encoding observed phenomena into discrete categories.
- With **rating scales,** observers rate phenomena along a dimension that is typically bipolar (e.g., passive/aggressive); ratings are made either at specific intervals (e.g., every 5 minutes) or after observations are completed.
- **Time sampling** involves the specification of the duration and frequency of observational periods and intersession intervals. **Event sampling** selects integral behaviors or events of a special type for observation.
- Observational methods are an excellent way to operationalize some constructs, but are subject to various biases. The greater the degree of observer inference, the more likely that distortions will occur. The most prevalent observer biases include the **enhancement of contrast effect, central tendency bias,** the **halo effect, assimilatory biases, errors of leniency,** and **errors of severity.**
- **Biophysiologic measures** comprise **in vivo measurements** (those performed within or on living organisms, like blood pressure measurement) and **in vitro measurements** (those performed outside the organism's body, such as blood tests).
- Biophysiologic measures are objective, accurate, and precise, but care must be taken in using such measures with regard to practical, technical, and ethical considerations.
- When researchers cannot collect the data without assistance, they should carefully select data collection staff and formally train them.

STUDY ACTIVITIES

Chapter 13 of the *Resource Manual for Nursing Research: Generating and Assessing Evidence for Nursing Practice, 9th edition,* offers exercises and study suggestions for reinforcing concepts presented in this chapter. In addition, the following study questions can be addressed:

1. Suppose you were planning to conduct a statewide study of the work plans and intentions of nonemployed registered nurses in your state. Would you ask mostly open-ended or closed-ended questions? Would you adopt an interview or questionnaire approach? If a questionnaire, how would you distribute it?
2. Suppose that the study of nonemployed nurses were done by a mailed questionnaire. Draft a cover letter to accompany it.
3. A nurse researcher is planning to study temper tantrums displayed by hospitalized children. Would you recommend using a time sampling approach? Why or why not?

STUDIES CITED IN CHAPTER 13

Akhar-Danesh, N., Baxter, P., Valaitis, R., Stanyon, W., & Sproul, S. (2009). Nurse faculty perceptions of simulation use in nursing education. *Western Journal of Nursing Research, 31,* 312–329.

Alpert, P., Miller, S., Wallmann, H., Havey, R., Cross, C., Chevalia, T., Gillis, C. B., & Kodandapari, K. (2009). The effect of modified jazz dance on balance, cognition, and mood in older adults. *Journal of the American Academy of Nurse Practitioners, 21,* 108–115.

Ayhan, H., Iyigun, E., Tastan, S., Orhan, M., & Ozturk, E. (2009). Comparison of two different oxygen delivery methods in the early postoperative period. *Journal of Advanced Nursing, 65,* 1237–1247.

Berger, A., Treat Marunda, H., & Agrawal, S. (2009). Influence of menopausal status on sleep and hot flashes throughout breast adjuvant chemotherapy. *Journal of Obstetric, Gynecologic, & Neonatal Nursing, 38,* 353–366.

Brown, L., Thoyre, S., Pridham, K., & Schubert, C. (2009). The Mother-Infant Feeding Tool. *Journal of Obstetric, Gynecologic, & Neonatal Nursing, 38*, 491–503.

Bryanton, J., Gagnon, A., Hatem, M., & Johnston, C. (2009). Does perception of the childbirth experience predict women's early parenting behaviors? *Research in Nursing & Health, 32*, 191–203.

Choi, S., & Rankin, S. (2009). Glucose control in Korean immigrants with type 2 diabetes. *Western Journal of Nursing Research, 31*, 347–363.

Choi, J. Y., & Hwang, S. Y. (2009). Factors associated with health-related quality of life among low-compliance asthmatic adults in Korea. *Research in Nursing & Health, 32*, 140–147.

Conrad, A., & Altmaier, E. (2009). Specialized summer camp for children with cancer: Social support and adjustment. *Journal of Pediatric Oncology Nursing, 26*, 150–157.

Dirksen, S. R., Epstein, D., & Hoyt, M. (2009). Insomnia, depression, and distress among outpatients with prostate cancer. *Applied Nursing Research, 22*, 154–158.

Dorsey, S., Leitch, C., Renn, C., Lessans, S., Smith, B., Wang, X., & Dionne, R. (2009). Genome-wide screen identifies drug-induced regulation of the gene giant axonal neuropathy in a mouse model of antiretroviral-induced painful peripheral neuropathy. *Biological Research for Nursing, 11*, 7–16.

Foreman, S. W., Thomas, K., & Blackburn, S. (2008). Individual and gender differences matter in preterm infant state development. *Journal of Obstetric, Gynecologic, & Neonatal Nursing, 37*, 657–665.

Griffin, R., Polit, D., & Byrne, M. (2007). The effects of children's gender, race, and attractiveness on nurses' pain management decisions. *Research in Nursing & Health, 30*, 655–666.

Gross-King, M., Booth-Jones, M., & Couluris, M. (2008). Neurocognitive impairment in children treated for cancer. *Journal of Pediatric Oncology Nursing, 25*, 227–232.

Johnston, C., Filion, F., Campbell-Yeo, M., Goulet, C., Bell, L., McNaughton, K., Byron, J., Aita, M., Finley, G. A., Walker, C. D. (2008). Kangaroo mother care diminishes pain from heel lance in very preterm neonates. *BMC Pediatrics, 8*, 13.

Kang, D., Weaver, M., Park, N., Smith, B., McArdle, T., & Carpenter, J. (2009). Significant impairment in immune recovery after cancer treatment. *Nursing Research, 58*, 105–114.

Kleiber, C., & McCarthy, A. M. (2006). Evaluating instruments for a study on children's responses to a painful procedure when parents are distraction coaches. *Journal of Pediatric Nursing, 21*, 99–107.

Kleiber, C., McCathy, A. M., Hanrahan, K., Myers, L., & Weathers, N. (2007). Development of the Distraction Coaching Index. *Children's Healthcare, 36*, 219–235.

Kupferer, E., Dormire, S., & Becker, H. (2009). Complementary and alternative medicine use for vasomotor symptoms among women who have discontinued hormone therapy. *Journal of Obstetric, Gynecologic, & Neonatal Nursing, 38*, 50–59.

Liaw, J., Yang, L., Yuh, Y., & Yin, T. (2006). Effects of tub bathing procedures on preterm infants' behavior. *Journal of Nursing Research, 14*, 297–305.

Lynn, M., Morgan, J., & Moore, K. (2009). Development and testing of the Satisfaction in Nursing Scale. *Nursing Research, 58*, 166–174.

Mathew, A., Gasline, T., Dunning, K., & Ying, J. (2009). Central catheter blood sampling: the impact of changing the needleless caps prior to collection. *Journal of Infusion Nursing, 32*, 212–218.

McCaffrey, R. (2009). The effect of music on acute confusion in older adults after hip or knee surgery. *Applied Nursing Research, 22*, 107–112.

McCarthy, A. M., Hanrahan, K., Kleiber, C., Zimmerman, M. B., Lutgendorf, S., & Tsalikian, E. (2009). Normative salivary cortisol values and responsivity in children. *Applied Nursing Research, 22*, 54–62.

Neira, C., Hartig, M., Cowan, P., & Velasquez-Mieyer, P. (2009). The prevalence of impaired glucose metabolism in Hispanics with two or more risk factors for metabolic syndrome in the primary care setting. *Journal of the American Academy of Nurse Practitioners, 21*, 173–178.

Nyamathi, A., Berg, J., Jones, T., & Leake, B. (2005). Predictors of perceived health status of tuberculosis-infected homeless. *Western Journal of Nursing Research, 27*, 896–910.

Polit, D. F., London, A. S., & Martinez, J. M. (2001). *The health of poor urban women.* New York: MDRC.

Rempusheski, V. F., & O'Hara, C. (2005). Psychometric properties of the Granparent Perceptions of Family Scale (GPFS). *Nursing Research, 54*, 419–427.

Robb, S., Clair, A., Watanabe, M., Monahan, P., Azzouz, F., Stouffer, J., Ebberts, A., Darsie, E., Whitmer, C., Walker, J., Nelson, K., Hanson-Abromeit, D., Lane, D., & Hannan, A. (2008). A non-randomized controlled trial of the active music engagement (AME) intervention on children with cancer. *Psycho-oncology, 17*, 699–708.

Sarna, L., Bialous, S., Wells, M., Kotlerman, J., Wewers, M., & Froelicher, E. (2009). Frequency of nurses' smoking cessation interventions: Report from a national survey. *Journal of Clinical Nursing, 18*, 2066–2077.

Uitterhoeve, R., de Leeuw, J., Bensing, J., Heaven, C., Borm, G., deMulder, P., &van Achterberg, T. (2008). Cue-responding behaviours of oncology nurses in video-simulated interviews. *Journal of Advanced Nursing, 61*, 71–80.

Weiss, S. J. (1992). Measurement of the sensory qualities in tactile interaction. *Nursing Research, 41*, 82–86.

Yeo, S. (2009). Adherence to walking or stretching, and risk of preeclampsia in sedentary pregnant women. *Research in Nursing & Health, 32*, 379–390.

Methodologic and nonresearch references cited in this chapter can be found in a separate section at the end of the book.

14

Measurement and Data Quality

An ideal data collection procedure is one that captures a construct in a way that is accurate, truthful, and sensitive. Biophysiologic methods have a higher chance of success in attaining these goals than self-report or observational methods, but no method is flawless. In this chapter, we discuss criteria for evaluating the quality of data obtained with structured instruments.

We begin by discussing principles of measurement. Our discussion is based primarily on **classical measurement theory (CMT)**, the leading theory with regard to the measurement of affective constructs (i.e., constructs such as self-esteem or depression). An alternative measurement theory (*item response theory* or *IRT*) has gained in popularity, especially for measuring cognitive constructs (e.g., knowledge). We discuss IRT briefly in Chapter 15.

MEASUREMENT

Quantitative studies derive data through the measurement of variables. **Measurement** involves assigning numbers to represent the amount of an attribute present in an object or person, using a specified set of rules. Quantification and measurement go hand in hand. Attributes are not constant; they vary from day to day or from one person to another. Variability is presumed to be capable of a numeric expression signifying *how much* of an attribute is present. The purpose of assigning numbers is to differentiate between people with varying degrees of the attribute.

Rules and Measurement

Measurement involves assigning numbers according to rules. Rules for measuring temperature, weight, and other physical attributes are familiar to us. Rules for measuring many variables for nursing studies, however, have to be invented. Whether the data are collected by observation, self-report, or some other method, researchers must specify criteria for assigning numeric values to the characteristic of interest.

As an example, suppose we were studying parental attitudes toward dispensing condoms in school clinics, and we asked parents their extent of agreement with the following statement:

Teenagers should have access to contraceptives in school clinics.
- ❏ Strongly disagree
- ❏ Disagree
- ❏ Slightly disagree
- ❏ Neither agree nor disagree
- ❏ Slightly agree
- ❏ Agree
- ❏ Strongly agree

Responses to this question can be quantified by developing a system for assigning numbers to them. Note that *any* rule would satisfy the definition of measurement. We could assign the value of 30 to "strongly agree," 28 to "agree," 20 to "slightly agree," and so on, but there is no justification for doing so. In measuring attributes, researchers strive to use good, meaningful rules. Without *a priori* knowledge of the "distance" between response options, the most practical approach is to assign a 7 to "strongly agree" and a 1 to "strongly disagree." This rule would quantitatively differentiate, in increments of one point, among people with seven different opinions. Researchers seldom know in advance if their rules are the best possible. New measurement rules reflect hypotheses about how attributes vary. The adequacy of the hypotheses—that is, the worth of the instruments—needs to be assessed empirically.

Researchers try to link numeric values to reality. To state this goal more technically, measurement procedures are ideally isomorphic to reality. The term *isomorphism* signifies equivalence or similarity between two phenomena. An instrument cannot be useful unless the measurements resulting from it correspond with the real world.

To illustrate the concept of isomorphism, suppose a standardized test was administered to 10 students, who obtained the following scores: 345, 395, 430, 435, 490, 505, 550, 570, 620, and 640. These values are shown at the top of Figure 14.1. Suppose that in

reality the students' true scores on a hypothetically perfect test were as follows: 360, 375, 430, 465, 470, 500, 550, 610, 590, and 670, shown at the bottom of Figure 14.1. Although not perfect, the test came close to representing true scores; only two people (H and I) were improperly ordered. This example illustrates a measure whose isomorphism with reality is high but improvable.

Researchers work with fallible measures. Instruments that measure psychosocial phenomena are less likely to correspond to reality than physical measures, but few instruments are error free.

Advantages of Measurement

What exactly does measurement accomplish? Consider how handicapped healthcare professionals would be in the absence of measurement. What would happen, for example, if there were no measures of blood pressure or temperature? Subjective evaluations of clinical outcomes would have to be used. A principal strength of measurement is that it removes subjectivity and guesswork. Because measurement is based on explicit rules, resulting information tends to be objective—that is, it can be independently verified. Two people measuring the weight of a person using the same scale would likely get identical results. Most measures incorporate mechanisms for minimizing subjectivity.

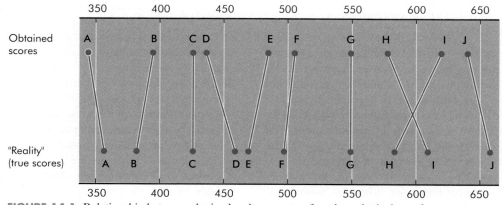

FIGURE 14.1 Relationship between obtained and true scores for a hypothetical set of test scores.

Measurement also makes it possible to obtain reasonably precise information. Instead of describing Nathan as "rather tall," we can depict him as being 6 feet 3 inches tall. With precise measures, researchers can differentiate among people with different degrees of an attribute.

Finally, measurement is a language of communication. Numbers are less vague than words and can communicate information more accurately. If a researcher reported that the average oral temperature of a sample of patients was "somewhat high," different readers might make different inferences about the sample's physiologic state. However, if the researcher reported an average temperature of 99.6°F, there would be no ambiguity.

Errors of Measurement

Procedures for obtaining measurements, as well as the objects being measured, are susceptible to influences that can alter the resulting data. Some influences can be controlled to a certain degree, and attempts should be made to do so, but such efforts are rarely completely successful.

Instruments that are not perfectly accurate yield measurements containing some error. Within classical measurement theory, an **observed** (or **obtained**) **score** can be conceptualized as having two parts— an error component and a true component. This can be written symbolically as follows:

Obtained score = True score ± Error

or

$$X_O = X_T \pm X_E$$

The first term in the equation is an observed score—for example, a score on an anxiety scale. X_T is the value that would be obtained with an infallible measure. The **true score** is hypothetical—it can never be known because measures are *not* infallible. The final term is the **error of measurement**. The difference between true and obtained scores is the result of factors that distort the measurement.

Decomposing obtained scores in this manner highlights an important point. When researchers measure an attribute, they are also *measuring* attributes that are not of interest. The true score component is what they hope to isolate; the error component is a composite of other factors that are also being measured, contrary to their wishes. This concept can be illustrated with an exaggerated example. Suppose a researcher measured the weight of 10 people on a spring scale. As participants step on the scale, the researcher places a hand on their shoulders and applies pressure. The resulting measures (the X_Os) will be biased upward because scores reflect both actual weight (X_T) and pressure (X_E). Errors of measurement are problematic because their value is unknown and also because they often are variable. In this example, the amount of pressure applied likely would vary from one person to the next. In other words, the proportion of true score component in an obtained score varies from one person to the next.

Many factors contribute to errors of measurement. Some errors are random while others are systematic, reflecting *bias*. Common influences on measurement error include the following:

1. *Situational contaminants.* Scores can be affected by the conditions under which they are produced. A participant's awareness of an observer's presence (reactivity) is one source of bias. Environmental factors, such as temperature, lighting, and time of day, are potential sources of measurement error.
2. *Transitory personal factors.* A person's score can be influenced by such personal states as fatigue or mood. In some cases, such factors directly affect the measurement, as when anxiety affects pulse rate measurement. In other cases, personal factors alter scores by influencing people's motivation to cooperate, act naturally, or do their best.
3. *Response-set biases.* Relatively enduring characteristics of people can interfere with accurate measurements. Response sets such as social desirability or acquiescence are potential biases in self-report measures, particularly in psychological scales (Chapter 13).
4. *Administration variations.* Alterations in the methods of collecting data from one person to the next can result in score variations unrelated

to variations in the target attribute. For example, if some physiologic measures are taken before a feeding and others are taken after a feeding, then measurement errors can potentially occur.

5. *Instrument clarity*. If the directions on an instrument are poorly understood, then scores may be affected. For example, questions in a self-report instrument may be interpreted differently by different respondents, leading to a distorted measure of the variable.

6. *Item sampling*. Errors can be introduced as a result of the sampling of items used in the measure. For example, a nursing student's score on a 100-item test of critical care nursing knowledge will be influenced by *which* 100 questions are included. A person might get 95 questions correct on one test but only 92 right on another similar test.

7. *Instrument format*. Technical characteristics of an instrument can influence measurements. For example, the ordering of questions in an instrument may influence responses.

⊃ **T I P :** The Toolkit section of Chapter 14 of the *Resource Manual* includes a list of suggestions for enhancing data quality and minimizing measurement error in quantitative studies.

RELIABILITY OF MEASURING INSTRUMENTS

The reliability of a quantitative instrument is a major criterion for assessing its quality. An instrument's **reliability** is the consistency with which it measures the target attribute. If a scale weighed a person at 120 pounds one minute and 150 pounds the next, it would be unreliable. The less variation an instrument produces in repeated measurements, the higher its reliability. Thus, reliability can be equated with a measure's stability, consistency, or dependability.

Reliability also concerns accuracy. An instrument is reliable to the extent that its measures reflect true scores—that is, to the extent that measurement errors are absent from obtained scores. Reliable measures

maximize the true score component and minimize error.

These two ways of explaining reliability (consistency and accuracy) are not so different as they might appear. Errors of measurement that impinge on an instrument's accuracy also affect its consistency. The example of the scale with variable weight readings illustrates this point. Suppose that the true weight of a person is 125 pounds, but that two independent measurements yielded 120 and 150 pounds. In terms of the equation presented in the previous section, we could express the measurements as follows:

$$120 = 125 - 5$$
$$150 = 125 + 25$$

The errors of measurement for the two trials (−5 and +25, respectively) resulted in scores that are inconsistent *and* inaccurate.

The reliability of an instrument can be assessed in various ways, and the appropriate method depends on the nature of the instrument and on the aspect of reliability of greatest concern. Three key aspects are stability, internal consistency, and equivalence.

Stability

The **stability** of an instrument is the extent to which similar scores are obtained on separate occasions. The reliability estimate focuses on the instrument's susceptibility to extraneous influences over time, such as participant fatigue.

Assessments of stability involve procedures that evaluate **test–retest reliability**. Researchers administer the same measure to a sample twice and then compare the scores. The comparison is performed objectively by computing a **reliability coefficient**, which is an index of the magnitude of the test's reliability.

To explain reliability coefficients, we must discuss a statistic called a **correlation coefficient**. We have pointed out that researchers seek to detect and explain relationships among phenomena. For example, is there a relationship between patients' gastric acidity levels and degree of stress? The correlation coefficient is a tool for quantitatively describing the magnitude and direction of a relationship between two variables. The computation of this index does not concern us here. It is more important to understand how to read a correlation coefficient.

Two variables that are obviously related are people's height and weight. Tall people tend to be heavier than short people. We would say that there was a **perfect relationship** if the tallest person in a population were the heaviest, the second tallest person were the second heaviest, and so forth. Correlation coefficients summarize how perfect a relationship is. The possible values for a correlation coefficient range from –1.00 through .00 to +1.00. If height and weight were perfectly correlated, the correlation coefficient expressing this relationship would be 1.00. Because the relationship exists but is not perfect, the correlation coefficient is in the vicinity of .50 or .60. The relationship between height and weight can be described as a **positive relationship** because *increases* in height tend to be associated with *increases* in weight.

When two variables are totally unrelated, the correlation coefficient equals zero. One might expect that women's dress sizes are unrelated to their intelligence. Large women are as likely to perform well on IQ tests as small women. The correlation coefficient summarizing such a relationship would presumably be in the vicinity of .00.

Correlation coefficients running from .00 to –1.00 express **inverse** or **negative relationships**. When two variables are inversely related, increases in one variable are associated with *decreases* in the second variable. Suppose that there is an inverse relationship between people's age and the amount of sleep they get. This means that, on average, the older the person, the fewer the hours of sleep. If the relationship were perfect (e.g., if the oldest person in a population got the least sleep, and so on), the correlation coefficient would be –1.00. In actuality, the relationship between age and sleep is probably modest—in the vicinity of –.15 or –.20. A correlation coefficient of this magnitude describes a weak relationship: older people *tend* to sleep fewer hours and younger people *tend* to sleep more, but nevertheless some younger people sleep few hours, and some older people sleep a lot.

Now, we can discuss the use of correlation coefficients to compute reliability estimates. With test–retest reliability, an instrument is administered twice to the same people. Suppose we wanted to assess the stability of a self-esteem scale. Self-esteem is a fairly stable attribute that does not fluctuate much from day to day, so we would expect a reliable measure of it to yield consistent scores on two occasions. To check the instrument's stability, we administer the scale 2 weeks apart to 10 people. Fictitious data for this example are presented in Table 14.1. It can be seen that, in general, differences in scores on the two testings are not large. The reliability coefficient for test–retest estimates is the correlation coefficient between the two sets of scores. In this example, the reliability coefficient is .95, which is high.

The value of the reliability coefficient theoretically can range between –1.00 and +1.00, like other correlation coefficients. A negative coefficient would have been obtained in our example if those with high self-esteem scores at time 1 had low scores at time 2, and vice versa. In practice, reliability coefficients usually range between .00 and 1.00. The higher the coefficient, the more stable the

TABLE 14.1	Fictitious Data for Test–Retest Reliability of Self-Esteem Scale	
PARTICIPANT NUMBER	**TIME 1**	**TIME 2**
1	55	57
2	49	46
3	78	74
4	37	35
5	44	46
6	50	56
7	58	55
8	62	66
9	48	50
10	67	63	$r = .95$

measure. Reliability coefficients above .80 usually are considered good.

The test–retest method is easy, and can be used with self-report, observational, and physiologic measures. Yet, this approach has certain disadvantages. One issue is that many traits *do* change over time, independently of the measure's stability. Attitudes, knowledge, perceptions, and so on can be modified by experiences between testings. Test–retest procedures confound changes from measurement error with true changes in the attribute. Still, there are many relatively enduring attributes for which a test–retest approach is suitable.

Stability estimates suffer from other problems, however. One possibility is that people's responses (or observers' coding) on the second administration will be influenced by their memory of initial responses, regardless of the actual values the second day. Such memory interference results in spuriously high reliability coefficients. Another difficulty is that people may actually change *as a result of* the first administration. Finally, people may not be as careful using the same instrument a second time. If they find the process boring on the second occasion, then responses could be haphazard, resulting in a spuriously low estimate of stability.

On the whole, reliability coefficients tend to be higher for short-term retests than for long-term retests (those greater than 1 month) because of actual changes in the attribute being measured. Stability indexes are most appropriate for relatively stable characteristics such as personality, abilities, or certain physical attributes such as adult height.

It might be noted that while most test–retest efforts involve the calculation of a standard correlation coefficient, as just described, other methods are sometimes used. For example, Yen and Lo (2002) describe how an *intraclass correlation* (ICC) approach offers advantages because of the ability of this index to detect systematic error.

Example of test–retest reliability: Kao and Lynn (2009) developed the Family Caregiver Medication Administration Hassles Scale for use with Mexican American family caregivers of older relatives. The 3-week test–retest reliability for the scale was .64.

Internal Consistency

Scales and tests that involve summing item scores are typically evaluated for their internal consistency. Scales designed to measure an attribute ideally are composed of items that measure that attribute and nothing else. On a scale to measure nurses' empathy, it would be inappropriate to include an item that measures diagnostic competence. An instrument may be said to be **internally consistent** or *homogeneous* to the extent that its items measure the same trait.

Internal consistency reliability is the most widely used reliability approach. Its popularity reflects the fact that it is economical (it requires only one administration) and is the best means of assessing an especially important source of measurement error in psychosocial instruments, the sampling of items.

➔ **T I P :** Many scales contain multiple **subscales**, each of which taps distinct but related concepts (e.g., a measure of fatigue might include subscales for mental and physical fatigue). The internal consistency of each subscale should be assessed. If subscale scores are summed for a total score, the scale's overall internal consistency is also computed.

The most widely used method for evaluating internal consistency is **coefficient alpha** (or **Cronbach's alpha**). Coefficient alpha can be interpreted like other reliability coefficients: the normal range of values is between .00 and +1.00, and higher values reflect higher internal consistency. It is beyond the scope of this text to explain this method in detail, but information is available in psychometric textbooks (e.g., Nunnally & Bernstein, 1994; Waltz, et al. 2010). Most statistical software can be used to calculate alpha. The research example at the end of Chapter 15 presents some computer output for a reliability analysis.

In summary, coefficient alpha is an index of internal consistency to estimate the extent to which different subparts of an instrument (i.e., items) are reliably measuring the critical attribute. Cronbach's alpha does not, however, evaluate fluctuations over time as a source of unreliability.

Example of internal consistency reliability: Villanueva and colleagues (2009) developed and evaluated a scale to measure nonpsychiatric health-care providers' attitudes toward pediatric patients with mental illness. The 18-item scale had good internal consistency, alpha = .85.

Equivalence

Equivalence, in the context of reliability assessment, primarily concerns the degree to which two or more independent observers or coders agree about scoring. If there is a high level of agreement, then the assumption is that measurement errors have been minimized. Nurse researchers are especially likely to use this approach with observational measures, although it can be used in other applications—for example, for evaluating the consistency of coding open-ended questions or the accuracy of extracting data from records.

The reliability of ratings and classifications can be enhanced by careful training and the specification of clearly defined, nonoverlapping categories. Even when such care is taken, researchers should assess the reliability of observational instruments and coding systems. In this case, "instrument" includes both the category or rating system *and* the observers or coders making the measurements.

Interrater (or *interobserver*) **reliability** can be assessed using various approaches, which can be categorized as consensus, consistency, and measurement approaches (Stemler, 2004). Many interrater reliability indexes used by nurse researchers are of the consensus type, in which the goal is to have observers share a common interpretation of a construct, and to reach consensus (exact agreement). Consensus measures of interrater reliability for observational coding involve having two or more trained observers watching an event simultaneously, and independently recording data. The data are then used to compute an index of agreement between observers. (For coders, information would be independently coded into categories and then intercoder agreement would be assessed.) When ratings are dichotomous, one procedure is to calculate the proportion of agreements, using the following equation:

$$\frac{\text{Number of agreement}}{\text{Number of agreement} + \text{disagreements}}$$

This formula unfortunately tends to overestimate agreements because it fails to account for agreement by chance. If a behavior being observed were coded for absence versus presence, the observers would agree 50% of the time by chance alone. A widely used statistic in this situation is Cohen's **kappa**, which adjusts for chance agreements. Different standards have been proposed for acceptable levels of kappa, but there is some agreement that a value of .60 is minimally acceptable, and that values of .75 or higher are very good.

For certain types of data (e.g., ratings on a multipoint scale), correlation techniques are suitable, and these typically capture consistency rather than consensus. For example, a correlation coefficient can be computed to demonstrate the strength of the relationship between one rater's scores and another's. The **intraclass correlation coefficient** (ICC) can also be used to assess interrater reliability (Shrout & Fleiss, 1979).

Example of interrater reliability: Voepel-Lewis and colleagues (2010) assessed the FLACC Behavioral Scale, an observational tool to assess pain in critically ill patients. Exact agreement, kappa values, and intraclass correlation coefficients suggested strong interrater reliability of the measure.

Interpretation of Reliability Coefficients

Reliability coefficients are important indicators of an instrument's quality. Unreliable measures reduce statistical power and hence affect statistical conclusion validity. If data fail to support a hypothesis, one possibility is that the instruments were unreliable—not necessarily that the expected relationships do not exist. Knowing an instrument's reliability thus is critical in interpreting research results, especially if hypotheses are not supported.

For group-level comparisons, coefficients in the vicinity of .70 may be adequate (especially for subscales), but coefficients of .80 or greater are highly desirable. By group-level comparisons, we mean that researchers compare scores of groups, such as male versus female or experimental versus control participants. The reliability coefficients for measures used for making decisions about individuals ideally should be .90 or better. For instance, if a test score was used as a criterion for admission to a nursing program, then the test's accuracy would be of critical importance to both the applicants and the school of nursing.

Reliability coefficients have a special interpretation that relates to our discussion of decomposing observed scores into error and true score components. Suppose we administered a scale that measures hopefulness to 50 patients with cancer. The scores would vary from one person to another—that is, some people would be more hopeful than others. Some variability in scores is true variability, reflecting real individual differences in hopefulness; some variability, however, is error. Thus,

$$V_O = V_T + V_E$$

where V_O = observed total variability in scores
V_T = true variability
V_E = variability owing to errors

A reliability coefficient is directly associated with this equation. *Reliability is the proportion of true variability to the total obtained variability,* or

$$r = \frac{V_T}{V_O}$$

If, for example, the reliability coefficient were .85, then 85% of the variability in obtained scores would represent true individual differences, and 15% of the variability would reflect extraneous fluctuations. Looked at in this way, it should be clear why instruments with reliability lower than .70 are risky to use.

Factors Affecting Reliability

Various things affect an instrument's reliability, and these factors are useful to keep in mind in selecting an instrument. First, the reliability of composite self-report and observational scales is partly a function of their length (i.e., number of items). To improve reliability, more items tapping the same concept should be added. Items that have no discriminating power (i.e., that elicit similar responses from everyone) should, however, be removed. Item analysis procedures for guiding decisions about item retention, modification, or deletion are outlined in Chapter 15.

With observational scales, reliability can be improved by greater precision in defining categories, or greater clarity in explaining the underlying construct for rating scales. The best means of enhancing reliability in observational studies, however, is thorough observer training.

An instrument's reliability is related in part to the heterogeneity of the sample with which it is used. The more homogeneous the sample (i.e., the more similar their scores), the lower the reliability coefficient will be. This is because instruments are designed to measure differences among those being measured. If the sample is homogeneous, then it is more difficult for the instrument to discriminate reliably among those who possess varying degrees of the attribute. For example, a depression scale will be less reliable when administered to a homeless sample than when it is used with a general population.

An instrument's reliability is not a fixed entity. *The reliability of an instrument is a property not of the instrument but rather of the instrument when administered to certain people under certain conditions.* A scale that reliably measures dependence in hospitalized adults may be unreliable with nursing homes residents. This means that in selecting an instrument, it is important to know the characteristics of the group with which it was developed. If the group is similar to the population for a new study, then the reliability estimate calculated by the scale developer is probably a reasonably good index of the instrument's accuracy in the new research.

➲ **TIP:** You should not be satisfied with an instrument that will *probably* be reliable in your study. The recommended procedure is to compute new estimates of reliability whenever research data are collected.

Finally, reliability estimates vary according to the procedures used to obtain them. A scale's test–retest reliability is rarely the same value as its internal consistency reliability. In selecting an instrument, researchers need to determine which aspect of reliability (stability, internal consistency, or equivalence) is relevant.

> **Example of different reliability estimates:** Schilling and colleagues (2009) developed a scale to measure self-management of type I diabetes among adolescents. They evaluated the scale's reliability using test–retest and internal consistency approaches. As an example of their findings, the coefficient alpha for the 7-item Goals subscale was .75. The subscale's test–retest reliability was .60 at 2 weeks and .59 at 3 months.

VALIDITY

A second key criterion for evaluating an instrument is its validity. **Validity** is the degree to which an instrument measures what it is supposed to measure. When researchers develop an instrument to measure hopelessness, they need to be sure that resulting scores validly reflect this construct and not something else, like depression.

Reliability and validity are not independent qualities of an instrument. *A measuring device that is unreliable cannot be valid.* An instrument cannot validly measure an attribute if it is inconsistent and inaccurate. An unreliable instrument contains too much error to be a valid indicator of the target variable. An instrument can, however, be reliable without being valid. Suppose we had the idea to assess patients' anxiety by measuring their height. We could obtain highly accurate, consistent measurements of their height, but such measures would not be valid indicators of anxiety. Thus, the high reliability of an instrument provides no evidence of its validity; low reliability *is* evidence of low validity.

Like reliability, validity has different aspects and assessment approaches, but unlike reliability, an instrument's validity is difficult to evaluate. There are no equations that can easily be applied to the scores of a hopelessness scale to estimate how good a job the scale is doing in measuring the critical variable. Validation is an evidence-building enterprise, in which the goal is to assemble sufficient evidence from which validity can be inferred. The greater the amount of evidence supporting validity, the more sound the inference.

> ⮕ **T I P :** Instrument developers usually gather evidence of the validity and reliability of their instrument in a **psychometric assessment** before making the instrument available for general use. If you use an existing instrument, choose one with demonstrated high reliability and validity.

Face Validity

Face validity refers to whether the instrument *looks* like it is measuring the target construct. Although face validity is not considered strong evidence of validity, it is helpful for a measure to have face validity if other types of validity have also been demonstrated. It might be easier to persuade people to participate in a study if the instruments have face validity, for example.

> **Example of face validity:** Jones and colleagues (2008) developed the Stroke Self-Efficacy Questionnaire for use by practitioners working in stroke care. Face validity was addressed through consultation with experts in stroke rehabilitation and self-efficacy theory, as well as with stroke survivors.

Content Validity

Content validity concerns the degree to which an instrument has an appropriate sample of items for the construct being measured and adequately covers the construct domain. Content validity is relevant for both affective measures (i.e., measures of psychological traits) and cognitive measures.

For cognitive measures, the content validity question is, how representative are the test questions of the universe of questions on this topic? For example, suppose we were testing students' knowledge about major nursing theories. The test would not be content valid if it omitted questions about, for example, Orem's Self-Care Theory.

Content validity is also relevant in developing affective measures. Researchers designing a new instrument should begin with a thorough conceptualization of the construct so the instrument can capture the full content domain. Such a conceptualization might come from a variety of sources, including rich first-hand knowledge, an exhaustive literature review, consultation with experts, or findings from a qualitative inquiry.

Example of using qualitative data to enhance content validity: Williams and Kristjanson (2009) developed a scale to measure hospitalized patients' perceptions of the emotional care they experienced. The items were based on the themes identified in a grounded theory study, which explored characteristics of interpersonal interactions patients perceived to be therapeutic.

An instrument's content validity is necessarily based on judgment. There are no completely objective methods of ensuring adequate content coverage on an instrument, but it is common to use a panel of experts to evaluate the content validity of new instruments.

There are various approaches to assessing content validity using an expert panel, but nurse researchers have been in the forefront in developing approaches that involve the calculation of a **content validity index (CVI)**. The experts are asked to evaluate individual items on the new measure as well as the overall instrument. Two key issues in such an evaluation are whether individual items are relevant and appropriate in terms of the construct, and whether the items taken together adequately measure all dimensions of the construct.

At the item level, a common procedure is to have experts rate items on a four-point scale of relevance. There are several variations of labeling the 4 points, but the scale used most often is as follows: 1 = *not relevant*, 2 = *somewhat relevant*, 3 = *quite relevant*, 4 = *highly relevant*. Then, for each item, the **item CVI (I-CVI)** is computed as the number of experts giving a rating of 3 or 4, divided by the

number of experts—that is, the proportion in agreement about relevance. For example, an item rated as "quite" or "highly" relevant by 4 out of 5 judges would have an I-CVI of .80, which is considered an acceptable value.

There are two approaches to calculating **scale CVIs (S-CVIs)**, and unfortunately, instrument development papers seldom indicate which approach was used (Polit & Beck, 2006). One approach is to calculate the percentage of items on the scale for which *all* judges agreed on content validity. In other words, if a 10-item scale had 6 items for which the I-CVIs were 1.00, then the S-CVI would be .60. We call this the S-CVI/UA (universal agreement) approach. Because disagreements (as well as agreements) can occur by chance, and because disagreements could reflect bias or misunderstanding, we find this approach too stringent.

A second method is to compute the S-CVI by averaging I-CVIs. We recommend the averaging approach, which we refer to as S-CVI/Ave, and suggest a value of .90 as the standard for establishing excellent content validity (Polit & Beck, 2006). Content validation should be done with at least 3 experts, but a larger group is preferable. Further guidance is offered in Chapter 15.

Example of using a content validity index: Chien and Chan (2009) tested the Chinese version of the Level of Expressed Emotion Scale, a scale used with families of people with schizophrenia. The item-level CVIs ranged from .86 to 1.00 and the scale-level CVI, using the averaging approach, was .993.

Criterion-Related Validity

An instrument is said to have **criterion-related validity** if its scores correlate highly with scores on an external criterion. For example, if scores on a scale of attitudes toward premarital sex correlate highly with subsequent loss of virginity in a sample of teenagers, then the attitude scale would have good validity. For criterion-related validity, the key issue is whether the instrument is a useful predictor of other behaviors, experiences, or conditions.

A requirement of this approach is the availability of a reliable and valid criterion with which measures on the instrument can be compared. This is, unfortunately, seldom easy. If we were developing an instrument to measure nursing students' clinical skills, we might use supervisory ratings as our criterion—but can we be sure that these ratings are valid and reliable? The ratings might themselves need validation. Criterion-related validity is most appropriate when there is a concrete, reliable criterion. For example, a scale to measure smokers' motivation to quit smoking has a clear-cut, objective criterion: subsequent smoking.

Once a criterion is selected, a criterion-related **validity coefficient** can be computed by correlating scores on the instrument and the criterion. The magnitude of the coefficient is a direct estimate of how valid the instrument is, according to this validation method. To illustrate, suppose we developed a scale to measure nurses' professionalism. We administer the instrument to a sample of nurses and also ask the nurses to indicate how many professional conferences they have attended. The conference variable was chosen as one of many potential objective criteria of professionalism. Fictitious data are presented in Table 14.2. The correlation coefficient of .83 indicates that the professionalism scale correlates fairly well with the number of conferences attended. Whether the scale is really measuring professionalism is a different issue—an issue that is a construct validation concern discussed in the next section.

A distinction is sometimes made between two types of criterion-related validity. **Predictive validity** refers to the adequacy of an instrument in differentiating between people's performance on a future criterion. When a school of nursing correlates incoming students' high school grades with subsequent grade-point averages, the predictive validity of the high school grades for nursing school performance is being evaluated.

Example of predictive validity: Chang and colleagues (2009) developed and tested the Chinese version of the Positive and Negative Suicide Ideation Inventory. To assess predictive validity, a subsample of students used in the original instrument development study was recruited 1 year later to see if scores on the scale were predictive of recent suicide attempts.

Concurrent validity reflects an instrument's ability to distinguish individuals who differ on a present criterion. For example, a psychological test to differentiate between patients in a mental institution who can and cannot be released could be correlated with current behavioral ratings of healthcare

TABLE 14.2	Fictitious Data for Criterion-Related Validity Example	
PARTICIPANT	**SCORE ON PROFESSIONALISM SCALE**	**NUMBER OF NURSING CONFERENCES**
1	25	2
2	30	4
3	17	0
4	20	1
5	22	0
6	27	2
7	29	5
8	19	1
9	28	3
10	15	1

$r = .83$

personnel. The difference between predictive and concurrent validity, then, is the difference in the timing of obtaining measurements on a criterion.

> **Example of concurrent validity:** Cha and colleagues (2008) assessed the concurrent validity of a condom self-efficacy scale in Korean college students by correlating scores on the scale with actual condom use.

Criterion-related validation is most often used in practically oriented research. Criterion-related validity is helpful in assisting decision makers by giving them some assurance that their decisions will be effective, fair, and, in short, valid.

Construct Validity

Construct validity is a key criterion for assessing the quality of a study. As noted in Chapter 10, construct validity concerns inferences from study particulars (such as measures used to operationalize variables) to higher-order constructs. The key construct validity question in measurement is: What is this instrument *really* measuring? Unfortunately, the more abstract the concept, the more difficult it is to establish construct validity; at the same time, the more abstract the concept, the less suitable it is to rely on criterion-related validity. It is really not just a question of suitability, but feasibility. What objective criterion is there for such concepts as empathy or separation anxiety?

Construct validation of an instrument is a challenging but vital task. Construct validation is a hypothesis-testing endeavor, typically linked to a theoretical perspective about the construct. In validating a measure of death anxiety, its relationship to a criterion would be less informative than its correspondence to a cogent conceptualization of death anxiety. Construct validation can be approached in several ways, but it always involves logical analysis and hypothesis tests. Constructs are explicated in terms of other abstract concepts; researchers develop hypotheses about the manner in which the target construct functions in relation to other constructs.

There are a number of ways to gather evidence about construct validity, which we discuss in this section. It should also be noted, however, that if an instrument developer has taken strong steps to ensure the content validity of the instrument, construct validity will also be strengthened.

Known Groups

One construct validation approach is the **known-groups technique**, which yields evidence of **contrast validity**. In this procedure, the instrument is administered to groups hypothesized to differ on the critical attribute because of a known characteristic. For instance, in validating a measure of fear of childbirth, we could contrast the scores of primiparas and multiparas. We would expect that women who had never given birth would be more anxious than women who had done so, and so we might question the instrument's validity if such differences did not emerge. We would not necessarily expect large differences; some primiparas would feel little anxiety, and some multiparas would express fears. We would, however, hypothesize differences in *average* group scores.

> **Example of the known-groups technique:** Gozum and Hacihasanoglu (2009) did a psychometric assessment of the Turkish version of the Medication Adherence Self-Efficacy Scale with a sample of hypertensive patients. Using the known-groups approach, they compared scale scores for those with controlled versus uncontrolled blood pressure.

Hypothesized Relationships

A similar method of construct validation involves testing hypothesized relationships, often on the basis of theory or prior research. This is really a variant of the known-groups approach, which involves hypotheses about the relationship between the measure of the construct and a variable representing group membership. A researcher might reason as follows:

- According to theory, construct X is positively related to construct Y.
- Instrument A is a measure of construct X; instrument B is a measure of construct Y.

- Scores on A and B are correlated positively, as predicted.
- Therefore, it is inferred that A and B are valid measures of X and Y.

This logical analysis does not constitute proof of construct validity, but yields important evidence. Construct validation is essentially an ongoing evidence-building enterprise.

Example of testing relationships: Simmons and colleagues (2009) developed and tested a scale to measure psychological adjustment in patients with an ostomy. In the construct validation efforts, they hypothesized that adjustment scores would be positively correlated with time elapsed since surgery and with scores on an acceptance of illness scale, and their hypotheses were supported.

Convergent and Discriminant Validity

The **multitrait–multimethod matrix method (MTMM)** is a significant construct validation tool (Campbell & Fiske, 1959). This procedure involves the concepts of convergence and discriminability. **Convergence** is evidence that different methods of measuring a construct yield similar results. Different measurement approaches should converge on the construct. **Discriminability** is the ability to differ-

entiate the construct from other similar constructs. Campbell and Fiske argued that evidence of both convergence and discriminability should be brought to bear in construct validation.

To help explain the MTMM approach, fictitious data from a study to validate a "need for autonomy" measure are presented in Table 14.3. In using this approach, researchers must measure the critical concept by two or more methods. Suppose we measured need for autonomy in nursing home residents by (1) giving a sample of residents a self-report scale (the measure we are attempting to validate), (2) asking nurses to rate residents after observing them in a task designed to elicit autonomy or dependence, and (3) having residents react to a pictorial stimulus depicting an autonomy-relevant situation (a so-called *projective* measure).

A second requirement of the full MTMM is to measure a differentiating construct, using the same measuring methods. In the current example, suppose we wanted to differentiate "need for autonomy" from "need for affiliation." The discriminant concept must be similar to the focal concept, as in our example: We would expect that people with high need for autonomy would tend to be relatively low on need for affiliation. The point of including both concepts in a single validation study is to gather evidence

TABLE 14.3 Multitrait–Multimethod Matrix

METHOD	TRAITS	SELF-REPORT (1)		OBSERVATION (2)		PROJECTIVE (3)	
		AUT$_1$	AFF$_1$	AUT$_2$	AFF$_2$	AUT$_3$	AFF$_3$
Self-report (1)	AUT$_1$	(.88)					
	AFF$_1$	−.38	(.86)				
Observation (2)	AUT$_2$	.60	−.19	(.79)			
	AFF$_2$	−.21	.58	−.39	(.80)		
Projective (3)	AUT$_3$	.51	−.18	.55	−.12	(.74)	
	AFF$_3$	−.14	.49	−.17	.54	−.32	(.72)

AUT = need for autonomy trait; AFF = need for affiliation trait.

that the two concepts are distinct, rather than two different labels for the same underlying attribute.

The numbers in Table 14.3 represent correlation coefficients between scores on six measures (two traits × three methods). For instance, the coefficient of −.38 at the intersection of AUT_1–AFF_1 is the correlation between self-report scores on the need for autonomy and need for affiliation measures. Recall that a minus sign before the correlation coefficient signifies an inverse relationship. In this case, the −.38 tells us that there was a slight tendency for people scoring high on the need for autonomy scale to score low on the need for affiliation scale. (The numbers in parentheses along the diagonal of this matrix are the reliability coefficients.)

Various parts of the MTMM matrix have a bearing on construct validity. The most direct evidence (**convergent validity**) comes from the correlations between two different methods measuring the same trait. In the case of AUT_1–AUT_2, the coefficient is .60, which is reasonably high. Convergent validity should be large enough to encourage further scrutiny of the matrix. Second, the convergent validity entries should be higher, in absolute magnitude,* than correlations between measures that have neither method nor trait in common. That is, AUT_1–AUT_2 (.60) should be greater than AUT_2–AFF_1 (−.21) or AUT_1–AFF_2 (−.19), as it is here. This requirement is a minimum one that, if failed, should cause researchers to have serious doubts about the measures. Third, convergent validity coefficients should be greater than coefficients between measures of different traits by a single method. Once again, the matrix in Table 14.3 fulfills this criterion: AUT_1–AUT_2 (.60) and AUT_2–AUT_3 (.55) are higher in absolute value than AUT_1–AFF_1 (−.38), AUT_2–AFF_2 (−.39), and AUT_3–AFF_3 (−.32). The last two requirements provide evidence for **discriminant validity**.

The evidence is seldom as clear-cut as in this contrived example. Indeed, a common problem with MTMM is interpreting the pattern of coefficients. Another issue is that there are no clear-cut criteria

for deciding whether MTMM requirements have been met—that is, there are no objective means of assessing the magnitude of similarities and differences within the matrix. The MTMM is nevertheless a valuable tool for exploring construct validity. Researchers sometimes decide to use MMTM concepts even when the full model is not feasible, as in focusing only on convergent validity.

Example of convergent and discriminant validity: Morea and colleagues (2008) developed and tested the Illness Self-Concept Scale, an instrument designed to predict adjustment in fibromyalgia. Their analyses provided some evidence that their construct, illness self-concept, is distinct from other similar constructs like depression (discriminant validity) and various analyses also supported evidence of convergent validity.

Factor Analysis

Another approach to construct validation uses a statistical procedure called factor analysis. Although factor analysis, which is discussed in Chapter 15, is computationally complex, it is conceptually rather simple. **Factor analysis** is a method for identifying clusters of related variables—that is, dimensions underlying a broad construct. Each dimension, or **factor**, represents a relatively unitary attribute. The procedure is used to identify and group together different items measuring an underlying attribute. In effect, factor analysis constitutes another means of testing hypotheses about the interrelationships among variables, and for looking at the convergent and discriminant validity of a large set of items. Indeed, a procedure known as **confirmatory factor analysis** (CFA) is sometimes used as a method for analyzing MTMM data (Ferketich, et al., 1991; Lowe & Ryan-Wenger, 1992).

Example of factor analysis in construct validation: Zheng and colleagues (2010) developed and tested the Dialysis Patient-Perceived Exercise Benefits and Barriers Scale. Responses to the scale's 24 items by a sample of 269 hemodialysis patients in China were factor analyzed to assess construct validity. Confirmatory factor analysis confirmed a 6-factor structure.

---

*Absolute value** refers to the value without a plus or minus sign. A value of −.80 is of a higher absolute magnitude than +.40.

Interpretation of Validity

Like reliability, validity is not an all-or-nothing characteristic of an instrument. An instrument does not possess or lack validity; it is a question of degree. An instrument's validity is not proved, established, or verified but rather is supported to a greater or lesser extent by evidence.

Strictly speaking, researchers do not validate an instrument but rather an application of it. A measure of anxiety may be valid for presurgical patients on the day of an operation but may not be valid for nursing students on the day of a test. Of course, some instruments may be valid for a wide range of uses with different types of samples, but each use requires new supporting evidence. The more evidence that can be gathered that an instrument is measuring what it is supposed to be measuring, the more confidence researchers will have in its validity.

➡ **TIP:** When you select an instrument, you should seek evidence of the scale's psychometric soundness by examining the instrument developers' report. However, you also should consider evidence from others who have used the scale. Each time the scale "performs" as hypothesized, this constitutes supplementary evidence for its validity. Conversely, if hypotheses involving the use of the scale are not supported, this suggests potential validity problems (although, of course, other factors may account for nonsupported hypotheses, such as a small sample).

SENSITIVITY, SPECIFICITY, AND LIKELIHOOD RATIOS

Reliability and validity are the two most important criteria for evaluating quantitative instruments, but researchers sometimes need to consider other qualities of an instrument. In particular, sensitivity and specificity are criteria that are important in evaluating instruments used as screening or diagnostic tools (e.g., a scale to measure risk of osteoporosis). Screening/diagnostic instruments can be self-report, observational, or biophysiologic measures.

Sensitivity is the ability of a measure to identify a "case" correctly, that is, to screen in or diagnosis a condition correctly. A measure's sensitivity is its rate of yielding "true positives." **Specificity** is the measure's ability to identify noncases correctly, that is, to screen *out* those without the condition. Specificity is an instrument's rate of yielding "true negatives." To evaluate an instrument's sensitivity and specificity, researchers need a reliable and valid criterion of "caseness" against which scores on the instrument can be assessed.

Calculating Sensitivity, Specificity, and Related Indicators

Suppose we wanted to evaluate whether adolescents' self-reports about their smoking were accurate, and we asked 100 teenagers about whether they had smoked a cigarette in the previous 24 hours. The "gold standard" for nicotine consumption is cotinine levels in a body fluid, so assume that we did a urinary cotinine assay. Some fictitious data are shown in Table 14.4.

Sensitivity, in this example, is calculated as the proportion of teenagers who said they smoked *and* who had high concentrations of cotinine, divided by all real smokers as indicated by the urine test. Put another way, it is the true positives divided by all positives. In this case, there was considerable under-reporting of smoking and so the sensitivity of the self-report was only .50. Specificity is the proportion of teenagers who accurately reported they did not smoke, or the true negatives divided by all negatives. In our example, specificity is .83. There was considerably less over-reporting of smoking ("faking bad") than under-reporting ("faking good"). Sensitivity and specificity are often reported as percentages rather than proportions, by multiplying the proportions by 100.

Often, other related indicators are calculated with such data. **Predictive values** are posterior probabilities—the probability of an outcome after the results are known. A **positive predictive value** (or PPV) is the proportion of people with a positive result who have the target outcome or disease. In our example, the PPV is the proportion of teens who

TABLE 14.4	Example Illustrating Sensitivity, Specificity, and Likelihood Ratios		
	URINARY COTININE LEVEL		
SELF-REPORTED SMOKING	**Positive (Cotinine > 200 ng/mL)**	**Negative (Cotinine ≤ 200 ng/mL)**	**Total**
Yes, smoked	A (true positive) 20	B (false positive) 10	A + B 30
No, did not smoke	C (false negative) 20	D (true negative) 50	C + D 70
Total	A + C 40	B + D 60	A + B + C + D 100

Sensitivity = A/(A + C)   = .50
Specificity = D/(B + D)   = .83
Positive predictive value (PPV) = A/(A + B)   = .67
Negative predictive value (NPV) = D/(C = D)   = .71
Likelihood ratio—positive (LR+) = sensitivity/(1 − specificity)   = 2.99
Likelihood ratio—negative (LR−) = (1 − sensitivity)/specificity   = .60

said they smoke who actually *do* smoke, according to the cotinine test results. Two out of three of those who reported smoking had high concentrations of cotinine, and so PPV = .67. A **negative predictive value** (NPV) is the proportion of people who have a negative test result who do not have the target outcome or disease. As shown in Table 14.4, 50 out of the 70 teenagers who reported not smoking actually were nonsmokers, and so NPV in our example is .71.

Example of sensitivity, specificity, and predictive values: Chichero and colleagues (2009) developed a dysphagia screening tool to triage patients at risk of dysphagia on admission to acute hospital wards. Sensitivity was 95% and specificity was 97%. Positive predictive value was 92% and negative predictive value was 98%.

In the medical community, reporting **likelihood ratios** has come into favor because it summarizes the relationship between specificity and sensitivity

in a single number. The likelihood ratio addresses the question, "How much more likely are we to find that an indicator is positive among those *with* the outcome of concern compared to those for whom the indicator is negative?" For a positive test result, then, the likelihood ratio (LR+) is the ratio of true-positive results to false-positive results. The formula for LR+ is sensitivity divided by 1 minus specificity. For the data in Table 14.4, LR+ is 2.99: We are about three times as likely to find that a self-report of smoking really *is* for a true smoker than it is for a nonsmoker. For a negative test result, the likelihood ratio (LR−) is the ratio of false-negative results to true-negative results. For the data in Table 14.4, the LR− is .60. In our example, we are about half as likely to find that a self-report of nonsmoking is false than we are to find that it reflects a true nonsmoker. When a test is high on both sensitivity and specificity (which is not especially true in our example), the likelihood ratio is high and discrimination is good.

Example of likelihood ratios: Novotny and Anderson (2008) tested an algorithm for predicting the probability of readmission (Pra) of medical inpatients within 41 days of discharge from the hospital, using hospital records data. Pra score values ranged from .16 to .75. With a Pra value of .45, the likelihood ratio was 1.6.

Receiver Operating Characteristic (ROC) Curves

All of the indicators that we calculated for the data in Table 14.4 are contingent upon the critical value that we established for cotinine concentration. Sensitivity and specificity would be quite different if we had used 100 ng/mL as indicative of smoking status, rather than 200 ng/mL. There is almost invariably a trade-off between the sensitivity and specificity of a measure. When sensitivity is increased to include more true positives, the proportion of true negatives declines. Therefore, a critical task in developing new diagnostic or screening measures is to develop the appropriate **cutoff point** (or *cutpoint*), that is, a score to distinguish cases and noncases.

To identify the best cutoff point, researchers often are guided by a **receiver operating characteristic curve** (**ROC curve**) (Fletcher, et al., 2005). To construct an ROC curve, the sensitivity of an instrument (i.e., the rate of correctly identifying a case vis-à-vis a well-established criterion) is plotted against the false-positive rate (i.e., the rate of incorrectly diagnosing someone as a case, which is the inverse of its specificity) over a range of different scores. The score (cutoff point) that yields the best balance between sensitivity and specificity can then be determined. The optimum cutoff is at or near the shoulder of the ROC curve.

ROC curves can best be explained with an illustration. Figure 14.2 presents an ROC curve from a study in which a goal was to establish cutoff points for scores on the Braden Q scale for predicting pressure ulcer risk in children (Curley et al., 2003). In this figure, sensitivity and one minus specificity are plotted for each possible score of the Braden Q scale. The upper left corner represents sensitivity at its highest possible value (1.0) and false positives at its lowest possible value (.00). Screening instruments that do an excellent job of discriminating

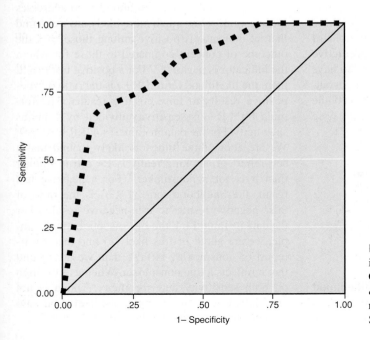

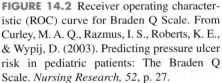

FIGURE 14.2 Receiver operating characteristic (ROC) curve for Braden Q Scale. From Curley, M. A. Q., Razmus, I. S., Roberts, K. E., & Wypij, D. (2003). Predicting pressure ulcer risk in pediatric patients: The Braden Q Scale. *Nursing Research, 52,* p. 27.

have points that crowd close to the upper left corner, which indicates that as sensitivity increases there is relatively little loss in specificity. ROC curves that are closer to a diagonal, from lower left to upper right, are indicative of an instrument with poor discriminatory power.

The overall accuracy of an instrument can be calculated as the proportion of the area under the ROC curve, an index referred to as **area under the curve**, or **AUC**. The larger the area, the more accurate the instrument. The AUC for the data portrayed in Figure 14.2 is .83. The cutoff score in this example was established at 16. At this cutoff value, the sensitivity was .88 and the specificity was .58. The researchers used these preliminary analyses to improve on the Braden Q scale and achieved even better results.

In selecting an appropriate cutoff point, the final decision is likely to be driven by clinical or economic factors and not just statistical ones. The financial and emotional costs of misclassifying people may be greater for false positives than false negatives, or vice versa.

OTHER CRITERIA FOR ASSESSING QUANTITATIVE MEASURES

Although we have already discussed the major criteria that are used to evaluate the quality of measuring instruments, we briefly mention a few others.

Efficiency

Instruments of comparable reliability and validity may differ in their efficiency. A depression scale that requires 5 minutes of people's time is efficient compared with a depression scale that requires 20 minutes to complete. In most studies, efficient instruments are desirable because they reduce participant burden.

One aspect of efficiency is the number of items on the instrument. Long instruments tend to be more reliable than shorter ones, but there is a point

of diminishing returns. As an example, consider a 40-item scale to measure social support that has an internal consistency reliability of .94. We can use a formula, known as the **Spearman-Brown formula**, to estimate how reliable the scale would be with fewer items. As an example, if we wanted to shorten the scale to 30 items, the formula would result in an estimated reliability of .92.** Thus, a 25% reduction in the instrument's length resulted in a negligible decrease in reliability, from .94 to .92. Most researchers likely would sacrifice a modest amount of reliability in exchange for reducing response burden and data collection costs. Other things being equal, it is desirable to select as efficient an instrument as possible.

Other Criteria

A few remaining qualities that sometimes are considered in assessing a quantitative instrument can be noted. Most of the following criteria are actually aspects of the reliability and validity:

1. *Comprehensibility*. Participants and researchers should be able to comprehend the behaviors required to secure accurate and valid measures.
2. *Precision*. An instrument should discriminate between people with different amounts of an attribute as precisely as possible.
3. *Range*. The instrument should be capable of achieving a meaningful measure from the smallest expected value of the variable to the largest.
4. *Linearity*. A researcher normally strives to construct measures that are equally accurate and sensitive over the entire range of values.
5. *Reactivity*. The instrument should, insofar as possible, avoid affecting the attribute being measured.

**The equation (and the worked-out example) for this situation is as follows:

$$r^1 = \frac{kr}{1 + [(k - 1)r]} = \frac{.75(.94)}{1 + [(-.25)(.94)]} = .92$$

where k = the factor by which the instrument is being decreased, in this case, $k = 30 \div 40 = .75$; r = reliability for the full scale, here, .94; and r^1 = reliability estimate for the shorter scale.

DATA QUALITY WITH SINGLE INDICATORS

The discussion in this chapter has primarily focused on methods of evaluating data quality for multi-item scales, which are widely used by nurse researchers. Textbooks on research methods or measurement rarely say much about reliability or validity for single questions (e.g., "What is your date of birth?") or single-item scales, such as visual analog scales.

The truth of the matter is that it is not easy to evaluate data quality in such situations. This is of great concern in large national surveys, such as the National Longitudinal Study of Adolescent Health. Population estimates of, say, average number of times adolescents have been hospitalized, or the percentage who have ever used marijuana, are based on reports in response to individual (nonscaled) questions, so the accuracy of the responses is vital. We touch briefly here on data quality assessment for single indicators.

The two basic strategies for estimating measurement error in such situations are a test–retest approach and external verification. In the former, the questions that are of interest are asked on two separate occasions. When this happens for the express purpose of assessing consistency (in what is called a *response variance reinterview*), the second administration typically involves a subsample of respondents and an abbreviated instrument with key questions. Survey researchers compute various statistical indexes (e.g., an *index of inconsistency*) to help them understand and interpret response differences—that is, measurement error—in the two administrations (Subcommittee on Measuring and Reporting the Quality of Survey Data, 2001). Although few nurse researchers would have the resources to undertake such an enterprise, there may be opportunities to use the underlying principle for critical pieces of information. For example, in a self-report instrument, it might be possible to ask the same question twice, early and later, for example, or to ask the question in slightly different ways in the same questionnaire or interview. Also, if a study is longitudinal, factual information (e.g., date of birth) could be gathered twice to assess any discrepancies.

The second approach is to verify information provided in the primary data gathering method against an external source—a form of criterion-related validation. For example, information from a question about birth date could be checked against birth records. Responses to questions about health status, diagnosis, or healthcare could be checked against medical records. Measurement errors are then estimated based on a comparison of the two types of information. It should not necessarily be assumed that records are free of error, but they may be less prone to certain types of bias. Other forms of external verification may be available. In particular, **proxy reports** (obtaining data from another person, such as a family member) might be an option. Patrician (2004) has offered additional guidance regarding single-item scales.

Researchers using biophysiologic measures should also give data quality some thought rather than assuming they will be error free. Instruments may not be properly calibrated, the person doing the tests may not follow laboratory protocols, and laboratory procedures can vary from one lab to the next. Measurement errors can also occur because of patient circumstances, such as insufficient sleep. Moreover, if physiologic measures are taken from charts, the possibility of error should be considered.

CRITIQUING DATA QUALITY IN QUANTITATIVE STUDIES

If data are seriously flawed, the study cannot contribute useful evidence. Therefore, in drawing conclusions about a study's evidence, it is important to consider whether researchers have taken appropriate steps to collect data that accurately reflect reality. Research consumers have the right—indeed, the obligation—to ask: Can I trust the data? Do the data accurately and validly reflect key constructs?

Information about data quality should be provided in every quantitative research report because it is not possible to come to conclusions about the quality of study evidence without such information. Reliability estimates are usually reported because they are

BOX 14.1 Guidelines for Critiquing Data Quality in Quantitative Studies

1. Is there congruence between the research variables as conceptualized (i.e., as discussed in the introduction of the report) and as operationalized (i.e., as described in the method section)?
2. If operational definitions (or scoring procedures) are specified, do they clearly indicate the rules of measurement? Do the rules seem sensible? Were data collected in such a way that measurement errors were minimized?
3. Does the report offer evidence of the reliability of measures? Does the evidence come from the research sample itself, or is it based on other studies? If the latter, is it reasonable to conclude that data quality would be similar for the research sample as for the reliability sample (e.g., are sample characteristics similar)?
4. If reliability is reported, which estimation method was used? Was this method appropriate? Should an alternative or additional method of reliability appraisal have been used? Is the reliability sufficiently high?
5. Does the report offer evidence of the validity of the measures? Does the evidence come from the research sample itself, or is it based on other studies? If the latter, is it reasonable to believe that data quality would be similar for the research sample as for the validity sample (e.g., are the sample characteristics similar)?
6. If validity information is reported, which validity approach was used? Was this method appropriate? Does the validity of the instrument appear to be adequate?
7. If there is no reliability or validity information, what conclusion can you reach about the quality of the data in the study?
8. If a diagnostic or screening tool was used, is information provided about its sensitivity and specificity, and were these qualities adequate?
9. Were the research hypotheses supported? If not, might data quality play a role in the failure to confirm the hypotheses?

easy to communicate. Ideally—especially for composite scales—the report should provide reliability coefficients based on data from the study itself, not just from previous research. Interrater or interobserver reliability is especially crucial for coming to conclusions about data quality in observational studies. The values of the reliability coefficients should be sufficiently high to support confidence in the findings. It is especially important to scrutinize reliability information in studies with nonsignificant findings because the unreliability of measures can undermine statistical conclusion validity.

Validity is more difficult to document in a report than reliability. At a minimum, researchers should defend their choice of existing measures based on validity information from the developers, and they should cite the relevant publication. If a study used a screening or diagnostic measure, information should also be provided about its sensitivity and specificity.

Box 14.1 ✪ provides some guidelines for critiquing aspects of data quality of quantitative

measures. The guidelines are available in the Toolkit of the accompanying *Resource Manual* for your use and adaptation.

RESEARCH EXAMPLE

In this section, we describe a study that used both self-report and observational measures. We focus on the researchers' excellent documentation of data quality in their study.

Study: Communication and outcomes of visits between older patients and nurse practitioners (Gilbert and Hayes, 2009)

Statement of Purpose: The purpose of this study was to examine relationships among patient–clinician communication, background characteristics of the patients and the clinicians (nurse practitioners or NPs), and both proximal outcomes (e.g., patient satisfaction) and longer-term outcomes (e.g., changes in patients' physical and mental health).

Design: Visits between 31 NPs and 155 patients were video recorded and various aspects of patient and NP behaviors were coded. Proximal outcomes were measured by self-report after the visits. Four weeks later, changes in patients' health outcomes were assessed using self-report measures.

Instruments and Data Quality: Communications during the visits were measured using the Roter Interaction Analysis System (RIAS) for verbal interaction and a checklist for nonverbal behaviors. The Roter system involves coding for both the content of the communication and relationship aspects, using a system of 69 categories for all utterances (only 43 were used in this study). The researchers noted that the predictive validity of the RIAS had considerable support. The average interrater reliability in the present study for the 43 coded behavior categories was .95. For the nonverbal behavior checklist, various actions (e.g., gazes, nods, smiles) were coded in 1-second segments over a 30-second sample. Two coders independently coded all segments and any discrepancies in coding were resolved by a third party. Several variables were measured by patients' self-report, including both 1-item measures (e.g., satisfaction with the visit) and multi-item scales (e.g., physical and mental health). For example, patient satisfaction with the NP visit was measured using one item, previously used in a large national survey, which asked for ratings of perceived quality of care on a 10-point scale from 1 (*worst care possible*) to 10 (*best care possible*). The authors noted that a correlation of .72 between the ratings and the average of several other satisfaction items provided some evidence for the reliability of the single item. Physical and mental health were measured with a 12-item scale called the SF-12 Health Survey, a widely used and well-validated instrument. The test developer had reported results indicating Cronbach alpha values of .89 for physical health and .82 for mental health among people 65 years and older. In the present study, the researchers computed the internal consistency reliability to be .87 and .72 for physical and mental health, respectively.

Key Findings: Among the many findings reported in this study, the researchers found that better patient outcomes were associated with a higher amount of communication content involving seeking and giving biomedical and psychosocial information, and with a relationships component of more positive talk and greater trust and receptivity.

SUMMARY POINTS

- **Measurement** involves assigning numbers to objects to represent the amount of an attribute, using a specified set of rules. Researchers strive to develop or use measurements whose rules are *isomorphic* with reality.

- Few quantitative measuring instruments are infallible. Sources of measurement error include situational contaminants, response-set biases, and transitory personal factors, such as fatigue.

- **Obtained scores** from an instrument consist of a **true score** component (the value that would be obtained for a hypothetical perfect measure of the attribute) and an error component, or **error of measurement**, that represents measurement inaccuracies.

- **Reliability**, one of two primary criteria for assessing an instrument, is the degree of consistency or accuracy with which an instrument measures an attribute. The higher an instrument's reliability, the lower the amount of error in obtained scores.

- There are different methods for assessing an instrument's reliability and for computing a **reliability coefficient**. A reliability coefficient typically is based on the computation of a **correlation coefficient** that indicates the magnitude and direction of a relationship between two variables.

- Correlation coefficients can range from −1.00 (a **perfect negative relationship**) through zero to +1.00 (a **perfect positive relationship**). Reliability coefficients usually range from .00 to 1.00, with higher values reflecting greater reliability.

- The **stability** aspect of reliability, which concerns the extent to which an instrument yields the same results on repeated administrations, is evaluated as **test–retest reliability**.

- The **internal consistency** aspect of reliability— the extent to which all the instrument's items are measuring the same attribute—is usually assessed by **Cronbach's alpha**.

- When the reliability assessment focuses on **equivalence** between observers in rating or coding behaviors, estimates of **interrater** (or interobserver) **reliability** are obtained. When a consensus measure capturing interrater agreement within a small number of categories is desired, the **kappa** statistic is often used.

- **Reliability coefficients** reflect the proportion of true variability in a set of scores to the total obtained variability.
- **Validity** is the degree to which an instrument measures what it is supposed to measure.
- **Face validity** refers to whether the instrument appears, on the face of it, to be measuring the appropriate construct.
- **Content validity** concerns the sampling adequacy of the content being measured. Expert ratings on the relevance of items can be used to compute **content validity index (CVI)** information. **Item CVIs (I-CVIs)** represent the proportion of experts rating each item as relevant. A **scale CVI** using the averaging calculation method (S-CVI/Ave) is the average of all I-CVI values.
- **Criterion-related validity** (which includes both **predictive validity** and **concurrent validity**) focuses on the correlation between the instrument and an outside criterion.
- **Construct validity**, an instrument's adequacy in measuring the focal construct, is a hypothesis-testing endeavor. One approach assesses **contrast validity**, using the **known-groups technique** to contrast scores of groups hypothesized to differ on the attribute; another approach is **factor analysis**, a statistical procedure for identifying unitary clusters of items or measures.
- Another construct validity approach is the **multitrait–multimethod (MTMM) matrix technique**, which is based on the concepts of convergence and discriminability. **Convergence** refers to evidence that different methods of measuring the same attribute yield similar results. **Discriminability** refers to the ability to differentiate the construct being measured from other, similar concepts.
- A **psychometric assessment** of a new instrument is usually undertaken to gather evidence about validity, reliability, and other assessment criteria.
- Sensitivity and specificity are important criteria for screening and diagnostic instruments. **Sensitivity** is the instrument's ability to identify a case

correctly (i.e., its rate of yielding true positives). **Specificity** is the instrument's ability to identify noncases correctly (i.e., its rate of yielding true negatives). Other related indexes include the measure's **positive predictive value (PPV), negative predictive value (NPV)**, and **likelihood ratios**.

- Sensitivity is sometimes plotted against specificity in a **receiver operating characteristic curve (ROC curve)** to determine the optimum **cutoff point** for caseness.

STUDY ACTIVITIES

Chapter 14 of the *Resource Manual for Nursing Research: Generating and Assessing Evidence for Nursing Practice*, 9th edition, offers exercises and study suggestions for reinforcing concepts presented in this chapter. In addition, the following study questions can be addressed:

1. Explain in your own words the meaning of the following correlation coefficients:
   a. The relationship between intelligence and grade-point average was found to be .72.
   b. The correlation coefficient between age and gregariousness was −.20.
   c. It was revealed that patients' compliance with nursing instructions was related to their length of stay in the hospital ($r = -.50$).
2. Use the critiquing guidelines in Box 14.1 to evaluate data quality in the study by Gilbert and Hayes (2009), referring to the original study if possible.

STUDIES CITED IN CHAPTER 14

Cha, E., Kim, K., & Burke, L. (2008). Psychometric validation of a condom self-efficacy scale in Korean. *Nursing Research, 57*, 245–251.

Chang, H., Lin, C., Chou, K., Ma, W., & Yang, C. (2009). Chinese version of the positive and negative suicide ideation: Instrument development. *Journal of Advanced Nursing, 65*, 1485–1496.

Chichero, J., Heaton, S., & Bassett, L. (2009). Triaging dysphagia: Nurses screening for dysphagia in an acute hospital. *Journal of Clinical Nursing, 18*, 1649–1659.

Chien, W. T., & Chan, S. (2009). Testing the psychometric properties of a Chinese version of the Level of Expressed Emotion Scale. *Research in Nursing & Health, 32*, 59–70.

Curley, M. A. Q., Razmus, I. S., Roberts, K. E., & Wypij, D. (2003). Predicting pressure ulcer risk in pediatric patients. *Nursing Research, 52*, 22–33.

Gilbert, D., & Hayes, E. (2009). Communication and outcomes of visits between older patients and nurse practitioners. *Nursing Research, 58*, 283–293.

Gozum, S., & Hacihasanoglu, R. (2009). Reliability and validity of the Turkish adaptation of Medication Adherence Self-Efficacy Scale in hypertensive patients. *European Journal of Cardiovascular Nursing, 8*, 129–136.

Jones, F., Partridge, C., & Reid, F. (2008). The Stroke Self-Efficacy Questionnaire: Measuring individual confidence in functional performance after stroke. *Journal of Clinical Nursing, 17*, 244–252.

Kao, H., & Lynn, M. (2009). Use of the measurement of medication administration hassles with Mexican American family caregivers. *Journal of Clinical Nursing, 18*, 2596–2603.

Morea, J., Friend, R., & Bennett, R. (2008). Conceptualizing and measuring illness self-concept. A comparison with self-esteem and optimism in predicting fibromyalgia adjustment. *Research in Nursing & Health, 31*, 563–575.

Novotny, N., & Anderson, M. A. (2008). Prediction of early readmission in medical inpatients using the probability of repeated admission instrument. *Nursing Research, 57*, 406–415.

Schilling, L., Dixon, J., Knafl, K., Lynn, M., Murphy, K., Dumser, S., & Grey, M. (2009). A new self-report measure of self-management of type I diabetes for adolescents. *Nursing Research, 58*, 228–236.

Simmons, K., Smith, J., & Maekawa, A. (2009). Development and psychometric evaluation of the Ostomy Adjustment Inventory-23. *Journal of Wound, Ostomy & Continence Nursing, 36*, 69–75.

Williams, A., & Kristjanson, L. (2009). Emotional care experienced by hospitalized patients: Development and testing of a measurement instrument. *Journal of Clinical Nursing, 18*, 1069–1077.

Villanueva, C., Scott, S., Guzzetta, C., & Foster, B. (2009). Development and psychometric testing of the Attitudes toward Mental Illness in Pediatric Patients Scale. *Journal of Child & Adolescent Psychiatric Nursing, 22*, 220–227.

Voepel-Lewis, T., Zanotti, J., Dammeyer, J., & Merkel, S. (2010). Reliability and validity of the Face, Legs, Activity, Cry, Consolability Behavioral Tool in assessing acute pain in critically ill patients. *American Journal of Critical Care, 19*, 55–61.

Zheng, J., You, L., Lou, T., Chen, N., Lai, D., Liang, Y., Li, Y. N., Gu, Y. M., Lv, S. F., & Zhai, C. Q. (2010). Development and psychometric evaluation of the Dialysis Patient-Perceived Exercise Benefits and Barriers Scale. *International Journal of Nursing Studies, 47*, 166–180.

Methodologic and nonresearch references cited in this chapter can be found in a separate section at the end of the book.

15

Developing and Testing Self-Report Scales

Researchers sometimes are unable to identify an appropriate instrument to operationalize a construct. This may occur when the construct is new, but often it is due to limitations of existing instruments. Because this situation occurs fairly often, this chapter provides an overview of the steps involved in the development of high-quality self-report scales.

The scope of this chapter is fairly narrow, but it covers instruments that nurse researchers often use. First, we focus on structured *self-report* measures rather than observational ones (although many steps would apply to observational scales). Second, we describe methods of developing *multi-item* scales (i.e., not 1-item visual analog scales). Third, we exclude infrequently used scale types, such as semantic differentials. Fourth, we focus on scales rooted in classical measurement theory rather than on item response theory. We use examples of scales to measure the *affective domain* (e.g., measures of attitudes, psychological traits, and so on) rather than scales to measure the *cognitive domain* (e.g., achievement, knowledge), but many principles apply to both domains.

➲ **TIP:** The development of high-quality scales is a lengthy, labor-intensive process that requires some statistical sophistication. We urge you to think carefully about embarking on a scale-development endeavor and to consider involving a psychometric consultant if you proceed.

BEGINNING STEPS: CONCEPTUALIZATION AND ITEM GENERATION

Conceptualizing the Construct

The importance of a sound, thorough conceptualization of the construct to be measured cannot be overemphasized. You will not be able to quantify an attribute adequately unless you thoroughly understand the **latent variable** (the underlying construct) you wish to capture. In measurement theory, the latent variable, which is not directly observable, is the *cause* of the scores on the measure. The strength of the latent variable is presumed to trigger a certain numeric value on the scale. You cannot develop items to produce the right score, and you cannot expect good content and construct validity if you are unclear about the construct, its dimensions, and its nuances.

Thus, the first step in scale development is to become an *expert* on the construct. This means being knowledgeable about relevant theory, research relating to the construct, and existing (albeit imperfect) instruments. Scale developers usually begin with a thorough review of relevant literature, on which they can base their conceptual definitions.

Most complex constructs have a number of different facets or dimensions, and it is important to identify and understand each one. In part, this is a content validity consideration: For the overall scale to be content valid, there must be items representing all facets of the construct. Identifying dimensions also has methodologic implications. All scales—or subscales of a broader scale—need to be unidimensional and internally homogeneous, so an adequate number of items (operational definitions) of each dimension needs to be developed.

During the early conceptualization, you also need to think about related constructs that should be differentiated from the target construct. If you are measuring, say, self-esteem, you have to be sure you can differentiate it from similar but distinct constructs, such as self-confidence. In thinking about the dimensions of the target construct, you should be sure that they are truly aspects of the construct and not a different construct altogether.

Before you begin, you should also have an explicit conceptualization of the population for whom the scale is intended. For example, an anxiety scale for a general population may not be suitable if your interest is in measuring childbearing anxiety in pregnant women. There are arguments for developing patient-specific scales, particularly with respect to the relevancy of items. On the other hand, developing a highly focused scale with low "bandwidth," while possibly enhancing "fidelity" (Cronbach, 1990), reduces the scale's generalizability and researchers' ability to make comparisons across populations. The point is that you should have a clear view of how and with whom the scale will be used.

Understanding the population for whom the scale is intended is critical for developing good items. Without a good grasp of the population, it will be difficult to consider such issues as reading levels and cultural appropriateness in wording the items.

For instruments that are being developed for use by others, it is advisable to establish an expert panel to review domain specifications in an early effort to ensure the content validity of the scale (AERA, APA, & NCME Joint Committee, 1999). An iterative, Delphi survey-type approach with opportunities for refinement by the expert panel is often useful (Berk, 1990).

Deciding on the Type of Scale

Before items can be generated, you need to decide on the type of scale you wish to create because item characteristics vary by scale type. Our focus is restricted to the most widely used scale types because this is not a textbook on psychometrics. For those interested in such scaling approaches as semantic differentials, Guttman or Thurstone scaling, multidimensional scaling, ipsative (forced choice) scaling, or other approaches, consult other references (e.g., Gable & Wolfe, 1993; Nunnally & Bernstein, 1994; Waltz, et al., 2010).

In this chapter, we concentrate on multi-item summated rating scales, which are also the focus of several other books on scale development that can be consulted for greater elaboration (DeVellis, 2003; Streiner & Norman, 2008). Two broad categories of scales fall into this category: traditional Likert scales and latent trait scales.

Traditional Likert scales (Chapter 13) are based in classical measurement theory (CMT). Items on Likert scales, it may be recalled, are declarative statements with a bipolar response scale that is often on an agree/disagree continuum. In CMT, the scale developer selects items that are presumed to be roughly comparable indicators of the underlying construct. The items gain strength in approximating a hypothetical true score through their aggregation. Traditional Likert scales, then, rely on items that are deliberately redundant, in the hope that multiple indicators of the construct will converge on the true score and balance out error.

Item response theory (IRT), an alternative to CMT, is widely used in creating cognitive tests, and its use in developing affective measures is growing. IRT methods differentiate error more finely than CMT methods, particularly with respect to item characteristics. The goal of IRT is to allow researchers to determine the characteristics of items independent of who completes them. **Latent trait scales** are developed using an IRT framework, and although it is beyond the scope of this book to elaborate on the complex statistical procedures involved in testing latent trait scales, we can provide a few brief comments and references for those who wish further guidance.

Latent trait scales can use items like the ones used in CMT, such as items with a Likert-type format—in fact, a person completing a Likert scale would likely not know whether it had been developed within the CMT or IRT framework. But a person *developing* a Likert-type scale must decide in advance which measurement approach is being used because the scale items would be different. Whereas the items on a CMT Likert scale are designed to be similar to each other to tap the underlying construct in a comparable manner, items on a latent-trait IRT scale are carefully chosen and refined to tap different degrees of the attribute being measured.

As an example, suppose we were developing a scale to measure risk-taking behavior in adolescents. In a CMT scale, the items might include statements about risk-taking of similar intensity, with which respondents would agree or disagree. The aggregate of responses would array respondents along a continuum indicating varying propensity to take risks. In an IRT scale, the items themselves would be chosen to reflect different levels of risk-taking (e.g., smoking cigarettes, using drugs, driving a car at 80 miles an hour while text messaging). Each item could be described as having a different *difficulty*. It is "easier" to agree with or admit to lower-risk items than higher-risk items. Item difficulty is one of several parameters that can be analyzed in IRT scale development. When item difficulty is the only parameter being considered in an IRT analysis, researchers often say that they are using a **Rasch model**.

IRT is a more sophisticated approach than CMT for assessing the strengths and weaknesses of individual items, but it is more complex and uses software that is not as readily available. DeVellis (2003) believes that CMT scaling approaches will continue to prevail for affective measures, but suggests that IRT scaling is especially appropriate when the scale involves items that are inherently hierarchical. Those interested in latent trait scales and IRT should consult Hambleton and colleagues (1991) or Embretson and Reise (2000).

Example of an IRT analysis: Gómez and colleagues (2007) analyzed the 20-item Death Anxiety Inventory within an IRT framework.

Developing an Item Pool: Getting Started

The next step is to develop a pool of possible items for the scale. Items—which collectively constitute the operational definition of the construct—need to be carefully crafted to reflect the latent variable they are designed to measure. This is often easier to do as a team effort, because different people articulate a similar idea in diverse ways. Regardless of whether you are doing this alone or with a team, you may be asking: Where do scale items come from? Here are some possible sources:

1. *Existing instruments.* Sometimes it is possible to adapt an existing instrument rather than starting from scratch. Adaptations often require adding and deleting items, but may involve rewording items—for example, to make them more culturally appropriate, or to simplify wording for a population with low reading skills. Permission from the author of the original scale should be sought because published scales are copyright protected.

2. *The literature.* Ideas for item content often come from a thorough understanding of the literature. Since at this point you would already be an "expert" on the construct, this is an obvious source of ideas for items.

3. *Concept analysis.* A related source of ideas is a concept analysis—which you may already have undertaken as a preliminary step. Walker and Avant (2004) offer concept analysis strategies that could be used to develop items for a scale.

4. *In-depth qualitative research.* In-depth inquiry relating to the key construct is a particularly rich source for scale items. A qualitative study can help you to understand the dimensions of a phenomenon, and can also give you actual words for items. Tilden and her colleagues (1990), Beck and Gable (2001), and Gilgun (2004) offer guidance on using qualitative research to enhance the content validity of a new scale. If you are unable to undertake an in-depth study yourself, be sure to pay particular attention to the verbatim quotes in published qualitative reports about your construct.

5. *Clinical Observations.* Patients in clinical settings may be an excellent source of items. Ideas for items may come from direct observation of patients' behaviors in relevant situations, or from listening to their comments and conversations.

Examples of sources of items: Jones and Gulick (2009) developed new items for a revised version of the Sexual Pressure Scale, using qualitative data from seven focus groups. Bu and Wu (2008) derived items for the Attitude Toward Patient Advocacy Scale from a literature review and consultation with experts.

DeVellis (2003) urged scale developers to get started writing scale items without a lot of editing and critical review in the early stages. Perhaps a good way to begin if you are struggling is to develop a simple statement with the key construct mentioned in it. For example, if the construct is test anxiety, you might start with, "I get anxious when I take a test." This could be followed by similar statement worded differently (e.g., "Taking tests makes me nervous").

Making Decisions about Item Features

In preparing to write items, you need to make decisions about such issues as the number of items to develop, the number and form of the response options, whether to include positively and negatively worded items, and how to deal with time.

Number of Items

In the CMT framework, a **domain sampling model** is assumed, which involves the random sampling of a homogeneous set of items from a hypothetical universe of items relating to the construct. Of course, sampling from a *universe* of all possible items does not happen in reality, but it is a principle worth keeping in mind. The idea is to generate a fairly exhaustive set of item possibilities, given the construct's theoretical demands. For a traditional Likert scale, redundancy (except for trivial word substitutions) is a good thing—the goal is to measure the construct of interest with a set of items that capture the central theme in slightly different ways so that irrelevant idiosyncrasies of individual items will cancel each other out.

There is no magic formula for how many items should be developed, but our advice is to generate a very large pool of items. As you proceed, many items will be discarded. Longer scales tend to be more reliable, so starting with a large number of items promotes the likelihood that you will eventually have an internally consistent scale. DeVellis (2003) recommended starting with 3 to 4 times as many items as you will have in your final scale (e.g., 30 to 40 items for a 10-item scale), but at a minimum there should be 50% more (e.g., 15 items for a 10-item scale).

Response Options

Scale items involve both a stem (usually a declarative statement), and a set of response options. Traditional Likert scales often involve response options on a continuum of agreement, but other continua are also possible, such as frequency (never/always), importance (very important/unimportant), quality (excellent/very poor), and likelihood(definitely/impossible).

How many response options should there be? There is no simple answer, but keep in mind the goal is to array people on a continuum, and so variability is essential. Variability can be enhanced by including a lot of items, by offering numerous response options, or both. However, there is not much merit in creating the illusion of precision when it does not exist. With a 0–100 range of scores, for example, the difference between a 96 and a 98 might not be meaningful. Also, it has been found that too many options can be confusing to people with limited education.

Most Likert scales have 5 to 7 options, with verbal descriptors attached to each option and—often—with numbers placed under the descriptors to facilitate coding and to further help respondents find an appropriate place on the continuum. An odd number of items gives respondents an opportunity to be neutral or ambivalent (i.e., to chose a midpoint), and so some scale developers prefer an even number (e.g., 4 or 6) to force even slight tendencies and to avoid equivocation. However, some respondents may actually *be* neutral or ambivalent, so a midpoint option allows them to express it. The midpoint can be labeled with such phrases as "neither agree nor disagree," "undecided," "agree and disagree equally," or simply "?".

➲ T I P : Here are some frequently used words for response options, with the midpoint term not listed:

- Strongly disagree, disagree, agree, strongly agree
- Disagree strongly, disagree moderately, disagree slightly, agree slightly, agree moderately, agree strongly
- Never, rarely (or seldom), occasionally (or sometimes), frequently (or usually), always
- Very important, important, somewhat important, of little importance, unimportant
- Definitely not, probably not, possibly, probably, very probably, definitely

---

Positive and Negative Stems

A generation ago, leading psychometricians advised scale developers to deliberately include both positively and negatively worded statements and to reverse-score negative items. As an example, consider these two items for a scale of depression: "I frequently feel blue," and "I am happy most of the time." The objective was to include items that would minimize the possibility of an acquiescence response set—the tendency to agree with statements regardless of their content.

There is now ample evidence that it is not prudent to include both types of items on a scale. Some respondents are confused by reversing polarities. Answering negative item stems appears to be an especially difficult cognitive task for younger respondents. Some research suggests that acquiescence can be minimized by putting the most positive response options (e.g., strongly agree) at the end of the list rather than at the beginning.

Item Intensity

In a traditional Likert scale, the intensity of the statements (stems) should be similar and fairly strongly worded. If items are worded such that almost anyone would agree with them, the scale will not be able to discriminate between people with different amounts of the underlying latent variable. For exam-

ple, an item such as "Good health is important" would generate almost universal agreement. On the other hand, statements should not be so extremely worded as to result in universal rejection. For example, "Nurses who do not have a Bachelor's degree should be fired," is obviously a poor measure of people's attitudes toward nursing credentials.

For a latent trait scale, scale developers seek a range of item intensities. Yet, even on an IRT-based scale there is no point in including items with which almost everyone would either agree or disagree.

Item Time Frames

Some items make an explicit reference to a time frame (e.g., "In the past few days, I have had trouble falling asleep"), but others do not (e.g., "I have trouble falling asleep"). Sometimes, instructions to a scale can designate a temporal frame of reference (e.g., "In answering the following questions, please indicate how you have felt in the past week"). And yet other scales ask respondents to respond in terms of a time frame: "In the past week, I have had trouble falling asleep: Every day, 5 to 6 days . . . Never".

A time frame should not emerge as a consequence of item development. You should decide in advance, based on your conceptual understanding of the construct and the needs for which the scale is being constructed, how to deal with time.

Example of handling time in a scale: The Postpartum Depression Screening Scale asks respondents to indicate their emotional state in the past 2 weeks—for example, over the last 2 weeks I: ". . .felt so all alone" or ". . . cried a lot for no reason" (Beck and Gable, 2000, 2001). The 2-week period was chosen because it parallels the duration of symptoms required for a diagnosis of major depressive episode according to the DSM-IV criteria.

Wording the Items

Items should be worded in such a manner that every respondent is answering the same question. Guidance in wording good items is offered by Fowler (1995) and Streiner and Norman (2008). In addition to the suggestions on question wording we provided in Chapter 13, some additional tips specific to scale items are as follows:

1. *Clarity.* Scale developers should strive for clear, unambiguous items. Words should be carefully chosen with the educational and reading level of the target population in mind. In most cases, this will mean developing a scale at the 6th- to 7th-grade reading level. But even beyond reading level, you should strive to select words that everyone understands, and to have everyone reach the same conclusion about what the words mean.

2. *Jargon.* Jargon should be avoided. Be especially cautious about using terms that might be well-known in healthcare circles (e.g., lesion) but not familiar to the average person.

3. *Length.* Avoid long sentences or phrases. Simple sentences are the easiest to comprehend. In particular, eliminate unnecessary words. For example, "It is fair to say that in the scheme of things I do not get enough sleep," could more simply be worded, "I usually do not get enough sleep."

4. *Double negatives.* It is often preferable to word things affirmatively ("I am usually happy") than negatively ("I am not usually sad"), but double negatives should always be avoided ("I am *not* usually *un*happy").

5. *Double-Barreled Items.* Avoid putting two or more ideas in a single item. For example, "I am afraid of insects and snakes" is a bad item because a person who is afraid of insects but not snakes (or vice versa) would not know how to respond.

Examples of well-worded items: Ellenbecker and colleagues (2008) revised a scale to measure job satisfaction among home healthcare nurses. Here are two items from their revised scale: "I am able to meet the demands of my job" and "I am satisfied with the amount of control I have over my work." Respondents indicate agreement or disagreement with items on a 5-point scale.

PRELIMINARY EVALUATION OF ITEMS

Internal Review

Once a large pool of items has been generated, it is time for critical appraisal. Care should be devoted to such issues as whether individual items capture the construct, and are grammatical and well worded. The initial review should also consider whether the items taken together adequately embrace the full nuances of the construct—that is, whether additional items need to be generated to enhance the scale's content validity.

It is also imperative to assess the scale's **readability**, unless the scale is intended for a population with known high literacy, such as people with advanced degrees. There are different approaches for assessing the reading level of written documents, but many methods are either time-consuming or require several hundreds of words of text, and thus are not suited to evaluating scale items (Streiner & Norman, 2008).

Many word-processing programs provide some information about readability. In Microsoft Word, for example, you could type your items on a list and then get readability statistics for the items as a whole or for individual items, as described in Chapter 7. For example, take the following two sets of items for tapping fatigue:

Set A	Set B
I am frequently exhausted.	I am often tired.
I invariably get insufficient sleep.	I don't get enough sleep.

The software tells us that the items in Set A have a *Flesch-Kincaid grade level* of 12.0 and a *Flesch reading ease score* of 4.8. (Reading ease scores rate text on a 100-point scale, with higher values associated with greater ease, using a formula that considers average sentence length and average number of syllables). Set B, by contrast, has a grade level of 1.8 and a reading ease score of 89.4. Streiner and Norman (2008) warn that word-processing–based readability scores be interpreted cautiously, but it is clear from the foregoing analysis that the second set of items would be superior for a population that includes people with limited education. A general principle is to avoid long sentences and words with four or more syllables.

Example of assessing readability: Schilling and colleagues (2009) developed the Self-Management of Type 1 Diabetes in Adolescents (SMOD-A) scale. The scale's readability was assessed using the Flesch-Kincaid grade level score, which was found to be at the 5.9 grade level.

Input from the Target Population

It is often productive to pretest the initial set of items with a sample of 10 to 20 people from the target population. These respondents can be asked some simple questions (e.g., Are there statements that confused you? Did you understand the meaning of each question? Were the directions clear?). *Cognitive questioning* is an excellent technique for discovering how others process the words and ideas presented to them in structured questions. (The Toolkit offers suggestions for cognitive questioning ⊗.) Streiner and Norman (2008) describe several other techniques that can be used to detect ambiguities and language problems in a pretest.

Example of cognitive questioning: Hamilton and colleagues (2009) developed a measure of preferred coping strategies for older African American cancer survivors. Cognitive questioning methods were used with a small sample to assess how each question was understood.

➲ **TIP:** When questioning pretest respondents about the clarity or meaning of the items, avoid using the word "item," which is research jargon (e.g., do not say, "Are there *items* that confused you?").

Additionally, it is a good idea to peruse the pretest answers to see if response patterns suggest the need for item revisions. For example, items with no variability (e.g., everyone agrees or disagrees) should be revised or omitted because they cannot contribute to

the scale's ability to discriminate among people with varying amounts of the underlying construct. Streiner and Norman (2008) warned that if the pretest fails to suggest any changes, this probably indicates a flaw in the pretest rather than problem-free items.

As an alternative or supplement to pretests, *focus groups* can also be used at this stage in scale development. Two or three groups can be convened to discuss whether, from the respondents' perspective, the items are understandable, linguistically and culturally appropriate, inoffensive, and relevant to the construct.

External Review by Experts

External review of the revised items by a panel of experts should be undertaken to assess the scale's content validity. It is advisable to undertake two rounds of review, if feasible—the first to refine or weed out faulty items or to add new items to cover the domain adequately, and the second to formally assess the content validity of the items and scale. We discuss some procedures in such a two-step strategy, although the two steps are sometimes combined.

Selecting and Recruiting the Experts

The panel of experts needs to include people with strong credentials with regard to the construct being measured. Criteria such as the following can be used in selecting substantive experts: clinical or personal experience, published papers in refereed journals, or an ongoing program of research on the topic. Experts should be knowledgeable about the key construct *and* the target population. In the first review, it is also desirable to include experts on scale construction.

In the initial phase of a two-part review, we advise having an expert panel of 8 to 12 members, with a good mix in terms of roles (e.g., clinicians, faculty, researchers) and disciplines. For example, for a scale designed to measure fear of dying in the elderly, the experts might include nurses, gerontologists, and psychiatrists. If the scale is intended for broad use, it might also be advantageous to recruit experts from various countries or areas of a country, because of possible regional variations in language.

The second panel for formally assessing the content validity of a more refined set of items should consist of 3 to 5 experts in the content area.

Example of an expert panel: Lin and colleagues (2008) developed and tested the Diabetes Self-Management Instrument in Taiwan. A panel of seven experts in diabetes and instrument development was assembled. The experts included three diabetes educators with doctorates, two physicians specializing in diabetes, and two nurse practitioners who worked in a diabetes clinic.

Experts are typically sent a packet of materials, including a strong cover letter, background information about the construct and target population, reviewer instructions, and a questionnaire soliciting their opinion (Grant & Davis, 1997). A critical component of the packet is a careful explanation of the conceptual underpinnings of the construct, including an explication of the various dimensions encompassed by the construct to be captured in subscales. The panel may also be given a brief overview of the literature, as well as a bibliography.

➔ **TIP:** The Toolkit section of the *Resource Manual* includes a sample cover letter and other material relating to expert review, as Word documents that can be adapted.

Preliminary Expert Review: Content Validation of Items

The experts' job is to evaluate individual items and the overall scale (and any subscales), using guidelines established by the scale developer. The first panel of experts is usually invited to rate each item along several dimensions. Among the dimensions often used are the following: clarity of wording, relevance of the item to the construct or to one of its dimensions, and appropriateness for the target population (e.g., developmental or cultural appropriateness). Experts could either be asked to make judgments dichotomously (e.g., ambiguous/clear) or along a continuum. As noted in the previous chapter, relevance is most often rated as follows: 1 = *not relevant*, 2 = *somewhat relevant*, 3 = *quite relevant*, 4 = *highly relevant*. Figure 15.1 ⊗ shows a possible format for a content validation assessment of relevance.

The scale items shown below have been developed to measure one dimension of the construct of safe sexual behaviors among adolescents, namely **assertiveness**. Please read each item and score it for its relevance in representing this concept.

Assertiveness is defined as the use of verbal and interpersonal skills to negotiate protection during sexual activities.

| | **Relevance Rating** | | | |
| | Not | Somewhat | Quite | Highly |
Item	Relevant	Relevant	Relevant	Relevant
1. I ask my partner about his/her sexual history before having intercourse.	1	2	3	4
2. I don't have sex without asking the person if he/she has been tested for HIV/AIDS.	1	2	3	4
3. When I am having sex with someone for the first time, I insist that we use a condom.	1	2	3	4
4. I don't let my partner talk me into having sex without knowing something about how risky it would be.	1	2	3	4

Please comment on any of these items, including possible revisions or substitutions, or your thoughts about why an item is not relevant to the concept of assertiveness. Please suggest any additional items you feel would improve the measurement of assertiveness relating to adolescents' safe sexual behaviors.

FIGURE 15.1 ⊗ Example of a portion of a content validation form.

The questionnaire usually asks for detailed comments about items judged to be unclear, not relevant, or not appropriate, such as how wording might be improved, or why the item is deemed to be not relevant. Another dimension that could be included for each item in a first phase evaluation concerns an overall recommendation—for example: retain the item exactly as worded, make major revisions to the item, make minor revisions to the item, and drop the item entirely.

In addition to evaluating each item, the initial expert panel should be asked to consider whether the items taken as a whole adequately cover the construct domain. The items on a scale constitute the operational definition of the construct, so it is important to assess whether the operational definition taps each dimension adequately. Experts should be asked for specific guidance on items or subdomains that should be added. For scales constructed within an IRT framework, the experts should also be asked whether the items as a whole span a continuum of difficulty (i.e., whether the underlying hierarchy is adequately captured).

If there is agreement among the experts, the next step is straightforward: Their opinion is used to guide decisions about retaining, revising, deleting, or adding items. When there is disagreement, however, it may require further investigation. Perhaps the experts did not understand the task, perhaps the conceptual definitions were ambiguous, and so on.

The typical formula for evaluating agreement among experts on individual items is the number agreeing, divided by the number of experts. When the dimension being rated is relevance, the standard method for computing a content validity index *at the item level* (I-CVI) is the number giving a rating of either 3 or 4 on the 4-point relevance scale, divided by the number of raters. For example, if five experts rated an item as 3 and one rated the item as 2, the I-CVI would be .83. Because of the risk of chance agreement when ratings are dichotomous—relevant versus not relevant—we recommend that I-CVIs should be .78 or higher (Polit, et al., 2007). This means that there must be 100% agreement among raters when there are 4 or fewer experts. When there are 5 to 8 experts, one rating of "not relevant" can be tolerated, and when

there are 9 or more experts, even more can disagree on relevance.

Items with lower-than-desired I-CVIs need careful scrutiny. It may be necessary to recontact the experts to better understand genuine differences of opinion or to strive for greater consensus. If there are legitimate disagreements among the experts on individual items (or if there is agreement about lack of relevance), the items should be revised or dropped.

Content Validation of the Scale

In the second round of content validation, a smaller group of experts (3 to 5) can be used to evaluate the relevance of the revised set of items and to compute the scale content validity (S-CVI). Although it is possible to use a new group of experts, we recommend using a subset from the first panel because then information from the first round can be used to select the most qualified judges. With information from round 1, for example, you can perhaps identify experts who did not understand the task, who had a tendency to give high (or low) ratings, who were not as familiar with the construct as you thought, or who otherwise seemed biased. In other words, data from the first round can be analyzed with a view toward evaluating the performance of the experts, not just the items. This analysis might also require discussion with some of the experts to fully understand the reason for incongruent or anomalous ratings.

In terms of selecting experts based on their ratings in the first round, here are some suggestions. First, it may be imprudent to select experts who rated every item as "highly relevant" (or "not relevant"). Second, it would not be wise to invite back an expert who gave high ratings to items that were judged by most others to not be relevant, or vice versa. Third, the proportion of items judged relevant should be computed for all judges. For example, if an expert rated 8 out of 10 items as relevant, the proportion for that judge would be .80. The pattern across experts can be examined for "outliers." If the average proportion across raters is, for example, .80, you might consider not inviting back for a second round experts whose average proportion was either very low (e.g., .50) or very high (e.g., 1.0). Qualitative feedback from an expert in round 1, in the form of useful comments, might indicate both content capability and a commitment to the project. Finally, items known not to be relevant can be included in the first round to identify judges who rate irrelevant items as relevant and thus may not really be experts after all.

After ratings of relevance are obtained for a revised set of items, the S-CVI can be computed. There is more than one way to compute an S-CVI, as noted in Chapter 14 (Polit & Beck, 2006). We recommend the approach that averages across I-CVIs. On a 10-item scale, for example, if the I-CVIs for 5 items were .80 and the I-CVIs for the remaining 5 items were 1.00, then the S-CVI/Ave would be .90. An S-CVI/Ave of .90 or higher is desirable.

In summary, we recommend that for a scale to be judged as having excellent content validity, it would be composed of items that had I-CVIs of .78 or higher and an S-CVI (using the averaging approach) of .90 or higher. This requires strong items, outstanding experts, and clear instructions to the experts regarding the underlying constructs and the rating task.

➔ **TIP:** When you describe content validation in a report, be specific about your criteria for accepting items (i.e., the cutoff value for your I-CVIs) and the scale (the S-CVI). The report should indicate the range of obtained I-CVI values and the method used to compute the S-CVI.

ADMINISTRATION TO A DEVELOPMENT SAMPLE

At this point, you will have whittled down and refined your items based on your own and others' careful scrutiny. The next step in scale development is to undertake a quantitative assessment of the items, which requires that they be administered to a fairly large development sample. As with content validation, this may involve a two-part process, with preliminary assessment occurring in the first phase and subsequent efforts to evaluate the scale's psychometric adequacy in the second.

Testing a new instrument is a full study in and of itself, and care must be taken to design the study to yield useful evidence about the scale's worth. Important steps include the development of a sampling plan and data collection strategy.

Developing a Sampling Plan

The sample for testing the scale should be representative of the population for whom the scale has been devised, and should be large enough to support complex analyses. If it is not possible to administer the items to a random sample (as is typical), it is advantageous to recruit a sample from multiple sites—preferably in different areas—to enhance representativeness and to assess geographic variation in interpreting items. Other strategies to enhance representativeness should be sought, as well—for example, making sure that the sample includes older and younger respondents, men and women, people with varying educational and ethnic backgrounds, and so on, if these characteristics are relevant. You should also consider taking steps to ensure that the sample includes the right subsets of people for a "known groups" analysis.

How large is a "large" sample? There is neither consensus among experts nor hard-and-fast rules. Some suggest that 300 is an adequate number to support a factor analysis (Nunnally & Bernstein, 1994), while others offer guidance in terms of a ratio of items to respondents. Recommendations range from 3 or 4 people per item to 40 or 50 per item, with 10 per item being the number most often recommended. That means that if you have 20 items, your sample should probably be at least 200. Having a sufficiently large sample is essential to ensure stability in the covariation among the items.

Developing a Data Collection Plan

Decisions have to be made concerning how to administer the instrument (e.g., by mailed or distributed questionnaires, over the Internet), and what to include in the instrument. In deciding on a mode of administration, you should choose an approach that best approximates how the scale typically would be administered after it is finalized. Thought should also be given to administration setting. For example, if the scale is designed as a screening tool for hospitalized patients, then hospitals should be the setting for collecting the development data.

The instrument should include the scale items and basic demographic information. Thought should also be given to including other measures on the instrument—which would be essential if you do not plan to undertake a separate study to evaluate the scale's validity.

Various types of validation measures are possible to evaluate the facets of construct and criterion-related validity discussed in Chapter 14. For example, you might include a measure of constructs similar to, but distinct from, the target construct to evaluate discriminant validity. Measures of other constructs hypothesized to be correlated with the target construct should be included. If the data confirm a relationship predicted by theory or prior research, this would lend evidence to the new scale's validity. Finally, it may be useful to include measures to assess response biases, especially social desirability. Item correlations with a measure of social desirability could suggest potentially biased items. (More complex approaches to evaluating and addressing the effects of social desirability and "faking bad" biases are discussed in Streiner and Norman, Chapter 6). Brief social desirability scales have been developed (e.g., Reynolds, 1982; Strahan & Gerbasi, 1972).

➲ **T I P :** In deciding on what other measures to include in the study, keep in mind that respondents' willingness to cooperate may decline as the instrument package gets longer.

Preparing for Data Collection

As in all data collection efforts, care should be taken to make the instrument attractive, professional looking, and easy to understand. Friends, colleagues, mentors, or family members should be asked to evaluate the appearance of the instrument before it is reproduced.

Instructions for completing the instrument should be clear, and a readability assessment of the instructions is useful. There should be no ambiguity about what is expected of respondents. Guidance in understanding the end points of response options should be provided if points along the continuum are not explicitly labeled. The instructions should encourage candor. Sometimes, social desirability can be minimized by stating that there are no right or wrong answers. Anonymity also reduces social desirability bias, and is recommended—unless the scale needs to be administered twice to estimate test–retest reliability. Pett and colleagues (2003) offer useful suggestions for laying out an instrument and for developing instructions to respondents.

One other consideration is how to sequence the items in the instrument. At issue is something that is called a *proximity effect*, the tendency to be influenced in responding to an item by the response given to the previous item. This effect would tend to artificially inflate estimates of internal consistency. One approach to deal with this is the random ordering of items. An alternative, for scales designed to measure several related dimensions, is to systematically alternate items that are expected to be scored into different subscales.

Example of item ordering: Lange and Yellen (2009), who refined a Spanish version of a scale to measure satisfaction with nursing care, deliberately placed two positively worded items at the beginning of the instrument, because Lange's previous work suggested that negatively worded items at the beginning confused people. After the first two items, negative items were positioned throughout the scale at random.

ANALYSIS OF SCALE DEVELOPMENT DATA

The analysis of data from multi-item scales is a topic about which entire books have been written. We provide only an overview here. We assume that readers of this section have basic familiarity with statistics. Those who need a refresher should consult Chapters 16 through 18.

Basic Item Analysis

The performance of each item on the preliminary scale needs to be evaluated empirically. Within classical measurement theory, what is desired is an item that has a high correlation with the true score of the underlying construct. We cannot assess this directly, but if each item is a measure of that latent variable, then the items should correlate with one another.

The degree of **inter-item correlation** can be assessed by inspecting the correlation matrix of all the items. If there are items with substantial negative inter-item correlations, some should perhaps be reverse-scored (e.g., NEWITEM = 8 – OLDITEM, for 7-point scales). Unless intentional, however, negative correlations are likely to reflect problems and may signal the desirability of removing some items. For items on the same subscale, inter-item correlations between .30 and .70 are often recommended (e.g., Ferketich, 1991), with correlations lower than .30 suggesting little congruence with the underlying construct and ones higher than .70 suggesting over-redundancy. However, the evaluation depends on the number of items in the scale. An average inter-item correlation of .57 is needed to achieve a coefficient alpha of .80 on a 3-item scale, but an average of only .29 is needed for a 10-item scale (DeVellis, 2003).

A next step is to compute preliminary total scale scores (or subscale scores) and then to calculate correlations between individual items and total scores on the scales they are intended to represent. If item scores do not correlate well with scale scores, it is probably measuring something else and will lower the reliability of the scale. There are two types of **item–scale correlations**, one in which the total score includes the item under consideration (*uncorrected*), and another in which the individual item is removed in calculating the total scale score. The latter (*corrected*) approach is preferable because the inclusion of the item on the scale inflates the correlation coefficients, and the inflation factor increases as the number of items on the scale decreases. The standard advice is to eliminate items whose item–scale correlation is less than .30 but some recommend a criterion as high as .50.

DeVellis (2003) also recommends looking at basic descriptive information for each item, as a double check. Items should have good variability—without it, they will not correlate with the total scale and will not fare well in a reliability analysis. Means for the items that are close to the center of the range of possible scores are also desirable (e.g., a mean near 4 on a 7-point scale). Items with means near one extreme or the other tend not to discriminate well among respondents.

Other item analysis techniques have been developed. Some scale developers compute item *p* levels or *difficulty levels*, which are indicators of how "difficult" each item is. For example, if 60 people agreed with an item and 40 disagreed with it, it could be said that the *p* level for the item was .60 because 60% found it "easy" to agree. Items in the mid-range of difficulty are most desirable. Another index that is too complex to explain here is the *discrimination index*, which examines the discriminative ability of each item. As mentioned earlier, item response theory has given rise to a number of excellent diagnostic tools for examining the performance of individual items. These and other item analysis techniques are described elsewhere (e.g., Gable & Wolfe, 1993; Nunnally & Bernstein, 1994; Waltz et al., 2010).

Example of item analysis: Heo and colleagues (2005) undertook several item analytic procedures with data from a sample of 638 patients in their evaluation of the Minnesota Living with Heart Failure Questionnaire. They computed item–total correlations, inter-item correlations, item *p* levels, and a discrimination index. As a result of these and other analyses, they recommended that 5 items be deleted.

Exploratory Factor Analysis

A set of items is not necessarily a scale—the items form a scale only if they have a common underlying construct. **Factor analysis** disentangles complex interrelationships among items and identifies items that "go together" as unified concepts. This section deals with a type of factor analysis known as **exploratory factor analysis (EFA)**, which essentially assumes no *a priori* hypotheses about dimensionality of a set of items. Another type—confirmatory factor analysis—uses more complex modeling and estimation procedures, as described later.

Suppose we developed 50 Likert-type items measuring women's attitudes toward menopause. We could form a scale by adding together scores from several individual items, but which items should be combined? Would it be reasonable to combine all 50 items? Probably not, because the 50 items are not all tapping the same thing—there are various *dimensions* to women's attitude toward menopause. One dimension may relate to aging and another to loss of reproductive ability. Other items may involve sexuality, and yet others may concern avoidance of monthly menstruation. These multiple dimensions to women's attitudes toward menopause should be captured on separate subscales. Women's attitude on one dimension may be independent of their attitude on another. Dimensions of a construct are usually identified during the conceptualization phase and when the items are being evaluated by experts. Preconceptions about dimensions, however, do not always "pan out" when tested against actual responses. Factor analysis offers an objective, empirical method of clarifying the underlying dimensionality of a large set of measures. Underlying dimensions thus identified are called **factors**, which are weighted combinations of items in the analysis.

⮕ **TIP:** Before undertaking an EFA, you should evaluate the *factorability* of your set of items. Procedures for a factorability assessment are described in Polit (2010).

Factor Extraction

EFA involves two phases. The first phase (**factor extraction**) condenses items into a smaller number of factors and is used to identify the number of underlying dimensions. The goal is to extract clusters of highly interrelated items from a correlation matrix. There are various methods of performing the first step, each of which uses different criteria for assigning weights to items. A widely used factor extraction method is **principal components analysis**

(**PCA**) and another is **principal-axis factor analysis**. The pros and cons of alternative approaches to factor extraction have been nicely summarized by Pett and colleagues (2003). Our discussion focuses mostly on PCA, although the two methods often (but not always) lead to the same conclusion about dimensionality.

Factor extraction yields an *unrotated factor matrix*, which contains coefficients or *weights* for all original items on each extracted factor. Each extracted factor is a weighted linear combination of all the original items. For example, with three items, a factor would be item 1 (times a weight) + item 2 (times a weight) + item 3 (times a weight). In the PCA method, weights for the first factor are computed such that the average squared weight is maximized, permitting a maximum amount of variance to be extracted by the first factor. The second factor, or linear weighted combination, is formed so that the highest possible amount of variance is extracted from what *remains* after the first factor has been taken into account. The factors thus represent independent sources of variation in the data matrix.

Factoring should continue until no further meaningful variance is left, so a criterion must be applied to decide when to stop extraction and move on to the next phase. There are several possible criteria, which makes factor analysis a semisubjective process. Several criteria can be described by illustrating information from a factor analysis. Table 15.1 presents fictitious values for eigenvalues, percentages of variance accounted for, and cumulative percentages of variance accounted for, for 10 factors. **Eigenvalues** are equal to the sum of the squared item weights for the factor. Many researchers establish as their cutoff point for factor extraction eigenvalues greater than 1.00. In our example, the first five factors meet this criterion. Some believe that the eigenvalue rule is too generous—that is, extracts too many factors (DeVellis, 2003). Another cutoff benchmark, called the *scree test,* is based on a principle of discontinuity: A sharp drop in the percentage of explained variance indicates the appropriate termination point. In Table 15.1, we might argue that there is considerable discontinuity

TABLE 15.1	Summary of Factor Extraction Results		
FACTOR	**EIGENVALUE**	**PERCENTAGE OF VARIANCE EXPLAINED**	**CUMULATIVE PERCENTAGE OF VARIANCE EXPLAINED**
1	12.32	29.2	29.2
2	8.57	23.3	52.5
3	6.91	15.6	68.1
4	2.02	8.4	76.5
5	1.09	6.2	82.7
6	.98	5.8	88.5
7	.80	4.5	93.0
8	.62	3.1	96.1
9	.47	2.2	98.3
10	.25	1.7	100.0

between the third and fourth factors—that is, that three factors should be extracted. Another guideline concerns the amount of variance explained by the factors. Some advocate that the number of factors extracted should account for at least 60% of the total variance and that for any factor to be meaningful it must account for at least 5% of the variance. In our table, the first three factors account for 68.1% of the total variance; 6 factors contribute 5% or more to the total variance.

So, should we extract 3, 5, or 6 factors? One approach is to see whether there is any convergence among these guidelines. In our example, two of them (the scree test and total variance test) suggest three factors. Another approach is to determine whether any of the rules yields a number consistent with our original conceptualization about dimensionality. In our example, if we had designed the items to represent three theoretically meaningful subscales, we might consider three factors to be the right number because there is sufficient empirical support for that conclusion. Indeed, some have argued that restricting the factor solution to a prespecified number of factors that is consistent with the original conceptualization can yield important information regarding how much variance is accounted for by the factors.

⊃ TIP: Polit (2010) provides a "walk-through" demonstration of how decisions are made in undertaking an exploratory factor analysis.

Factor Rotation

The second phase of factor analysis—**factor rotation**—is performed on factors that have met extraction criteria, to make the factors more interpretable. The concept of rotation can be best explained graphically. Figure 15.2 shows two coordinate systems, marked by axes A1 and A2 and B1 and B2. The primary axes (A1 and A2) represent factors I and II, respectively, as defined *before* rotation. Points 1 through 6 represent six items in this two-dimensional space. The weights for each item can be determined in reference to these axes. For instance, before rotation, item 1 has a weight of .80 on factor I and .85 on factor II, and item 6 has a weight of −.45 on factor I and .90 on factor II. Unrotated axes account for a maximum amount of variance but may not provide a structure with conceptual meaning. Interpretability is enhanced by rotating the axes so that clusters of items are distinctly associated with a factor. In the figure, B1 and B2 represent rotated factors. After rotation, items 1, 2, and 3 have large weights on factor I and

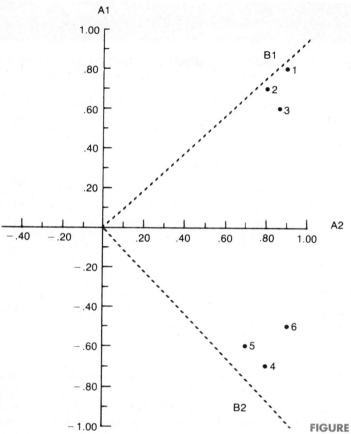

FIGURE 15.2 Illustration of factor rotation.

small weights on factor II, and the reverse is true for items 4, 5, and 6.

Researchers choose from two types of rotation. Figure 15.2 illustrates **orthogonal rotation**, in which factors are kept at right angles to one another. Orthogonal rotations maintain the independence of factors—that is, orthogonal factors are uncorrelated with one another. **Oblique rotations** permit rotated axes to depart from a 90-degree angle. In our figure, an oblique rotation would have put axis B1 between items 2 and 3 and axis B2 between items 5 and 6. This placement strengthens the clustering of items around an associated factor, but results in correlated factors. Some writers argue that orthogonal rotation leads to greater theoretical clarity; others claim that it is unrealistic. Advocates of oblique rotation point

out that if the concepts *are* correlated, then the analysis should reflect this fact. In developing a scale with multiple dimensions, we likely would expect the dimensions to be correlated, so oblique rotation might well be more theoretically meaningful. This can be assessed empirically: If an oblique rotation is specified, the correlation between factors is calculated. If the correlations are low (e.g., less than .15 or .20), an orthogonal rotation may be preferred because it yields a simpler model.

Researchers work with a **rotated factor matrix** in interpreting the factor analysis. As an example, the matrix in Table 15.2 shows information from a factor analysis of the School-Age Temperament Inventory (SATI) for 12 of the scale's 38 items (McClowry, et al., 2003). The entries under each

TABLE 15.2	Factor Loadings: School-Age Temperament Inventory			
ITEM	**FACTOR 1**	**FACTOR 2**	**FACTOR 3**	**FACTOR 4**
1. Does not complete homework[a]	.04	**.82**	−.01	.07
2. Is shy with adults he (she) doesn't know	.02	.00	**.78**	.00
3. Runs when entering or leaving	.16	.03	.00	**.79**
4. Is bashful when meeting new children	.09	.01	**.80**	−.01
5. Stays with homework until finished	.04	**.84**	.00	.06
6. Yells or snaps at others when angry	**.79**[b]	.05	.04	.12
7. Runs or jumps when going down stairs	.18	.11	.05	**.74**
8. Is moody when corrected for misbehavior	**.75**	.10	.13	.02
9. Runs to where he (she) wants to go	.09	.07	−.10	**.77**
10. Responds intensely to disapproval	**.78**	.11	.06	.12
11. Has difficulty completing assignments[a]	.08	**.78**	.01	.04
12. Seems uncomfortable at someone's house	.11	.06	**.75**	.06

[a]Item was reverse-coded before factor analysis.

[b]Bolded entries represent high loadings on a factor and are used to name and interpret the factor.

Adapted from Table 1 of McClowry, S. G., Halverson, C. F., & Sanson, A. (2003). A re-examination of the validity and reliability of the School-Age Temperament Inventory. *Nursing Research, 52*(3), p. 180.

factor are the weights, or **factor loadings**. For orthogonally rotated factors, factor loadings can range from −1.00 to +1.00 and can be interpreted like correlation coefficients—they express the correlation between items and factors. In this example, item 1 is highly correlated with Factor 2, .82. By examining factor loadings, we can find which items "belong" to a factor. For example, items 6, 8, and 10 have sizable loadings on factor 1. Loadings with an absolute value of .40 or higher often are used as cutoff values, but somewhat smaller values may be acceptable if it makes theoretical sense to do so. The underlying dimensionality of the items can then be interpreted. By inspecting the content of items 6, 8, and 10, we can search for a common theme that makes the items go together. The developers of the SATI called this first factor *Negative Reactivity*. Items 1, 5, and 11 have high loadings on Factor 2, which they named *Task Persistence*. Factor 3 and 4 are called *Approach/Withdrawal* and *Activity*, respectively. The naming of factors is a process of identifying underlying constructs—and this naming often would have occurred during the conceptualization phase.

The results of the factor analysis can be used not only to identify the dimensionality of the construct, but also to make decisions about item retention and deletion. If items have low loadings on all factors, they may be good candidates for deletion (or revision, if you can detect wording problems that may have caused different respondents to infer different meaning from the item). Items with fairly high loadings on multiple factors may also be candidates for deletion. Items with marginal loadings (e.g., .34) but that had good content validity probably should be retained for the reliability analysis.

Example of exploratory factor analysis:
Heaman and Gupton (2009) developed a scale called the Perception of Pregnancy Risk Questionnaire. The 9-item scale was tested with 199 women in the third trimester of pregnancy. Exploratory factor analysis resulted in a 2-factor solution: Risk for Baby (5 items with loadings ranging from .40 to .99) and Risk for Self (4 items with loadings from .51 to .92).

Reliability Analysis

After a final set of items is selected based on the item analysis and factor analysis, a reliability analysis should be undertaken to calculate coefficient alpha. Alpha, it may be recalled, provides an estimate of the proportion of variance in the scale scores that is attributable to the true score and thus is a key indicator of the scale's quality.

Most computer programs for doing reliability analysis provide extensive information, including many item analysis diagnostics we described earlier. Especially important at this point in scale development is information about the value of coefficient alpha for the scale—and for a hypothetical scale with each individual item removed. If the overall alpha is extremely high, it may be prudent to eliminate redundancy by deleting items that do not make a sizeable contribution to alpha. (Sometimes removal of a faulty item actually *increases* alpha.) A modest reduction in reliability is sometimes worth the benefit of lowering respondent burden. Scale developers must consider the best trade-off between brevity and reliability.

One thing that should be kept in mind is that reliabilities tend to capitalize on chance factors in a sample of respondents and will often be lower in a new sample. Thus, you should aim for reliabilities a bit higher in the development sample than ones you would consider minimally acceptable so that if the alphas deteriorate they will still be adequate. This is especially true if the development sample is small.

➲ TIP: If you have the good fortune to have a very large sample, you should consider dividing the sample in half, running the factor analysis and reliability analysis with one subsample, and then rerunning them with the second as a cross-validation of factor structure and scale reliabilities.

FINAL STEPS: SCALE REFINEMENT AND VALIDATION

In some scale development efforts, the bulk of work is over at this point. For example, if you developed a scale as part of a larger substantive project because you were unable to identify a good measure of a key construct, you may be ready to pursue your substantive analyses. If, however, you are developing a scale for others to use, a few more steps remain.

Revising the Scale

The analyses undertaken in the development study often suggest the need to revise or add items. For example, if subscale alpha coefficients are lower than .80 or so, consideration should be given to adding items for subsequent testing. In thinking about new items, a good strategy is to examine items that had high factor loadings. Such items presumably correlate most strongly with the latent variable and so may offer powerful clues for additional items.

There may be other reasons for adding new items. For example, if a confirmatory factor analysis is envisioned as part of a scale validation effort, there should be at least 4 items for each factor (subscale) because of technical problems with dimensions having three or fewer items.

Finally, you should carefully examine the content of the items remaining in your scale. Sometimes alphas are inflated by items that have similar wording, so it is wise to make decisions about retaining or removing items based not only on their contribution to alpha, but also on content validity considerations. It may prove worthwhile to re-examine the I-CVIs of each item in making final decisions.

Scoring and Transforming the Scale

Scoring the scale is often easy with Likert-type items: Item scores are typically just added together (with reverse scoring of items, if appropriate) to form subscale scores, and subscale scores are sometimes added together to form total scale scores. Scoring in this manner should, however, be a conscious decision.

When individual items are simply added together, the implicit assumption is that all of the items are equally important indicators of the latent variable. If there are theoretical or empirical reasons for suspecting otherwise, a system of weighting the items (so that more important items are given more weight in the total score) might be considered. For example, a scale to assess a person's risk of a disease or condition (e.g., risk of cardiovascular disease) might benefit from weighting some items (e.g., high blood pressure) more heavily than others. Weighting is sometimes accomplished empirically, for example, by using factor loadings from a PCA to weight items. Weighting is discussed more extensively in Streiner and Norman (2008), and Pett and colleagues (2003) provide detailed information about factor scores.

A related consideration is whether the scores should be *transformed*. If, for example, subscales have different numbers of items, the means will almost surely vary even if the average intensity is similar across dimensions—making it difficult to make comparisons across dimensions. For this reason, some scale developers deliberately try to construct scales that have an equal number of items per subscale. Another approach is to transform scores, most typically through the use of *standard scores* or *z scores* (see Streiner & Norman, 2008).

Conducting a Validation Study

Scale developers ideally should take steps to gather new data about the worth of their instrument in a validation study. Those who are not able to undertake a second study should strive to undertake many of the activities described in this section with data from the original development sample. Designing a validation study entails much of the same issues (and advice) as designing a development study, in terms of sample composition, sample size, data collection strategies, and so on. Thus, we focus here on analyses undertaken in a validation study. Internal consistency reliability should be recomputed in the validation sample.

Confirmatory Factor Analysis

Confirmatory factor analysis (CFA) is playing an increasingly important role in validation studies. CFA is preferable to EFA as an approach to construct validity because CFA is a hypothesis testing approach—testing the hypothesis that the items belong to specific factors, rather than having the dimensionality of a set of items emerge empirically, as in EFA.

CFA is a subset of an advanced class of statistical techniques known as **structural equation modeling** (SEM). CFA differs from EFA in a number of respects, many of which are quite technical. One concerns the estimation procedure. As we explain in Chapter 18, many statistical procedures used by nurse researchers employ *least-squares estimation*. In SEM, the most frequently used estimation procedure is *maximum likelihood estimation*. (Maximum likelihood estimators are ones that estimate the parameters most likely to have generated the observed measurements.) Least-squares procedures have several stringent assumptions that are generally untenable—for example, the assumption that variables are measured without error. SEM approaches can accommodate measurement error and avoid other restrictions as well.

CFA involves the testing of a **measurement model**, which stipulates the hypothesized relationships among underlying latent variables and the *manifest variables*—that is, the items. The measurement model is essentially a factor analytic model that seeks to confirm a hypothesized factor structure. Loadings on the factors (the *latent variables*) provide a method for evaluating relationships between observed variables (the items) and unobserved variables (the factors or dimensions of a construct).

We illustrate with a simplified example involving a scale designed to measure two aspects of fatigue: physical fatigue and mental fatigue. In the example shown in Figure 15.3, both types of fatigue are captured by five items each: items I1 to I5 for physical fatigue and items I6 to I10 for mental fatigue. According to the model, respondents' item responses are *caused by* their physical and mental fatigue (and thus the straight arrows indicating hypothesized causal paths) and are also affected by error (e_1 through e_{10}). Moreover, it is hypothesized that the error terms are correlated, as indicated by the curved lines connecting the errors. Correlated measurement errors on the items might arise as a result of the person's desire to "look good" or to acquiesce—factors that would systematically affect all item scores. The figure also shows that the two latent fatigue variables are hypothesized to be correlated.

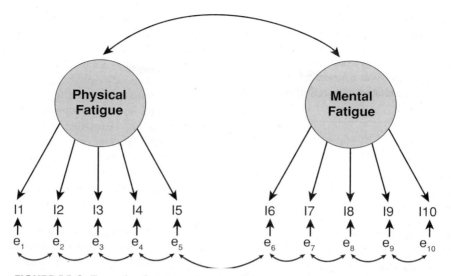

FIGURE 15.3 Example of a measurement model.

The hypothesized measurement model would be tested against actual data. The analysis would yield loadings of observed variables on the latent variables, the correlation between the two latent variables, and correlations among the error terms. The analysis would also indicate whether the overall model fit is good, based on a **goodness-of-fit statistic**. If the hypothesized model is *not* a good fit to the data, the measurement model could be respecified and retested.

CFA is a complex topic, and we have described only basic characteristics. Further reading on the topic is imperative for those wishing to pursue it (e.g., Brown, 2006; Harrington, 2008).

Example of confirmatory factor analysis:
Kalisch and colleagues (2010) undertook a psychometric assessment of the Nursing Teamwork Survey with a sample of over 1,700 nurses in acute care facilities. Exploratory factor analysis with a randomly selected half of the sample revealed five factors. Confirmatory factor analysis with the other half of the sample confirmed the factor structure.

Other Validation Activities

A validation effort would not be complete without undertaking additional activities designed to pro-

vide evidence of the scale's validity, such as ones described in Chapter 14. The assessment of criterion or construct validity primarily relies on correlational evidence. In criterion-related validity, scores on the new scale are correlated with an external criterion. In construct validity, scores on the scale can, for example, be correlated with measures of constructs hypothesized to be related to the target construct, or supplementary measures of the same construct (convergent validity), or measures of a closely related but distinguishable construct (divergent validity). Contrast validity using a known-groups approach requires selecting people with membership in groups expected to be different, on average, on the scale. It is desirable to produce as much validity evidence as possible.

If a CFA is not possible (perhaps because of lack of training in using it), it is nevertheless advisable to undertake a "confirmatory" factor analysis using the more traditional methods, such as PCA, with the validation sample. Comparisons between the original and new factor analyses can be made with respect to factor structure, loadings, variance explained, eigenvalues, and so on. In the new analysis, the number of factors to be extracted and rotated can be prespecified, since this is now the working hypothesis about the underlying dimensionality of the construct.

➡ **TIP:** Scale development and validation activities should be reported in the nursing literature so that others can benefit. An editorial in the journal *Research in Nursing & Health* provides guidance regarding information to include in an instrument development paper (Froman & Schmitt, 2003), and further guidance is offered by DeVon and colleagues (2007).

Establishing Cutoff Points

Scales produce scores along a continuum, but there are constructs for which it is important to dichotomize scale scores. A familiar example is classroom and licensing examinations: There must be a score (cutoff point) that distinguishes those who pass and those who fail. Diagnostic and screening scales need to provide information about whether there is "caseness" or not.

Various methods—both empirical and subjective—have been developed for establishing cutoff points on scales (Streiner & Norman, 2008). As described in Chapter 14, the method that has the most credibility is the construction of receiver operating characteristic (ROC) curves and its associated indicators. Data for undertaking such an analysis typically come from a validation study. Scale developers who intend to develop ROC curves need to select highly reliable criteria for dividing people into groups (e.g., those with and those without the condition being screened), and the criteria must be independent of participants' responses on the scale.

Establishing Norms

In some cases, it might be desirable to *standardize* a new scale and establish norms. This typically occurs if the expectation is that (a) the scale will be widely used, and used by people who will rely on solid comparative information to help them evaluate scores, and (b) average scale scores vary markedly by members of well-defined subpopulations. Norms are most commonly established for key demographic characteristics, such as age and gender.

Sampling is the most critical aspect of a standardization effort. The sample used to establish norms should be geographically dispersed (within the desired scope) and representative of the population for whom the scale is intended. In most cases, this means using probability sampling. A large standardization sample is required so that subgroup values are stable.

After the scale is administered to a standardization sample, various descriptive statistics are computed. Norms are often expressed in terms of percentiles. For example, an adult male with a score of 72 on the scale might be at the 80th percentile, but a female with the same score might be at the 85th percentile. Guidelines for norming instruments have been developed by Waltz and her colleagues (2010) and Nunnally and Bernstein (1994).

➡ **TIP:** If you expect the scale to be used by others, you should develop a manual for its use. The manual should include the items; the underlying conceptual rationale; the process used to develop, refine, and evaluate items; instructions for using the scale, including scoring and interpretation; information about norms and cutoff points, if relevant; and information about the scale's psychometric properties. Guidelines for preparing manuals are published in *Standards for Educational and Psychological Testing* (AERA, APA, & NCME Joint Committee, 1999). Scale developers should consider registering a copyright, even if they do not plan to publish the scale commercially.

TRANSLATING SCALES INTO OTHER LANGUAGES

Scales are increasingly being used with people from various linguistic and cultural backgrounds. Developing equivalent scales in other languages requires nearly as much care and effort as developing an original scale. We provide a brief overview and offer suggestions for further reading on this important topic.

Centered Versus Decentered Translations

Translation is often approached in a "centered" way, in which the scale is translated into another language, with no effect on the wording of the original instrument. In a *centered* (or asymmetric) *translation*, loyalty to the original scale items is maintained. Such translations typically occur after-the-fact, that is, after the original scale has been validated and used, and has been identified as a candidate for translation because it has desirable features.

By contrast, a *decentered translation* involves the possibility of modifications to items on the original scale. Such decentered (or symmetric) translations often reflect the goal of replacing culturally exclusive language with more universally understood language. This approach is often adopted when the developer knows in advance that the scale will be used in two languages, so translation activities are built into the scale development process.

⇨ **T I P :** When a translation is anticipated upfront, scale developers should consider the following as they are crafting items: (1) avoid metaphors, idioms, and colloquialisms; (2) use specific words rather than ones open to interpretation, such as "daily" rather than "frequently"; (3) avoid pronouns—repeat nouns if necessary to avoid ambiguity; (4) write in the present tense and avoid the subjunctive mode, such as "should"; and (5) use words with a Latin root if the target language is a Romance language such as Spanish or French (Hilton & Skrutkowski, 2002; Lange, 2002).

Example of a decentered translation: Coffman (2008) translated the Diabetes Self-Efficacy Scale into Spanish using a decentered translation approach.

Conceptual Equivalence

The goal of a translation is to achieve equivalence between an original version of a scale and a translated version. *Equivalence*, however, is itself a complex concept. Over a dozen different types of equivalencies have been suggested, although only a few are given consideration in a typical translation (Beck, et al., 2003; Streiner & Norman, 2008).

A particularly important consideration early in a translation concerns *conceptual equivalence.* Do people in the two cultures view the construct in the same way? As an example, consider *obesity.* A person who is obese in some western cultures might not be considered obese elsewhere. A related question is, does the construct even have *meaning* in the other culture? For example, does the construct of *pleasure* or *enjoyment* have meaning in devastatingly poor societies in which daily survival is a struggle? (Note that conceptual equivalence is an important issue even among subcultures that speak the same language.) Thus, one of the first tasks in a translation effort is to ascertain whether the meaning of the construct as defined in the scale reflects the meaning of the construct within the "target" culture. Experts knowledgeable about the culture in question are often consulted in this early step.

Semantic Equivalence: Back Translations

Semantic equivalence is the extent to which each item's *meaning* is the same in the target culture after translation as it was in the original. Literal translations are rarely satisfactory. The translation needs to preserve the underlying meaning of the original wording rather than the exact wording.

The most respected translation process for achieving semantic equivalence involves **back-translation** (Brislin, 1970), in which an instrument is translated from an original *source language* into a *target language*, and then translated back into the source language by translators who are unfamiliar with the original wording. The process typically involves several important steps.

Selecting and Preparing Translators

The first step is to select translators. At a minimum, two translators are needed, but four or more working as a team is usually desirable. For example, for translations from English to Spanish, it is important to include native Spanish speakers from various regions because of regional linguistic and cultural variations (e.g., Mexico, Puerto Rico, Central America, etc.). Translations are typically done *into* the native tongue of the translator. So, for example, for an English-to-French translation, the items would first be translated by a native French speaker and the back translation would be translated by a native English speaker. Being bilingual is not a sufficient qualification for doing a translation; ideally, translators would have some professional training and experience and have first-hand familiarity with both cultures and be capable of understanding the conceptual underpinnings of the construct.

The scale developer needs to carefully explain the construct and the intent of each item to the translators. Translators should also be given guidance about expectations for their performance—for example, they need to be told what reading level to aim for, whether colloquialisms are discouraged, the importance of semantic equivalence, and so on.

➡ **T I P :** It is sometimes productive to have two independent translations, a procedure that was used by Wang and colleagues (2006) in their translation of the High School Questionnaire: Profile of Experiences into Chinese. One translation was done by a person who taught English in Taiwan, and the second version was done by a graduate student majoring in English.

Undertaking an Iterative Process

The translation/back-translation process is often an iterative one, requiring multiple rounds of translation, review, and group discussion to arrive at consensus. It begins with the translation of items, followed by the back translation by translators blinded to the original wording. Then a comparison is made between the wording of original items and their back-translated counterparts to detect any possible alterations resulting from the translation. The theory is that if the original and back-translated versions are identical, the translated item is equivalent in meaning.

➡ **T I P :** Some back translators infer the original item wording (even when the translation is poor), rather than actually translating from the target language back to the source language, so it is advisable to instruct back translators to treat the target-language version as the original.

More often than not, the original and back-translated versions are *not* identical. If there are serious differences, it may be fruitful to have a group discussion among the translators, and then begin the process anew with a second group of translators after making changes to either the qualifications of the translators, item wording in the source language, or instructions to the translators (or some combination of these).

Example of a Back-Translated Item: Beck and colleagues (2003) provided the following example from the development of the Spanish version of the Postpartum Depression Screening Scale:

Original item: I was afraid that I would never be my normal self again
Translated item: Temia no volver a ser otra vez la misma de antes
Back-translated item: I was afraid I was not going to be the same person as before

When the original and back-translated items are reasonably close, it is time to involve a committee to review what has transpired and to arrive at a consensus about the translated version of the scale items. The committee may be the team of translators but may also be three or more bilingual persons who have not participated in the translation process. Committee members are given complete information on each item—the original version, translated versions, and back-translated versions. They may also be given supplementary information, such as the desired reading level and the *actual* reading level of the various versions. Committee work may require several hours of discussion before consensus is reached.

The committee may conclude that a back-translated item is a better match to the translated item than the original wording. In such a case, if a decentering approach has been used, the wording of the original item can be changed to reflect a more universally understood construction.

Testing the Translated Version

Translated scales need to be tested in a manner analogous to testing the original scale. Pretesting with a small sample from the target culture is important, and cognitive questioning is especially valuable with a translated instrument.

A good way to further evaluate semantic equivalence is to pretest both versions with a sample of bilingual people. Two forms of the instrument should be prepared (source language first on one, target language first on the other), with forms distributed randomly to the pretest sample. Responses on the two versions then can be compared, at both the scale and item level.

Finally, the translated scale should be submitted to a full psychometric evaluation with a large sample of respondents. These efforts not only provide evidence of the soundness of the translated scale, but also support inferences about equivalence. For example, if the internal consistency of the translated scale is substantially lower than the original, there is something wrong with the translation. Confirmatory factor analysis is another strategy that is useful in facilitating conclusions about both the conceptual and semantic equivalence of the scales. Other construct validation procedures ideally would also be used with a sample from the new culture (e.g., known groups).

Example of a scale translation study: Pinar and colleagues (2009) undertook a translation of the Health-Promoting Lifestyle Profile II (HPLPII). The scale was translated from English into Turkish by three translators and back-translated by three independent translators. An expert panel of 10 health professionals reviewed the process. The instrument was pretested with 30 monolingual Turkish speakers. Then cultural equivalence was assessed by administering both the English and Turkish versions to 109 bilingual people. Psychometric evaluation of the translated scale's reliability and validity was undertaken with a sample of 920 people. Validation efforts (including both EFA and CFA) indicated good construct validity of the translated scale. Test–retest and internal consistency reliability were high.

CRITIQUING SCALE DEVELOPMENT STUDIES

Articles on scale development appear regularly in many nursing journals. If you are planning to use a scale in a substantive study, you should carefully review the methods used to construct and validate the scale—and to translate it, if a translated version is under consideration. You should also evaluate whether the evidence regarding the scale's psychometric adequacy is sufficiently sound to merit its use. Remember that you run the risk of undermining the statistical conclusion validity of your study (i.e., of having insufficient power for testing your hypotheses) if you use a scale with weak reliability. And you can run the risk of poor construct validity in your study if your measures are not strong proxies for key constructs.

Box 15.1 ⚙ provides guidelines for evaluating a research report on the development and validation of a scale.

BOX 15.1 Guidelines for Critiquing Scale Development and Validation Reports

1. Does the report offer a clear definition of the construct? Does it provide sufficient context for the study through a summary of the literature and discussion of relevant theory? Is the population for whom the scale intended adequately described?
2. Does the report indicate how items were generated? Do the procedures seem sound? Is information provided about the reading level for the scale items?
3. Does the report describe content validation efforts, and was the description thorough? Is there evidence of good content validity?
4. Were appropriate efforts made to refine the scale (e.g., through pretests, item analysis)?
5. Was the development or validation sample of participants appropriate in terms of representativeness and size?
6. Was factor analysis used to examine or validate the scale's dimensionality? If yes, does the report offer evidence to support the factor structure and the naming of factors?
7. Were appropriate methods used to assess the scale's reliability? Were reliability estimates sufficiently high?
8. Were appropriate methods used to assess the scale's criterion or construct validity? Is the evidence about the scale's validity persuasive? What other validation methods would have strengthened inferences about the scale's worthiness?
9. Does the report provide information for scoring the scale and interpreting scale scores—for example, means and standard deviations, cutoff scores, norms?
10. If the study involves a translation, were appropriate procedures (e.g., back translation, a committee approach, validation efforts) used to ensure scale equivalency?

RESEARCH EXAMPLE

Studies: Postpartum Depression Screening Scale: Development and psychometric testing (Beck & Gable, 2000); Further validation of the Postpartum Depression Screening Scale (Beck & Gable, 2001); Postpartum Depression Screening Scale: Spanish version (Beck & Gable, 2003).

Background: Beck studied postpartum depression (PPD) in a series of qualitative studies, using both a phenomenological approach (1992, 1996) and a grounded theory approach (1993). Based on her in-depth understanding of PPD, she began in the late 1990s to develop a scale that could be used to screen for PPD, the Postpartum Depression Screening Scale (PDSS).

Statement of Purpose: Beck and an expert psychometrician undertook methodologic studies to develop, refine, and validate a scale to screen women for postpartum depression, and to translate the scale into Spanish.

Scale Development: The PDSS is a Likert scale designed to tap seven dimensions, such as sleeping/eating disturbances and mental confusion. A 56-item pilot form of the PDSS was initially developed with 8 items per dimension, using a 5-point response scale. Beck's program of research on PPD and her knowledge of the literature were the basis for specifying the domain. Themes from Beck's qualitative research were used to develop 7 dimensions, and to craft the items to operationalize those dimensions. The reading level of the final PDSS was assessed to be at the third-grade level and the Flesch reading ease score was 92.7.

Content Validity: Content validity was enhanced by using direct quotes from the qualitative studies as items on the scale (e.g., "I felt like I was losing my mind"). The pilot form was subjected to two content validation procedures with a panel of five content experts. Feedback from these procedures led to some item revisions.

Construct Validity: The PDSS was administered to a sample of 525 new mothers in six states (Beck & Gable, 2000). Preliminary item analyses resulted in the deletion of several items, based on item–total correlations. The PDSS was finalized as a 35-item scale with seven subscales, each with 5 items. This version of the PDSS was subjected to confirmatory factor analyses, which involved a validation of Beck's hypotheses about how individual items mapped onto

underlying constructs, such as cognitive impairment. Item response theory was also used, and provided supporting evidence of the scale's construct validity. In a subsequent study, Beck and Gable (2001) administered the PDSS and two other depression scales to 150 new mothers and tested hypotheses about how scores on the PDSS would correlate with scores on other scales. The results indicated good convergent validity.

Criterion-Related Validity: In the second study, Beck and Gable correlated scores on the PDSS with an expert clinician's diagnosis of PPD for each woman. The validity coefficient was .70, which was higher than the correlations between the diagnosis and scores on other depression scales, indicating its superiority as a screening instrument.

Internal Consistency Reliability: In both studies, Beck and Gable evaluated the internal consistency reliability of the PDSS and its subscales. Subscale reliability was high, ranging from .83 to .94 in the first study and from .80 to .91 in the second study. Figure 15.4 shows a reliability analysis printout (from the Statistical Package for the Social Sciences, or SPSS, Version 17.0) for the five items on the Mental Confusion subscale from the first study. In Panel A, we see that the reliability for the 5-item subscale is high, .912. The first column of Panel B (Item Statistics) identifies subscale items by number: Item 11, Item 18, and so on. Item 11, for example, is the item "I felt like I was losing my mind." The item means and standard deviations for the 522 cases suggest a good amount of variability on each item. Panel C presents intercorrelations among the 5 items. The correlations are fairly high, ranging from .601 for item 25 with 53, to .814 for item 11 with 25. Panel D (Summary Item Statistics) presents various descriptive statistics about the items. In Panel E, the fourth column ("Corrected Item–Total Correlation") presents correlation coefficients for the relationship between women's score on an item and their score on the total subscale, after removing the item from the scale. Item 11 has a corrected item–total correlation of .799, which is very high; all five items have excellent correlations with the total subscale score. The final column shows what the internal consistency would be if an item were deleted. If Item 11 were removed from the subscale and only four items remained, the reliability coefficient would be .888—less than the reliability for all 5 items (.912). Deleting any of the items on the subscale would reduce its internal consistency, but only by a rather small amount.

A   **Reliability Statistics**

Cronbach's Alpha	Cronbach's Alpha Based on Standardized Items	N of Items
.912	.912	5

B   **Item Statistics**

	Mean	Std. Deviation	N
Item11	2.36	1.424	522
Item 18	2.21	1.270	522
Item 25	2.21	1.374	522
Item 39	2.40	1.351	522
Item 53	2.28	1.349	522

C   **Inter-Item Correlation Matrix**

	Item11	Item 18	Item 25	Item 39	Item 53
Item11	1.000	.654	.814	.646	.649
Item 18	.654	1.000	.603	.659	.751
Item 25	.814	.603	1.000	.652	.601
Item 39	.646	.659	.652	1.000	.724
Item 53	.649	.751	.601	.724	1.000

D   **Summary Item Statistics**

	Mean	Minimum	Maximum	Range	Maximum / Minimum	Variance	N of Items
Item Means	2.292	2.205	2.399	.194	1.088	.008	5
Item Variances	1.835	1.612	2.029	.416	1.258	.023	5
Inter-Item Correlations	.675	.601	.814	.213	1.354	.006	5

E   **Item-Total Statistics**

	Scale Mean if Item Deleted	Scale Variance if Item Deleted	Corrected Item-Total Correlation	Squared Multiple Correlation	Cronbach's Alpha if Item Deleted
Item11	9.09	21.371	.799	.715	.888
Item 18	9.24	23.006	.770	.623	.895
Item 25	9.25	22.097	.769	.691	.894
Item 39	9.06	22.290	.869	.610	.894
Item 53	9.18	22.176	.781	.666	.891

[1] In 2010, SPSS, Inc. was acquired by IBM and the software (starting with version 18.0) is now called PASW Statistics (or IBM SPSS).

FIGURE 15.4 SPSS reliability analysis for the Mental Confusion subscale of the Postpartum Depression Screening Scale.

Sensitivity and Specificity: In the second validation study, ROC curves were constructed to examine the sensitivity and specificity of the PDSS at different cutoff points, using the expert diagnosis to establish PPD caseness. In the validation study, 46 of the 150 mothers had a diagnosis of major or minor depression. To illustrate the trade-offs the researchers made, the ROC curve (Figure 15.5) revealed that with a cutoff

score of 95 on the PDSS to screen in PPD cases, the sensitivity would be only .41, meaning that only 41% of the women actually diagnosed with PPD would be identified. A score of 95 has a specificity of 1.00, meaning that all cases *without* an actual PPD diagnosis would be accurately screened out. At the other extreme, a cutoff score of 45 would have 1.00 sensitivity but only .28 specificity (i.e., 72% false positive),

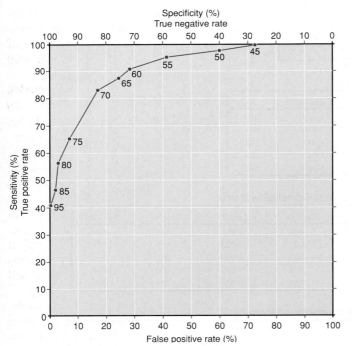

FIGURE 15.5 Receiver operating characteristic (ROC) curve for Postpartum Depression Screening Scale (PDSS): Major or minor postpartum depression. Area = 0.91 (SD = 0.03). Used with permission from Beck, C. T., & Gable, R. K. (2001). Further validation of the Postpartum Depression Screening Scale. *Nursing Research, 50,* p. 161.

an unacceptable rate of overdiagnosis. Beck and Gable recommended a cutoff score of 60, which would accurately screen in 91% of true PPD cases, and would mistakenly screen in 28% who do not have PPD. Beck and Gable found that using this cutoff point would have correctly classified 85% of their sample. In their ROC analysis, the area under the curve was excellent, .91.

Spanish Translation: Beck collaborated with translation experts to develop a Spanish version of the PDSS. Eight bilingual translators from four backgrounds (Mexican, Puerto Rican, Cuban, and South American) translated and back-translated the items. The translators met as a committee to review each others' wordings and to arrive at a consensus. The English and Spanish versions were then administered, in random order, to a bilingual sample. Scores on the two versions correlated highly (e.g., .98 on the "Sleeping/Eating Disturbances" subscale). The alpha reliability was .95 for the total Spanish scale, and ranged from .76 to .90 for subscales. Confirmatory factor analysis yielded information that was judged to indicate an adequate fit with the hypothesized measurement model, and screening performance was found to be good (Beck & Gable, 2005).

SUMMARY POINTS

- Scale development begins with a sound conceptualization of the construct (the **latent variable**) to be measured, including its dimensionality.
- After deciding on the type of scale to construct, items must be generated; common sources for items include existing instruments, the research literature, concept analyses, qualitative studies, focus groups, and clinical observations.
- In classical measurement theory, a **domain sampling model** is assumed; the basic notion is to sample a homogeneous set of items from a hypothetical universe of items.
- In generating items, a number of decisions must be made, including how many items to generate (typically a large number initially), what to use as the continuum for the response options, how many response options there should be, whether to include positive and negative item stems, how

intensely worded the items should be, and what to do about references to time.
- Items should be inspected for clarity, length, inappropriate use of jargon, and good wording; the scale's **readability** should also be assessed.
- External review of the preliminary pool of items should also be undertaken, including review by members of the target population (e.g., via a small pretest that could include **cognitive questioning**).
- Content validity should be built into the scale through careful efforts to conceptualize the construct, and through content validation by a panel of experts—including the calculation of a quantitative index such as the CVI to summarize the experts' judgments of the relevance of scale items.
- Once content validity has been established at a satisfactory level, the scale must be administered to a development sample—typically 300 or more respondents who are representative of the target population.
- Data collected from the development sample are then analyzed using a number of techniques, including **item analysis** (e.g., a scrutiny of **inter-item correlations** and **item–scale correlations**); **exploratory factor analysis (EFA)**, and reliability analysis.
- EFA is used to reduce a large set of variables into a smaller set of underlying dimensions, called **factors**. Mathematically, each factor is a linear combination of variables in a data matrix.
- The first phase of EFA (**factor extraction**) identifies clusters of items that are strongly intercorrelated and is used to define the number of underlying dimensions in the items empirically; a widely used factor extraction method is **principal components analysis (PCA)**, but another important alternative is **principal axis factor analysis**.
- The second phase of factor analysis involves **factor rotation**, which enhances the interpretability of the factors by aligning items more distinctly with a particular factor. Rotation can be either **orthogonal** (which maintains the independence of the factors) or **oblique** (which allows correlated factors). **Factor loadings** of the items on the rotated factor matrix are used to interpret and name the factors.

- After the scale is finalized based on the preliminary analyses, a second study is often undertaken to validate the scale, using a variety of validation techniques; one widely used approach is **confirmatory factor analysis (CFA)**.
- CFA involves tests of a **measurement model**, which stipulates the hypothesized relationship between latent variables and *manifest variables*. CFA is a subset of sophisticated statistical techniques called **structural equation modeling**.
- Well-constructed scales with good psychometric properties are increasingly likely to be translated for use in other cultures. Translations are often **centered** on the original language, but a **decentered approach**, which would allow modifications to the wording of items in the original scale, may be preferred when it is anticipated during the development phase that the scale will be used in two languages.
- Both *conceptual equivalence* and *semantic equivalence* are critical to the success of a translated effort. The "gold standard" for semantic equivalence involves **back-translation**, in which the scale is first translated from the *source language* into the *target language*, and then translated back to the source language by translators blind to the original wording. The next step typically involves a committee that convenes with the goal of arriving at a consensus translation.
- The translated version is then tested in a manner similar to the original scale. Evidence for semantic equivalence and psychometric soundness comes from pretests of both original and translated scale with a sample of bilingual people, and comparison of reliabilities, factor structures, and other validity estimates between the two scales.

●○●○●○●○●○●○●○●○●○●○●○●○●○

STUDY ACTIVITIES

Chapter 15 of the *Resource Manual for Nursing Research*: *Generating and Assessing Evidence for Nursing Practice*, *9th edition*, offers exercises and study suggestions for reinforcing concepts presented in this chapter. In addition, the following study questions can be addressed:

1. Read a recent scale development paper and see how many of the steps discussed in this chapter were followed. Do omitted steps (if any) jeopardize the evidence about the scale's quality?
2. Use the critiquing guidelines in Box 15.1 to evaluate scale development procedures in the studies by Beck and Gable, referring to the original studies if possible.

⬤⬤⬤⬤⬤⬤⬤⬤⬤⬤⬤⬤⬤⬤⬤⬤⬤⬤⬤⬤⬤⬤

STUDIES CITED IN CHAPTER 15

Beck, C. T. (1992). The lived experience of postpartum depression: A phenomenological study. *Nursing Research, 41*, 166–170.

Beck, C. T. (1993). Teetering on the edge: A substantive theory of postpartum depression. *Nursing Research, 42*, 42–48.

Beck, C. T. (1996). Postpartum depressed mothers interacting with their children. *Nursing Research, 45*, 98–104.

Beck, C. T., & Gable, R. K. (2000). Postpartum Depression Screening Scale: Development and psychometric testing. *Nursing Research, 49*, 272–282.

Beck, C. T., & Gable, R. K. (2001). Further validation of the Postpartum Depression Screening Scale. *Nursing Research, 50*, 155–164.

Beck, C. T., & Gable, R. K. (2003). Postpartum Depression Screening Scale: Spanish version. *Nursing Research, 52*, 296–306.

Beck, C. T., & Gable, R. K. (2005). Screening performance of the Postpartum Depression Screening Scale—Spanish version. *Journal of Transcultural Nursing, 16*, 331–338.

Bu, X., & Wu, Y. (2008). Development and psychometric evaluation of the instrument: Attitude toward patient advocacy. *Research in Nursing & Health, 31*, 63–75.

Coffman, M. (2008). Translation of a Diabetes Self-Efficacy Instrument: Assuring content and semantic equivalence. *The Journal of Theory Construction & Testing, 12*, 58–62.

Ellenbecker, C. H., Byleckie, J., & Samia, L. (2008). Further psychometric testing of the Home Healthcare Nurse Job Satisfaction Scale. *Research in Nursing & Health, 31*, 152–164.

Gómez, J., Hidalgo, M., & Tomás-Sábado, J. (2007). Using polytomous item response models to assess death anxiety. *Nursing Research, 56*, 89–96.

Hamilton, J., Stewart, B., Crandell, J., & Lynn, M. (2009). Development of the Ways of Helping Questionnaire: A measure of preferred coping strategies for older African American cancer survivors. *Research in Nursing & Health, 32*, 243–259.

Heaman, M., & Gupton, A. (2009). Psychometric testing of the Perception of Pregnancy Risk Questionnaire. *Research in Nursing & Health, 32*, 493–503.

Heo, S., Moser, D. K., Riegel, B., Hall, L. A., & Christman, N. (2005). Testing the psychometric properties of the Minnesota Living with Heart Failure Questionnaire. *Nursing Research, 54*, 265–272.

Jones, R., & Gulick, E. (2009). Reliability and validity of the Sexual Pressure Scale for Women—Revised. *Research in Nursing & Health, 32*, 71–85.

Kalisch, B., Lee, H., & Salas, E. (2010). The development and testing of the nursing teamwork survey. *Nursing Research, 59*, 42–50.

Lange, J. W., & Yellen, E. (2009). Measuring satisfaction with nursing care among hospitalized patients: Refinement of a Spanish version. *Research in Nursing & Health, 32*, 31–37.

Lin, C. C., Anderson, R., Chang, C., Hagerty, B., & Loveland-Cherry, C. (2008). Development and testing of the Diabetes Self-Management Instrument. *Research in Nursing & Health, 31*, 370–380.

McClowry, S. G., Halverson, C. F., & Sanson, A. (2003). A re-examination of the validity and reliability of the School-Age Temperament Inventory. *Nursing Research, 52*, 176–182.

Pinar, R., Celik, R., & Bahcecik, N. (2009). Reliability and construct validity of the Health-Promoting Lifestyle Profile II in an adult Turkish population. *Nursing Research, 58*, 184–193.

Schilling, L., Dixon, J., Knafl, K., Lynn, M., Murphy, K., Dumser, S., & Grey, M. (2009). A new self-report measure of self-management of type I diabetes for adolescents. *Nursing Research, 58*, 228–236.

Methodologic and nonresearch references cited in this chapter can be found in a separate section at the end of the book.

16

Descriptive Statistics

Statistical analysis enables researchers to organize, interpret, and communicate numeric information. Mathematic skill is not required to grasp statistics—only logical thinking ability is needed. In this book, we underplay computation in any event. We focus on how to use statistics in different situations, and how to understand what statistical results mean.

Statistics are either descriptive or inferential. **Descriptive statistics** are used to describe and synthesize data. Averages and percentages are examples of descriptive statistics. Actually, when such indexes are calculated from population data, they are called **parameters**. A descriptive index from a sample is a **statistic**. Research questions are about parameters, but researchers calculate statistics to estimate them and use **inferential statistics** to make inferences about the population. This chapter discusses descriptive statistics, and Chapter 17 focuses on inferential statistics. First, however, we discuss levels of measurement because the analyses that can be performed depend on how variables are measured.

LEVELS OF MEASUREMENT

Scientists have developed a system for classifying measures. The four **levels of measurement** are nominal, ordinal, interval, and ratio.

Nominal Measurement

The lowest level of measurement is **nominal measurement**, which involves assigning numbers to classify characteristics into categories. Examples of variables amenable to nominal measurement include gender, blood type, and marital status.

The numbers assigned in nominal measurement have no quantitative meaning. If we code males as 1 and females as 2, the number 2 does not mean "more than" 1. The numbers are merely symbols representing different values of gender. We easily could use 1 for females and 2 for males. It may strike you as odd to think of such categorization as measurement, but nominal measurement does involve assigning numbers to attributes according to rules.

Nominal measurement provides no information about an attribute except equivalence and nonequivalence. If we were to "measure" the gender of Nate, Alan, Norah, and Lauren by assigning them the codes 1, 1, 2, and 2, respectively, this means Nate and Alan are equivalent on the gender attribute but are not equivalent to Norah and Lauren.

Nominal measures must have categories that are mutually exclusive and collectively exhaustive. For example, if we were measuring marital status, we might use the following codes: 1 = married, 2 = separated or divorced, 3 = widowed. Each person must be classifiable into one and only one category. The requirement for collective exhaustiveness would not be met if, for example, there were participants who had never been married.

Numbers in nominal measurement cannot be treated mathematically. It is not meaningful to calculate the average gender of a sample, but we can state percentages. In a sample of 50 patients with 30 men and 20 women, we could say that 60% were male and 40% were female.

Ordinal Measurement

Next in the measurement hierarchy is **ordinal measurement**, which involves sorting people based on their relative ranking on an attribute. This measurement level goes beyond categorization: Attributes are *ordered* according to some criterion. Ordinal measurement captures information about not only equivalence, but also about relative rank.

Consider this scheme for coding ability to perform activities of daily living: (1) completely dependent, (2) needs another person's assistance, (3) needs mechanical assistance, (4) completely independent. In this case, measurement is ordinal. The numbers signify incremental ability to perform activities of daily living. People coded 4 are equivalent to each other with regard to functional ability *and*, relative to those in the other categories, have more of that attribute.

Ordinal measurement does not, however, tell us anything about how much greater one level is than another. We do not know if being completely independent is twice as good as needing mechanical assistance. Nor do we know if the difference between needing another person's assistance and needing mechanical assistance is the same as that between needing mechanical assistance and being completely independent. Ordinal measurement tells us only the relative ranking of the attribute's levels.

As with nominal measures, mathematic operations with ordinal-level data are restricted—for example, averages are usually meaningless. Frequency counts, percentages, and several other

statistics to be discussed later are appropriate for ordinal-level data.

Interval Measurement

Interval measurement occurs when researchers can specify rank ordering on an attribute and can assume equivalent distance between them. The Fahrenheit temperature scale is an example: A temperature of 60°F is 10°F warmer than 50°F. A 10°F difference similarly separates 40°F and 30°F, and the two differences in temperature are equivalent. Interval measures are more informative than ordinal ones, but interval measures do not communicate absolute magnitude. For example, it cannot be said that 60°F is twice as hot as 30°F, or three times as hot as 20°F. The Fahrenheit scale uses an arbitrary zero point. Zero on the thermometer does not signify an absence of heat. In interval scales, there is no real, rational zero point. Most psychological and educational tests yield interval-level data.

Interval scales expand analytic possibilities—in particular, interval-level data can be averaged meaningfully. It is reasonable, for example, to compute an average daily temperature for hospital patients. Many statistical procedures require interval measurements.

Ratio Measurement

Ratio measurement is the highest measurement level. Ratio measures provide information about ordering on the critical attribute, the intervals between objects, *and* the absolute magnitude of the attribute because they have a rational, meaningful zero. Many physical measures provide ratio-level data. A person's weight, for example, is measured on a ratio scale. It is meaningful to say that someone who weighs 200 pounds is twice as heavy as someone who weighs 100 pounds.

Because ratio scales have an absolute zero, all arithmetic operations are permissible. One can meaningfully add, subtract, multiply, and divide numbers on a ratio scale. All the statistical procedures suitable for interval-level data are also appropriate for ratio-level data.

Example of different measurement levels:
Bozak and colleagues (2010) tested the effects of an Internet physical activity intervention for adults with metabolic syndrome. Race and gender were measured as nominal-level variables. Alcohol consumption was measured on an ordinal scale. Participants' self-efficacy was measured on an interval scale using the Cardiac Exercise Self-Efficacy Instrument. Many outcome variables, such as lipid biomarkers, physical activity duration, and energy expenditure, were measured on a ratio-level scale.

➡ **TIP:** Nominal-level measures are often called categorical. Variables measured on an interval- or ratio-level scale may be referred to as continuous variables.

Comparison of the Levels

The four levels of measurement form a hierarchy, with ratio scales at the top and nominal measurement at the base. Moving from a higher to a lower level of measurement results in an information loss, as we demonstrate with an example of people's weight. Table 16.1 presents fictitious data for 6 people. The second column shows their actual weight in pounds—ratio-level data. In the third column, ratio data have been converted to interval measures by assigning a score of 0 to the lightest person (Alaine), a score of 5 to the person 5 pounds heavier than the lightest person (Caitlin), and so on. The resulting interval values are still equally far apart, but they are at different parts of the scale.

The data no longer tell us anything about actual weights. Alaine could be a 10-pound infant or a 130-pound adult.

In the fourth column of Table 16.1, people were rank ordered from the lightest (assigned the score of 1) to the heaviest (assigned the score of 6), yielding an ordinal measure. Now more information is missing. The ordinal data provide no indication of how much heavier Alex is than Alaine. The difference separating them could be 5 pounds or 150 pounds.

The final column presents nominal measurements in which people were classified as either *heavy* or *light*. The criterion used to categorize people was weight greater than, or less than or equal to, 150 pounds. Within a category, there is no information as to who is heavier than whom. With this level of measurement, Alex, Derek, and James are equivalent with regard to the attribute heavy/light, as defined by the classification criterion.

This example illustrates that at every successive level in the measurement hierarchy, information is lost. It also illustrates another point: With information at one level, it is possible to convert data to a lower level, but the converse is not true. If we were given only the nominal measurements, we could not reconstruct actual weights.

It is not always easy to identify a variable's level of measurement. Nominal and ratio measures usually are discernible, but the distinction between ordinal and interval measures is more problematic. Some methodologists argue that most psychological

TABLE 16.1	Fictitious Data, Four Levels of Measurement: Participants' Weight (Pounds)			
(1) **PARTICIPANTS**	**(2)** **RATIO-LEVEL**	**(3)** **INTERVAL-LEVEL**	**(4)** **ORDINAL-LEVEL**	**(5)** **NOMINAL**
Alex	180	70	6	2
Alaine	110	0	1	1
Derek	165	55	4	2
Andrea	125	20	3	1
James	175	65	5	2
Caitlin	115	5	2	1

TABLE 16.2		Patients' Anxiety Scores							
22	27	25	19	24	25	23	29	24	20
26	16	20	26	17	22	24	18	26	28
15	24	23	22	21	24	20	25	18	27
24	23	16	25	30	29	27	21	23	24
26	18	30	21	17	25	22	24	29	28
20	25	26	24	23	19	27	28	25	26

measures that are treated as interval measures are really only ordinal measures. Although instruments such as Likert scales produce data that are, strictly speaking, ordinal, many analysts believe that treating them as interval measures results in too few errors to warrant using less powerful statistical procedures.

➔ **TIP:** In operationalizing variables, it is usually best to use the highest measurement level possible. Higher levels of measurement yield more information and are amenable to more powerful analyses than lower levels. Sometimes, however, group membership is more informative than continuous scores, especially for clinicians who need meaningful "cut points" for making decisions. For example, for some purposes, it may be more relevant to designate infants as being of low versus normal birth weight (nominal level) than to use actual birth weight values (ratio level). But it is best to *measure* at the higher level and then convert to a lower level, if appropriate.

FREQUENCY DISTRIBUTIONS

When quantitative data are unanalyzed, it is not even possible to discern general trends. Consider the 60 numbers in Table 16.2. Let us assume that these are the scores of 60 preoperative patients on a six-item measure of anxiety—scores that we will consider as interval level. Inspection of the numbers does not help us understand patients' anxiety.

A set of data can be described in terms of three characteristics: the shape of the distribution of values, central tendency, and variability. Central tendency and variability are dealt with in subsequent sections.

Constructing Frequency Distributions

Frequency distributions are used to organize numeric data. A **frequency distribution** is a systematic arrangement of values from lowest to highest, together with a count of the number of times each value was obtained. Our 60 anxiety scores are shown in a frequency distribution in Table 16.3. We can readily see the highest and lowest scores, the most common score, where the bulk of scores clustered, and how many patients were in the sample (total sample size is typically depicted as N). None of this was apparent before the data were organized.

Frequency distributions consist of two parts: observed values (the Xs) and the frequency of cases at each value (the fs). Values are listed in numeric order in one column, and corresponding frequencies are listed in another. Table 16.3 shows the step of tallying, using four vertical bars and a slash for the fifth observation. In frequency distributions, values must be mutually exclusive and collectively exhaustive. The sum of numbers in the frequency column must equal the sample size. In less verbal terms, $\Sigma f = N$, which means the sum of (signified by Greek sigma, Σ) the frequencies (f) equals the sample size (N).

It is usually useful to display percentages for each value, as shown in the fourth column of Table 16.3. Just as the sum of all frequencies should equal N, the sum of all percentages should equal 100.

Sometimes researchers display frequency data in graphs, which communicate a lot of information

TABLE 16.3	Frequency Distribution of Patients' Anxiety Scores		
SCORE (X)	**TALLIES**	**FREQUENCY (f)**	**PERCENTAGE (%)**
15	I	1	1.7
16	II	2	3.3
17	II	2	3.3
18	III	3	5.0
19	II	2	3.3
20	IIII	4	6.7
21	III	3	5.0
22	IIII	4	6.7
23	JHT	5	8.3
24	JHT IIII	9	15.0
25	JHT II	7	11.7
26	JHT I	6	10.0
27	IIII	4	6.7
28	III	3	5.0
29	III	3	5.0
30	II	2	3.3
		$N = 60 = \Sigma f$	$\Sigma\% = 100.0\%$

quickly. Graphs for displaying interval- and ratio-level data include **histograms** and **frequency polygons**, which are constructed in a similar fashion. First, score values are arrayed on a horizontal dimension, with the lowest value on the left, ascending to the highest value on the right. Frequencies or percentages are displayed vertically. A histogram is constructed by drawing bars above the score classes to the height corresponding to the frequency for that score. Figure 16.1 shows a histogram for the anxiety score data. Frequency polygons are similar, but they use dots connected by straight lines to show frequencies. A dot corresponding to the frequency is placed above each score (Figure 16.2).

Shapes of Distributions

Frequency polygons can assume many shapes. A distribution is **symmetric** if, when folded over, the two halves are superimposed on one another. All the distributions in Figure 16.3 are symmetric. With real data sets, distributions are rarely perfectly symmetric, but minor discrepancies are ignored in characterizing a distribution's shape.

In **skewed** (asymmetric) distributions, the peak is off center and one tail is longer than the other.

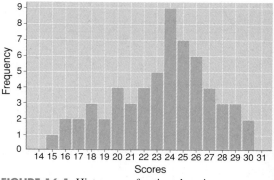

FIGURE 16.1 Histogram of patients' anxiety scores.

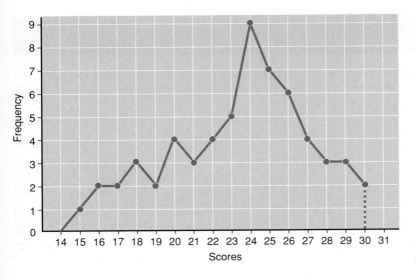

FIGURE 16.2 Frequency polygon of patients' anxiety scores.

When the longer tail points to the right, the distribution is **positively skewed** (Figure 16.4A). Personal income, for example, is positively skewed. Most people have low to moderate incomes, with relatively few people with high incomes in the tail. If the tail points to the left, the distribution is **negatively skewed** (Figure 16.4B). Age at death is an example of a negatively skewed attribute: Most people are at the upper end of the distribution, with

relatively few dying at an early age. Patients' anxiety scores (Figure 16.2) were negatively skewed, with high scores more common than low ones.

A second aspect of a distribution's shape is **modality**. A **unimodal distribution** has only one peak (i.e., a value with high frequency), whereas a **multimodal distribution** has two or more peaks. A distribution with two peaks is **bimodal**. Figure 16.3A is unimodal, and multimodal distributions are illustrated in Figure 16.3B and D. Symmetry and modality are independent aspects of a distribution. Skewness is unrelated to how many peaks the distribution has.

Some distributions have special names. Of particular importance is the **normal distribution** (sometimes called a *Gaussian distribution* or *bell-shaped curve*). A normal distribution is symmetric, unimodal, and not too peaked, as shown in Figure 16.3A. Many human attributes approximate a normal distribution. Examples include height and intelligence. The normal distribution plays a key role in inferential statistics.

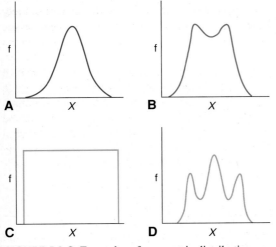

FIGURE 16.3 Examples of symmetric distributions.

CENTRAL TENDENCY

Frequency distributions are a good way to organize data and clarify patterns. Often, however, a pattern

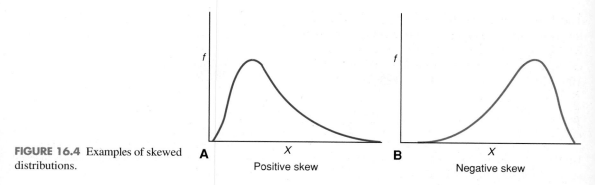

FIGURE 16.4 Examples of skewed distributions.

is of less interest than an overall summary. Researchers usually ask such questions as, "What is the average body temperature of infants during bathing?" or "What is the average weight loss of patients with cancer?" Such questions seek a single number that best represents a distribution of values. Because an index of typicalness is more likely to come from the center of a distribution than from an extreme, such indexes are called measures of **central tendency**. Lay people use the term *average* to designate central tendency. Researchers avoid this term because there are three indexes of central tendency: the mode, the median, and the mean.

The Mode

The **mode** is the most frequently occurring score value in a distribution. In the following distribution, we can readily see that the mode is 53:

50 51 51 52 53 53 53 53 54 55 56

The score of 53 occurred four times, a higher frequency than for any other number. The mode of patients' anxiety scores (Table 16.3) is 24. In multimodal distributions, there is more than one score value that has high frequencies.

Modes are a quick way to determine a "popular" score, but are rather unstable. By *unstable*, we mean that modes tend to fluctuate from sample to sample drawn from the same population. The mode is used primarily to describe typical values for nominal-level measures. For instance, researchers

may characterize their samples by stating modal information on nominal-level demographics, as in the following example: "The typical (modal) participant was a married white woman."

The Median

The **median** is the point in a distribution above which and below which 50% of cases fall. As an example, consider the following set of values:

2 2 3 3 4 5 6 7 8 9

The value that divides the cases exactly in half is 4.5, the median for this set of numbers. The point that has 50% of the cases above and below it is halfway between 4 and 5. For the patient anxiety scores, the median is 24. An important characteristic of the median is that it does not take into account the quantitative values of scores—it is an index of average *position* in a distribution and is thus insensitive to extremes. In the above set of numbers, if the value of 9 were changed to 99, the median would remain 4.5. Because of this property, the median is often the preferred index of central tendency when a distribution is skewed. In research reports, the median may be abbreviated as **Md** or **Mdn**.

The Mean

The **mean**—often symbolized as *M* or $\overline{X}$—is the sum of all scores, divided by the number of scores.

The mean is what people usually refer to as the *average*. The mean of the patients' anxiety scores is 23.4 (1405 ÷ 60). Let us compute the mean weight of eight people with the following weights: 85, 109, 120, 135, 158, 177, 181, and 195:

$$\overline{X} = \frac{85 + 109 + 120 + 135 + 158 + 177 + 181 + 195}{8} = 145$$

Unlike the median, the mean is affected by every score. If we were to exchange the 195-pound person in this example for one weighing 275 pounds, the mean would increase from 145 to 155. Such a substitution would leave the median unchanged.

The mean is the most widely used measure of central tendency. Many important tests of statistical significance, described in Chapter 17, are based on the mean. When researchers work with interval-level or ratio-level measurements, the mean, rather than the median or mode, is usually the statistic reported.

Comparison of the Mode, Median, and Mean

The mean is the most stable index of central tendency. If repeated samples were drawn from a population, means would fluctuate less than modes or medians. Sometimes, however, the primary interest is to understand what is typical, in which case a median might be preferred. If we wanted to know about the economic well-being of U.S. citizens, for example, we would get a distorted impression by considering mean income, which would be inflated by the wealth of a minority. The median would better reflect how a typical person fares financially.

When a distribution of scores is symmetric and unimodal, the three indexes of central tendency coincide. In skewed distributions, the values of the mode, median, and mean differ. The mean is always pulled in the direction of the long tail, as shown in Figure 16.5. A variable's level of measurement plays a role in determining the appropriate index of central tendency to use. In general, the mode is most suitable for nominal measures,

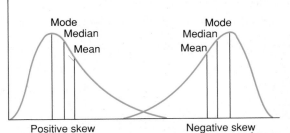

FIGURE 16.5 Relationships of central tendency indexes in skewed distributions.

the mode or median is appropriate for ordinal measures, and the mean is appropriate for interval and ratio measures.

VARIABILITY

Two distributions with identical means could differ in **variability**—how spread out or dispersed the data are. Consider the two distributions in Figure 16.6, which represent fictitious scores for students from two schools on an IQ test. Both distributions have a mean of 100, but the score patterns differ. School A has a wide range of scores, from below 70 to above 130. In school B, by contrast, there are few low scores but also few high scores. School A is more **heterogeneous** (i.e., more variable) than school B, and school B is more **homogeneous** than school A.

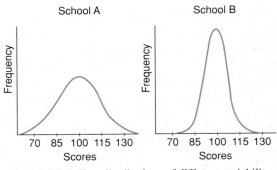

FIGURE 16.6 Two distributions of different variability.

Researchers compute an index of variability to express the extent to which scores in a distribution differ from one another. Two common indexes are the range and standard deviation.

The Range

The **range** is simply the highest score minus the lowest score in a distribution. In the example of patients' anxiety scores, the range is 15 (30 – 15). In the examples shown in Figure 16.6, the range for school A is about 80 (140 – 60), and the range for school B is about 50 (125 – 75).

The chief virtue of the range is computational ease but, being based on only two scores, the range is unstable. From sample to sample from the same population, the range tends to fluctuate widely. Another limitation is that the range ignores variations in scores between the two extremes. In school B of Figure 16.6, suppose one student obtained a score of 60 and another obtained a score of 140. The range of both schools would then be 80, despite clear differences in heterogeneity. For these reasons, the range is used largely as a gross descriptive index.

➲ **T I P :** Another index of variability is called the *interquartile range (IQR)*, which is calculated on the basis of *quartiles*. The IQR indicates the range of scores within which the middle 50% of score values lie. IQRs are rarely reported, but play a role in the detection of extreme values (*outliers*). For more detailed information, see Polit (2010).

Standard Deviation

With interval- or ratio-level data, the most widely used measure of variability is the standard deviation. The **standard deviation** indicates the *average amount* of deviation of values from the mean and is calculated using every score. In research reports, the standard deviation is often abbreviated as *s* or *SD*.

A variability index needs to capture the degree to which scores deviate from one another. This concept of deviation is represented in the range by the minus sign, which produces an index of deviation, or difference, between two score points. The standard deviation is also based on score differences. In fact, the first step in calculating a standard deviation is to compute deviation scores. A **deviation score** (symbolized as *x*) is the difference between an individual score and the mean, that is, $x = X - \bar{X}$. If a person weighed 150 pounds and the sample mean were 140, then the person's deviation score would be +10.

Because we want an *average* deviation, you might think that a good variability index could be computed by summing deviation scores and then dividing by the number of cases. This gets us close to a good solution, but the problem is that the sum of a set of deviation scores is always zero. Table 16.4 presents an example of deviation scores computed for nine numbers. As shown in the second column, the sum of the *x*s is zero. Deviations above the mean always balance exactly deviations below the mean.

The standard deviation overcomes this problem by squaring each deviation score before summing. After dividing by the number of cases, the square root is taken to bring the index back to the original

TABLE 16.4	Computation of a Standard Deviation	
X	**$x = X - \bar{X}$**	**$x^2 = (X - \bar{X})^2$**
4	−3	9
5	−2	4
6	−1	1
7	0	0
7	0	0
7	0	0
8	1	1
9	2	4
10	3	9
$\Sigma X = 63$	$\Sigma x = 0$	$\Sigma x^2 = 28$
$\bar{X} = 7$		

$$SD = \sqrt{\frac{28}{9}} = \sqrt{3.11} = 1.76$$

unit of measurement. The formula for the standard deviation is

$$SD = \sqrt{\frac{\Sigma x^2}{N}}$$

➡ **TIP:** Statistical texts often indicate that the formula for an unbiased estimate of the population *SD* uses *N* − 1 rather than *N* in the denominator. *N* is appropriate when the researcher is interested in *describing* variation in sample data (Knapp, 1970). Statistical programs use *N* − 1 in computing *SD*s. Differences in the results from the two formulas are negligible unless the sample size is small.

A standard deviation has been worked out for the data in Table 16.4. First, a deviation score is calculated for each of the nine raw scores by subtracting the mean ($\overline{X}$ = 7) from them. Each deviation score is squared (column 3), converting all values to positive numbers. The squared deviation scores are summed (Σx^2 = 28), divided by 9 (*N*), and a square root taken to yield an *SD* of 1.76.

➡ **TIP:** The standard deviation often is shown in relation to the mean without a formal label. For example, patients' anxiety scores might be shown as *M* = 23.4 (3.7) or *M* = 23.4 ± 3.7, where 23.4 is the mean and 3.7 is the standard deviation.

A related index of variability is the **variance**, which is the value of the standard deviation before a square root has been taken. In other words, Variance = SD^2. In our example, the variance is 1.76^2, or 3.11. The variance is rarely reported because it is not in the same unit of measurement as the original data, but it is important in statistical tests we discuss later.

A standard deviation is more difficult to interpret than other statistics, like the mean or range. In our example, we calculated an *SD* of 1.76. One might well ask, 1.76 *what*? What does the number mean? First, the standard deviation is a variability index for a set of scores. If two distributions had a mean of 25.0, but one had an *SD* of 7.0 and the other had an *SD* of 3.0, we would know that the first sample was more heterogeneous.

Second, think of a standard deviation as an average of deviations from the mean. The mean tells us the single best value for summarizing a distribution;

a standard deviation tells us how much, on average, scores deviate from that mean. A standard deviation can thus be interpreted as our degree of error when we use a mean to describe the entire sample.

The standard deviation can also be used to interpret individual scores in a distribution. Suppose we had weight data from a sample whose mean weight was 150.0 pounds with *SD* = 10.0. The *SD* provides a *standard* of variability. Weights greater than 1 SD away from the mean (i.e., greater than 150 or less than 130 pounds) are greater than the average for that distribution in terms of variability.

In normal and near-normal distributions, there are roughly 3 *SD*s above and 3 *SD*s below the mean. To illustrate, suppose we had normally distributed scores with a mean of 50 and an *SD* of 10 (Figure 16.7). In a normal distribution, a fixed percentage of cases falls within certain distances from the mean. Sixty-eight percent of cases fall within 1 *SD* of the mean (34% above and 34% below the mean). In our example, nearly 7 out of 10 scores fall between 40 and 60. Ninety-five percent of scores in a normal distribution fall within 2 *SD*s from the mean. Only a handful of cases—about 2% at each extreme—lie more than 2 *SD*s from the mean. In the figure, we

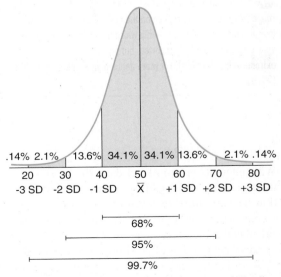

FIGURE 16.7 Standard deviations in a normal distribution.

can see that a person with a score of 70 had a higher score than about 98% of the sample.

In summary, the *SD* is a useful variability index for describing a distribution and interpreting individual scores. Like the mean, the standard deviation is a stable estimate of a parameter and is the preferred index of a distribution's variability.

➡ **TIP:** Descriptive statistics (e.g., percentages, means, standard deviations) are used for various purposes, but are most often used to summarize sample characteristics, describe key research variables, and document methodologic features (e.g., response rates). They are seldom used to answer research questions—inferential statistics (Chapter 17) are usually used for this purpose. The Toolkit section of the accompanying *Resource Manual* includes some table templates for displaying descriptive information that can be "filled in" with descriptive results.

Example of descriptive statistics: Nyamathi and colleagues (2009) examined factors related to hospitalization for health problems among methadone maintenance therapy clients with a history of alcohol abuse. Sophisticated statistical analyses were performed, but the researchers also presented a wealth of descriptive information about participants' risk factors. For example, the mean score on a depression scale was 17.3 (*SD* = 5.6), 90.2% were cigarette smokers, and 18.4% reported multiple sex partners.

BIVARIATE DESCRIPTIVE STATISTICS

The mean, mode, and standard deviation are **univariate** (one-variable) **descriptive statistics** that describe one variable at a time. Most research is about relationships between variables, and **bivariate** (two-variable) **descriptive statistics** describe such relationships. Two commonly used methods of describing two-variable relationships are through contingency tables and correlation indexes.

Contingency Tables

A **contingency table** (or **crosstabs table**) is a two-dimensional frequency distribution in which the frequencies of two variables are *crosstabulated*. Suppose we had data on patients' gender and whether they were nonsmokers, light smokers (<1 pack of cigarettes a day), or heavy smokers (≥1 pack a day). The question is whether there is a tendency for men to smoke more heavily than women, or vice versa (i.e., whether there is a relationship between smoking and gender). Fictitious data on these two variables are shown in a contingency table in Table 16.5. Six **cells** are created by placing one variable (gender) along one dimension and the other variable (smoking status) along the other.

TABLE 16.5 Contingency Table for Gender and Smoking Status Relationship

| | GENDER | | | | | |
| | WOMEN | | MEN | | TOTAL | |
SMOKING STATUS	*n*	%	*n*	%	*n*	%
Nonsmoker	10	45.4	6	27.3	16	36.4
Light smoker	8	36.4	8	36.4	16	36.4
Heavy smoker	4	18.2	8	36.4	12	27.3
TOTAL	22	100.0	22	100.0	44	100.0

After participants' data are allocated to the appropriate cells, percentages are computed. The crosstab allows us to see that, in this sample, women were more likely than men to be nonsmokers (45.4% versus 27.3%) and less likely to be heavy smokers (18.2% versus 36.4%). Contingency tables are used with nominal data or ordinal data with few ranks. In the present example, gender is nominal, and smoking status, as defined, is ordinal.

Contingency tables are easily constructed by hand or (more often) by commands to a computer. A key issue is which variable to put in the rows and which in the columns. Contingency tables are often set up such that the percentages in a column add to 100%, as in Table 16.5. However, cell percentages can be computed based on either row totals or column totals. In Table 16.5, the number 10 in the first cell (nonsmoking women) was divided by the *column* total (i.e., total number of women—22) to arrive at the percentage of women who were nonsmokers (45.4%). This cell *could* have shown 62.5%—the percentage of nonsmokers who were women (10 ÷ 16). Thus, care must be taken in interpreting crosstabs tables.

Example of crosstabulations: Bellini and Damato (2009) studied nurses' knowledge and attitudes about do-not-resuscitate (DNR) status for hospitalized neonates. They presented tables showing responses to specific items crossed with nurses' years of NICU experience and educational background. For example, the item "DNR means withholding CPR only" was correctly answered yes by 19% of nurses with 5 or more years of NICU experience, but by 50% of those with less than 2 years of experience.

Correlation

Relationships between two variables are usually described through **correlation** procedures. Correlation coefficients, briefly described in Chapter 14, can be computed with two variables measured on the ordinal, interval, or ratio scale. The correlation question is: To what extent are two variables related to each other? For example, to what degree are anxiety scores and blood pressure readings related?

Correlations between two variables can be graphed on a **scatter plot** (*scatter diagram*) using a coordinate graph, with the two variables laid out at right angles. Values for one variable (*X*) are scaled on the horizontal axis, and values for the second variable (*Y*) are scaled vertically, as shown in Figure 16.8. This graph presents data for 10 people (a–j). For person *a*, the values for *X* and *Y* are 2 and 1, respectively. To graph person *a*'s position, we go two units to the right along the *X* axis, and one unit up on the *Y* axis. This procedure is followed for all participants. The letters on the plot are shown to help identify people, but normally only dots appear.

In a scatter plot, the direction of the slope of points indicates the direction of the correlation. As noted in Chapter 14, a positive correlation occurs when high values on one variable are associated with high values on a second variable. If the slope of points begins at the lower left corner and extends to the upper right corner, the relationship is positive. In the current example, *X* and *Y* are positively related. People with high scores on variable *X* tended to have high scores on variable *Y*, and low scorers on *X* tended to score low on *Y*.

A negative relationship is one in which high values on one variable are related to low values on the other. Negative relationships on a scatter plot are depicted by points that slope from the upper left corner to the lower right corner, as in Figure 16.9A and D.

When relationships are perfect, it is possible to predict perfectly the value of one variable by knowing the value of the second. For instance, if all people who were 6 feet 2 inches tall weighed 180 pounds, and all people who were 6 feet 1 inch tall weighed 175 pounds, and so on, then weight and height would be perfectly, positively related. In such a situation, we would only need to know a person's height to know his or her weight, or vice versa. On a scatter plot, a perfect relationship is represented by a sloped straight line (Figure 16.9C). When a relationship is not perfect, as is usually the case, one can interpret the *degree* of correlation by seeing how closely the points cluster around a straight line. The closer the points are around a diagonal slope, the stronger the correlation. When the points are scattered all over the graph, the relationship is low or nonexistent. Various degrees and directions of relationships are shown in Figure 16.9.

It is more efficient to express relationships by computing a correlation coefficient, an index with

Subject	X	Y
a	2	1
b	5	7
c	10	10
d	8	7
e	10	9
f	4	3
g	1	2
h	7	6
i	4	5
j	9	10

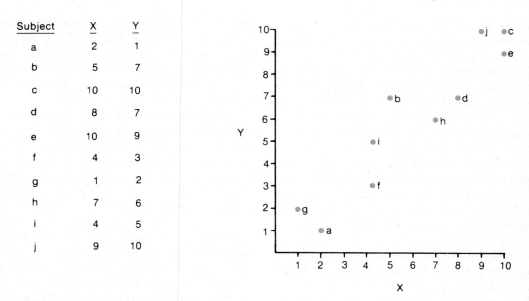

FIGURE 16.8 Construction of a scatter plot.

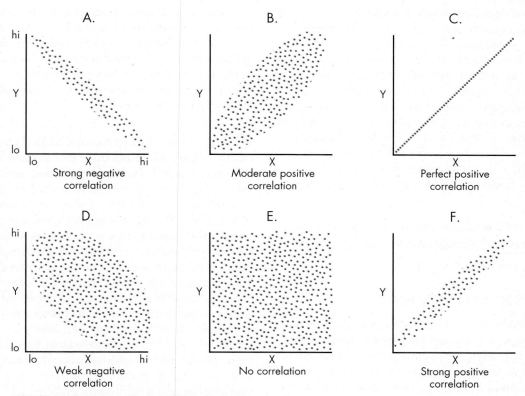

FIGURE 16.9 Various relationships graphed on scatter plots.

values ranging from −1.00 for a perfect negative correlation, through zero for no relationship, to +1.00 for a perfect positive correlation. All correlations that fall between .00 and −1.00 are negative, and ones that fall between .00 and +1.00 are positive. The higher the absolute value of the coefficient (i.e., the value disregarding the sign), the stronger the relationship. A correlation of −.30, for instance, is stronger than a correlation of +.20.

The most widely used correlation index is the **product-moment correlation coefficient**, also called **Pearson's** *r*. This coefficient is computed with variables measured on an interval or ratio scale. **Spearman's rho (ρ)** is a correlation index for ordinal-level data. The calculation of these correlation statistics is laborious and seldom performed by hand. (Computational formulas are available in statistics textbooks, such as that by Polit, 2010.)

It is difficult to offer guidelines on what to interpret as strong or weak relationships because it depends on the variables. If we measured patients' body temperatures orally and rectally, a correlation (*r*) of .70 between the two values would be low. For most psychosocial variables (e.g., stress and illness severity), an *r* of .70 is high; correlations between such variables are typically in the .20 to .40 range. Perfect correlations (+1.00 and –1.00) are rare.

Correlation coefficients are often reported in tables displaying a two-dimensional **correlation matrix**, in which every variable is displayed in both a row and a column and coefficients are displayed at the intersections. An example of a correlation matrix is presented at the end of this chapter.

⬇ **TIP:** Many statistics discussed in this chapter *can* be used for inferential as well as descriptive purposes, as we discuss in Chapter 17.

RISK INDEXES

The EBP movement has made clinical decision making based on research findings an important issue. There are a number of descriptive statistical indexes that can be used to interpret findings and facilitate such decision making. These indexes reflect the growing realization that risks (and risk reduction)

must be interpreted within a context. If an intervention reduces the risk of an adverse event three times over, but the initial risk is miniscule, the intervention may have too high a cost/benefit ratio to be practical. Both absolute change and relative change in risks are important in clinical decision making.

The indexes described in this section are often not reported in nursing journal articles, but can be calculated by potential users of research information. Further information about the use and interpretation of these indexes can be found in DiCenso and colleagues (2005), Guyatt and colleagues (2008), and Polit (2010).

We focus in this section on describing risk for dichotomous outcomes (e.g., alive/dead, had a fall/did not have a fall) in relation to exposure versus nonexposure to a treatment. This situation results in a 2×2 contingency table with four cells, as depicted in Table 16.6, which shows labels for the four cells so that computations can be explained. *Cell a* is the number with an undesirable outcome (e.g., death) in an intervention group, *cell b* is the number with a desirable outcome (e.g., survival) in an intervention group, and *cells c and d* are the two outcome possibilities for a nontreated (control) group. We can now explain the meaning and calculation of several indexes that are of particular interest to clinicians.

⬇ **TIP:** Note that the computations shown in Table 16.6 specifically reflect risk indexes that assume that the intervention exposure will be beneficial, and that information for the *undesirable* outcome (risk) will be in cells a and c. If good outcomes rather than risks are put in cells a and c, formulas would have to be modified. For example, AR_E would then be b/(a + b), and so on. Similarly, if the research question involved the association between an adverse outcome and a hypothesized risk factor (e.g., the risk that high cholesterol is associated with a cardiovascular accident), the group exposed to the risk factor (e.g., those with high cholesterol) should be in the *bottom* row (cells c and d) and not the top row—or, again, the formulas would need to be adapted. As a general rule, to use the formulas shown in Table 16.6, the cell in the lower left corner (cell c) should be expected to reflect the highest number of undesirable outcomes. Note that some software packages, such as the widely used Statistical Package for the Social Sciences (SPSS), calculate the indexes with *cell a* as the one where risk is expected to be highest (Norušis, 2008).

TABLE 16.6	Indexes of Risk and Association in a 2 × 2 Table for an Intervention Study		

EXPOSURE TO AN INTERVENTION	OUTCOME		TOTAL
	Yes (Undesirable Outcome)	No (Desirable Outcome)	
Yes (Exposed to the intervention)	a	b	a + b
No (Not exposed to the intervention)	c	d	c + d
TOTAL	a + c	b + d	a + b + c + d

Absolute risk, exposed group (AR_E) $= a/(a + b)$

Absolute risk, non-exposed group (AR_{NE}) $= c/(c + d)$

Absolute risk reduction (ARR) $= (c/(c + d)) - (a/(a + b))$ or $AR_{NE} - AR_E$

Relative risk (RR) $= \dfrac{a/(a + b)}{c/(c + d)}$ or $\dfrac{AR_E}{AR_{NE}}$

Relative risk reduction (RRR) $= \dfrac{(c/(c + d)) - (a/(a + b))}{c/(c + d)}$ or $\dfrac{ARR}{AR_{NE}}$

Odds ratio (OR) $= \dfrac{ad}{bc}$ or $\dfrac{a/b}{c/d}$

Number needed to treat $= \dfrac{1}{(c/(c + d)) - (a/(a + b))}$ or $\dfrac{1}{ARR}$

Absolute Risk

Absolute risk can be computed for both those exposed to an intervention or risk factor, and for those not exposed. **Absolute risk** is simply the proportion of people who experienced an undesirable outcome in each group. We illustrate this and other indexes with fictitious data from a hypothetical intervention study in which 200 smokers were randomly assigned to a smoking cessation intervention or to a control group (Table 16.7). Smoking status 3 months after the intervention is the outcome variable. In this example, the absolute risk of continued smoking was .50 in the intervention group and .80 in the control group. The risk of an

undesirable outcome for a treatment group is sometimes called the *experimental event rate (EER)* and the risk of an adverse outcome for untreated people is sometimes called the *baseline risk rate,* or the *control event rate (CER).* In the absence of the intervention, 20% of those in the experimental might have stopped smoking anyway, but the intervention boosted the rate to 50%.

Absolute Risk Reduction

The **absolute risk reduction (ARR),** sometimes called the *risk difference* or *RD,* represents a comparison of the two risks. It is computed by

TABLE 16.7	Hypothetical Data for Smoking Cessation Example Illustrating Risk Index Calculation			
EXPOSURE TO SMOKING CESSATION INTERVENTION	**OUTCOME**			**TOTAL**
	Continued Smoking	**Stopped Smoking**		
Yes, Exposed (Experimental Group)	50	50		100
No, Not Exposed (Control Group)	80	20		100
TOTAL	130	70		200

Absolute risk, exposed group (AR$_E$)	=	50/100	= .50
Absolute risk, nonexposed group (AR$_{NE}$)	=	80/100	= .80
Absolute risk reduction (ARR)	=	.80 − .50	= .30
Relative risk (RR)	=	.50/.80	= .625
Relative risk reduction (RRR)	=	.30/.80	= .375
Odds ratio (OR)	=	$\dfrac{(50/50)}{(80/20)}$	= .25
Number needed to treat	=	1/.30	= 3.33

subtracting the absolute risk for the treated group from the absolute risk for the untreated group. This index indicates the estimated proportion of people who would be spared from the undesirable outcome through exposure to the intervention. In our example, the value of ARR is .30: 30% of the control group participants would presumably have stopped smoking if they had received the intervention, over and above the 20% who stopped without the intervention.

Relative Risk

Relative risk (RR), or the *risk ratio*, represents the estimated proportion of the original risk of an adverse outcome (in our example, continued smoking) that persists when people are exposed to the intervention. To compute an RR, the absolute risk for exposed people is divided by the absolute risk

for nonexposed people. In our fictitious example, the RR is .625. This means that the risk of continued smoking after the smoking cessation intervention is estimated to be 62.5% of what it would have been in its absence.

Relative Risk Reduction

Relative risk reduction (RRR) is another useful index for evaluating the effectiveness of an intervention. RRR is the estimated proportion of baseline (untreated) risk that is reduced through exposure to the intervention. This index is computed by dividing the ARR by the absolute risk for the control group. In our example, RRR = .375. This means that the smoking cessation intervention decreased the relative risk of continued smoking by 37.5%, compared to not having had the intervention.

Odds Ratio

The **odds ratio (OR)** is a widely reported index, even though it is less intuitively meaningful than RR as an index of risk. The **odds**, in this context, are the proportion of people *with* the adverse outcome relative to those *without* it. In our example, the odds of continued smoking for the experimental group is 50 (the number who continued smoking) divided by 50 (the number who stopped), or 1. The odds for the control group are 80 divided by 20, or 4. The **odds ratio** is the ratio of these two odds, or .25 in our example. The estimated odds of continuing to smoke are one fourth as high among those in the intervention group as among those in the control group Turned around, we could say that the estimated odds of continued smoking are 4 times higher among smokers who do not get the intervention as among those who do.

➡ **TIP:** Odds ratios can be computed when the independent variable is not dichotomous, using a statistical procedure described in Chapter 18. For example, we could estimate the odds ratio for obesity among adults in 4 different ethnic groups, using one of the groups as a reference.

Number Needed to Treat

A final index of interest is the **number needed to treat (NNT)**, which represents an estimate of how many people would need to receive a treatment or intervention to prevent one undesirable outcome. NNT is computed by dividing 1 by the value of the absolute risk reduction. In our example, ARR = .30, and so NNT is 3.33. About three smokers would need to be exposed to the intervention to avoid one person's continued smoking. The NNT is inversely related to the RRR. An intervention that is twice as effective with regard to relative risk reduction will cut the number needed to treat in half. The NNT is especially valuable for decision makers because it can be integrated with monetary information to determine if an intervention is cost-effective.

Example of RR and NNT: Nakagami and colleagues (2007) conducted a clinical trial to evaluate the effectiveness of a new dressing for preventing persistent erythema. The dressing was randomly assigned to the right or left greater trochanter for 3 weeks in a sample of bedridden older patients in a Japanese hospital. The incidence of persistent erythema was lower in the intervention area than the control area, RR = .18. The number needed to treat was 4.11.

➡ **TIP:** Various tools on the Internet facilitate the calculation of indexes described in this section, including the website for the Centre for Evidence-Based Medicine's EBM toolbox (*www.cebm.net/index.aspx?o=1160*) and the University of British Columbia's Clinical Significance Calculator (*http://spph.ubc.ca/sites/healthcare/files/calc/clinsig.html*). These and other useful websites are available in the Toolkit for you to "click" on directly.

THE COMPUTER AND DESCRIPTIVE STATISTICS

Researchers almost invariably use a computer to calculate statistics. This section aims to familiarize you with printouts from a widely used computer program called Statistical Package for the Social Sciences (SPSS), which is now sometimes called IBM-SPSS or PASW.

Suppose we were evaluating the effectiveness of an intervention for low-income pregnant adolescents. The intervention is a program of healthcare, nutrition education, and contraceptive counseling. Thirty young women are randomly assigned to either the special program or usual care. Two key outcomes are infant birth weight and repeat pregnancy within 18 months of delivery. Fictitious data are presented in Table 16.8.

Figure 16.10 presents information from an SPSS frequency distribution printout for the variable, infant birth weight. Several descriptive statistics are shown in panel A. The *Mean* is 104.70, the *Median* is 102.50, and the *Mode* is 99.00, suggesting a modestly skewed distribution. The *SD* (*Std Deviation*) is 10.95, and the *Variance* is 120.01

(10.95²). The *Range* is 52.00, which is equal to the *Maximum* of 128.00 minus the *Minimum* of 76.00.

The frequency distribution is shown in panel B. Each birth weight is listed in the first column, from the low value of 76 to the high value of 128. The

next column, *Frequency*, shows the number of occurrences of each birth weight. There was one 76-ounce baby, two 89-ounce babies, and so on. The next column, *Percent*, indicates the percentage of infants in each birth weight category: 3.3%

TABLE 16.8	Fictitious Data on Low-Income Pregnant Adolescents				
GROUP*	INFANT BIRTH WEIGHT	REPEAT PREGNANCY†	MOTHER'S AGE (YEARS)	NO. OF PRIOR PREGNANCIES	SMOKING STATUS‡
1	107	1	17	1	1
1	101	0	14	0	0
1	119	0	21	3	0
1	128	1	20	2	0
1	89	0	15	1	1
1	99	0	19	0	1
1	111	0	19	1	0
1	117	1	18	1	1
1	102	1	17	0	0
1	120	0	20	0	0
1	76	0	13	0	1
1	116	0	18	0	1
1	100	1	16	0	0
1	115	0	18	0	0
1.	113	0	21	2	1
0	111	1	19	0	0
0	108	0	21	1	0
0	95	0	19	2	1
0	99	0	17	0	1
0	103	1	19	0	0
0	94	0	15	0	1
0	101	1	17	1	0
0	114	0	21	2	0
0	97	0	20	1	0
0	99	1	18	0	1
0	113	0	18	0	1
0	89	0	19	1	0
0	98	0	20	0	0
0	102	0	17	0	0
0	105	0	19	1	1

*Group: 1 = experimental; 0 = control.
†Repeat pregnancy: 1 = yes; 0 = no.
‡Smoking status: 1 = smokes; 0 = does not smoke.

A   **Statistics**

Infant birth weight in ounces

N	Valid	30.00
	Missing	.00
	Mean	104.70
	Median	102.50
	Mode	99.00
	Std. Deviation	10.95
	Variance	120.01
	Range	52.00
	Minimum	76.00
	Maximum	128.00

B   **Infant birth weight in ounces**

		Frequency	Percent	Valid Percent	Cumulative Percent
Valid	76	1	3.3	3.3	3.3
	89	2	6.7	6.7	10.0
	94	1	3.3	3.3	13.3
	95	1	3.3	3.3	16.7
	97	1	3.3	3.3	20.0
	98	1	3.3	3.3	23.3
	99	3	10.0	10.0	33.3
	100	1	3.3	3.3	36.7
	101	2	6.7	6.7	43.3
	102	2	6.7	6.7	50.0
	103	1	3.3	3.3	53.3
	105	1	3.3	3.3	56.7
	107	1	3.3	3.3	60.0
	108	1	3.3	3.3	63.3
	111	2	6.7	6.7	70.0
	113	2	6.7	6.7	76.7
	114	1	3.3	3.3	80.0
	115	1	3.3	3.3	83.3
	116	1	3.3	3.3	86.7
	117	1	3.3	3.3	90.0
	119	1	3.3	3.3	93.3
	120	1	3.3	3.3	96.7
	128	1	3.3	3.3	100.0
	Total	30	100.0	100.0	

FIGURE 16.10 SPSS printout or a frequency distribution for infant birth weight.

weighed 76 ounces, 6.7% weighed 89 ounces, and so on. The next column, *Valid Percent*, indicates the percentage in each category after removing any missing values. In this example, birth weights were obtained for all 30 infants, but if one birth weight had been missing, the valid percent for the 76-ounce baby would have been 3.4% (1 ÷ 29 rather than 30). The last column, *Cumulative Percent*, adds the percentage for a given birth weight value to the percentage for all preceding values. Thus, we can tell by looking at the shaded row for 99 ounces that, cumulatively, 33.3% of the babies weighed less than 100 ounces.

Many computer programs also produce graphs. Figure 16.11 shows a histogram for maternal age. The age values (ranging from 13 to 21) are on the horizontal axis, and frequencies are on the vertical axis. The histogram shows at a glance that the modal age is 19 ($f = 7$) and that age is negatively skewed (i.e., there are few very young mothers). Descriptive statistics to the left of the histogram indicate that the mean age for this group is 18.17, with an SD of 2.09.

To compare the repeat pregnancy rate of experimental versus control group mothers, we instructed the computer to crosstabulate the two variables, as shown in the contingency table in Figure 16.12. This crosstabulation resulted in four main cells: (1) control mothers with no repeat pregnancy (upper left cell), (2) experimental mothers with no repeat pregnancy, (3) control mothers with a repeat pregnancy, and (4) experimental mothers with a repeat pregnancy. Each cell contains four pieces of information. The first is number of people in the cell (*Count*). In the first cell, 11 control participants did not have a repeat pregnancy within 18 months of delivery. Below the 11 is the *row* percentage or *% within Repeat pregnancy*: 52.4% of the women who did not become pregnant again were controls (11 ÷ 21). The next entry is the *column* percentage or *% within Treatment group*: 73.3% of the controls did not become pregnant (11 ÷ 15). Last is the *overall* percentage of participants who were in that cell (11 ÷ 30 = 36.7%). Figure 16.12 indicates that a somewhat higher percentage of experimental (33.3%) than control participants (26.7%) had an early repeat pregnancy. The row totals on the far right indicate that, overall, 30.0% of the sample ($N = 9$) had a subsequent pregnancy. The column totals at the bottom indicate that 50.0% of the participants were in the

Frequencies

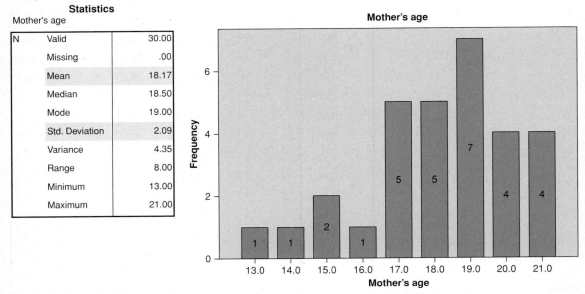

Statistics

Mother's age

N	Valid	30.00
	Missing	.00
	Mean	18.17
	Median	18.50
	Mode	19.00
	Std. Deviation	2.09
	Variance	4.35
	Range	8.00
	Minimum	13.00
	Maximum	21.00

FIGURE 16.11 SPSS printout: Descriptive statistics and histogram for maternal age.

Crosstabs

Repeat pregnancy * Treatment group Crosstabulation

			Treatment group		
			Control	Experimental	Total
Repeat pregnancy	No	Count	11	10	21
		% within Repeat pregnancy	52.4%	47.6%	100.0%
		% within Treatment group	73.3%	66.7%	70.0%
		% of Total	36.7%	33.3%	70.0%
	Yes	Count	4	5	9
		% within Repeat pregnancy	44.4%	55.6%	100.0%
		% within Treatment group	26.7%	33.3%	30.0%
		% of Total	13.3%	16.7%	30.0%
Total		Count	15	15	30
		% within Repeat pregnancy	50.0%	50.0%	100.0%
		% within Treatment group	100.0%	100.0%	100.0%
		% of Total	50.0%	50.0%	100.0%

FIGURE 16.12 SPSS printout: Crosstabulation of repeat pregnancy and treatment group status.

control group, and 50.0% were in the experimental group.

CRITIQUING DESCRIPTIVE STATISTICS

Descriptive statistics help to set the stage for understanding quantitative research evidence. Descriptive statistics are particularly useful for communicating information about the study sample. Readers of reports cannot draw inferences about the study's external validity without understanding who the participants were, especially with regard to key demographic characteristics and health-related attributes.

In addition to describing sample characteristics, descriptive statistics are useful in communicating information about the baseline values of key outcome variables in longitudinal or intervention studies, or correlations between a set of independent variables. Methodologic information about study quality also typically relies on descriptive statistics—for example, response rates and attrition rates are typically shown as percentages, and means are used to characterize such things as time elapsed between two interviews.

Descriptive statistics are sometimes used to directly address research questions in studies that are primarily descriptive. However, when only descriptive statistics are presented, readers should think about whether the inclusion of inferential statistics would have been appropriate.

In critiquing the researcher's use of descriptive statistics, readers can consider whether the information was adequate, whether the correct statistical indexes were used, and whether it was presented in a clear and efficient manner. Box 16.1 ⊗ presents some guiding questions for critiquing the descriptive statistics in a research report.

BOX 16.1 Guidelines for Critiquing Descriptive Statistics

1. Did the report include descriptive statistics? Do these statistics sufficiently describe major characteristics of the dataset?
2. Were descriptive statistics used appropriately—for example, were descriptive statistics used to describe sample characteristics, key variables, and methodologic features of the study, such as response rate or attrition rate? Were they used to answer research questions when inferential statistics would have been more appropriate?
3. Were the correct descriptive statistics used—for example, was a mean presented when percentages would have been more informative? Was the mean used without information about the median even though the distribution was severely skewed?
4. Was the descriptive information presented in a useful format—for example, were tables used effectively? Is information in the text and the tables redundant? Were the tables clear, with a good title and carefully labeled headings?
5. Were any risk indexes computed? If not, should they have been, to increase the clinical utility of the findings?

RESEARCH EXAMPLE

Study: Testing a theoretical model of perceived self-efficacy for cancer-related fatigue self-management and optimal physical function status (Hoffman et al., 2009).

Statement of Purpose: The overall purpose of this study was to test the theory-driven hypothesis that, in patients with cancer, physical functional status can be predicted on the basis of cancer-related fatigue (CRF), perceived self-efficacy, other symptoms, and patient characteristics.

Methods: The study design was a secondary analysis of data gathered at baseline in two RCTs. The combined data set included 298 patients undergoing chemotherapy. Sophisticated multivariate modeling techniques were used for the primary analyses, but the researchers presented considerable descriptive data to help contextualize their main findings.

Analysis and Findings: One table showed descriptive statistics for continuous study variables (e.g., age). The table showed the means, *SDs*, the potential range for scaled variables (i.e., the lowest and highest score theoretically possible), and coefficient alpha. A separate table showed frequency information for nominal-level variables (e.g., sex) and ordinal-level variables (e.g., educational level). To conserve space, we have collapsed some of the data from these two tables into Table 16.9. This table shows, for example, that 70% of the participants were female and that 87% were

white. The participants had a wide range of comorbid conditions, with 45% being hypertensive and 28% having emotional problems. On average, sample members had 2.0 comorbid conditions.

Participants were also asked to report their symptoms, in terms of both frequency and severity. The researchers presented a summary table that shows the percentage of people reporting each symptom, the average severity score, and what the rank order of the symptoms were. We do not reproduce that table here, but as an example, fatigue was the highest ranked symptom for frequency (100% reported the symptom) and 5th for severity, with a mean severity rating of 5.2 ± 2.3 (on a 0 to 10 scale).

Another table presented a correlation matrix for main study variables. An adapted version of this matrix is presented in Table 16.10.* This table lists, on the left, six variables: age (variable 1), number of comorbid conditions, fatigue severity, total symptom severity, scores on a scale of perceived self-efficacy for fatigue self-management, and physical function scores. The numbers in the top row correspond to the six variables: 1 is age, and so on. The correlation matrix shows, in the first column, the correlation coefficient between age with all six variables. At the intersection of row 1 and column 1, we find the value 1.00, which simply indicates that age values are perfectly correlated with

---

*Although we present only descriptive information, Hoffman and her colleagues also presented inferential statistical information in their correlation matrix table.

TABLE 16.9	Selected Demographic Characteristics and Clinical Variables for Study Sample (N = 298)*	
SAMPLE CHARACTERISTIC	**FREQUENCY (N)**	**PERCENT OR MEAN (SD)**
Sex		
Men	89	30%
Women	209	70%
Race		
Caucasian	259	87%
Other	39	13%
Comorbid conditions (selected)		
Hypertension	134	45%
Emotional problems	82	28%
Heart problem	52	17%
Diabetes	41	14%
Arthritis	29	10%
Number of comorbid conditions		2.0 (1.6)
Age		57.1 (11.9)
Cancer-Related Fatigue Severity		5.8 (2.2)
Total Symptom Severity		4.6 (1.6)
Self-Efficacy for Fatigue Self-Management		6.4 (2.3)
Physical Function Status		58.1 (27.1)

*Adapted from Tables 1 and 3 of Hoffman et al. (2009)

TABLE 16.10	Correlation Matrix for Selected Main Study Variables: Cancer-Related Fatigue*					
VARIABLE	**1**	**2**	**3**	**4**	**5**	**6**
1 Age	1.00					
2 Comorbid conditions	.41	1.00				
3 Cancer-related fatigue severity	−.08	.14	1.00			
4 Total symptom severity	−.03	.09	.51	1.00		
5 Self-efficacy for fatigue self-management	.06	−.06	−.39	−.14	1.00	
6 Physical function status	−.16	−.38	−.50	−.36	.32	1.00

*Adapted from Table 2 of Hoffman et al. (2009)

themselves. The next entry in the first column is the correlation between age and comorbid conditions. The value of .41 indicates a moderate positive relationship between these variables. The next entry (−.08) indicates a modest negative relationship between age and cancer-related fatigue severity: the older the patient, the *less* severe the fatigue, but only marginally so. The strongest relationship is the positive correlation between fatigue severity and total symptom severity. As the coefficient of .51 indicates, the more severe the level of fatigue, the more severe the overall symptoms experienced. And, the more severe the fatigue, the lower the score on the physical function scale (−.50).

SUMMARY POINTS

- There are four **levels of measurement**: (1) **nominal measurement**—the classification of characteristics into mutually exclusive categories; (2) **ordinal measurement**—the ranking of objects based on their relative standing on an attribute; (3) **interval measurement**—indicating not only the ranking of objects but also the amount of distance between them; and (4) **ratio measurement**—distinguished from interval measurement by having a rational zero point.
- **Descriptive statistics** enable researchers to summarize and describe quantitative data.
- **Frequency distributions** impose order on raw data. Numeric values are ordered from lowest to highest, accompanied by a count of the number (or percentage) of times each value was obtained.
- **Histograms** and **frequency polygons** are two common methods of displaying frequency information graphically.
- Data for a variable can be completely described in terms of the shape of the distribution, central tendency, and variability.
- A distribution is **symmetric** if its two halves are mirror images of each other. A **skewed distribution**, by contrast, is asymmetric, with one tail longer than the other.
- In **positively skewed distributions**, the long tail points to the right (e.g., personal income); in **negatively skewed distributions**, the long tail points to the left (e.g., age at death).

- The **modality** of a distribution refers to the number of peaks: A **unimodal** distribution has one peak, and a **multimodal** distribution has more than one peak.
- A **normal distribution** (or *Gaussian distribution, bell-shaped curve*) is symmetric, unimodal, and not too peaked.
- Measures of **central tendency** are indexes—expressed as a single number—that represent the average or typical value of a set of scores. The **mode** is the value that occurs most frequently in a distribution; the **median** is the point above which and below which 50% of the cases fall; and the **mean** is the arithmetic average of all scores. The mean is usually the preferred measure of central tendency because of its *stability*.
- Measures of **variability**—how spread out the data are—include the range and standard deviation. The **range** is the distance between the highest and lowest scores. The **standard deviation** indicates how much, on average, scores deviate from the mean.
- The *SD* is calculated by first computing **deviation scores**, which represent the degree to which each person's score deviates from the mean. The **variance** is equal to the *SD* squared. In a normal distribution, 95% of scores fall within 2 *SD*s above and below the mean.
- **Bivariate descriptive statistics** describe relationships between two variables.
- A **contingency table (crosstabs table)** is a two-dimensional frequency distribution in which the frequencies of two nominal- or ordinal-level variables are **crosstabulated**.
- Correlation coefficients describe the direction and magnitude of a relationship between two variables. The most frequently used correlation coefficient is the **product–moment correlation coefficient (Pearson's r)**, used with interval- or ratio-level variables. The **Spearman rho coefficient** is used with ordinal-level variables.
- Graphically, the relationship between two variables can be displayed on a **scatter plot**.
- Several risk indexes describe outcomes in relation to exposures (to risks or interventions) for a two-group (e.g., experimental versus control)

situation with dichotomous outcomes (e.g., alive/dead). These indexes provide useful information for making clinical decisions.

- **Absolute risk reduction (ARR)** expresses the estimated proportion of people who would be spared from an adverse outcome through exposure to an intervention. **Relative risk (RR)** is the estimated proportion of the original risk of an adverse outcome that persists among people exposed to the intervention. **Relative risk reduction (RRR)** is the estimated proportion of untreated risk that is reduced through exposure to the intervention. The **odds ratio (OR)** is the ratio of the odds for the treated versus untreated group, with the **odds** reflecting the proportion of people with the adverse outcome relative to those without it. The **number needed to treat (NNT)** is an estimate of how many people would need to receive the intervention to prevent one adverse outcome.

STUDY ACTIVITIES

Chapter 16 of the *Resource Manual for Nursing Research: Generating and Assessing Evidence for Nursing Practice*, 9th edition, offers exercises and study suggestions for reinforcing concepts presented in this chapter. In addition, the following study questions can be addressed:

1. What are the mean, median, and mode for the following set of data?

   13 12 9 15 7 10 16 9 6 10

   Compute the range and standard deviation.

2. Suppose that 400 subjects (200 per group) were in the intervention study described in connection with Table 16.8 and that 60% of those in the experimental group and 90% of those in the control group continued smoking. Compute the various risk indexes for this scenario.
3. Apply relevant questions in Box 16.1 to the research example at the end of the chapter (Hoffman et al., 2009), referring to the full journal article as necessary.

STUDIES CITED IN CHAPTER 16

Bellini, S., & Damato, E. (2009). Nurses' knowledge, attitudes/beliefs, and care practices concerning do not resuscitate status for hospitalized neonates. *Journal of Obstetric, Gynecologic, & Neonatal Nursing, 38*, 195–205.

Bozak, K., Yates, B., & Pozehl, B. (2010). Effects of an Internet physical activity intervention in adults with metabolic syndrome. *Western Journal of Nursing Research, 32*, 5–22.

Hoffman, A., von Eye, A., Gift, A., Given, B., Given, C., & Rothert, M. (2009). Testing a theoretical model of perceived self-efficacy for cancer-related fatigue self-management and optimal physical function status. *Nursing Research, 58*, 32–41.

Nakagami, G., Sanada, H., Konya, C., Tadaka, E., & Matsuyama, Y. (2007). Evaluation of a new pressure ulcer prevention dressing containing cermaide 2 with low frictional outer layer. *Journal of Advanced Nursing, 59*, 520–529.

Nyamathi, A., Compton, P., Cohen, A., Marfisse, M., Shoptaw, S., Greengold, B., de Castro, V., Reaves, M., Hasson, A., George, D., & Leake, B. (2009). Correlates of hospitalization for alcohol-using methadone-maintained persons with physical health problems. *Western Journal of Nursing Research, 31*, 525–543.

Methodologic and nonresearch references cited in this chapter can be found in a separate section at the end of the book.

17

Inferential Statistics

I nferential statistics, based on the **laws of probability**, provide a means for drawing conclusions about a population, given data from a sample. Inferential statistics would help us with such questions as, "What can I infer about 3-minute Apgar scores of premature babies (the population) after calculating a mean Apgar score of 7.5 in a sample of 300 premature babies?"

Researchers use inferential statistics to estimate population parameters from sample statistics. Inferential statistics provide a framework for making objective judgments about the reliability of sample estimates. Different researchers applying inferential statistics to the same data are likely to draw the same conclusions.

SAMPLING DISTRIBUTIONS

To estimate population parameters, it is advisable to use representative samples, and probability samples are the best way to get representative samples (Chapter 12). Inferential statistics assume random sampling from populations, an assumption that is widely violated. The validity of statistical calculations does depend, however, on the extent to which results from the sample are similar to what you would have obtained had you randomly selected people from the population.

Even when random sampling *is* used, sample characteristics are seldom identical to population characteristics. Suppose we had a population of 50,000 nursing school applicants whose mean score on a standardized entrance exam was 500.0 with a standard deviation (*SD*) of 100.0. Suppose we had to estimate the population mean from the scores of a random sample of 25 students. Would we expect a mean of *exactly* 500 for the sample? Obtaining the exact population value is unlikely. Let us say the sample mean is 505. If a new random sample were drawn, we might obtain a mean of, say, 497. The tendency for statistics to fluctuate from one sample to another reflects **sampling error**. The challenge is to decide whether sample values are good estimates of population parameters.

Researchers compute statistics with only *one* sample, but to understand inferential statistics, we must perform a mental exercise. Consider drawing a sample of 25 students from the population of 50,000, calculating a mean, replacing the students, and drawing a new sample. Each mean is one datum. If we drew 10,000 such samples, we would have 10,000 means (data points) that could be used to construct a frequency polygon (Figure 17.1). This distribution is a **sampling distribution of the mean**. A sampling distribution is a theoretical rather than actual distribution because in practice no one draws consecutive samples from a population

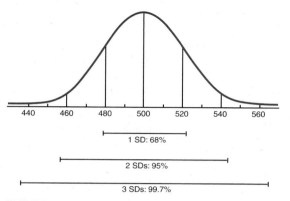

FIGURE 17.1 A sampling distribution.

and plots their means. Sampling distributions are the basis of inferential statistics.

Characteristics of Sampling Distributions

When an infinite number of samples is drawn from a population, the sampling distribution of the mean has certain characteristics. (Our example of 10,000 samples is large enough to approximate these characteristics.) Sampling distributions of means are normally distributed, and the mean of a sampling distribution with an infinite number of sample means always equals the population mean. In the example shown in Figure 17.1, the mean of the sampling distribution is 500, the same as the population mean.

Remember that when data are normally distributed, 68% of values fall between ±1 *SD* from the mean. Because a sampling distribution of means is normally distributed, we can say that the probability is 68 out of 100 that any randomly drawn sample mean lies between +1 *SD* and −1 *SD* of the population mean. Thus, if we knew the standard deviation of the sampling distribution, we could interpret the accuracy of a sample mean.

Standard Error of the Mean

The standard deviation of a sampling distribution of the mean is called the **standard error of the mean** (**SEM**). The word *error* signifies that the various

means in the sampling distribution have some error as estimates of the population mean. The smaller the *SEM*—that is, the less variable the sample means— the more accurate are the means as estimates of the population value.

No one actually constructs a sampling distribution, so how can its standard deviation be computed? Fortunately, there is a formula for estimating the *SEM* from a single sample, using two pieces of information: the sample's standard deviation and sample size. The equation for the SEM is: $SD / \sqrt{N}$. In our example, if we use this formula to calculate the *SEM* for an *SD* of 100 with a sample of 25 students we obtain:

$$SEM = \frac{100}{\sqrt{25}} = 20.0$$

The standard deviation of the sampling distribution in our example is 20, as shown in Figure 17.1. This *SEM* is an estimate of how much sampling error there is from one sample mean to another when samples of 25 are randomly drawn and the *SD* is 100.0.

Given that a sampling distribution of means follows a normal curve, we can estimate the probability of drawing a sample with a certain mean. With a sample size of 25 and a population mean of 500, the chances are about 95 out of 100 that any sample mean will fall between 460 and 540 (i.e., 2 *SDs* above and below the mean). Only 5 times out of 100 would the mean of a randomly selected sample exceed 540 or be less than 460. Only 5 times out of 100 would we get a sample whose mean deviated from the population mean by more than 40 points.

Because the *SEM* is partly a function of sample size, we need only increase sample size to increase the accuracy of our estimate. If we used a sample of 100 applicants, rather than 25, the SEM would be 10 (i.e., $100 / \sqrt{100} = 10.0$). In this situation, the chances are about 95 out of 100 that a sample mean will be between 480 and 520. The chances of drawing a sample with a mean very different from the population mean is reduced as sample size increases because large numbers promote the likelihood that extreme cases will cancel each other out.

ESTIMATION OF PARAMETERS

Statistical inference consists of two techniques: estimation of parameters and hypothesis testing. Parameter estimations are infrequently presented in nursing research reports, but that situation is changing. The emphasis on evidence-based practice (EBP) has heightened interest among practitioners in learning not only whether a hypothesis was supported (via traditional hypothesis tests), but also the estimated value of a population parameter and the level of accuracy of the estimate (via parameter estimation). Many medical research journals *require* that estimation information be reported because it is more useful to clinicians, reflecting the view that this approach offers information about both clinical and statistical significance (e.g., Braitman, 1991; Sackett et al., 2000). In this section, we present general concepts relating to parameter estimation and offer some examples based on one-variable descriptive statistics. We expand on this discussion throughout the chapter within the context of specific bivariate statistical tests.

Confidence Intervals

Parameter estimation is used to estimate a parameter—for example, a mean, a proportion, or a mean difference between two groups (e.g., experimental and control participants). Estimation can take two forms: point estimation or interval estimation. *Point estimation* involves calculating a single descriptive statistic to estimate the population parameter. To continue with the earlier example, if we calculated the mean entrance exam score for a sample of 25 applicants and found that it was 510, then this would be the point estimate of the population mean.

Point estimates convey no information about margin of error, however, so inferences about the accuracy of the parameter estimate cannot objectively be made. *Interval estimation* is useful because it indicates a range of values within which the parameter has a specified probability of lying. With interval estimation, researchers construct a **confidence interval** (**CI**) around the estimate; the upper and lower limits are **confidence limits**. Constructing a confidence interval around a sample mean establishes a range of values for the population value as well as the probability of being right—the estimate is made with a certain degree of confidence. Researchers usually use either a 95% or a 99% confidence interval, purely by convention.

> **➡ TIP:** Confidence intervals address one of the key EBP questions for appraising evidence (Box 2.2): How precise is the estimate of effects?

Confidence Intervals around a Mean

Calculating confidence limits around a mean involves using the *SEM*. In a normal distribution, 95% of the scores lie within about 2 *SD*s (more precisely, 1.96 *SD*s) from the mean. In our example, suppose the point estimate for mean entrance exam scores is 510, and the *SD* is 100. The *SEM* for a sample of 25 would be 20.0. We can build a 95% confidence interval with the following formula:

$$CI\ 95\% = (\overline{X} \pm 1.96 \times SEM)$$

That is, confidence is 95% that the population mean lies between the values equal to 1.96 times the *SEM*, above and below the sample mean. In the example at hand, we would obtain the following:

$$CI\ 95\% = (510.0 \pm (1.96 \times 20.0))$$
$$CI\ 95\% = (510.0 \pm (39.2))$$
$$CI\ 95\% = (470.8 \leq \mu \leq 549.2)$$

The final statement may be read as follows: the confidence is 95% that the population mean (symbolized by the Greek letter mu [μ] by convention) is between 470.8 and 549.2. This would be stated in a research report as 95% CI = 470.8 to 549.2, or 95% CI (470.8, 549.2).

Confidence intervals reflect the researchers' risk of being wrong. With a 95% CI, researchers accept the probability that they will be wrong five times out of 100. A 99% CI sets the risk at only 1% by allowing a wider range of possible values. The formula is as follows:

$$CI\ 99\% = (\overline{X} \pm 2.58 \times SEM)$$

The 2.58 reflects the fact that 99% of all cases in a normal distribution lie within ±2.58 *SD* units from the mean. In the example, the 99% confidence interval would be:

CI 99% = (510.0 ± (2.58 × 20.0))
CI 99% = (510.0 ± (51.6))
CI 99% = (458.4 ≤ μ ≤ 561.6)

In random samples with 25 subjects, 99 out of 100 confidence intervals so constructed would contain the population mean. The price of having a reduced risk of being wrong is reduced precision. With a 95% interval, the range of the CI was about 80 points; with a 99% interval, the range is more than 100 points. The acceptable risk of error depends on the nature of the problem. In research that could affect the health of individuals, a stringent 99% confidence interval might be used; for most studies, a 95% confidence interval is sufficient.

Confidence Intervals around Proportions and Risk Indexes

Calculating confidence intervals around a proportion or percentage is important in certain types of research, especially with regard to risk estimates. Consider, for example, this question: "What percentage of people exposed to a certain hazard will contract a disease?" This question calls for an estimated proportion (an absolute risk index, as described in Chapter 16) that is more useful if it is reported within a 95% confidence interval.

For proportions based on dichotomous variables, as implied in the above question (positive/negative for a disease), the applicable theoretical distribution is not a normal distribution, but rather a **binomial distribution**. A binomial distribution is the probability distribution of the number of "successes" (e.g., heads) in a sequence of independent yes/no trials (e.g., a coin toss), each of which yields "success" with a specified probability.

Using binomial distributions to build confidence intervals around a proportion is computationally complex, so we do not provide formulas here (see Motulsky, 1995). Certain features of confidence

intervals around proportions are, however, worth noting. First, the CI is rarely symmetric around a sample proportion. For example, if 3 out of 30 sample members were "positive" for an outcome, such as hospital readmission, the estimated population proportion would be .10 and the 95% CI for the proportion would be from .021 to .265. Second, the width of the CI depends on both the value of the proportion and the sample size. The larger the sample, the smaller the CI. Also, the closer the sample proportion is to .50, the wider the CI. For example, with a sample size of 30, the range for a 95% CI for a proportion of .50 is .374 (.313, .687), while that for a proportion of .10 is only .188 (.021, .265). Finally, the CI for a proportion never extends below 0 or above 1.0, but a CI can be constructed around an *obtained* proportion of 0 or 1.0. For example, if 0 out of our 30 participants were readmitted to the hospital, the estimated proportion would be 0.0 and the 95% CI would be from 0.0 to .116.

It is possible—and advisable—to construct confidence intervals around all of the indexes of risk described in the previous chapter, such as the ARR, RRR, OR, and NNT. The computed value of these indexes from study data represents a single "best estimate," but confidence intervals convey important information about the precision of the estimate. Clearly, clinical inference is enhanced when information about a plausible range of values for risk indexes is presented. Formulas for constructing CIs around the major risk indexes are presented in an appendix of DiCenso and colleagues (2005), but an easier method for constructing 95% CIs around major risk indexes is to use the University of British Columbia's "Clinical Significance Calculator" on the Internet (*http://spph.ubc.ca/sites/healthcare/files/calc/clinsig.html*).

Example of CIs around proportions: Arderko and colleagues (2010) explored the contribution of smoking exposure to prevalence of a childhood learning disability, as reported by parents. One finding was that 19.4% of children whose mothers smoked during pregnancy had a learning disability (95% CI = 15.4, 24.2), compared with 8.5% of children of nonsmoking mothers (95% CI = 7.3, 9.9).

HYPOTHESIS TESTING

Statistical hypothesis testing provides objective criteria for deciding whether hypotheses are supported by data. Suppose we hypothesized that participation in a stress-management program would reduce anxiety levels among patients with cancer. The sample is 25 patients in the control arm who do not participate in the program and 25 experimental patients who do. The mean posttreatment anxiety score for experimentals is 15.8 and that for controls is 17.9. Should we conclude that the hypothesis is correct? Group differences are in the predicted direction, but the results might reflect sampling fluctuations. With a new sample, group means might be nearly identical. Statistical hypothesis testing allows researchers to make objective decisions about whether study results likely reflect chance sample differences or true population differences.

The Null Hypothesis

Hypothesis testing is based on negative inference. In our example, patients participating in the intervention had lower mean anxiety scores than control group patients. There are two possible explanations: (1) the intervention was successful in reducing anxiety, or (2) the differences resulted from chance factors, such as group differences in anxiety even before the treatment. The first explanation is our research hypothesis, and the second is the null hypothesis. The **null hypothesis**, it may be recalled, states that there is no relationship between variables. Statistical hypothesis testing is basically a process of rejection. It cannot be demonstrated directly that

the research hypothesis is correct but, using theoretical sampling distributions, it can be shown that the null hypothesis has a high probability of being incorrect. Researchers seek to reject the null hypothesis through various **statistical tests**.

The null hypothesis in our example can be stated formally as follows:

$$H_0: \mu_E = \mu_C$$

The null hypothesis (H_0) is that the mean population anxiety score for experimental patients (μ_E) is the same as that for controls (μ_C). The **alternative**, or research, **hypothesis** (H_A) is that the means are *not* the same:

$$H_A: \mu_E \neq \mu_C$$

Null hypotheses are accepted or rejected based on sample data, but hypothesis testing is used to make inferences about the population.

Type I and Type II Errors

Researchers decide whether to accept or reject a null hypothesis by determining how *probable* it is that observed results are due to chance. Researchers cannot know with certainty whether a null hypothesis is or is not true. They can only conclude that hypotheses are *probably* true or *probably* false, and there is always a risk of error.

Researchers can make two types of statistical error: rejecting a true null hypothesis or accepting a false null hypothesis. Figure 17.2 summarizes possible outcomes of researchers' decisions. Researchers make a **Type I error** by rejecting a null hypothesis that is, in fact, true. For instance, if we concluded

		The actual situation is that the null hypothesis is:	
		True	False
The researcher calculates a test statistic and decides that the null hypothesis is:	True (Null accepted)	Correct decision	Type II error (False negative)
	False (Null rejected)	Type I error (False positive)	Correct decision

FIGURE 17.2 Outcomes of statistical decision making.

that a drug was more effective than a placebo in reducing cholesterol, when in fact observed differences in cholesterol levels resulted from sampling fluctuations, we would be making a Type I error—a false positive conclusion. Conversely, if we concluded that group differences in cholesterol resulted by chance, when in fact the drug *did* reduce cholesterol, we would be committing a **Type II error**—a false negative conclusion. In the context of drug testing, a good way to think about statistical error can be expressed as follows: A Type I error might allow an ineffective drug to come onto the market, but a Type II error might *prevent* an effective drug from coming onto the market.

Level of Significance

Researchers never know when they have made an error in statistical decision making. The validity of a null hypothesis could be known only by collecting data from the population. Researchers control the *risk* of a Type I error by selecting a **level of significance**, which signifies the probability of incorrectly rejecting a true null hypothesis.

The two most frequently used significance levels (referred to as **alpha** or α) are .05 and .01. With a .05 significance level, we accept the risk that out of 100 samples drawn from a population, a true null hypothesis would be rejected 5 times. With a .01 significance level, the risk of a Type I error is *lower*: in only 1 sample out of 100 would we erroneously reject the null hypothesis. The minimum acceptable level for α usually is .05. A stricter level (e.g., .01 or .001) may be needed when the decision has important consequences.

Naturally, researchers want to reduce the risk of committing both types of error, but unfortunately lowering the risk of a Type I error increases the risk of a Type II error. The stricter the criterion for rejecting a null hypothesis, the greater the probability of accepting a false null hypothesis. Researchers must deal with trade-offs in establishing criteria for statistical decision making, but the simplest way of reducing the risk of a Type II error is to increase sample size. Type II errors are discussed later in this chapter.

Critical Regions

By selecting a significance level, researchers establish a decision rule. That rule is to reject the null hypothesis if the test statistic falls at or beyond the limits that establish a **critical region** on an applicable theoretical distribution and to accept the null hypothesis otherwise. The critical region indicates whether the null hypothesis is *improbable*, given the results.

An example from our study of gender bias in nursing research (Polit & Beck, 2009) illustrates the statistical decision-making process. We examined whether males and females are equally represented as participants in nursing studies—that is, whether the average percentage of females across studies in eight leading journals was 50.0. The null hypothesis is H_0: $\mu = 50.0$, and the alternate hypothesis is H_A: $\mu \neq 50.0$. We found, using a consecutive sample of 834 studies published over a 2-year period, that the mean percentage of females was 71.0. Using statistical procedures, we tested the hypothesis that the mean of 71.0 was not merely a chance fluctuation from a population mean of 50.0.

In hypothesis testing, researchers assume the null hypothesis is true and then gather evidence to disprove it. Assuming a mean percentage of 50.0 for the population of nursing studies, a theoretical sampling distribution can be constructed. For simplicity, let us say that the standard error of the mean in this example is 2.0 (in our study, the *SEM* was less than 2.0), as shown in Figure 17.3.

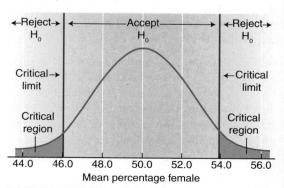

FIGURE 17.3 Critical regions in the sampling distribution for a two-tailed test: gender bias example.

Based on normal distribution characteristics*, we can determine *probable* and *improbable* values of sample means from the population of nursing studies. If, as is assumed in the null hypothesis, the population mean is 50.0, then 95% of all sample means would fall between 46.0 and 54.0, that is, within about 2 *SD*s above and below the mean of 50.0. The obtained sample mean of 71.0 lies in the critical region considered *improbable* if the null hypothesis were correct—in fact, any value greater than 54.0% female would be improbable if a true population mean of 50.0 is assumed and the criterion of improbability is an alpha of .05. The *improbable* range beyond 2 *SD*s corresponds to only 5% (100% to 95%) of the sampling distribution. In our study, the probability of obtaining a value of 71.0% female by chance alone was less than 1 in 10,000. We thus rejected the null hypothesis that the mean percentage of females in nursing studies was 50.0. We would not be justified in saying that we had *proved* the research hypothesis because the possibility of having made a Type I error remains—but the possibility is, in this case, remote. We can thus *accept* the alternative hypothesis that the population mean is not 50.0—that is, that males and females are not equally represented in nursing studies.

> ⮕ **TIP:** Levels of significance are analogous to the CI values described earlier—an alpha of .05 is analogous to the 95% CI, and an alpha of .01 is analogous to the 99% CI. In our example of gender bias, the 95% CI around the mean of 71.0 was 69.2 to 72.8.

Statistical Tests

Researchers do not compute critical regions. Rather, they compute **test statistics** with their data. For every test statistic, there is a related theoretical distribution. Researchers compare the value of the computed test statistic to values of the critical limits for the applicable distribution.

---

*Strictly speaking, the appropriate theoretical distribution in this example is the *t* distribution, but with a large *N*, the *t* and normal distribution are highly similar.

When researchers calculate a test statistic that is beyond the critical limit, the results are said to be **statistically significant**. The word *significant* does not mean *important* or *clinically relevant*. In statistics, *significant* means that obtained results are not likely to have been the result of chance, at a specified level of probability. A **nonsignificant result** means that an observed result could reflect chance fluctuations.

> ⮕ **TIP:** When the null hypothesis is retained (i.e., when results are nonsignificant), this is sometimes referred to as a *negative result*. Negative results are often disappointing to researchers and may lead to rejection of a manuscript by journal editors. Research reports with negative results are not rejected because editors are prejudiced against certain types of outcomes; they are rejected because negative results are usually inconclusive and difficult to interpret. A nonsignificant result indicates that the result *could* have occurred as a result of chance, and offers no evidence that the research hypothesis is or is not correct.

One-Tailed and Two-Tailed Tests

In most hypothesis-testing situations, researchers use **two-tailed tests**. This means that both tails of the sampling distribution are used to determine improbable values. In Figure 17.3, for example, the critical region that contains 5% of the sampling distribution's area involves 2½% in one tail of the distribution and 2½% at the other. If the significance level were .01, the critical regions would involve ½% in each tail.

When researchers have a strong basis for a directional hypothesis (Chapter 4), they sometimes use a **one-tailed test**. For example, if we did an RCT study involving a program to improve prenatal practices among rural women, we would expect birth outcomes for the two groups not to just be *different*, but we would expect program participants to *benefit*. It might make little sense to use the tail of the distribution signifying *worse* outcomes in the intervention group.

In one-tailed tests, the critical region of improbable values is in only one tail of the distribution— the tail corresponding to the direction of the hypothesis, as illustrated in Figure 17.4. Using our earlier gender bias example, the research hypothesis being tested might be that the population mean is *greater than* 50.0—in other words that, on average,

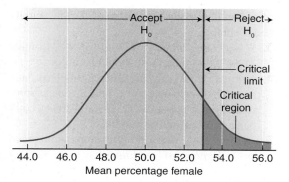

FIGURE 17.4 Critical region in the sampling distribution for a one-tailed test: gender bias example.

females are overrepresented in nursing studies. When a one-tailed test is used, the critical 5% area of "improbability" covers a bigger area of the specified tail, so one-tailed tests are less conservative. Thus, it is easier to reject the null hypothesis with a one-tailed test than with a two-tailed test. In our example, with an alpha of .05, a sample mean of 53.0 or greater would result in rejecting the null hypothesis for a one-tailed test, rather than 54.0 for a two-tailed test.

One-tailed tests are controversial. Most researchers use a two-tailed test even if they have a directional hypothesis. In reading research reports, one can assume that two-tailed tests were used unless one-tailed tests are specifically mentioned. When there is a strong theoretical reason for a directional hypothesis and for assuming that findings in the opposite direction are virtually impossible, however, a one-tailed test might be warranted. In the remainder of this chapter, the examples are for two-tailed tests.

TIP: You should choose a one-tailed test only if you state a directional hypothesis in advance of statistical testing. And, you must be prepared to attribute group differences in the "wrong" direction to chance, even if the group differences are large.

Parametric and Nonparametric Tests

There are two broad classes of statistical tests, parametric and nonparametric. **Parametric tests** involve estimation of a parameter, require measure-

ments on at least an interval scale, and involve several assumptions, such as the assumption that the variables are normally distributed in the population. **Nonparametric tests**, by contrast, do not estimate parameters. They involve less restrictive assumptions about the shape of the variables' distribution than do parametric tests. For this reason, nonparametric tests are sometimes called *distribution-free statistics*.

Parametric tests are more powerful than nonparametric tests and are usually preferred, but there is some disagreement about the use of nonparametric tests. Purists insist that if the requirements of parametric tests are not met, they are inappropriate. Statistical studies have shown, however, that statistical decision making is not affected when the assumptions for parametric tests are violated if sample sizes are large. Nonparametric tests are most useful when data cannot in any manner be construed as interval level, when the distribution is markedly non-normal, or when the sample size is very small.

TIP: Some statisticians advise that when *N* is 50 or greater, it may not be necessary to use nonparametric statistics, unless the population has a markedly unusual distribution. Such advice invokes the **central limit theorem**, which, briefly, concerns the fact that when samples are large, the theoretical distribution of sample *means* tends to follow a normal distribution—*even if* the variable itself is not normally distributed in the population. With small *N*s, you cannot rely on the central limit theorem, so probability values could be wrong if a parametric test is used.

Between-Subjects Tests and Within-Subjects Tests

Another distinction in statistical tests concerns the nature of the comparisons. When comparisons involve different people (e.g., men versus women), the study uses a between-subjects design, and the statistical test is a **test for independent groups**. Other designs involve one group of people —for example, with a crossover design, participants are exposed to two or more treatments. In within-subjects designs, comparisons are not independent because the same people are used in all conditions, and the appropriate statistical tests are **tests for dependent groups**.

Overview of Hypothesis-Testing Procedures

This chapter describes several bivariate statistical tests. The discussion emphasizes applications rather than computations, but we urge you to consult other references (e.g., Gravetter & Wallnau, 2007; Polit, 2010) for fuller explanations if you are conducting a statistical analysis. In this research methods textbook, our main interest is to provide an overview of the use and interpretation of some common statistical tests.

Each statistical test has a particular application, but the process of testing hypotheses is basically the same. The steps are as follows:

1. *Select an appropriate test statistic.* Figure 17.5 provides a quick reference guide for selecting many widely used bivariate statistical tests. (Multivariate tests are discussed in Chapter 18). Researchers must consider such factors as which levels of measurement were used, whether a parametric test is justified, whether a dependent test is needed, and whether the focus is correlations or group comparisons—and how many groups are being compared.
2. *Establish the level of significance.* Researchers establish the criterion for accepting or rejecting the null hypothesis. An α of .05 is usually acceptable.
3. *Select a one-tailed or two-tailed test.* In most cases, a two-tailed test should be used.
4. *Compute a test statistic.* Using collected data, researchers calculate a test statistic using appropriate computational formulas, or instruct a computer to calculate the statistic.
5. *Determine the degrees of freedom* (symbolized as *df*). **Degrees of freedom** refers to the number of observations free to vary about a parameter. The concept is too complex for full elaboration here, but *df* is easy to compute.
6. *Compare the test statistic with a tabled value.* The theoretical distributions for test statistics enable researchers to determine whether obtained values of the test statistic (Step 4) are beyond the range of what is *probable* if the null hypothesis were true. Researchers compare the value of the computed test statistic to values in a table. If the absolute value of the test statistic is larger than the tabled value, the results are statistically significant. If the computed value is smaller, the results are nonsignificant.

Level of Measurement of Dependent Variable	Group Comparisons: Number of groups (the independent variable)				Correlational analyses (to examine relationship strength)
	2 Groups		3+ Groups		
	Independent Groups Tests	Dependent Groups Tests	Independent Groups Tests	Dependent Groups Tests	
Nominal (categorical)	χ^2 (or Fisher's exact test)	McNemar's test	χ^2	Cochran's Q	Phi coefficient (dichotomous) or Cramér's V (not restricted to dichotomous)
Ordinal (rank)	Mann-Whitney test	Wilcoxon signed ranks test	Kruskal-Wallis H test	Friedman's test	Spearman's rho (or Kendall's tau)
Interval or ratio (continuous)*	Independent group t-test	Paired t-test	ANOVA	RM-ANOVA	Pearson's r
	Multifactor ANOVA for 2+ independent variables				
	RM-ANOVA for 2+ groups x 2+ measurements over time				

*For distributions that are markedly non-normal or samples that are small, the nonparametric tests in the row above may be needed.

FIGURE 17.5 Quick guide to bivariate statistical tests.

When analyses are done by a computer, as is usually the case, researchers follow only the first three steps and then give commands to the computer. The computer calculates the test statistic, degrees of freedom, and the *actual* probability that the null hypothesis is true. For example, the computer may show that the two-tailed probability (p) of an intervention group being different from a control group by chance alone is .025. This means that only 25 times out of 1,000 would a group difference as large as the one obtained reflect haphazard differences rather than true intervention effects. The computed probability can then be compared with the desired significance level. If the significance criterion were .05, then the results would be significant, because .025 is more stringent than .05. By convention, any computed probability greater than .05 (e.g., .20) indicates nonsignificance (sometimes abbreviated *NS*)—that is, a result that could have occurred by chance in more than 5 out of 100 samples.

➡ **TIP:** The reference guide in Figure 17.5 does not include every test you may need, but it does include bivariate tests most often used by nurse researchers. There are many resources now available on the Internet to help with selecting an appropriate test, including interactive decision-tree tools. Useful websites include the following: *http://graphpad.com/www/book/Choose.htm* or *http://www.socialresearchmethods.net/selstat/ssstart.htm*. Links to these websites are included in the Toolkit of the *Resource Manual* for you to click on directly.

In the sections that follow, several of the most common bivariate statistical tests and their applications are described. Computer examples are provided at the end of the chapter.

TESTING DIFFERENCES BETWEEN TWO GROUP MEANS

A common research situation involves comparing two groups of participants on a continuous dependent variable. For instance, we might compare an experimental and control group of patients with regard to their mean blood pressure. Or, we might contrast men and women with regard to mean cholesterol levels.

The parametric procedure for testing differences in group means is the *t*-test. A *t*-test can be used when there are two independent groups (e.g., experimental versus control), and when the sample is dependent (e.g., pretreatment and posttreatment scores for the same people).

➡ **TIP:** A **one-sample *t*-test** can be used to compare mean values of a single group to a hypothesized value. One-sample *t*-tests were used in Polit and Beck's (2009) study of gender bias in nursing studies, which tested obtained mean values to a hypothesized population value of 50.0.

t-Tests for Independent Groups

Suppose we wanted to test the effect of early discharge of maternity patients on perceived maternal competence. We administer a scale of perceived maternal competence at discharge to 20 primiparas who had a vaginal delivery: 10 who remained in the hospital 25 to 48 hours (regular discharge group) and 10 who were discharged within 24 hours of delivery (early discharge group). In Table 17.1, we

TABLE 17.1	Fictitious Data for *t*-Test Example: Scores on a Perceived Maternal Competence Scale for Regular-Discharge and Early-Discharge Mothers

REGULAR-DISCHARGE MOTHERS	EARLY-DISCHARGE MOTHERS
30	23
27	17
25	22
20	18
24	20
32	26
17	16
18	13
28	21
29	14
Mean = 25.0	Mean = 19.0
$t = 2.86$: $df = 18$; $p = .011$	

see that mean scores for these two groups are 25.0 and 19.0, respectively. Are these differences *reliable* (i.e., would they be found in the population of early-discharge and later-discharge mothers?), or do group differences reflect chance fluctuations?

Note that the 20 scores in Table 17.1—10 per group—vary from one person to another. Some variability reflects individual differences in perceived maternal competence. Some variability might be due to measurement error (e.g., the scale's low reliability), some could result from participants' moods on a particular day, and so forth. The research question is: Can a portion of the variability reliably be attributed to the independent variable—time of discharge from the hospital? The *t*-test allows us to answer this question objectively. The hypotheses are:

$$H_0: \mu_A = \mu_B \qquad H_A: \mu_A \neq \mu_B$$

To test these hypotheses, we would compute a *t*-statistic. The formula for the *t*-statistic uses group means, variability, and sample size to calculate a value for *t*. When the data from Table 17.1 are used in the formula, the value of *t* is 2.86. Next, degrees of freedom are calculated. In this situation, degrees of freedom equal the total sample size minus 2 (*df* = 20 − 2 = 18). A table of critical *t* values is shown in Table A-1, Appendix A. Degrees of freedom are listed in the left column, and different alpha values are shown in the top rows. The shaded column shows values for $\alpha = .05$ for a two-tailed test. We find in this column that for *df* = 18, the tabled value of *t* is 2.10. *This value establishes an upper limit to what is probable if the null hypothesis is true.* Thus, the calculated *t* of 2.86, which is larger than the tabled value of the statistic*, is improbable (i.e., statistically significant). We can now say that the primiparas discharged early had significantly lower perceptions of maternal competence than those who were not discharged early. The group difference in perceived maternal competence is sufficiently large enough that it is unlikely to reflect merely chance fluctuations. If a computer were

used to analyze the data, the output would show the *exact* probability, which is .011. This means that in only 11 out of 1,000 samples would we expect a group difference of 6.0 points by chance alone.

Example of independent *t*-tests: Lee and colleagues (2009) used data from a multinational sample (from the United States, Australia, and Thailand) to study gender differences in heart failure self-care. In their overall sample of more than 2,000 adults with chronic heart failure, men had higher scores on a self-care maintenance scale (71.5) than women (68.0) (*t* = 4.29, *df* = 2081, *p* < .001).

When multiple tests are run with the same data—that is, when there are multiple dependent variables—the risk of a Type I error increases. One *t*-test with an $\alpha = .05$ has a 5% probability of a Type I error. Two *t*-tests with the same data set, however, have a probability of 9.75% of one spurious significant result, and with three tests, the risk goes up to 14.3%. Researchers sometimes apply a **Bonferroni correction** when they run multiple tests to establish a more conservative alpha level. For example, if the desired α is .05, and there are three separate tests, the corrected alpha needed to reject the null hypothesis for *all* tests would be .017, not .05. The correction is computed by dividing the desired α by the number of tests—for example, .05/3 = .017. If we concluded that mean group differences were significant for three tests at or below *p* = .017, there would be only a 5% probability of wrongly rejecting the null across all three comparisons. The Bonferroni correction can, however, be problematic in that it tends to increase the risk of a Type II error—incorrectly concluding there is no statistical association when in fact there is one.

Confidence Intervals for Mean Differences

Confidence intervals can be constructed around the difference between two means, and the results provide information about both statistical significance (i.e., whether the null hypothesis should be

---

* The tabled *t* values should be compared to the absolute value of the calculated *t*. Thus, if the calculated *t* were −2.86, then the results would still be significant.

rejected) and precision of the estimated difference. Because CI information is richer and more useful in clinical applications than *p* values, it is sometimes preferred—although nursing journals have not yet required it, as many medical journals have.

In the example in Table 17.1, the mean maternal competence scores were 25.0 in the regular discharge group and 19.0 in the early discharge group. Using a formula to compute the *standard error of the difference*, CIs can be constructed around the mean difference of 6.0. For a 95% CI, the confidence limits in our example are 1.6 and 10.4. This means that we can be 95% confident that the true difference in population means for early- and regular-discharge mothers lies somewhere between these limits.

In the *t*-test analysis, we obtained an estimate of mean group differences (6.0) and the probability that group differences were spurious ($p = .011$). With CI information, we learn the range within which the mean difference probably lies. We can see from the CI that the mean difference is significant at the .05 level *because the range does not include 0*. Given that there is a 95% probability that the mean difference is not lower than 1.6, this means that there is less than a 5% probability that there is no difference at all—thus, the null hypothesis can be rejected.

Because the CI does not give exact probabilities about the plausibility of the null hypothesis, it is often useful to present both parameter estimation and hypothesis testing information in reports. In the current example, the results could be reported as follows: "Mothers who were discharged early had significantly lower maternal competence scores (19.0) than mothers with a regular discharge (26.0) ($t = 2.86$, $df = 18$, $p = .011$); the mean difference of 6.0 had a 95% CI of 1.6 to 10.4." Such information is more conveniently displayed in tables when there are multiple dependent variables.

➲ **TIP:** The Toolkit section of the accompanying *Resource Manual* has some table templates that may be useful for presenting findings from analyses described in this chapter.

Paired *t*-Tests

Researchers sometimes obtain two measures from the same people, or measures from paired sets of participants (e.g., siblings). When means for two sets of scores are not independent, researchers should use a **paired *t*-test**—a *t*-test for dependent groups.

Suppose we were studying the effect of a special diet on the cholesterol level of elderly men. A sample of 50 men is randomly selected, and their cholesterol levels are measured before and again after 2 months on the diet. The hypotheses being tested are:

$$H_0: \mu_{x_1} = \mu_{x_2} \qquad H_A: \mu_{x_1} \neq \mu_{x_2}$$

where X_1 = pretreatment cholesterol levels
X_2 = posttreatment cholesterol levels

A *t*-statistic then would be computed from pretest and posttest data, using a different formula than for the independent group *t*-test. The obtained *t* would be compared with tabled *t*-values. For this type of *t*-test, degrees of freedom equal the number of paired observations minus 1 ($df = N - 1$). Confidence intervals can be constructed around mean differences for paired as well as independent means. For example, in the McFarlane and colleagues (2006) study described earlier, for the two groups of women combined, the mean decline in threats of assault from baseline to follow-up was 14.5, 95% CI = 12.6 to 16.4.

Nonparametric Two-Group Tests

In certain two-group situations, a nonparametric test may be needed—for example, if the dependent variable is on an ordinal scale, or if the distribution is markedly non-normal. The **Mann-Whitney U test**, the nonparametric analog of an independent group's t-test, involves assigning ranks to the two groups of scores. The sum of the ranks for the two groups can be compared by calculating the U statistic. When ordinal-level data are paired (dependent), the Wilcoxon signed-rank test can be used. The **Wilcoxon signed-rank test** involves taking the difference between paired scores and ranking the absolute difference.

TESTING MEAN DIFFERENCES WITH THREE OR MORE GROUPS

Analysis of variance (ANOVA) is the parametric procedure for testing differences between means when there are three or more groups. The statistic computed in ANOVA is the **F-ratio**. ANOVA decomposes total variability in a dependent variable into two parts: (1) variability attributable to the independent variable and (2) all other variability, such as individual differences, measurement error, and so on. Variation *between* groups is contrasted with variation *within* groups to get an F-ratio. When differences between groups are large relative to variation within groups, the probability is high that the independent variable is related to, or has caused, group differences.

One-Way ANOVA

Suppose we were comparing the effectiveness of different interventions to help people stop smoking. One group of smokers receives intensive nurse counseling (group A), a second group is treated by a nicotine patch (group B), and a third control group receives no special treatment (group C). The dependent variable is 1-day cigarette consumption measured 1 month after the intervention. Thirty smokers who wish to quit smoking are randomly assigned to one of the three conditions. **One-way ANOVA** tests the following hypotheses:

$$H_0: \mu_A = \mu_B = \mu_C \qquad H_A: \mu_A \neq \mu_B \neq \mu_C$$

The null hypothesis is that the population means for posttreatment cigarette smoking are the same for all three groups, and the alternative (research) hypothesis is inequality of means. Table 17.2 presents

TABLE 17.2	Fictitious Data for a One-Way ANOVA: Number of Cigarettes Smoked in 1 Day, 1 Month Postintervention in Three Treatment Groups				
GROUP A **NURSE COUNSELING**		**GROUP B** **NICOTINE PATCH**		**GROUP C** **UNTREATED CONTROL**	
28	19	0	27	33	35
0	24	31	0	54	0
17	0	26	3	19	43
20	21	30	24	40	39
35	2	24	27	41	36
$\bar{X}_A = 16.6$		$\bar{X}_B = 19.2$		$\bar{X}_C = 34.0$	

$F = 4.98$, $df = 2, 27$, $p = .01$

fictitious data for each participant. The mean numbers of posttreatment cigarettes consumed are 16.6, 19.2, and 34.0 for groups A, B, and C, respectively. These means are different, but are they significantly different—or do differences reflect random fluctuations?

In calculating an F-statistic, total variability in the data is broken down into two sources. The portion of the variance due to group status (i.e., exposure to different treatments) is reflected in the **sum of squares between groups**, or SS_B. The SS_B is the sum of squared deviations of individual group means from the overall **grand mean** for all participants. SS_B reflects variability in scores attributable to the independent variable, that is, group membership.

The second component is the **sum of squares within groups**, or SS_W. This index is the sum of the squared deviations of each individual score from its *own* group mean. SS_W indicates variability attributable to individual differences, measurement error, and so on.

Recall from Chapter 16 that the formula for calculating a variance is $\Sigma x^2 \div N$. The two sums of squares are like the numerator of this variance equation: both SS_B and SS_W are sums of squared deviations from means. So, to compute variance within and variance between groups, we must divide the sums of squares by something similar to N, namely degrees of freedom for each sum of squares. For between groups, $df_B = G - 1$ (number of groups minus 1). For within groups, df_W is the number of participants less 1, for each group.

In an ANOVA context, the variance is conventionally referred to as the **mean square** (MS). The formulas for the mean square between groups and the mean square within groups are:

$$MS_B = \frac{SS_B}{df_B} \qquad MS_W = \frac{SS_W}{df_W}$$

The F-ratio statistic is the ratio of these mean squares, or

$$F = \frac{MS_B}{MS_W}$$

The ANOVA summary table (Table 17.3) shows that the calculated F-statistic in our example is 4.98. For $df = 2$ and 27 and $\alpha = .05$, the tabled F value is 3.35 (see Table A-2 in Appendix A for values from the theoretical F distribution). Because our obtained F-value of 4.98 exceeds 3.35, we reject the null hypothesis that the population means are equal. The *actual* probability, calculated by computer, is .014. Group differences in posttreatment cigarette smoking are beyond chance expectations. In only 14 samples out of 1,000 would differences this great be obtained by chance alone.

The data support the research hypothesis that different treatments were associated with different cigarette smoking, but we cannot tell from the test whether treatment A was significantly more effective than treatment B. Statistical analyses known as **multiple comparison procedures** (or **post hoc tests**) are needed. Their function is to isolate the differences between group means that are responsible for rejecting the overall ANOVA null hypothesis. Note that it is *not* appropriate to use a series of t-tests (group A versus B, A versus C, and B versus C) because this would increase the risk of a Type I error. Multiple comparison methods are described

TABLE 17.3	ANOVA Summary Table for Posttreatment Smoking Example				
SOURCE OF VARIANCE	**SS**	**df**	**MEAN SQUARE**	**F**	**p**
Between groups	1761.9	2	880.9	4.98	.014
Within groups	4772.0	27	176.7		
TOTAL	6533.9	29			

in most intermediate statistical textbooks, such as that by Polit (2010).

Example of a one-way ANOVA: Shin and colleagues (2009) conducted a pilot study to assess the effects of two alternative treatments, compared with no treatment, on menstrual symptom severity in Korean women. Using ANOVA, they found that post-treatment symptom severity differed significantly among women in the control group ($M = 17.5$), the hand acupuncture therapy group ($M = 3.9$), and the hand moxibustion therapy group ($M = 3.4$) ($F = 124.6$, $df = 2, 22$, $p < .001$).

Two-Way ANOVA

One-way ANOVA is used to test the relationship between one categorical independent variable (e.g., different interventions) and a continuous dependent variable. Data from studies with multiple factors, as in a factorial design, are sometimes analyzed by **multifactor ANOVA**. In this section, we describe some principles underlying **two-way ANOVA**.

Suppose we wanted to determine whether the two smoking cessation treatments (nurse counseling and a nicotine patch) were equally effective for men and women. We randomly assign women and men, separately, to the two treatment conditions. One month after the intervention, participants report the number of cigarettes they smoked the previous day. Fictitious data for this example are shown in Table 17.4.

With two independent variables, three hypotheses are tested. First, we are testing the effectiveness, for both men and women, of nurse counseling versus the nicotine patch. Second, we are testing whether postintervention smoking differs for men and women, regardless of treatment approach. These are tests for **main effects**. Third, we are testing for **interaction effects** (i.e., differential treatment effects on men and women). Interaction concerns whether the effect of one independent variable is consistent for all levels of a second independent variable.

TABLE 17.4	Fictitious Data for a Two-Way (2 × 2) ANOVA: Number of Cigarettes Smoked in 1 Day, 1 Month Postintervention for Gender × Two Treatment Groups				
	FACTOR A—TREATMENT				
FACTOR B—GENDER	**Nurse Counseling (1)**		**Nicotine Patch (2)**		
Female (1)	24	25	27	23	
	28	38	0	18	
	2	21	45	20	
	19	0	29	12	
	27	36	22	4	Female $\bar{X}_{B1} = 21.0$
	$\bar{X}_{A1B1} = 22.0$		$\bar{X}_{A2B1} = 20.0$		
Male (2)	10	16	36	27	
	21	18	41	0	
	17	3	28	49	Male
	0	25	37	35	
	33	17	5	42	$\bar{X}_{B2} = 23.0$
	$\bar{X}_{A1B2} = 16.0$		$\bar{X}_{A2B2} = 30.0$		
Total	Treatment 1 $\bar{X}_{A1} = 19.0$		Treatment 2 $\bar{X}_{A2} = 25.0$		$\bar{X}_{T} = 22.0$

The data in Table 17.4 reveal that participants in the Nurse Counseling group smoked less, on average, than those in Nicotine Patch group (19.0 versus 25.0), that women smoked less than men after treatment (21.0 versus 23.0), and that men smoked less when exposed to nurse counseling, but women smoked less when exposed to the nicotine patch. By performing a two-way ANOVA on these data, we could learn whether the differences were statistically significant.

Multifactor ANOVA is not restricted to two-way analyses. In theory, any number of independent variables is possible, but in practice, studies with more than two factors are rare. Other statistical techniques typically are used with three or more independent variables, as we discuss in Chapter 18.

Example of a two-way ANOVA: Rew and colleagues (2008) studied the effects of duration of homelessness (less than 6 months versus 1 year or more) and gender on sexual health outcomes among homeless youth. Using two-way ANOVAs, the researchers found that, regardless of gender, youth who had been homeless more than 1 year reported significantly more sexual risk taking—there was no interaction of gender and duration on risk-taking behavior. Newly homeless young men, however, reported higher levels of social connectedness than chronically homeless young men, whereas duration of homelessness was unrelated to connectedness in young women, indicating an interaction.

Repeated-Measures ANOVA

Repeated-measures ANOVA (*RM-ANOVA*) is used in several situations, one of which is when there are three or more measures of the same dependent variable for each participant. For instance, in some studies, physiologic measures such as blood pressure or heart rate might be collected before, during, and after a medical procedure. In this situation, a one-way RM-ANOVA is an extension of a paired *t*-test. It can be used with a single group studied longitudinally, or in a crossover design with 3 or more different conditions. (In Chapter 18, we discuss RM-ANOVA for mixed designs).

As an example, suppose we wanted to compare three interventions for preterm infants, with regard to effects on infants' feeding rates: (1) nonnutritive

sucking, (2) nonnutritive sucking plus music, or (3) music alone. Using an experimental repeated-measures design, the infants participating in the study are randomly assigned to different orderings of the three treatments. Bottle feeding rate, the dependent variable, is measured after each treatment. The null hypothesis for this study is that type of intervention is unrelated to feeding rate (i.e., $\mu_1 = \mu_2 = \mu_3$). The alternative hypothesis is that feeding rate and type of intervention are related (i.e., that the three population means are not all equal).

We would find in such a study that there was variability in feeding rates both across infants within each condition and across the three treatment conditions within infants. As was true with other ANOVA situations, total variability in the dependent variable is represented by the total sum of squares, which can be partitioned into contributing components. In RM-ANOVA, three sources of variation contribute to total variability:

$$SS_{total} = SS_{treatments} + SS_{subjects} + SS_{error}$$

Conceptually, *sum of squares–treatments* is analogous to *sum of squares–between* in regular ANOVA: It represents the effect of the independent variable. (When measurements are taken at multiple points without an intervention, it may be called *sum of squares–time*). The *sum of squares–error* is similar to the *sum of squares–within* in regular ANOVA: Both represent variations associated with random fluctuations. The third component, *sum of squares–subjects*, has no counterpart in a simple ANOVA, because those being compared in regular ANOVA are not the same people. The $SS_{subjects}$ term captures individual differences, the effects of which are consistent across conditions. That is, some infants tend to have high feeding rates and others tend to have low feeding rates, regardless of conditions. Because individual differences can be statistically isolated from the error term (random fluctuation), RM-ANOVA yields a more sensitive test of the relationship between the independent and dependent variables than between-subjects ANOVA. By statistical isolation, we mean that variability attributable to individual differences is removed from the denominator in computing the *F* statistic.

Example of RM-ANOVA: Dougherty and Thompson (2009) studied changes in the physical and mental health of partners of patients receiving an implantable cardioverter defibrillator. Data on physical functioning, depression, and healthcare use were gathered at hospital discharge and at 1, 3, 6, and 12 months, and then analyzed using RM-ANOVA. One finding was that scores on a physical functioning scale declined significantly over the year ($F (4, 94) = 3.78$, $p = .007$).

Nonparametric "Analysis of Variance"

Nonparametric tests do not, strictly speaking, analyze variance, but there are nonparametric analogs to ANOVA when a parametric test is inappropriate. The **Kruskal-Wallis test** is a generalized version of the Mann-Whitney U test, based on assigning ranks to the scores of various groups. This test is used when the number of groups is greater than two and a one-way test for independent samples is desired. When multiple measures are obtained from the same subjects, the **Friedman test** for "analysis of variance" by ranks can be used. Both tests are described in Polit (2010) and other statistics textbooks.

TESTING DIFFERENCES IN PROPORTIONS

Tests discussed thus far involve dependent variables measured on an interval or ratio scale, when group means are being compared. In this section, we examine tests of group differences when the dependent variable is on a nominal scale.

The Chi-Square Test

The **chi-square** (χ^2) **test** is used to test hypotheses about group differences in proportions, as when a contingency table has been created. Suppose we were studying the effect of nursing instruction on patients' compliance with a self-medication regimen. Nurses implement a new instructional strategy with 100 randomly assigned experimental patients, while 100 control group patients are cared for using usual instruction. The research hypothesis is that a higher proportion of people in the treatment than in the control condition will be compliant.

The chi-square statistic is computed by comparing observed frequencies (i.e., values observed in the data) and expected frequencies. **Observed frequencies** for our example are shown in Table 17.5. As this table shows, 60 experimental participants (60%), but only 40 controls (40%), reported self-medication compliance after the intervention. The chi-square test enables us to decide whether a difference in proportions of this magnitude is likely to reflect a real treatment effect or only chance fluctuations. **Expected frequencies** are the cell frequencies that would be found if there was no relationship

| TABLE 17.5 | Observed Frequencies for Chi-Square Example: Patient Compliance in Two Treatment Groups |

PATIENT COMPLIANCE	GROUP		TOTAL
	CONTROL	EXPERIMENTAL	
Compliant	40	60	100
Noncompliant	60	40	100
TOTAL	100	100	200

$\chi^2 = 8.00$, $df = 1$, $p = .005$

between the two variables. In this example, if there were no relationship between the two groups, the expected frequency would be 50 people per cell because, overall, exactly half the participants (100 out of 200) complied.

The chi-square statistic is computed by summarizing differences between observed and expected frequencies for each cell. In our example, $\chi^2 = 8.00$. For chi-square tests, df equals the number of rows minus 1 times number of columns minus 1. In the current case, $df = 1 \times 1 = 1$. With 1 df, the tabled value (Table A-3 of Appendix A) from a theoretical chi-square distribution that must be exceeded to establish significance at the .05 level is 3.84. The obtained value of 8.00 is much larger than would be expected by chance (actual $p = .005$). We can conclude that a significantly larger proportion of experimental patients than control patients were compliant.

Example of chi-square test: Soltani and Arden (2009) studied breastfeeding behavior in mothers with three types of diabetes—type I, type II, and gestational. Using chi-square tests, they found, for example, that higher percentages of mothers with gestational diabetes (92.5%) and type II diabetes (81.8%) than those with type I diabetes (66.7%) breastfed at birth ($p = .02$).

Confidence Intervals for Differences in Proportion

As with means, it is possible to construct confidence intervals around the difference between two proportions. To do this, we would need to calculate the *standard error of the difference of proportions*. In the example used to explain the chi-square statistic, the difference in proportions was .20 ($p < .01$), and the *SE* of the difference is .069. The 95% CI in this example is .06 to .34. We can be 95% confident that the true population difference in compliance rates between those exposed to the intervention and those not exposed is between 6% and 34%. This interval does not include 0%, indicating that we can be 95% confident that group differences are "real."

Other Tests of Proportions

Sometimes a chi-square test is not appropriate. When the total sample size is small (total N of 30 or less) or when there are cells with small frequencies (5 or fewer), **Fisher's exact test** should be used to test the significance of differences in proportions. When the proportions being compared are from two paired groups (e.g., when a pretest–posttest design is used to compare changes in proportions on a dichotomous variable), the appropriate test is **McNemar's test**.

TESTING CORRELATIONS

The statistical tests discussed thus far are used to test differences between *groups*—they involve situations in which the independent variable is a nominal-level variable. In this section, we consider statistical tests used when the independent variable is ordinal, interval, or ratio.

Pearson's r

Pearson's r, the correlation coefficient calculated when two variables are measured on at least the interval scale, is both descriptive and inferential. Descriptively, the correlation coefficient summarizes the magnitude and direction of a relationship between two variables. As an inferential statistic, r tests hypotheses about population correlations, which are symbolized as ρ, the Greek letter rho. The null hypothesis is that there is no relationship between two variables:

$$H_0: \rho = 0 \qquad H_A: \rho \neq 0$$

For instance, suppose we studied the relationship between patients' self-reported level of stress and the pH level of their saliva. In a sample of 50 people, we find that $r = -.29$, indicating a modest tendency for people with high stress scores to have low-pH levels. But can we generalize this finding to the population? Does the coefficient of $-.29$ reflect a random fluctuation, observable only for the people in our sample, or is the relationship *real?* We can compare our computed r to a tabled value from a theoretical distribution for r. Degrees of freedom for r equal the number of participants minus 2, or $(N - 2)$. With $df = 48$, the tabled value for r for a two-tailed test with $\alpha = .05$ (Table A-4 in Appendix A) is .2803. Because the absolute value of the calculated r is .29, the null hypothesis can be rejected. We accept the research hypothesis that the correlation between stress and saliva acidity in the population is not zero.

Pearson's r can be used in both within-group and between-group situations. The example about the relationship between stress scores and the pH levels is a between-group situation: The question is whether people with high stress scores tend to have significantly lower-pH levels than *different* people with low stress scores. If stress scores were obtained both before and after surgery, however, the correlation between the two scores would be a within-group situation.

Example of Pearson's r: Simpson (2009) tested the hypothesis that medical-surgical nurses' scores on a work engagement scale would be correlated with job satisfaction, turnover cognitions, and job search behavior. She found that work engagement was, as predicted, positively correlated with job satisfaction ($r = .53$, $p < .001$), and negatively correlated with turnover cognitions ($r = -.44$, $p < .001$) and job search behavior ($r = -.25$, $p < .001$) in her sample of 167 nurses.

⮕ **TIP:** CIs can be constructed around Pearson's rs. In our example, the 95% CI around the r of .29 for stress levels and saliva pH, with a sample of 50 subjects, is (.01, .53).

Other Tests of Bivariate Relationships

Pearson's r is a parametric statistic. When the assumptions for a parametric test are violated, or when the data are ordinal level, then the appropriate coefficient of correlation is either **Spearman's rho** (r_S) or, less often, **Kendall's tau**. The values of these statistics range from -1.00 to $+1.00$, and their interpretation is similar to that of Pearson's r.

Measures of the magnitude of relationships can also be computed with nominal-level data. For example, the **phi coefficient** (Φ) is an index describing the relationship between two dichotomous variables. **Cramér's *V*** is an index of relationship applied to contingency tables larger than 2×2. Both statistics are based on the chi-square statistic and yield values that range between .00 and 1.00, with higher values indicating a stronger association between variables.

POWER ANALYSIS AND EFFECT SIZE

Many published nursing studies (and even more *un*published ones) have nonsignificant findings—many of which could reflect Type II errors. As indicated earlier, researchers set the probability of committing a Type I error (a false positive) as the significance level, alpha (α). The probability of a Type II error (a false negative) is **beta** (β). The complement of beta $(1 - \beta)$ is the *probability of detecting a true relationship or group difference* and is the **power** of a statistical test. Polit and Sherman (1990) found that many published nursing studies have insufficient power, placing them at risk for Type II errors. Although many years have elapsed since their analysis was undertaken, a glance through nursing research reports suggests that many studies continue to be **underpowered**.

Power analysis is used to reduce the risk of Type II errors and strengthen statistical conclusion validity by estimating in advance how big a sample is needed. There are four components in a power analysis, three of which must be known or estimated:

1. *The significance criterion*, α. Other things being equal, the more stringent this criterion, the lower the power.
2. *The sample size, N*. As sample size increases, power increases.
3. *The effect size* (ES). ES is an estimate of how wrong the null hypothesis is, that is, how strong the relationship between the independent variable and the dependent variable is in the population.
4. *Power, or $1 - \beta$*. This is the probability of rejecting a false null hypothesis.

Researchers typically use power analysis at the outset of a study to estimate the sample size needed to avoid a Type II error. To estimate needed sample size (N), researchers must specify α, ES, and $1 - \beta$. Researchers usually establish the risk of a Type I error (α) as .05. The conventional standard for $1 - \beta$ is .80. With power equal to .80, there is a 20% risk of committing a Type II error. Although this risk may seem high, a stricter criterion requires sample sizes much larger than most researchers could afford.

With α and $1 - \beta$ specified, the information needed to solve for N is ES, the estimated population effect size. The **effect size** is the magnitude of the relationship between the research variables. When relationships (effects) are strong, they can be detected at significant levels even with small samples. When relationships are modest, large sample sizes are needed to avoid Type II errors.

In using power analysis to estimate sample size needs, the population effect size is not *known*; if it were known, there would be no need for a new study. Effect size must be estimated using available evidence. Sometimes evidence comes from a pilot study, which can be a good approach when the main study is costly. More often, an effect size is calculated based on findings from earlier studies on a similar problem. When there are *no* relevant earlier findings, researchers use conventions based on expectations of a *small, medium,* or *large* effect. Most nursing studies have modest (small-to-medium) effects.

➲ TIP: One problem with using pilot data to estimate sample size needs for the main study is that pilot studies are small, and sample values are thus unstable. One solution is to calculate the 95% CI around a key effect size estimate from the pilot, and use a conservative estimate of needed sample size. Another approach is to supplement pilot ES information with estimates from other studies. Researchers can usually find more than one study from which the effect size can be estimated. In such a case, the estimate should be based on the study with the most reliable results. Researchers can also estimate effect size by combining information from multiple high-quality studies through averaging or weighted averaging. If you are studying a problem that has been the focus of a meta-analysis, ES estimates will likely be readily available in the report.

Procedures for estimating effects and sample size needs vary from one statistical situation to another. We focus mainly on a two-group situation for which we can estimate mean values.

Sample Size Estimates for Testing Differences between Two Means

Suppose we were testing the hypothesis that cranberry juice reduces the urinary pH of diet-controlled patients. We plan to assign some patients randomly to a control condition (no cranberry juice) and others to an experimental condition in which they will be given 300 mL of cranberry juice for 5 days. How large a sample is needed for this study, given a desired α of .05 and power of .80?

To answer this, we must first estimate ES. In a two-group situation in which mean differences are of interest, ES is usually designated as **Cohen's *d***, the formula for which is:

$$d = \frac{\mu_1 - \mu_2}{\sigma}$$

That is, the effect size (d) is the difference between the two population means, divided by the population standard deviation. These values are not known in advance, but must be estimated. For example, suppose we found an earlier nonexperimental study that compared the urinary pH of people who had or had not ingested cranberry juice in the previous 24 hours. The earlier and current studies are different in many respects, but the earlier study is a reasonable starting point. Suppose the results were as follows:

$$\overline{X}_1 (\text{no cranberry juice}) = 5.70$$
$$\overline{X}_2 (\text{cranberry juice}) = 5.50$$
$$\text{SD} = .50$$

Thus, the estimated value of d would be .40:

$$d = \frac{5.70 - 5.50}{.50} = .40$$

Table 17.6 presents approximate sample size requirements for various effect sizes and powers, for $\alpha = .05$ (for two-tailed tests), in a two-group

| TABLE 17.6 | Approximate Sample Sizes* Necessary To Achieve Selected Levels of Power as a Function of Estimated Effect Size for Test of Difference of Two Means, with $\alpha = .05$ | | | | | | | | | | |

	ESTIMATED EFFECT SIZE (d)†										
POWER	.10	.15	.20	.25	.30	.35	.40	.50	.60	.70	.80
.60	979	435	245	157	109	80	62	40	28	20	16
.70	1233	548	309	198	137	101	78	50	35	26	20
.80	1576	701	394	253	176	129	99	64	44	33	25
.90	2103	935	526	337	234	172	132	85	59	43	33
.95	2594	1154	649	416	289	213	163	105	73	53	41

*Sample size requirements for each group; total sample size would be twice the number shown.

†Estimated effect size (d) is the estimated population mean group difference divided by the estimated population standard deviation or $(\mu_1 - \mu_2)/\sigma$.

mean-difference situation. We find in this table that the estimated n (number per group) to detect an effect size of .40 with power equal to .80 is 99 people. Assuming that the earlier study provided a good estimate of the population effect size, the total number of people needed in the new study would be about 200, with half assigned to the control group (no cranberry juice) and the other half assigned to the experimental group. With a sample size smaller than 200, there would be a greater than 20% chance of a false negative conclusion, that is, a Type II error. For example, a sample size of 128 (64 per group) would result in an estimated 40% chance of incorrect nonsignificant results.

If there is no prior research, researchers can, as a last resort, estimate whether the expected effect is small, medium, or large. By convention (Cohen, 1988), the value of ES in a two-group test of mean differences is estimated at .20 for small effects, .50 for medium effects, and .80 for large effects. With an α value of .05 and power of .80, the n (number of participants per group) for studies with expected small, medium, and large effects would be 394, 64, and 25, respectively. Most nursing studies cannot expect effect sizes in excess of .50; those in the range of .20 to .40 are most common. In Polit and

Sherman's (1990) analysis of effect sizes for all studies published in *Nursing Research* and *Research in Nursing & Health* in 1989, the average effect size for *t*-test situations was .35. Cohen (1988) noted that in new areas of research inquiry, effect sizes are likely to be small. A medium effect should be estimated only when the effect is so substantial that it can be detected by the naked eye (i.e., without formal research procedures).

TIP: Performing a power analysis based on estimates of an effect size is an *evidence-based* approach to designing a new study — that is, the new study uses evidence from earlier studies to estimate how many sample members will be needed to achieve an effect that seems plausible in light of what is already known. A useful supplementary approach is to ask how big an effect would be needed to be clinically relevant? If effect-size estimates are both evidence-based and clinically meaningful, the study will be stronger.

Sample Size Estimates for Other Bivariate Tests

Power analysis can be undertaken for the other statistical tests described in this chapter. It is relatively easy to do a power analysis online (we suggest

TABLE 17.7	Approximate Sample Sizes Necessary To Achieve Selected Levels of Power as a Function of Estimated Population Correlation, with $\alpha = .05$

ESTIMATED POPULATION CORRELATION COEFFICIENT (ρ)*

POWER	.10	.15	.20	.25	.30	.35	.40	.50	.60	.70	.80
.60	489	217	122	78	54	39	30	19	13	9	7
.70	614	272	152	97	67	49	37	23	16	11	8
.80	785	347	194	123	85	62	47	29	19	13	10
.90	1047	463	258	164	112	81	61	37	25	17	12
.95	1296	575	322	204	141	101	80	50	32	22	18

*Estimated effect size (r) is the estimated population correlation coefficient (ρ)

several relevant websites in the Toolkit with the *Resource Manual* 😊). Here, we discuss only a few basic features for situations in which ANOVA, Pearson's *r*, or a chi-square situation would be the basis for doing the power analysis.

There are alternative approaches to doing a power analysis in an ANOVA context. The simplest approach is to estimate **eta-squared** (η^2), which is an ES index indicating the proportion of variance explained in ANOVA. Eta-squared equals the sum of squares between (SS_B) divided by the total sum of squares (SS_T), and can be used directly as the estimate of effect size if sum of square information is available. (For the data in Table 17.2 and shown in an ANOVA summary table in Table 17.3, $\eta^2 = .27$, a large effect). When eta-squared cannot be estimated, researchers can estimate whether effects are likely to be small, medium, or large. For ANOVA situations, the conventional estimates for small, medium, and large effects would be values of η^2 equal to .01, .06, and .14, respectively. Assuming $\alpha = .05$ and power = .80, this corresponds to sample size requirements of about 319, 53, or 22 subjects *per group* in a three-group study, and about 272, 44, and 19 *per group* in a four-group study.*

---

* When analysis of covariance (see Chapter 18) is used in lieu of *t*-tests or ANOVA, sample size requirements are smaller— sometimes appreciably so—because of reduced error variance.

For Pearson correlations, the estimated value of ES is ρ, the population correlation coefficient. Thus, the value of the correlation coefficient (*r*) from a relevant earlier study can be used directly as the estimated effect size. Table 17.7 shows sample size requirements in situations in which Pearson's *r* is used for various effect sizes and powers when $\alpha = .05$. For example, if our estimated population correlation was .25, we would need a sample size of 123 for power = .80. With a sample this size, we can expect that we would wrongly reject a true null hypothesis 5 times out of 100 and wrongly retain a false null hypothesis 20 times out of 100. When prior estimates of effect size are unavailable, the conventional values of small, medium, and large effect sizes in a bivariate correlation situation are .10, .30, and .50, respectively (i.e., samples of 785, 85, and 29 for a power of .80 and a significance level of .05). In Polit and Sherman's (1990) study, the average correlation in nursing studies was found to be around .20.

Estimating sample size requirements for testing differences in proportions between groups is complex. The effect size for contingency tables is influenced not only by expected differences in proportions (e.g., 60% in one group versus 40% in another, a 20-percentage point difference), but also by the absolute values of the proportions. Effect sizes are *larger* (and thus sample size needs are *smaller*) at the extremes than near the midpoint. A 20-percentage point difference is easier to detect if the percentages are 10% and 30% than if they are near the middle, such as 60% and 40%. Because of this fact, it is difficult to offer information on values for small, medium, and large effects in this context. We can, however, give *examples* of differences in proportions that conform to the conventions in a 2 × 2 situation:

Small: .05 versus .10, .20 versus .29, .40 versus .50, .60 versus .70, .80 versus .87
Medium: .05 versus .21, .20 versus .43, .40 versus .65, .60 versus .82, .80 versus .96
Large: .05 versus .34, .20 versus .58, .40 versus .78, .60 versus .92, .80 versus .96

As an example, if the expected proportion for a control group were .40, the researcher would need about 385, 70, and 24 per group if higher values were expected for the experimental group and the effect was expected to be small, medium, and large, respectively. As in other situations, researchers are encouraged to avoid using the conventions, if possible, in favor of more precise estimates based on empirical evidence. If the conventions cannot be avoided, conservative estimates should be used to minimize the risk of obtaining nonsignificant results.

Example of a power analysis: Gao and colleagues (2009) compared first-time Chinese mothers and fathers with regard to psychological outcomes in the postpartum period. Power calculations to estimate sample size needs were based on an assumed medium effect ($d = .50$). With a power of .80 and $\alpha = .05$, the power analysis indicated a need for 126 dyads. A total of 130 couples completed the study.

Effect Size Calculations in Completed Studies

Power analysis concepts are sometimes used *after* analyses are completed to calculate estimated population effects based on *actual N*s. In this situation, power, alpha, and *N* are known, and so the task is to solve for ES. Effect sizes provide readers and clinicians with estimates about the magnitude of effects—an important issue in EBP (see Table 2.1). Effect size information can be crucial because, with large samples, even tiny effects can be statistically significant at dramatic levels. *P* values tell you whether results are likely to be *real*, but effect sizes can suggest whether they are important. Effect size estimates are needed in doing meta-analyses (see Chapter 27), and so when these values are presented directly in a report, they are helpful to meta-analysts.

Example of calculated effect size: Mackenzie and colleagues (2006) tested a mindfulness-based stress reduction intervention for nurses and nurse aides. They presented a table of results that showed the values of both *F*-ratio statistics, *p* values, and effect sizes (the values of η^2) for seven outcome variables.

THE COMPUTER AND BIVARIATE INFERENTIAL STATISTICS

We have emphasized the logic and uses of various statistical tests rather than computational formulas.[*] Because computers are almost always used for statistical analysis, and because it is important to know how to read a computer printout, we include examples of computer analyses for two statistical tests. We return to the example described in Chapter 16, which involved a randomized trial to test the effects of a prenatal program for young low-income women. Raw data for the 30 participants in this example were presented in Table 16.8. Given these data, let us test some hypotheses.

Hypothesis One: *t*-Test

Our first research hypothesis is that experimental group infants have higher birth weights than control

---

[*]This introduction to inferential statistics is simplified, and has neglected important issues such as specific assumptions underlying various tests. We urge readers to have a good grasp of statistical principles before undertaking quantitative analyses.

group infants. The *t*-test for independent samples is used to test the hypothesis of mean group differences. The null and alternative hypotheses are:

$$H_0: \mu \text{ experimental} = \mu \text{ control}$$
$$H_A: \mu \text{ experimental} \neq \mu \text{ control}$$

Figure 17.6 presents the SPSS printout for the *t*-test. Panel A presents some descriptive statistics (mean, standard deviation, and standard error of the mean) for the birth weight variable, separately for the two groups. The mean birth weight of the babies in the experimental group is 107.5333 ounces, compared with 101.8667 ounces for those in the control group. The data are consistent with the research hypothesis—that is, the average weight of babies in the experimental group is higher than that of controls. But is the difference attributable to the intervention, or does it reflect random fluctuations?

Panel B of Figure 17.6 first presents results of **Levene's test** for equality of variances. An assumption underlying use of the *t*-test is that the population variances for the two groups are equal. In Panel A, we can see that the standard deviations (and thus the variances) are quite different, with substantially more variability among experimentals ($SD = 13.38$)

than controls ($SD = 7.24$). Levene's test tells us that the two variances are, in fact, significantly different (Sig. = .046).

Panel B then presents two rows of *t*-test information. The top row is for the **pooled variance *t*-test**, which is used when equality of variances can be assumed. Given the significantly different variances in this sample, however, we should use information in the second row, which uses a different (**separate variance *t*-test**) formula. The mean group difference in birth weights is -5.66667 ounces. The value of the *t* statistic is -1.443, and the two-tailed probability (Sig.) for the differences in group means is .163. This means that in about 16 samples out of 100, we could expect a mean difference in weights this large as a result of chance. Therefore, because $p > .05$ (a nonsignificant result), we cannot conclude that the intervention was effective in improving the birth weights of experimental group infants. Note that we cannot conclude that it was *not* effective, either. Failure to reject the null hypothesis does not mean that there is evidence that the null is true.

The last two columns of Panel B show the 95% confidence intervals for the population mean difference. We can conclude with 95% confidence that the mean difference in birth weights for the population

A Group Statistics

	Treatment group	N	Mean	Std. Deviation	Std. Error Mean
Infant birth weight in ounces	Control	15	101.8667	7.23944	1.86922
	Experimental	15	107.5333	13.37838	3.45428

B Independent Samples Test

		Levene's Test for Equality of Variances		*t*-test for Equality of Means						
		F	Sig.	t	df	Sig. (2-tailed)	Mean Difference	Std. Error Difference	95% Confidence Interval of the Difference Lower	Upper
Infant birth weight in ounces	Equal variances assumed	4.370	.046	−1.443	28	.160	−5.66667	3.92760	−13.71199	2.37865
	Equal variances not assumed			−1.443	21.552	.163	−5.66667	3.92760	−13.82185	2.48851

FIGURE 17.6 SPSS *t*-test printout: Testing group differences in infant birth weight.

of young mothers exposed and not exposed to the intervention lies between -13.8218 ounces and $+2.4885$ ounces. Zero is within this interval, indicating the possibility that there are no group differences in the population. This is consistent with the fact that we could not reject the null hypothesis of equal means on the basis of the t-test.

It was noted earlier than power analysis can be used to estimate effect size. In our example, the effect size estimate is as follows:

$$ES = (107.5333 - 101.8667) \div 10.955 = .52$$

The estimated effect size is the experimental mean minus the control mean, divided by the overall (pooled) standard deviation, which is 10.955. The obtained effect size of .52 is moderate, but an examination of Table 17.6 indicates that with a sample size of only 15 per group, our power to detect a true population difference is less (actually *far* less) than .60. This means that we had a very high risk of a Type II error. We can also see that with an effect size of .52, we would have needed about 60 mothers in each group to achieve a power of .80.

Hypothesis Two: Pearson Correlation

Our second research hypothesis is as follows: Older mothers have babies of higher birth weight than younger mothers. In this case, both birth weight and maternal age are measured on the ratio scale, so the appropriate test statistic is Pearson's product-moment correlation. The hypotheses are:

$$H_0: \rho \text{ birth weight—age} = 0$$
$$H_A: \rho \text{ birth weight—age} \neq 0$$

The SPSS printout for the hypothesis test is presented in Figure 17.7. The correlation matrix shows, in row one, the correlation of infant birth weight with infant birth weight and of birth weight with mother's age; and in row two, the correlation of mother's age with infant birth weight and of age with age. In the shaded cell at the intersection of age and birth weight, we find three numbers. The first is the correlation coefficient ($r = .594$), which indicates a moderately strong positive relationship: The older the mother, the higher the baby's weight tended to be, consistent with the research hypothesis. The second number in the cell shows the probability that the correlation occurred by chance: Sig. (for significance level) $= .001$ for a two-tailed test. In other words, a relationship this strong would be found by chance in fewer than 1 out of 1,000 samples of 30 young mothers. Therefore, the research hypothesis is accepted. The final number in the shaded cell is 30, the total sample size (N).

→ TIP: You may find it helpful to consult the glossary of statistical symbols in the inside back cover if you find a symbol in a research report that you do not recognize. Note that not all symbols in this glossary are described in this book, so it may be necessary to refer to a statistics textbook, such as that of Polit (2010) for further information.

CRITIQUING INFERENTIAL STATISTICAL ANALYSES

It is difficult to critique researchers' data analysis decisions without adequate training in statistics and

Correlations

		Infant birth weight in ounces	Mother's age
Infant birth weight in ounces	Pearson Correlation	1.000	.594**
	Sig. (2-tailed)		.001
	N	30.000	30
Mother's age	Pearson Correlation	.594**	1.000
	Sig. (2-tailed)	.001	
	N	30	30.000

**Correlation is significant at the 0.01 level (two-tailed).

FIGURE 17.7 SPSS correlation matrix printout: Testing the relationship between maternal age and infant birth weight.

data analysis. Nevertheless, there are certain things you can do to critically appraise the statistical analysis even if your background in statistics is modest.

You can begin by asking whether the report presents the results of statistical tests for all study hypotheses, and whether the researchers undertook analyses to address questions about the study's internal validity. For example, in an RCT, was the baseline comparability of the treatment groups assessed (i.e., were analyses undertaken to test for selection biases)? Did groups differ with regard to attrition? As noted in Chapter 10, statistical analyses and design issues are sometimes intertwined, in the sense that both analytic and design decisions can affect statistical conclusion validity. When sample size is small, when an independent variable is weakly defined (or when participation in an intervention is low), and when a weak statistical procedure is used in lieu of a more powerful one, then the risk of drawing the wrong conclusion about the research hypotheses is heightened. Risks to statistical conclusion validity should be considered when research hypotheses are not supported.

Other issues important in a thorough critique are whether the researcher used the right statistical tests, whether the statistical information reported is adequate to meet readers' information needs, and whether the results were presented in a clear and thoughtful manner, with a judicious combination of information reported in the text and in well–laid-out tables. ⊗ Box 17.1 presents some guiding questions for critiquing the use of bivariate inferential statistics in a research report.

BOX 17.1 Guidelines for Critiquing Bivariate* Inferential Analyses

1. Does the report include any bivariate inferential statistics? Was a statistical test performed for each hypothesis or research question? If inferential statistics were not used, should they have been?
2. Were statistical tests used to strengthen inferences about the study's internal validity (e.g., to test for selection bias or attrition bias)? If not, should they have been?
3. Were the selected statistical tests appropriate, given the level of measurement of the variables and the nature of the hypotheses?
4. Were parametric tests used? Does it appear that the use of parametric tests was appropriate? If nonparametric tests were used, was a rationale provided, and does the rationale seem sound? Should more powerful parametric procedures have been used instead?
5. Was information provided about both hypothesis testing and estimation of parameters? Were effect sizes reported? Overall, did the statistical results provide readers and potential users of the study results with sufficient information about the evidence the study yields?
6. Were the results of any statistical tests significant? What do the tests tell you about the plausibility of the research hypotheses? Were effects sizeable? What do the effects suggest about the clinical importance of the findings?
7. Were the results of any statistical tests nonsignificant? Is it plausible that these reflect Type II errors? What factors might have undermined the study's statistical conclusion validity?
8. In general, does the report provide a rationale for the use of the selected statistical tests? Does the report contain sufficient information for you to judge whether appropriate statistics were used?
9. Was an appropriate amount of statistical information reported? Are the findings clearly and logically organized?
10. Were tables used judiciously to summarize large amounts of statistical information? Are the tables clearly presented, with good titles and carefully labeled column headings? Is the information presented in the text consistent with the information presented in the tables? Is the information totally redundant?

---

*Most of these questions are equally appropriate for critiquing the use of multivariate statistics, as described in Chapter 18.

RESEARCH EXAMPLE

Study: Neonatal neurobehavioral organization after exposure to maternal epidural analgesia in labor (Bell et al., 2010).

Statement of Purpose: The purpose of this study was to explore relationships between exposure to epidural analgesia in labor to measures of neurobehavioral organization in infants at the initial feeding 1 hour after birth.

Methods: A sample of 52 mothers (18 who were unmedicated and 34 who opted for an epidural) and their term infants were recruited for the study. A nutritive sucking apparatus yielded data on the infants' total number of sucks over a 5-minute period and sucking pressure. Video recordings of the infants before and after the first feeding were coded for frequency of alertness over a 15-minute period by raters blinded to mothers' use of epidural analgesia.

Analysis and Findings: The researchers presented a table summarizing key demographic and clinical characteristics of the two groups. Group differences were tested using *t*-tests for continuous variables (e.g., maternal age) and chi-square tests for categorical variables (e.g., infant gender). The two groups were found to be significantly different in many respects. For example, the unmedicated group was significantly older ($p = .03$), more likely to be multiparous ($p = .03$), and had a shorter mean duration of labor ($p = .03$). The groups were similar with regard to gestational age ($p = .87$), infant birth weight ($p = .83$), and pitocin dosage ($p = .14$).

The mean number of sucks was 37.6 (95% CI = 28.8, 46.3) in the unmedicated group and 34.4 (95% CI = 26.0, 42.9) in the epidural group. The two groups were not significantly different with regard to mean number of sucks ($t = .51$, $p = .61$), nor in terms of mean sucking pressure ($t = -.16$, $p = .87$).

Two-way ANOVA was used to compare three medication groups (unmedicated, high dose, and low dose epidural) and infant girls versus boys (a 3 × 2 analysis) in terms of total number of sucks. A post hoc test indicated that girls in the unmedicated group had a significantly higher number of sucks than girls in the high-dose group. Chi-square tests were used to compare the three groups (unmedicated, low dose, and high dose), separately by infant gender, in terms of having a low versus high number of sucks. Unmedicated girls (but not boys) were significantly more likely to be classified in the high-number group, while girls in the high epidural dosage group were more likely to be in the low-number group ($\chi^2 = 10.80$, $p = .005$).

Because of highly skewed data, the researchers used the Mann-Whitney U test to examine differences between the no medication and epidural groups with regard to infants' frequency of alertness. No significant differences were found either before feeding ($p = .40$) or after feeding ($p = .79$).

SUMMARY POINTS

- **Inferential statistics**, which are based on **laws of probability**, allow researchers to make inferences about a population based on data from a sample; they offer a framework for deciding whether the **sampling error** that results from sampling fluctuations is too high to provide reliable population estimates.

- The **sampling distribution of the mean** is a theoretical distribution of the means of an infinite number of samples drawn from a population. The sampling distribution of means follows a normal curve, so the probability that a specified sample value will be obtained can be ascertained.

- The **standard error of the mean** (**SEM**)—the standard deviation of this theoretical distribution—indicates the degree of average error of a sample mean; the smaller the *SEM*, the more accurate are the sample estimates of the population mean.

- Statistical inference consists of two approaches: estimating parameters and testing hypotheses. **Parameter estimation** is used to estimate a population parameter.

- **Point estimation** provides a single descriptive value of the population estimate (e.g., a mean or odds ratio). **Interval estimation** provides the upper and lower limits of a range of values— the **confidence interval (CI)**—between which the population value is expected to fall, at a specified probability. Researchers establish the degree of confidence that the population value lies within this range. A 95% CI indicates a 95% probability that the true population value lies between the upper and lower **confidence limits**.

- **Hypothesis testing** through statistical procedures enables researchers to make objective decisions about the validity of their hypotheses.

- The **null hypothesis** states that there is no relationship between research variables, and that any observed relationship is due to chance. Rejection of the null hypothesis lends support to the research hypothesis.

- A **Type I error** occurs when a null hypothesis is incorrectly rejected (a false positive). A **Type II error** occurs when a null hypothesis is wrongly accepted (a false negative).

- Researchers control the risk of a Type I error by establishing a **level of significance** (or **alpha** level), which is the probability that such an error will occur. The .05 level means that in only 5 out of 100 samples would the null hypothesis be rejected when it should have been accepted.

- In testing hypotheses, researchers compute a **test statistic** and then determine whether the statistic falls at or beyond the **critical region** on the relevant theoretical distribution. If the value of the test statistic indicates that the null hypothesis is "improbable," the result is **statistically significant** (i.e., obtained results are not likely to result from chance fluctuations at the specified level of probability).

- Most hypothesis testing involves **two-tailed tests**, in which both ends of the sampling distribution are used to define the region of improbable values; a **one-tailed test** may be appropriate if there is a strong rationale for an *a priori* directional hypothesis.

- **Parametric tests** involve the estimation of at least one parameter, the use of interval- or ratio-level data, and assumptions of normally distributed variables; **nonparametric tests** are used when the data are nominal or ordinal or when a normal distribution cannot be assumed—especially when samples are small.

- **Tests for independent groups** compare separate groups of people, and **tests for dependent groups**

compare the same group of people over time or conditions (within-subjects designs).

- Two common statistical tests are the **t-test** and **analysis of variance** (**ANOVA**), both of which are used to test the significance of the difference between group means; ANOVA is used when there are three or more groups (**one-way ANOVA**) or when there is more than one independent variable (e.g. **two-way ANOVA**). **Repeated measures ANOVA (RM-ANOVA)** is used when there are multiple means being compared over time.

- Nonparametric analogs of *t*-tests and ANOVA include the **Mann-Whitney** U **test** and the **Wilcoxon signed-rank test** (two-group situations), and the **Kruskal-Wallis** and **Friedman tests** (three-group or more situations).

- The **chi-square test** is used to test hypotheses about differences in proportions. For small samples or small cell sizes, **Fisher's exact test** should be used.

- Statistical tests to measure the magnitude of bivariate relationships and to test whether the relationship is significantly different from zero include Pearson's *r* for interval-level data, Spearman's rho and **Kendall's tau** for ordinal-level data, and the **phi coefficient** and **Cramér's V** for nominal-level data.

- Confidence intervals can be constructed around almost any computed statistic, including differences between means, differences between proportions, and correlation coefficients. CI information is valuable to clinical decision-makers, who need to know more than whether differences are probably *real*.

- **Power analysis** is a method of estimating either the likelihood of committing a Type II error or sample size requirements. Power analysis involves four components: desired significance level (α), **power** ($1 - \beta$), sample size (N), and estimated **effect size** (ES). Effect size estimates convey important information about the magnitude of effects in a study and are a useful supplement to *p* values and CI values. **Cohen's** *d* is a widely used effect size index summarizing mean-difference effects between two groups.

STUDY ACTIVITIES

Chapter 17 of the *Resource Manual for Nursing Research: Generating and Assessing Evidence for Nursing Practice, 9th edition*, offers exercises and study suggestions for reinforcing concepts presented in this chapter. In addition, the following study questions can be addressed:

1. Which inferential statistics would you choose for the following sets of variables? Explain your answers (refer to Figure 17.5.).
   a. Variable 1 represents the weights of 100 patients; variable 2 is the patients' resting heart rate.
   b. Variable 1 is the patients' marital status; variable 2 is the patients' level of preoperative stress on a 10-item scale.
   c. Variable 1 is whether an amputee has a leg removed above or below the knee; variable 2 is whether or not the amputee shows signs of aggressive behavior during rehabilitation.
2. Apply relevant questions in Box 17.1 to the research example at the end of the chapter (Bell et al., 2010), referring to the full journal article as necessary.

STUDIES CITED IN CHAPTER 17

Arderko, L., Braun, J., Auinger, P. (2010). Contribution of tobacco smoke exposure to learning disabilities. *Journal of Obstetric, Gynecologic, & Neonatal Nursing, 39*, 111–117.

Bell, A., White-Traut, R., & Medoff-Cooper, B. (2010). Neonatal neurobehavioral organization after exposure to maternal epidural analgesia in labor. *Journal of Obstetric, Gynecologic, & Neonatal Nursing, 39*, 178–190.

Dougherty, C., & Thompson, E. (2009). Intimate partner physical and mental health after sudden cardiac arrest and receipt of an implantable cardioverter defibrillator. *Research in Nursing & Health, 32*, 432–442.

Gao, L., Chan, S., & Mao, Q. (2009). Depression, perceived stress, and social support among first-time Chinese mothers and fathers in the postpartum period. *Research in Nursing & Health, 32*, 50–58.

Lee, C., Riegel, B., Driscoll, A., Suwanno, J., Moser, D., Lennie, T., Dickson, W., Cameron, J., & Worrall-Carter, L. (2009). Gender differences in heart failure: A multinational cross-sectional study. *International Journal of Nursing Studies, 46*, 1485–1495.

Mackenzie, C., Poulin, P., & Seidman-Carlson, R. (2006). A brief mindfulness-based stress reduction intervention for nurses and nurse aides. *Applied Nursing Research, 19*(2), 105–109.

McFarlane, J., Groff, J., O'Brien, J., & Watson, K. (2006). Secondary prevention of intimate partner violence. *Nursing Research, 55*, 52–61.

Polit, D. F., & Beck, C. T. (2009). International gender bias in nursing research, 2005-2006: A quantitative content analysis. *International Journal of Nursing Studies, 46*, 1102–1110.

Rew, L., Grady, M., Whittaker, T., & Bowman, K. (2008). Interaction of duration of homelessness and gender on adolescent sexual health indicators. *Journal of Nursing Scholarship, 40*, 109–115.

Shin, K., Ha, J., Park, H., & Heitkemper, M. (2009). The effect of hand acupuncture therapy and hand moxibustion therapy on premenstrual syndrome among Korean women. *Western Journal of Nursing Research, 31*, 171–186.

Simpson, M. R. (2009). Predictors of work engagement among medical-surgical registered nurses. *Western Journal of Nursing Research, 31*, 44–65.

Soltani, H., & Arden, M. (2009). Factors associated with breastfeeding up to 6 months postpartum in mothers with diabetes. *Journal of Obstetric, Gynecologic, & Neonatal Nursing, 38*, 586–594.

VandeVusse, L., Hanson, L., Berner, M., & Winters, J. (2010). Impact of self-hypnosis in women on select physiologic and psychological parameters. *Journal of Obstetric, Gynecologic, & Neonatal Nursing, 39*, 159–168.

Methodologic and nonresearch references cited in this chapter can be found in a separate section at the end of the book.

18

Multivariate Statistics

P henomena of interest to nurse researchers usually are complex. Phenomena such as patients' spirituality or abrupt elevations of patients' temperature are multiply determined. Scientists, in efforts to explain or predict phenomena, have recognized that two-variable studies are often inadequate. The classic approach to data analysis and research design, which involved studying the effect of a single independent variable on a single dependent variable, is being replaced by sophisticated **multivariate* procedures**.

Multivariate statistics are computationally formidable. Our purpose is to provide a general understanding of how, when, and why multivariate statistics are used, without working out computations. Nevertheless, we must present more formulas than we did in the previous two chapters because, to read and create tables with results from multivariate procedures, you must understand underlying components. This chapter introduces a few frequently used multivariate techniques. Those needing more comprehensive coverage should consult books such as those by Tabachnick and Fidell (2007) or Hair and colleagues (2009).

One widely used multivariate procedure is multiple regression analysis, which is used to analyze the effects of two or more independent variables on a continuous dependent variable. The terms **multiple correlation** and **multiple regression** will be used almost interchangeably, consistent with the strong bond between correlation and regression. To comprehend this bond, we first explain simple (i.e., bivariate) regression.

SIMPLE LINEAR REGRESSION

Regression analysis is used to make predictions. In simple regression, one independent variable (X) is used to predict a dependent variable (Y). For instance, we could use simple regression to predict stress from noise levels. An important feature of regression is that the higher the correlation between two variables, the more accurate the prediction. If the correlation between diastolic and systolic blood pressure were perfect (i.e., if $r = 1.00$), we would need to measure only one to know the value of the other. Few variables are perfectly correlated, and so predictions made through regression analysis usually are imperfect.

---

*We use the term *multivariate* in this chapter to refer to analyses with at least three variables.

The basic linear regression equation is:

$$Y' = a + bX$$

where Y' = predicted value of variable Y
  a = intercept constant
  b = regression coefficient
  X = actual value of variable X

Regression analysis solves for a and b, and so a prediction about Y can be made for any value of X. You may remember from high school algebra that the preceding equation is the algebraic equation for a straight line. **Linear regression** is used to determine a straight-line fit to the data that minimizes deviations from the line.

As an illustration, consider the data in Table 18.1, for five people on two strongly correlated variables, X and Y ($r = .90$). If we used the five pairs of X and Y values to solve for a and b in a regression equation, we would be able to predict Y values for a *new* group of people about whom we will have information on variable X only.

We do not show the formulas for computing the values of a and b here, but suffice it to say they are straightforward calculations involving deviation scores from X and Y values. As shown at the bottom of Table 18.1, the solution to the regression equation is $Y' = 1.5 + .9X$. Now suppose that the X values in column 1 are the only data we have, and

we want to predict values for Y. For the first person, $X = 1$; we would predict that $Y = 1.5 + (.9)(1)$, or 2.4. Column 3 shows Y' values for each X. These numbers show that Y' does not exactly equal the actual values obtained for Y (column 2). Most **errors of prediction** (*e*) are small, as shown in column 4. Errors of prediction occur because the correlation between X and Y is not perfect. Only when $r = 1.00$ or -1.00 does $Y' = Y$. The regression equation solves for a and b in a way that minimizes such errors. More precisely, the solution minimizes the sums of squares of prediction errors, so standard regression analysis is said to use a **least-squares** criterion. Indeed, standard regression is sometimes called **ordinary least squares**, or **OLS**, **regression**. In column 5 of Table 18.1, the error terms—called **residuals**—have been squared and summed to yield a value of 7.60. Any values of a and b other than 1.5 and .9 would have yielded a larger sum of squared residuals.

Figure 18.1 shows the solution to this regression analysis graphically. Actual X and Y values are plotted on the graph with circles. The line running through these points represents the regression solution. The intercept (a) is the point at which the line crosses the Y axis, which in this case is 1.5. The slope (b) is the angle of the line. With $b = .90$, the line slopes so that for every 4 units on the X axis, we must go up 3.6 units ($.9 \times 4$) on the Y axis. The

TABLE 18.1	Example of Simple Linear Regression			
(1) X	**(2)** Y	**(3)** Y'	**(4)** e	**(5)** e^2
1	2	2.4	−.4	.16
3	6	4.2	1.8	3.24
5	4	6.0	−2.0	4.00
7	8	7.8	.2	.04
9	10	9.6	.4	.16
$\overline{X} = 5.0$	$\overline{Y} = 6.0$		0.0	$\Sigma e^2 = 7.60$

$r = .90$
$Y' = a + bX = 1.5 + .9X$

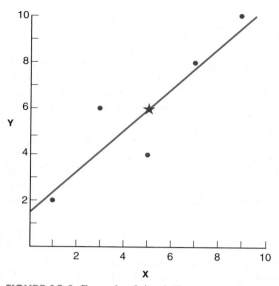

FIGURE 18.1 Example of simple linear regression.

line, then, embodies the regression equation. To predict a value for Y, we would go to the point on the X axis for an obtained X value, go up vertically to the point on the regression line directly above the X score, and then read the predicted Y' value horizontally on the Y axis. For example, for an X value of 5, we would predict a Y' of 6, indicated by the star.

Correlation coefficients express how variation in one variable is associated with variation in another. The square of r (r^2) tells us the proportion of variance in Y that is accounted for by X. In our example, $r = .90$, so $r^2 = .81$. This means that 81% of the variability in Y values can be understood in terms of variability in X values. The remaining 19% is variability due to other factors. Thus, the stronger the correlation, the better the prediction; the stronger the correlation, the greater the percentage of variance explained.

MULTIPLE LINEAR REGRESSION

The correlation between two variables is rarely perfect, so researchers often try to improve predictions of Y by including multiple independent variables—

which are often called **predictor variables** in a multiple regression context.

Basic Concepts for Multiple Regression

Suppose we wanted to predict graduate nursing students' grade point averages (GPA). Not all applicants can be accepted, so we want to select those with the greatest chance of success. Suppose we had previously found that students with high scores on the verbal portion of an entrance exam (EE-V) tended to get better grades than those with lower EE-V scores. The correlation between EE-V and graduate GPAs is .50. With only 25% ($.50^2$) of the variance of graduate GPA accounted for, there will be many errors of prediction: Many admitted students will not perform as well as expected, and many rejected applicants would have made good students. It may be possible, by adding information, to make more accurate predictions through multiple regression. The basic multiple regression equation is:

$$Y' = a + b_1X_1 + b_2X_2 + \ldots b_kX_k$$

where Y' = predicted value for variable Y
a = intercept constant
k = number of predictor (independent) variables
b_1 to b_k = regression coefficients for the k variables
X_1 to X_k = scores or values on the k independent variables

In our example of predicting graduate nursing students' GPAs, suppose we hypothesized that undergraduate GPA (GPA-U) and scores on the quantitative portion of the entrance exam (EE-Q) would improve our ability to predict graduate GPA. Suppose the resulting equation were:

$Y' = .4 + .05(GPA-U) + .003(EE-Q) + .002(EE-V)$

For instance, suppose an applicant had an EE-V score of 600, an EE-Q score of 550, and a GPA-U of 3.2. The predicted graduate GPA would be:

$Y' = .4 + (.05)(3.2) + .003(550) + .002(600) = 3.41$

We can assess the degree to which adding two independent variables improved our ability to predict graduate school performance through the multiple correlation coefficient. In bivariate correlation, the index is Pearson's r. With two or more independent variables, the index is the **multiple correlation coefficient**, or R. Unlike r, R does not have negative values. R varies from .00 to 1.00, showing the *strength* of relationship between several independent variables and a dependent variable but not *direction*. R, when squared (R^2), indicates the proportion of variance in Y accounted for by the combined, simultaneous influence of the independent variables.

R^2 provides a way to evaluate the accuracy of a prediction equation. Suppose that with the three predictors in the current example, the value of $R = .71$. This means that 50% ($.71^2$) of the variation in graduate GPA can be explained by verbal and quantitative EE scores and undergraduate grades. Adding two predictors doubled the variance accounted for by EE-V alone, from .25 to .50.

The multiple correlation coefficient is never less than the highest bivariate correlation between a predictor and the dependent variable. Table 18.2 presents a correlation matrix with the correlation coefficients for all pairs of variables in this example. The predictor most strongly correlated with graduate grades is GPA-U, $r = .60$. The value of R could not be less than .60.

R is more readily increased when predictors have low correlations among themselves. In the current case, the correlations range from .40 (between EE-Q and GPA-U) and .70 (EE-Q and EE-V). All correlations are fairly substantial, which helps to explain why R is not much higher than the r between the GPA-GRAD and GPA-U alone (.71 compared with .60). This somewhat puzzling phenomenon reflects redundancy of information among predictors. When correlations among independent variables are high, they add little predictive power to each other. With low correlations among predictors, each can contribute something unique to predicting a dependent variable. In our example, GPA-U predicts 36% of Y's variance ($.60^2$). The remaining two independent variables do not contribute as much as we would expect by considering their bivariate correlation with graduate GPA. In fact, their *combined* added contribution is only 14% ($.50 - .36 = .14$), which is small because the two test scores have redundant information with undergraduate grades.

As more independent variables are added to the regression equation, increments to R tend to decrease. It is rare to find predictor variables that correlate well with a dependent variable but modestly with one another. Redundancy is difficult to avoid as more and more variables are added to the equation. The inclusion of independent variables beyond the first three or four typically does little to improve the proportion of variance accounted for or the accuracy of prediction.

Dependent variables in multiple regression analysis, as in ANOVA, should be measured on an interval or ratio scale. Independent variables, on

TABLE 18.2	Correlation Matrix for Graduate Nursing Student Grade Example			
	GPA-GRAD	**GPA-U**	**EE-Q**	**EE-V**
GPA-GRAD	1.00			
GPA-U	.60	1.00		
EE-Q	.55	.40	1.00	
EE-V	.50	.50	.70	1.00

GPA, grade point average; EE, entrance examination; GPA-GRAD, graduate GPA; GPA-U, undergraduate GPA; EE-Q, entrance examination quantitative score; EE-V, entrance examination verbal score.

the other hand, can be either interval- or ratio-level variables *or* categorical variables. Categorical variables usually are coded as dichotomous **dummy variables**, with the code of 1 designating the presence of an attribute and 0 designating its absence. For example, if males were coded 1 and females were coded 0, the code of 1 would represent "maleness." A text such as that by Polit (2010) can be consulted for information on how to use and interpret dichotomous dummy variables.

Tests of Significance

Multiple regression analysis is not used solely (or even primarily) to develop prediction equations. Researchers typically ask inferential questions about relationships in the analysis (e.g., Does R reflect chance fluctuations, or does it reflect true relationships in the population?) There are several significance tests that address different questions.

Tests of the Overall Equation and R

The basic null hypothesis in multiple regression is that the population multiple correlation coefficient equals zero. The test for the significance of R is based on principles analogous to those for ANOVA. With ANOVA, the F-ratio statistic is the ratio of the mean squares between divided by mean squares within. In multiple regression, the form is similar:

$$F = \frac{SS_{\text{due to regression}}/df_{\text{regression}}}{SS_{\text{of residuals}}/df_{\text{residuals}}}$$

$$= \frac{\text{Mean Square}_{\text{due to regression}}}{\text{Mean Square}_{\text{of residuals}}}$$

As in ANOVA, variance from independent variables is contrasted with variance attributable to other factors, or error. In our example of predicting graduate GPAs, suppose a multiple correlation coefficient of .71 ($R^2 = .50$) was calculated for a sample of 100 graduate students. The computed value of the F-statistic in this example is 32.05. The tabled value of F (with $df = 3$ and 96) for a significance level of .01 is about 4.00; thus, the proba-

bility that $R = .71$ resulted from chance fluctuations is considerably less than .01.

Example of multiple regression: Lau-Walker and colleagues (2009) studied the relationship between heart disease patients' characteristics at the time of hospitalization and their physical and mental health outcomes 3 years later. Using multiple regression, they found, for example, that lower perceived number of symptoms, belief that their disease was controllable, admission as an emergency, and no prior history of cardiac illness were significant predictors of physical health 3 years after discharge. Overall, the R^2 between predictor variables and physical health scores was .43, $p < .001$.

Tests for Adding Predictors

Another question researchers may want to answer is: Does *adding* X_k to the regression significantly improve the prediction of Y over that achieved with X_{k-1}? For example, does a third predictor increase our ability to predict Y after two predictors have been used? An F-statistic can be computed to answer this question.

Let us number each independent variable in the current example: $X_1 = $ GPA-U; $X_2 = $ EE-Q; and $X_3 = $ EE-V. We can then symbolize various correlation coefficients as follows:

$R_{y.1}$ = the correlation of Y with GPA-U = .60
$R_{y.12}$ = the correlation of Y with
    GPA-U *and* EE-Q = .71
$R_{y.123}$ = the correlation of Y with
    all three predictors = .71

These figures indicate that EE-V scores made no independent contribution to the multiple correlation coefficient. The value of $R_{y.12}$ is identical to the value of $R_{y.123}$. We cannot tell at a glance, however, whether adding X_2 to X_1 *significantly* increased the prediction of Y. What we want to know is whether X_2 would improve predictions in the population, or if its added predictive power in this sample resulted from chance. In the current example, the value of the F-statistic for testing whether adding EE-Q scores significantly improves our prediction of Y is 27.16. If we consulted a table for the theoretical distribution of F

with $df = 1$ and 97 and a significance level of .01, we would find that the critical value is about 6.90. Therefore, adding EE-Q to the regression equation with GPA-U significantly improved the accuracy of predicting graduate GPA, beyond the .01 level.

Tests of the Regression Coefficients

When a regression coefficient (b) is divided by its standard error, the result is a value for the t statistic, which can be used to assess the significance of individual predictors. A significant t indicates that the regression coefficient (b) is significantly different from zero.

In simple regression, the value of b indicates the amount of change in predicted values of Y, for a specified rate of change in X. In multiple regression, the coefficients represent the number of units the dependent variable is predicted to change for each unit change in a given independent variable *when the effects of other predictors are held constant.* "Holding constant" other variables means that they are statistically controlled, a feature that can enhance a study's internal validity. If a regression coefficient is significant and confounding variables are included in the regression equation, it means that the variable associated with the coefficient contributed significantly to the regression, even after confounding variables are taken into account.

Strategies for Handling Predictors in Multiple Regression

Three alternative strategies for entering predictor variables into regression equations are simultaneous, hierarchical, and stepwise regressions.

Simultaneous Multiple Regression

The most basic strategy, **simultaneous multiple regression**, enters all predictor variables into the regression equation at the same time. One regression equation is developed, and statistical tests indicate the significance of R and of individual regression coefficients. This strategy is most appropriate when there is no basis for considering any particular predictor as causally prior to another and

when the predictors are of comparable importance to the research problem.

Hierarchical Multiple Regression

Many researchers use **hierarchical multiple regression**, which involves entering predictors into the equation in a series of steps. Researchers control the order of entry, with the order typically based on theoretical considerations. For example, some predictors may be thought of as causally or temporally prior to others, in which case they could be entered in an early step. Another important reason for using hierarchical regression is to examine the effect of a key independent variable after first removing (controlling) the effect of confounding variables.

> **Example of hierarchical multiple regression:** Hays and colleagues (2010) studied factors that predicted exercise adoption among older women at risk for cardiovascular disease. They used hierarchical regression to enter predictor variables in a series of steps. Demographic variables (e.g., age, race) were entered first, health status variables were entered next, and then other variables in their theoretical model (e.g., self-efficacy, outcome expectations) were entered in the third block.

With hierarchical regression, researchers determine the number of steps and the number of predictors included in each step. When several variables are added as a block, as in the Hays example, the analysis is a simultaneous regression for those variables at that stage. Thus, hierarchical regression can be considered a controlled sequence of simultaneous regressions.

Stepwise Multiple Regression

Stepwise multiple regression involves *empirically* selecting the combination of independent variables with the most predictive power. In stepwise multiple regression, predictors enter the regression equation in the order that produces the greatest increments to R^2. The first step selects the single best predictor of the dependent variable, that is, the independent variable with the highest bivariate correlation with Y. The second variable to enter the equation is the one that produces the largest

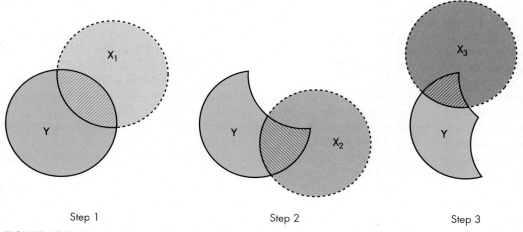

FIGURE 18.2 Visual representation of stepwise multiple regression analysis.

increase to R^2 when used simultaneously with the variable selected in the first step. The procedure continues until no additional predictor significantly increases the value of R^2.

Figure 18.2 illustrates stepwise multiple regression. Suppose that the first variable (X_1) has a correlation of .60 with Y ($r^2 = .36$). Variable X_1 accounts for the portion of the variability of Y represented by the hatched area in step 1 of the figure. This hatched area is, in effect, removed from further consideration, because this portion of Y's variability is explained. The variable chosen in step 2 is not always the X variable with the second largest correlation with Y. The selected predictor is the one that explains the largest portion of what *remains* of Y's variability after X_1 has been taken into account. Variable X_2, in turn, removes a second part of Y so that the independent variable selected in step 3 is the one that accounts for the most variability in Y after *both* X_1 and X_2 are removed.

Example of stepwise multiple regression:
Kong and Bernstein (2009) used stepwise regression to explore the ability of several types of childhood trauma (e.g., emotional abuse, physical abuse) to predict eating disorders in a sample of Korean patients. Emotional abuse, physical neglect, and sexual abuse were found to be significant predictors of eating psychopathology.

➔ **TIP:** Stepwise regression is controversial because variables are entered into the regression equation based on statistical rather than theoretical criteria. If stepwise regression is used, cross-validation is recommended (e.g., by dividing the sample in half and running two independent series of regressions).

Relative Contribution of Predictors

Scientists want not only to predict phenomena, but also to explain them. Predictions can be made in the absence of understanding. For instance, in our graduate school example, we could predict performance moderately well without explaining *why* the factors contributed to students' success. For practical applications, it may be sufficient to make accurate predictions, but scientists typically want to understand phenomena.

In multiple regression, one approach to understanding a phenomenon is to explore the relative importance of independent variables. Unfortunately, the determination of the relative contributions of independent variables in predicting a dependent variable is a thorny issue. When independent variables are correlated, as they usually are, there is no ideal way to disentangle the effects of variables in the equation.

It may appear that the solution is to compare the contributions of the Xs to R^2. In our graduate school example, GPA-U accounted for 36% of Y's variance; EE-Q explained an additional 14%. Should we conclude that undergraduate grades are more than twice as important as EE-Q scores in explaining graduate school grades? This conclusion would be inaccurate because the order of entry of variables in a regression equation affects their apparent contribution. If these two predictor variables were entered in reverse order (i.e., EE-Q first), R^2 would remain unchanged at .50; however, EE-Q's contribution would be .30 ($.55^2$), and GPA-U's contribution would be .20 ($.50 - .30$). This is because whatever variance the independent variables have in common is attributed to the first variable entered in the analysis.

Another approach to assessing the relative importance of the predictors is to compare regression coefficients. Earlier, we presented an equation for multiple regression that included a (the constant) and bs (regression coefficients) for each predictor. The b values cannot be directly compared because they are in the units of original scores, which differ from one X to another. X_1 might be in milliliters, X_2 in degrees Fahrenheit, and so forth. The use of **standard scores**[*] (or z **scores**) eliminates this problem by transforming all variables to scores with a mean of 0.0 and a standard deviation (SD) of 1.00. Transforming regular scores to z scores is easy—they are the difference between a score and the mean of that score divided by the standard deviation, or:

$$z_x = \frac{X - \overline{X}}{SD_x}$$

In standard score form, the regression equation uses standard scores (zs) instead of raw scores (Xs), and the regression coefficients for each z are standardized regression coefficients, called **beta** [β] **weights**. With all the βs in the same measurement units, can their relative size shed light on the

relative importance of predictors? Many researchers have interpreted beta weights in this fashion, but there are problems in doing so. These regression coefficients will be the same no matter what the order of entry of the variables. The difficulty, however, is that regression weights are unstable. The values of β tend to fluctuate from sample to sample. Moreover, when a variable is added to or subtracted from the regression equation, beta weights change. Because values of the regression coefficients fluctuate, it is difficult to attach theoretical importance to them.

One of the best solutions is to compare the **squared semipartial correlation coefficients (sr^2)** of the predictors. It is beyond the scope of this book to explain this index in detail, but we note that the sr^2 is useful because it indicates a predictor's unique contribution to variability in the dependent variable—that is, the contribution after other predictors are controlled.

Regression Results

There are no standard table formats for presenting regression results, and different formats are relevant depending on whether standard, hierarchical, or stepwise regression has been performed. The most frequently reported elements are values of β, R^2, and p values. We illustrate a table of regression results using a study of predictors of sleep disturbance among patients with heart failure in Taiwan (Chen et al., 2009). These researchers used hierarchical regression. Table 18.3 shows results for the final model in which all predictors were in the equation.

The first column of Table 18.3 shows that the analysis used five independent variables to predict scores on a sleep quality scale. The next column shows values for bs, that is, the raw regression coefficients for each predictor, and for the intercept constant. With the information in this column, we could predict sleep quality scores for a new sample. The next column shows the standard error (SE) of the regression coefficients. In this table, t values are not shown, but some regression tables *do* present them. We can compute them, though,

---

[*]Further discussion of standard scores can be found in statistics textbooks, such as that by Polit (2010).

TABLE 18.3	Multiple Regression Analysis Results: Sleep Disturbance Scores[a] among Patients with Heart Failure, Regressed on Five Predictor Variables ($N = 125$)			
PREDICTOR	**b**	**SE b**	**BETA**	
(Constant)	18.65	3.77		
Educational attainment	−.06	.23	−.02	
Functional classification, NY Heart Association	.20	.96	.01	
Perceived health[b]	−.78	.35	−.18*	
Social functioning[b]	−.05	.02	−.28*	
Physical symptoms[b]	−.05	.02	−.22*	

$R^2 = .27$, Adjusted $R^2 = .24$, $F(5, 119) = 8.74$, $p < .001$
*$p < .05$

[a]Higher scores on the sleep quality scale indicate greater sleep disturbance
[b]Higher scores reflect better health status and life quality
Adapted from Table 4 of Chen et al., 2009

from information in the table; for example, the value of t for the predictor *perceived health* would be −2.23 (i.e., *b/SE* or −.78 ÷ .35 = −2.23). This is significant ($p < .05$), as shown by the asterisk in the last column: The probability (p) is less than 5 in 100 that the relationship between perceived health and sleep quality is spurious. The results suggest that lower perceived health is associated with higher sleep disturbance scores, as indicated by the negative regression coefficient. This relationship was found to be significant, even with the other four predictors controlled. Two other predictor variables were significantly related to sleep quality: The better a person's social functioning and the better the physical health status in terms of symptoms, the lower the sleep disturbances. Other predictors in the analysis (e.g., education and functional classification) were not related significantly to sleep quality once other factors were taken into account.

The fourth column of Table 18.3 shows the value of the beta (β) coefficients for each predictor. In this particular sample, and with these particular predictors, the variable *social functioning* was the best predictor of sleep quality scores (β = −.28). Indeed, in the hierarchical regression, social functioning scores

were added in the fourth step, and the increment to R^2 at that point was .07, which was a significant increment ($p < .01$), not shown in the table.

At the bottom of the table, we see that the F for the overall regression equation was 8.74 ($df = 5$, 119), which was highly significant, $p < .001$. The value of R^2 was .27, but after adjusting for sample size and number of predictors, the value is reduced to .24. Thus, 24% of the variance in sleep quality scores was explained by the combined effect of the 5 predictors. The remaining 76% of variation is explained by factors not included in the regression model.

TIP: Knapp (1994) offered suggestions for reporting regression results. Also, some table templates for presenting multivariate results are included in the Toolkit of the accompanying *Resource Manual*.

Power Analysis for Multiple Regression

Small samples are especially problematic in multiple regression and other multivariate procedures. Inadequate sample size can lead to Type II errors, and can also yield erratic and misleading regression coefficients.

One approach to estimating sample size needs concerns the ratio of predictor variables to total number of cases. Tabachnick and Fidell (2007) suggest this guideline: *N* should be greater that $50 + 8$ times the number of predictors. So, with 5 predictors, the sample size should be at least 90 ($50 + [8 \times 5]$). Some experts recommend a ratio of 20 to 1 for simultaneous and hierarchical regression and a ratio of 40 to 1 for stepwise. More cases are needed for stepwise regression because this procedure capitalizes on the idiosyncrasies of a specific data set.

A better way to estimate sample size needs is to perform a power analysis. The number of participants needed to reject the null hypothesis that *R* equals zero is estimated based on effect size, number of predictors, desired power, and the significance criterion. In multiple regression, the estimated effect size is a function of the value of R^2. Researchers must either predict the value of R^2 on the basis of earlier research, or use the convention that effect size will be small ($R^2 = .02$), moderate ($R^2 = .13$), or large ($R^2 = .30$).

Table 18.4 presents sample size estimates for 2 to 10 predictors and various values of R^2, for power $= .80$ and alpha $= .05$. As an example, suppose we were planning a study to predict functional ability in nursing home residents using five predictor variables. We estimate a moderate effect size ($R^2 = .13$) and want to achieve a power of .80 and $\alpha = .05$. A sample of about 92 nursing home residents is needed to detect a population R^2 of .13 with five predictors, with a 5% chance of a Type I error and a 20% chance of a Type II error.

➲ **TIP:** Several websites (many of which are in the Toolkit for you to click on) do instantaneous power calculations and sample size estimates for many multivariate procedures. An especially useful link, from which you can be directed to many others, is *http://statpages.org/*.

ANALYSIS OF COVARIANCE

Analysis of covariance (**ANCOVA**) has much in common with multiple regression, but it also has features of ANOVA. Like ANOVA, ANCOVA is

| TABLE 18.4 | Power Analysis Table for Multiple Regression: Sample Size Estimates to Test the Null Hypothesis that $R^2 = .00$, for Power $= .80$ and $\alpha = .05$ with 2–10 Predictor Variables |

NO. OF PREDICTORS	ESTIMATED POPULATION R^2										
	.02	.04	.06	.08	.10	.13	.15	.20	.25	.30	.40
2	478	230	152	113	89	67	58	42	32	26	18
3	543	261	173	128	102	77	66	48	37	30	21
4	597	287	190	141	112	85	73	53	41	33	24
5	643	309	205	153	121	92	79	57	45	36	26
6	684	329	218	163	129	98	84	61	48	39	28
7	721	347	231	172	136	104	89	65	51	41	30
8	755	375	242	180	143	109	94	69	54	44	32
9	788	380	252	188	150	114	98	72	56	46	33
10	818	395	262	196	156	119	102	75	59	48	35

Shaded columns indicate conventions for small, medium, and large effect sizes.

used to compare the means of two or more groups, and the central question for both is the same: Are mean group differences likely to be *real* or spurious? Like multiple regression, however, ANCOVA allows researchers to control confounding variables statistically.

Uses of Analysis of Covariance

ANCOVA is especially useful in certain situations. For example, if a nonequivalent control group design is used to test an intervention, researchers must consider whether obtained results are influenced by pre-existing group differences. When experimental control through randomization is lacking, ANCOVA offers post hoc statistical control. Even in true experiments, ANCOVA can result in more precise estimates of group differences because, even with randomization, there are typically slight differences between groups. ANCOVA adjusts for initial differences so that the results more precisely reflect the effect of an intervention.

Strictly speaking, ANCOVA should not be used with existing groups because randomization is an underlying assumption of ANCOVA. This assumption is often violated, however. Random assignment to the groups being compared should be done whenever possible, but when randomization is not feasible, ANCOVA can often improve the internal validity of a study.

ANCOVA Procedures

Suppose we were testing the effectiveness of biofeedback therapy on patients' anxiety. A group in one hospital is exposed to the treatment, and a comparison group in another hospital is not. Patients' anxiety levels are measured both before and after the intervention, so pretest anxiety scores can be statistically controlled through ANCOVA. In such a situation, the dependent variable is the posttest anxiety scores, the independent variable is experimental/comparison group status, and the **covariate** is pretest anxiety scores. Covariates are usually continuous variables (e.g., anxiety scores), but can sometimes be dichotomous variables (male/female); the independent variable is a nominal-level variable.

Analysis of covariance is used to test the significance of differences between group means after adjusting scores on the dependent variable to remove the effect of covariates. In essence, the first step in ANCOVA is the same as the first step in hierarchical multiple regression. Variability in the dependent measure that can be explained by the covariate is removed from further consideration. ANOVA is performed on what remains of Y's variability to see whether, once the covariate is controlled, significant differences between group means exist.

Let us consider another example to explore further aspects of ANCOVA. Suppose we were testing the effectiveness of weight-loss diets, and we randomly assigned 30 people to one of three groups. ANCOVA, using pretreatment weight as the covariate, permits a more sensitive analysis of weight change than simple ANOVA. Some hypothetical data for such a study are shown in Table 18.5. Two aspects of the weight values in this table are discernible. First, despite random assignment to treatment groups, initial group means are different. Participants in Diet B differ from those in Diet C by an average of 10 pounds (175 versus 185 pounds). This difference, reflecting chance fluctuations, is not significant ($F = .45$, $p = .64$). Second, posttreatment means are also different by a maximum of only 10 pounds (160 to 170). However, the mean number of pounds *lost* ranged from 10 pounds for Diets A and B to 25 pounds for Diet C.

When we perform an ordinary analysis of variance testing group differences in posttreatment weights, we get an F of 0.55, indicating nonsignificant mean group differences. Based on ANOVA, we would conclude that all three diets had comparable effects on weight loss.

Now, let us use ANCOVA to analyze the data. The first step breaks total variability in posttreatment weights into two components: (1) variability explained by the covariate (pretreatment weights)

TABLE 18.5	Fictitious Data for ANCOVA Example: Comparison of Pre- and Posttreatment Weights for Three Diet Interventions			
	DIET A	**DIET B**	**DIET C**	**TOTAL**
Pretreatment weight, mean (SD)	180.0 (23.5)	175.0 (22.5)	185.0 (24.6)	180.0 (23.1)
Posttreatment weight, mean (SD)	170.0 (21.7)	165.0 (22.0)	160.0 (20.3)	165.0 (20.0)
ANOVA $F_{(2, 27)}$ for mean group differences in posttreatment weight = 0.55, p = .58				
ANCOVA $F_{(1, 26)}$ for covariate = 309.88, $p < .001$ ANCOVA $F_{(2, 26)}$ for mean group differences in posttreatment weight = 17.54, $p < .001$				

and (2) residual variability. The covariate accounts for a significant amount of variance, which is not surprising because there is a strong relationship between pretreatment and posttreatment weights: People who started out especially heavy tended to stay that way, relative to others in the sample. In the second step, residual variance is broken down to reflect between-group and within-group contributions. The resulting F of 17.54, with $df = 2$ and 26, is significant beyond the .001 level. The conclusion is that, after controlling for initial weight, there is a significant difference in weight attributable to exposure to different diets.

This fictitious example was contrived so that an ANOVA result of "no difference" would be altered by adding a covariate. Most actual results are less dramatic. Nonetheless, ANCOVA yields a more sensitive statistical test than ANOVA because the covariate reduces the error term (within-group variability), against which treatment effects are compared.

Theoretically, it is possible to use any number of covariates. It is seldom advisable, however, to use more than three or four. For one thing, a large number of covariates is often unnecessary because of the typically high degree of redundancy beyond the first few. Moreover, each covariate uses up a degree of freedom; fewer degrees of freedom means that a higher F is required for significance.

For instance, with 2 and 26 df, an F of 5.53 is required for significance at the .01 level, but with 2 and 23 df (i.e., adding three covariates), an F of 5.66 is needed.

Selection of Covariates

Useful covariates are almost always available. Background characteristics, such as age and education, are good candidates, for example. Covariates should be variables that you suspect are correlated with the dependent variable. Background characteristics are especially important to control when there are significant differences on confounding background characteristics between groups being compared. The literature is a good source of information about correlates of the dependent variable that should be controlled.

A pretest measure (i.e., an early measure of the dependent variable) is another good covariate, although in such a situation RM-ANOVA is an alternative when analyzing data from studies with pretest–posttest designs. Propensity scores, discussed briefly in Chapter 9, can be very powerful covariates. Propensity scores capture group differences on a broad range of attributes because they represent an attempt to model group differences using available data. The use of propensity scores as covariates is described by Qin and colleagues (2008). In general, it is important to select covariates that have strong reliability. Measurement errors can lead to either overadjustments or underadjustments of the mean and can contribute to Type I or Type II errors.

> **TIP:** In many situations, ANCOVA is preferable to ANOVA or *t*-tests, although in recent versions of SPSS, it is somewhat more difficult to run these analyses than bivariate tests. (They must be run within the procedure called General Linear Model, or GLM). ANCOVA can, however, enhance both statistical conclusion and internal validity in a study and is a useful analytic tool.

> **TIP:** For ANCOVA, an eta squared can be computed to summarize the magnitude of the *adjusted* relationship between the independent and dependent variables. Estimates of eta squared can be used in a power analysis to estimate sample size needs when planning a study. In general, when ANCOVA is used with carefully selected covariates, the analysis of group differences is more powerful than with ANOVA because error variance is reduced. In our example of the three diets, the value of adjusted eta squared is .57.

Example of ANCOVA: Paradis and colleagues (2010) tested the efficacy of a motivational nursing intervention on self-care in heart failure patients. ANCOVA was used to compare patients in the experimental and control groups on self-care outcomes, using baseline values as covariates.

Adjusted Means

In our example of the three diets, the significant ANCOVA *F* test indicates that at least one of the three groups had a posttreatment weight that is significantly different from the overall grand mean, after adjusting for pretreatment weights. It sometimes is useful to examine **adjusted means**, that is, group means on the dependent variable after adjusting for (i.e., removing the effect of) covariates. Adjusted means allow researchers to determine **net effects** (i.e., group differences on the dependent variable that are *net* of the effect of covariates). In our example of posttreatment weights for participants in three diet interventions, the adjusted means for Diets A, B, and C were 170.0, 169.4, and 155.6, respectively—values that more clearly indicate differences among those exposed to the different diets.

When ANCOVA results in a significant group *F* test, researchers can reject the null hypothesis that the adjusted group means are equal. As with ANOVA, further analysis is needed to assess which pairs of adjusted group means are significantly different from one another. In our example, post-hoc tests revealed that Diet C is significantly different from both Diets A and B, but A and B are not significantly different from each other.

OTHER LEAST-SQUARES MULTIVARIATE TECHNIQUES

Many of the multivariate statistics we have discussed thus far are related. For example, ANOVA and multiple regression are very similar. Both techniques analyze total variability in a continuous dependent measure and contrast variability due to independent variables with that attributable to individual differences or error. By tradition, experimental data typically are analyzed by ANOVA, and correlational data are analyzed by regression. Yet, *any data for which ANOVA is appropriate can be analyzed by multiple regression*, although the reverse is not true.

A broad class of statistical techniques are subsumed under the **general linear model (GLM)**, which include techniques that fit data to straight-line (linear) solutions. The GLM is the foundation for such procedures as the *t*-test, ANOVA, and multiple regression. The GLM is an important model because of its generality and applicability to numerous research situations, but a thorough understanding of the GLM requires advanced statistical training. In this section, other GLM methods are briefly introduced. The intent is to acquaint you with research situations for which these methods are appropriate.

Repeated Measures ANOVA for Mixed Designs

In Chapter 17, we discussed one-way repeated-measures ANOVA (RM-ANOVA). This procedure is appropriate when one group of people is measured at multiple points. Many RCTs involve randomly assigning participants to different treatment groups, and then collecting data multiple times. When there are only two data collection points (e.g., a pretest and a posttest), ANCOVA is often used to test the null hypothesis that groups means are equal, after removing the effect of pretest scores. When data are collected three or more times, the appropriate analysis usually is a **repeated measures ANOVA for mixed designs**.

As an example, suppose we collected heart rate data at 2 hours (Time 1 or T1), 4 hours (T2), and 6 hours (T3) postsurgery for people in an experimental and control group. Structurally, the ANOVA for analyzing these data would look similar to a 2 × 3 multifactor ANOVA, but calculations would differ in this mixed design (mixed because it involves both a within-subject and a between-subject factor). An *F*-statistic would be computed to test for a *between-subjects effect* (i.e., differences between experimentals and controls). This statistic would indicate whether, across all time periods, mean heart rate differed in the two groups. Another *F*-statistic would be computed to test for a *within-subjects effect* or time factor (i.e., differences at T1, T2, and T3). This statistic would indicate whether, across both groups, mean heart rates differed over time. Finally, an interaction effect would be tested to assess whether group differences varied across time. In mixed design RM-ANOVA, the interaction effect typically is of primary importance. When people are randomized to treatment groups, we would expect their mean values at baseline to be equivalent—but if there are treatment effects, group means would differ at subsequent points of data collection, thus resulting in a time × treatment interaction.

The various procedures within the GLM have several basic assumptions, all of which are fully described in statistics textbooks. Assumptions such as normality of the distributions and the equality of variances apply to most GLM procedures, but ANOVA and most of its variants are fairly **robust** to violation of assumptions (i.e., violations tend not to affect the accuracy of statistical decision making). However, RM-ANOVA has some unique assumptions—the assumption of *sphericity* and the related assumption of *compound symmetry*, both of which are too complex to elaborate here. RM-ANOVA is not, unfortunately, robust to violations of these assumptions. Furthermore, there are different opinions about how to detect and address violations. Thus, RM-ANOVA tends to be more complex than many procedures discussed thus far. Polit (2010) and advanced statistical texts offer suggestions on using RM-ANOVA.

> **Example of mixed design RM-ANOVA:** Baird and colleagues (2010) used mixed design RM-ANOVA to test the efficacy of a guided imagery intervention for symptoms of osteoarthritis. Pain and medication use were compared for those in the intervention and control groups at multiple points in time.

Multivariate Analysis of Variance

Multivariate analysis of variance (**MANOVA**) is the extension of ANOVA to more than one dependent variable. MANOVA is used to test the significance of differences in group means for multiple dependent variables, considered simultaneously. For instance, if we wanted to examine the effect of two methods of exercise on diastolic *and* systolic blood pressure, MANOVA would be appropriate. Researchers often analyze such data by performing two separate ANOVAs. Strictly speaking, this practice is not appropriate. Separate ANOVAs imply that the dependent variables have been obtained independently when, in fact, they have been obtained from the same people and are correlated. MANOVA takes the intercorrelations of dependent variables into account. ANOVA is, however, a more widely understood procedure than MANOVA, and thus, its results may be more easily communicated to a broad audience.

MANOVA can be readily extended in ways analogous to ANOVA. For example, it is possible to perform **multivariate analysis of covariance (MANCOVA)**, which allows for the control of confounding variables (covariates) when there are two or more dependent variables.

➲ **T I P :** If you opt to use simpler analyses to enhance the usefulness of the evidence to clinical audiences (e.g., three separate ANOVAs rather than a MANOVA), you should run the analyses both ways. Then, you could present bivariate results (e.g., from ANOVAs) in the report, but note whether the more complex test (e.g. MANOVA) changed the conclusions.

Example of MANCOVA: Good and Ahn (2008) tested the effect of a music intervention on pain among Korean women who had had gynecologic surgery. Women in the treatment group chose between several types of music, and those in the control group had no music. Both a sensory component and an affective (distress) component of pain were measured. The groups were compared on the two postintervention pain measures using MANCOVA with baseline pain levels controlled.

Discriminant Analysis

In multiple regression, the dependent variable is an interval or ratio measure. The regression makes predictions about continuous values, such as scores on a depression scale or heart rate. **Discriminant analysis**, in contrast, makes predictions about membership in groups. For instance, we may wish to predict membership in such groups as compliant versus noncompliant cancer patients, or patients who do or do not survive a medical treatment.

Discriminant analysis develops an equation—called a **discriminant function**—for a categorical dependent variable, with independent variables that are either dichotomous or continuous. Researchers begin with data from people whose group membership is known and develop an equation to predict membership when only measures of the independent variables are available. The discriminant function indicates to which group each person would likely belong.

Discriminant analysis for predicting membership into only two groups (e.g., survived versus died) can be interpreted in much the same way as multiple regression. When there are more than two groups, the calculations and interpretations are more complex. With three or more groups (e.g., very–low-birth-weight, low-birth-weight, and normal-birth-weight infants), the number of discriminant functions is either the number of groups minus 1 or the number of independent variables, whichever is smaller. The first discriminant function is the linear combination of predictors that maximizes the ratio of between-group to within-group variance. The second function is the linear combination that maximizes this ratio, after the effect of the first function is removed. Because independent variables have different weights on the various functions, it is possible to develop theoretical interpretations based on the knowledge of which predictors are important in discriminating among different groups.

Discriminant analysis produces an index designating the proportion of variance in the dependent variable accounted for by predictor variables. The index is **Wilks' lambda** (λ), which actually indicates the proportion of variance *unaccounted for* by predictors, or $\lambda = 1 - R^2$.

Example of discriminant analysis: Zachariah (2009) used discriminant analysis to evaluate risk factors for pregnancy complications in low-income women. The dependent variables were having versus not having complications. Predictors included various risk factors such as maternal anxiety, emotional support, and negative life events. State anxiety and total functional social support were especially strong predictors of prenatal complications (overall Wilks' lambda = .79, p = .02).

LOGISTIC REGRESSION

Logistic regression is a widely used multivariate technique. Like multiple regression, logistic regression analyzes the relationship between multiple independent variables and a dependent variable and yields a predictive equation. Like discriminant analysis, logistic regression is used to predict categorical dependent variables. Logistic regression, however, relies on an estimation procedure that has less restrictive assumptions than multivariate procedures within the GLM, which use least-squares estimation.

Basic Concepts for Logistic Regression

Logistic regression uses **maximum likelihood estimation** (**MLE**). Maximum likelihood estimators are ones that estimate the parameters most likely to have generated the observed data. Confirmatory factor analysis, discussed in Chapter 15, also uses MLE.

Because logistic regression has fewer assumptions about the underlying distribution of variables, it is often more technically appropriate than discriminant analysis. Logistic regression is also well suited to many clinical questions because it models the probability of an outcome rather than predicting group membership. For example, we might be interested in modeling the probability of engaging in breast self-examination, or the probability of smoking cessation.

Logistic regression transforms the probability of an event occurring (e.g., that a woman will practice breast self-examination) into its odds. As discussed briefly in Chapter 16, **odds** reflect the ratio of two probabilities: the probability of an event occurring, to the probability that it will not occur. For example, if 40% of women practice breast self-examination, the odds would be .40 divided by .60, or .667.

Probabilities, which range between zero and one, are then transformed into continuous variables that range between zero and infinity. Because this range is still restricted, a further transformation is performed, namely calculating the logarithm of the odds. The range of this new variable (the **logit**, short for *log*istic probability un*it*) is from minus to plus infinity. Using the logit as the dependent variable, a maximum likelihood procedure estimates the coefficients of the independent variables, with the logit as a continuous dependent variable.

The solution yields an equation that predicts the logit from a weighted combination of independent variables, plus a constant, much like a multiple regression equation. The interpretation, however, is different because the equation does not predict *actual* values of the dependent variable. In logistic regression, a regression coefficient (b) can be interpreted as the change in the log odds associated with a one-unit change in the associated predictor variable.

The Odds Ratio

The meaning of the logistic regression equation is hard to comprehend because we do not think in terms of log odds. However, the equation can be transformed back to yield information in terms of odds rather than log odds. The factor by which the odds change is the *odds ratio* (OR), the risk index we discussed in Chapter 16.

For example, suppose that we used logistic regression to predict the probability of performing breast self-examination. One of the independent variables might be whether or not the woman has had a close family member (e.g., a sister) who had breast cancer. A logistic regression analysis might indicate that the *OR* was 12.1, with all other predictors in the equation held constant. (This is often called an *adjusted odds ratio*) As noted previously, the odds ratio provides an estimate (around which confidence intervals can be built) of relative risk—the risk of an event occurring given one condition, versus the risk of it occurring given a different condition. In our example, we would estimate that the "risk" of performing breast self-examination is about 12 times greater if a woman has a family history of breast cancer than if she does not, with other factors in the model held constant (controlled).

➲ **T I P :** Just as there is simple regression with least-squares estimation—that is, the prediction of a dependent variable based on a single independent variable—**bivariate logistic regression** is also possible. This is often done to produce estimates of *unadjusted* (or *crude*) odds ratios—that is, odds ratios without controlling other variables.

Variables in Logistic Regression

The dependent variable in binary logistic regression is a dichotomous variable. The dependent variable is typically coded 1 to represent an event or a characteristic (e.g., had a fall, is obese), and 0 to represent the absence of the event or characteristic (no fall, no obesity). Predictor variables can be continuous variables, categorical variables, or interaction terms. Although there are no strict limits to the number of predictors that can be included, it is best to achieve a parsimonious model with strong predictive power using a small set of good predictors.

When continuous variables are the predictors, the odds ratio is interpreted somewhat differently than with categorical variables. For example, suppose we were predicting whether a nursing home resident would or would not have a fall, and one predictor variable was age. Suppose we found, for example, that the *OR* associated with age was 1.15. This means that for every additional year of age, the odds of having a fall increased by 15%, with everything else in the model held constant.

Dummy-coded variables, also called *indicator variables*, are a common method of representing dichotomous predictors, such as smokes cigarettes (1) versus does not smoke cigarettes (0). For variables with more than two categories, a series of dummy variables is needed. If, for example, marital status was a predictor variable in a logistic regression for predicting breast self-examination, a bivariate logistic analysis could provide estimates of the relative risk of different marital statuses (e.g., never married, married, formerly married) on breast self-examination. In such an analysis, one group would be the **reference group**, with an *OR* of 1.0, and the other two groups would have *OR*s in relation to the reference group. As a hypothetical example, if the *OR* for a never-married reference group was 1.0 and the *OR* for married was 1.23, this means that married women were 23% more likely to perform breast self-examination than never-married women.

As with multiple regression, predictors in multiple regression can be entered into the equation in different ways. The options include simultaneous, hierarchical, and stepwise entry.

⮕ **TIP:** When a categorical dependent variable is not dichotomous (e.g., 3 different types of chronic illness), *multinomial logistic regression* can be used (Kwak & Clayton-Matthews, 2002).

Significance Tests in Logistic Regression

Researchers usually want to assess the overall reliability of the model, that is, whether the set of predictors, taken as a whole, is significantly better than chance in predicting the probability of the outcome event. Unfortunately, assessing the goodness of fit of a logistic regression model can be confusing because there are several different tests, and different authors use different names for the tests. Another potential source of confusion is that some tests indicate goodness of fit by a significant result, and others indicate goodness of fit by a *non*significant result. We briefly describe two approaches, but recommend further reading in advanced textbooks, such as Tabachnick & Fidell (2007) or Hosmer and Lemeshow (2000).

One index in logistic regression is called the **likelihood index**, which is the probability of the observed results, given parameters estimated in the analysis. If the overall model fits the data perfectly, the likelihood index is 1.0. Because the likelihood index is typically a small decimal, it is usually transformed by multiplying it by -2 times the log of the likelihood. The transformed index ($-2LL$) is a small number when the fit is good; in a perfect fit, the value is zero. The chi-square statistic is then used to test the null hypothesis that all of the *b* regression coefficients are zero, in what is sometimes called a **likelihood ratio test**. A **goodness-of-fit statistic**, which has a chi-squared distribution, is the analog of the overall *F* test in multiple regression. This statistic is based on the residuals for all cases in the analysis—which, in logistic regression is the difference between the observed probability of an event and the predicted probability. This statistic is thus a mechanism for evaluating the fit of the predictive model.

The likelihood ratio test also can be used to evaluate the significance of *improvement* to $-2LL$ with successive entry of predictors, when hierarchical or stepwise regression is performed.

An alternative approach to testing the overall model is the **Hosmer-Lemeshow test**, which compares the prediction model to a hypothetically "perfect" model. In brief, the perfect model is one that contains the exact set of predictors needed to duplicate the observed frequencies in the dependent variable. The full model can be tested against the perfect model by computing differences between observed frequencies and expected frequencies—that is, those expected in the perfect model. With this test, a *nonsignificant* chi-square is desired. A nonsignificant result indicates that the model being tested is not reliably different from the perfect model. In other words, nonsignificance supports the inference that the model adequately duplicates the observed frequencies of the outcome.

➲ **TIP:** There is no consensus on which approach for an overall model test is better, but most logistic regression software programs can perform both tests, and some researchers present both results.

It is also possible to test the significance of individual predictors in the model—just as the t statistic is used in multiple regression. A frequently used statistic for this purpose is the **Wald statistic**, which is distributed as a chi-square. Significance is also sometimes assessed by examining the confidence intervals around the odds ratios. If the 95% CI includes the value of 1.0, this indicates that the *OR* was not statistically significant at the .05 level.

Effect Size in Logistic Regression

Statisticians have worked on developing an effect size index for logistic regression that is analogous to R^2 in multiple regression. The main problem, however, is that R^2 in multiple regression can be interpreted as the percentage of variance in the dependent variable explained by the predictors, but this is more complex with a dichotomous outcome. Despite difficulties in achieving a good analog to

least squares-based R^2, several **pseudo R^2** measures have been proposed for logistic regression. These indexes should be reported as approximations to an R^2 from least-squares regression rather than as the percentage of variance explained. A statistic called the **Nagelkerke R^2** is the most frequently reported pseudo R^2 index.

Example of logistic regression: Griffith (2009) studied biologic, psychological/behavioral, and social variables that predicted timely screening for colorectal cancer in African Americans. In her hierarchical logistic regression model, she found that biologic factors (age and gender) did not contribute significantly to the model ($\chi^2 = 6.26$, $p = .39$). The psychological and behavioral block (e.g., smoking, activity level) also was nonsignificant ($\chi^2 = 10.81$, $p = .09$). The social system block was, however, significant ($\chi^2 = 189.83$, $p < .001$). This block included such predictors as education, employment, and insurance. Among those whose healthcare provider had recommended screening, having healthcare insurance was an especially strong predictor ($OR = 3.25$, 95% CI = 1.14, 9.31).

SURVIVAL AND EVENT HISTORY ANALYSIS

Some dependent variables are time related. **Survival analysis** is widely used by epidemiologists when the dependent variable is a time interval between an initial event (e.g., onset of a disease) and a terminal event (e.g., death). Survival analysis calculates a survival score, which compares survival time for one participant with that for others. When researchers are interested in group comparisons—for example, comparing the survival function of people in an experimental group versus a control group—a statistic can be computed to test the null hypothesis that the groups are sampled from the same survival distribution.

Survival analysis can be applied to many situations unrelated to mortality. For example, survival analysis could be used to analyze such time-related phenomena as length of time in labor, length of stay in hospital, or length of time breastfeeding. Survival analysis can be used when time-related data are **censored**, that is, the observation period does not cover all possible events. As an example, if the outcome were hospital readmission and data are collected 2 years after release, the data are censored because there will be readmissions beyond the 2-year period, and some will never be readmitted. Further information about survival analysis can be found in Hosmer and colleagues (2008).

Extensions of survival analysis have been developed that allow researchers to examine determinants of survival-type transitions in a multivariate (regression) framework. In these analyses, independent variables are used to model the risk (or hazard) of experiencing an event at a given point in time, given that one has not experienced the event before that time. The most common specification of the hazard is known as the **Cox proportional hazards model**. Further information may be found in O'Quigley (2008).

Example of Cox regression: One of this book's authors (Polit) and colleagues in Australia used Cox regression to test the effects of an intervention to reduce hospital admissions among residents of long-term care facilities presenting to an emergency room. Using Cox regression, they found that those in the intervention group had significantly shorter lengths of in-hospital stay than those in a usual care group, even after controlling for age, sex, and acuity (Crilly et al., 2010).

CAUSAL MODELING

Causal modeling involves testing a hypothesized causal explanation of a phenomenon, typically with data from nonexperimental studies. In a causal model, researchers posit causal linkages among three or more variables, and then test whether hypothesized pathways from the causes to the effect are consistent with the data. We briefly describe some features of two approaches to causal modeling without discussing analytic procedures.

Path Analysis

Path analysis, which relies on regression using least-squares estimation, is a method for studying causal patterns among variables. Path analysis is not a method for discovering causes; rather, it is a method applied to a prespecified model formulated on the basis of prior knowledge and theory.

In reports, path analytic results are usually displayed in a **path diagram**, and we use such a diagram (Figure 18.3) to illustrate key concepts. This model postulates that the dependent variable, patients' functional ability (V4), is the result of patients' capacity for self-care (V3); this, in turn, is affected by nursing actions (V1) and the severity of

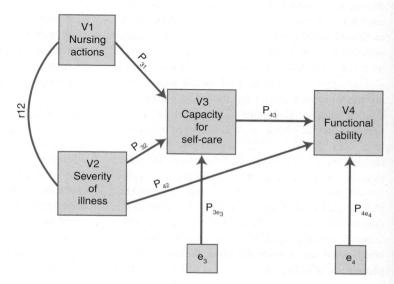

FIGURE 18.3 Example of a path diagram.

their illness (V2). This model is a **recursive model**, which means that the causal flow is unidirectional: It is assumed that variable 2 is a cause of variable 3, and that variable 3 is *not* a cause of variable 2.

Path analysis distinguishes exogenous and endogenous variables. Determinants of an **exogenous variable** lie outside the model. In Figure 18.3, nursing actions (V1) and illness severity (V2) are exogenous; no attempt is made in the model to elucidate what causes different nursing actions or different degrees of illness. An **endogenous variable**, by contrast, is one whose variation is hypothesized to be affected by other variables in the model. In our example, self-care capacity (V3) and functional ability (V4) are endogenous.

Causal linkages are shown on a path diagram by arrows drawn from presumed causes to presumed effects. In our illustration, severity of illness is hypothesized to affect functional ability both directly (path p_{42}) and indirectly through the *mediating variable* self-care capacity (paths p_{32} and p_{43}). Correlated exogenous variables are indicated by curved lines, as shown by the curved line between nursing actions and illness severity.

Ideally, the model would totally explain the outcome, but this almost never happens because there are other determinants, which are **residual variables**. The two boxes labeled *e* in Figure 18.3 denote a composite of all determinants of self-care capacity (e_3) and functional ability (e_4) that are not in the model. If we could identify and measure additional causes and incorporate them into the theory, they should be in the model if possible.

Path analysis solves for **path coefficients**, which are the weights representing the effect of one variable on another. In Figure 18.3, causal paths indicate that one variable (e.g., V3) is caused by another (e.g., V2), yielding a path labeled p_{32}. In research reports, path symbols would be replaced by actual path coefficients, which are derived through regression procedures. Path coefficients are standardized partial regression slopes. For example, path p_{32} is equal to $\beta_{32.1}$—the beta weight between variables 2 and 3, holding variable 1 constant. Because path coefficients are in standard form, they indicate the proportion of a standard deviation difference in the

caused variable that is directly attributable to a $1SD$ difference in the specified causal variable. Thus, the path coefficients give us indication about the relative importance of various determinants. Kline (2005) and Olobatuyi (2006) offer further guidance on path analysis.

Example of path analysis: Whiteside-Mansell and colleagues (2009) used path analysis to test a mediation model in which the effect of family conflict was hypothesized to affect preschool children's social behavior via the effect of conflict on mothers' harsh discipline and maternal warmth.

Structural Equations Modeling

A drawback of path analysis using OLS regression is that the method's validity is based on a set of restrictive assumptions, most of which are virtually impossible to meet. First, it is assumed that variables are measured without error, but most measures *do* contain error. Second, it is assumed that residuals (error terms) in the different regression equations are uncorrelated. This assumption is seldom tenable, because error terms often represent unmeasured individual differences—differences that are not random. Third, traditional path analysis assumes that the causal flow is unidirectional (recursive). In reality, causes and effects are often reciprocal.

Structural equations modeling (SEM) using maximum likelihood estimation is a more powerful approach that avoids these problems. SEM can accommodate measurement errors, correlated residuals, and **nonrecursive models** that allow for reciprocal causation. Another attractive feature of SEM is that it can be used to analyze causal models involving latent variables. A *latent variable*, as discussed in Chapter 15, is an unmeasured variable corresponding to an abstract construct. For example, factor analysis yields information about underlying, latent dimensions that are not measured directly. In SEM, latent variables are captured by two or more measured (manifest) variables that are indicators of the underlying construct.

SEM proceeds in two phases. In the first phase, which corresponds to a confirmatory factor analysis (CFA), a measurement model is tested (Chapter 15). When there is evidence of an adequate fit of the data to the hypothesized measurement model, the theoretical causal model is tested by structural equation modeling. SEM yields information about the hypothesized causal parameters—that is, path coefficients that are presented as beta weights. The coefficients indicate the expected amount of change in the latent endogenous variable that is caused by a change in the latent causal variable. SEM programs yield information on the significance of individual paths. The overall fit of the causal model to the research data can be tested by means of several statistics, such as the **goodness-of-fit index** (**GFI**) and **adjusted goodness-of-fit index** (**AGFI**). For both indexes, a value of .90 or greater indicates a good fit of the model to the data.

SEM has gained considerable popularity among nurse researchers, but is a highly complex procedure. Readers interested in further information on SEM can consult Loehlin (2003) or Kline (2005).

Example of SEM: Lou and Chen (2009) used data from 823 Taiwanese adolescents to test a causal model of factors affecting their sexual health. A structural equations model was used to test the relationships among sexual knowledge, sexual attitudes, and safe sex behavior.

THE COMPUTER AND MULTIVARIATE STATISTICS

Multivariate analyses are invariably done by computer because computations are complex. To illustrate computer analyses for three multivariate techniques, we return to the example described in Chapters 16 and 17, involving a prenatal intervention for low-income young women. Data for these examples were presented in Table 16.8, page 396.

Example of Multiple Regression

In Chapter 17, we tested the hypothesis that older mothers in the sample had infants with higher birth weights than younger mothers, using Pearson's r. The calculated value of r (.594) was highly significant, thereby supporting the research hypothesis.

Suppose that we want to test whether we can significantly *improve* our ability to predict infant birth weight by adding two predictor variables in a multiple regression: whether the mother smoked while pregnant and her number of prior pregnancies. Figure 18.4 presents part of the Statistical Package for the Social Sciences (SPSS) printout for a multiple regression analysis in which infant birth weight is the dependent variable and maternal age, smoking status, and number of prior pregnancies are predictor variables. We will explain a few noteworthy aspects of this printout.

Panel A of Figure 18.4 shows that we used hierarchical regression to predict infant birth weight (footnote b). Mother's age was entered first (Model 1), and then smoking status and prior pregnancies were entered in a second block (Model 2).

Panel B (Model Summary) indicates that, in Model 1, $R = .594$—the same as the bivariate correlation shown in Figure 17.7. The value of R^2 is .353 ($.594^2$), which represents the proportion of variance in birth weight accounted for by mother's age. The *adjusted R^2* of .330 in Model 1 is the R^2 after it has been adjusted to reflect more closely the goodness of fit the regression model in the population, through a formula that involves sample size and number of predictors. Next, the standard error of the estimate (8.9702) is shown. The next few columns present information about changes to R^2. In Model 1, the change is from 0.0 to .353—which yields an F (15.252) that, with $df = 1$ and 28, is significant ($p = .001$). In Model 2, the value of R is higher (.598), but the F for change (.109) with 2 and 26 df is not significant ($p = .897$).

Panel C (ANOVA) shows, for Model 1, the F-ratio in which variability due to regression (for the relationship between birth weight and age) is contrasted with residual variability. Again, it shows that the value of F (15.252) is significant at the .001

Regression

A

Variables Entered/Removed[b]

Model	Variables Entered	Variables Removed	Method
1	Mother's age[a]	.	Enter
2	Smoking status, No. of prior pregnancies[a]	.	Enter

a. All requested variables entered.
b. Dependent Variable: Infant birth weight in ounces

B

Model Summary

Model	R	R Square	Adjusted R Square	Std. Error of the Estimate	Change Statistics				
					R Square Change	F Change	df1	df2	Sig. F Change
1	.594[a]	.353	.330	8.97022	.353	15.252	1	28	.001
2	.598[b]	.358	.284	9.26997	.005	.109	2	26	.897

a. Predictors: (Constant), Mother's age
b. Predictors: (Constant), Mother's age, Smoking status, No. of prior pregnancies

C

ANOVA[c]

Model		Sum of Squares	df	Mean Square	F	Sig.
1	Regression	1227.283	1	1227.283	15.252	.001[a]
	Residual	2253.017	28	80.465		
	Total	3480.300	29			
2	Regression	1246.061	3	415.354	4.834	.008[b]
	Residual	2234.239	26	85.932		
	Total	3480.300	29			

a. Predictors: (Constant), Mother's age
b. Predictors: (Constant), Mother's age, Smoking status, No. of prior pregnancies
c. Dependent Variable: Infant birth weight in ounces

D

Coefficients[a]

Model		Unstandardized Coefficients		Standardized Coefficients	t	Sig.	95% Confidence Interval for B	
		B	Std. Error	Beta			Lower Bound	Upper Bound
1	(Constant)	48.040	14.600		3.290	.003	18.133	77.947
	Mother's age	3.119	.799	.594	3.905	.001	1.483	4.755
2	(Constant)	52.170	18.398		2.836	.009	14.354	89.987
	Mother's age	2.916	1.021	.555	2.855	.008	.817	5.016
	No. of prior pregnancies	.394	2.410	.030	.163	.872	−4.561	5.349
	Smoking status	−1.643	3.610	−.076	−.455	.653	−9.064	5.778

a. Dependent Variable: Infant birth weight in ounces

E

Excluded Variables[b]

Model		Beta In	t	Sig.	Partial Correlation	Collinearity Statistics
						Tolerance
1	No. of prior pregnancies	.020[a]	.108	.915	.021	.727
	Smoking status	−.072[a]	−.446	.659	−.086	.910

a. Predictors in the Model: (Constant), Mother's age.
b. Dependent Variable: Infant birth weight in ounces.

FIGURE 18.4 SPSS printout for hierarchical multiple regression of infant birth weight.

level. The information for Model 2 is for all *three* predictors that are in the model when variables in the second block are entered. Here, the value of F (4.834) with 3 and 26 *df* is statistically significant at $p = .008$.

Regression equations are presented in Panel D (Coefficients). If we wanted to predict new values of birth weight based on maternal age at birth, the equation from Model 1 would be:

$$\text{Birth weight'} = (3.119 \times \text{age}) + 48.040$$

The predicted birth weights in a new sample of young mothers would equal the regression coefficient ($b = 3.119$) times the value of maternal age (X_1), plus the value of the intercept constant ($a = 48.040$). When values of b are divided by the standard error (.799 for maternal age in Model 1), the result is a t statistic, which indicates the significance of each predictor. In Model 1, $t = 3.905$, which is significant ($p = .001$). The standardized beta weight (β) for maternal age is .594. In the far right, we see that the 95% CI for the regression coefficient b is 1.483 and 4.755—which indicates statistical significance: The interval does not include 0.0.

If we wanted to use all three predictors to predict infant birth weight, the equation for Model 2 shows the b coefficients for each of the three predictors. In Model 2, neither number of prior pregnancies nor smoking status is significant: $p = .872$ and .653, respectively. The 95% CI for both these predictors *does* include 0.0. When we compare the standardized coefficients (the βs) for the three variables, we see that Beta for maternal age is substantial (.555), while those for the other two predictors are negligible (.030 and $-.076$).

Panel E (Excluded Variables) shows the two predictors not yet in the equation in Model 1, that is, number of prior pregnancies and smoking status. The printout shows that the t values associated with the regression coefficients for the two predictors are both nonsignificant ($p = .915$ and .659, respectively), once variation due to maternal age is taken into account. This reinforces what we have already learned—that neither of the two predictors in Block 2 would significantly add to the prediction

of birth weight, over and above what was already achieved with maternal age.

An additional piece of information in the Panel E concerns **multicollinearity**, which is a problem that can occur when predictors are too highly intercorrelated. When multicollinearity is present, the computations required for regression coefficients are compromised and results tend to be unstable. Multicollinearity can be diagnosed by computing an index of **tolerance**. If predictors are totally uncorrelated, tolerance is 1.0, and if they are perfectly intercorrelated, tolerance is 0.0. Thus, higher values are more desirable. The computer can be instructed to exclude predictors whose tolerance falls below a specified level (e.g., .10). In our example, tolerance values of .727 and .910 for the two variables not yet in the model are acceptable.

Example of Analysis of Covariance

In Chapter 17, we tested the hypothesis that infants in the experimental group would have higher birth weights than infants in the control group, using a t-test. The computer calculated t to be 1.44, which was nonsignificant with 28 *df*. The research hypothesis was therefore rejected.

Through ANCOVA, we can test the same hypothesis controlling for maternal age, which, as we have just seen, is significantly correlated with birth weight. Figure 18.5 presents the printout for ANCOVA for this analysis, with birth weight as the dependent variable, maternal age (Age) as the covariate, and Group (experimental versus control) as the independent variable. Panel A shows that the treatment group variable involves 15 experimentals and 15 controls. Panel B (Descriptive Statistics) presents means and *SD*s for the two groups and the overall sample of 30 mothers.

In Panel C (Tests of Between-Subjects Effects), the F-value for the overall model is highly significant (14.088, $p = .000$). The value of F for the covariate Age is 24.358, significant at the .000 level (i.e., beyond the .001 level). The value of partial (adjusted) eta squared for age (i.e., the effect size) is .474, and observed power to detect this effect, for

Univariate Analysis of Variance

A   **Between-Subjects Factors**

		Value Label	N
Treatment group	0	Control	15
	1	Experimental	15

B   **Descriptive Statistics**

Dependent Variable: Infant birth weight in ounces

Treatment group	Mean	Std. Deviation	N
Control	101.8667	7.23944	15
Experimental	107.5333	13.37838	15
Total	104.7000	10.95492	30

C   **Tests of Between-Subjects Effects**

Dependent Variable: Infant birth weight in ounces

Source	Type III Sum of Squares	df	Mean Square	F	Sig.	Partial Eta Squared	Observed Power[b]
Corrected Model	1777.228[a]	2	888.614	14.088	.000	.511	.997
Intercept	572.734	1	572.734	9.080	.006	.252	.828
Age	1536.395	1	1536.395	24.358	.000	.474	.997
Group	549.945	1	549.945	8.719	.006	.244	.812
Error	1703.072	27	63.077				
Total	332343.000	30					
Corrected Total	3480.300	29					

a. R Squared = .511 (Adjusted R Squared = .474).
b. Computed using alpha = .05.

Estimated Marginal Means

D   **1. Grand Mean**

Dependent Variable: Infant birth weight in ounces

Mean	Std. Error	95% Confidence Interval	
		Lower Bound	Upper Bound
104.700[a]	1.450	101.725	107.675

a. Covariates appearing in the model are evaluated at the following values: Mother's age = 18.1667.

E   **2. Treatment group**

Dependent Variable: Infant birth weight in ounces

Treatment group	Mean	Std. Error	95% Confidence Interval	
			Lower Bound	Upper Bound
Control	100.320[a]	2.074	96.063	104.576
Experimental	109.080[a]	2.074	104.824	113.337

a. Covariates appearing in the model are evaluated at the following values: Mother's age = 18.1667.

FIGURE 18.5 SPSS printout for ANCOVA.

$\alpha = .05$, is quite high, .997. After controlling for Age, the F-value for the independent variable Group is 8.719, which is significant at the .006 level. In other words, once Age is controlled, the research hypothesis about experimental versus control differences in infant birth weight is supported rather than rejected. Moreover, the effect size for the intervention (.244) is fairly high. The unadjusted R^2 for predicting birth weight (footnote a), based on both Age and Group, is .511—substantially more than the R^2 between maternal age and birth weight alone (.352).

Panel D shows the overall mean (104.70) for the sample, the standard error (1.45), and the 95% confidence interval for the estimated population mean (95% CI = 101.725, 107.675). Finally, Panel E shows group means *after they are adjusted for maternal age*. The original, unadjusted means for the experimental and control groups were 107.53 and 101.87, respectively (panel B). After adjusting for maternal age, however, the experimental mean is 109.08, and the control mean is 100.32, a more sizable difference.

Example of Logistic Regression

The output for a logistic regression analysis in SPSS is complex, and so we include only a few key panels from an analysis in which we used three predictors (smoking status, maternal age, and number of prior pregnancies) to predict whether or not the young mother had a repeat pregnancy within 18 months of delivering the index infant.

Panel A of Figure 18.6 presents the results of the chi-square goodness of fit test for the overall model with three predictors (i.e., the test based on the likelihood ratio). The chi-square of 1.107 ($df = 3$) was not significant, $p = .775$, suggesting that the null hypothesis should be retained. In Panel B, we see that $-2LL = 35.544$ and that the value of Nagelkerke R squared is .051. In Panel C, the Hosmer-Lemeshow test was nonsignificant ($p = .587$), a result that conflicts with the earlier chi-square goodness of fit test in terms of our ability to infer that the model was adequate in predicting likeli-

hood of a repeat pregnancy. The next two panels suggest that the model is, in fact, disappointing. Panel D indicates how cases would have been classified using the logistic regression equation in terms of having a repeat pregnancy, compared to the women's actual status. Only 66.7% of cases were correctly classified, and the model did not predict a repeat pregnancy for a single case where one was observed.

Panel E shows the logistic regression equation—that is, the value of the b weights and the constant—in the column headed B. The Wald statistics indicate that none of the three predictors was significant. For example, the Wald statistic for predicting a repeat pregnancy based on the number of prior pregnancies (Priors) was .027, $p = .870$. The column headed Exp(B) is a particularly important one—the values in this column are the adjusted odds ratios associated with each predictor. The *OR* of .458 for the smoking status variable, for example, indicates that those who smoked were 46% less likely to have a repeat pregnancy, with age and prior pregnancies controlled. However, this *OR* was not significant. The 95% CI extends from .079 to 2.645 and, because this encompasses the value of 1.0, this means that we cannot reject the null hypothesis that smokers and nonsmokers were equally likely to have a repeat pregnancy.

CRITIQUING MULTIVARIATE STATISTICS

As we advised in the previous chapter, it is difficult to critique researchers' statistical analysis without statistical skills. This caution is even more relevant when it comes to complex multivariate analyses.

As with bivariate statistics, one issue is whether the researcher selected the right tests. The selection of a multivariate procedure depends on several factors, including the nature of the research question and the measurement level of the variables. (It also depends on whether the data conformed to various assumptions underlying the tests—an issue we did

Logistic Regression
Block 1: Method = Enter

A Omnibus Tests of Model Coefficients

		Chi-square	df	Sig.
Step 1	Step	1.107	3	.775
	Block	1.107	3	.775
	Model	1.107	3	.775

B Model Summary

Step	-2 Log likelihood	Cox & Snell R Square	Nagelkerke R Square
1	35.544	.036	.051

a. Estimation terminated at iteration number 5 because parameter estimates changed by less than .001.

C Hosmer and Lemeshow Test

Step	Chi-square	df	Sig.
1	6.540	8	.587

D Classification Table[a,b]

			Predicted		
			Repeat pregnancy		
Observed			No (0)	Yes (1)	Percentage Correct
Step 1	Repeat pregnancy	No (0)	20	1	95.2
		Yes (1)	9	0	.0
		Overall Percentage			66.7

a Constant is included in the model.
b The cut value is .500

E Variables in the Equation

	B	S.E.	Wald	df	Sig.	Exp(B)	95.0% C.I.for EXP(B) Lower	Upper
Step 1[a] Age	−.131	.239	.298	1	.585	.878	.549	1.402
Priors	−.097	.593	.027	1	.870	.907	.284	2.901
Smoke	−.781	.895	.762	1	.383	.458	.079	2.645
Constant	1.891	4.283	.195	1	.659	6.628		

[a]Variable(s) entered on step 1: AGE, PRIORS, SMOKE.

FIGURE 18.6 Partial SPSS printout for logistic regression.

not address in this brief chapter.) Table 18.6, which summarizes some of the major features of multivariate statistics discussed in this chapter, may be helpful in assessing the appropriateness of an analytic approach. It might also be noted that studies in which multivariate statistics were *not* used might

well be critiqued in terms of whether or not they *should* have been used. As we illustrated, results from an ANOVA or *t*-test can sometimes be altered by controlling confounding variables. Conversely, some researchers apply multivariate statistics when their sample size is too small to justify their use.

| TABLE 18.6 | Guide to Selected Multivariate Analyses |

TEST NAME	PURPOSE	MEASUREMENT LEVEL OF VARIABLES			NUMBER OF VARIABLES†		
		IV	DV	CV	IVs	DVs	CV
Multiple regression/ correlation	To test the relationship between 2 + IVs and 1 DV; to predict a DV from 2 + IVs	N, I, R	I, R	—	2+	1	—
Analysis of covariance (ANCOVA)	To test the difference between the means of 2 + groups, while controlling for 1+ covariate	N	I, R	N, I, R	1+	1	1+
Mixed design RM-ANOVA	To test mean differences for 2+ groups for outcomes measured multiple times	N	I, R		1+	1	—
Multivariate analysis of variance (MANOVA)	To test the difference between the means of 2+ groups for 2+ DVs simultaneously	N	I, R	—	1+	2+	—
Multivariate analysis of covariance (MANCOVA)	To test the difference between the means of 2+ groups for 2+ DVs simultaneously, while controlling for 1+ covariate	N	I, R	N, I, R	1+	2+	1+
Discriminant function analysis	To test the relationship between 2+ IVs and 1 DV; to predict group membership; to classify cases into groups	N, I, R	N	—	2+	1	—
Logistic regression	To test the relationship between 2+ IVs and 1 DV; to predict the probability of an event; to estimate relative risk	N, I, R	N	—	2+	1	—

*Variables: IV, independent variables; DV, dependent variable; CV, covariate.
†Measurement levels: N, nominal; I, interval; R, ratio.

No specific critiquing guidelines for multivariate statistics are presented in this chapter, but most of the questions presented in Box 17.1 (p. 429) are also relevant for researchers' use of the statistics discussed in this chapter.

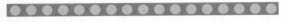

RESEARCH EXAMPLE

Study: Predictors of implantable cardioverter defibrillator shocks during the first year (Dougherty & Hunziker, 2009)

Statement of Purpose: This study used demographic and clinical characteristics to predict whether a patient would experience a shock in the first year after receiving an implantable cardioverter defibrillator (ICD) for secondary prevention of cardiac arrest.

Methods: A prospective design was used to follow 168 first-time ICD recipients over a 1-year period. Data on ICD shock were obtained from ICD interrogation reports over the 12 months. The outcome variable for the analysis was ever having received a shock. Demographic and clinical data used as predictors were obtained from medical records at the time of ICD implantation. Predictors included such variables as age, sex, ethnicity, anxiety scores, smoking status, reason for initial ICD implantation, and presence of other medical problems such as COPD, congestive heart failure, and diabetes.

Analysis and Findings: Overall, 33.3% of the patients experienced at least one shock in the first year after ICD insertion. The researchers first tested bivariate relationships between having had a shock and a broad range of baseline characteristics, using chi-squared tests. Many characteristics were unrelated to shock in these bivariate analyses. For example, men (31.8%) were not significantly more likely than women (34.4%) to have experienced a shock ($p = .47$). In the logistic regression model, predictors were omitted from the final model if they failed to meet certain statistical criteria. The final model included three predictors. The Hosmer-Lemshow test suggested that the model fit the data adequately ($\chi^2 = 0.52, p = .77$), and the goodness of fit test was significant ($p < .001$). The three significant predictors (all with significant Wald statistics values) were: a history of COPD ($OR = 3.10$, 95% CI = $1.08-8.91$), chronic heart failure ($OR = 2,28$, 95% CI = $1.14-4.56$), and having had the ICD implanted for unmonitored syncope with ventricular tachycardia

lasting more than 10 seconds ($OR = 4.45$, 95% CI = $1.32-14.98$). The pseudo R^2 for the model was .09.

SUMMARY POINTS

- **Multivariate statistical procedures** are increasingly being used in nursing research to untangle complex relationships among three or more variables.
- Simple **linear regression** makes predictions about the values of one variable based on values of a second variable. **Multiple regression** is a method of predicting a continuous dependent variable on the basis of two or more independent (**predictor**) variables.
- The **multiple correlation coefficient** (R) can be squared (R^2) to estimate the proportion of variability in the dependent variable accounted for by the predictors. The F statistic is used to test the overall regression model, as well as changes to R^2 as new predictors are introduced.
- The regression equation yields **regression coefficients** (***b***s) for each predictor that, when standardized, are called **beta weights** (βs).
- **Simultaneous multiple regression** enters all predictor variables into the regression equation at the same time. **Hierarchical multiple regression** enters predictors into the equation in a series of steps controlled by researchers. **Stepwise multiple regression** enters predictors in steps using a statistical criterion for order of entry.
- **Analysis of covariance** (**ANCOVA**), an extension of ANOVA, removes the effect of confounding variables (**covariates**) before testing whether mean group differences on the outcome variable are statistically significant.
- **Mixed design RM-ANOVA** is used to test mean differences between groups (between-subjects factor) over time (within-subjects factor). RM-ANOVA is not **robust** to the unique assumptions for RM-ANOVA, which include *sphericity* and *compound symmetry*. In mixed-design RM-ANOVAs, the interaction term (time × group) usually is of primary interest.

- **Multivariate analysis of variance (MANOVA)** is the extension of ANOVA to situations in which there is more than one dependent variable.
- **Discriminant analysis** is used to make predictions about dependent variables that are categorical (i.e., predictions about membership in groups) on the basis of two or more predictor variables.
- The **general linear model (GLM)** encompasses a broad class of frequently used statistical techniques that fit data to straight-line (linear) solutions, including *t*-tests, ANOVA, ANCOVA, and multiple regression.
- **Least-squares estimation** used within GLM minimizes the square of **errors of prediction** (the **residuals**). An alternative is **maximum likelihood estimation (MLE)**, which estimates the parameters most likely to have generated observed data.
- **Logistic regression**, which is based on MLE, is used to predict the probability of an outcome. Logistic regression yields an **odds ratio** that is an index of relative risk for each predictor, that is, the risk of an outcome occurring given one condition, versus the risk of it occurring given a different condition, while controlling other predictors.
- The overall logistic regression model can be tested with a **likelihood ratio test** that uses a **goodness-of-fit chi-square** statistic. An alternative is the **Hosmer-Lemeshow** test that tests how close the model is to a perfect model. Individual predictors can be tested with the **Wald statistic**. Statisticians have devised several **pseudo** R^2 indexes to summarize overall effect size for logistic regression; the most widely reported is the **Nagelkerke** R^2.
- **Survival analysis** and other related event history methods such as **Cox regression** are used when the dependent variable of interest is a time interval (e.g., length of time in hospital).
- **Causal modeling** involves the development and testing of a hypothesized causal explanation of a phenomenon.
- **Path analysis**, a regression-based method for testing causal models, involves the preparation

of a **path diagram** that stipulates hypothesized causal links among variables. Path analysis tests **recursive models** in which causation is presumed to be unidirectional.
- **Structural equations modeling (SEM)**, an MLE approach to causal modeling, does not have as many assumptions and restrictions as path analysis. SEM can accommodate measurement errors, **nonrecursive models** that allow for reciprocal causal paths, and correlated errors.

STUDY ACTIVITIES

Chapter 18 of the *Resource Manual for Nursing Research*: *Generating and Assessing Evidence for Nursing Practice*, *9th edition*, offers exercises and study suggestions for reinforcing concepts presented in this chapter. In addition, the following study questions can be addressed:

1. A researcher has examined the relationship between preventive healthcare attitudes on the one hand and the person's educational level, age, and gender on the other. The multiple correlation coefficient is .62. Explain the meaning of this statistic. How much variation in attitudinal scores is explained by the three predictors? How much is *unexplained*? What other variables might improve the power of the prediction?
2. Using power analysis, determine the sample size needed to achieve power = .80 for α = .05, when (a) estimated R^2 = .15, and k = 5; and (b) estimated R^2 = .08, and k = 3.

STUDIES CITED IN CHAPTER 18

Baird, C., Murawski, M., & Wu, J. (2010). Efficacy of guided imagery with relaxation for osteoarthritis symptoms and medication intake. *Pain Management Nursing, 11*, 56–65.

Chen, H., Clark, A., Tsai, L., & Chao, Y. (2009). Self-reported sleep disturbance of patients with heart failure in Taiwan. *Nursing Research, 58*, 63–71.

Crilly, J., Chaboyer, W., Wallis, M., Thalib, L., & Polit, D. (2010). An outcomes evaluation of an Australian Hospital in the Nursing Home admission avoidance programme. *Journal of Clinical Nursing, 19,* 3010–3018.

Dougherty, C., & Hunziker, J. (2009). Predictors of implantable cardioverter defibrillator shocks during the first year. *Journal of Cardiovascular Nursing, 24,* 21–28.

Good, M., & Ahn, S. (2008). Korean and American music reduces pain in Korean women after gynecologic surgery. *Pain Management Nursing, 9,* 96–103.

Griffith, K. (2009). Biological, psychological and behavioral, and social variables influencing colorectal cancer screening in African Americans. *Nursing Research, 58,* 312–320.

Hays, L., Pressler, S., Damush, T., Rawl, T., & Clark, D. (2010). Exercise adoption among older, low-income women at risk for cardiovascular disease. *Public Health Nursing, 27,* 79–88.

Kong, A., & Bernstein, K. (2009). Childhood trauma as a predictor of eating psychopathology and its mediating variables in patients with eating disorders. *Journal of Clinical Nursing, 18,* 1897–1907.

Lau-Walker, M., Cowie, M., & Roughton, M. (2009). Coronary heart disease patients' perceptions of their symptoms and sense of control are associated with their quality of life three years following hospital discharge. *Journal of Clinical Nursing, 18,* 63–71.

Lous, J., & Chen, S. (2009). Relationships among sexual knowledge, sexual attitudes, and safe sex behaviour among adoelescents. *International Journal of Nursing Studies, 46,* 1595–1603.

Paradis, V., Cossette, S., Frasure-Smith, N., Heppell, S., & Guertin, M. (2010). The efficacy of a motivational nursing intervention based on the stages of change on self-care in heart failure patients. *Journal of Cardiovascular Nursing, 25,* 130–141.

Whiteside-Mansell, L., Bradley, R., McKelvey, L., & Fussell, J. (2009). Parenting: Linking impacts of interpartner conflict to preschool children's social behavior. *Journal of Pediatric Nursing, 24,* 389–400.

Zachariah, R. (2009). Social support, life stress, and anxiety as predictors of pregnancy complications in low-income women. *Research in Nursing & Health, 32,* 391–404.

Methodologic and nonresearch references cited in this chapter can be found in a separate section at the end of the book.

19

Processes of Quantitative Data Analysis and Interpretation

I n this chapter, we offer an overview of steps that are normally taken in analyzing quantitative data, including interpretation of the results. Figure 19.1 shows what the flow of tasks might look like, organized in phases. Progress in analyzing quantitative data is not always as linear as this figure suggests, but it provides a framework for discussing key steps in the analytic process.

PREANALYSIS PHASE

The first phase involves various clerical and administrative tasks, such as logging in forms, reviewing data for completeness and legibility, retrieving pieces of missing information, and assigning identification (ID) numbers. Another task involves selecting statistical software for doing the data analyses. Two widely used statistical software packages are the Statistical Package for the Social Sciences (SPSS, now called PASW) and the Statistical Analysis System (SAS). Next, researchers must code the data and enter them onto computer files to create a **data set** (the total collection of data for all sample members) for analysis.

Coding Quantitative Data

Coding is the process of transforming data into symbols—usually numbers. Certain variables are inherently quantitative (e.g., age, body temperature) and may not require coding, unless the data are gathered in categories (e.g., younger than 30 years of age versus 30 or older). Even with "naturally" quantitative data, researchers need to inspect their data. All responses should be of the same form and precision. For example, for the variable *height* in the nonmetric system, researchers need to decide whether to record feet and inches or to convert the information entirely to inches. Whichever method is adopted, it must be used consistently for all participants. There must also be consistency in handling information reported with different degrees of precision (e.g., coding a response such as 5 feet 2½ inches).

Most data from structured instruments can be precoded, with codes designated before data are collected. For example, questions with fixed response alternatives can be preassigned a numeric code that is printed on the data collection form, such as under age 30 = 1 and 30 and older = 2. Codes are often arbitrary, as in the case of the variable gender. Whether a female subject is coded 1 or 2 has no analytic importance so long as females are consistently assigned one code and males another code.

Respondents sometimes can check off more than one response to a question, as in the following:

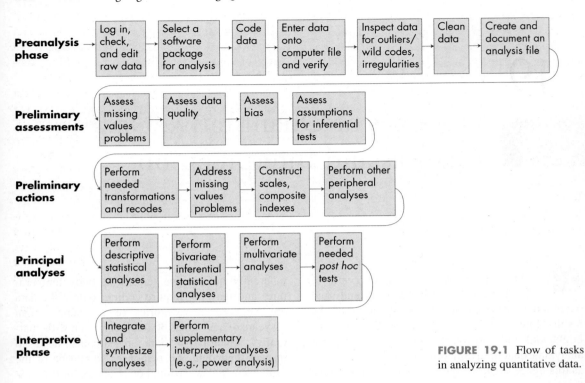

FIGURE 19.1 Flow of tasks in analyzing quantitative data.

To which of the following journals do you subscribe? Check all that apply.

❏ *International Journal of Nursing Studies*
❏ *Journal of Advanced Nursing*
❏ *Nursing Research*
❏ *Research in Nursing & Health*
❏ *Western Journal of Nursing Research*

With questions of this type, a 1-2-3-4-5 coding scheme cannot be used. Responses must be coded as though there were five separate questions: Do you subscribe to the *International Journal of Nursing Studies*? Do you subscribe to the *Journal of Advanced Nursing*? And so on. Each check is treated as a "yes." The question yields five variables, with one code (e.g., 1) signifying "yes" and another code (e.g., 0) signifying "no."

If data from open-ended questions are going to be used in quantitative analysis, they must be coded. Sometimes researchers can develop codes ahead of time, but usually unstructured data are collected because responses cannot be anticipated. In such situations, researchers typically review a sizable portion of the data to understand content and then develop a coding scheme.

A code is needed for each variable for every sample member, even if there is no response. **Missing values** can be of various types. A person answering a question may be undecided, refuse to answer, or say, "Don't know." When skip patterns are used, there is missing information for those questions that are irrelevant to some respondents. A single missing values code may suffice, but it may be important to distinguish different types of missing data using different codes (e.g., distinguishing refusals and *don't know*s).

The choice of what code to use for missing data is often arbitrary, but missing values codes must be ones that have not been used for actual pieces of information. Some researchers use blanks, periods, or negative values for missing information. Others use 9 as the missing code because this value is out of the range of real codes for most variables.

Precise coding instructions should be documented in a coding manual. Coders, like observers and interviewers, must be properly trained, and intercoder reliability checks are recommended.

Entering, Verifying, and Cleaning Data

Coded data typically are transferred onto a data file via keyboard entry, but other options (e.g., scanning of forms) are also available. Various programs can be used for data entry, including spreadsheets or databases. Major software packages for statistical analysis also have data editors that make data entry fairly easy.

Figure 19.2 shows a portion of a data file for the Statistical Package for the Social Sciences (SPSS), for data we used in analytic examples in the last three chapters (see Table 16.8). The entire data file is a 30 × 7 matrix, with 30 rows (1 for each person) and 7 columns for the variables. This figure displays data for only the first 5 people to conserve space. Each variable had to be named (group, weight, and so on). The participants' unique ID should be entered along with actual data, which allows researchers to go back to original sources if need be. The ID number normally is entered as the first variable of the record, as in Figure 19.2.

Data entry is prone to error, so it is essential to verify entries and correct mistakes. One method is to compare visually the numbers on a printout of the data file with codes on the original source and another is to double enter data. There are also special verifying programs designed to perform comparisons during direct data entry.

Even verified data need to be cleaned. **Data cleaning** involves two types of checks. The first is a check for outliers and wild codes. **Outliers** are values that lie outside the normal range. Outliers can be found by inspecting frequency distributions, paying special attention to the lowest and highest values. (Most researchers begin data analysis by constructing frequency distributions for all variables in their data set.) Some outliers are true, legitimate values (e.g., an income of $1 million in a distribution where the mean is $50,000), but sometimes they result from data entry errors. Another problem is a **wild code**—that is, a code that is not possible. For example, the variable gender might have these three codes: 1 = female, 2 = male, and 9 = missing. If someone was coded 3 for gender, there is an error. The computer could show the ID number of the faulty record, and the correct code could then be tracked down.

TIP: Such checks will never reveal all errors. If a male were incorrectly coded 1 for gender, the mistake might not be detected. Errors can have a big effect on the analysis and interpretation of data, so it is important to code, enter, verify, and clean data with care.

A second data-cleaning procedure involves **consistency checks**, which focus on internal data consistency. In this task, researchers check for errors

	id	group	bweight	repeat	age	priors	smokstat
1	1	1	107	1	17	1	1
2	2	1	101	0	14	0	0
3	3	1	119	0	21	3	0
4	4	1	128	1	20	2	0
5	5	1	89	0	15	1	1

FIGURE 19.2 Portion of an SPSS data file.

by testing compatibility of data within a case. For example, one question in a survey might ask current marital status, and another might ask number of marriages. If the data were internally consistent, respondents who answered "Single, never married" to the first question should have a zero (or a missing values code) for the second. Researchers should search for opportunities to check the consistency of entered data.

> **Example of data verification and cleaning:**
> Minnick and Needleman (2009) studied anesthesia provider models in over 1,000 hospitals with regard to their association with obstetric outcomes. Here is how they described data management: "Data were subjected to standard cleaning programs for outliers and repeated entry (detected coding error of less than 1%)" (p. 807).

Creating and Documenting the Analysis Files

The decisions that researchers make about coding and variable naming should be fully documented. Memory should not be trusted; several weeks after coding, researchers may no longer remember if males were coded 1 and females were coded 2, or vice versa. Moreover, colleagues may wish to borrow the data for a secondary analysis. Documentation should always be sufficiently thorough that someone unfamiliar with the original study could use the data.

Documentation primarily involves preparing a codebook. A **codebook** is essentially a listing of each variable together with information about placement in the file, codes associated with the values of the variable, and other basic information. Codebooks can be generated by statistical or data entry programs.

PRELIMINARY ASSESSMENTS AND ACTIONS

Researchers typically undertake several preanalytic activities before they test their hypotheses. Several preparatory activities are discussed next.

Assessing and Handling Missing Values Problems

Researchers strive to have data values for all participants on all key variables—but usually find their data sets have some missing values. Before they can deal with this problem, researchers must first understand their missing values. An appropriate solution depends on such factors as the extent of missing data, the role of the variable with missing data, and the pattern of missingness.

There are three missing values patterns. The first, and most desirable, is **missing completely at random (MCAR)**, which occurs when cases with missing values are just a random subsample of all cases. When data are MCAR, analyses remain unbiased—but missing values are seldom MCAR. Data are considered **missing at random (MAR)** if missingness is related to other variables (e.g., gender)—but *not* related to the value of the variable that has the missing values. The third pattern is **missing not at random (MNAR)**, a pattern in which the value of the variable that is missing *is* related to its missingness (e.g., those declining to report their income tend to be either rich or poor). Missing values that are MAR or MNAR can result in biased results, but solutions are most readily accomplished when missing data are MAR and not MNAR—though it is difficult to know for sure which of these two patterns applies.

A first step in analyzing missing data is to assess the extent of the problem by examining frequency distributions on a variable-by-variable basis. Another step is to examine the cumulative extent of missing values (e.g., what percentage of cases had no variables missing, one variable missing, and so on). Another task is to evaluate the randomness of missing values. A simple procedure is to divide the sample into two groups—those with and without missing data on a specified variable. The two groups can then be compared in terms of their characteristics to assess whether the two groups are comparable—for example, were men more likely than women to leave certain questions blank?

Until recently, examining patterns of missingness was a tedious process, which may explain why many researchers simply ignore the problem of missing data (and therefore ignore the risk of bias that can be introduced). Now, however, programs in widely used statistical software have greatly simplified this important task. For example, the Missing Values Analysis (MVA) module within SPSS offers powerful means of detecting and addressing missing values. Approaches to assessing missing values problems using both traditional methods and MVA are described in Polit (2010).

Once researchers have assessed the extent and patterning of missing values, they must decide how to address the problem. There are three basic types of solutions: deletions, imputations, and mixed modeling with repeated measures. We discuss the first two here; information about sophisticated hierarchical modeling solutions are discussed in Shin (2009).

Missing Data and Deletions

Listwise deletion (also called *complete case analysis*) is simply the analysis of those cases for which there are no missing data. Listwise deletion is based on an implicit assumption of MCAR. Researchers who use this method typically have not made a formal assessment of the extent to which MCAR is probable, but rather are simply disregarding the problem of missing data.

Perhaps the most widely used (but not the best) approach is to delete cases selectively, on a variable-by-variable basis by means of **pairwise deletion** (also called *available case analysis*). For example, in a test of an intervention to reduce patient anxiety, the dependent variables might be blood pressure and self-reported anxiety. If 10 people from the sample 100 failed to complete the anxiety scale, we might base the analyses of anxiety data on the 90 people who completed the scale, but use the full sample of 100 in the blood pressure analysis. If the number of cases fluctuates widely across outcomes, the results are difficult to interpret because the sample is essentially a "moving target."

> ➲ **T I P :** Computer programs like SPSS use either listwise or pairwise deletion as the **default** (i.e., the option that will be used in the analysis unless there are specific instructions to the contrary).

Researchers sometimes use pairwise deletion in analyses involving a correlation matrix. From one pair of variables in the matrix to another, the number of cases can vary substantially. Although such correlation matrixes may provide useful descriptive information, it is imprudent to use pairwise deletion for correlation-based multivariate analyses such as multiple regression or factor analysis because the correlations are calculated on nonidentical subsets of people.

Another deletion option is to delete a variable for all participants. This option may be suitable when a high percentage of cases have missing values on a variable that is not central to the analysis. Recommendations for how much missing data should drive this decision range from 15% to 40% of cases (Fox-Wasylyshyn & El-Masri, 2005).

Missing Data and Imputations

Preferred methods for addressing missing values involve **imputation**—that is, "filling in" missing data with values believed to be good estimates of what the values would have been, had they not been missing. An attractive feature of imputation is that it allows researchers to maintain full sample size, and thus statistical power is not compromised. The risk is that the imputations will be poor estimates of real values, leading to biases of unknown magnitude and direction.

The simplest imputation procedure is **mean substitution** or *median substitution*, which involves using "typical" sample values to replace missing data that are continuous. For example, if a person's age were missing and if the average age of sample members were 45.2 years, we could substitute the value 45.2 in place of the missing values code. Mean substitution is, like listwise deletion, popular because of its simplicity. Yet, even though mean substitution increases sample size and leaves variable means unchanged, it is rarely the best approach. Regardless of what the underlying pattern of missingness is, mean imputation underestimates variance, and variance is what most statistical analyses are all about.

A refinement on mean substitution is to use the mean value for a relevant subgroup—called a **subgroup** (or *conditional*) **mean substitution.** The assumption is that a better estimate of the missing value can be obtained by making the substitution conditional on participants' characteristics. For example, rather than replacing a missing age value with 45.2, we could replace a man's missing value with men's mean age, and a woman's mean value with women's mean age. This is a better option than mean substitution because the substituted values are presumably closer to the real values, and also because variance is not reduced as much. Nevertheless, conditional (subgroup) mean substitution is not a preferred approach, except when overall missingness is low.

⇨ **TIP:** When data are missing for individual items on a multi-item scale, it is often appropriate to replace a missing value with the mean of other similar items from the person with the missing value, an approach that assumes that people are "internally consistent" across similar questions. Such **case mean substitution**, which uses person-specific information to inform the estimate, has the advantage of not throwing out data altogether (listwise deletion), and not assuming that a person is similar to all others in a sample or subgroup (mean substitution). Case mean substitution has been found to be an acceptable method of imputation at the item level, even compared to more sophisticated methods.

Researchers are increasingly using imputation methods that make more extensive use of data in the data set. One example is to use regression analysis to "predict" the correct value of missing data. Suppose we found that participants' age was correlated with gender, education, and health status. Based on data from those with complete data, age could be regressed on these three variables to predict age for people with missing age data, but whose values for the three other variables were not missing. Regression-based imputation is more

accurate than previously discussed strategies, although variability remains underestimated using regression.

Even more sophisticated solutions have been developed. Maximum likelihood estimation is useful because it uses all data points in a dataset to construct estimated replacement values. **Expectation (EM) maximization** involves using an iterative procedure with a maximum-likelihood–based algorithm to produce the best parameter estimates. An approach called **multiple imputation (MI)** is currently considered one of the best methods of addressing missing values problems. MI addresses a fundamental issue—the uncertainty of any given estimate—by imputing several (m) estimates of the missing data, each of which has an element of randomness introduced. Results from analyses across the m imputations are later pooled. MI has not often been used because of its complexity and the limited availability of appropriate software, but recent versions of the SPSS MVA module (version 17.0 and higher) do offer multiple imputation. Procedures for dealing with missing data are discussed at greater length in McKnight and colleagues (2007) and Polit (2010).

⇨ **TIP:** The "gold standard" for analyzing data from randomized controlled trials (RCTs) is to use an **intention-to-treat (ITT) analysis**, which involves analyzing outcome data from all participants who were randomized, regardless of whether they dropped out of the study. A true ITT analysis is achieved only if there are no missing outcome data, or if missing values are accounted for in the analysis, such as through imputation. A resource for advice on how to achieve ITT is offered in Polit and Gillespie (2010). Polit and Gillespie (2009) found, in their analysis of 124 nursing randomized trials, that 75% of the RCTs had missing outcome data, and one out of four had 20% or more missing values. Listwise and pairwise deletion were the most common approaches; only about 10% of the studies used imputation or mixed effects modeling in their ITT analyses. The approach most often used to impute values for missing outcome variables in RCTs is a now discredited procedure called **last observation carried forward (LOCF)**, which imputes the missing outcome using the previous measurement of that same outcome.

Example of handling missing values: Kim and colleagues (2009) studied the relationship between nursing practice environments on the one hand and nurse-perceived quality of geriatric care on the other. Of the 206 nurses who completed a survey, 14 nurses had extensive missing data and were dropped. Of the remaining 192 cases, 96 had no missing data, and other cases had modest amounts of missing data. Different patterns of missingness were detected. They used a variant of multiple imputation to impute estimated values for these cases.

Assessing Data Quality

Assessing data quality is another early analytic task. For example, when composite scales are used, researchers should assess internal consistency reliability (Chapter 14). The distribution of data values for key variables also should be examined to assess any anomalies, such as limited variability, extreme skewness, or the presence of ceiling or floor effects. For example, a vocabulary test for 10-year-olds likely would yield a clustering of high scores in a sample of 11-year-olds, creating a **ceiling effect** that would reduce correlations between test scores and other characteristics of the children. Conversely, there likely would be a clustering of low scores on the test with a sample of 9-year-olds, resulting in a **floor effect** with similar consequences.

Earlier we discussed outliers in connection with efforts to clean a data set to ensure the accuracy of data entered into a file. Legitimate outliers—extreme scores that are true values—are a data quality issue. Outliers can distort study results and cause errors in statistical decision making, so outliers should be scrutinized. By convention, a value is considered an **extreme outlier** if it is greater than 3 times the *interquartile range (IQR)* above the third quartile or below the first quartile. The IQR, as noted briefly in Chapter 16, is an index of variability. Methods for detecting and addressing outlier problems are discussed in Polit (2010).

➡ TIP: For those using the Statistical Package for the Social Sciences (SPSS), the "Explore" routine is invaluable in making assessments of data quality.

Assessing Bias

Researchers often undertake preliminary analyses to assess biases, including the following:

- *Nonresponse (volunteer) bias.* If possible, researchers should assess whether a biased subset of people participated in a study. If there is information about the characteristics of all people who were asked to participate (e.g., demographic information from hospital records), researchers should compare the characteristics of those who did and did not participate to assess the nature and direction of any biases and to inform conclusions about the study's generalizability.
- *Selection bias.* When nonrandomized comparison groups are used (e.g., in quasi-experimental studies), researchers should check for selection biases by comparing the groups' baseline characteristics. Detected differences should, if possible, be controlled—for example, through analysis of covariance or regression. Even when an experimental design has been used, researchers should check the success of randomization.
- *Attrition bias.* In studies with multiple points of data collection, it is important to check for attrition biases by comparing people who did and did not continue to participate in later waves of data collection, based on baseline characteristics.

In performing any of these analyses, significant group differences are an indication of bias, and such bias must be taken into consideration in interpreting and discussing the results. Whenever possible, the biases should be controlled in testing the main hypotheses.

Example of assessing bias: Downe-Wamboldt (2007) conducted an RCT to test the effectiveness of individualized counseling on depression in patients with cancer. They tested volunteer bias by comparing characteristics of patients who consented to participate with those of people who refused. They compared those in the experimental and control groups on baseline traits to assess selection bias. Finally, they compared those who stayed in the study to those who did not to assess attrition bias.

Testing Assumptions for Statistical Tests

Most statistical tests are based on a number of assumptions—conditions that are presumed to be true and, when violated, can lead to erroneous conclusions. For example, parametric tests assume that variables are distributed normally. Frequency distributions, scatter plots, and other assessment procedures provide researchers with information about whether or not underlying assumptions for statistical tests have been upheld.

Graphic displays of frequency distributions can show whether the distribution of values is severely skewed, multimodal, too peaked, or too flat. There are statistical indexes of skewness or peakedness that test whether the shape of the distribution is significantly skewed or peaked or flat. Many software programs also include the *Kolmorogov-Smirnov test*, which tests that a distribution does not deviate significantly from a normal distribution.

Example of testing assumptions: Shellman and colleagues (2009) tested the effects of integrative reminiscence on depressive symptoms in older African Americans. Before undertaking their primary analyses, "preliminary analyses were conducted to ensure that there were no violations of the assumptions of normality, linearity, homogeneity of variances, homogeneity of regression slopes, and reliable measurement of the covariates" (p. 780).

Performing Data Transformations

Raw data often need to be modified or transformed before hypotheses can be tested. Various **data transformations** can easily be handled through commands to the computer. For example, the scoring direction of some items on multi-item scales might need to be reversed before item scores can be summed. Some guidance on **item reversals** was presented in Chapter 15.

Sometimes researchers want to create a variable that is a cumulative **count** based on other variables in the dataset. For example, suppose we asked people to indicate which types of illegal drug they had used in the past month, from a list of 10 options.

Use of each drug would be answered independently in a yes (e.g., coded 1) or no (e.g., coded 0) fashion. We could create a new variable of number of different drugs used that represented a count of all the "1" codes for the 10 drug items. Other transformations involve **recodes** of original values. Recoding is often used to create *dummy variables* for multivariate analyses.

Transformations also can be undertaken to render data appropriate for statistical tests. For example, if a distribution is non-normal, a transformation can sometimes help to make parametric procedures appropriate. A logarithmic transformation, for example, tends to normalize positively skewed distributions.

⊗ **T I P :** The Toolkit in the accompanying *Resource Manual* includes a table with data transformations that may help to correct skewed distributions. The table also identifies the SPSS functions that would be used for the transformations.

When you do transformations, it is important to check that they were done correctly by examining a sample of values for the original and transformed variables. This can be done by instructing the computer to list, for a sample of cases, the values of the newly created variables and the original variables used to create them.

Example of transforming variables: Groër and Shelton (2009) explored the relationship between exercise in postpartum women and concentrations of cytokines and secretory immunoglobulin A in their milk. All of the cytokine measures were logarithmically transformed to correct for positive skewness.

Performing Additional Peripheral Analyses

Depending on the study, additional peripheral analyses may be needed before proceeding to substantive analyses. It is impossible to catalog all such analyses, but we offer a few examples to alert readers to the kinds of issues that need to be given some thought.

Data Pooling

Researchers sometimes obtain data from more than one source, as when researchers recruit participants from multiple sites. The risk is that participants from different sites may not really be drawn from the same population, so it is wise to evaluate whether **pooling** of data (combining data across sites) is warranted. This involves comparing participants from the different sites in terms of key research variables, or comparing the extent to which correlations between key variables are similar across sites.

> **Example of testing for pooling:** Mullin and colleagues (2009) studied how patients who had undergone a coronary artery bypass graft surgery described sensations experienced during removal of epicardial pacing wires. They used data from two existing datasets, one from the United States and one from Canada, and undertook analyses to assess whether pooling was justified.

Testing Cohort Effects

Nurse researchers sometimes accumulate a sample over an extended period of time to achieve adequate sample sizes. This can result in **cohort effects,** that is, differences in participant characteristics over time. This might occur because of changes in community characteristics or in healthcare services, for example. If the research involves an intervention, it may also be that the treatment itself changes—for example, if those administering the treatment get better at doing it. Thus, researchers with a long period of *sample intake* should consider testing for cohort effects because such effects can confound the results or even mask relationships. This activity usually involves examining correlations between entry dates and key variables.

> **Example of testing for cohort effects:** Polit and colleagues (2001), in their study of health problems among low-income mothers, analyzed survey data that were collected over a 12-month period from a sample of 4,000 women. They discovered that women interviewed later were significantly more disadvantaged than those interviewed early. In their analyses, timing of the interview was statistically controlled.

Testing Ordering (Carryover) Effects

When a crossover design is used (i.e., people are randomly assigned to different orderings of treatments), researchers should assess whether outcomes are different for people in the different treatment-order groups. That is, did getting A before B yield different outcomes than getting B before A? In essence, such tests offer evidence that it is legitimate to pool the data from alternative orderings.

> **Example of testing for ordering effects:** Mackereth and colleagues (2009) compared the effects of reflexology versus progressive muscle relaxation training for people with multiple sclerosis, using a crossover design. Despite having a 4-week washout period, outcome measures such as salivary cortisol and blood pressure did not return to baseline levels, and an ordering effect was detected.

PRINCIPAL ANALYSES

At this point in the analysis process, researchers have a cleaned data set, with missing data problems resolved and transformations completed; they also have some understanding of data quality and biases. They can now proceed with more substantive data analyses.

Planning the Substantive Data Analysis

In many studies, researchers collect data on dozens of variables. They cannot analyze every variable in relation to all others, so a plan to guide data analysis must be developed. One approach is to prepare a list of the analyses to be undertaken, specifying both the variables and the statistical test to be used. Another approach is to develop table shells. **Table shells** are layouts of how researchers envision presenting their findings, without numbers filled in. Once a table shell is prepared, researchers can do the analyses needed to complete the table. (The table templates in the Toolkit of the accompanying *Resource Manual*, for Chapters 16 through 18, can be used as a basis for table shells. ✸) Researchers do not need to adhere rigidly to table shells, but they provide a good mechanism for organizing the analysis of large amounts of data.

Substantive Analyses

Substantive analyses typically begin with descriptive analyses. Researchers usually develop a descriptive profile of the sample, and may look descriptively at correlations among variables. These initial analyses may suggest further analyses or further data transformations that were not originally envisioned. They also give researchers an opportunity to become familiar with their data.

➲ **T I P :** When you explore your data, resist the temptation of going on a "fishing expedition," that is, hunting for *any* significant relationships. The facility with which computers can generate statistics makes it easy to run analyses indiscriminately. The risk is that you will serendipitously find significant correlations between variables as a function of chance. For example, in a correlation matrix with 10 variables—which results in 45 nonredundant correlations—there are likely to be two to three *spurious* significant correlations when alpha = .05 (i.e., .05 × 45 = 2.25).

Researchers then perform statistical analyses to test their hypotheses. Researchers whose data analysis plan calls for multivariate analyses (e.g., MANOVA) often begin with bivariate analyses (e.g., a series of ANOVAs). The primary statistical analyses are complete when all research questions are addressed and when table shells have the applicable numbers in them.

Supplementary Analyses

Sometimes supplementary analyses can facilitate interpretation of the results. For example, suppose our analyses revealed that an exercise intervention was successful in lowering blood pressure in hypertensive patients. In scrutinizing sample characteristics, however, we find that women were underrepresented, which might lead critics to suggest that the evidence for effectiveness in a mixed-gender population is weak. In this situation, we

could examine experimental-control group differences for men and women separately. If the results are similar, it would strengthen inferences about the potential benefits of the intervention for both genders.

Another strategy is to undertake **sensitivity analyses**, which are analyses that test research hypotheses using different assumptions or different strategies. A major example concerns testing alternative strategies to address missing values problems. Some strategies are appropriate under varying conditions, so sensitivity analyses to understand how different strategies affect substantive results are valuable. Another example of sensitivity analyses is running analyses with and without legitimate outliers to see if the results change.

Example of sensitivity analysis: Groom and colleagues (2010) evaluated the costs and effects of a nutrient-based skin care program, compared to usual care, regarding the prevention of skin tears. For cost analyses, there was some uncertainty regarding assumptions (e.g., usual healing time for skin tears). The researchers undertook sensitivity analyses, using different estimates of healing time.

INTERPRETATION OF QUANTITATIVE RESULTS

The analysis of research data provides the **results** of the study. These results need to be evaluated and interpreted, giving thought to the aims of the study, its theoretical basis, the body of related research evidence, and limitations of the adopted research methods. Interpretations of statistical results form the basis for the Discussion section of quantitative research reports.

Issues in Interpretation

The interpretive task is complex, requiring strong methodologic and substantive skills and an appropriate viewpoint. Although interpretation is difficult to teach, we offer some advice about ways of making sound inferences from the study results.

The Interpretive Mindset

Evidence-based practice (EBP) encourages clinicians to make decisions based on a careful assessment of "best evidence." Thinking critically and demanding evidence are also part of a research interpreter's job. Just as clinicians must ask, what *evidence* is there that this intervention or strategy will be beneficial? So too must interpreters ask, what *evidence* is there that the results are real and true? Evidence for *clinical decisions* involves making judgments about study results, which relies on inferences from the evidence on *methodologic decisions* in a body of studies.

To be a good interpreter of research results, it is reasonable to adopt a skeptical attitude, much like in hypothesis testing, which begins with a null hypothesis that researchers want to reject. *The "null hypothesis" to be rejected in interpretation is that the results are wrong.* The "research hypothesis" in interpretation is that the evidence can be trusted and used in practice because the results reflect the truth. The greater the evidence that your design and methods were sound, the less plausible is the null hypothesis of erroneous results.

⊃ **TIP:** You should ask such questions as, is it *plausible* that my results were affected by selection biases? Is it *plausible* that if participants had been blinded to the treatment, the results would have been different? Is it *plausible* that if I had used a different instrument, or had gotten a larger sample, or had less attrition, my results would change? You hope that the answers to such questions are "no," but should start with the working assumption that the answer is "yes" until you have satisfied yourself that this is not true.

Aspects of Interpretation

Interpreting the results of a study involves attending to six different but overlapping considerations:

- The credibility and accuracy of the results
- The precision of the estimate of effects
- The magnitude of effects and importance of the results
- The meaning of the results, especially with regard to causality
- The generalizability of the results

- The implications of the results for nursing practice, theory development, or further research

Credibility of Quantitative Results

One of the most important interpretive tasks is to assess whether the results are *right*. This corresponds to the first EBP question we posed in Chapter 2 (Box 2.2): "What is the quality of the evidence—that is, how rigorous and reliable is it?" If the results are not credible, the remaining interpretive issues (meaning, magnitude, precision, generalizability) are not likely to be relevant.

Research findings are meant to reflect "truth in the real world." The findings are intended to be proxies for the true state of affairs in actual community or healthcare settings. Inference is the vehicle for linking results to the real world. Inferences about the real world are valid, however, to the extent that the researchers have made rigorous methodologic decisions. To come to a conclusion about whether the results closely approximate "truth in the real world," each aspect of the study—its research design, intervention design, sampling plan, measurement and data collection plan, and analytic approach—must be subjected to critical scrutiny.

There are various ways to approach the issue of credibility, including the use of the critiquing guidelines we have offered throughout this book. Here we share some additional perspectives.

Proxies and Credibility

Researchers begin with abstract constructs, and then devise ways to operationalize them. Constructs are linked to actual realities in a series of approximations, each of which affects interpretation because at each step there is a potential for error. The better the proxies, the more credible results are likely to be. In this section, we illustrate successive proxies using sampling concepts to highlight the potential for inferential challenges.

When researchers formulate research questions or hypotheses, the population is typically broad and abstract. Population specifications are delineated later, when eligibility criteria are defined. For

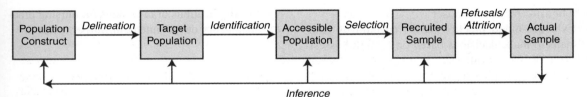

FIGURE 19.3 Inferences about populations: From the analysis sample to the population construct.

example, suppose we wanted to test the effectiveness of an intervention to increase physical activity in low-income women. Figure 19.3 shows the series of steps between the abstract population construct (low-income women) and the *actual* women who participated in the study. Using data from the actual sample on the far right, the researcher would like to make inferences about the effectiveness of the intervention for a broader group, but each proxy along the way represents a potential problem for achieving the desired inference. In interpreting a study,

readers must consider how *plausible* it is that the actual sample reflects the recruited sample, the accessible population, the target population, and then the population construct.

Table 19.1 presents a description of a hypothetical scenario in which the researchers moved from a population construct of low-income women, to an actual sample of 161 women who participated in the study. The table shows some questions that a person trying to make inferences about the study results might ask. Answers to these questions

TABLE 19.1	Successive Proxies in Sampling Example: From The Population Construct to the Analysis Sample	
ELEMENT	**DESCRIPTION**	**POSSIBLE INFERENTIAL CHALLENGES**
Population construct	Low-income women	
Target population	All women who receive public assistance (cash welfare) in California	• Why only welfare recipients—why not the working poor? • Why California?
Accessible population	All women who receive public assistance in Los Angeles and who speak English or Spanish	• Why Los Angeles? • What about non-English/non-Spanish speakers?
Recruited sample	A consecutive sample of 300 female welfare recipients (English or Spanish speaking) who applied for benefits in January, 2011 at two randomly selected welfare offices in Los Angeles	• Why only new applicants—what about women with long-term receipt? • Why only two offices? Are these representative? • Is January a typical month?
Actual sample	161 women from the recruited sample who fully participated in the study	• Who refused to participate (or was too ill, and so on) and why? • Who dropped out of the study, and why?

would affect the interpretation of whether the intervention *really* is effective with low-income women, or only with motivated, cooperative welfare recipients from two neighborhoods of Los Angeles who recently got approved for public assistance.

As Figure 19.3 suggests, researchers in our example made a series of methodologic decisions that affect inferences, and these decisions must be carefully scrutinized in assessing study credibility. However, participant behavior and external circumstances also affect the results and need to be considered in the interpretation. In our example in Table 19.1, 300 women were recruited, but only 161 provided usable data for analysis. The final sample of 161 almost surely would differ in important ways from the 139 who were not in the study, and these differences affect inferences about the value of the study evidence.

We illustrated how successive proxies in a study, from the abstract to the concrete, can affect inferences with regard to sampling, but we could have chosen other aspects of a study. As another example, Figure 19.4 considers successive proxies for an intervention. As with our previous illustration, researchers move from an abstraction on the left (here, a theory about why an intervention might have beneficial outcomes), through the design of protocols that purport to operationalize the theory, to the actual implementation and use of the intervention on the right. Researchers want the right side to be a good proxy for the left side—and they must assess the plausibility that they were successful in the transformation in interpreting results.

Credibility and Validity

Studies inherently involve making inferences. We *infer* that scores on a depression scale are, in fact, cap-turing the depression construct. We *infer* that a sample can tell us something about a population. We use inferential statistics to make inferences about relationships observed in the data. Inference and validity are inextricably linked. Indeed, research methodology experts Shadish and colleagues (2002) defined validity as "the approximate truth of an inference" (p. 34). To be careful interpreters, researchers must seek evidence within their study that desired inferences are, in fact, valid. Part of this process involves considering alternative and potentially competing hypotheses about the credibility and meaning of the results.

In Chapter 10, we discussed four types of validity that play a central role in assessing the credibility of quantitative study results: statistical conclusion validity, internal validity, external validity, and construct validity. Let us use our sampling example (Figure 19.3 and Table 19.1) to demonstrate the relevance of methodologic decisions to all four types of validity—and hence to inferences about study results.

First, let us consider construct validity—a term that has relevance not only for the measurement of research constructs, but also for many aspects of a study. In our example, the population construct was *low-income women*, which led to population eligibility criteria stipulating public assistance recipients in California. There are, however, other alternative operationalizations of the population construct (e.g., women living in families below the official poverty level). Construct validity, it may be recalled, involves inferences from the particulars of the study to higher-order constructs. So, it is fair to ask, do the specified eligibility criteria adequately capture the population construct, low-income women?

Statistical conclusion validity—the extent to which correct inferences can be made about the existence of "real" relationships between key

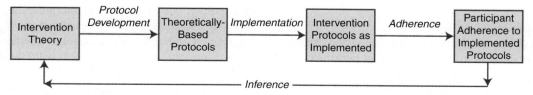

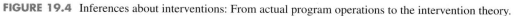

FIGURE 19.4 Inferences about interventions: From actual program operations to the intervention theory.

variables—is also affected by sampling decisions. Ideally, researchers should do an upfront power analysis to estimate how large a sample is needed. In our example, let us say we estimated (based on previous research) a small-to-moderate effect size for the intervention, $d = .40$. For a power of .80, with risk of a Type I error set at .05, we would need a sample of about 200 participants. The actual sample of 161 yields a nearly 30% risk of a Type II error, that is, falsely concluding that the intervention was not successful.

External validity—the generalizability of the results—is clearly affected by sampling decisions and outcomes. To whom would it be safe to generalize the results in this example? To the population construct of low-income women? To all welfare recipients in California? To all new welfare recipients in Los Angeles who speak English or Spanish? Inferences about the extent to which the study results correspond to "truth in the real world" must take sampling decisions and sampling problems (e.g., recruitment and retention difficulties) into account.

Finally, internal validity (the extent to which a causal connection between variables can be inferred) is also affected by sample composition. In particular (in this example), differential attrition would be a concern. Were those in the intervention group more likely (or less likely) than those in the control group to drop out of the study? If so, any observed differences in physical activity outcomes could be caused by individual differences in the groups (e.g., differences in motivation), rather than by the intervention itself.

Methodologic decisions and the careful implementation of those decisions—whether they be about sampling, intervention design, measurement, research design, or analysis—inevitably affect study validity and the interpretation of the results.

Credibility and Bias

Part of a researcher's job in designing and conducting a study is to translate abstract constructs into plausible and meaningful proxies. Another job is to eliminate, reduce, or control biases—or, as a last resort, to detect and understand them. In interpret-

ing results, the risk for various biases should be assessed and factored into conclusions.

Biases are factors that create distortions and undermine researchers' efforts to capture and reveal "truth in the real world." Biases are pervasive. It is not so much a question of whether there *are* biases in a study, so much as what types of bias are present, and how extensive and systematic the biases are. We have discussed many types of bias—some reflect design inadequacies (e.g., selection bias), others reflect recruitment or sampling problems (nonresponse bias), others are related to measurement (social desirability bias). To our knowledge, there is no comprehensive listing of biases that might arise in a study, but Table 19.2 presents a list of some of the biases and errors mentioned in this book. This list is not all inclusive, but is meant to serve as a reminder of some of the problems to consider in interpreting study results.

> **TIP:** The Toolkit on the accompanying *Resource Manual* includes a longer list of biases, with definitions and notes. It is important to recognize that different disciplines may use different names for the same or similar biases. The actual names are not important—what is important is to understand how different forces can distort the results and affect inferences.

Credibility and Corroboration

Earlier we noted that research interpreters should seek evidence to disconfirm the interpretive "null hypothesis" that the research results were inaccurate. Some evidence to discredit the null hypothesis comes from the plausibility that proxies were good stand-ins for abstractions or idealized methods. Other evidence involves ruling out validity threats and biases. Yet another strategy is to seek corroboration for results.

Corroboration can come from both internal and external sources, and the concept of *replication* is an important one in both cases. Interpretations are aided by considering prior research on the topic, for example. Interpreters can examine whether the study results replicate (are congruent with) those of other studies. Discrepancies in study results may lend support to the "null hypothesis" of erroneous results, while consistency across studies discredits it.

TABLE 19.2	Selected List of Major Potential Biases or Errors in Quantitative Studies		

RESEARCH DESIGN	SAMPLING	MEASUREMENT	ANALYSIS
Expectation bias	Sampling error	Social desirability bias	Type I error
Hawthorne effect	Volunteer bias	Acquiescence bias	Type II error
Performance bias	Non-response bias	Nay-sayers bias	
Detection bias		Extreme response set bias	
Contamination of treatments		Recall/memory bias	
Carryover (ordering) effects		Ceiling effects	
Noncompliance bias		Floor effects	
Selection bias		Reactivity	
Attrition bias		Observer biases	
History bias			

Researchers can pursue opportunities for replication themselves. For example, in multisite studies, if results are similar across sites, this suggests that something "real" is occurring with some regularity. Triangulation can be another form of replication and sometimes can help to corroborate results. For example, if results are similar across different measures of an outcome, then there can perhaps be greater confidence that the results are "real" and do not reflect some peculiarity of an instrument. If results are different, this could provide support for the null hypothesis of erroneous results—but it could also reflect a problem with one of the measures. When mixed results occur, interpreters must dig deeper to uncover the reason.

Finally, we are strong advocates of mixed methods studies, a special type of triangulation (Chapter 25 and 26). When findings from the analysis of qualitative data are consistent with the results of statistical analyses, internal corroboration can be especially powerful and persuasive.

Precision of the Results

The results of statistical tests indicate whether an observed relationship or group difference is probably real and replicable with another sample. A p value in hypothesis testing indicates how strong the evidence is that the null hypothesis is false—it is not an estimate of a numeric value of direct relevance to clinicians. A p value offers information that is important, but incomplete.

Confidence intervals, by contrast, communicate information about how precise (or imprecise) the study results are. Dr. David Sackett, a founding father of the EBP movement, had this to say about confidence intervals: "P values on their own are . . . not informative . . . By contrast, CIs indicate the strength of evidence about quantities of direct interest, such as treatment benefit. They are thus of particular relevance to practitioners of evidence-based medicine" (2000, p. 232). It seems likely that nurse researchers will increasingly report CI information in the years ahead because of its value for interpreting study results and assessing their potential utility for nursing practice.

Magnitude of Effects and Importance

In quantitative studies, results that support the researcher's hypotheses are described as *significant*. A careful analysis of study results involves evaluating whether, in addition to being statistically significant, the effects are large and clinically important.

Attaining statistical significance does not necessarily mean that the results are meaningful to nurses and clients. Statistical significance indicates that the results are unlikely to be due to chance—not that they are necessarily important. With large samples, even modest relationships are statistically significant. For instance, with a sample of 500, a correlation coefficient of .10 is significant at the .05 level, but a relationship this weak may have little practical value. When assessing the importance of findings, interpreters of research results must pay attention to actual numeric values and also, if available, to effect sizes. We expect that, like CIs, effect size information will increasingly be reported in nursing reports to address the important EBP question (Box 2.2): "What *is* the evidence—what is the magnitude of effects?"

The absence of statistically significant results, conversely, does not always mean that the results are unimportant, although because nonsignificant results could reflect a Type II error, the case is more complex. Suppose we compared two alternative procedures for making a clinical assessment (e.g., body temperature). Suppose further that we retained the null hypothesis—that is, we found no statistically significant differences between the two methods. If an effect size analysis suggested a very small effect size for the differences *despite a large sample size*, we might be justified in concluding that the two procedures yield equally accurate assessments. If one of these procedures is less painful or costly than the other, nonsignificant findings could indeed be clinically important. Nevertheless, corroboration through replication would be needed before firm conclusions could be reached.

Meaning of the Results

In quantitative studies, statistical results are in the form of test statistic values, *p* levels, effect sizes, and confidence intervals, to which researchers must attach meaning if they have concluded that these results are credible. Many questions about the meaning of statistical results reflect a desire to interpret causal connections.

Interpreting what results mean usually is not challenging in descriptive studies. For example, suppose we found that among patients undergoing electroconvulsive therapy (ECT), the percentage who experience an ECT-induced headache is 59.4% (95% CI = 56.3, 63.1). This result is directly meaningful and interpretable. But if we found that headache prevalence is significantly lower in a cryotherapy intervention group than among patients given acetaminophen, we would need to interpret what the results mean. In particular, we need to interpret whether it is plausible that cryotherapy *caused* reductions in headaches. Even if the results are deemed to be "real," that is, statistically significant, interpretation involves coming to conclusions about internal validity when a causal inference is sought.

In this section, we discuss the interpretation of various research outcomes within a hypothesis-testing context, with an emphasis on causal interpretations. In thinking about causal interpretations, we encourage you to review the criteria for causal relationships (Chapter 9).

Interpreting Hypothesized Results

Interpreting the meaning of statistical results is often easiest when hypotheses are supported. Such interpretations have been partly accomplished beforehand because, in developing hypotheses, researchers have already brought together prior findings, a theoretical framework, and logical reasoning. This groundwork forms the context within which more specific interpretations are made. Nevertheless, a few caveats should be kept in mind.

First, it is important to be conservative in drawing conclusions from the results and to avoid the temptation of going beyond the data to explain what results mean. An example might help to explain what we mean by "going beyond" the data. Suppose we hypothesized that pregnant women's anxiety level about labor and delivery is correlated with the number of children they have borne. The data reveal that a significant negative relationship between anxiety levels and parity ($r = -.30$) exists. We interpret this to mean that increased experience with childbirth results in decreased anxiety. Is this conclusion supported by the data? The conclusion appears to be logical, but in fact, there is nothing in the data that leads directly to this interpretation. An important, indeed critical, research precept is: *correlation does not prove causation*. The finding that two variables are related offers no evidence suggesting which of the two variables—if either—caused the other. In our example, perhaps causality runs in the opposite direction, that is, a woman's anxiety level influences how many children she bears. Or perhaps a third variable not examined in the study, such as the woman's relationship with her husband, influences both anxiety and number of children. Inferring causality is especially difficult in studies that have not used an experimental design.

Alternative explanations for the findings should always be considered. Researchers sometimes can test rival hypotheses directly. If competing interpretations can be ruled out, so much the better, but every angle should be examined to see if one's own explanation has been given adequate competition. Threats to internal validity reflect competing explanations for what the results might mean and need thorough consideration.

Empirical evidence supporting research hypotheses never constitutes *proof* of their veracity. Hypothesis testing is probabilistic. There is always a possibility that observed relationships resulted from chance—that is, that a Type I error occurred. Researchers must be tentative about their results and about interpretations of them. Even when the results are in line with expectations, researchers should draw conclusions with restraint and should give due consideration to limitations identified in assessing the credibility of the results.

Example of corroboration of a hypothesis: Coleman (2007) used the Health Belief Model to guide his cross-sectional study of factors related to high-risk sexual behaviors in HIV-infected African American men. Consistent with the model, Coleman found (among other things) that self-efficacy about condom use was significantly related to condom use, and stated that self-efficacy and other factors "were observed to be key determinants of condom use during sexual activity" (p. 113).

This study is a good example of the challenges of interpreting findings in correlational studies. The researchers' interpretation was that self-efficacy was a factor that *determined* ("caused") whether an HIV-infected man would use a condom. This is a conclusion

supported by earlier research and consistent with a well-respected theory of health behavior. Yet nothing in the data rules out the possibility that a person's use of condoms *determined* self-efficacy, or that a third factor caused both condom use and higher self-efficacy. Coleman's interpretation is plausible, and even likely to be correct, but his cross-sectional design makes it difficult to rule out other explanations. A major threat to the internal validity of the inference in this study is temporal ambiguity.

Interpreting Nonsignificant Results

Nonsignificant results pose interpretative problems because statistical tests are geared toward disconfirmation of the null hypothesis. Failure to reject a null hypothesis can occur for many reasons, and the real reason is usually difficult to discern. The null hypothesis *could* actually be true, for example. A nonsignificant result could accurately reflect the absence of a relationship among research variables. On the other hand, the null hypothesis could be false, in which case a Type II error has been committed.

Retention of a false null hypothesis can result from a variety of methodologic problems, such as poor internal validity, an anomalous sample, a weak statistical procedure, or unreliable measures. In particular, failure to reject null hypotheses is often a consequence of insufficient power resulting from too small a sample size.

In any event, a retained null hypothesis should not be considered as proof of the *absence* of relationships among variables. *Nonsignificant results provide no evidence of the truth or the falsity of the hypothesis*. Interpreting the meaning of nonsignificant results can, however, be aided by considering such factors as sample size and effect size estimates.

Example of nonsignificant results: Griffin and colleagues (2007) hypothesized that nurses' stereotypes (based on patients' gender, race, and attractiveness) would influence nurses' pain treatment recommendations. The hypotheses were not supported (there was no evidence of stereotyping). The conclusion that stereotyping did not occur was bolstered by the fact that the sample was fairly large ($N = 334$), and nurses were blinded to the manipulation (child characteristics). Extremely low effect sizes offered additional support for concluding that stereotyping was absent.

Because statistical tests provide support for rejecting null hypotheses, they are not well suited for testing *actual* research hypotheses about the absence of relationships or about equivalence between groups. Yet, sometimes this is exactly what researchers want to do—and this is especially true in clinical situations in which the goal is to assess if one practice is as effective than another (an *equivalence trial*) or not less effective as another (a *noninferiority trial*). When the actual research hypothesis is null (i.e., a prediction of no group difference or no relationship), additional strategies must be used to provide supporting evidence. In particular, it is important to compute effect sizes and confidence intervals to show that the risk of a Type II error was small. There may also be clinical standards that can be used to corroborate that nonsignificant—but predicted—results are plausible. In noninferiority and equivalence trials, clinical parameters must be stipulated for undertaking a power analysis (da Silva et al., 2009).

Example of support for a hypothesized non-significant result: Gouchon and colleagues (2010) conducted a noninferiority trial to test that skin-to-skin contact between caesarean-delivered babies and their mothers did not result in worse outcomes than usual care in terms of the infants' body temperature. The mean temperature of both groups was nearly identical.

Interpreting Unhypothesized Significant Results

Unhypothesized significant results can occur in two situations. The first involves exploring relationships that were not considered during the design of the study. For example, in examining correlations among variables in the data set, a researcher might notice that two variables that were not central to the research questions were nevertheless significantly correlated—and interesting. To interpret serendipitous findings, it is wise to consult the literature to see if similar relationships had been previously observed.

Example of a serendipitous significant finding: Landis and colleagues (2009) conducted a descriptive correlational study to examine relationships among hunger, satiety, food cravings, caloric intake, and total amount of sleep in healthy adolescents. They unexpectedly found a significant relationship between increased *daytime* sleep and food-craving scores.

The second situation is more perplexing, and it does not happen often: obtaining results *opposite* to those hypothesized. For instance, a researcher might hypothesize that individualized teaching about AIDS risks is more effective than group instruction, but the results might indicate that group instruction was significantly better. Some researchers view such situations as awkward, but research should not be undertaken primarily to corroborate researchers' predictions, but rather to arrive at truthful evidence. Study results cannot be said to have "come out wrong" if they reflect the truth.

When significant findings are opposite to what was hypothesized, it is less likely that the methods are flawed than that the reasoning or theory is problematic. The interpretation of such findings should involve comparisons with other research, a consideration of alternative theories, and a critical scrutiny of the research methods.

Example of unhypothesized significant results: Peters and Templin (2008) tested new scales to measure blood pressure knowledge and self-care behaviors among African Americans. Although they found considerable evidence supporting the psychometric adequacy of their scales, one unexpected finding was that higher scores on the knowledge and self-care scales were associated with *higher* blood pressure. They speculated that the effects could reflect the fact that those with hypertension are more motivated to learn and do more about this health risk.

Interpreting Mixed Results

Interpretation is often complicated by *mixed results*: some hypotheses are supported by the data, but others are not. Or a hypothesis may be accepted with one measure of the dependent variable, but rejected with a different measure. When only some results run counter to a theoretical prediction, the research methods are the first aspect of the study deserving critical scrutiny. Differences in the validity and reliability of the various measures may account for such discrepancies, for example. On the other hand, mixed results may suggest that a theory needs to be qualified, or that certain constructs within the theory need to be reconceptualized. Mixed results sometimes present opportunities for making conceptual advances because efforts to make sense of disparate pieces of evidence may lead to a breakthrough.

In summary, interpreting the meaning of research results is a demanding task, but it offers the possibility of intellectual rewards. Interpreters must in essence play the role of scientific detectives, trying to make pieces of the puzzle fit together so that a coherent picture emerges.

Generalizability of the Results

Researchers are rarely interested in discovering relationships among variables for a specific group of people at a specific point in time. If a new nursing intervention is found to be successful, others will want to adopt it. Thus, an important interpretive question is whether the intervention will "work" or whether relationships will "hold" in other settings, with other people. Part of the interpretive process involves asking the question, "To what groups, environments, and conditions can the results of the study reasonably be applied?"

In interpreting the study with regard to the generalizability of the results, it is useful to consider our earlier discussion about proxies. For which higher-order constructs, which populations, which settings, or which versions of an intervention were the study operations good "stand-ins"?

Implications of the Results

Once you have reached conclusions about the credibility, precision, importance, meaning, and generalizability of the results, you are ready to think about their implications. You might consider the implications with respect to future research (What should other researchers working in this area do—what is the right "next step?") or theory development (What are the implications for nursing theory?). Finally, you should carefully consider the implications of the evidence for nursing practice. How do the results contribute to a base of evidence to improve nursing? Specific suggestions for implementing the results of the study in a real

nursing context are extremely valuable in the EBP process.

All of the dimensions of interpretation that we have discussed are critical in evidence-based nursing practice. With regard to generalizability, it may not be enough to ask a broad question about to whom the results could apply—you need to ask, are these results relevant to *my* particular clinical situation, or to a clinical situation of practicing nurses in my community?

➲ **TIP :** In interpreting your data, remember that others will be reviewing your interpretation with a critical and perhaps even a skeptical eye. The job of consumers is to make decisions about the credibility and utility of the evidence, which is likely to be affected by how much support you offer for the validity and meaning of your results.

CRITIQUING INTERPRETATIONS

Researchers offer their interpretation of the findings and discuss what the findings might imply for nursing in the discussion section of research reports. When critiquing a study, your own interpretation and inferences can be contrasted against those of the researchers.

As a reviewer, you should be wary if a discussion section fails to point out any limitations. Researchers are in the best position to detect and assess the impact of sampling deficiencies, practical constraints, data quality problems, and so on, and it is a professional responsibility to alert readers to these difficulties. Moreover, when researchers note methodologic shortcomings, readers have some confidence that these limitations were considered in interpreting the results. Of course, researchers are unlikely to note all relevant shortcomings of their own work. The task of reviewer is to develop independent interpretations and assessments of limitations, to challenge conclusions that do not appear to be warranted by the results, and to indicate how the study's evidence could have been enhanced.

In addition to comparing your interpretation with that of the researchers, your critique should

BOX 19.1 Guidelines for Critiquing Interpretations in Discussion Sections of Quantitative Research Reports

Interpretation of the Findings

1. Are all important results discussed?
2. Did the researchers discuss the limitations of the study and their possible effects on the credibility of the research evidence? In discussing limitations, were all key threats to the study's validity and biases noted? Did the interpretations take limitations into account?
3. What types of evidence were offered in support of the interpretation, and was that evidence persuasive? If results were "mixed," were possible explanations offered? Were results interpreted in light of findings from other studies?
4. Were any supplementary analyses undertaken to facilitate interpretation? If not, should they have been?
5. Did the researchers make any unwarranted causal inferences? Were alternative explanations for the findings considered? Were the rationales for rejecting these alternatives convincing?
6. Did the interpretation take into account the precision of the results and/or the magnitude of effects? Did the researchers distinguish between clinical and statistical significance?
7. Did the researchers discuss the generalizability of the findings? Did they draw any unwarranted conclusions about generalizability?

Implications of the Findings and Recommendations

8. Did the researchers discuss the study's implications for clinical practice ("clinical significance"), nursing theory, or future nursing research? Did they make specific recommendations?
9. If yes, are the stated implications appropriate, given the study's limitations and the magnitude of the effects—as well as evidence from other studies? Are there important implications that the report neglected to include?

also draw conclusions about the stated implications of the study. Some researchers make grandiose claims or offer unfounded recommendations on the basis of modest results. Some guidelines for evaluating researchers' interpretation and implications are offered in Box 19.1.

RESEARCH EXAMPLE

We conclude this chapter with an example of a study that provided considerable detail about their data management and analyses.

Study: Randomized clinical trial of a school-based academic and counseling program for older school-age students (Kintner & Sikorskii, 2009).

Statement of Purpose: The purpose of this feasibility study was to gather preliminary evidence about the efficacy of an academic and counseling program for older elementary students with asthma, in terms of cognitive, behavioral, psychosocial, and quality of life outcomes.

Method: The researchers used a two-group cluster randomized design with a sample of fourth- to sixth-grade students aged 9 to 12 years. Three schools were randomly assigned to receive the SHARP (Staying Healthy—Asthma Responsible and Prepared) program and two schools were assigned to a control group, in an effort to reduce contamination of treatments among students at a given school. A total of 66 students were included in the sample. Students in the SHARP program met weekly for 10 weeks during school hours to discuss asthma management. There was also a community component for family members, friends, and others. Data were collected at baseline and after the intervention for such outcomes as knowledge of asthma, asthma health behaviors, acceptance of asthma, participation in life activities, and illness severity.

Analyses: The researchers collected and managed their data using laptop computers: "The system included quality-control methods to restrict field ranges and values, to provide internal consistency checks, to prevent entry of erroneous data, and to track missing data" (p. 326). Virtually no missing data were found in completed surveys. There were, however, four dropouts (all in the intervention group) before the Time 2 data collection, and data for one control group member could not be used. Reasons for all participant loss were reported. The researchers noted that "an intention-to-treat approach was adopted for analysis" (p. 326). The researchers looked at distributions for all variables to assess data quality and evaluate whether assumptions for statistical tests had been met. Reliability coefficients were computed for all scales. The baseline characteristics of students in the two groups were compared to assess selection biases. Because the groups differed in terms of some baseline measures, baseline values were statistically controlled to estimate program effects. The researchers also compared the characteristics of those who completed the study and those who did not, and found no significant differences. Postintervention outcomes for the two groups were assessed using complex hierarchical models. The researchers computed adjusted mean scores, as well as effect size indexes, for all outcomes.

Results: Compared with students in the control group, students in the SHARP program had statistically significant improvements in asthma knowledge, use of risk reduction behaviors, and other outcomes, with sizeable effect sizes of *d* greater than .70. Moderate (but not statistically significant) effects (*d* between .30 and .50) were observed for two other outcomes.

Discussion: Here are a few excerpts from the Discussion section of this report:

"Evaluation of the SHARP Student and Community Components confirmed preliminary efficacy, with large effect sizes for statistically significant asthma knowledge, reasoning about asthma, use of risk reduction behaviors, and participation in life activities and medium effects for clinically significant use of episode management behaviors and acceptance of asthma in taking control and vigilance. A larger sample size is needed to reach statistical significance where observed effect sizes were medium. Clinical significance in scores with improvements more

than 30% warrants further testing with large samples . . . More research is needed to assess the impact of SHARP on lessening condition severity, use of healthcare services, and school or work absenteeism due to asthma symptoms" (pp. 328–239).

"All outcomes were derived from self-report of individuals participating in the intervention. Self-report measures have been found to contain inherent limitations . . . However, self-report measures capture personal dynamics, convey perceptions of experiences, have value, and are of interest to health researchers" (p. 329).

"Caution should be taken in generalizing findings to larger populations due to limited sample drawn from one moderate size Midwest community. Large sample sizes drawn from more diverse communities are needed to evaluate the efficacy and effect of the program fully" (p. 330).

SUMMARY POINTS

- Researchers who collect quantitative data typically progress through a series of steps in the analysis and interpretation of their data. Careful researchers lay out a data analysis plan in advance to guide that progress.
- Quantitative data typically must be **coded** into numerical values; codes need to be developed for legitimate data and for **missing values**. Decisions about coding and variable naming are documented in a **codebook**.
- **Data entry** is an error-prone process that requires verification and **data cleaning**. Cleaning involves checks for **outliers** (values that lie outside the normal range of values) and **wild codes** (codes that are not legitimate), and **consistency checks** (checks for internally consistent information).
- Steps must almost always be taken to evaluate missing data problems. Decisions on handling missing values must be based on the amount of missing data and how missing data are patterned (i.e., the extent to which missingness is random). Addressing missing data is especially important for undertaking **intention-to-treat analyses**.

- The three missing values patterns are: (1) **missing completely at random** (MCAR), which occurs when cases with missing values are just a random subsample of all cases in the sample; (2) **missing at random** (MAR), which occurs if missingness is related to other variables but *not* related to the value of the variable that has the missing values; and **missing not at random** (MNAR), a pattern in which the value of the variable that is missing is related to its missingness.
- Two basic missing values strategies involve **deletion** or **imputation**. Deletion strategies include deleting cases with missing values (i.e., **listwise deletion**), selective **pairwise deletion** of cases, or deleting variables with missing values. Imputation strategies include **mean substitution**, regression-based estimation of missing values, **expectation maximization (EM) imputation**, and **multiple imputation (MI)**, which is considered the "gold standard."
- Raw data entered onto a computer file often need to be transformed for analysis. Examples of **data transformations** include reversing the coding of items, recoding the values of a variable (e.g., for dummy variables), and transforming data to meet statistical assumptions (e.g., through logarithmic transformations).
- Before the main analyses can proceed, researchers usually undertake additional steps to assess data quality, such as evaluating scale reliability, examining distributions for anomalies or **extreme outliers** that are legitimate values, and analyzing the magnitude and direction of any biases.
- Sometimes peripheral analyses involve tests to determine whether **pooling** of participants is warranted, and tests for **cohort effects** or **ordering effects**.
- Once the data are fully prepared for substantive analysis, researchers should develop a formal analysis plan, to reduce the temptation to go on a "fishing expedition." One approach is to develop **table shells**, that is, fully laid-out tables without numbers in them.

- Supplementary statistical analyses (e.g., testing competing hypotheses or doing **sensitivity analyses**) can sometimes facilitate interpretation.
- The interpretation of quantitative research **results** (the outcomes of the statistical analyses) typically involves consideration of: (1) the credibility of the results, (2) precision of estimates of effects, (3) magnitude of effects, (4) underlying meaning of the results, (5) generalizability of results, and (6) implications for future research, theory development, and nursing practice.
- Inference is central to interpretation. The particulars of the study—especially the methodologic decisions made by researchers—affect the inferences that can be made about the correspondence between study results and "truth in the real world." A cautious and even skeptical outlook is appropriate in drawing conclusions about the credibility and meaning of study results.
- An assessment of a study's credibility can involve various approaches, one of which involves an evaluation of the degree of congruence between abstract constructs or idealized methods on the one hand, and the proxies actually used on the other. Credibility assessments can also involve a careful assessment of study rigor through an analysis of validity threats and various biases that could undermine the accuracy of the results. Corroboration (replication) of results, through either internal or external sources, is another approach in a credibility assessment.

STUDY ACTIVITIES

Chapter 19 of the *Resource Manual for Nursing Research: Generating and Assessing Evidence for Nursing Practice, 9th edition*, offers exercises and study suggestions for reinforcing concepts presented in this chapter. In addition, the following study questions can be addressed:

1. Read an article in a recent nursing research journal. Write out a brief interpretation of the

results based on the report's "Results" section and then compare your interpretation with that of the researchers.

2. Use the critiquing guidelines in Box 19.1 to critique the study used as the research example at the end of the chapter (Kintner & Sikorskii, 2009), referring to the full study as necessary.

⦿⦿⦿⦿⦿⦿⦿⦿⦿⦿⦿⦿⦿⦿⦿⦿⦿⦿⦿⦿⦿

STUDIES CITED IN CHAPTER 19

Coleman, C. (2007). Health beliefs and high-risk sexual behaviors among HIV-infected African American men. *Applied Nursing Research, 20,* 110–115.

Downe-Wamboldt, B., Butler, L., Melanson, P., Coulter, L., Singleton, J., Keefe, J., & Bell, D. (2007). The effects and expense of augmenting usual cancer clinic care with telephone problem-solving counseling. *Cancer Nursing, 30,* 441–453.

Gouchon, S., Gregori, D., Picotto, A., Patrucco, G., Nangeroni, M., & DiGiulio, P. (2010). Skin-to-skin contact after caesarean delivery. *Nursing Research, 59,* 78–84.

Griffin, R., Polit, D., & Byrnes, M. (2007). Stereotyping and nurses' treatment of children's pain. *Research in Nursing & Health, 30,* 655–666.

Groër, M., & Shleton, M. (2009). Exercise is associated with elevated proinflammatory cytokines in human milk. *Journal of Obstetric, Gynecologic, & Neonatal Nursing, 38,* 35–41.

Groom, M., Shannon, R., Chakravarthy, D., & Fleck, C. (2010). An evaluation of costs and effects of a nutrient-based skin care program as a component of prevention of skin tears in an extended convalescence center. *Journal of Wound, Ostomy, & Continence Nursing, 37,* 46–51.

Kim, H., Capezuti, E., Boltz, M., & Fairchild, S. (2009). The nursing practice environment and nurse-perceived quality of geriatric care in hospitals. *Western Journal of Nursing Research, 31,* 480–495.

Kintner, E., & Sikorskii, A. (2009). Randomized clinical trial of a school-based academic and counseling program for older school-age students. *Nursing Research, 58,* 321–331.

Landis, A., Parker, K., & Dunbar, S. (2009). Sleep, hunger, food cravings, and caloric intake in adolescents. *Journal of Nursing Scholarship, 41,* 115–123.

Mackereth, P., Booth, K., Hillier, V., & Caress, A. (2009). Reflexology and progressive muscle relaxation training for people with multiple sclerosis: A crossover trial. *Complementary Therapies in Clinical Practice, 15,* 14–21.

Minnick, A., & Needleman, J. (2009). Methodological issues in explaining maternal outcomes. *Western Journal of Nursing Research, 30,* 801–816.

Mullin, M., Roschkov, S., Jensen, L., Moore, G., & Smith, A. (2009). Sensations during removal of epicardial pacing wires after coronary bypass graft surgery. *Heart & Lung, 38,* 377–381.

Peters, R., & Templin, T. (2008). Measuring blood pressure knowledge and self-care behaviors of African Americans. *Research in Nursing & Health, 31,* 543–552.

Polit, D. F., London, A. S., & Martinez, J. M. (2001). *The health of poor urban women.* New York: MDRC (available at *www.mdrc.org*).

Shellman, J., Mokel, M., & Hewitt, N. (2009). The effects of integrative reminiscence on depressive symptoms in older African Americans. *Western Journal of Nursing Research, 31,* 772–786.

Methodologic and nonresearch references cited in this chapter can be found in a separate section at the end of the book.

PART 4

DESIGNING AND CONDUCTING QUALITATIVE STUDIES TO GENERATE EVIDENCE FOR NURSING

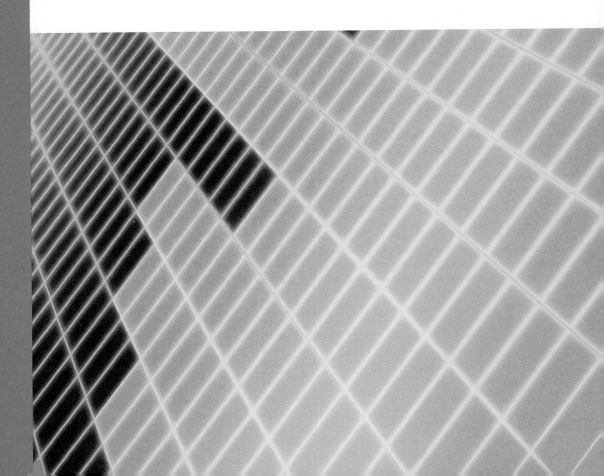

20 | Qualitative Research Design and Approaches

THE DESIGN OF QUALITATIVE STUDIES

Quantitative researchers specify a research design before collecting their data and rarely depart from that design once the study is underway. In qualitative research, by contrast, the design typically evolves over the course of the study. Decisions about how best to obtain data and whom to include are made as the study unfolds. Qualitative studies use an **emergent design** that evolves as researchers make ongoing decisions reflecting what has already been learned. An emergent design is not the result of sloppiness or laziness on the part of qualitative researchers, but rather a reflection of their desire to have the inquiry based on the realities and viewpoints of participants—realities and viewpoints that are not known at the outset (Lincoln & Guba, 1985).

Characteristics of Qualitative Research Design

Qualitative inquiry has been used in many different disciplines, and each has developed methods for addressing questions of particular interest. However, some characteristics of qualitative research design tend to apply across disciplines. In general, qualitative design:

- Often involves merging together various data collection strategies (i.e., triangulation)
- Is flexible, capable of adjusting to new information during the course of data collection
- Tends to be holistic, striving for an understanding of the whole
- Requires researchers to become intensely involved
- Requires researchers to become the research instrument
- Involves ongoing analysis of the data to formulate subsequent strategies and to determine when data collection is done.

With regard to the first characteristic, qualitative researchers often put together a complex array of data, derived from a variety of sources and using a variety of methods. This tendency has sometimes been described as *bricolage*, and the qualitative researcher has been referred to as a *bricoleur*, a person who "is adept at performing a large number of diverse tasks, ranging from interviewing to intensive reflection and introspection" (Denzin & Lincoln, 2000, p. 6).

Qualitative Design and Planning

Although design decisions are not specified in advance, qualitative researchers typically do advance planning that supports their flexibility in pursuing an emergent design. In the total absence of planning, design choices might actually be constrained. For example, researchers initially might anticipate a 6-month period for data collection, but may need to be prepared (financially and emotionally) to spend even longer periods of time in the field to pursue data collection opportunities that could not have been foreseen. In other words, qualitative researchers plan for broad contingencies that may be expected to pose decision opportunities once the study has begun. Advanced planning is especially useful with regard to the following:

- Selecting a broad framework or tradition (described in the next section) to guide design decisions
- Determining the maximum amount of time available for the study, given costs and other constraints
- Developing a broad data collection strategy, and identifying opportunities for enhancing trustworthiness (e.g., through triangulation)
- Collecting relevant site materials (e.g., maps, organizational charts, resource directories)
- Identifying the types of equipment that could aid in the collection and analysis of data in the field (e.g., audio and video recording equipment, computers, personal digital assistants)
- Identifying personal biases, views, and presuppositions vis-à-vis the phenomenon or the study site, as well as ideological stances (reflexivity)

Thus, qualitative researchers need to plan for a variety of circumstances, but decisions about how to deal with them must be resolved when the social context of time, place, and human interactions is better understood. By both allowing for and anticipating an evolution of strategies, qualitative researchers seek to make their research design responsive to the situation and to the phenomenon under study. In planning their qualitative studies, nurse researchers should also reflect on how the findings might be useful to practicing nurses and, if possible, seek opportunities to enhance the EBP-potential of the research.

➔ **TIP:** Davies and colleagues (2009) offered numerous excellent suggestions for planning a qualitative culture study and addressing numerous challenges that arise. One broad recommendation that is relevant to most qualitative research was to "allow generous time" (p. 14)—even more time than you might expect—for every phase of the project.

Qualitative Design Features

In Chapter 8, we discussed three design features that are relevant to qualitative research—comparisons, settings, and timeframes. Here we briefly review these features as a reminder of aspects of qualitative design that should be kept in mind in undertaking qualitative research.

Qualitative researchers seldom explicitly plan a comparative study (e.g., comparing children who have or do not have cancer). Nevertheless, patterns emerging in the data often suggest that certain comparisons are relevant and illuminating. Indeed, as Morse (2004b) noted in an editorial in *Qualitative Health Research*, "All description requires comparisons" (p. 1323). Inevitably in coding qualitative information and in evaluating whether categories are saturated, there is a need to compare "this" to "that." Morse pointed out that qualitative comparisons are often not dichotomous: "life is usually on a continuum" (p. 1324). Of course, comparisons sometimes *are* planned in qualitative studies (e.g., a comparison of nurses' and patients' perspectives about a phenomenon). Moreover, qualitative researchers can sometimes plan for the *possibility* of comparisons by selecting a richly diverse group of people as participants.

Example of comparisons in a qualitative study: Black and colleagues (2009) studied the phenomenon of becoming a mother of a medically fragile preterm infant. They wrote, "Each woman's experience had unique features; however, early in the analysis, differences emerged between experienced mothers and those with no previous mothering experience . . . Subsequently, within-group comparisons of experienced and inexperienced mothers were made to examine similarities and divergence in their experiences . . . Later, between-group comparisons were made" (p. 42).

In terms of research settings, qualitative researchers usually collect their data in real-world, naturalistic settings. And, whereas a quantitative researcher usually strives to collect data in one type of setting to maintain control over the environment (e.g., conducting all interviews in participants' homes), qualitative researchers may deliberately strive to study phenomena in a variety of natural contexts.

With regard to timeframes, qualitative research can be either cross-sectional, with one data collection point, or longitudinal, with multiple data collection points over an extended time period, to observe the evolution of some phenomenon. Sometimes qualitative researchers plan in advance for a longitudinal design, but, in other cases, the decision to study a phenomenon longitudinally may be made after preliminary data have been collected and analyzed.

Example of a longitudinal qualitative study: Sarenmalm and colleagues (2009) explored how women with recurrent cancer adjusted to their illness. To describe the evolution of the process, the researchers conducted between two and five interviews with 12 women over a 2-year period following the recurrence of their breast cancer.

Causality and Qualitative Research

In evidence hierarchies that rank evidence in terms of its ability to support causal inferences (e.g., Figure 2.1), qualitative inquiry is usually near the base—a fact that has led some to criticize the current EBP environment. The issue of causality, which has been controversial throughout the history of science, is especially contentious in qualitative research.

Some qualitative researchers think that causality is not an appropriate construct within the constructivist paradigm. For example, Lincoln and Guba (1985) devoted an entire chapter of their book to a critique of causality and argued that it should be replaced with a concept that they called *mutual shaping*. According to their view of mutual and simultaneous shaping, "Everything influences everything else, in the here and now. Many elements are implicated in any given action, and each element interacts with all of the others in ways that change them

all while simultaneously resulting in something that we . . . label as outcomes or effects" (p. 151).

Others, however, believe that causal explanation is not only a legitimate pursuit in qualitative research, but also that qualitative methods are especially well suited to understanding causal relationships. Huberman and Miles (1994) argued that qualitative studies "can look directly and longitudinally at the local processes underlying a temporal series of events and states, showing how these led to specific outcomes, and ruling out rival hypotheses" (p. 434).

In attempting to not only describe but to explain phenomena, qualitative researchers who undertake in-depth studies will inevitably reveal patterns and processes suggesting causal interpretations. These interpretations can be (and often are) subjected to more systematic testing using more controlled methods of inquiry.

OVERVIEW OF QUALITATIVE RESEARCH TRADITIONS

Despite some features common to many qualitative research designs, there is nevertheless a wide variety of approaches—but no readily agreed-upon classification system for these approaches. One useful system, as noted in Chapter 3, is to describe qualitative research according to disciplinary traditions. These traditions vary in their conceptualization of what types of questions are important to ask and in the methods they consider appropriate for answering them. This section provides an overview of several qualitative research traditions, some of which we have previously introduced.

The research traditions that have provided a theoretical underpinning for qualitative studies come primarily from the disciplines of anthropology, psychology, and sociology. As shown in Table 20.1, each discipline has tended to focus on one or two broad domains of inquiry.

The discipline of anthropology is concerned with human cultures. **Ethnography** (discussed more fully later in this chapter) is the primary research

TABLE 20.1	Overview of Qualitative Research Traditions		
DISCIPLINE	**DOMAIN**	**RESEARCH TRADITION**	**AREA OF INQUIRY**
Anthropology	Culture	Ethnography Ethnoscience (cognitive anthropology)	Holistic view of a culture Mapping of the cognitive world of a culture; a culture's shared meanings, semantic rules
Psychology/ philosophy	Lived experience	Phenomenology Hermeneutics	Experiences of individuals within their lifeworld Interpretations and meanings of individuals' experiences
Psychology	Behavior and events	Ethology Ecological psychology	Behavior observed over time in natural context Behavior as influenced by the environment
Sociology	Social settings	Grounded theory Ethnomethodology Semiotics	Social structural process within a social setting Manner by which shared agreement is achieved in social settings Manner by which people make sense of social interactions
Sociolinguistics	Human communication	Discourse analysis	Forms and rules of conversation
History	Past behavior, events, and conditions	Historical analysis	Description and interpretation of historical events

tradition in anthropology. Ethnographers study cultural patterns and experiences in a holistic fashion. **Ethnoscience** (sometimes referred to as **cognitive anthropology**) focuses on the cognitive world of a culture, with particular emphasis on the semantic rules and shared meanings that shape behavior. Cognitive anthropologists assume that a group's cultural knowledge is reflected in its language.

Example of an ethnoscientific study: Hirst (2002) used ethnoscientific methods to articulate a definition of resident abuse as perceived by nurses working in long-term care settings. She focused on the linguistic symbols and "folk terms" of the culture in long-term care institutions.

Phenomenology has its disciplinary roots in both philosophy and psychology. As noted in Chapter 3, phenomenology focuses on the meaning of lived experiences of humans. A closely related research tradition is **hermeneutics**, which uses lived experiences as a tool for better understanding the social, cultural, political, or historical context in which those experiences occur. Hermeneutic inquiry almost always focuses on meaning and interpretation—how socially and historically conditioned individuals interpret their world within their given context.

The discipline of psychology has several other qualitative research traditions that focus on *behavior*. Human **ethology**, sometimes described as the biology of human behavior, studies behavior as it evolves in its natural context. Human ethologists use primarily observational methods in an attempt to discover universal behavioral structures. Warnock and Allen (2003) have urged nurse researchers to consider using ethological methods and used neonatal pain to illustrate how ethology can be used to develop nursing knowledge and mid-range theory.

Example of an ethological study: Spiers (2006) used ethological methods to study pain-related interactions between patients and home-care nurses. Spiers analyzed micropatterns of videotaped communication in the patients' homes over multiple home-nurse visits.

Ecological psychology focuses on the influence of the environment on human behavior, and attempts to identify principles that explain the interdependence of humans and their environmental context. Viewed from an ecological context, people are affected by (and affect) a multilayered set of systems, including family, peer group, and neighborhood as well as the more indirect effects of healthcare and social services systems, and the larger cultural belief and value systems of the society in which individuals live.

Example of an ecological study: Robertson and colleagues (2007) used an ecological framework to study Latino construction workers' experiences with occupational noise and hearing protection. Their risk perceptions were examined with regard to environmental and personal factors.

Sociologists study the social world in which we live and have developed several research traditions of importance to qualitative researchers. The *grounded theory* tradition (elaborated upon later in this chapter) seeks to describe and understand key social psychological and structural processes in social settings.

Ethnomethodology seeks to discover how people make sense of their everyday activities and interpret their social worlds, so as to behave in socially acceptable ways. Within this tradition, researchers attempt to understand a social group's norms and assumptions that are so deeply ingrained that members no longer think about the underlying reasons for their behaviors.

Example of an ethnomethodologic study: Ozeki (2008) used an ethnomethodologic approach in studying transcultural stress among Japanese mothers living in the United Kingdom.

Symbolic interaction (or *interactionism*) is a sociological and social-psychological tradition with roots in American pragmatism and is sometimes associated with grounded theory research. As noted in Chapter 6, symbolic interaction focuses on the manner in which people make sense of social interactions and the interpretations they attach to social symbols, such as language. Symbolic interactionists sometimes use **semiotics**, which is the study of signs and their meanings. A sign is any entity or object that carries information (e.g., a diagram, map, or picture).

Example of a semiotic analysis: Giarelli (2006) did a semiotic analysis of the manifest and latent meanings in editorial cartoons published in the United States between 2001 and 2004 relating to cloning and stem cell research.

The domain of inquiry for sociolinguists is human communication. The tradition referred to as **discourse analysis** (sometimes called *conversation analysis*) seeks to understand the rules, mechanisms, and structure of conversations and texts. Discourse analysts seek to understand the action that a given kind of talk "performs." The data for discourse analysis often are transcripts from naturally occurring conversations, such as those between nurses and their patients. In discourse analysis, the texts are situated in their social, cultural, political, and historical context.

Example of a discourse analysis: Plumridge and colleagues (2009) used conversation analysis to examine the elements of partnership and collaboration between nurses and parents during children's vaccinations.

Finally, **historical research**—the systematic collection and critical evaluation of data relating to past occurrences—is a tradition that relies primarily on qualitative data. Nurses have used historical research methods to examine a wide range of phenomena in both the recent and more distant past.

Researchers in each of these traditions have developed methodologic strategies for the design and conduct of relevant studies. Thus, once a researcher has identified what aspect of the human experience is of greatest interest, there is typically a wealth of advice available about methods likely to be productive in designing and undertaking the study.

⮕ **TIP:** Sometimes a research report identifies more than one tradition as having provided the framework for a qualitative inquiry (e.g., a phenomenological study using the grounded theory method). Such "method slurring" (Baker et al., 1992) has been criticized because each research tradition has different intellectual assumptions and methodologic prescriptions. However, as noted by Nepal (2010), echoing some of the sentiments expressed in an editorial by Janice Morse (2009), mixed qualitative methods may be viable when "the researcher has ascertained, from the beginning . . ., that the research questions cannot be answered in their entirety unless and until there are two different qualitative methods used" (p. 281).

ETHNOGRAPHY

Ethnography involves the description and interpretation of cultural behavior. Ethnographies are a blend of a process and a product, fieldwork, and a written text. Fieldwork is the process by which the ethnographer comes to understand a culture, and the ethnographic text is how that culture is communicated and portrayed. Because culture is, in itself, not visible or tangible, it must be constructed through ethnographic writing. Culture is inferred from the words, actions, and products of members of a group.

Ethnographic research is sometimes concerned with broadly defined cultures (e.g., an Afghan village culture), in a **macroethnography**. Ethnographies often focus on more narrowly defined cultures in a **microethnography** or **focused ethnography**. Microethnographies are exhaustive, fine-grained studies of either small units in a group or culture (e.g., the culture of homeless shelters), or of specific activities in an organizational unit (e.g., how nurses communicate with children in an emergency department). An underlying assumption of the ethnographer is that every human group eventually evolves a culture that guides the members' view of the world and the way they structure their experiences.

Example of a focused ethnography:
Smallwood (2009) used a focused ethnographic approach to study the roles of nurses in the culture established in a cardiac assessment team in the United Kingdom. Analysis of data from interviews, observation, and a field journal revealed four main roles: gatekeeper, catalyst, diplomat, and specialist consultancy practice.

Ethnographers seek to learn from members of a cultural group—to understand their world view. Ethnographic researchers sometimes refer to "emic" and "etic" perspectives (terms from linguistics, i.e., phon*emic* versus phon*etic*). An **emic perspective** is the way the members of the culture envision their world—it is the insiders' view. The emic is the local language, concepts, or means of expression used by members of the group under study to characterize their experiences. The **etic perspective** is the outsiders' interpretation of the experiences of that culture; it is the language used by those doing the research to refer to the same phenomena. Ethnographers strive to acquire an emic perspective of a culture. Moreover, they strive to reveal **tacit knowledge**, information about the culture that is so deeply embedded in cultural experiences that members do not talk about it or may not even be consciously aware of it.

Ethnographers typically undertake extensive fieldwork to learn about a cultural group. Ethnographic research typically is labor intensive, requiring long periods (months or even years) in the field. Researchers usually strive to participate actively in cultural activities. The study of a culture requires a certain level of intimacy with members of the cultural group, and such intimacy can be developed only over time and by working directly with those members as active participants. The concept of **researcher as instrument** is frequently used by anthropologists to describe the significant role ethnographers play in analyzing and interpreting a culture.

Three broad types of information are usually sought by ethnographers: cultural behavior (what members of the culture do), cultural artifacts (what people make and use), and cultural speech (what people say). This implies that ethnographers rely on a wide variety of data sources, including observations, in-depth interviews, records, charts, and physical evidence such as photographs, diaries, and letters. Ethnographers typically use a **participant observation** strategy in which they make observations of the culture while participating in its activities. Ethnographers observe people day after day in their natural environments to observe behavior in a wide array of circumstances. Ethnographers also enlist the help of **key informants** to help them understand and interpret the events and activities being observed.

Some ethnographers undertake an **egocentric network analysis**, which focuses on the pattern of relationships and networks of individuals. Each person has his or her own network of relationships that are presumed to contribute to the person's behaviors and attitudes. In studying these networks, researchers develop lists of a person's network members (called *alters*) and seek to understand the scope and nature of interrelationships and social supports. Network data from such efforts are often quantified and analyzed statistically. Egocentric network analysis is used to understand features of personal networks, and has been used to explain such phenomena as longevity, coping with crisis, and risk taking.

Example of an egocentric network analysis: Kelley (2005) studied gendered approaches to elder care in a Caribbean village using an egocentric network analysis.

The product of ethnographic research usually is a rich and holistic description of the culture. Ethnographers also make interpretations of the culture, describing normative behavioral and social patterns. Among healthcare researchers, ethnography provides access to the health beliefs and health practices of a culture or subculture. Ethnographic inquiry can thus help to facilitate understanding of behaviors affecting health and illness.

In addition to written reports about ethnographic findings, ethnographers have recently used their research as the basis for performance ethnographies. **A performance ethnography** has been described as a scripted and staged re-enactment of ethnographically derived notes that reflect an interpretation of the culture. Denzin (2000) noted that "we inhabit a performance-based, dramaturgical culture. The dividing line between performance and audience blurs, and culture itself becomes a dramatic performance" (p. 903).

A rich array of ethnographic methods have been developed and cannot be fully explicated in this general textbook, but more information may be found in Atkinson and colleagues (2001), Fetterman (2010), and Gobo (2008). Three variants of ethnographic research (ethnonursing research, institutional ethnography, and auto-ethnography) are described here, and a fourth (critical ethnography) is described later in this chapter.

Ethnonursing Research

Many nurse researchers have undertaken ethnographic studies. Indeed, Leininger coined the phrase **ethnonursing research**, which she defined as "the study and analysis of the local or indigenous people's viewpoints, beliefs, and practices about nursing care behavior and processes of designated cultures" (1985, p. 38). In conducting an ethnonursing study, the investigator uses a broad theoretical framework to guide the research, such as Leininger's Theory of Culture Care.

Leininger and McFarland (2006) described a number of enablers to support researchers' efforts in conducting ethnonursing research. *Enablers* are ways to discover complex phenomena like human care. Some of her enablers include her Stranger–Friend Model, Observation–Participation–Reflection Model, and Acculturation Enabler Guide. The stranger–friend enabler guides researchers in mapping their progress and becoming more aware of their feelings, behaviors, and responses as they transition from stranger to trusted friend. The phases of Leininger's observation–participation–reflection enabler go from (1) primary observation and active listening, (2) primary observation with limited participation, (3) primary participation with continuing observations, to (4) primary reflection and reconfirmation of results with informants. The acculturation enabler guide was designed to aid researchers in assessing the degree of acculturation of a person or group with regard to the specific culture under study.

> **Example of an ethnonursing study:** Aga and colleagues (2009) conducted an ethnonursing study focusing on the conceptions of care among family caregivers of persons living with HIV/AIDS in Ethiopia. Four themes emerged using Leininger's phases of ethnonursing analysis: nourishing the ill family member while struggling with poverty, maintenance of cleanliness and hygiene of the ill family member and the surroundings, comforting, and sacrificing self to care for the relative with HIV/AIDS.

Institutional Ethnography

A type of ethnographic approach called **institutional ethnography** was pioneered by Dorothy Smith, a Canadian sociologist (1999). Institutional ethnography has been used in such fields as nursing, social work, and community health to study the organization of professional services, examined from the perspective of those who are clients or front-line workers. Institutional ethnography seeks to understand the social determinants of people's everyday experiences, especially institutional work processes. The focus in institutional ethnography is on social organization and institutional processes, and so research findings have the potential to play a role in organizational change.

> **Example of institutional ethnography:** Riley and Manias (2006) conducted an institutional ethnography to examine how time is controlled and governed in operating rooms through communication between nurses and doctors.

Autoethnography

Ethnographers are often "outsiders" to the culture under study. A type of ethnography that involves self-scrutiny (including study of groups or cultures to which researchers belong) is **autoethnography**, but other terms such as *insider research*, and *peer research* also have been used. Autoethnography offers numerous advantages, the most obvious being ease of access, ease of recruitment, and the ability to get particularly candid, in-depth data based on pre-established trust and rapport. Another potential advantage is the researcher's ability to detect subtle nuances that an outsider might miss or take months to uncover. A potential limitation, however, is the researcher's inability to be objective about group (or self) processes, which can result in unsuspected myopia about important but sensitive issues. Autoethnography demands that researchers maintain consciousness of their role and monitor their internal state and their interactions with others during the study. Various methodologic strategies have been developed for autoethnographic work and are summarized by Ellis and Bochner (2000).

> **Example of a performance autoethnography:** Schneider (2005) described an autoethnography that explored how mothers of adults with schizophrenia talk about their children. Schneider herself was the mother of a schizophrenic person. Her report presented the script for a performance autoethnography based on her research.

PHENOMENOLOGY

Phenomenology, rooted in a philosophical tradition developed by Husserl and Heidegger, is an approach to understanding people's everyday life experiences.

Phenomenological researchers ask: What is the *essence* of this phenomenon as experienced by these people and what does it *mean?* Phenomenologists assume there is an *essence*—an essential invariant structure—that can be understood, in much the same way that ethnographers assume that cultures exist. Essence is what makes a phenomenon what it is, and without which it would not be what it is. Phenomenologists investigate subjective phenomena in the belief that critical truths about reality are grounded in people's lived experiences. The phenomenological approach is especially useful when a phenomenon has been poorly defined or conceptualized. The topics appropriate to phenomenology are ones that are fundamental to the life experiences of humans; for health researchers, these include such topics as the meaning of suffering, the experience of domestic violence, and the quality of life with chronic pain.

Phenomenologists believe that lived experience gives meaning to each person's perception of a particular phenomenon. The goal of phenomenological inquiry is to understand lived experience and the perceptions to which it gives rise. Four aspects of lived experience of interest to phenomenologists are *lived space*, or spatiality; *lived body*, or corporeality; *lived time*, or temporality; and *lived human relation*, or relationality.

Phenomenologists view human existence as meaningful and interesting because of people's consciousness of that existence. The phrase **being-in-the-world** (or *embodiment*) is a concept that acknowledges people's physical ties to their world—they think, see, hear, feel, and are conscious through their bodies' interaction with the world.

In phenomenologic studies, in-depth conversations are the main data source, with researchers and informants as co-participants. Researchers help informants to describe lived experiences without leading the discussion. Through in-depth conversations, researchers strive to gain entrance into the informants' world, to have full access to their experiences as lived. Multiple interviews or conversations are sometimes needed. Typically, phenomenological studies involve a small number of study participants—often 10 or fewer. For some phenomenological researchers, the inquiry includes not only gathering information from informants, but also efforts to experience the phenomenon through participation, observation, and introspective reflection.

Phenomenologists share their insights in rich, vivid reports. A phenomenological text describing study results should help readers "see" something in a different way that enriches their understanding of experiences. Van Manen (1997) warned that if a phenomenological text is flat and boring, it "loses power to break through the taken-for-granted dimensions of everyday life" (p. 346). A wealth of resources is available on phenomenological methods. Interested readers may wish to consult such classic sources as Giorgi (1985, 2005), Colaizzi (1973, 1978), or Van Manen (1990).

There are several variants and methodologic interpretations of phenomenology. The two main schools of thought are descriptive phenomenology and interpretive phenomenology (hermeneutics). Lopez and Willis (2004) provided a useful discussion about the need to differentiate the two and laid out underlying philosophical assumptions in nursing studies.

Descriptive Phenomenology

Descriptive phenomenology was developed first by Husserl (1962), who was primarily interested in the question: What do we know as persons? His philosophy emphasized descriptions of human experience. Descriptive phenomenologists insist on the careful description of ordinary conscious experience of everyday life—a description of "things" as people experience them. These "things" include hearing, seeing, believing, feeling, remembering, deciding, evaluating, and acting.

Descriptive phenomenological studies often involve the following four steps: bracketing, intuiting, analyzing, and describing. **Bracketing** is the process of identifying and holding in abeyance preconceived beliefs and opinions about the phenomenon under study. Bracketing can never be achieved totally, but researchers strive to bracket out the world and any presuppositions in an effort to confront the data in pure form. Bracketing is an iterative process that involves preparing, evaluating, and providing systematic ongoing feedback about the effectiveness of the bracketing. Phenomenological researchers (as well as other qualitative researchers) often maintain a **reflexive journal** in their efforts to bracket. Ahern (1999) provided 10 tips to help qualitative researchers with bracketing through notes in a reflexive journal:

1. Make note of interests that, as a researcher, you may take for granted.
2. Clarify your personal values and identify areas in which you know you are biased.
3. Identify areas of possible role conflict.
4. Recognize gatekeepers' interest and make note of the degree to which they are favorably or unfavorably disposed toward your research.
5. Identify any feelings you have that may indicate a lack of neutrality.
6. Describe new or surprising findings in collecting and analyzing data.

7. Reflect on and profit from methodologic problems that occur during your research.
8. After data analysis is complete, reflect on how you write up your findings.
9. Reflect on whether the literature review is truly supporting your findings, or whether it is expressing the similar cultural background that you have.
10. Consider whether you can address any bias in your data collection or analysis by interviewing a participant a second time or reanalyzing the transcript in question.

Intuiting, the second step in descriptive phenomenology, occurs when researchers remain open to the meanings attributed to the phenomenon by those who have experienced it. Phenomenological researchers then proceed to the analysis phase (i.e., extracting significant statements, categorizing, and making sense of the essential meanings of the phenomenon). Chapter 23 provides further information regarding the analysis of data collected in phenomenological studies. Finally, the descriptive phase occurs when researchers come to understand and define the phenomenon.

Example of a descriptive phenomenological study: Flinck and Paavilainen (2010) studied women's perceptions of their own violent behavior in heterosexual partnerships. They noted that their approach involved "bracketing our preunderstandings and meeting the phenomenon with open minds" (p. 309). Their goal was one of "standing before an experience with an attitude of unknowing so that different possibilities could emerge" (p. 309).

Interpretive Phenomenology

Heidegger, a student of Husserl, moved away from his professor's philosophy into **interpretive phenomenology** or hermeneutics. To Heidegger (1962), the critical question is: What is *being*? He stressed interpreting and understanding—not just describing—human experience. His premise is that the lived experience is inherently an interpretive process. Heidegger argued that hermeneutics is a basic characteristic of human existence. Indeed, the term hermeneutics refers to the art and philosophy of interpreting the

meaning of an object (such as a *text*, work of art, and so on). The goals of interpretive phenomenological research are to enter another's world and to discover the practical wisdom, possibilities, and understandings found there.

Gadamer (1976), another influential interpretive phenomenologist, described the interpretive process as a circular relationship known as the **hermeneutic circle** where one understands the whole of a text (e.g., a transcribed interview) in terms of its parts and the parts in terms of the whole. In his view, researchers enter into a dialogue with the text, in which the researcher continually questions its meaning.

One distinction between descriptive and interpretive phenomenology is that in an interpretive phenomenological study, bracketing does not necessarily occur. For Heidegger, it was not possible to bracket one's being-in-the-world. Hermeneutics presupposes prior understanding on the part of the researcher. Gearing (2004), who developed a typology of bracketing, described one type as *reflexive bracketing*—in which researchers attempt to identify internal suppositions to facilitate greater transparency, but without bracketing them out—as a tool for hermeneutic inquiry. Interpretive phenomenologists ideally approach each interview text with openness—they must be open to hearing what it is the text is saying. As Heidegger (1971) stated, "We never come to thoughts. They come to us" (p. 6).

Example of an interpretive phenomenological study: Ellett and colleagues (2009) studied fathers' experiences living with a colicky infant using interpretive phenomenology. In-depth interviews with 10 fathers of colicky infants were conducted. The overall experience reported was one of "falling into and arising from the crying abyss together as a family" (p. 164).

Interpretive phenomenologists, like descriptive phenomenologists, rely primarily on in-depth interviews with individuals who have experienced the phenomenon of interest, but they may go beyond a traditional approach to gathering and analyzing data. For example, interpretive phenomenologists sometimes augment their understandings of the phenomenon through an analysis of supplementary texts, such as novels, poetry, or other artistic expressions— or they use such materials in their conversations with study participants. Guidance in undertaking a hermeneutic phenomenological nursing study is offered by Cohen and colleagues (2000).

> **Example of a hermeneutic study using artistic expression:** Lauterbach (2007) studied the phenomenon of maternal mourning over the death of a wished-for-baby. She increased her "attentive listening" to this phenomenon by turning to examples of infant death experiences illustrated in the arts, literature, and poetry. For example, she included a poem written by Robert Frost on home burial for an infant death. She also explored cemeteries to discover memorial art in babies' gravestones. She used the examples of memorial art and of literature to validate the themes of mothers' experiences in her research.

In several recent health studies, researchers have cited the work of a group of psychological phenomenologists, who have described an approach called **interpretive phenomenological analysis** or **IPA** (Smith and colleagues, 2009). The focus of IPA is on the subjective experiences of people—their *lifeworld*. Studying individuals' experiences requires interpretation on the part of the researcher and the participant because it is not possible to directly access a person's lifeworld. There are three key principles to IPA: (1) it investigates the phenomenon of experience of a person, (2) it requires intense interpretation and engagement with the data obtained from the person, and (3) it is examined in detail.

➲ TIP: As Mackey (2005) has pointed out, nurse researchers undertaking interpretive phenomenological studies should fully understand the philosophical and methodologic underpinnings of this tradition so that the results will be coherent. The same caution is true for other qualitative traditions, and we urge you to read original sources before undertaking a study.

The Parse Phenomenological-Hermeneutic Research Method

Many nurse researchers use an approach that has been formulated by Rosemary Parse (2001), based on her Theory of Human Becoming. Parse's approach has elements of both phenomenology and hermeneutics. The aim of Parse's research method is to uncover the meaning of universal human health experiences by studying descriptions of people's experiences. The data are interpreted through the lens of Parse's theory. Parse's research methods consist of three processes: dialogical engagement, extraction-synthesis, and heuristic interpretation (Parse, 2001).

Dialogical engagement, the first process, is the data-gathering process. Parse stressed that this is not an interview but a unique dialogue where the researcher is a true presence with the participant, who is asked to talk about the experience under study. The second process calls for *extraction-synthesis* during which the descriptions are moved out of the participant's language into the language of science, a higher level of abstraction. The six steps in her extraction-synthesis process include the following:

a. Constructing a story that captures core ideas about the phenomenon from each person's dialogue.

b. Extracting and synthesizing *essences* from participants' descriptions. Essences are succinct expressions of the core ideas about the phenomenon.

c. Synthesizing and extracting essences as conceptualized in the researcher's language at a higher level of abstraction.

d. Formulating a *proposition* from each participant's essences. A proposition is a nondirectional statement conceptualized by joining core ideas of the essences that arise from the participant's description in the researcher's language.

e. Extracting and synthesizing *core concepts* from the propositions of all participants. Core concepts are ideas that capture the central meaning of the propositions.

f. Synthesizing a *structure* of the lived experience from the core concepts. A structure involves a conceptualization in which the researcher joins the core concepts.

Heuristic interpretation, the third and final process, entails structural transposition and conceptual integration. By means of structural transposition, the structure of the description of the experience is moved to a higher level of abstraction. Finally, the structure of the experience is connected with the concepts of Parse's human becoming theory through conceptual integration.

Example of Parse's phenomenological method: Naef and Bournes (2009) investigated the lived experience of waiting. Eleven persons who were waiting for a lung transplant participated in the study and shared their experiences. Using the three processes of Parse's method, the central finding was that "the lived experience of waiting is arduous constraint arising with anticipating the cherished in fortifying engagements" (p. 147).

GROUNDED THEORY

Grounded theory, an important method for the study of nursing phenomena, has contributed to the development of many middle-range nursing theories. Grounded theory was formulated in the 1960s as a systematic method of qualitative inquiry by two sociologists, Glaser and Strauss (1967). An early grounded theory study (Glaser & Strauss, 1965) focused on dying in hospitals.

Grounded theory tries to account for actions in a substantive area from the perspective of those involved. Grounded theory researchers seek to understand actions by focusing on the main concern or problem that the individuals' behavior is designed to resolve (Glaser, 1998). The manner in which people resolve this main concern is called the **core variable**. One type of core variable is called a **basic social process (BSP)**. The goal of grounded theory is to discover this main concern and the basic social process that explains how people continually resolve it. The main concern must be discovered from the data.

Conceptualization is a key aspect of grounded theory (Glaser, 2003). Grounded theory researchers generate emergent conceptual categories and their properties and integrate them into a substantive theory grounded in the data. Through this conceptual process, the generated grounded theory represents

an abstraction based on participants' actions and their meanings. The grounded theorist uncovers and names latent patterns (categories) from the participants' accounts. Glaser (2003) emphasized that concepts transcend time, place, and person. "In grounded theory, behavior is a pattern that a person engages in; it is not the person. People are not categorized, behavior is" (p. 53).

Grounded theory methods constitute an entire approach to the conduct of field research. For example, a study that follows Glaser and Strauss's precepts does not begin with a focused research problem; the problem emerges from the data. In a grounded theory study, both the research problem and the process used to resolve it are discovered.

A fundamental feature of grounded theory research is that data collection, data analysis, and sampling of participants occur simultaneously. The grounded theory process is recursive: Researchers collect data, categorize them, describe the emerging central phenomenon, and then recycle earlier steps. In-depth interviews and observation are the most common data source in grounded theory studies, but other data sources such as documents may also be used.

A procedure called **constant comparison** is used to develop and refine theoretically relevant categories. Categories elicited from the data are constantly compared with data obtained earlier so that commonalities and variations can be determined. As data collection proceeds, the inquiry becomes increasingly focused on emerging theoretical concerns. Data analysis in a grounded theory framework is described in greater depth in Chapter 23.

Example of a grounded theory study: Kohara and Inoue (2010) used a grounded theory approach to study the decision-making process in patients considering participation in cancer phase I clinical trials. Using data from both interviews and observations, the researchers identified the core problem as "searching for a way to live to the end."

Like most theories, a grounded theory is modifiable as the researcher (or other researchers) collect new data. Modification is an ongoing process and is the method by which theoretical completeness is enhanced (Glaser, 2001). As more data are found and more qualitative studies are published in the substantive area, the grounded theory can be modified to accommodate new or different dimensions.

Example of a modification of a grounded theory study: In 2007, Beck first modified her 1993 grounded theory study, "Teetering on the Edge," which was a substantive theory of postpartum depression. Five years later, Beck (2012) again modified her grounded theory to include 17 qualitative studies of postpartum depression in other cultures published after the first modification. The results from these 17 transcultural studies were compared with the findings from her 2007 modification. Maximizing differences among comparative groups is a powerful method for enhancing theoretical properties and extending the theory.

TIP: Glaser and Strauss (1967) distinguished two types of grounded theory: substantive and formal. **Substantive theory** is grounded in data on a specific substantive area, such as postpartum depression. It can serve as a springboard for **formal grounded theory**, which is at a higher level of conceptualization and is abstract of time, place, and persons. The goal of formal grounded theory is not to discover a new core variable but to develop a theory that goes beyond the substantive grounded theory and extends the general implications of the core variable. Kearney (1998) likened formal grounded theory to ready-to-wear clothing, in contrast to substantive grounded theory, which is personally tailored.

Alternate Views of Grounded Theory

In 1990, Strauss and Corbin published what was to become a controversial book, *Basics of Qualitative Research: Grounded Theory Procedures and Techniques.* The authors stated that the book's purpose was to provide beginning grounded theory researchers with basic procedures involved for building theory at the substantive level.

Glaser, however, disagreed with some of the procedures advocated by Strauss (his original coauthor) and Corbin (a nurse researcher). Glaser published a rebuttal in 1992, *Emergence versus Forcing: Basics of Grounded Theory Analysis.* Glaser believed that Strauss and Corbin developed a method that is not grounded theory but rather what he called

"full conceptual description." According to Glaser, the purpose of grounded theory is to generate concepts and theories about their relationships that explain, account for, and interpret variation in behavior in the substantive area under study. *Conceptual description,* in contrast, is aimed at describing the full range of behavior of what is occurring in the substantive area, "irrespective of relevance and accounting for variation in behavior" (Glaser, 1992, p. 19). In Corbin and Strauss' latest edition (2008), they stated that they use grounded theory "in a more generic sense to denote theoretical constructs derived from qualitative analysis of data" (p. 1).

Nurse researchers have conducted grounded theory studies using both the original Glaser and Strauss and the Strauss and Corbin approaches. Heath and Cowley (2004) provided a comparison of the two approaches. We describe differences between the two in greater detail in Chapter 23.

Example of Strauss and Corbin's grounded theory methods: In their study of daughters advocating for a parent with dementia in a Canadian long-term care facility, Legault and Ducharme (2009) used Corbin and Strauss' grounded theory approach. Analysis revealed that daughters' advocacy role centered around three processes: developing trust in the care setting, integrating of the setting, and evaluating quality of care.

Constructivist Grounded Theory

Strauss and Glaser had different training and backgrounds. Strauss, trained at the University of Chicago, had a background in symbolic interactionism and pragmatist philosophy. Glaser, by contrast, came from a tradition of positivism and quantitative methods at Columbia University. In one of Glaser's (2005) later publications, in which he discussed the takeover of grounded theory by symbolic interaction, he argued that "grounded theory is a general inductive method possessed by no discipline or theoretical perspective or data type" (p. 141).

In recent years, an approach called **constructivist grounded theory** has emerged. A leading advocate is sociologist Kathy Charmaz, who has sought to bring the Chicago School antecedents of grounded theory into the forefront again. "Returning to the pragmatist foundation encourages us to construct an interpretive rendering of the worlds we study rather than an external reporting of events and statements" (Charmaz, 2006, p. 184). Charmaz (2000) viewed Glaser and Strauss' grounded theory as being based in the positivist tradition. Her position is that what is missing from their more objective grounded theory method is the researcher's influence on the data collected and analyzed and interactions between the researcher and participants. Charmaz (2006) also placed Strauss and Corbin's (1998) version of grounded theory in a positivist tradition.

In Charmaz's approach, the developed grounded theory is viewed as an interpretation. The data collected and analyzed are acknowledged to be constructed from shared experiences and relationships between the researcher and the participants. A grounded theory "depends on the researcher's view; it does not and cannot stand outside of it" (p. 130). Reflexivity of both the researcher's own interpretations and the interpretations of the participants is important. Data and analyses are viewed as social constructions.

Example of a constructivist grounded theory: Kean (2010) used constructivist grounded theory methods to explore the experience of families of brain-injured ICU patients. Data from nine family interviews revealed that "ambiguous loss" reflects the loss of a family member who is physically present but psychologically absent.

➡ **TIP:** Beginning qualitative researchers should be aware that a grounded theory study is a much lengthier and more complex process than a phenomenological study. This may be an important consideration if there are constraints in the amount of time that can be devoted to a study.

HISTORICAL RESEARCH

Historical research is the systematic collection, critical evaluation, and interpretation of historical evidence—that is, data relating to past occurrences. In general, historical research is undertaken to answer questions about causes, effects, or trends in past events that may shed light on present behaviors or practices. Historians seek to explain why events happen. An understanding of contemporary nursing theories, practices, or issues can often be enhanced by a study of phenomena in the past. Historical data are usually qualitative, but quantitative data are sometimes used (e.g., historical census data).

Historical research can take many forms. For example, many nurse researchers have undertaken *biographical histories* that study the lives and contributions of individuals, such as nursing leaders. Currently, some historians are focusing on the experiences of the ordinary person, often studying such issues as gender, race, and class. Other historical researchers undertake *social histories* that focus on a particular period in attempts to understand prevailing values that may have helped to shape subsequent developments. Still others undertake *intellectual histories*, where historical ideas or ways of thinking are scrutinized. *Technological histories* are another form that has emerged recently in nursing (Sandelowski, 1997).

Historical research should not be confused with a review of the literature about historical events. Like other types of research, historical inquiry has as its goal discovering *new* knowledge, not summarizing existing knowledge. One important difference between historical research and a literature review is that historical researchers, in addition to being guided by specific questions focused on explaining and interpreting past events or conditions, are often guided by a theoretical orientation or ideology (e.g., feminism). Social, cultural, and policy frameworks emerged in the 20th century (Buck, 2008). Buck, for example, used a combination of social and policy history frameworks for her research on the American hospice movement.

After research questions are developed, researchers must ascertain what types of data are available. Historical researchers typically devote considerable effort to identifying and evaluating data sources on events and situations that occurred in the past.

Collecting Historical Data

Data for historical research are usually in the form of written records: diaries, letters, notes, newspapers, minutes of meetings, medical or legal documents, and so on. Nonwritten materials may also be of interest. For example, physical remains and objects are potential sources of information. Visual materials, such as photographs and films, are forms of data, as are audio materials, such as records and tapes. In some cases, it is possible to conduct interviews with people who participated in historical events (e.g., nurses who served in the Vietnam War).

Many historical materials are difficult to obtain and, in many cases, have been discarded. Historically significant materials are not always conveniently indexed by subject or author. The identification of appropriate historical materials usually requires a considerable amount of time, effort, and detective work. Fortunately, there are several archives of historical nursing documents, such as the collections at various universities. The website of the American Association for the History of Nursing provides information about archives in the United States and several other countries (*www.aahn.org*). Useful sources for identifying other archives in the United States include the *National Inventory of Documentary Sources in the United States* and the *Directory of Archives and Manuscript Repositories in the United States*.

Example of nursing archives: The Archives of Nursing Leadership are housed in the Thomas J. Dodd Research Center at the University of Connecticut. The archives include papers and records of Connecticut organizations that support nursing and personal papers of people who contributed significantly to nursing in Connecticut. Letters written by Ella Louise Wolcott, a Connecticut native who was a nurse during the Civil War, are in the Josephine Dolan Collection within the archives.

◆ TIP: Archives contain unpublished materials that are accessed through **finding aids**, resources that tell researchers what is in the archive. Archival materials do not circulate; researchers are almost always required to use the material on site. Typically, because of the fragile nature of the material, it cannot be photocopied, so researchers must take detailed notes (laptop computers are invaluable). Sometimes gloves are required when touching original materials. Access to archives may be limited to researchers who present a description of a proposed project to archivists.

Historical materials are classified as either primary or secondary sources. A **primary source** is first-hand information, such as original documents, relics, or artifacts. Examples are diaries and writings of historically important nurses, minutes of American Nurses Association meetings, and so forth. Primary source documents are authored by people directly *involved* in a focal event. Primary sources represent the most direct link with historical events or situations: Only the narrator (in the case of written materials) intrudes between original events and the historical researcher. Multiple primary sources are usually needed for comparison.

Secondary sources are second- or third-hand accounts of historical events or experiences. For example, textbooks, other reference books, and newspaper articles are secondary sources. Secondary sources, in other words, are discussions of events written by individuals who did not participate in them, but are summarizing or interpreting primary source materials. Secondary sources may be historical (e.g., newspaper accounts contemporaneous with the events under study), or more modern interpretations of past events.

Primary sources should be used whenever possible in historical research. The further removed from the historical event the information is, the less reliable, objective, and comprehensive the data are likely to be. However, secondary sources can be useful in identifying primary sources. It is particularly important in reading secondary source material to pay careful attention to footnotes, which often provide important clues about primary sources. Secondary sources also provide context for evaluating events.

Example of primary and secondary sources: Leifer and Glass (2008) studied nurses' involvement in mass disaster preparations during the Cold War era, focusing on the role of Harriet Werley and the Army Nurse Corps. The researchers described their sources as follows: "Primary sources included memos, speeches, letters, reports, photos, and publication in the Harriet H. Werley papers at the Golda Meir Library, University of Wisconsin-Milwaukee. Secondary sources included professional and popular literature regarding Werley, the ANC, and Army Medical Service; nursing research; and disaster planning in the Cold War era. Werley's publications from 1941 to 1964 were also studied. Other materials were obtained at the Walter Reed Army Medical Center Library in Washington, DC" (p. 238).

One issue that needs consideration in historical research conducted in the United States is the effect of the Health Insurance Portability and Accountability Act (HIPAA) of 1996. HIPAA has resulted in the creation of new barriers between nurse historians and archival resources (Lusk & Sacharski, 2005). Historians face potential restrictions to accessing collections. These access restrictions vary from archive to archive. In addition to problems of access, nurse historians may lose some of the context for their historical analysis if individual identities are protected. Nurse historians may also face constraints on their ability to use photographs, such as images of patients. Researchers conducting historical research must gain permission to access patient records from, for example, the 18th century, in the same way as those attempting to gain access from current records in the beginning of the 21st century. Waivers of authorization are options that may be obtained from IRBs. Lusk and Sacharski noted that HIPAA'a privacy rule was not developed with historical research in mind, and so areas of confusion need to be clarified.

Evaluating Historical Data

Historical evidence is subjected to two types of evaluation, external and internal criticism. **External criticism** concerns the data's authenticity. For example, a nurse historian might have a diary presumed to be written by Dorothea Dix. External criticism would involve asking such questions as: Is this the handwriting of Ms. Dix? Is the diary's paper of the right age? Are the writing style and ideas expressed consistent with her other writings? Various scientific techniques are available to assess the age of materials, such as x-ray and radioactive procedures. Other problems may be less easy to detect. For example, there is the possibility that material may have been written by a ghostwriter, that is, by someone other than the person of interest. There are also potential problems of mechanical errors associated with transcriptions, translations, or typed versions of historical materials.

Internal criticism of historical data refers to an evaluation of the worth of the evidence. The focus of internal criticism is not on the physical aspects of the materials but on their content. The key issue is the accuracy or truth of the data. For example, researchers must question whether a writer's representations of historical events are unbiased. It may also be appropriate to ask if a document's author was in a position to make a valid report of an event or occurrence, or whether the writer was competent as a recorder of fact. Evidence bearing on the accuracy of historical data comes from comparisons with other people's accounts of the same event, evaluation of *when* the document was produced (reports of events or situations tend to be more accurate if they are written immediately after the event), and an assessment of the writers' biases and competence to record events authoritatively and accurately.

➲ **TIP:** Tuchman (1994) offered this useful advice: "Ask questions of all data, primary and secondary sources. Do not assume anything about the data is 'natural,' inevitable, or even true. To be sure, a datum has a physical presence: One may touch the page . . . one has located. But that physical truth may be radically different from the interpretive truth . . . " (p. 321).

Analyzing and Interpreting Historical Data

In historical research, data analysis and data collection are usually ongoing, concurrent activities. The analysis of historical data is broadly similar to other approaches to qualitative analysis (see Chapter 23), in that researchers search for themes. In historical research, however, the thematic analysis is often guided by underlying theoretical frameworks. Within the selected framework, researchers concentrate on particular issues present in the data.

Historical research is usually interpretive. Historical researchers try to describe what happened, and also how and why it happened. Relationships between events and ideas, between people and organizations, are explored and interpreted within their historical context and within the context of new viewpoints about what is historically significant. Resources available for those interested in undertaking historical nursing research include Lewenson (2003) and Lundy (2012).

OTHER TYPES OF QUALITATIVE RESEARCH

Qualitative studies often can be characterized in terms of the disciplinary research traditions discussed in the previous section. However, several other important types of qualitative research also deserve mention. This section discusses qualitative research that is not associated with any particular discipline.

Case Studies

Case studies are in-depth investigations of a single entity (or small number of entities), which could be an individual, family, group, institution, community, or other social unit. In a case study, researchers obtain a wealth of descriptive information and may examine relationships among different phenomena, or may examine trends over time. Case study researchers attempt to analyze and understand issues that are important to the history, development, or circumstances of the entity under study.

One way to think of a case study is to consider what is center stage. In most studies, whether qualitative or quantitative, a certain phenomenon or variable (or set of variables) is the core of the inquiry. In a case study, the *case* itself is central. As befits an intensive analysis, the focus of case studies is typically on understanding *why* an individual thinks, behaves, or develops in a particular manner rather than on *what* his or her status, progress, or actions are. It is not unusual for probing research of this type to require detailed study over a considerable period. Data are often collected that relate not only to the person's present state, but also to past experiences and situational factors relevant to the problem being examined.

There are four basic types of designs for case studies: single-case, holistic; single-case, embedded; multiple-case, holistic; and multiple-case, embedded (Yin, 2009). A **single-case study** is an appropriate design when (1) it is a critical case in testing a well-formulated theory, (2) it represents an extreme or unique case, (3) it is a representative or typical case, (4) it is a revelatory case, and (5) it is a longitudinal case. A **multiple-case design** is a study that involves more than a single case. Single and multiple case studies can be either holistic or embedded. In a **holistic design**, the global nature of a case—be it an individual, community, or organization—is examined. An **embedded design** involves more than one unit of analysis. Attention is given to subunits. A wide variety of data can be used in case studies, including data from interviews, observations, documents, and artifacts.

A distinction is sometimes drawn between an intrinsic and instrumental case study. In an *intrinsic case study*, researchers do not have to select the case. For instance, an evaluation of the process of implementing an innovation is often a case study of a particular institution; the "case" is a given. In an *instrumental case study*, researchers begin with a research question or problem, and seek out a case that offers illumination. The aim of such a case study is to use the case to understand a phenomenon of interest. In such a situation, a case is usually selected not because it is typical, but rather because it can maximize what can be learned about the phenomenon (Stake, 1995). Case studies can also be layered, which involves having a large case study built out of smaller ones (Patton, 2002).

Although understanding a particular case is the central concern of case studies, they are sometimes a useful way to explore phenomena that have not been rigorously researched. The information obtained in case studies can be used to develop hypotheses to be tested more rigorously in subsequent research. The intensive probing that characterizes case studies often leads to insights concerning previously unsuspected relationships. Furthermore, case studies may serve the important role of clarifying concepts or of elucidating ways to capture them.

➲ TIP : Sometimes thematic maps or models are created in case study research to help understand and interpret the case's experiences. For example, in Donna Zucker's case study of two men with coronary heart disease (CHD), creating a map "contributed to my ability to visualize the *aha* necessary to make meaning of Bernie's and Ed's experiences" (Hunter et al., 2002, p. 392).

The greatest strength of case studies is the depth that is possible when a limited number of individuals, institutions, or groups are being investigated. Case studies provide researchers with opportunities of having an intimate knowledge of a person's condition, thoughts, actions (past and present), intentions, and environment. On the other hand, this same strength is a potential weakness because researchers' familiarity with the person or group may make objectivity more difficult. Perhaps the biggest concern about case studies is generalizability: If researchers discover important relationships, it is difficult to know whether the same relationships would occur with others. However, case studies can often play a critical role in challenging generalizations based on other types of research.

It is important to recognize that case study *research* is not simply anecdotal descriptions of a particular incident or patient, such as a case report. Case study research is a disciplined process and typically requires an extended period of data collection. Two excellent resources for further reading on case study methods are the books by Yin (2009) and Stake (1995, 2005).

Example of a multiple case study: Green and colleagues (2008) conducted a multiple case study of nursing students' experiences studying abroad in two schools, one in the United Kingdom and one in Sweden. Individual and group interviews were conducted and documents (e.g., minutes of meetings) were analyzed.

➲ TIP : Although most case studies involve the collection of in-depth qualitative information, some case studies are quantitative and use statistical methods to analyze data.

Narrative Analysis

Narrative analysis focuses on *story* as the object of inquiry, to examine how individuals make sense of events in their lives. Narratives are viewed as a type of "cultural envelope" into which people pour their experiences (Riessman, 1991). What distinguishes narrative analysis from other types of qualitative research designs is its focus on the broad contours of a narrative; stories are not fractured and dissected. The broad underlying premise of narrative research is that people most effectively make sense of their world—and communicate these meanings— by constructing, reconstructing, and narrating stories. Individuals construct stories when they wish to understand specific events and situations that require linking an inner world of desire and motive to an external world of observable actions. Narrative analysts explore *form* as well as content, asking, "Why was the story told that way?" (Riessman, 2008).

A number of approaches can be used to analyze stories. The choice depends on the fit between the structural approach and the types of narrative to be analyzed. Three popular structural approaches include those of Gee (1996), Labov and Waletzky (1967) and Burke (1969). Gee offers a linguistic approach for narrative analysis. His method draws on oral rather than text-based tradition and attends to how the story is told. For example, he pays attention to changes in pitch, loudness, stress, and syllable length, as well as to hesitations and pauses. He also examines the cohesion of each sentence, and how they form larger units (stanzas). His analysis examines the rhetorical function of each stanza in relation to other stanzas. Stanzas are then organized into larger units (strophes), which are analyzed to see how the themes of the text are organized.

Example of a narrative analysis, Gee's approach: Crepeau (2000) analyzed the stories that a geropsychiatric team, which included nurses, social workers, a psychiatrist, and a dietician, told about "Gloria" in the construction of an image of the patient during team meetings. Crepeau based her methods on Gee's approach, and presented numerous stanzas in her report.

Labov and Waletzky's (1967) view narratives as a social phenomenon. Their structural approach proposes that a complete narrative consists of the following 6 components: the abstract (summary), orientation (time, place, individuals), complicating action (sequence of events), evaluation (significance of the action), result or resolution (what occurred at the end), and coda (perspective returned back to the present). As a social phenomenon, narratives vary by social context (hospital, home, and so on), and evaluative data extracted from the narratives vary by the social context in which they were collected.

Example of a narrative analysis, Labov and Waletzky's approach: Montgomery and colleagues (2009) conducted a narrative analysis of "my husband" stories narrated by women with postpartum depression. They used a modified Labov-Waletzky approach in their analysis of interview data from 27 Canadian women.

Burke's (1969) **pentadic dramatism** is another approach to narrative analysis. For Burke there are five key elements of a story: act, scene, agent, agency, and purpose. Analysis of a story "will offer some kind of answers to these five questions: what was done (act), when or where it was done (scene), who did it (agent), how he did it (agency), and why (purpose)" (p. xv). The five terms of Burke's pentad are meant to be understood paired together as ratios such as, act: agent, act: scene, agent: agency, purpose: agent. The analysis focuses on the internal tensions of these 5 terms and their relationships to each other. Each pairing in the pentad provides a different way of directing the researcher's attention. What drives the narrative analysis is not just the interaction of the pentadic terms, but also an imbalance between two or more terms. Bruner (1991) modified Burke's pentad with the addition of a sixth term that he called Trouble with a capital T. Bruner included this sixth element to provide more focus in narrative analysis on Burke's imbalance between the terms in his pentad.

Example of a narrative analysis, Burke's approach: One of the authors of this textbook (Beck, 2006) conducted a narrative analysis of birth trauma. Eleven mothers sent her their stories of traumatic childbirth via the Internet. Burke's pentad of terms was used to analyze these narratives. The most problematic ratio imbalance was between act and agency. Frequently in the mothers' narratives, it was the "How" an act was carried out by the labor and delivery staff that led to the women perceiving their childbirth as traumatic.

Descriptive Qualitative Studies

Many qualitative researchers acknowledge a link to one of the research traditions discussed in this chapter. Many other qualitative studies, however, claim no particular disciplinary or methodologic roots. The researchers may simply indicate that they have conducted a qualitative study or a naturalistic inquiry, or they may say that they have done a *content analysis* of their qualitative data (i.e., an analysis of themes and patterns that emerge in the narrative content). We refer to the many qualitative studies that do not have a formal name as **descriptive qualitative studies**.

Sandelowski (2000), in a widely read article, noted that in doing such descriptive qualitative studies, researchers tend not to penetrate their data in any interpretive depth. These studies present comprehensive summaries of a phenomenon or of events. Qualitative descriptive designs tend to be eclectic and are based on the general premises of constructivist inquiry. These studies often borrow or adapt methodologic techniques from other qualitative traditions, such as constant comparison.

In a more recent article, Sandelowski (2010) warned researchers not to name their studies as *qualitative description* "after the fact to give a name to poorly conceived and conducted studies" (p. 80). She noted that qualitative descriptive studies produce findings closer to the data ("data-near") than studies within such traditions as phenomenology or grounded theory, but that good qualitative descriptions are still interpretive products. She recognized that her 2000 article had provided justification for studies that primarily reproduce raw data and stated that she "never intended to communicate . . . that qualitative description removes the researcher's obligation to do any analyzing or interpreting at all" (p. 79). Rather than being a distinct methodologic classification, qualitative description is perhaps viewed as a "distributed residual category" (p. 82) that signals a "confederacy" of diverse qualitative inquirers.

➲ TIP: In their study of international differences in nursing research, Polit and Beck (2009) analyzed data from about 450 qualitative studies published in 8 nursing journals over a 2-year period. More than half were descriptive, without naming a specific tradition. The tradition with the highest representation was phenomenological, accounting for 20% of the qualitative studies.

Example of a descriptive qualitative study:
Fritzell and colleagues (2010) undertook a descriptive qualitative study to explore and describe how familial adenomatous polyposis, a condition that requires surgery and a lifetime program of surveillance, affects patients' lives.

Sally Thorne (2008) recently expanded qualitative description into a realm she called **interpretive description**. Her book outlined an approach that extends "beyond mere description and into the domain of the 'so what' that drives all applied disciplines" (p. 33) such as nursing. While acknowledging that her approach is neither novel nor distinctive, Thorne noted that it emphasizes the importance of having a disciplinary conceptual frame (such as nursing): "Interpretive description becomes a conceptual maneuver whereby a solid and substantive logic derived from the disciplinary orientation justifies the application of specific techniques and procedures outside of their conventional context" (p. 35). An important thrust of her approach is that it requires integrity of purpose from an actual practice goal; it, therefore, seeks to generate new insights that can help shape applications of qualitative evidence to practice.

Example of an interpretive descriptive study: Johansson and colleagues (2010) used an interpretive descriptive approach in their study of patients' symptoms before, during, and 14 months after beginning treatment for lymphoma.

RESEARCH WITH IDEOLOGICAL PERSPECTIVES

Some qualitative researchers conduct inquiries within an ideological framework, typically to draw attention to social problems or the needs of certain groups and to effect change. These approaches, which are sometimes described as being within a **transformative paradigm** (Mertens, 2007), represent important investigative avenues and are briefly described in this section.

Critical Theory

Critical theory originated with a group of Marxist-oriented German scholars in the 1920s, referred to as the Frankfurt School. Essentially, a critical researcher is concerned with a critique of society and with envisioning new possibilities.

Critical social science is typically action oriented. Its broad aim is to integrate theory and practice such that people become aware of contradictions and disparities in their beliefs and social practices, and become inspired to change them. Critical researchers reject the idea of an objective and disinterested inquirer, and are oriented toward a transformation process. An important feature of critical theory is that it calls for inquiries that foster enlightened self-knowledge and sociopolitical action. Critical theory also involves a self-reflective aspect. To prevent a critical theory of society from becoming yet another self-serving ideology, critical theorists must account for their own transformative effects.

The design of critical research often begins with a thorough analysis of aspects of the problem. For example, critical researchers might analyze and critique taken-for-granted assumptions that underlie the problem, the language used to depict the situation, or the biases of prior researchers studying the problem. Critical researchers often triangulate multiple methodologies and emphasize multiple perspectives (e.g., alternative racial or social class perspectives) on problems. They typically interact with study participants in ways that emphasize participants' expertise. Some of the features that distinguish more

TABLE 20.2 Comparison of Traditional Qualitative Research and Critical Research

ISSUE	TRADITIONAL QUALITATIVE RESEARCH	CRITICAL RESEARCH
Research aims	Understanding; reconstruction of multiple constructions	Critique; transformation; consciousness raising; advocacy
View of knowledge	Transactional/subjective; knowledge is created in interaction between investigator and participants	Transactional/subjective; value-mediated and value-dependent; importance of historical insights
Methods	Dialectic: truth is arrived at logically through conversations	Dialectic and didactic: dialogue designed to transform naivety and misinformation
Evaluative criteria for inquiry quality	Authenticity; trustworthiness	Historical situatedness of the inquiry; erosion of ignorance; stimulus for change
Researcher's role	Facilitator of multivoice reconstruction	Transformative agent; advocate; activist

traditional qualitative research and critical research are summarized in Table 20.2.

Critical theory has been applied in a number of disciplines, and has played an especially important role in ethnography. **Critical ethnography** focuses on raising consciousness and aiding emancipatory goals in the hope of effecting social change. Critical ethnographers address the historical, social, political, and economic dimensions of cultures and their value-laden agendas. An assumption in critical ethnographic research is that actions and thoughts are mediated by power relationships (Hammersley, 1992). Critical ethnographers attempt to increase the political dimensions of cultural research and undermine oppressive systems—there is an explicit political purpose. Cook (2005) has argued that critical ethnography is especially well suited to health promotion research because both are concerned with enabling people to take control of their own situation.

Carspecken (1996) developed a 5-stage approach to critical ethnography that has been found useful in nursing studies (e.g., Hardcastle et al., 2006) and in health-promotion research. Morrow and Brown (1994) also provide guidance about critical theory methodology.

Example of a critical ethnography: Gardezi and colleagues (2009) conducted a critical ethnography of communication, silence, and power in the operating room between physicians and nurses in Canada. Three forms of recurring silences were observed: absence of communication, not responding to questions, and speaking quietly. These silences may be influenced by institutional and structural power dynamics.

TIP: Denzin (1997) has described ethnography as having passed through five "historical moments": (1) traditional ethnography (1900 to World War II), (2) modernist ethnography (World War II to middle of the 1970s), (3) blurred genres (1970–1986), (4) crisis of representation (1986 to present), and (5) the present. In the traditional period, ethnographers wrote objective accounts of their fieldwork, whereas in the second, modernist phase, researchers focused on formalizing qualitative methods based in the language of positivism. By the middle of the 1980s, ethnographers' writings became more reflexive, and gender, social class, and ethnicity became key concerns. Denzin described ethnography at the beginning of the 21st century as a time of intense reflection, experiments with autoethnography, performance texts, ethnographic poetics, and narratives of self.

Feminist Research

Feminist research is similar to critical theory research, but the focus is on gender domination and discrimination within patriarchal societies. Like critical researchers, feminist researchers seek to establish collaborative and nonexploitative relationships with their informants, to place themselves within the study to avoid objectification, and to conduct research that is transformative.

Gender is the organizing principle in feminist research, and investigators seek to understand how gender and a gendered social order have shaped women's lives and their consciousness. The aim is to ameliorate the "invisibility and distortion of female experience in ways relevant to ending women's unequal social position" (Lather, 1991, p. 71).

Although feminist researchers agree on the importance of focusing on women's diverse situations and the relationships that frame those situations, there are many variants of feminist inquiry. Three broad models (within each of which there is diversity) have been identified: (1) *feminist empiricism*, whose adherents usually work within fairly standard norms of qualitative inquiry but who seek to portray more accurate pictures of the social realities of women's lives; (2) *feminist standpoint research*, which holds that inquiry ought to begin in and be tested against the lived everyday sociopolitical experiences of women, and that women's views are particular and privileged; and (3) *feminist postmodernism*, which stresses that "truth" is a destructive illusion, and views the world as endless stories, texts, and narratives. In nursing and healthcare, feminist empiricism and feminist standpoint research have been most prevalent.

The scope of feminist research ranges from studies of the subjective views of individual women to studies of social movements, structures, and broad policies that affect (and often exclude) women. Olesen (2000), a sociologist who studied nurses' career patterns and definitions of success, has noted that some of the best feminist research on women's subjective experiences has been done in the area of women's health.

Feminist research methods typically include in-depth, interactive, and collaborative individual or group interviews that offer the possibility of reciprocally educational encounters. Feminists usually seek to negotiate the meanings of the results with those participating in the study, and to be self-reflective about what they themselves are experiencing and learning.

Feminist research, like other research that has an ideological perspective, has raised the bar for the conduct of ethical research. With the emphasis on trust, empathy, and nonexploitative relationships, proponents of these newer modes of inquiry view any type of deception or manipulation as abhorrent. As Punch (1994) noted in speaking about ethics and feminist research, "you do not rip off your sisters" (p. 89). Those interested in feminist methodologies may wish to consult such writers as Hesse-Biber (2007) or Romazanoglu and Holland (2002).

> **Example of feminist research:** Using feminist methods and theory, Van den Tillaart and colleagues (2009) studied Canadian women's experiences of living with a mental health diagnosis, and the interpersonal and organizational challenges they confronted as women interfacing with the healthcare system.

> **TIP:** Plummer and Young (2010) argued that there is a strong affinity between feminist inquiry and grounded theory. They identified areas where the underpinnings of grounded theory are enriched by a feminist perspective when the research question focuses on women.

Participatory Action Research

A type of research known as participatory action research is closely allied to both critical research and feminist research. **Participatory action research** (PAR), one of several types of *action research* that originated in the 1940s with social psychologist Kurt Lewin, is based on a recognition that the production of knowledge can be political and can be used to exert power. Action researchers typically work with groups or communities that are vulnerable to the control or oppression of a dominant group or culture.

Participatory action research is, as the name implies, participatory. Researchers and study participants collaborate in defining the problem, selecting research methods, analyzing the data, and deciding on the use to which findings are put. The aim of PAR is to produce not only knowledge, but action and consciousness raising as well. Researchers seek to empower people through the process of constructing and using knowledge. The PAR tradition has as its starting point a concern for the powerlessness of the group under study. Thus, a key objective is to produce an impetus that is directly used to make improvements through education and sociopolitical action.

In PAR, research methods take second place to emergent processes of collaboration and dialogue that can motivate, increase self-esteem, and generate community solidarity. "Data-gathering" strategies are not only the traditional methods of interview and observation (including both qualitative and quantitative approaches), but may also include storytelling, sociodrama, drawing and painting, plays and skits, and other activities designed to encourage people to find creative ways to explore their lives, tell their stories, and recognize their own strengths. Koch and Kralik (2006) offer a useful resource for learning more about PAR.

Example of PAR: Nomura and colleagues (2009) conducted a PAR project designed to empower older persons with early dementia and their family caregivers in Japan. The PAR lasted 5 years and consisted of three cycles: one focused on an individual level, the second on a group level, and the third at community levels.

⬆ TIP: Research within the transformative paradigm most often involves the collection and analysis of qualitative data, but may well involve the use of quantitative data as well. Mixed methods are not unusual within the transformative paradigm (Teddlie & Tashakkori, 2009).

CRITIQUING QUALITATIVE DESIGNS

Evaluating a qualitative design is often difficult. Qualitative researchers do not always document design decisions and are even less likely to describe the process by which such decisions were made. Researchers often do, however, indicate whether the study was conducted within a specific qualitative tradition, and this information can be used to come to some conclusions. For example, if a report indicated that the researcher conducted 1 month of fieldwork for an ethnographic study, there would be reason to suspect that insufficient time had been spent in the field to obtain an emic perspective of the culture under study. Ethnographic studies may also be critiqued if their only source of information was from interviews, rather than from a broader range of data sources, particularly observations.

In a grounded theory study, look for evidence about when the data were collected and analyzed. If all the data were collected before analysis, you might question whether constant comparison was used correctly. Glaser and Strauss (1967) offered four properties on which a grounded theory should be evaluated: fitness, understanding, generality, and control. The theory should fit the substantive area for which the data were collected. A grounded theory should increase the understanding of persons working in that substantive area. Also, the categories in the grounded theory should be abstract enough to allow the theory to be a general guide to changing situations—but not so abstract to decrease their sensitizing features. Lastly, the substantive theory must allow individuals who apply it to have some control in daily situations.

In critiquing a phenomenological study, you should first determine if the study is descriptive or interpretive. This will help you to assess how closely the researcher kept to the basic tenets of that qualitative research tradition. For example, in a descriptive phenomenological study, did the researcher bracket? When critiquing phenomenological studies, in addition to critiquing the methodology, you should also look at the power of the studies to show and present the meaning of the phenomena being studied. Van Manen (1997) called for phenomenological researchers to address five textual features in their reports: lived thoroughness (placing the phenomenon concretely in the lifeworld), evocation (phenomenon is vividly brought into presence),

---

BOX 20.1 Guidelines for Critiquing Qualitative Designs

1. Is a research tradition for the qualitative study identified? If none is identified, can one be inferred? If more than one is identified, is this justifiable or does it suggest "method slurring"?
2. Is the research question congruent with a qualitative approach and with the specific research tradition (i.e., is the domain of inquiry for the study congruent with the domain encompassed by the tradition)? Are the data sources, research methods, and analytic approach congruent with the research tradition?
3. How well is the research design described? Are design decisions explained and justified? Does it appear that the researcher made all design decisions up-front, or did the design emerge during data collection, allowing researchers to capitalize on early information?
4. Is the design appropriate, given the research question? Does the design lend itself to a thorough, in-depth, intensive examination of the phenomenon of interest? What design elements might have strengthened the study (e.g., a longitudinal perspective rather than a cross-sectional one)?
5. Did the researcher spend a sufficient amount of time doing fieldwork or collecting the research data?
6. Is there appropriate evidence of reflexivity in the design?
7. Was the study undertaken with an ideological perspective? If so, is there evidence that ideological methods and goals were achieved? (e.g., was there evidence of full collaboration between researchers and participants? Did the research have the power to be transformative or is there evidence that a transformative process occurred?)

---

intensification (give key phrases their full value), tone (let the text speak to the reader), and epiphany (sudden grasp of the meaning).

The guidelines in Box 20.1 are designed to assist you in critiquing the designs of qualitative studies.

RESEARCH EXAMPLES

Nurse researchers have conducted studies in all of the qualitative research traditions described in this chapter, and several actual examples have been cited. In the following sections, we present more detailed descriptions of three qualitative nursing studies.

Research Example of an Ethnography

Study: Cervical screening in Canadian First Nation Cree women (O'Brien et al., 2009).

Statement of Purpose: The purpose of this study was to describe attitudes toward cervical cancer screening and belief about cervical cancer in First Nation (indigenous) Cree women.

Setting: The research was conducted in a rural First Nation Cree reserve community in western Canada.

Method: A focused ethnography was conducted to explore cultural values that influenced women's attitudes toward cervical cancer and cervical cancer screening. The third author is a First Nation woman who was a healthcare provider in the community. She conducted the interviews and was also a participant observer who was able to observe women's responses to screening and illness. A sample of eight women who had experience with cervical cancer screening was recruited. The women were interviewed in-depth for 60 to 90 minutes. In the interviews, participants were invited to share their attitudes, health beliefs, and experiences concerning cervical cancer screening. Interviews were tape recorded, transcribed, and analyzed. Data analysis took place concurrently with data collection and the recording of field notes.

Key Findings: Women had vivid recollections of their healthcare encounters related to cervical cancer screening. Women did not believe they had adequate information, and were resistant to screening because of both embarrassment and fear of cancer, which they viewed as a "death sentence." The results highlighted the need for nursing sensitivity to the needs of the First Nation Cree women.

Research Example of a Phenomenological Study

Study: Cognitive deficits in heart failure: Re-cognition of vulnerability as a strange new world (Sloan & Pressler, 2009).

Statement of Purpose: The purpose of this phenomenological study was to describe how persons with heart failure and cognitive deficits manage self-care in their daily lives.

Setting and Sample: Study participants were recruited from three heart failure clinics in midwestern United States. Twelve participants who had low scores on neuropsychological tests comprised the sample. Interviews were conducted in settings chosen by the participants, which was mostly in their own homes.

Method: In-depth face-to-face interviews lasting from 1 to 1½ hours were conducted with each participant. Interviews were unstructured, allowing participants to tell their own stories of heart failure and its effect in their daily lives as a means of eliciting their interpretation of their situation. Broad guiding questions included: "Tell me about finding out you had heart failure," and "Tell me about the changes in your life since you found out you had heart failure" (p. 242). Information about managing medications, diet, and symptoms was obtained, as well as perceptions relating to cognition (e.g., "Tell me about how you remember everything," p. 242). Interviews were tape recorded and transcribed. Investigators read each interview several times to gain an understanding of what participants were experiencing. Data analysis for recurring themes was undertaken.

Key Findings: The data analysis revealed one overarching theme—re-cognition of vulnerability—a strange new world. This theme had three components: (1) not recognizing cognitive deficits, (2) recognizing cognitive deficits, and (3) recognizing vulnerability, explained by perceptions of cognitive, physical, and social vulnerabilities. The third theme was influenced by participants' perception of nearness of death.

Research Example of a Grounded Theory Study

Study: The substantive theory of surviving on the margin of a profession (Etowa et al., 2009).

Statement of Purpose: The purpose of this grounded theory study was to examine the work life experiences of black registered nurses in Nova Scotia, Canada.

Setting and Sample: Twenty black nurses working in Nova Scotia were recruited. Sampling was guided by what was learned in earlier interviews.

Method: Data were collected primarily by means of individual interviews and observations during the interviews. Analysis began soon after completing the first interview, and constant comparative methods were used throughout. As the research evolved, new aspects of the experiences of black nurses emerged, and new hypotheses were constructed and pursued in subsequent interviews. The generated hypotheses guided continuation of the sampling process until no new information was discovered. Once interviews were completed, two group discussions were held with the black nurses to validate key findings.

Key Findings: Analysis revealed the core variable of *surviving on the margin of a profession*. This basic social process consisted of three phases: realizing, surviving, and thriving. There were three conditions that influenced surviving on the margin: racism, diversity, and quality of professional experiences, such as healthy work environment.

SUMMARY POINTS

- Qualitative research involves an **emergent design**—a design that emerges in the field as the study unfolds. Although qualitative design is flexible, qualitative researchers plan for broad contingencies that pose decision opportunities for study design in the field.
- As *bricoleurs*, qualitative researchers tend to be creative and intuitive, putting together an array of data drawn from many sources to arrive at a holistic understanding of a phenomenon.
- Qualitative research traditions have their roots in anthropology (e.g., **ethnography** and **ethnoscience**), philosophy (**phenomenology** and **hermeneutics**), psychology (**etiology** and **ecological** psychology), sociology (**grounded theory, ethnomethodology**, and **semiotics**), sociolinguistics (**discourse analysis**), and history (**historical research**).
- Ethnography focuses on the culture of a group of people and relies on extensive fieldwork that

usually includes **participant observation** and in-depth interviews with **key informants**. Ethnographers strive to acquire an **emic** (insider's) perspective of a culture rather than an **etic** (outsider's) perspective.

- The concept of **researcher as instrument** is used by ethnographers to describe the researcher's significant role in analyzing and interpreting a culture. The product of ethnographic research is typically a holistic description of the culture, but sometimes the products are **performance ethnographies** (interpretive scripts that can be performed).

- Nurses sometimes refer to their ethnographic studies as **ethnonursing research**. Other types of ethnographic work include **institutional ethnographics** (which focus on the organization of professional services from the perspective of the front-line workers or clients) and **autoethnographies** or *insider research* (which focus on the group or culture to which the researcher belongs).

- Phenomenology seeks to discover the *essence* and *meaning* of a phenomenon as it is experienced by people, mainly through in-depth interviews with people who have had the relevant experience.

- In **descriptive phenomenology**, which seeks to describe lived experiences, researchers strive to **bracket** out preconceived views and to **intuit** the essence of the phenomenon by remaining open to meanings attributed to it by those who have experienced it.

- **Interpretive phenomenology (hermeneutics)** focuses on interpreting the meaning of experiences, rather than just describing them.

- **Grounded theory** aims to discover theoretical precepts grounded in the data. Grounded theory researchers try to account for people's actions by focusing on the main concern that the behavior is designed to resolve. The manner in which people resolve this main concern is the **core variable**. The goal of grounded theory is to discover this main concern and the **basic social process (BSP)** that explains how people resolve it.

- Grounded theory uses **constant comparison**: Categories elicited from the data are constantly compared with data obtained earlier.

- A controversy among grounded theory researchers concerns whether to follow the original Glaser and Strauss procedures or to use the adapted procedures of Strauss and Corbin; Glaser argued that the latter approach does not result in *grounded theories* but rather in *conceptual descriptions*.

- More recently, Charmaz's **constructivist grounded theory** has emerged as a method to emphasize interpretive aspects in which the grounded theory is constructed from shared experiences and relationships between the researcher and study participants.

- **Historical research** is the systematic attempt to establish facts and relationships about past events. Historical data are normally subjected to **external criticism**, which is concerned with the authenticity of the source, and **internal criticism**, which assesses the worth of the evidence.

- **Case studies** are intensive investigations of a single entity or a small number of entities, such as individuals, groups, organizations, or communities; such studies usually involve collecting data over an extended period. Case study designs can be **single** or **multiple**, and **holistic** or **embedded**.

- **Narrative analysis** focuses on *story* in studies in which the purpose is to explore how people make sense of events in their lives. Several different structural approaches can be used to analyze narrative data, including, for example, Burke's **pentadic dramatism**.

- **Descriptive qualitative studies** do not fit into any disciplinary tradition. Such studies may be referred to as qualitative studies, naturalistic inquiries, or as qualitative content analyses. Qualitative description has been expanded into a realm called **interpretive description**, which is emphasizes the importance of having a disciplinary conceptual frame, such as nursing.

- Research is sometimes conducted within an ideological perspective, and such research tends to rely primarily on qualitative research.

- **Critical theory** entails a critique of existing social structures; critical researchers strive to conduct inquiries that involve collaboration with participants and foster enlightened self-knowledge and transformation. **Critical ethnography** applies the principles of critical theory to the study of cultures.

- **Feminist research**, like critical research, is designed to be transformative, but the focus is on how gender domination and discrimination shape women's lives and their consciousness.
- **Participatory action research** (PAR) produces knowledge through close collaboration with groups or communities that are vulnerable to control or oppression by a dominant culture; in PAR research, methods take second place to emergent processes that can motivate people and generate community solidarity.

STUDY ACTIVITIES

Chapter 20 of the *Resource Manual for Nursing Research: Generating and Assessing Evidence for Nursing Practice, 9th edition*, offers exercises and study suggestions for reinforcing concepts presented in this chapter. In addition, the following study questions can be addressed:

1. Which of the following topics is best suited to a phenomenological inquiry? To an ethnography? To a grounded theory study? Provide a rationale for each response.
   a. The passage through menarche among Haitian refugees
   b. The process of coping among AIDS patients
   c. The experience of having a child with leukemia
   d. Rituals relating to dying among nursing home residents
   e. The experience of waiting for service in a hospital emergency department
   f. Decision-making processes among nurses regarding do-not-resuscitate orders
2. Apply the questions in Box 20.1 to one of the three studies described at the end of the chapter, referring as necessary to the full research report for additional information. Also, do you think this study could have been undertaken with a critical or feminist perspective? Why or why not?

STUDIES CITED IN CHAPTER 20

Aga, F., Kylma, J., & Nikkonen, M. (2009). The conceptions of care among family caregivers of persons living with HIV/AIDS in Addis Ababa, Ethiopia. *Journal of Transcultural Nursing, 20*, 37–50.

Beck, C. T. (2006) Pentadic cartography: Mapping birth trauma narratives. *Qualitative Health Research, 16*, 453–466.

Beck, C. T. (2012). Exemplar: Teetering on the edge: A second grounded theory modification. In P. Munhall (Ed.), *Nursing research: A qualitative perspective* (5th ed., pp. 225–256). Sudbury, Ma: Jones & Bartlett Publishers.

Black, B. P., Holditch-Davis, D., & Miles, M. (2009). Life course theory as a framework to examine becoming a mother of a medically fragile preterm infant. *Research in Nursing & Health, 32*, 38–49.

Crepeau, E. B. (2000). Reconstructing Gloria: A narrative analysis of team meetings. *Qualitative Health Research, 10*, 766–787.

Ellett, M. L., Appleton, M. M., & Sloan, R. S. (2009). Out of the abyss of colic: A view through the fathers' eyes. *MCN: The American Journal of Maternal Child Health, 34*, 164–171.

Etowa, J., Sethi, S., & Thompson-Isherwood, R. (2009). The substantive theory of surviving on the margin of a profession. *Nursing Science Quarterly, 22*, 174–181.

Flinck, A., & Paavilainen, E. (2010). Women's experience of their violent behavior in an intimate partner relationship. *Qualitative Health Research, 20*, 306–318.

Fritzell, K., Persson, C., Bjork, J., Hultcrantz, R., & Wttergren, L. (2010). Patients' views of surgery and surveillance for familial adenomatous polyposis. *Cancer Nursing, 33*, 17–23.

Gardezi, F., Lingard, L., Espin, S., Whyte, S., Orser, B., & Baker, R. (2009). Silence, power and communication in the operating room. *Journal of Advanced Nursing, 65*, 1390–1399.

Giarelli, E. (2006). Images of cloning and stem cell research in editorial cartoons in the United States. *Qualitative Health Research, 16*, 61–78.

Glaser, B., & Strauss, A. (1965). *Awareness of dying.* Chicago: Aldine.

Green, B. F., Johansson, I., Rosser, M., Tengnah, C., & Segrolt, J. (2008). Studying abroad: A mulitiple case study of nursing students' international experiences. *Nurse Education Today, 28*, 981–992.

Hallett, C. (2009). Russian romances: Emotionalism and spirituality in the writing of "Eastern Front" nurses, 1914–1918. *Nursing History Review, 17*, 101–128.

Hardcastle, M., Usher, K., & Holmes, C. (2006). Carspecken's five-stage critical qualitative research method: An application to nursing research. *Qualitative Health Research, 16*, 151–161.

Hirst, S. P. (2002). Defining resident abuse within the culture of long-term care institutions. *Clinical Nursing Research, 11*, 267–284.

Johansson, E., Wilson, B., Brunton, L., Tishelman, C., & Molassiotis, A. (2010). Symptoms before, during, and 14 months after the beginning of treatment as perceived by patients with lymphoma. *Oncology Nursing Forum, 37*, 105–113.

Kean, S. (2010). The experience of ambiguous loss in families of brain-injured ICU patients. *Nursing in Critical Care, 15*, 66–75.

Kelley, L. (2005). Gendered elder care exchanges in a Caribbean village. *Western Journal of Nursing Research, 27*, 73–92.

Kohara, I., & Inoue, T. (2010). Searching for a way to live to the end: decision-making process in patients considering participation in cancer phase I clinical trials. *Oncology Nursing Forum, 37*, E124–132.

Lauterbach, S. S. (2007). Meanings in mothers' experience with infant death: Three phenomenological inquiries: In another world; five years later; and what forever means. In P. L. Munhall (Ed.), *Nursing research: A qualitative perspective* (4th ed., pp. 211–238). Sudbury, MA: Jones & Bartlett Publishers.

Legault, A., & Ducharme, F. (2009). Advocating for a patient with dementia in a long-term facility: The process experienced by daughters. *Journal of Family Nursing, 15*, 198–219.

Leifer, S., & Glass, L. (2008). Planning for mass disaster in the 1950s. *Nursing Research, 57*, 237–244.

Montgomery, P., Bailey, P., Johnson-Purdon, S., Snelling, S., & Kauppi, C. (2009). Women with postpartum depression: "My husband" stories. *BMC Nursing, 8*, 8.

Naef, R., & Bournes, D. A. (2009). The lived experience of waiting: A Parse method study. *Nursing Science Quarterly, 22*, 141–153.

Nomura, M., Makimoto, K., Kato, M., Shiba, T., Matsuura, C., Shigenobu, K., Ishikawa, T., Matsumoto, N., & Ikeda, M. (2009). Empowering older people with early dementia and family caregivers: A participatory action research study. *International Journal of Nursing Studies, 46*, 431–441.

O'Brien, B., Mill, J., & Wilson, T. (2009). Cervical screening in Canadian First Nation Cree women. *Journal of Transcultural Nursing, 20*, 83–92.

Ozeki, N. (2008). Transcultural stress factors of Japanese mothers living in the United Kingdom. *Journal of Transcultural Nursing, 19*, 47–54.

Polit, D. & Beck, C. T. (2009). International differences in nursing research, 2005-2006. *Journal of Nursing Scholarship, 41*, 44–53.

Plumridge, E., Goodyear-Smith, F., & Ross, J. (2009). Nurse and parent partnership during children's vaccinations: A conversation analysis. *Journal of Advanced Nursing, 65*, 1187–1194.

Riley, R., & Manias, E. (2006). Governing time in operating rooms. *Journal of Clinical Nursing, 15*, 546–553.

Robertson, C., Kerr, M., Garcia, C., & Halterman, E. (2007). Noise and hearing protection: Latino construction workers' experiences. *AAOHN Journal, 55*, 153–160.

Sarenmalm, E., Thorén-Jönsson, A. L., Gaston-Johansson, F., & Öhlén, J. (2009). Making sense of living under the shadow of death: Adjusting to recurrent breast cancer illness. *Qualitative Health Research, 19*, 1116–1130.

Schneider, B. (2005). Mothers talk about their children with schizophrenia: A performance autoethnography. *Journal of Psychiatric & Mental Health Nursing, 12*, 333–340.

Sloan, R., & Pressler, S. (2009). Cognitive deficits in heart failure: Re-cognition of vulnerability as a strange new world. *Journal of Cardiovascular Nursing, 24*, 241–248.

Smallwood, A. (2009). Cardiac assessment teams: A focused ethnography of nurses' roles. *British Journal of Cardiac Nursing, 4*, 132–139.

Spiers, J. (2006). Expressing and responding to pain and stoicism in home-care nurse-patient interactions. *Scandinavian Journal of Caring Science, 20*, 293–301.

Van den Tillaart, S., Kurtz, D., & Cash, P. (2009). Powerlessness, marginalized identity, and silencing of health concerns: Voiced realities of women living with a mental health diagnosis. *International Journal of Mental Health Nursing, 18*, 153–163.

Methodologic and nonresearch references cited in this chapter can be found in a separate section at the end of the book.

21

Sampling in Qualitative Research

In Chapter 12, we presented technical terms and concepts relating to sampling in quantitative research. Sampling in qualitative studies is quite different. Qualitative studies almost always use small, nonrandom samples. This does not mean that qualitative researchers are unconcerned with the quality of their samples, but rather that they use different considerations in selecting participants. This chapter describes sampling approaches used by qualitative researchers.

THE LOGIC OF QUALITATIVE SAMPLING

Quantitative research is concerned with measuring attributes and relationships in a population; therefore, a representative sample is desired to ensure that the measurements accurately reflect and can be generalized to the population. The aim of most qualitative studies is to discover *meaning* and to uncover multiple realities, not to generalize to a target population.

Qualitative researchers begin with the following types of sampling question in mind: Who would be an information-rich data source for my study? Whom should I talk to or observe to maximize my understanding of the phenomenon? A critical first step in qualitative sampling is selecting settings

with high potential for information richness. As the study progresses, new sampling questions emerge, such as the following: Who can confirm my understandings? Challenge or modify my understandings? Enrich my understandings? Thus, as with the overall design in qualitative studies, sampling is emergent and capitalizes on early learning to guide subsequent direction.

Another point worth mentioning is that individuals are not always the *unit of analysis* in qualitative studies. For example, Glaser and Strauss (1967) have noted that "incidents" or experiences are often the basis for analysis. An information-rich informant can therefore contribute dozens of incidents, so even a small number of informants can generate a large sample for analysis.

Example of a sample of incidents in a qualitative study: Gunnarsson and Warrén-Stomberg (2009) studied factors that influence decision making among Swedish ambulance nurses in emergency care situations. They interviewed 14 nurses, who described 30 incidents that were the focus of the analysis.

Qualitative researchers do not articulate an explicit population to whom results are intended to be generalized, but they do establish the kinds of people who are eligible to participate in their research. A prime criterion is whether a person has experienced the phenomenon (or culture) that is under study. Practical issues, such as costs, accessibility, health problems, and researcher-participant language compatibility, also affect who can be included in the sample.

Example of eligibility criteria in a qualitative study: In their descriptive qualitative study, Williams and colleagues (2009) studied how irrational thinking affects adherence to medicines prescribed to manage diabetic kidney disease. Patients from the nephrology department of an Australian hospital were eligible if they had coexisting diabetes and kidney disease, were 18 or older, were cognitively intact, and were English speaking. Exclusion criteria included pregnancy, impending commencement of dialysis, diagnosis of an aggressive form of cancer, and mental illness that was not stabilized.

TYPES OF QUALITATIVE SAMPLING

There are many different approaches to sampling in qualitative research, which we review in this section. Despite differences, however, a few key features that characterize most sampling strategies have been distilled from an analysis of the qualitative literature (Curtis et al., 2000).

- Participants are not selected randomly. A random sample is not considered the best method of selecting people who will make good informants, that is, people who are knowledgeable, articulate, reflective, and willing to talk at length with researchers.
- Samples tend to be small and studied intensively, with each participant provided a wealth of data. Typically, qualitative studies involve fewer (and sometimes much fewer) than 50 participants.
- Sample members are not wholly prespecified; their selection is emergent.
- Sample selection is driven to a great extent by conceptual requirements rather than by a desire for representativeness.

Convenience Sampling

Qualitative researchers often begin with a convenience sample, which is sometimes referred to in qualitative studies as a *volunteer sample*. Volunteer samples are especially likely to be used when researchers need to have potential participants come forward and identify themselves. For example, if we wanted to study the experiences of people with frequent nightmares, we might have difficulty readily identifying potential participants. In such a situation, we might recruit sample members by placing a notice on a bulletin board, in a newspaper, or on the Internet, requesting people with frequent nightmares to contact us. In this situation, we would be less interested in obtaining a representative sample of people with nightmares, than in obtaining a diverse group representing various experiences with nightmares.

Sampling by convenience is easy and efficient, but it is not a preferred sampling approach, even in qualitative studies. The key in qualitative studies is to extract the greatest possible information from the few cases in the sample, and a convenience sample may not provide the most information-rich sources. However, a convenience sample may be an economical and easy way to begin the sampling process, relying on other methods as data are collected.

Convenience sampling may also work well with participants who need to be recruited from a particular clinical setting or from a specific organization. Thorne (2008), however, advised that in such situations the researcher should carefully reflect on and understand any peculiarities of the study context. In essence, researchers must consider whether participants' narrations reflect the experience of the healthcare or organizational setting to a greater extent than the experience of the phenomenon under study.

Example of a convenience sample: Early and colleagues (2009) conducted in-depth interviews with Latino and Caucasian clients with type 2 diabetes about their dietary self-management goal behaviors. Participants were sampled by convenience from a community/migrant health clinic in rural Washington State.

Snowball Sampling

Qualitative researchers, like quantitative researchers, sometimes use snowball (or chain) sampling, asking early informants to refer other study participants. Snowball sampling has distinct advantages over convenience sampling from a broad population or community group. The first is that it may be more cost-efficient and practical. Researchers may spend less time screening people to determine if they are appropriate for the study, for example. Furthermore, with an introduction from the referring person, researchers may have an easier time establishing a trusting relationship with new participants. Finally, researchers can more readily specify the characteristics that they want new participants to have. For example, in the study of people with nightmares, we could ask early respondents if they knew anyone else who had the same problem *and* who was articulate. We could also ask for referrals to people who would add other dimensions to the sample, such as people who vary in age, race, and socioeconomic status.

A weakness of this approach is that the eventual sample might be restricted to a rather small network of acquaintances. Moreover, the quality of the referrals may be affected by whether the referring sample members trusted the researcher and truly wanted to cooperate.

⮕ **TIP:** Researchers should be careful about protecting the rights of the individuals whom early participants refer. It is wise to suggest that early informants first check with the potential referrals to make sure they are interested in participating before their names are shared with the researcher. This is especially true if the study focuses on sensitive issues (e.g., drug use, suicide attempts).

Example of snowball sampling: Weinberg and colleagues (2009) studied the quality of communication and interactions between nurses and medical residents from the residents' perspective. They relied on snowball sampling to recruit their sample of 20 medical and surgical residents.

Purposive Sampling

Qualitative sampling may begin with volunteer informants and may be supplemented with new participants through snowballing, but many qualitative studies eventually evolve to a purposive (or

purposeful) sampling strategy—that is, selecting cases that will most benefit the study.

More than a dozen purposive sampling strategies have been identified (Patton, 2002). We briefly describe many of these strategies to illustrate the diverse approaches qualitative researchers have used to meet the conceptual and substantive needs of their research. As an organizing structure, we have adapted the typology of purposive sampling proposed by Teddlie and Tashakkori (2009).

⮕ **TIP:** Note that researchers themselves do not necessarily refer to their sampling plans with the labels suggested by Patton or categorized by Teddlie and Tashakkori.

Sampling for Representativeness or Comparative Value

The first broad category of purposive sampling involves two general goals: (1) sampling to find examples that are representative or typical of a broader group on some dimension of interest or (2) sampling to set up the possibility of comparisons or replications across different types of cases on a dimension of interest. The latter goal is the more common one in this category of purposive sampling.

Maximum variation sampling is perhaps the most widely used method of purposive sampling. It involves purposefully selecting persons (or settings) with a wide range of variation on dimensions of interest. By selecting participants with diverse perspectives and backgrounds, researchers invite enrichments of and challenges to emerging conceptualizations. Maximum variation sampling might involve ensuring that people with diverse backgrounds are represented in the sample (ensuring that there are men and women, poor and affluent people, and so on). It might also involve deliberate attempts to include people with different viewpoints about the phenomenon under study. For example, researchers might use snowballing to ask early participants for referrals to people who hold different points of view. One major advantage of maximum variation sampling is that any common patterns emerging despite the diversity of the sample are of particular value in capturing core experiences.

Maximum variation sampling is often an emergent approach: Information from initial participants helps to guide the subsequent selection of a diverse group of participants. However, there may be an advantage to having some up-front insights into the dimensions of variation that will likely prove productive. The factors that affect the health or wellness experience under scrutiny can often be anticipated or identified in advance, and having a mental list of such factors can be useful in ensuring sufficient diversity in the sample.

Example of maximum variation sampling: Petersen and colleagues (2009) explored barriers to communication between midwives and pregnant women in Capetown (South Africa) regarding smoking during pregnancy. The study involved in-depth interviews with 12 pregnant women, sampled so as to maximize variation in terms of their smoking behavior, age, and marital status.

At the other end of the spectrum, **homogeneous sampling** deliberately reduces variation and permits a more focused inquiry. Researchers may use this approach if they wish to understand a particular group of people especially well. Homogeneous sampling is often used to select people for group interviews.

Example of homogeneous sampling: Sabuni (2007) explored people's perceptions of the cause of illnesses in the Democratic Republic of Congo using focus groups and case studies. She selected persons of the same generation and gender with experience of home remedies so that groups would be constituted according to gender and generation. Sabuni called her approach purposive sampling, noting that "other authors have called this homogeneous sampling" (p. 1282).

Typical case sampling involves selecting cases that illustrate or highlight what is typical, average, normal, or representative. Identifying typical cases can help the researcher understand key aspects of a phenomenon as they are manifested under ordinary circumstances. The data resulting from this sampling strategy can be used to create a qualitative profile illustrating typical manifestations of the phenomenon being studied. Such profiles can be especially helpful to those not familiar with the social setting or culture.

Example of typical case sampling: Lash and colleagues (2006) studied nursing and midwifery students' experiences with verbal abuse in clinical settings in Turkey. Typical case sampling was used to capture the students' most typical experiences of verbal abuse.

Typical case sampling can be expanded by selecting a **stratified purposive sample** of average, above average, and below average cases. This strategy approaches maximum variation sampling, but is typically done along a single dimension (e.g., income or illness severity). In this approach, each "stratum" would comprise a fairly homogeneous sample.

Example of stratified purposive sampling: Ward and colleagues (2009) explored African American women's beliefs about and barriers to seeking mental health services. The used a stratified purposive sample, using age as the stratifier, to recruit 15 women from three age groups: young, aged 25 to 45; middle-aged, aged 46 to 65; and older, aged 66 to 85.

Extreme (deviant) case sampling is also sometimes called *outlier sampling*. This approach provides opportunities for learning from the most unusual and extreme informants—cases that at least on the surface seem like "exceptions to the rule" (e.g., outstanding successes and notable failures). The assumption underlying this approach is that extreme cases are rich in information because they are special in some way. In some circumstances, more can be learned by intensively studying extreme cases, but extreme cases can also distort understanding of a phenomenon. Most often, this approach is a supplement to other sampling strategies—the extremes are sought out to develop a richer or more nuanced understanding of the phenomenon under study.

Example of extreme case sampling: Riegel and colleagues (2007) explored factors associated with the development of expertise in heart failure self-care. They used extreme case sampling to identify 29 chronic heart failure patients who were either particularly poor or good in self-care.

Intensity sampling is similar to extreme case sampling, but with less emphasis on the extremes.

Intensity samples involve information-rich cases that manifest the phenomenon of interest intensely, but not as extreme or potentially distorting manifestations. Thus, the goal in intensity sampling is to select rich cases that offer *strong* examples of the phenomenon. Intensity sampling is well suited as an adjunct method of sampling. For example, a researcher could collect data from 20 or so participants, using (for example) maximum variation or typical case sampling. Then, a subset set of intense cases could be sampled for more in-depth questioning or analysis.

Reputational case sampling, a variant of purposive sampling not included in Patton's (2002) list, involves selecting cases based on a recommendation of an expert or key informant. This approach, most often used in ethnographies, is useful when researchers have little information about how best to proceed with sampling and must rely on recommendations from others.

Many of the sampling strategies discussed thus far require that researchers have some knowledge about the context in which the study is taking place. For example, to choose extreme cases, typical cases, or homogenous cases, researchers must have information about the range of variation of the phenomenon and how it manifests itself. Early participants may be helpful in implementing these sampling strategies.

⮕ **T I P :** Quantitative researchers design sampling plans that avoid sampling bias, but Morse (2003a) has argued that "biasphobia" can undermine good qualitative research. She noted that the goal of sampling should be to actively and purposefully pursue the *best*, rather than the average, case. Her advice was to start with excellent examples of the phenomenon being studied, and then—once the phenomenon is better understood and there is a sense of what to look for—to examine "weaker instances and average occurrences" of the phenomenon.

Sampling Special or Unique Cases

The second broad category of purposive sampling involves selecting special or unique cases. In these approaches, individual cases or a specific group of cases are the focus of the investigation. Several of these approaches are especially likely to be used in case study research.

Critical case sampling involves selecting important cases regarding the phenomenon of interest. With this approach, researchers look for the particularly good story that illuminates critical aspects of the phenomenon, and then intensely explore that story. To identify critical cases, the researcher must be able to identify the factors that make a case critical.

Example of critical case sampling: Speraw (2009) explored the concept of personhood and its relationship to healthcare delivery in the context of a case study of a 16-year-old girl disfigured by multiple cancer treatments. The case study was part of a larger phenomenological study of children and adolescents with disabilities or special needs. Speraw wrote that "Kelly's case is selected for presentation here both because of the striking clarity in description of life experience and its unique and articulate emphasis on the dilemmas associated with striving to express the fullness of humanity" (p. 736).

Criterion sampling involves selecting cases that meet a predetermined criterion of importance. For example, in studying patient satisfaction with nursing care, researchers might sample only those patients whose responses to questions upon discharge expressed a complaint about some aspect of nursing care. Criterion sampling is another approach that has the potential for identifying and understanding cases that are fertile with experiential information on the phenomenon of interest.

Example of criterion sampling: Stevens and Hildebrant (2009), in their longitudinal study of HIV-infected women's experiences with antiretroviral (ARV) regimens, focused on a subsample of 14 out of the full sample of 55 women who persistently had difficulties taking their medication as prescribed and who were vulnerable to ARV treatment failure.

Yin (2009), whose work on case study research is widely cited, described **revelatory case sampling**. This approach involves identifying and gaining access to a single case representing a phenomenon that was previously inaccessible to research scrutiny.

Example of revelatory case sampling: Beck (2009) used revelatory case sampling to choose the participant for the single, holistic case study of an adult survivor of child sexual abuse and her breast-feeding experience.

A final type of special-case sampling is **sampling of politically important cases**. This approach is used to select or search for politically sensitive cases (or sites) for analysis. Sometimes, politically salient cases or sites can enhance the visibility of a study, or increase the likelihood that it has an impact. In some cases, the approach is used to select *out* politically sensitive locales or individuals to avoid attracting unwanted attention.

Sampling Sequentially

Several of the purposive strategies already described can be combined in a single study. For example, extreme case sampling could occur after an initial strategy such as maximum variation sampling. The strategies in this third broad category of purposive sampling involve a gradual, and often planned, sequence of sampling. One such strategy, theory-based or theoretical sampling, is discussed separately in the next section.

A type of sampling called **opportunistic sampling** (or *emergent sampling*) involves adding new cases to a sample based on changes in research circumstances as data are being collected, or in response to new leads and opportunities that may develop in the field. As the researcher gains greater knowledge of a setting or a phenomenon, on-the-spot sampling decisions can take advantage of unfolding events. This approach, although seldom labeled as opportunistic sampling, is used regularly in qualitative research because of its flexible and emergent nature.

Sampling confirming and disconfirming cases tends to be used toward the end of data collection. This approach involves testing ideas and assessing the viability of emergent findings and conceptualizations with new data. **Confirming cases** are additional cases that fit researchers' conceptualizations and offer enhanced credibility, richness, and depth to the analysis and conclusions. **Disconfirming cases** (or **negative cases**) are

examples that do not fit and serve to challenge researchers' interpretations. These negative cases may simply be "exceptions that prove the rule," but they may be exceptions that disconfirm earlier insights and suggest rival explanations about the phenomenon. These cases can bring to light how the original conceptualization needs to be revised or expanded.

Example of sampling negative cases: Ching and colleagues (2009) explored how Chinese women cope with breast cancer and concluded that "reframing" was the core feature of the early adjustment process. One of the strategies they adopted to validate their explanation was to sample negative cases.

TIP: Some qualitative researchers appear to call their sample *purposive* simply because they "purposely" selected people who experienced the phenomenon of interest. However, exposure to the phenomenon is an eligibility criterion—the group of interest comprises people with that exposure. If the researcher then recruits *any* person with the desired experience, the sample is selected by convenience, not purposively. Purposive sampling implies an intent to choose *particular* exemplars or *types* of people who can best enhance the researcher's understanding of the phenomenon.

Theoretical Sampling

Patton (2002) described **theoretical sampling** (or *theory-based sampling*) as a strategy involving the selection of "incidents, slices of life, time periods, or people on the basis of their potential manifestation or representation of important theoretical constructs" (p. 238). Although Patton categorized this type of sampling as purposive sampling, we devote a separate subsection to this sampling strategy because of its importance in grounded theory.

TIP: In Patton's (2002) scheme, theory-based sampling is viewed as a focused approach that could be based on an *a priori* theory that is being examined qualitatively, so it is a different approach to linking sampling decisions to theoretical constructs than is found in grounded theory studies.

Glaser (1978, p. 36) defined theoretical sampling as "the process of data collection for generating theory whereby the analyst jointly collects, codes, and analyzes his data and decides what data to collect next and where to find them, in order to develop his theory as it emerges." The process of theoretical sampling is guided by the developing grounded theory. Theoretical sampling is not envisioned as a single, unidirectional line. This complex sampling technique requires researchers to be involved with multiple lines and directions as they go back and forth between data and categories in the emerging theory.

Glaser stressed that theoretical sampling is not the same as purposive sampling. Theoretical sampling's purpose is to discover categories and their properties and to offer interrelationships that occur in the substantive theory. "The basic question in theoretical sampling is: what groups or subgroups does one turn to next in data collection?" (Glaser, 1978, p. 36). These groups are not chosen before the research begins but only as they are needed for their theoretical relevance for developing further emerging categories.

Example of a theoretical sampling: Beck (2002) used theoretical sampling in her grounded theory study of mothering twins during the first year of life. A specific example of theoretical sampling concerned what the mothers kept referring to as the "blur period" — the first few months of caring for the twins. Initially, Beck interviewed mothers whose twins were around 1 year of age. Her rationale was that these mothers would be able to reflect back over the entire first year of mothering the multiples. When these mothers referred to the "blur period," Beck asked them to describe this period more fully. The mothers said they could not provide many details about this period because "it was such a blur!" Beck then chose to interview mothers whose twins were 3 months of age or younger, to ensure that mothers were still immersed in the "blur period" and would be able to provide rich detail about what this phase of mothering twins was like.

➡ **TIP:** No matter what type of qualitative sampling you use, you should keep a journal or notebook to jot down ideas and reminders regarding the sampling process (e.g., whom you should interview next). Memos to yourself will help you remember valuable ideas about your sample.

SAMPLE SIZE IN QUALITATIVE RESEARCH

There are no fixed rules for sample size in qualitative research. In qualitative studies, sample size should be based on informational needs. Hence, a guiding principle in sampling is **data saturation**— that is, sampling to the point at which no new information is obtained and redundancy is achieved. The key issue is to generate enough in-depth data that can illuminate the patterns, categories, and dimensions of the phenomenon under study. Redundancy, and hence sample size, can be affected by the purpose of the inquiry, the quality of the informants, and the type of sampling strategy used. For example, a larger sample is likely to be needed with maximum variation sampling than with typical case sampling.

Morse (2000) noted that the number of participants needed to reach saturation depends on a number of factors. One factor concerns the scope of the research question: The broader the scope, the more participants will likely be needed. A broader scope may mean not only more interviews with people who have experienced the phenomenon, but also a search for supplementary data sources. Researchers should consider this issue of scope and its implications for data needs before embarking on a study.

Data quality can also affect sample size. If participants are good informants who are able to reflect on their experiences and communicate effectively, saturation can be achieved with a relatively small sample. For this reason, convenience sampling may require more cases to achieve saturation than purposive or theoretical sampling.

Another issue that can affect sample size is the sensitivity of the phenomenon being studied. If the topic is one that is deeply personal or perhaps embarrassing, participants may be more reluctant to fully share their thoughts. Thus, to obtain sufficient data for a deep understanding of sensitive or controversial phenomena, more data may be required.

Greater amounts of data can be created by increasing the sample size, but sometimes depth and richness in the data can be achieved by longer, more intense interviews (or observations), or by going back to the same participants more than once. Multiple interviews often have the advantage of not only generating more data, but also yielding better-quality data if participants are more forthcoming in later sessions because of increased trust. In qualitative studies that are longitudinal, fewer participants may be needed because each will provide a greater amount of information.

Also, Morse (2000) noted that sample size can also be affected by the availability of what she called *shadowed data.* These are data provided by participants who are able to discuss not only their own experiences, but also the experiences of others. Morse noted that shadowed data can provide researchers "with some idea of the range of experiences and the domain of the phenomena beyond the single participant's personal experience" (p. 4). Such shadowed data can help inform decisions relevant to purposive and theoretical sampling.

The skills and experience of the researcher also can affect sample size. Researchers with strong interviewing or observational skills often require fewer participants because they are more successful in putting participants at ease, encouraging candor, and soliciting important revelations. Thus, students who are just starting out on a qualitative project are likely to require a larger sample size to achieve data saturation than their more experienced mentors.

One final suggestion that may be especially important for beginning researchers is to "test" whether data saturation has been achieved. Essentially, this involves adding one or two cases after achieving informational redundancy to ensure that no new information emerges.

Example of data saturation: Pugh (2009) conducted an in-depth qualitative study of how Australian nurses deal with an allegation of unprofessional conduct. A sample of 21 nurses who had been reported to a regulatory authority was interviewed. Pugh stated that "All 21 eligible respondents were interviewed, even though data saturation, i.e., a sense that no new concepts were being identified, occurred at the 19th interview. The reason for interviewing all respondents was to ensure that saturation was obtained" (p. 2029).

⬛ **TIP:** Sample size estimation can create practical dilemmas if you are seeking approval or funding for a project. Patton (2002) recommended that, in a proposal, researchers should specify *minimum* samples that would reasonably be adequate for understanding the phenomenon. Additional cases can then be added, as necessary, to achieve saturation.

SAMPLING IN THE THREE MAIN QUALITATIVE TRADITIONS

There are similarities among the various qualitative traditions with regard to sampling: samples are small, probability sampling is not used, and final sampling decisions usually take place during data collection. However, there are some differences as well.

Sampling in Ethnography

Ethnographers may begin by adopting a "big net" approach—that is, mingling with and having conversations with as many members of the culture under study as possible. Although they may converse with many people (usually 25 to 50), they often rely heavily on a smaller number of key informants. *Key informants* (or *cultural consultants*) are individuals who are highly knowledgeable about the culture or organization and who develop special, ongoing relationships with the researcher. These key informants are often the researcher's main link to the "inside."

Key informants are chosen purposively, guided by the ethnographer's informed judgments. Developing a pool of potential key informants often depends on ethnographers' prior knowledge to construct a relevant framework. For example, an ethnographer might make decisions about different types of key informants to seek out based on roles (e.g., physicians, nurse practitioners) or on some other substantively meaningful distinction. Once a pool of potential key informants is developed, the primary considerations for final selection are their level of knowledge about the culture and their willingness to collaborate with the ethnographer in revealing and interpreting the culture.

➲ TIP : Be careful not to choose your key informants too quickly. The first participants who want to be key informants may be "deviant" members of the culture being studied. If ethnographers align themselves with marginal members of the culture, this may prevent gaining access to other valuable informants (Bernard, 2006).

Sampling in ethnography typically involves more than selecting informants because observation and other means of data collection play an important role in helping researchers understand a culture. Ethnographers have to decide not only *whom* to sample, but *what* to sample as well. For example, ethnographers have to make decisions about observing *events* and *activities*, about examining *records* and *artifacts*, and about exploring *places* that provide clues about the culture. Key informants can play an important role in helping ethnographers decide what to sample.

Example of an ethnographic sample:
Sobralske (2006) conducted an ethnographic study exploring healthcare-seeking beliefs and behaviors of Mexican American men living in Washington state. The researchers participated in activities within the Mexican American community, and then recruited participants through community organizations, religious groups, schools, and personal contacts. The sample consisted of eight key informants who varied in terms of acculturation, occupation, educational levels, and interests. The sample also included 28 secondary research participants, who were men and women with insight into healthcare-seeking beliefs and actions of Mexican American men. The secondary participants helped to validate the findings from the key informants.

Sampling in Phenomenological Studies

Phenomenologists tend to rely on very small samples—typically 10 or fewer participants. There is one guiding principle in selecting the sample for a phenomenological study: All participants must have experienced the phenomenon and must be able to articulate what it is like to have lived that experience. It might thus be said that phenomenol-

ogists use a criterion sampling method, the criterion being experience with the phenomenon under study. Although phenomenological researchers seek participants who have had the targeted experiences, they also want to explore diversity of individual experiences. Thus, they may specifically look for people with demographic or other differences who have shared a common experience (Porter, 1999).

Example of a sample in a phenomenological study: Wåhlin and colleagues (2009) studied empowerment from the perspective of family members of patients in intensive care units (ICUs) in two Swedish hospitals. The researchers used maximum variation sampling to select 10 families, to obtain a wide range of the phenomenon. "This strategy aimed at capturing and describing the central themes that cut across a great deal of variation . . . Next of kin . . . of different ages, genders and relationships to the ICU patients were selected in collaboration with ICU nurses in each department" (pp. 2581–2582).

Sampling in Grounded Theory Studies

Grounded theory research is typically done with samples of about 20 to 30 people, using theoretical sampling. The goal in a grounded theory study is to select informants who can best contribute to the evolving theory. Sampling, data collection, data analysis, and theory construction occur concurrently. Study participants are selected serially and contingently (i.e., contingent on the emerging conceptualization). Sampling might evolve as follows:

1. The researcher begins with a general notion of where and with whom to start. The first few cases may be solicited purposively, by convenience, or through snowballing.
2. In the early part of the study, a strategy such as maximum variation sampling might be used, to gain insights into the range and complexity of the phenomenon under study.
3. The sample is adjusted in an ongoing fashion. Emerging conceptualizations help to inform the sampling process.
4. Sampling continues until saturation is achieved.

5. Final sampling may include a search for confirming and disconfirming cases to test, refine, and strengthen the theory.

Draucker and colleagues (2007) have provided particularly useful guidance with regard to actual implementation of theoretical sampling, based on strategies used in their study of responses to sexual violence. Their article included a model for a "theoretical sampling guide."

Example of a sample in a grounded theory study: Mordoch and Hall (2009) studied the process by which children manage their experiences of living with a parent with mental illness. Their study involved interviews with 22 children from 14 families. Initially, purposive sampling was used, but "as the categories were developed from codes, theoretical sampling was used to increase the conditions and properties associated with the categories" (p. 1128). Ten children were interviewed a second time, several months to a year after the initial interview. All 10 of these second-round participants were sampled theoretically, "which provided incidents to develop properties of the categories" (p. 1129).

SAMPLING AND GENERALIZABILITY IN QUALITATIVE RESEARCH

Qualitative research, perhaps because of its richly diverse disciplinary and philosophical roots, is beleaguered by many dilemmas and debates. Several important controversies concern the issue of study integrity and validity, which we discuss in Chapter 24. We focus in this chapter on the controversial issue of generalizability because of its relevance to sampling strategies.

Qualitative researchers seldom worry explicitly about the issue of generalizability. The goal of most qualitative studies is to provide a contextualized understanding of human experience through the intensive study of particular cases. Sampling decisions are not guided by a desire to generalize to a target population. Qualitative researchers are not in full agreement, however, about the importance or attainability of generalizability. At one extreme are

those who challenge the possibility of generalizability in any type of research. In this view, knowledge is to be found in the particulars. Generalization requires extrapolation that can never be fully justified because findings are never free from context. On the other hand, some believe that in-depth qualitative inquiry is particularly well suited for revealing higher-level concepts that are not unique to a particular person or setting (Glaser, 2002; Misco, 2007). It might also be argued that the rich, highly detailed nature of qualitative findings make them especially suitable for extrapolation.

Many who have written about generalizability in qualitative research take a middle ground and attempt to find a balance between the generalizable and the particular through "reasonable extrapolation" (Patton, 2002, p. 489). A position that we think is sensible has been advanced by leading thinkers in both quantitative research (Lee Cronbach) and qualitative research (Egon Guba), both of whom asserted that any generalization represents a *working hypothesis*. Cronbach (1975) noted that, "When we give proper weight to local conditions, any generalization is a working hypothesis, not a conclusion" (p. 125). Guba (1978) concurred, writing that "in the spirit of naturalistic inquiry (the researcher) should regard each possible generalization only as a working hypothesis, to be tested again in the next encounter and again in the encounter after that" (p. 70).

In the current evidence-based practice environment, the issue of the applicability of research findings beyond the particular people who took part in a study is a critical one. Indeed, Groleau and colleagues (2009), in discussing generalizability, have argued that an important goal of qualitative studies is to shape the opinion of decision makers whose actions affect people's health and well-being. They noted that "it is not qualitative data itself that must have a direct impact on decision makers but the insights they foster in relation to the problem under investigation" (p. 418).

Firestone (1993) developed a useful typology depicting three models of generalizability. The first model is extrapolating from a sample to a population, the model that guides most sampling designs in quantitative research, as discussed in Chapter 12. The second model is analytic or conceptual generalization, and the third is case-to-case translation, which is more often referred to as transferability.

Analytic Generalization

In **analytic generalization**, researchers strive to generalize from particulars to a broader theory. Curtis and colleagues (2000) viewed analytic generalization as a key feature of qualitative samples, which they believe are often selected expressly on the basis of how selected cases "fit" with general constructs. Miles and Huberman (1994), who wrote an influential book on analyzing qualitative data, argued that qualitative sampling can provide the opportunity to select and analyze observations of generic processes that are key to understanding and developing theory about the phenomenon being studied. In their view, theory and conceptualization should drive the selection of cases, and the careful analysis of data from these cases can then result in elaboration, refinement, or reformulation of the theory.

Firestone (1993) noted that generalizing to a theory or conceptualization is a matter of identifying evidence that supports (but does not definitely prove) that conceptualization. Qualitative researchers use analytic generalization to increase confidence that the conceptualizations are cogent. In essence, analytic generalization involves the concept of *replication*. Firestone argued that "When conditions vary, successful replication contributes to generalizability. Similar results under different conditions illustrate the robustness of the finding" (p. 17).

In this model of generalization, several sampling approaches can be profitably used to advance the conceptualization. Critical case sampling, for example, can be used for contrasting alternative conceptualizations. Deviant case sampling can help to refine or revise a conceptualization, but can also help to understand extreme conditions under which the conceptualization holds. Maximum variation sampling can also help to strengthen generalization by including cases that vary on attributes likely to affect the conceptualization of the key phenome-

non. In grounded theory, theoretical sampling is clearly geared to using particular cases to develop a theory grounded in personal experiences.

In short, analytic generalization concerns the conceptual power of the inquiry. As noted by Thorne and colleagues (2009), "When articulated in a manner that is authentic and credible to the reader, (findings) can reflect valid descriptions of sufficient richness and depth that their products warrant a degree of *generalizability in relation to a field of understanding*" (p. 1385, emphasis added).

➔ **TIP:** Analytic generalization is particularly well exemplified in metasyntheses of multiple qualitative studies, which we describe in Chapter 27.

Transferability

The third model of generalizability proposed by Firestone (1993) is what he called *case-to-case translation*. Case-to-case transfer involves judgments about whether findings from an inquiry can be extrapolated to a different setting or group of people. This model is more widely referred to as **transferability** (Lincoln and Guba, 1985), but has also been called *reader generalizability* (Misco, 2007).

Transferability is inherently a collaborative endeavor. The researcher's job is to provide detailed descriptive information that allows readers to make inferences about extrapolating the findings to other settings. The main work of transferability, however, is done by readers and consumers. Their job is to assess the extent to which the conceptualizations and findings apply to new situations. It is the readers of research who "transfer" the results.

Transferability has close connections to concepts developed by research methodologist Donald Campbell (1986), who suggested an approach to generalizability called the **proximal similarity model**. (Indeed, Campbell thought that proximal similarity was a more suitable term than external validity—a term he himself had coined—for considering how research might be extrapolated). Within the proximal similarity model, researchers and consumers develop a conceptualization about which contexts are more or less like the one in the study. His model, depicted graphically in Figure 21.1, involves conceptualizing a *gradient of similarity* for people, settings, times, and sociopolitical contexts. Although generalizations can never be made with certainty, this model of proximal similarity supports transferability to those people, places, and contexts that are most like (i.e., most proximally similar to) those in the focal study.

In discussing how researchers can support the transferability of their findings, most writers discuss the need for thick description. **Thick description** refers to a rich and thorough description of the research setting, study participants, and observed transactions and processes. Readers can only make good judgments about the proximal similarity of the contexts in the study and their own environments if researchers provide high-quality descriptive information. (Of course, thick description serves other functions in a qualitative inquiry, such as allowing the depiction of a phenomenon, process, or culture to "ring true" and seem credible).

Because researchers are familiar with only the "sending contexts" of their study and not the "receiving contexts" of potential users (Lincoln & Guba, 1985, p. 297), some argue that the researcher's responsibility is solely to provide thorough description of the sending contexts. The proximal similarity model suggests, however, that researchers can do a bit more. In developing thick descriptions, researchers can think conceptually rather than simply descriptively about their study contexts. That is, they can develop (and communicate) a theoretical perspective about essential contextual features that might make their findings transferable so that readers can make theoretically informed judgments about which contexts are most proximally similar. The goal is not so much to have a formal theory about contexts and gradients of similarity, but to have a framework that is abstract and conceptual in deciding on the types of descriptive information to share. For example, if a prominent feature of the phenomenon under study relates to participants' *vulnerability*, what characteristics need to be described to effectively communicate ways in which that vulnerability is manifested or factors that contribute to it?

Qualitative researchers use various means of describing the contexts of their inquiries and their study participants. In studies with diverse and relatively large samples, qualitative reports sometimes include a table with demographic information, much like in a quantitative report. For example, such a table might present participants' average age, gender, socioeconomic information, and clinical information. When samples are small, key characteristics of the study participants are often described in a paragraph or two in the text. Sometimes, however, qualitative researchers present a table that shows information about each individual participant in terms of characteristics deemed to be important—although care must taken in ensuring

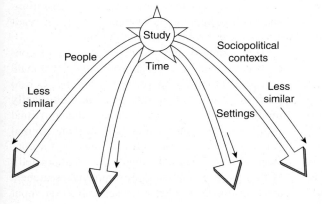

FIGURE 21.1 Graphical representation of the proximal similarity model and gradients of similarity.

that such a table does not compromise participants' confidentiality.

➡ **TIP:** The issue of transferability has been mainly discussed in connection with qualitative research, but it is also an appropriate construct for quantitative research (Polit & Beck, 2010). Using sampling methods such as those described in Chapter 12, researchers make inferences about whether findings from the sample can be generalized to the population. However, findings from a generalizable study may also be transferable. For example, findings about intervention effects in three hospitals in Boston can perhaps be *generalized* to patients in the Boston area, or to those in northeastern United States — but perhaps they are *transferable* to similar patients in Hong Kong.

CRITIQUING SAMPLING PLANS

Qualitative researchers do not always describe in much detail their method of identifying, recruiting, and selecting participants. Yet, readers will have difficulty drawing conclusions about the study findings without knowing something about researchers' sampling strategies. Indeed, there have been increased demands for making sampling decisions and processes in qualitative research more "public" (Onwuegbuzie & Leech, 2007). In keeping with the goal of thick description, qualitative reports should ideally describe the following:

- The type of sampling approach used (e.g., snowball, purposive, theoretical), together with an indication of how variation was dealt with (e.g., in maximum variation sampling, the dimensions chosen for diversification)
- Eligibility criteria for inclusion in the study
- The nature of the setting or community
- The time period during which data were collected
- The number of participants, and a rationale for the sample size, such as an explicit statement that data saturation was achieved
- The main characteristics of participants (e.g., age, gender, length of illness, and so on)

Inadequate description of the researcher's sampling strategy can be an impediment to assessing

whether the strategy was productive. Moreover, if the description is vague, it will be difficult for readers to come to a conclusion about whether the evidence can be applied in their clinical practice. Thus, in critiquing a report you should see whether the researcher provided an adequately thick description of the sample and the context in which the study was carried out so that someone interested in transferring the findings could make an informed decision.

Various writers have proposed criteria for evaluating sampling in qualitative studies. Morse (1991b), for example, advocated two criteria: adequacy and appropriateness. *Adequacy* refers to the sufficiency and quality of the data the sample yielded. An adequate sample provides data without any "thin" spots. When the researcher has truly obtained data saturation, informational adequacy has been achieved, and the resulting description or theory is richly textured and complete.

Appropriateness concerns the methods used to select a sample. An appropriate sample is one resulting from the identification and use of participants who can best supply information according to the conceptual requirements of the study. Researchers should use a strategy that yields the fullest possible understanding of the phenomenon of interest. A sampling approach that excludes negative cases or that fails to include participants with unusual experiences may not meet the information needs of the study.

Curtis and colleagues (2000) proposed six criteria for evaluating qualitative sampling strategies, which they adapted from Miles and Huberman (1994). These strategies are in some cases more relevant for a self-evaluation by qualitative researchers themselves than for a critique by readers. First, the sampling strategy should be relevant to the tradition, conceptual framework, and research question addressed by the research. Second, the sample should yield rich information on the phenomenon under study. Third—and this relates to our earlier discussion—the sample should enhance the analytic generalizability of the findings. Fourth, the sample should produce believable descriptions, in the sense of being true to real life. Fifth, the sampling strategy should be ethical. Finally, the sampling plan should be

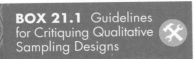

BOX 21.1 Guidelines for Critiquing Qualitative Sampling Designs

1. Is the setting or context adequately described? Is the setting appropriate for the research question?
2. Are the sample selection procedures clearly delineated? What type of sampling strategy was used?
3. Are the eligibility criteria for the study specified? How were participants recruited into the study? Did the recruitment strategy yield information-rich participants?
4. Given the information needs of the study—and, if applicable, its qualitative tradition—was the sampling approach appropriate? Are dimensions of the phenomenon under study adequately represented?
5. Was the sample size adequate and appropriate for the qualitative tradition of the study? Did the researcher indicate that saturation had been achieved?
6. Do the findings suggest a richly textured and comprehensive set of data without any apparent "holes" or thin areas? Did the sample contribute sufficiently to analytic generalization?
7. Are key characteristics of the sample described (e.g., age, gender)? Is a rich description of participants and context provided, allowing for an assessment of the transferability of the findings?

feasible in terms of resources, time, and researcher's skills—and in terms of the researcher's or participants' ability to cope with the data collection process.

Some specific questions that can be used to critique sampling in a qualitative study are presented in Box 21.1.

RESEARCH EXAMPLE

Examples of various approaches to sampling in qualitative research have been presented through-out this chapter. In this section, we describe in some detail the sampling plan of an ethnographic study. (This study appears in its entirety in the appendix to the *Resource Manual*.)

Study: Formative infant feeding experiences and education of NICU nurses (Cricco-Lizza, 2009).

Purpose: The researcher explored in detail the formative infant feeding experiences and understandings of nurses working in neonatal intensive care units (NICUs).

Method: Cricco-Lizza used ethnographic methods to collect contextually rich and detailed information about NICU nurses and infant feeding. The research was undertaken over a 14-month period in a level IV NICU in a pediatric hospital in northeastern United States. Data were collected primarily through observations and interviews.

Sampling Strategy: Approximately 250 nurses worked in the NICU, and 114 of them participated as general informants. These nurses were observed or informally interviewed during routine NICU activities, and they provided a broad overview of infant feeding on the unit. From these 114 nurses, 18 nurses with a variety of professional experiences and educational backgrounds were purposefully sampled to be key informants. These key informants, who were followed more intensively over the course of the fieldwork, were chosen from different expertise levels (novice to clinical expert), to obtain varied views of the NICU culture with regard to infant feeding practices. The researcher observed nurses during the usual course of their activities in the NICU. The observational sessions, which lasted for an hour or 2, involved sampling of activities on varying days, work shifts, and times of the week. Cricco-Lizza also made observations during breastfeeding committee meetings, psychosocial rounds, and nurse-run breastfeeding support groups for parents. General informants were observed and informally interviewed an average of 3.5 times each over the study period. Key informants agreed to a formal interview and were also observed and informally interviewed a total of 3 to 43 times each, with an average of 13.1 interactions over the study. The repeated contacts "allowed for deeper exploration about infant feeding in the NICU" (p. 238).

Key Findings: The nurses recounted minimal exposure to breastfeeding in nursing school. Their personal experiences with breastfeeding were emotionally laden and intertwined with their feelings about motherhood. Cricco-Lizza suggested the possible transferability of her findings by noting that breastfeeding education programs for nurses should include reflective components so that they could identify barriers to breastfeeding support.

SUMMARY POINTS

- Qualitative researchers use the conceptual demands of the study to select articulate and reflective informants with certain types of experience in an emergent way, typically capitalizing on early learning to guide subsequent sampling decisions. Qualitative samples tend to be small, nonrandom, and intensively studied.
- Sampling in qualitative inquiry may begin with a convenience (or volunteer) sample. Snowball (chain) sampling may also be used.
- Qualitative researchers often use **purposive sampling** to select data sources that enhance information richness. Various purposive sampling strategies have been used by qualitative researchers, and can be loosely categorized as (1) sampling for representativeness or comparative value, (2) sampling special or unique cases, or (3) sampling sequentially.
- An important purposive strategy in the first category is **maximum variation sampling**, which entails purposely selecting cases with a wide range of variation. Other strategies used for comparative purposes or representativeness include **homogeneous sampling** (deliberately reducing variation), **typical case sampling** (selecting cases that illustrate what is typical), **extreme case sampling** (selecting the most unusual or extreme cases), **intensity sampling** (selecting cases that are intense but not extreme), **stratified purposeful sampling** (selecting average, above average, and below average cases), and **reputational case sampling** (selecting cases based on a recommendation of an expert or key informant).
- Purposive sampling in the "special cases" category include **critical case sampling** (selecting

cases that are especially important or illustrative), **criterion sampling** (studying cases that meet a predetermined criterion of importance), **revelatory case sampling** (identifying and gaining access to a case representing a phenomenon that was previously inaccessible to research scrutiny), and **sampling politically important cases** (searching for and selecting or deselecting politically sensitive cases or sites).
- Although many qualitative sampling strategies unfold while in the field, purposive sampling in the "sequential" category involve deliberative emergent efforts and include **theory-based sampling** (selecting cases on the basis of their representation of important constructs) and **opportunistic sampling** (adding new cases based on changes in research circumstances or in response to new leads that develop in the field). Another important sequential strategy is **sampling confirming and disconfirming cases**—that is, selecting cases that enrich and challenge the researchers' conceptualizations.
- A guiding sample size principle is **data saturation**—sampling to the point at which no new information is obtained and redundancy is achieved. Factors affecting sample size include data quality, researcher skills and experience, and scope and sensitivity of the problem.
- Ethnographers make numerous sampling decisions, including not only *whom* to sample, but also *what* to sample (e.g., activities, events, documents, artifacts); decision making is often aided by their *key informants* who serve as guides and interpreters of the culture.
- Phenomenologists typically work with a small sample of people (10 or fewer) who meet the criterion of having lived the experience under study.
- Grounded theory researchers typically use **theoretical sampling** in which sampling decisions are guided in an ongoing fashion by the emerging theory. Samples of about 20 to 30 people are typical in grounded theory studies.
- Generalizability in qualitative research is a controversial issue, with some writers claiming it to be unattainable because of the highly

contextualized nature of qualitative findings. Yet, most qualitative researchers strive to have their findings be relevant and meaningful beyond the confines of their particular study participants and settings.

- Two models of generalizability have relevance for qualitative research. In **analytic generalization**, researchers strive to generalize from particulars to broader conceptualizations and theories. Such generalizing involves identifying evidence in particular experiences or events that supports a broader conceptualization of a phenomenon.

- A widely used model of generalizability is **transferability**, which involves judgments about whether findings from an inquiry can be extrapolated to a different setting or group of people. Transferability is a collaborative effort between researchers (who must provide **thick description** about their research contexts) and potential users of qualitative evidence.

- Transferability has close connections to the **proximal similarity model**, which involves a conceptualization about which contexts are more or less like the one in the study in terms of a *gradient of similarity* for people, settings, times, and contexts.

STUDY ACTIVITIES

Chapter 21 of the *Resource Manual for Nursing Research: Generating and Assessing Evidence for Nursing Practice*, *9th edition*, offers exercises and study suggestions for reinforcing concepts presented in this chapter. In addition, the following study questions can be addressed:

1. Read a qualitative study involving a patient population that is personally relevant or interesting to you. Where would your own setting map onto the various dimensions of similarity (Figure 21.1)? How "proximally similar" is your setting to the setting described in the study?

2. Answer relevant questions from Box 21.1 with regard to the grounded theory study by Mordoch and Hall (2009), briefly described in this chapter.

STUDIES CITED IN CHAPTER 21

Beck, C. T. (2002). Releasing the pause button: Mothering multiples during the first year of life. *Qualitative Health Research 12*, 593–608.

Beck, C. T. (2009). An adult survivor of child sexual abuse and her breastfeeding experience: A case study. *MCN: The American Journal of Maternal/Child Nursing, 34*, 91–97.

Ching, S., Martinson, I., & Wong, T. (2009). Reframing: Psychological adjustment of Chinese women at the beginning of the breast cancer experience. *Qualitative Health Research, 19*, 339–351.

Cricco-Lizza, R. (2009). Formative infant feeding experiences and education of NICU nurses. *MCN: The American Journal of Maternal/Child Nursing, 34*, 236–242.

Early, K., Shultz, J., & Corbett, C. (2009). Assessing diabetes dietary goals and self-management based on in-depth interviews with Latino and Caucasian clients with type 2 diabetes. *Journal of Transcultural Nursing, 20*, 371–381.

Gunnarsson, B., & Warrén-Stomberg, M. (2009). Factors influencing decision-making among ambulance nurses in emergency care situations. *International Emergency Nursing, 17*, 83–89.

Lash, A., Kulakac, O., Buldukoglu, K., & Kukulu, K. (2006). Verbal abuse of nursing and midwifery students in clinical settings in Turkey. *Journal of Nursing Education, 45*, 396–403.

Mordoch, E., & Hall, W. (2009). Children's perception of living with a parent with a mental illness: Finding the rhythm, and maintaining the frame. *Qualitative Health Research, 19*, 1127–1144.

Petersen, Z., Nilsson, M., Everett, K., & Emmelin, M. (2009). Possibilities for transparency and trust in the communication between midwives and pregnant women: The case of smoking. *Midwifery, 25*, 382–391.

Pugh, D. (2009). The phoenix process: A substantive theory about allegations of unprofessional conduct. *Journal of Advanced Nursing, 65*, 2027–2037.

Riegel, B., Vaughan Dickson, V., Goldberg, L., & Deatrick, J. (2007). Factors associated with the development of expertise in heart failure self-care. *Nursing Research, 56*, 235–243.

Sabuni, L. P. (2007). Dilemma with the local perception of causes of illnesses in Central Africa: Muted concept but prevalent in everyday life. *Qualitative Health Research, 17*, 1280–1291.

Sobralske, M. C. (2006). Health care seeking among Mexican American men. *Journal of Transcultural Nursing, 17*, 129–138.

Speraw, S. (2009). "Talk to me—I'm human": The story of a girl, her personhood, and the failures of health care. *Qualitative Health Research, 19*, 732–743.

Stevens, P., & Hildebrandt, E. (2009). Pill taking from the perspective of HIV-infected women who are vulnerable to antiretroviral treatment failure. *Qualitative Health Research, 19*, 593–604.

Thorne, S., Armstrong, E., Harris, S., Hislop, T., Kim-Sung, C., Oglov, V., Oliffe, J. L., & Stajduhar, K. I. (2009). Patient real-time and 12-month retrospective perceptions of difficult communications in the cancer diagnostic period. *Qualitative Health Research, 19*, 1383–1394.

Wåhlin, I., Ek, A., & Idvall, E. (2009). Empowerment from the perspective of next of kin in intensive nursing. *Journal of Clinical Nursing, 18*, 2580–2587.

Ward, E., Clark, L., & Heidrich, S. (2009). African American women's beliefs, coping behaviors, and barriers to seeking mental health services. *Qualitative Health Research, 19*, 1589–1601.

Weinberg, D., Miner, D., & Rivlin, L. (2009). "It depends": Medical residents' perspectives on working with nurses. *American Journal of Nursing, 109*, 34–43.

Williams, A., Manias, E., & Walker, R. (2009). The role of irrational thought in medicine adherence: People with diabetic kidney disease. *Journal of Advanced Nursing, 65*, 2108–2117.

Methodologic and nonresearch references cited in this chapter can be found in a separate section at the end of the book.

Data Collection in Qualitative Research

T his chapter provides an overview of unstructured data collection approaches and strategies used in qualitative research.

DATA COLLECTION ISSUES IN QUALITATIVE STUDIES

In qualitative studies, data collection usually is more fluid than in quantitative research, and decisions about what to collect evolve in the field. For example, as researchers gather and digest information, they may realize that it would be fruitful to pursue an unanticipated line of questioning. Even while allowing for and profiting from this flexibility, however, qualitative researchers make a number of up-front decisions about data collection. Moreover, qualitative researchers need to be prepared for problematic situations that may arise in the field. Creativity for workable solutions and new strategies are often needed.

Example of need for flexibility in a qualitative study: Irwin and Johnson (2005) did a study that involved interviews with 6-year-old children about their health. The researchers described how they had to be creative and had to individualize interviews with the child participants. They used several forms of play (drawing, role-playing) to enhance children's comfort and build rapport. They also noted the need to be flexible and to "think outside the box" when it came to selecting a setting for the interview.

Types of Data for Qualitative Studies

Qualitative researchers typically go into the field knowing the most likely sources of data, while not ruling out other possible data sources that might come to light as data collection progresses. The primary method of collecting qualitative data is by interviewing study participants. Observation is often a part of many qualitative studies as well. Physiologic data are rarely collected in a constructivist inquiry, except perhaps to describe participants' characteristics or to ascertain eligibility for the sample.

Table 22.1 compares the types of data used by researchers in the three main qualitative traditions, as well as other aspects of the data collection process for each tradition. As noted in Chapter 20, ethnographers typically collect a wide array of data, with observation and interviews being the primary methods. Ethnographers also gather or examine products of the culture under study such as documents, records, artifacts, photographs, and so on. Phenomenologists and grounded theory researchers rely primarily on in-depth interviews, although observation also plays a role in grounded theory studies.

TABLE 22.1	Comparison of Data Collection Issues in Three Qualitative Traditions		
ISSUE	**ETHNOGRAPHY**	**PHENOMENOLOGY**	**GROUNDED THEORY**
Types of data	Primarily observation and interviews, plus artifacts, documents, photographs, genealogies, maps, social network diagrams	Primarily in-depth interviews, sometimes diaries, other written materials	Primarily individual interviews, sometimes group interviews, observation, participant journals, documents
Unit of data collection	Cultural systems	Individuals	Individuals
Data collection points	Mainly longitudinal	Mainly cross-sectional	Cross-sectional or longitudinal
Length of time for data collection	Typically long, many months or years	Typically moderate	Typically moderate
Data recording	Field notes, logs, interview notes/recordings	Interview notes/ recordings	Interview notes/ recordings, memoing, observational notes
Salient field issues	Gaining entrée, reactivity, determining a role, learning how to participate, encouraging candor and other interview logistics, loss of objectivity, premature exit, reflexivity	Bracketing one's views, building rapport, encouraging candor, listening while preparing what to ask next, keeping "on track," handling emotionality	Building rapport, encouraging candor, listening while preparing what to ask next, keeping "on track," handling emotionality

The research tradition also has implications for how the researcher as "self" is used (Lipson, 1991). Phenomenological researchers use "self" to collect rich descriptions of human experiences and to develop relationships in intensive interviews with a small number of people. Grounded theorists use themselves not only to collect data, but also to process the data and generate categories for the emerging theory. Ethnographers use themselves as observers who collect data not only through interviews, but also through active participation in field settings.

Field Issues in Qualitative Studies

The collection of qualitative data in the field often gives rise to several important issues, which are particularly salient in ethnographies. Ethnographic researchers, in addition to matters discussed in this section, must deal with such issues as gaining entrée, negotiating for space and privacy for interviewing and recording data, deciding on an appropriate role (i.e., the extent to which they will actually participate in the culture's activities), and taking care not to exit from the field prematurely. Ethnographers also need to be able to cope with culture shock and should have a high tolerance for uncertainty and ambiguity.

Gaining Trust

Researchers who do qualitative research must, to an even greater extent than quantitative researchers, gain and maintain a high level of trust with participants.

Researchers need to develop strategies in the field to establish credibility among those being studied. This may be a delicate balancing act, because researchers must try to "be like" the people being studied while at the same time keeping a certain distance. "Being like" participants means that researchers should be sensitive to such issues as styles of dress, modes of speech, customs, and schedules. In ethnographic research, it is important not to take sides on any controversial issue and not to appear too strongly affiliated with a particular subgroup of the culture—especially with leaders or prominent members of the culture. It is often impossible to gain the trust of the group if researchers appear close to those in power.

The Pace of Data Collection

In qualitative studies, data collection is often an intense and exhausting experience, especially if the phenomenon being studied concerns an illness experience or other stressful life event (e.g., domestic violence). Collecting high-quality qualitative data requires deep concentration and energy. The process can be an emotional strain for which researchers need to prepare. One way to deal with this is to collect data at a pace that minimizes stress. For example, it may be prudent to limit interviewing to no more than once a day, and to engage in emotionally releasing activities (e.g., exercising) between interviews. It may also be helpful to debrief about any feelings of distress with a co-researcher, colleague, or advisor.

Emotional Involvement with Participants

Qualitative researchers need to guard against getting too emotionally involved with participants, a pitfall that has been called "**going native**." Researchers who get too close to participants run several risks, including compromising their ability to collect meaningful and trustworthy data, and becoming overwhelmed with participants' suffering. It is important, of course, to be supportive and to listen carefully to people's concerns, but it usually is not advisable to intervene and try to solve participants' problems, or to share personal problems with them. If participants need help, it is better to give advice about where they can get it than to give it directly.

Reflexivity

As noted in Chapter 8, reflexivity is an important concept in qualitative data collection. Reflexivity refers to researchers' awareness of themselves as part of the data they are collecting. Researchers need to be conscious of the part they play in their own study and reflect on their own behavior and how it can affect the data they obtain.

Example of reflexivity: Egerod (2009) explored Danish physicians' perceptions of sedation in ICU settings. She interviewed seven informants, asking such questions as, "What is the role of the nurse in relation to sedation, in your view?" (p. 688) Here is what Egerod said about reflexivity: "As the sole investigator, I wished to come to terms with my motives, background, perspectives, and preliminary hypotheses . . . This included attending systematically to the context of knowledge construction, especially to the effect of my preconceptions." (p. 689)

Recording and Storing Qualitative Data

In addition to thinking about the types of data to be gathered, qualitative researchers need to plan ahead for how data will be recorded and stored. Interview data can be recorded by taking detailed notes of what participants say, or by audio or video recording. To ensure that interview data are participants' actual verbatim responses, we strongly recommend that qualitative interviews be recorded and subsequently transcribed, rather than relying on interviewer notes. Notes tend to be incomplete, and may be biased by the interviewer's memory or personal views. Moreover, note taking can distract researchers, whose main job is to listen intently and direct the flow of questioning based on what has already been said.

TIP: In addition to traditional audiotaping equipment, new technologies are emerging to facilitate recording in the field. For example, digital voice recorders with transcription capabilities allow researchers to record and transfer voice data to a personal computer using a USB interface. Some digital voice recorders come bundled with voice recognition software (see Chapter 23).

Environmental distractions are a common pitfall in recording interviews. A quiet setting without disruptions is ideal, but is not always possible. The second author of this book (Beck) has conducted many challenging interviews. As one example, a mother of three children was interviewed in her home about her experience with postpartum depression. The interview was scheduled during the toddlers' normal naptime, but when Beck arrived, the toddlers had already taken their nap. The television was on to occupy the toddlers, but they kept trying to play with the tape recorder. The 6-week-old baby was fussy, crying through most of the interview. The background noise level on the tape made accurate transcription difficult.

When observations are made, detailed observational notes must be maintained, unless it is possible to videotape. Observational notes should be made shortly after an observational session and are often entered onto a computer file. Whatever method is used to record observations, researchers need to go into the field with the equipment or supplies needed to record their data and to be sure that the equipment is functioning properly.

Grounded theory researchers write *analytic memos* that document researchers' ideas about how the theory is developing (e.g., how some themes are interrelated). These memos can vary in length from a sentence to multiple pages. Montgomery and Bailey (2007) offer some guidance and examples of grounded theory notes and memos.

If assistants are used to collect the data, qualitative researchers need to be as concerned as quantitative researchers about hiring appropriate staff and training them to collect high-quality data. In particular, the data collectors must be trained to elicit rich and vivid descriptions. Qualitative interviewers need to be good listeners; they need to hear all that is being said, rather than trying to anticipate what is coming next. A good data collector must have both self-awareness and an awareness of participants (e.g., by paying attention to nonverbal behavior). Qualitative data collectors must be able to create an atmosphere that safely allows for the sharing of experiences and feelings. Respect and authentic caring for participants are critical.

TIP: In qualitative studies, data are often collected by a single researcher working alone, in which case self-training and self-preparation are important. When a team of researchers works together on a qualitative study, attention needs to be paid to team issues related to fieldwork and to group decision making and planning in general (Hall et al., 2005).

Storage of data while in the field can be problematic because researchers may not have safe or secure storage space. When this happens, they often keep the data physically with them at all times until it can be secured (e.g., in a fanny pack). All data tapes or forms should be carefully labeled with an identification number, the date the data were collected, and (if relevant) the name or identification number of the data collector.

TIP: It is a wise strategy to have back-up copies of your data. Backing up files is imperative (and easy) for data stored on computers, but if computers are not being used, photocopies of written or transcribed materials should be maintained in a separate location. If you expect a delay between taping and transcribing an interview, you should also consider making back-up copies of the tapes, which can sometimes get erased through static electricity.

QUALITATIVE SELF-REPORT TECHNIQUES

Unstructured or loosely structured self-report methods provide narrative data for qualitative analysis. Most qualitative self-report data are collected through interviews rather than by questionnaire.

Types of Qualitative Self-Reports

Researchers use various approaches in collecting qualitative self-report data. The main methods are described here.

Unstructured Interviews
Researchers who do not have a preconceived view of the content or flow of information to be gathered may conduct completely **unstructured interviews**.

Unstructured interviews are conversational and interactive and are the mode of choice when researchers do not have a clear idea of what it is they do not know. Researchers using unstructured interviews do not have a set of prepared questions because they do not yet know what to ask or even where to begin—they let participants tell their stories, with little interruption. Phenomenological, grounded theory, and ethnographic studies often involve unstructured interviews.

Researchers using a completely unstructured approach often begin by informally asking a broad question (sometimes called a **grand tour question**) relating to the research topic, such as, "What happened when you first learned you had AIDS?" Subsequent questions are more focused and are guided by responses to the broad question. Some respondents may request direction after the initial broad question is posed, perhaps asking, "Where should I begin?" Respondents should be encouraged to begin wherever they wish.

Van Manen (1990) provided suggestions for guiding a phenomenological interview in a manner likely to produce rich descriptions of the experience under study:

- "Describe the experience from the inside, as it were; almost like a state of mind: the feelings, the mood, the emotions, etc.
- Focus on a particular example or incident of the object of experience: specific events, an adventure, a happening, a particular experience.
- Try to focus on an example of the experience which stands out for its vividness, or as it was the first time.
- Attend to how the body feels, how things smell(ed), how they sound(ed), etc." (pp. 64–65)

Kahn (2000), discussing unstructured interviews in hermeneutic phenomenological studies, recommended interviews that resemble conversations. If the experience under study is an ongoing one, Kahn suggested obtaining as much detail as possible about the participant's daily life. For example, a question that can be used is, "Pick a normal day for you and tell me what happened." (p. 62) If the experience being studied is primarily in the past, then Kahn advocated a retrospective approach. The interviewer would begin with a general question such as, "What does this experience mean to you?" (p. 63). The interviewer would then probe for more detail until the experience is thoroughly described.

Example of unstructured interviews: Rice (2009) studied the issue of violence among women diagnosed with schizophrenia. Unstructured interviews with women's case managers were initiated with the following statement: "I am interested in hearing your experiences as a case manager who works with women who have been diagnosed with schizophrenia and live with violence." (p. 843) Interviews, which were audiotaped, lasted between 1 and 2 hours each.

In grounded theory, questioning changes as the theory is developed. At the outset, interviews are similar to open-ended conversations using unstructured interviews. Glaser and Strauss (1967) suggested that researchers initially should just sit back and listen to participants' stories. Later, as the theory emerges, researchers ask more direct questions related to categories in the grounded theory. The more direct questions can be answered rather quickly, so the interviews tend to get shorter as the grounded theory develops.

Ethnographic interviews are also unstructured. Spradley (1979) describes three types of question used to guide interviews: descriptive, structural, and contrast questions. *Descriptive questions* ask participants to describe their experiences in their own language, and are the backbone of ethnographic interviews. *Structural questions* are more focused and help to develop the range of terms in a category or domain. Last are *contrast questions*, which are asked to distinguish differences in the meaning of terms and symbols.

Example of ethnographic interviewing: Storesund and McMurray (2009) conducted an ethnographic study of nursing practice in an Australian intensive care unit (ICU). An example of a descriptive question was, "How would you describe quality in your work in the ICU?" An example of a structural question was, "Can you describe how you organise your shift, and then what happens?" An example of a contrast question was, "Can you give me an example of a time you felt that the quality of your work was not as good as you would have preferred? How was this situation different to other times when your work was high quality?" (p. 122)

Completely unstructured methods most typically are used in face-to-face interview situations in naturalistic settings. It is, however, possible to use the Internet for collecting unstructured data, and this is particularly advantageous for "interviewing" respondents who are geographically distant. Mann and Steward (2001) offer advice about Internet interviewing.

Example of unstructured Internet interviewing:
Beck (2009) conducted a phenomenological study via the Internet about mothers' experiences caring for children with brachial plexus injuries. A recruitment notice was posted on the website of the United Brachial Plexus Network, a support organization. Women who were interested e-contacted Beck. Each mother was asked to respond to the following statement: "Please describe in as much detail as you wish to share your experience of caring for your child with a brachial plexus injury." Women sent Beck their stories by email attachment.

➔ **TIP:** An advantage of Internet interviewing is that participants' narratives are already typed, thus avoiding the expense of transcribing taped interviews. In an Internet environment, however, researchers need to devote time and effort to crafting individual email responses to make sure all participants feel valued and understand that their narratives made a contribution to the study.

Semistructured Interviews

Researchers sometimes want to be sure that a specific set of topics is covered in their qualitative interviews. They know what they want to ask, but cannot predict what the answers will be. Their role in the process is somewhat structured, whereas the participants' is not. In such **focused** or **semistructured interviews**, researchers prepare a written **topic guide**, which is a list of areas or questions to be covered with each participant. The interviewer's job is to encourage participants to talk freely about all the topics on the guide, and to tell stories in their own words. This technique ensures that researchers will obtain all the information required, and it gives people the freedom to provide as many illustrations and explanations as they wish.

In preparing the topic guide, questions should be ordered in a logical sequence—perhaps chronolog-

ically, or perhaps from the general to the specific. Interviewers need to be attentive, however, because respondents often volunteer information about questions that are later on the list. The topic guide might include suggestions for *probes* designed to elicit more detailed information. Examples of such probes include, "What happened next?" and "When that happened, how did you feel?" Questions that require one- or two-word responses, such as "yes" or "no," should be avoided. Questions should give people an opportunity to provide rich, detailed information about the phenomenon under study.

Example of a semistructured interview:
Arnaert and colleagues (2010) studied the role that a retreat weekend played in helping cancer patients' relatives to heal. Semistructured interviews, conducted with eight relatives after attendance at a retreat, included such questions as: "How did you experience the retreat weekend?" and "What is your perception of the concept of healing?" (p. 199)

Focus Group Interviews

Focus group interviews have become popular in the study of health problems. In a focus group interview, a group of five or more people is assembled for a discussion. The interviewer (or **moderator**) guides the discussion according to a written set of questions or topics to be covered, as in a semistructured interview. Focus group sessions are carefully planned discussions that take advantage of group dynamics for accessing rich information in an economical manner.

Typically, the people selected are a fairly homogeneous group, to promote a comfortable group dynamic. People usually feel more at ease expressing their views when they share a similar background with other group members. Thus, if the overall sample is diverse, it is best to organize focus groups for people with similar characteristics (e.g., in terms of age or gender).

Several writers have suggested that the optimal group size for focus groups is 6 to 12 people, but Côté-Arsenault and Morrison-Beedy (1999) advocated smaller groups of about 5 participants when the topic is emotionally charged or sensitive. Groups of four or fewer may not generate sufficient interaction, however, particularly because not everyone is equally comfortable in expressing their views.

⮕ **TIP:** In recruiting group members, it is usually wise to recruit one or two more people than is considered optimal, because of the risk of no-shows. Monetary incentives can help reduce this risk. It is also important to call recruits the night before the session to remind them of the appointment and confirm attendance.

The setting for the focus group sessions should be selected carefully and, ideally, should be a neutral one. Churches, hospitals, or other settings that are strongly identified with particular values or expected behaviors may not be suitable, depending on the topic. The location should be comfortable, accessible, easy to find, and acoustically amenable to audio-tape recording.

Moderators play a critical role in the success of focus group interviews. They must take care to solicit input from all group members, and not let a few vocal people dominate the discussion. Researchers other than the moderator should be present, to take detailed observational notes about each session.

A major advantage of a group format is that it is efficient—researchers obtain the viewpoints of many people in a short time. Moreover, focus groups capitalize on the fact that members react to what is being said by others, thereby potentially leading to deeper expressions of opinion. Focus group interviews are also usually stimulating to respondents, but one problem is that some people are uncomfortable about expressing their views in front of a group. Another concern is that the dynamics of the session may foster a group culture that could inhibit individual expression as "group think" takes hold. Studies of focus groups suggest that they are similar to individual interviews in terms of number and quality of ideas generated (Kidd & Parshall, 2000), but some critics have worried about whether data from focus groups are as "natural" as data obtained from individual interviews (Morgan, 2001).

Key to an effective focus group is the researcher's *questioning route,* that is, the series of questions used to guide the interview. Krueger and Casey (2008) provide guidelines for developing a good questioning

route. A typical 2-hour focus group session should include about 12 questions. A good strategy for question sequence is to move from general to specific.

Focus groups have been used by researchers in many qualitative research traditions and can play an important role in feminist, critical theory, and participatory action research. Nurse researchers have offered excellent guidance on studies with focus groups (e.g., Côté-Arsenault & Morrison-Beedy, 2005; Morrison-Beedy et al., 2001) and books on how to do focus group research are available (e.g., Bader & Rossi, 2002; Krueger & Casey, 2008). The Toolkit in the accompanying *Resource Manual* also has additional resources on focus groups. ⊗

Example of focus group interviews: Wu and colleagues (2010) studied the experience of cancer-related fatigue among Chinese children with leukemia. A total of 14 children aged 7 to 18, divided into age groups, participated in one of four focus groups held at a clinical setting. An example of one of the nine questions from the interview guide is: "Could you describe what it feels like to be tired and lacking in energy?" (p. 52)

Joint Interviews

Nurse researchers are sometimes interested in phenomena that involve interpersonal relationships, or that require understanding the perspective of more than one person. For example, the phenomenon might be the grief that mothers *and* fathers experience on losing a child, or the experiences of AIDS patients *and* their caretakers. In such cases, it can be productive to conduct **joint (dyadic) interviews** in which two or more people are simultaneously questioned, using either an unstructured or a semistructured format. Unlike focus group interviews, which typically involve group members who do not know each other, joint interviews involve respondents who are intimately related.

Joint interviews usually supplement rather than replace individual interviews, because there are things that cannot readily be discussed in front of the other party (e.g., criticisms of the other person's behavior). Joint interviews can be especially helpful, however, when researchers want to *observe* the dynamics between two key actors. Morris (2001) raised important issues to consider in the conduct of joint interviews.

Example of joint interviews: Chang and Mu (2008) studied family stress among infertile couples undergoing treatment for ovarian hyperstimulation syndrome in Taiwan. Ten married couples participated in joint interviews shortly before or after hospital discharge. Interviews began with two questions: "Tell me how you felt during your/your wife's admission to the hospital?" and "How has that experience affected your family life?" (p. 533)

Life Histories

Life histories are narrative self-disclosures about individual life experiences. Ethnographers frequently use individual life histories to learn about cultural patterns. A famous example of this is Oscar Lewis' life history of poor Mexican families, which gave rise to the concept of *culture of poverty*.

With a life history approach, researchers ask respondents to provide, often in chronological sequence, a narration of their experiences, either orally or in writing. Life histories may take months to record, with researchers providing only gentle guidance in the telling of the story. Narrated life histories are often backed up by intensive observation of the person, interviews with friends or family members, or a scrutiny of letters, photographs, or other materials.

Leininger (1985) noted that comparative life histories are especially valuable for the study of the patterns and meanings of health and healthcare, especially among elderly people. Her highly regarded essay provides a protocol for obtaining a life health-care history.

Example of life histories: Patching and Lawler (2009) used a life history approach to study the experiences of 20 women who had recovered from an eating disorder (anorexia or bulimia).

Oral Histories

Researchers use the technique known as **oral history** to gather personal recollections of events and their perceived causes and consequences. Oral histories, unlike life histories, typically focus on describing important themes rather than individuals. Oral histories are a method for connecting individual experiences with broader social and cultural contexts.

Oral histories are an important method for historical researchers when the topic under study is the not-too-distant past, and people who experienced the event can still be asked about those experiences. Oral histories are also a tool used by feminist researchers and other researchers with an ideological perspective because oral histories are a way to reach groups that have been ignored or oppressed.

Depending on the focus of the oral history, researchers can conduct interviews with a number of persons or concentrate on multiple interviews with one individual. Researchers usually use unstructured interviews to collect oral history data.

Example of oral histories: Dunlop and colleagues (2009) analyzed the oral histories of several nurses in Canada who provided anesthesia at the beginning of the 20th century. The oral history data were maintained in a collection at the College of Registered Nurses of the British Columbia Library.

Critical Incidents

The **critical incidents technique** is a method of gathering information about people's behaviors by examining specific incidents relating to behavior under investigation (Flanagan, 1954). The technique focuses on a factual incident, which may be defined as an observable and integral episode of human behavior. The word *critical* means that the incident must have had a discernible impact on some outcome; it must make either a positive or negative contribution to the accomplishment of some activity of interest. For example, if we were interested in understanding the use of humor in clinical practice, we might ask a sample of nurses the following questions: "Think of the last time you used humor in your interactions with a patient. What led up to the situation? Exactly what did you do? What happened next? Why did you feel it would be appropriate to use humor?"

The technique differs from other self-report approaches in that it focuses on something specific about which respondents can be expected to testify as expert witnesses. Usually, data on 100 or more critical incidents are collected, but this typically involves interviews with a much smaller number of people because participants can often describe multiple incidents. The critical incident technique has been used in both individual and focus group interviews.

Example of a critical incidents study: Using the critical incidents technique, Donohue and Endacott (2010) studied nurses' perceptions of managing patients who deteriorate in acute wards, focusing on how such deterioration is recognized and communicated.

Diaries and Journals

Personal **diaries** have long been used as a source of data in historical research. It is also possible to generate new data for a nonhistorical study by asking study participants to maintain a diary or journal over a specified period—or by asking them to share a diary they wrote. Diaries can be useful in providing an intimate and detailed description of a person's everyday life.

The diaries may be completely unstructured; for example, individuals who have undergone organ transplantation could be asked simply to spend 10 to 15 minutes a day jotting down their thoughts and feelings. Frequently, however, participants are requested to make entries into a diary regarding a specific aspect of their experience, sometimes in a semistructured format (e.g., about their appetite or sleeping). Nurse researchers have used health diaries to collect information about how people prevent illness, maintain health, experience morbidity, and treat health problems.

Although diaries are a useful means of learning about ongoing experiences, one limitation is that they can be used only by people with adequate literacy skills, although there are examples of studies in which diary entries were audiotaped rather than written out. Diaries also require a high level of participant cooperation.

Example of diaries: In many European countries, nurses maintain diaries for critically ill patients while they are in the ICU. Egerod and Christenson (2009) analyzed 25 such patient diaries written by critical care nurses in Denmark. Their analysis identified three stages of the ICU experience: crisis, turning point, and normalization.

The Think-Aloud Method

The **think-aloud method** is a technique for collecting data about cognitive processes, such as thinking, problem solving, and decision making. This method involves having people use audio recording devices to talk about decisions as they are being made or while problems are being solved, over an extended period (e.g., throughout a shift). The method produces an inventory of decisions as they occur in a naturalistic context, and allows researchers to analyze sequences of thoughts, and the contexts in which they occur (Fonteyn et al., 1993). Think-aloud procedures have been used in several studies of clinical nurses' decision-making and reasoning processes.

The think-aloud method has been used in both naturalistic and simulated settings. Although simulated settings offer the opportunity of controlling context (e.g., presenting people with a common problem to be solved), naturalistic settings offer the best opportunity for understanding clinical processes.

Think-aloud sessions are sometimes followed up with personal interviews or focus group interviews in which the tape may be played (or excerpts from the transcript quoted). Participants are then questioned about aspects of their reasoning and decision making.

Example of the think-aloud method: Hoffman and colleagues (2009) used the think-aloud method to explore differences between novice and expert nurses in the range and type of cues used in making clinical decisions regarding care for postoperative patients in the intensive care unit.

Photo Elicitation Interviews

Photo elicitation involves an interview stimulated and guided by photographic images. This procedure, most often used in ethnographies, is a method that can break down barriers between researchers and study participants, and promote a collaborative discussion (Frith & Harcourt, 2007). The photographs sometimes are ones that researchers have made of the participants' world, through which researchers can gain insights into a new culture. Participants may need to be continually reassured that their taken-for-granted explanations of the photos are providing new and useful information.

Photo elicitation can also be used with photos that participants have in their homes, although in such case researchers have less time to frame useful questions, and no opportunity to select the photos that will be the stimulus for discussion. Researchers have also used the technique of asking participants to take photographs themselves and then interpret them, a method sometimes called **photovoice**. Oliffe and colleagues (2008) offered useful suggestions for a four-part strategy of analyzing participant-produced photographs.

Example of photo elicitation: Fleury and colleagues (2009) used photo elicitation to explore the cultural, social, and contextual resources for physical activity among Hispanic women. Each participant was given a 24-print disposable camera with instructions to take pictures of resources for engaging in physical activity.

Self-Report Narratives on the Internet

In addition to the possibility of gathering narrative data on the Internet through structured or semistructured "interview" methods, a potentially rich data source for qualitative researchers involves narrative self-reports available directly on the Internet. For example, researchers can enter into long conversations with other users in a chat room. Also, some data that can be analyzed qualitatively are simply "out there," as when a researcher enters a chat room or blog site and analyzes the content of existing, unsolicited messages.

Using the Internet to access narrative data has obvious advantages. This approach is economical and allows researchers to obtain information from geographically dispersed and perhaps remote Internet users (Fitzpatrick & Montgomery, 2004). However, a number of ethical concerns have been raised, and authenticity and other methodologic challenges need to be considered (Kralik et al., 2006; Moloney et al., 2003; Robinson, 2001).

Example of Internet data use: Hall and Irvine (2009) analyzed email messages from 40 mothers participating in an online community-based support group for mothers of infants and toddlers in Canada.

Gathering Qualitative Self-Report Data

The purpose of gathering narrative self-report data is to enable researchers to construct reality in a way that is consistent with the constructions of the people being studied. This goal requires researchers to take steps to overcome communication barriers and to enhance the flow of meaning. Asking good questions and eliciting good narrative data are far more difficult than it appears. This section offers some suggestions about gathering qualitative self-report data through in-depth interviews. Further suggestions are offered by Fontana and Frey (2003), Rubin and Rubin (2005), and Gubrium and Holstein (2001).

Preparing for the Interview

Although qualitative interviews are conversational, this does not mean that they are entered into casually. The conversations are purposeful ones that require advance preparation. For example, careful thought should be given to the wording of questions. To the extent possible, the wording should make sense to respondents and reflect their world view. Researchers and respondents should, for example, have a common vocabulary. If the researcher is studying a different culture or a group that uses distinctive terms or slang, efforts should be made before data collection begins to understand those terms and their nuances.

Researchers usually prepare for the interview by developing, mentally or in writing, the broad questions to be asked (or the initial questions, in unstructured interviews). Sometimes it is useful to do a practice interview with a stand-in respondent. If there are sensitive questions, it is a good idea to ask them late in the interview when rapport has been established.

TIP: Memorize central questions if you have written them out, so that you will be able to maintain eye contact with participants.

It is important to decide in advance how to present yourself—as a researcher, as a nurse, as an ordinary person like participants, as a humble "learner," and so on. An advantage of assuming the nurse role is that people often trust nurses. Yet, people may be overly deferential if nurses are perceived as better educated or more knowledgeable than they are. Moreover, participants may use the interview as an opportunity to ask health questions, or to solicit opinions about particular health practitioners. Jack (2008) provided some guidelines to support nurse researchers in their reflection on this role conflict in qualitative interviewing.

A decision must also be made about where the interviews will take place. In-home interviews are often preferred because interviewers can then observe the participants' world and take observational notes. When in-home interviews are not desired by participants (e.g., if they prefer more privacy), it is wise to have alternative suggestions, such as an office, coffee shop, and so on. The important thing is to select places that offer some privacy, that protect insofar as possible against interruptions, and that are adequate for recording the interview. Warren (2001) advocated letting participants select the setting, but in some cases, the setting will be dictated by circumstances, as when interviews take place while participants are hospitalized.

Most qualitative interviews are conducted in person, but new technologies have opened up other options. For example, video conferencing makes it possible to conduct face-to-face interviews with participants remotely—a particular advantage for interviewing people in rural areas. Video conferencing is also advantageous from the perspective of having both a visual and auditory record of the interview. In-depth telephone interviews are also possible, but are relatively rare. Indeed, Novick (2008) has speculated about a bias against telephone interviews among qualitative researchers. The argument against telephone interviews concerns the absence of visual cues, but these cues are also absent in interviews conducted over the Internet.

Example of video interviews: Sevean and colleagues (2009) studied patients' and families' experiences with video telehealth in rural communities in northern Canada. Hour-long in-depth video interviews were conducted with 10 patients and 4 family members.

For interviews done in the field, researchers must anticipate needed equipment and supplies. Preparing a checklist of all such items is helpful. The checklist typically would include recording equipment, batteries, tapes, consent and demographic forms, notepads, and pens. Other possibilities include laptop computers, incentive payments, cookies or donuts to help break the ice, and distracting toys or books if children will be home. It may be necessary to bring proper identification to assure participants of the legitimacy of the visit. And, if the topic under study is likely to elicit emotional narratives, tissues should be readily at hand.

➲ **TIP:** It is wise to use high-quality equipment and tapes to ensure proper recording. For example, for recording interviews, make sure that the microphone is adequately sensitive for the acoustics of the environment, or use lapel microphones for both respondents and interviewers. Also, make sure that the size of the tape corresponds to the size used in the transcription equipment.

Conducting the Interview

Qualitative interviews are typically long, sometimes lasting hours. Researchers often find that the respondents' construction of their experience begins to emerge after lengthy, in-depth dialogues. Interviewers must prepare respondents for the interview by putting them at ease. Part of this process involves sharing pertinent information about the study (e.g., about confidentiality), and another part is using the first few minutes for ice-breaking exchanges of conversation before actual questioning begins. Upfront "small talk" can help to overcome stage fright, which can occur for both interviewers and respondents. Participants may be particularly nervous when interviews are being tape-recorded. They typically forget about the tape recorder after the interview is underway, so the first few minutes should be used to help both parties "settle in."

➲ **TIP:** If possible, place the actual tape recording equipment on the floor or somewhere out of sight.

Study participants will not share much information with interviewers they do not trust. Close rapport with respondents provides access to richer information and to intimate details of their stories. Interviewer personality plays a role in developing rapport: Good interviewers are usually congenial people who have the ability to see the situation from the respondent's perspective. Nonverbal communication can be critical in conveying concern and interest. Facial expressions, nods, and so on, help to set the tone for the interview. Gaglio and colleagues (2006) offered some insights concerning the development of rapport in primary care settings.

The most critical interviewing skill for in-depth interviews is being a good listener. It is especially important not to interrupt respondents, to "lead" them, to offer advice or opinions, or to counsel them. The interviewer's job is to listen intently to the respondents' stories. Only by attending carefully to what respondents are saying can interviewers develop appropriate follow-up questions. Even when a topic guide is used, interviewers must not let the flow of dialogue be bound by those questions.

⮕ **TIP:** In-depth interviewers must be comfortable with pauses and silences, and should let participants set the pace. Interviewers can encourage respondents with nonspecific prompts, such as "Mmhm."

Interviewers need to be prepared for strong emotions, such as anger, fear, or grief, to surface. Narrative disclosures can "bring it all back" for respondents, which can be a cathartic or therapeutic experience if interviewers create an atmosphere of concern and caring—but it can also be stressful.

Interviewers may need to manage potential crises during the interviews (MacDonald & Greggans, 2008). One frequent problem is the failed or improper recording of the interview. Thus, even when interviews are tape-recorded, notes should be taken immediately after the interview to ensure the highest possible reliability of data and to prevent total information loss. Interruptions (usually the telephone) and other distractions are another common problem when interviewing in participants' homes. If respondents are willing, telephones can be controlled by unplugging them or turning them off in the case of cell phones. Interruptions by personal intrusions of friends or family members may be more difficult to

manage. In some cases, the interview may need to be terminated and rescheduled—for example, when a woman is discussing domestic violence and the perpetrator enters and stays in the room.

Interviewers should strive for positive closure to interviews. The last questions in in-depth interviews should usually be along these lines: "Is there anything else you would like to tell me?" or "Are there any other questions that you think I should have asked you?" Such probes can often elicit a wealth of important information. In closing, interviewers normally ask respondents whether they would mind being contacted again, in the event that additional questions come to mind after reflecting on the information, or in case interpretations of the information need to be verified.

⮕ **TIP:** It is usually unwise to schedule back-to-back interviews. It is important not to rush or cut short the first interview to be on time for the next one, and you may be too emotionally drained to do a second interview in 1 day. It is also important to have an opportunity to write out notes, impressions, and analytic ideas, and it is best to do this when an interview is fresh in your mind.

Postinterview Procedures

Tape-recorded interviews should be listened to and checked for audibility and completeness soon after the interview is over. If there have been problems with the recording, the interview should be reconstructed in as much detail as possible. Listening to the interview may also suggest possible follow-up questions that could be asked if respondents are recontacted. Morse and Field (1995) recommend that interviewers listen to the tapes objectively and critique their own interviewing style, so that improvements can be made in subsequent interviews.

Steps also need to be taken to ensure that the transcription of interviews is done with rigor. It is prudent to hire experienced transcribers, to check the quality of initial transcriptions, and to give the transcribers feedback. Transcribers can sometimes unwittingly change the meaning of data by misspelling words, omitting words, or not adequately entering information about pauses, laughter, crying, or speech volume. Transcriptionists, like interviewers, can be affected by hearing heart-wrenching interviews. Regular contact between the researcher and transcriptionist may be necessary to warn about upcoming interviews that are particularly stressful and to allow the transcriber the opportunity to talk about his or her reaction to the interview (Lalor et al., 2006).

⮕ **TIP:** Transcriptions can be the most expensive part of a study. It generally takes about 3 hours of transcription time for every hour of interviewing. New and improved voice recognition computer software may help with transcribing interviews.

Evaluation of Qualitative Self-Report Approaches

In-depth interviews are an extremely flexible approach to gathering data and, in many research contexts, offer distinct advantages. In clinical situations, for example, it is often appropriate to let people talk freely about their problems and concerns, allowing them to take much of the initiative in directing the flow of information. Unstructured self-reports may allow investigators to ascertain what the basic issues or problems are, how sensitive or controversial the topic is, how individuals conceptualize and talk about the problems, and what range of opinions or behaviors exist relevant to the topic. In-depth interviews may also help elucidate the underlying meaning of a pattern or relationship repeatedly observed in more structured research. On the other hand, qualitative methods are extremely time-consuming and demanding of researchers' skills in gathering, analyzing, and interpreting the resulting data.

UNSTRUCTURED OBSERVATION

Qualitative researchers sometimes collect loosely structured observational data, often as an important supplement to self-report data. The aim of such observations is to understand the behaviors and experiences of people as they actually occur in naturalistic settings. Qualitative researchers seek to observe people and their environments with a minimum of structure and interference.

Unstructured observational data are most often gathered in field settings through **participant observation**. Participant observers participate in the functioning of the social group under investigation and strive to observe, ask questions, and record information within the contexts and structures that are relevant to group members. Participant observation is characterized by prolonged periods of intense social interaction between the researcher and the participants, in the participants' sociopolitical and cultural milieu.

Example of participant observation: Rasmussen and colleagues (2010) studied how breast cancer survivors experience physical changes to their bodies and how it affects their encounters with other people. Participant observation was undertaken at a cancer rehabilitation center.

Not all qualitative observational research is *participant* observation (i.e., with observations occurring from *within* the group under study). Some unstructured observations involve watching and recording behaviors without the observers participating in activities.

Example of unstructured nonparticipant observation: Martinsen and colleagues (2009) studied "sensitive cooperation" in the assisted feeding of patients with spinal cord injury. Participants, recruited from two spinal cord injury centers in Denmark, were interviewed twice in their homes. The second interview was followed by nonparticipant observation of a meal, to observe the physical aspect of assisted feeding.

Nevertheless, if a key research objective is to learn how group interactions and activities give meaning to human behaviors and experiences, then participant observation is an appropriate method. The members of any group or culture are influenced by assumptions they take for granted, and observers can, through active participation as members, gain access to these assumptions. Participant observation is most often used by ethnographers, grounded theory researchers, and researchers with ideological perspectives.

The Observer—Participant Role in Participant Observation

The role that observers play in the groups under study is important because the observers' social position determines what they are likely to see. That is, the behaviors that are likely to be available for observation depend on observers' position in a network of relations.

Leininger and McFarland (2006) describe a participant observer's role as evolving through a four-phase sequence:

1. Primarily observation and active listening
2. Primarily observation with limited participation
3. Primarily participation with continued observation
4. Primary reflection and reconfirmation of findings with informants

In the initial phase, researchers observe and listen to those under study to obtain a broad view of the situation. This phase allows both observers and the observed to "size up" each other, to become acquainted, and to become comfortable interacting. This first phase involves "learning the ropes." In the next phase, observation is enhanced by a modest degree of participation. By participating in the group's activities, researchers can study not only people's behaviors, but also people's reactions to them. In Phase 3, researchers become more active participants, learning by the actual experience of doing rather than just by watching and listening. In Phase 4, researchers reflect on what transpired and how people interacted with and reacted to them.

Junker (1960) described a somewhat different continuum that does not assume an evolving process: complete participant, participant as observer, observer as participant, and complete observer. Complete participants conceal their identity as researchers, entering the group ostensibly as regular members. For example, a nurse researcher might accept a job as a clinical nurse with the express intent of studying, in a concealed fashion, some aspect of the clinical environment. At the other extreme, complete observers do not attempt participation in the group's activities, but rather make observations as outsiders. At both extremes, observers may have difficulty asking probing questions—albeit for different reasons. Complete participants may arouse suspicion if they make inquiries not congruent with a total participant role, and complete observers may not have personal access to, or the trust of, those being observed. Most observational field work lies in between these two extremes and usually shifts over time.

> **Example of participant–observer roles:**
> Dupuis-Blanchard and colleagues (2009) conducted an ethnographic study about social engagement in elders relocated to senior-designated apartments. Here is what they said about their participant observation: " . . . The researcher observed the senior-designated apartment building's environment for day-to-day transactions . . ., followed by the observation of events in the environment. In a low-key manner, the researcher tried to become part of the subculture being studied . . . by engaging in participant observation of older adults during specific events or activities to identify attributes and behaviors of the culture" (p. 1189)

⊃ **TIP:** Being a fully participating member of a group does not *necessarily* offer the best perspective for studying a phenomenon—just as being an actor in a play does not offer the most advantageous view of the performance.

Getting Started

Observers must overcome at least two initial hurdles: gaining entrée into the social group or culture under study, and establishing rapport and developing trust within the social group. Without gaining entrée, the study cannot proceed; without the group's trust, researchers could be restricted to "front stage" knowledge (Leininger, 1985), that is, information distorted by the group's protective facades. The observer's goal is to "get back stage"—to learn about the realities of the group's experiences and behaviors. This section discusses some practical and interpersonal aspects of getting started in the field.

Gaining an Overview

Before fieldwork begins, or in the earliest stage of fieldwork, it is usually useful to gather some written or pictorial descriptive information that provides an overview of the setting. In an institutional setting, for example, it is helpful to obtain a floor plan, an organizational chart, an annual report, and so on. Then, a preliminary personal tour of the setting should be undertaken to gain familiarity with its ambiance and to note major activities, social groupings, and transactions.

In community studies, ethnographers sometimes conduct a **windshield survey** (or *windshield tour*), which involves an intensive exploration (sometimes in an automobile, and hence the name) to "map" important features of the community under study. Such community mapping can include documenting community resources (e.g., churches, businesses, public transportation, community centers), community liabilities (e.g., vacant lots, empty stores, dilapidated buildings), and social and environmental characteristics (e.g., condition of streets and buildings, traffic patterns, types of signs, children playing in public places). A protocol for a windshield survey is included in the Toolkit of the accompanying *Resource Manual.* ✖

Example of a windshield survey: Winters and colleagues (2007) studied rural nurses and their use of research in various communities in western United States. A windshield survey was undertaken in each community to provide context about where the nurses lived and practiced.

Establishing Rapport

After gaining entrée into a setting and obtaining permissions and suggestions from gatekeepers, the next step is to enter the field. In some cases, it may be possible just to "blend in" or ease into a social group, but often researchers walk into a "head-turning" situation in which there is considerable curiosity because they stand out as strangers. Participant observers often find that, for their own comfort level and also for that of participants, it is best to have a brief, simple explanation about their presence. Except in rare cases, deception is neither necessary nor recommended, but vagueness has many advantages. People rarely want to know *exactly* what researchers are studying, they simply want an introduction and enough information to

satisfy their curiosity and erase any suspicions about the researchers' ulterior motives.

After initial introductions with members of the group, it is usually best to keep a fairly low profile. At the beginning, researchers are not yet familiar with the customs, language, and norms of the group, and it is critical to learn these things. Politeness and friendliness are essential, but ardent socializing is not appropriate at the early stages of fieldwork.

⊃ **T I P :** Your initial job is to listen intently and learn what it takes to fit into the group, that is, what you need to do to become accepted as a member. To the extent possible, you should downplay any expertise you might have, because you do not want to distance yourself from participants. Your overall goal is to gain people's trust and to move relationships to a deeper level.

As rapport is developed and trust is established, researchers can play a more active participatory role and collect observational data in earnest.

Gathering Unstructured Observational Data

Participant observers typically place few restrictions on the nature of the data collected, in keeping with the goal of minimizing observer-imposed meanings and structure. Nevertheless, participant observers often have a broad plan for the types of information to be gathered. Among aspects likely to be considered relevant are the following:

1. *The physical setting*. What are key features of the setting? What is the context within which human behavior unfolds? What behaviors and characteristics are promoted (or constrained) by the physical environment?
2. *The participants*. What are the characteristics of the people being observed? How many people are there? What are their roles? Who is given free access to the setting—who "belongs"? What brings these people together?
3. *Activities and interactions*. What are people doing and saying? Is there a discernible progression of activities? How do people interact

with one another? How—and how often—do they communicate? What type of emotions do they show during their interactions? How are participants interconnected to one another or to activities underway?

4. *Frequency and duration*. When did the activity or event begin, and when is it scheduled to end? How much time has elapsed? Is the activity a recurring one, and if so, how regularly does it recur? How typical of such activities is the one that is under observation?

5. *Precipitating factors*. Why is the event or interaction happening? What contributes to how the event or interaction unfolds?

6. *Organization*. How is the event or interaction organized? How are relationships structured? What norms or rules are in operation?

7. *Intangible factors*. What did *not* happen (especially if it ought to have happened)? Are participants saying one thing verbally but communicating different messages nonverbally? What types of things were disruptive to the activity or situation?

Clearly, this is far more information than can be absorbed in a single session (and not all categories may be relevant to the research question). However, this framework provides a starting point for thinking about observational possibilities while in the field. (This list of features amenable to in-depth observation is included in the Toolkit ⊗ as a Word document.)

➲ **TIP:** When we enter a social setting in our everyday lives, we unconsciously process many of the questions on this list. Usually, however, we do not consciously *attend* to our observations and impressions in any systematic way, and are not careful about making note of the details that contribute to our impressions. This is precisely what participant observers must learn to do.

Spradley (1980) distinguished three levels of observation that typically occur during fieldwork. The first level, **descriptive observation**, tends to be broad and helps observers figure out what is going on. During these descriptive observations, researchers make every attempt to observe as much

as possible. Later in the inquiry, observers do **focused observations** on more carefully selected events and interactions. Based on the research aims and on what has been learned from descriptive observations, participant observers begin to focus more sharply on key aspects of the setting. From these focused observations, they may develop a system for organizing observations, such as a taxonomy or category system. **Selective observations** are the most highly focused, and are undertaken to facilitate comparisons between categories or activities. Spradley describes these levels as analogous to a funnel, with an increasingly narrow and more systematic focus.

While in the field, participant observers have to decide how to sample observations and select observational locations. **Single positioning** means staying in a single location for a period to observe behaviors and transactions in that location. **Multiple positioning** involves moving around the site to observe behaviors from different locations. **Mobile positioning** involves following a person throughout a given activity or period. It is usually useful to use a combination of positioning approaches in selecting observational locations.

Because participant observers cannot spend a lifetime in one site and because they cannot be in more than one place at a time, observation is almost always supplemented with information from unstructured interviews or conversations. For example, key informants may be asked to describe what went on in a meeting that the observer was unable to attend, or to describe events that occurred before the observer entered the field. In such a case, the informant functions as the observer's observer.

Recording Observations

Participant observers may be tempted to put more emphasis on the *participation* and *observation* parts of their research than on the recording of those activities. Without systematic recording of observational data, however, the project will flounder. Observational information cannot be trusted to memory; it must be diligently recorded as soon after the observations as possible.

Types of Observational Records

The most common forms of record keeping in participant observation are logs and field notes, but photographs and videotapes may also be used. A **log** (or **field diary**) is a daily record of events and conversations in the field. A log is a chronological listing of how researchers have spent their time and can be used for planning, for keeping track of expenses, and for reviewing what work has already been completed. Box 22.1 presents an example of a log entry from Beck's (2002) study of mothers of multiples (i.e., twins).

Field notes are broader, more analytic, and more interpretive than a simple listing of occurrences. Field notes represent the participant observer's efforts to record information and also to synthesize and understand the data.

➲ **TIP:** Field notes are important in many types of studies, not just in studies involving participant observation. For example, field notes are critical in grounded theory studies, process evaluations, and in inquiries relating to intervention fidelity.

The Content of Field Notes

Participant observers' field notes contain a narrative account of what is happening in the field; they serve as the data for analysis. Most "field" notes are not written while observers are literally in the field but rather are written after an observational session in the field has been completed.

Field notes are usually lengthy and time consuming to prepare. Observers need to discipline themselves to provide a wealth of detail, the meaning and importance of which may not emerge for weeks. Descriptions of what has transpired must include enough contextual information about time, place, and actors to portray the situation fully. *Thick description* is the goal for participation observers' field notes.

➲ **TIP:** Especially in the early stages of fieldwork, a general rule of thumb is this: When in doubt, write it down.

Field notes are both descriptive and reflective. **Descriptive notes** (or **observational notes**) are objective descriptions of observed events and conversations; information about actions, dialogue, and context are recorded as completely and objectively as possible. Sometimes descriptive notes are recorded on loosely structured forms analogous to topic guides to ensure that key information is captured. ✖

BOX 22.1 Example of a Log Entry: Mothering Multiples Grounded Theory Study

Log entry for Mothers of Multiples Support Group Meeting (Beck, 2002)
July 15, 1999 10–11:30 AM

This is my fourth meeting that I have attended. Nine mothers came this morning with their twins. One other woman attended. She was pregnant with twins. She came to the support group for advice from the other mothers regarding such issues as what type of stroller to buy, etc. All the moms sat on the floor with their infants placed on blankets on the floor next to them. Toddlers and older children played together off to the side with a box of toys. I sat next to a mom new to the group with her twin 4-month-old girls. I helped her hold and feed one of the twins. On my other side was a mom who had signed up at the last meeting to participate in my study. I hadn't called her yet to set up an appointment. She asked how my research was going. We then set up an appointment for next Thursday at 10 AM at her home for me to interview her. The new mother that I sat next to also was eager to participate in the study. In fact, she said we could do the interview right after the meeting ends today, but I couldn't due to another meeting. We scheduled an interview appointment for next Thursday at 1 PM. I also set up a third appointment for an interview for next week with I.K. for Monday at 1 PM. She had participated in an earlier study of mine. She came right over to me this morning at the support group meeting.

Reflective notes, which document the researcher's personal experiences, reflections, and progress while in the field, can serve a number of different purposes:

- **Methodologic notes** are reflections about observational strategies. Sometimes participant observers do things that do not "work," and methodologic notes document thoughts about new approaches or about why a strategy was especially effective. Methodologic notes also can provide instructions or reminders about how subsequent observations will be made.
- **Theoretical notes** (or **analytical notes**) document researchers' thoughts about how to make

sense of what is going on. These notes serve as a starting point for subsequent analysis.

- **Personal notes** are comments about researchers' own feelings in the field. Almost inevitably, field experiences give rise to personal emotions and challenge researchers' assumptions. It is essential to reflect on such feelings, because there is no other way to know whether the feelings are influencing what is being observed or what is being done in the participant role. Personal notes can also contain reflections relating to ethical dilemmas.

Box 22.2 presents examples of various types of field notes from Beck's (2002) study of mothering multiples.

BOX 22.2 Example of Field Notes: Mothering Multiples Grounded Theory Study

Observational Notes: O.L. attended the mothers of multiples support group again this month but she looked worn out today. She wasn't as bubbly as she had been at the March meeting. She explained why she wasn't doing as well this month. She and her husband had just found out that their house has lead-based paint in it. Both twins do have increased lead levels. She and her husband are in the process of buying a new home.

Theoretical Notes: So far, all the mothers have stressed the need for routine in order to survive the first year of caring for twins. Mothers, however, have varying definitions of routine. I.R. had the firmest routine with her twins. B.L. is more flexible with her routine, i.e., the twins are always fed at the same time but aren't put down for naps or bed at night at the same time. Whenever one of the twins wants to go to sleep is fine with her. B.L. does have a daily routine in regards to housework. For example, when the twins are down in the morning for a nap, she makes their bottles up for the day (14 bottles total).

Methodologic Notes: The first sign-up sheet I passed around at the Mothers of Multiples Support Group for women to sign up to participate in interviews for my grounded theory study only consisted of two columns: one for the mother's name and one for her telephone number. I need to revise this sign-up sheet to include extra columns for the age of the multiples, the town where the mother lives, and older siblings and their ages. My plan is to start interviewing mothers with multiples around 1 year of age so that the moms can reflect back over the process of mothering their infants for the first 12 months of their lives.

Right now, I have no idea of the ages of the infants of the mothers who signed up to be interviewed. I will need to call the nurse in charge of this support group to find out the ages.

Personal Notes: Today was an especially challenging interview. The mom had picked the early afternoon for me to come to her home to interview her because that is the time her 2-year-old son would be napping. When I arrived at her house, her 2-year-old ran up to me and said hi. The mom explained that he had taken an earlier nap that day and that he would be up during the interview. So in the living room with us during our interview were her two twin daughters (3 months old) swinging in the swings and her 2-year-old son. One of the twins was quite cranky for the first half hour of the interview. During the interview, the 2-year-old sat on my lap and looked at the two books I had brought as a little present. If I didn't keep him occupied with the books, he would keep trying to reach for the microphone of the tape recorder.

From Beck, C.T. (2002). Releasing the pause button: Mothering twins during the first year of life. *Qualitative Health Research, 12*, 593–608.

Reflective notes are typically not integrated into the descriptive notes, but are kept separately as parallel notes; they may be maintained in a journal or series of self-memos. Strauss and Corbin (1990) argue that these reflective memos or journals help researchers to achieve analytic distance from the actual data, and, therefore, play a critical role in the project's success.

➲ **T I P :** Personal notes should begin even before entering the field. By recording your feelings, assumptions, and expectations, you will have a baseline against which to compare feelings and experiences that emerge in the field.

The Process of Writing Field Notes

The success of participant observation depends on the quality of the field notes, and timing is important to quality. Field notes should be written as soon as possible after an observation is made. The longer the interval between an observation and field note preparation, the greater the risk of forgetting or distorting the data. If the delay is long, intricate details will be lost; moreover, memory of what was observed may be biased by things that happened subsequently.

➲ **T I P :** Be sure not to talk to anyone about your observation before you have had a chance to write up the observational notes. Such discussions could color what you record.

Participant observers cannot usually write their field notes while they are in the field, in part because this would distract them from their job of being keen observers, and also because it would undermine their role as ordinary group members. Researchers must develop the skill of making detailed mental notes that can later be committed to a permanent record. In addition, observers usually try to jot down unobtrusively a phrase or sentence that will later serve as a reminder of an event, conversation, or impression. Many experienced field workers use the tactic of frequent trips to the bathroom to record these **jottings**, either in a small notebook, into a recording device, or onto a PDA.

With the widespread use of cell phones, researchers can also excuse themselves to make a call and "phone in" their jottings to an answering machine. Observers use jottings and mental recordings to develop more extensive field notes.

➲ **T I P :** It is important to schedule enough time to record field notes after an observation. An hour of observation can take 3 or 4 hours to record, so advance planning is essential. Try to find a quiet place for recording field notes, preferably a location where you can work undisturbed for several hours. Most researchers now record field notes onto computers, so the place will probably need to accommodate computer equipment.

Observational field notes need to be as complete and detailed as possible. This means that hundreds of pages of field notes typically will be created, so systems need to be developed for managing them. For example, each entry should have the date and time the observation was made, the location, and the name of the observer (if several are working as a team). It is useful to give observational sessions a name that will trigger a memory (e.g., "Emotional Outburst by a Patient with Ovarian Cancer").

Thought also needs to be given to how to record participants' dialogue. The goal is to record conversations as accurately as possible, but it is not always possible to maintain verbatim records because tape recordings are seldom made if researchers are trying to maintain a stance as regular participating group members. Procedures need to be developed to distinguish different levels of accuracy in recording dialogue (e.g., by using quotation marks and italics for true verbatim recordings and a different designation for paraphrasings).

➲ **T I P :** Observation, participation, and record keeping are exhausting, labor-intensive activities. It is important to establish the proper pace of these activities to ensure the highest possible quality notes for analysis.

Evaluation of Participant Observation

Participant observation can provide a deeper and richer understanding of human behaviors and social situations than is possible with structured procedures. Participant observation is particularly valuable for its ability to "get inside" a situation and provide understanding of its complexities. Furthermore, this approach is inherently flexible and, therefore, gives observers the freedom to reconceptualize problems after becoming more familiar with the situation. Participant observation is a good method for answering questions about phenomena that are difficult for insiders to explain because these phenomena are taken for granted (e.g., group norms).

Like all research methods, however, participant observation faces potential problems. Observer bias and observer influence are prominent risks. Observers may lose objectivity in viewing and recording observations; they may also inappropriately sample events and situations to be observed. Once researchers begin to participate in a group's activities, the possibility of emotional involvement becomes a salient concern. Researchers in their member role may fail to attend to scientifically relevant aspects of the situation or may develop a myopic view on issues of importance to the group. Participant observation may thus be an unsuitable approach when the risk of identification is strong. Another important issue concerns the ethical dilemmas that often emerge in participant observation studies. Finally, the success of participant observation depends on the observer's observational and interpersonal skills—skills that may be difficult to cultivate.

On the whole, participant observation and other unstructured observational methods are extremely profitable for in-depth research in which researchers wish to develop a comprehensive description and conceptualization of phenomena within a social setting or culture.

⭢ **TIP:** Although this chapter emphasized the two most frequently used methods of collecting unstructured data (self-reports and observation), we encourage you to think about other data sources, such as documents. Miller and Alvarado (2005) offer useful suggestions for incorporating documents into qualitative nursing research.

CRITIQUING THE COLLECTION OF UNSTRUCTURED DATA

It is usually not easy to critique the decisions that researchers have made in collecting qualitative data because details about those decisions are seldom spelled out in research reports. In particular, there is often scant information about participant observation. It is not uncommon for a report to simply say that the researcher undertook participant observation, without descriptions of how much time was spent in the field, what exactly was observed, how observations were recorded, and what level of participation was involved. In fact, we suspect that many projects described as having used a participant observation approach were unstructured observations with little actual participation. Thus, one aspect of a critique is likely to involve an appraisal of how much information the research report provided about the data collection methods used. Even though space constraints in journals make it impossible for researchers to fully elaborate their methods, researchers have a responsibility to communicate basic information about their approach so that readers can assess the quality of evidence that the study yields. Researchers should provide examples of questions asked and types of observations made.

As we discuss more fully in Chapter 24, triangulation of methods provides important opportunities for qualitative researchers to enhance the quality of their data. Thus, an important issue to consider in evaluating unstructured data is whether the types and amount of data collected are sufficiently rich to support an in-depth, holistic understanding of the phenomena under study. Box 22.3 ✪ provides guidelines for critiquing the collection of unstructured data.

BOX 22.3 Guidelines for Critiquing Unstructured Data Collection Methods

1. Was the collection of unstructured data appropriate to the study aims?
2. Given the research question and the characteristics of study participants, did the researcher use the best method of capturing study phenomena (i.e., self-reports, observation)? Should supplementary data collection methods have been used to enrich the data available for analysis?
3. If self-report methods were used, did the researcher make good decisions about the specific method used to solicit information (e.g., focus group interviews, critical incident interviews, and so on)? Was the modality of obtaining the data appropriate (e.g., in-person interviews, telephone interviews, Internet questioning, and so on)?
4. If a topic guide was used, did the report present examples of specific questions? Were the questions appropriate and comprehensive? Did the wording minimize the risk of biases? Did the wording encourage full and rich responses?
5. Were interviews tape-recorded and transcribed? If interviews were not tape-recorded, what steps were taken to ensure the accuracy of the data?
6. Were self-report data gathered in a manner that promoted high-quality responses (e.g., in terms of privacy, efforts to put respondents at ease, and so on)? Who collected the data, and were they adequately prepared for the task?
7. If observational methods were used, did the report adequately describe what the observations entailed? What did the researcher actually observe, in what types of setting did the observations occur, and how often and over how long a period were observations made? Were decisions about positioning described? Were risks of observational bias addressed?
8. What role did the researcher assume in terms of being an observer and a participant? Was this role appropriate?
9. How were observational data recorded? Did the recording method maximize data quality?

RESEARCH EXAMPLE

This section provides an example of a qualitative study that collected a rich variety of unstructured data.

Study: Reconciling the good patient persona with problematic and non-problematic humour: A grounded theory (McCreaddie and Wiggins, 2009)

Statement of Purpose: The purpose of this study was to develop a theory about the use of humor in interactions between patients and clinical nurse specialists (CNS) in the United Kingdom. The researchers sought to understand the antecedents of humor, describe the use of humor, and explore its use within clinical interactions in relation to existing humor theories.

Design: The researchers used a constructivist grounded theory approach to investigate humor as a complex and dynamic phenomenon within situated contexts. The researchers argued that this approach "attempts

to address the difficulties of capturing and making sense" of a phenomenon (p. 1081). The researchers adopted an open interpretation of humor and applied an interpretive framework. The focus of the inquiry was on naturally occurring CNS–patient interactions. Theoretical sampling was used, which drove decisions about types of interactions to sample and types of data to collect.

Data Collection: A wide range of data was collected and was nicely summarized in a figure, which categorized data sources as either nonresearcher provoked or researcher-provoked. In the first category, there were 20 audiotaped CNS–patient interactions lasting 20 or more minutes, from 12 CNSs. The CNSs were asked to identify patients who were fairly typical of their caseload. Some of the 20 interaction sessions included patients' family members. One session of a negative case was observed, resulting in 10.5 hours of field note observations. There were also field notes based on observations of focus groups. In terms of researcher-provoked data, each CNS recorded an "audio diary" both prior to and after each interaction. In the preinteraction diaries, the

CNSs discussed details of the patient and purpose of the meeting. In the postinteraction diaries, they answered questions about the setting of the interaction, the environment, and their awareness of humor use. Finally, the researchers also conducted and audiotaped several unstructured interviews with both patients and CNSs. The researchers spent a total of 18 months in the field collecting their data.

Key Findings: The grounded theory developed from these data purports that patients use humor to reconcile a good patient persona and establish and maintain a meaningful and therapeutic interaction with their CNSs.

SUMMARY POINTS

- Qualitative studies typically adopt flexible data collection plans that evolve as the study progresses. Self-reports are the most frequently used type of data in qualitative studies, followed by observation. Ethnographies are likely to combine these two data sources with others such as the products of the culture (e.g., photographs, documents, artifacts).

- Qualitative researchers often confront such fieldwork issues as gaining participants' trust, pacing data collection to avoid being overwhelmed by the intensity of data, avoiding emotional involvement with participants ("**going native**"), and maintaining reflexivity (awareness of the part they play in the study and possible effects on their data).

- Qualitative researchers need to plan in advance for how their data will be recorded and stored. If technical equipment is used (e.g., audio recorders, video recorders), care must be taken to select high-quality equipment that functions properly in the field.

- Unstructured and loosely structured self-reports, which offer respondents and interviewers latitude in their questions and answers, yield rich narrative data for qualitative analysis.

- Methods of collecting qualitative self-report data include the following: (1) **unstructured interviews**, which are conversational discussions on the topic of interest; (2) **semistructured** (or focused) **interviews**, in which interviewers are guided by a **topic guide** of questions to be asked; (3) **focus group interviews**, which involve discussions with small, homogeneous groups; (4) **joint interviews**, which involve simultaneously talking with members of a dyad; (5) **life histories**, which encourage respondents to narrate their life experiences chronologically; (6) **oral histories**, which are used to gather personal recollections of events; (7) **critical incidents interviews**, which involve probes about the circumstances surrounding an incident that is critical to an outcome of interest; (8) **diaries** and journals, in which respondents maintain ongoing records about some aspects of their lives; (9) the **think-aloud method**, which involves having people use audio recording devices to talk about decisions as they make them; (10) **photo elicitation interviews**, which are stimulated and guided by photographic images; and (11) narrative communications available on the Internet.

- In preparing for in-depth interviews, researchers learn about the language and customs of participants, formulate broad questions, make decisions about how to present themselves, develop ideas about interview settings, and take stock of equipment needs.

- Conducting good in-depth interviews requires considerable skill in putting people at ease, developing trust, listening intently, and managing possible crises in the field.

- Qualitative researchers sometimes collect unstructured observational data, often through **participant observation**. Participant observers obtain information about the dynamics of social groups or cultures within members' own frame of reference.

- In the initial phase of participant observation studies, researchers are primarily observers gaining an understanding of the site. Researchers later become more active participants.

- Observations tend to become more focused over time, ranging from **descriptive observation** (broad observations) to **focused observation** of more carefully selected events or interactions, and then to **selective observations** designed to facilitate comparisons.

- Participant observers usually select events to be observed through a combination of **single positioning** (observing from a fixed location), **multiple positioning** (moving around the site to observe in different locations), and **mobile positioning** (following a person around a site).
- **Logs** of daily events and **field notes** are the major methods of recording unstructured observational data. Field notes are both descriptive and reflective.
- Descriptive notes (or **observational notes**) are detailed, objective accounts of what transpired in an observational session. Observers strive for detailed, thick description.
- **Reflective notes** include **methodologic notes** that document observers' thoughts about their strategies, **theoretical notes** (or **analytic notes**) that represent ongoing efforts to make sense of the data, and **personal notes** that document observers' feelings and experiences.
- In-depth unstructured data collection methods tend to yield data of considerable richness and are useful in gaining an understanding about little-researched phenomena, but they are time-consuming and yield a volume of data that are challenging to analyze.

○○○○○○○○○○○○○○○○○○○○○

STUDY ACTIVITIES

Chapter 22 of the *Resource Manual for Nursing Research: Generating and Assessing Evidence for Nursing Practice*, *9th edition*, offers exercises and study suggestions for reinforcing concepts presented in this chapter. In addition, the following study questions can be addressed:

1. Identify which qualitative self-report methods might be appropriate for the following research problems and provide a rationale:
   a. What are the coping strategies of parents whose child has a brain tumor?
   b. How do nurses in emergency departments make decisions about their activities?

   c. What are the health beliefs and practices of Filipino immigrants in the United States?
   d. What is it like to experience having a family member undergo open heart surgery?
2. Suppose you were interested in observing fathers' behavior in the delivery room during the birth of their first child. Identify the observer–observed relationship that you would recommend adopting for such a study, and defend your recommendation. What are the possible drawbacks of your approach, and how might you deal with them?
3. Apply relevant questions in Box 22.3 to the research example at the end of the chapter (McCreadie & Wiggins, 2009), referring to the full journal article as necessary.

○○○○○○○○○○○○○○○○○○○○○

STUDIES CITED IN CHAPTER 22

Arnaert, A., Gabos, T., Ballenas, V., & Rutledge, R. (2010). Contributions of a retreat weekend to the healing and coping of cancer patients' relatives. *Qualitative Health Research, 20,* 197–208.

Beck, C. T. (2002). Releasing the pause button: Mothering twins during the first year of life. *Qualitative Health Research, 12,* 593–608.

Beck, C. T. (2009). The arm: There is no escaping the reality for mothers of children with obstetric brachial plexus injuries. *Nursing Research, 58,* 237–245.

Chang, S., & Mu, P. (2008). Infertile couples' experience of family stress while women are hospitalized for ovarian hyperstimulation syndrome during infertility treatment. *Journal of Clinical Nursing, 17,* 531–538.

Donohue, L., & Endacott, R. (2010). Track, trigger and teamwork: Communication of deterioration in acute medical and surgical wards. *Intensive & Critical Care Nursing, 26,* 10–17.

Dunlop, J., Boschma, G., & Jefferson, R. (2009). Nursing and anesthesia: Historical developments in Canada. *Canadian Operating Room Nursing Journal, 27,* 16–27.

Dupuis-Blanchard, S., Neufeld, A., & Strang, V. (2009). The significance of social engagement in relocated older adults. *Qualitative Health Research, 19,* 1186–1195.

Egerod, I. (2009). Cultural changes in ICU sedation management. *Qualitative Health Research, 19,* 687–696.

Egerod, I., & Christensen, D. (2009). Analysis of patient diaries in Danish ICUs: A narrative approach. *Intensive and Critical Care Nursing, 25,* 268–277.

Fleury, J., Keller, C., & Perez, A. (2009). Exploring resources for physical activity in Hispanic women, using photo elicitation. *Qualitative Health Research, 19*, 677–686.

Hall, W., & Irvine, V. (2009). E-communication among mothers of infants and toddlers in a community-based cohort. *Journal of Advanced Nursing, 65*, 175–183.

Hoffman, K., Aitken, L., & Duffield, C. (2009). A comparison of novice and expert nurses' cue collection during clinical decision-making: Verbal protocol analysis. *International Journal of Nursing Studies, 46*, 1335–1344.

Irwin, L.G., & Johnson, J. (2005). Interviewing young children: Explicating our practices and dilemmas. *Qualitative Health Research, 15*, 821–831.

Martinsen, B., Harder, I., & Biering-Sorensen, F. (2009). Sensitive cooperation: A basis for assisted feeding. *Journal of Clinical Nursing, 18*, 708–715.

McCreaddie, M., & Wiggins, S. (2009). Reconciling the good patient persona with problematic and non-problematic humour: A grounded theory. *International Journal of Nursing Studies, 46*, 1079–1091.

Patching, J., & Lawler, J. (2009). Understanding women's experiences of developing an eating disorder and recovering: A life history approach. *Nursing Inquiry, 16*, 10–21.

Rasmussen, D., Hansen, H., & Elverdam, B. (2010). How cancer survivors experience their changed body encountering others. *European Journal of Oncology Nursing, 14*, 154–159.

Rice, E. (2009). Schizophrenia and violence: Accepting and forsaking. *Qualitative Health Research, 19*, 840–849.

Sevean, P., Dampier, M., Strickland, S., & Pilatzke, S. (2009). Patients and families experiences with video teleheatlh in rural/remote communities in Northern Canada. *Journal of Clinical Nursing, 18*, 2573–2579.

Storesund, A., & McMurray, A. (2009). Quality of practice in an intensive care unit (ICU): A mini-ethnographic case study. *Intensive and Critical Care Nursing, 25*, 120–127.

Winters, C., Lee, H., Besel, J., Strand, A., Echeverri, R., Jorgensen, K., & Dea, J. E. (2007). Access to and use of research by rural nurses. *Rural and Remote Health, 7*, 758.

Wu, M., Hsu, L., Zhang, B., Shen, N., Lu, H., & Li, S. (2010). The experiences of cancer-related fatigue among Chinese children with leukaemia. *International Journal of Nursing Studies, 47*, 49–59.

Methodologic and nonresearch references cited in this chapter can be found in a separate section at the end of the book.

23

Qualitative Data Analysis

Qualitative data take the form of such narrative materials as verbatim dialogue between an interviewer and a respondent, field notes of participant observers, or diaries kept by study participants. This chapter describes methods for analyzing such qualitative data.

INTRODUCTION TO QUALITATIVE ANALYSIS

The purpose of data analysis is to organize, provide structure to, and elicit meaning from data. In qualitative studies, data collection and data analysis often occur simultaneously, rather than after data are collected. The search for important themes and concepts begins from the moment data collection gets underway.

Qualitative analysis is a labor-intensive activity that requires creativity, conceptual sensitivity, and sheer hard work. First, we discuss some general considerations relating to qualitative analysis.

Qualitative Analysis Challenges

Qualitative data analysis is a particularly challenging enterprise. There are no universal rules for analyzing qualitative data, and the absence of standard procedures makes it difficult to explain how to do such analyses. It is also difficult for researchers to describe how their analysis was done in a report and to present findings in a way that their validity is apparent. Some of the procedures described in the next chapter are important tools for enhancing the trustworthiness of the analysis.

A second challenge of qualitative analysis is the enormous amount of work required. Qualitative analysts must organize and make sense of pages and pages of narrative materials. In a study by one of us (Polit), the data consisted of transcribed interviews with 100 poor women discussing life stressors and health problems. The transcriptions ranged from 30 to 50 pages, resulting in more than 3,000 pages that had to be read, reread, and then analyzed and interpreted.

A final challenge comes in reducing data for reporting purposes. Quantitative results can often be summarized in a few tables. Qualitative researchers, by contrast, must balance the need to be concise with the need to maintain the richness and evidentiary value of their data.

⊃ TIP: Qualitative analyses are more difficult to *do* than quantitative ones, but qualitative findings are easier to understand than quantitative ones because the stories are told in everyday language. Qualitative analyses are often harder to evaluate critically than quantitative analyses, however, because readers cannot know if researchers adequately captured thematic patterns in the data.

The Qualitative Analysis Process

The analysis of qualitative data is an active and interactive process. Qualitative researchers typically scrutinize their data carefully and deliberatively, often reading the data over and over in search of meaning and understanding. Insights and theories cannot emerge until researchers become completely familiar with their data. Morse and Field (1995) noted that qualitative analysis is a "process of fitting data together, of making the invisible obvious, of linking and attributing consequences to antecedents. It is a process of conjecture and verification, of correction and modification, of suggestion and defense" (p. 126).

QUALITATIVE DATA MANAGEMENT AND ORGANIZATION

Qualitative analysis is supported by several tasks that help to manage the mass of narrative data.

Transcribing Qualitative Data

Audiotaped interviews and field notes are major data sources in qualitative studies. Verbatim transcription of the tapes is a critical step in preparing for data analysis, and researchers need to ensure that transcriptions are accurate and that they validly reflect the interview experience.

Transcription conventions are essential. For example, transcribers have to indicate, through symbols in the written text, who is speaking (e.g., "I" for interviewer, "P" for participant), overlaps in speaking turns, time elapsed between utterances when there are gaps, nonlinguistic utterances (e.g., sighs, sobs, laughter), emphasis of words, and so on. Silverman (2001) offered guidance regarding transcription conventions.

Transcription errors are almost inevitable, which means that researchers need to check the accuracy of transcribed data. Poland (1995) noted that there are three categories of error:

1. *Deliberate alterations of the data.* Transcribers may intentionally "fix" data to make the transcriptions look more like what they "should" look like. Such alterations are not done out of malice, but rather reflect a desire to be helpful. For example, transcribers may alter profanities, omit sounds such as phones ringing, or "tidy up" the text by deleting "ums" and "uhs." It is crucial to impress on transcribers the importance of verbatim accounts.

2. *Accidental alterations of the data.* Inadvertent transcription errors are more common. One pervasive problem concerns proper punctuation. The insertion or omission of commas, periods, or question marks can alter the interpretation of the text. Another error is misinterpreting words. For example, the actual words might be, "this was totally moot," but the transcription might read, "this was totally mute." Researchers should take steps to verify accuracy before analysis gets underway.

3. *Unavoidable alterations.* Data are unavoidably altered by the fact that transcriptions capture only a portion of an interview experience. For example, transcriptions will inevitably miss nonverbal cues such as body language, intonation, and so on.

➲ **TIP:** When checking the accuracy of transcribed data, it is critical to listen to the taped interview while doing the cross-check. This is also a good time to insert in the transcription any nonverbal behavior you recorded in your field notes.

Researchers should begin data analysis with the best possible quality data, which requires careful training of transcribers, ongoing feedback, and continuous efforts to verify accuracy. MacLean and colleagues (2004) offered suggestions for improving the accuracy of transcripts. One suggestion is to work with a transcriptionist at the start of the project to establish guidelines for handling potential problems. For example, how will the researcher be alerted that the transcriptionist was unable to understand certain portions of the tape recording? Researchers should explain their notation preferences for inaudible sections (e.g., cannot hear, poor tape quality, too much background noise) and provide transcriptionists with lists of terms and acronyms that might be unfamiliar. Transcriptionists also need to be prepared for emotionally difficult material. Transcribing emotional-laden interviews can result in inaccuracies if transcriptionists deny or "mis-hear" the words.

Lapadat (2000) offered other strategies to enhance transcription rigor. She suggested keeping a log of decision points while transcribing (e.g., What has the transcriber chosen not to transcribe?) Lapadat also suggested developing a codebook to record transcription conventions that were adopted or newly created for the project.

Developing a Category Scheme

Qualitative analysis begins with data organization—that is, by classifying and indexing the data. Researchers must be able to gain access to parts of the data, without having repeatedly to reread the data set in its entirety. This phase of data analysis is essentially reductionist—data must be converted to smaller, more manageable units that can be retrieved and reviewed.

The most widely used procedure is to develop a category scheme and then to code data according to the categories. A preliminary category system (called a *template*) is sometimes drafted before data collection, but more typically, qualitative analysts develop categories based on a scrutiny of actual data. There are no straightforward or easy guidelines for this task. Developing a high-quality category scheme involves a careful reading of the data, with an eye to identifying underlying concepts and clusters of concepts. The nature of the categories may vary in level of detail or specificity, as well as in level of abstraction.

Researchers whose aims are primarily descriptive tend to use categories that are fairly concrete. For example, the category scheme may focus on differentiating various types of actions or events, or different phases in a chronologic unfolding of an experience.

Example of a descriptive category scheme: Perry and colleagues (2008) did a descriptive qualitative study about factors influencing women's participation in a 12-week walking program. Data from field notes and focus group sessions were coded into two broad descriptive categories, barriers, and motivators to adopting a walking program. For example, the three main "barrier" subcategories were (1) balancing family and self, (2) chronic illness, and (3) illness or injury breaking the routine.

Studies that are designed to develop a theory are more likely to involve abstract, conceptual categories. In creating conceptual categories, researchers must break the data into segments, closely examine them, and compare them to other segments for similarities and dissimilarities to determine what the meaning of those phenomena are. (This is part of the *constant comparison* process espoused in grounded theory research.) The researcher asks questions such as the following about discrete events, incidents, or statements:

What is this?
What is going on?
What does it stand for?
What else is like this?
What is this distinct from?

Important concepts that emerge from close examination of the data are then given a label that forms the basis for a category. These labels are necessarily abstractions, but they should be sufficiently graphic that the nature of the material to which they refer is clear—and, often, provocative.

Example of a conceptual category scheme: Box 23.1 shows the category scheme developed by Beck (2006) to code data from her Internet interviews on the anniversary of birth trauma. The coding scheme included four major categories with subcodes. For example, an excerpt that described a mother's feelings of dread and anxiety during the days leading up to the anniversary of her traumatic birth would be coded 1A, the category for "plagued with an array of distressing thoughts and emotions."

Additional suggestions on categorizing and coding qualitative data are offered by Saldaña (2009).

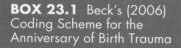

BOX 23.1 Beck's (2006) Coding Scheme for the Anniversary of Birth Trauma

Theme 1. The Prologue: An Agonizing Time
A. Plagued with an array of distressing thoughts and emotions
B. Physically taking a toll
C. Clocks, calendars, and seasons playing key roles
D. Ruminating about the day their babies had been born

Theme 2: The Actual Day: A Celebration of a Birthday or Torment of an Anniversary
A. Concept of time taking center stage
B. Not knowing how to celebrate her child's birthday
C. Tormented by powerful emotions
D. Scheduled birthday party on a different day
E. Consumed with technical details of the birthday party
F. Need to physically get away on the birthday

Theme 3: The Epilogue: A Fragile State
A. Surviving the actual anniversary took a heavy toll
B. Needed time to recuperate
C. Crippling emotions lingered
D. Sense of relief

Theme 4: Subsequent Anniversaries: For Better or Worse
A. Each birthday slightly easier to cope with
B. No improvement noted
C. Worrying about future birthdays
D. Each anniversary is a lottery; a time bomb.

spondence to the categories—a task that is seldom easy. Researchers may have difficulty deciding the most appropriate code, or may not fully comprehend the underlying meaning of some aspect of the data. It may take a second or third reading of the material to grasp its nuances.

Also, researchers often discover during coding that the initial categories were incomplete. It is common for categories to emerge that were not initially identified. When this happens, it is risky to assume that the category was absent in materials that have already been coded. A concept might not be identified as salient until it has emerged a few times. In such a case, it would be necessary to reread all previously coded material to have a truly complete grasp of that category. Making changes midway is often vexing, but a comprehensive category system is vital.

Another issue is that narrative materials usually are not linear. For example, paragraphs from transcribed interviews may contain elements relating to three or four different categories, embedded in a complex fashion.

Example of a multitopic segment: An example of a multitopic segment of an interview from Beck's (2006) phenomenological study of the anniversary of birth trauma is shown in Figure 23.1. The codes in the margin represent codes from the scheme presented in Box 23.1.

It is sometimes recommended that a single person code the entire data set to ensure the highest possible coding consistency across interviews or observations. Nevertheless, at least a portion of the interviews should be coded by two or more people early in the coding process, if possible, to evaluate and enhance reliability.

⭢ **TIP:** A good category scheme is critical to a thoughtful analysis, so a substantial sample of the data should be read before the scheme is drafted. To the extent possible, you should read materials that vary along key dimensions, to capture a range of content. The dimensions might be informant characteristics (e.g., men versus women) or aspects of the data collection experience (e.g., data from different sites).

Coding Qualitative Data

Once a category scheme has been developed, the data are read in their entirety and coded for corre-

⭢ **TIP:** It is wise to develop a codebook—written documentation describing the exact definition of the various categories used to code the data. Good qualitative codebooks usually include one or more actual excerpts that typify materials coded in each category. The Toolkit section of the accompanying *Resource Manual* includes an example of a codebook from Beck's work.

"I have experienced one anniversary of the trauma of Anna's birth. During the summer I remember looking at the calendar, fearing her birthday would take place on the same day of her birth (Wednesday). Hearing the word "October" or seeing the word in writing gave me chills.	1C
Prior to the anniversary I grew very sentimental about our hospital experience and would delve into piles of photos, hospital memorabilia and reading birth stories. Instead of feeling validated or better, it seemed to kick the grief into high gear. I felt very alone. My closet contained all the hospital stuff and when I was sad or alone I would go there, ironically, to feel even more alone. I didn't feel anyone would ever understand.	1A
Time was definitely a traumatic concept during the anniversary. There is sooo much emphasis on time in the birthing process, so this seemed to carry and surface on and around her birthday. I found myself linking the time of day to what happened that evening,	1C
driving to the hospital, number of dilation to the minute and when my water was broken. I	1D
would see commercials for a television show and feel scared, knowing it played during the time of my laboring. Even today, a clock reading 8:47 will turn my stomach upside down."	1C,1A

FIGURE 23.1 Coded excerpt from Beck's (2006) study on the anniversary of birth trauma.

Manual Methods of Organizing Qualitative Data

Traditional manual methods of organizing qualitative data are becoming less common as a result of the widespread use of software that can perform indexing functions. Here, we briefly describe some manual methods of data management; the next section describes computer methods.

When a category system is simple, researchers sometimes use colored paper clips or Post-It Notes to code narrative content. For example, if we were analyzing interviews about women's concerns about menopause, we might use blue paper clips for text relating to loss of fertility, red clips for text on menopausal side effects, yellow clips for text relating to aging, and so on. Then we could pull out all material with a certain color clip to examine one issue at a time.

Phenomenological researchers sometimes use a file card system, placing significant statements from interviews on a file card of its own. The file cards are then sorted into piles representing themes. Some researchers use different colored file cards for each person's data.

Before the advent of computer software for managing qualitative data, a typical procedure was to develop **conceptual files**. In this approach, researchers create a physical file folder for each category, and insert material relating to that category into the file. Researchers first go through all the data, writing relevant codes in the margins, as in Figure 23.1. Then they cut up a copy of the material by category area, and place the excerpts into the file for that category. All of the content on a particular topic then can be retrieved by going to the applicable file folder.

Creating such files is cumbersome, especially when segments of the narrative materials have multiple codes, as in Figure 23.1. For example, there would need to be three copies of the bottom paragraph, corresponding to the three codes. Researchers must also provide enough context that the cut-up material can be understood (e.g., including material preceding or following the directly relevant materials). Finally, researchers must usually include pertinent administrative information. For example, for interview data, each excerpt would need to include the ID number for the participant so that researchers could, if necessary, obtain additional information from the master copy.

Computer Programs for Managing Qualitative Data

Computer assisted qualitative data analysis software (CAQDAS) removes the work of cutting up pages of narrative material. These programs allow researchers to enter the entire data file onto the computer, code each portion of the narrative, and then retrieve and display text for specified codes for analysis. The software can also be used to examine relationships between codes. Software cannot, however, *do* the coding, and it cannot tell researchers how to analyze the data. Researchers must continue to be analysts and critical thinkers.

Dozens of CAQDAS have been developed. The main types of software packages that are available to handle and manage qualitative data include: text retrievers, code and retrieve, theory building, concept maps and diagrams, and data conversion/collection (Taylor, 2005; Lewins & Silver, 2007). *Text retrievers* are programs that help researchers locate text and terms in databases and documents. *Code-and-retrieve packages* permit researchers to code text.

More sophisticated *theory building software,* the most frequently used type of CAQDAS, permits researchers to examine relationships between concepts, develop hierarchies of codes, diagram, and create hyperlinks to create nonhierarchical networks. Examples of theory building packages include ATLAS/TI, HyperRESEARCH, MaxQDA, and NVivo8. NVivo8, software from Qualitative Solutions and Research (QSR), combines the best of two earlier packages (NVivo2 and NUD*IST 6). NVivo8 helps researchers find patterns in their data and explore hunches and enables them to display and analyze relationships in the data.

Software for *concept mapping* permits researchers to construct more sophisticated diagrams than theory building software. Concept maps are a means for organizing and representing knowledge (Novak & Canas, 2006). Concept maps include concepts (enclosed in circles or boxes) and relationships between them (indicated by connecting lines). CmapTools, an example of concept mapping software (*www.ihmc*), was developed at the Institute for Human and Machine Cognition. It is available at no cost for educational and not-for-profit organizations.

Data conversion/collection software converts audio into text. Voice recognition software can convert spoken voice into text and is attractive because of the time and expense needed to transcribe audiotaped interviews. Voice recognition software is designed for a single user. The software must be "trained" to recognize the voice of the user, typically an *oral transcriptionist*. Estimates of the time required to train software for voice recognition have averaged about 10 hours (Fogg & Wightman, 2000).

Voice recognition programs are available from a number of vendors. Their performance is variable and depends on such factors as the capability of the computer on which the software is installed, the quality of the microphone, and the amount of background noise. One disadvantage is voice recognition software's inability to automatically punctuate. The oral transcriptionist must specifically state the punctuation, such as "period" and "comma." Oral transcriptionists also still need to edit the text to correct errors.

MacLean and colleagues (2004) used voice recognition software to transcribe their interviews in their research on health promotion initiatives and discussed some problems they encountered. For instance, the voice recognition program consistently misinterpreted common homonyms like "here" and "hear," "to," "too," and "two," resulting in inaccuracies in the transcript. Thus, the time-saving advantages in using voice recognition software may be modest.

Computer programs offer many advantages for managing qualitative data, but some people prefer manual methods because they allow researchers to get closer to the data. Others have raised objections to having a process that is basically cognitive turned into an activity that is mechanical. Despite concerns, many researchers have switched to computerized data management. Proponents insist that it frees up their time and permits them to pay greater attention to important conceptual issues. CAQDAS is constantly revised and upgraded so it is important to stay current on this topic.

➲ **TIP:** Articles that describe the application of specific qualitative data analysis software are helpful to read before starting your own project. For example, Bringer and colleagues (2004) described in detail their use of the software program NVivo in a grounded theory study. A number of print screens from their analysis are included in the article as illustrations.

Example of using computers to manage qualitative data: Nordfjaern and colleagues (2010) studied perceptions of treatment and recovery from the perspective of patients with substance addiction. NVivo 8 was used to manage the transcribed data from semistructured interviews with 13 patients.

ANALYTIC PROCEDURES

Data *management* in qualitative research is reductionist in nature: It involves converting masses of data into smaller, manageable segments. By contrast, qualitative data *analysis* is constructionist: It involves putting segments together into meaningful conceptual patterns. Qualitative analysis involves discovering pervasive ideas and searching for general concepts (i.e., analytic generalization, Chapter 21) through an inductive process. Although there are various approaches to qualitative data analysis, some elements are common to several of them, yet it is also true that qualitative analysis is eclectic and nonprescriptive. We provide some general strategies, followed by a description of procedures favored by ethnographers, phenomenologists, and grounded theory researchers.

A General Analytic Overview

The analysis of qualitative materials typically begins with a search for broad categories or themes. In their thorough review of how the term *theme* is used among qualitative researchers, DeSantis and Ugarriza (2000) offered this definition: "A **theme** is an abstract entity that brings meaning and identity to a current experience and its variant manifestations. As such, a theme captures and unifies the nature or basis of the experience into a meaningful whole" (p. 362).

Thematic analysis often relies on what Spradley (1979) called the similarity principle and the contrast principle. The *similarity principle* involves looking for units of information with similar content, symbols, or meanings. The *contrast principle* guides efforts to find out how content or symbols differ from other content or symbols—that is, to identify what is distinctive about emerging themes or categories.

During analysis, qualitative researchers must distinguish between ideas that apply to all (or many) people and aspects of the experience that are unique to particular participants. Ayres and colleagues (2003) argued cogently for the importance of doing both across-case analysis and within-case analysis. The analysis of individual cases "enables the researcher to understand those aspects of experience that occur not as individual 'units of meaning' but as part of the pattern formed by the confluence of meanings within individual accounts" (p. 873). Themes that have explanatory or conceptual power both in individual cases and across the sample have the best potential for analytic generalization. Ayres and colleagues illustrated how within-case and across-case analyses were integrated in three nursing studies.

Themes emerge from the data. They often develop within categories of data, but may also cut across them. For example, in Beck's anniversary of birth trauma (2006) study (Box 23.1), one theme that emerged was mothers' fragile state after the actual day of the anniversary was over, which included codes 3B (needing time to recuperate) and 3D (sense of relief).

Thematic analysis involves not only discovering commonalities across participants, but also seeking natural variation. Themes are never universal. Researchers must attend not only to what themes arise, but also to how they are patterned. Does the theme apply only to certain types of people? In certain contexts? At certain periods? What are the conditions that precede the observed phenomenon, and what are the apparent consequences of it? In other words, the qualitative analyst must be sensitive to *relationships* within the data.

Researchers' search for themes and patterns sometimes can be facilitated by charting devices that enable them to summarize the evolution of behaviors, events, and processes. For example, for qualitative studies that focus on dynamic experiences—such as decision making—it is sometimes useful to develop flow charts or timelines that highlight time sequences, major decision points and events, and factors affecting the decisions.

Example of a timeline: In her grounded theory study of mothering twins during the first year of life, Beck (2002) found that timelines highlighting mothers' 24-hour schedule were helpful. For example, one mother had twins who had stayed in the neonatal intensive care unit for 2 months. When the twins were discharged, the mother maintained the twins on the same feeding schedule as they had been on in the hospital (every 3 hours) for several months. The timeline for this mother illustrated the mothers' heavy caretaking demands and her brief, interrupted sleep pattern.

Two-dimensional matrices to array thematic material is another frequently used method of displaying thematic material (Miles & Huberman, 1994). Traditionally, each row of a matrix is allocated to individual participants, and columns are used to enter either raw data or themes. Although matrices can be done by hand, computer spreadsheets may be preferred to enhance opportunities for sorting the data in various ways.

Identifying key themes and categories is seldom a tidy, linear process—iteration is almost always necessary. That is, researchers derive themes from the narrative materials, go back to the materials with the themes in mind to see if the materials really do fit, and then refine the themes as necessary. Sometimes apparent insights early in the process have to be abandoned.

Example of abandoning an early conceptualization: In their study of the experiences of family caregivers of relatives with dementia, Strang and colleagues (2006) commented as follows: "We coded data categories in stages with each stage representing a higher level of conceptual complexity . . . the interplay within the caregiver dyad reminded us of *dancing*. As the analysis progressed, the dance metaphor failed to fully represent the increasingly complex nature of the interactions between caregiver and the family member with dementia. We abandoned it completely" (p. 32).

Some qualitative researchers—especially phenomenologists—use metaphors as an analytic strategy, as the preceding example suggests. A **metaphor** is a symbolic comparison, using figurative language to evoke a visual analogy. Metaphors can be a powerfully expressive tool for qualitative analysts. As a literary device, metaphors can permit greater insight and understanding in qualitative analysis and can

help link together parts to the whole. Thorne and Darbyshire (2005) have, however, criticized the overuse of metaphors. In their view, metaphoric allusions can be a compelling approach to articulating human experience, but they can run the risk of "supplanting creative insight with hackneyed cliché masquerading as profundity" (p. 1111). Carpenter (2008) also warned that when researchers mix metaphors, fail to follow through with metaphors, or use metaphors that do not fit, they can misrepresent the data.

Example of a metaphor: Logsdon and Hines-Martin (2009) studied barriers to depression treatment in low-income, unmarried, adolescent mothers. Nine participants enrolled in a teen parent program were interviewed in a focus group. The researchers used the metaphor of a merry-go-round to describe the ups and downs that adolescent mothers experienced as they tried to adjust to motherhood. On the upside, adolescent mothers experienced pride in their babies, and on the down side, they experienced negative feelings such as sadness, anxiety, and frustration.

A further step involves validation. In this phase, the concern is whether the themes accurately represent the perspectives of the participants. Several validation procedures are discussed in Chapter 24. If more than one researcher is working on the study, sessions in which the themes are reviewed and specific cases discussed can be highly productive. Such investigator triangulation cannot ensure thematic integrity, but it can minimize idiosyncratic biases.

In validating and refining themes, some researchers introduce **quasi-statistics**—a tabulation of the frequency with which certain themes or insights are supported by the data. The frequencies cannot be interpreted in the same way as frequencies generated in survey studies because of imprecision in the enumeration of the themes, but, as Becker (1970) pointed out, "Quasi-statistics may allow the investigator to dispose of certain troublesome null hypotheses. A simple frequency count of the number of times a given phenomenon appears may make untenable the null hypothesis that the phenomenon is infrequent." (p. 81).

Sandelowski (2001) expressed her belief that numbers are underutilized in qualitative research because of two myths: first, that real qualitative researchers *do not* count and second, that qualitative researchers *cannot* count. Numbers can be helpful in highlighting the complexity and work of qualitative research. Numbers may also be useful in documenting and testing interpretations and conclusions and in describing events and experiences (although Sandelowski warned of the pitfalls of over counting). We discuss this issue at greater length in the chapter on mixed methods research (Chapter 25).

> **Example of tabulating data:** Hawkins and colleagues (2009) studied changes in sexuality and intimacy after treatment for cancer, based on in-depth interviews with informal carers who were the patients' sexual partners. The researchers tabulated different patterns of changes. For example, cessation or severely decreased frequency was reported by 59% of the women and 79% of the men. Renegotiation of intimacy and sex was reported by 19% of the women and 14% of the men. The report provided excerpts from participants with the various patterns.

In the final analysis stage, researchers strive to weave thematic pieces together into an integrated whole. The various themes need to be interrelated to provide an overall structure (such as a theory or integrated description) to the data. The integration task is a difficult one, because it demands creativity and intellectual rigor if it is to be successful.

Qualitative Content Analysis

In the remainder of this section, we discuss analytic procedures used by ethnographers, phenomenologists, and grounded theory researchers. Qualitative researchers who conduct descriptive qualitative studies not based in a specific tradition may, however, simply say that they performed a content analysis. **Qualitative content analysis** is the analysis of the content of narrative data to identify prominent themes and patterns among the themes. Qualitative content analysis involves breaking down data into smaller *units*, coding and naming the units according to the content they represent, and grouping coded material based on shared concepts.

Krippendorff (2005) identified five definitions of units: physical, syntactical, categorical, proposi-

tional, and thematic distinctions. These definitions refer to the types of cognitive operations coders needed to do to identify units within a text. Physical units are defined by time, length, or size—but not by type of information. Syntactical distinctions are based on grammatical divisions within the data—that is, words, sentences, paragraphs. Categorical distinctions define units by identifying something they have in common, that is, membership in a category. Propositional distinctions divide units based on specific constructions, such as a proposition or a clause. Lastly, thematic distinctions delineate units according to themes.

Krippendorff (2005) suggested *clustering* as a way to represent the results of content analyses. Clustering is based on similarities among units of analysis and hierarchies that conceptualize the text on different levels of abstraction. The steps of clustering can be displayed in *dendrograms*, which are treelike diagrams. Dendrograms indicate when and which units are merged. Hsieh and Shannon (2005) offered a good discussion of three different approaches to content analysis.

> **Example of a content analysis:** Beck (2005) undertook a content analysis of the benefits of women participating in Internet interviews regarding traumatic childbirths. Her paper included an example of a dendrogram.

Ethnographic Analysis

Analysis begins from the moment ethnographers set foot in the field. Ethnographers are continually looking for *patterns* in the behavior and thoughts of participants, comparing one pattern against another, and analyzing many patterns simultaneously (Fetterman, 2010). As they analyze patterns of everyday life, ethnographers acquire a deeper understanding of the culture being studied. Maps, flowcharts, and organizational charts are useful tools that help to crystallize and illustrate the data. Matrices (two-dimensional displays) can also help to highlight a comparison graphically, to cross-reference categories, and to discover emerging patterns.

Spradley's (1979) research sequence can be used for data analysis in ethnographies. His method is based on the premise that language is the primary means that relates cultural meaning in a culture. The task of ethnographers is to describe cultural symbols and to identify their coding rules. His sequence of 12 steps, which includes data collection and data analysis, is as follows:

1. Locating an informant
2. Interviewing an informant
3. Making an ethnographic record
4. Asking descriptive questions
5. Analyzing ethnographic interviews
6. Making a domain analysis
7. Asking structural questions
8. Making a taxonomic analysis
9. Asking contrast questions
10. Making a componential analysis
11. Discovering cultural themes
12. Writing the ethnography

Thus, in Spradley's method there are four levels of data analysis, the first of which is **domain analysis**. Domains, which are units of cultural knowledge, are broad categories that encompass smaller ones. During this first level of data analysis, ethnographers identify relational patterns among terms in the domains that are used by members of the culture. The ethnographer focuses on the cultural meaning of terms and symbols (objects and events) used in a culture and their interrelationships.

In **taxonomic analysis**, the second level of data analysis, ethnographers decide how many domains the analysis will encompass. Will only one or two domains be analyzed in depth, or will a number of domains be studied less intensively? After making this decision, a **taxonomy**—a system of classifying and organizing terms—is developed to illustrate the internal organization of a domain and the relationship among the subcategories of the domain.

In **componential analysis**, relationships among terms in the domains are examined. The ethnographer analyzes data for similarities and differences among cultural terms in a domain. Finally, in **theme analysis**, cultural themes are uncovered. Domains are connected in cultural themes, which help to provide a holistic view of the culture being studied. The discovery of cultural meaning is the outcome.

Example using Spradley's method: Fraser and colleagues (2009) conducted an ethnographic study of a pediatric home care program in Canada. Data sources included interviews with case managers, program leaders, and participant observation over a 5-month period. Data analysis included domain, taxonomic, and componential analysis. A key product was a taxonomy of factors that influence case managers' resource allocation decisions.

Other approaches to ethnographic analysis have been developed. For example, in their ethnonursing research method, Leininger and McFarland (2006) provided ethnographers with a four-phase ethnonursing data analysis guide. In the first phase, ethnographers collect, describe, and record data. The second phase involves identifying and categorizing descriptors. In Phase 3, data are analyzed to discover repetitive patterns in their context. The fourth and final phase involves abstracting major themes and presenting findings.

Example using Leininger's method: Aga and colleagues (2009) studied conceptions of care among family caregivers of people living with HIV or AIDS in Addis Ababa, Ethiopia. The researchers interviewed 6 key informants and 12 additional informants. Using Leininger's phases of ethnonursing analysis, four major cultural themes were identified.

Phenomenological Analysis

Many qualitative analysts use what might be called "fracturing" strategies that break down the data and rearrange them into categories that facilitate comparisons across cases (e.g., grounded theory researchers). Phenomenologists often prefer holistic, "contextualizing" strategies that involve interpreting the narrative data within the context of a "whole text."

Three frequently used methods for descriptive phenomenology are the methods of Colaizzi (1978), Giorgi (1985), and Van Kaam (1966), all of whom are from the Duquesne school of phenomenology, based on Husserl's philosophy.

Phenomenological analysis using all three methods involves a search for common patterns, but there are some important differences among these approaches, as summarized in Table 23.1. The basic outcome of

TABLE 23.1 Comparison of Three Phenomenological Analytic Methods

COLAIZZI (1978)	GIORGI (1985)	VAN KAAM (1966)
1. Read all protocols to acquire a feeling for them.	1. Read the entire set of protocols to get a sense of the whole.	1. List and group preliminarily the descriptive expressions that must be agreed upon by expert judges. Final listing presents percentages of these categories in that particular sample.
2. Review each protocol and extract significant statements.	2. Discriminate units from participants' description of phenomenon being studied.	2. Reduce the concrete, vague, and overlapping expressions of the participants to more descriptive terms. (Intersubjective agreement among judges needed.)
3. Spell out the meaning of each significant statement (i.e., formulate meanings).	3. Articulate the psychological insight in each of the meaning units.	3. Eliminate elements not inherent in the phenomenon being studied or that represent blending of two related phenomena.
4. Organize the formulated meanings into clusters of themes. a. Refer these clusters back to the original protocols to validate them. b. Note discrepancies among or between the various clusters, avoiding the temptation of ignoring data or themes that do not fit.	4. Synthesize all of the transformed meaning units into a consistent statement regarding participants' experiences (referred to as the "structure of the experience"); can be expressed on a specific or general level.	4. Write a hypothetical identification and description of the phenomenon being studied.
5. Integrate results into an exhaustive description of the phenomenon under study.		5. Apply hypothetical description to randomly selected cases from the sample. If necessary, revise the hypothesized description, which must then be tested again on a new random sample.
6. Formulate an exhaustive description of the phenomenon under study in as unequivocal a statement of identification as possible.		6. Consider the hypothesized identification as a valid identification and description once preceding operations have been carried out successfully.
7. Ask participants about the findings thus far as a final validating step.		

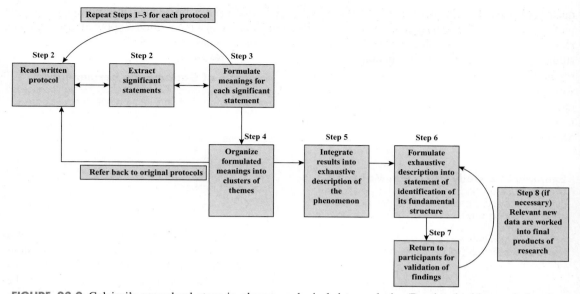

FIGURE 23.2 Colaizzi's procedural steps in phenomenological data analysis. (Reprinted with permission from Beck, C. T. (2009). The arm: There is no escaping the reality for mothers of children with obstetric brachial plexus injuries. *Nursing Research, 58*, 237–245.)

all three methods is the description of the meaning of an experience, often through the identification of essential themes. Colaizzi's method, however, is the only one that calls for a validation of results by returning to study participants. Figure 23.2 provides an illustration of the steps involved in data analysis using Colaizzi's approach. Giorgi's analysis relies solely on researchers. His view is that it is inappropriate either to return to participants to validate findings or to use external judges to review the analysis. Van Kaam's method requires that intersubjective agreement be reached with other expert judges.

Example of a study using Colaizzi's method: Beck and Watson (2008) explored the impact of birth trauma on mothers' breastfeeding experiences using Internet interviews with 52 women. Mothers' descriptions were analyzed using Colaizzi's method. Eight themes emerged that revealed the essence of women's experiences of the impact of a traumatic birth on their breastfeeding experiences. For example, one theme was, proving oneself as a mother: sheer determination to succeed.

A second school of phenomenology is the Utrecht School. Phenomenologists using this

approach combine characteristics of descriptive and interpretive phenomenology. Van Manen's (1990) method is an example of this approach, in which researchers try to grasp the essential meaning of the experience being studied. According to Van Manen, thematic aspects of experience can be uncovered or isolated from participants' descriptions of the experience by three methods: (1) the holistic approach, (2) the selective (highlighting) approach, and (3) the detailed (line-by-line) approach. In the **holistic approach**, researchers view the text as a whole and try to capture its meanings. In the **selective approach**, researchers highlight or pull out statements or phrases that seem essential to the experience under study. In the **detailed approach**, researchers analyze every sentence. Once themes have been identified, they become the objects of reflection and interpretation through follow-up interviews with participants. Through this process, essential themes are discovered.

Van Manen (2006) stressed that this phenomenological method cannot be separated from the practice of writing. In writing up the results of qualitative analysis the phenomenological researcher participates in an active struggle to understand and recognized the lived meanings of the phenomena studied. The text written by a phenomenological researcher must lead readers to a "questioning wonder." The words chosen by the writer need to take the reader into a "wondrous landscape" as the reader is drawn into the textual meaning (Van Manen, 2002, p. 4).

Example of a study using Van Manen's method: Jessup and Parkinson (2010) explored living with cystic fibrosis from the perspective of children, young adults, and parents. The researchers analyzed interview transcripts holistically for themes in line with Van Manen's approach of using four lifeworld existentials (space, time, body, and relationship).
From their original fright, through ongoing dynamics of "fear, fight, flight, form, familiarity, and philosophy" (p. 355), people with CF were found to pursue a future that is threatened and perpetually redefined.

In addition to identifying themes from participants' words, Van Manen also called for gleaning thematic descriptions from artistic sources. Van Manen urged qualitative researchers to keep in mind that literature, music, painting, and other art forms can provide a wealth of experiential information that can increase insights as the phenomenologist tries to grasp the essential meaning of the experience being studied. Experiential descriptions in literature and art help challenge and stretch phenomenologists' interpretive sensibilities.

A third school of phenomenology is an interpretive approach called Heideggerian hermeneutics. As noted in Chapter 20, a key notion in a hermeneutic study is the *hermeneutic circle*. The circle signifies a methodologic process in which, to reach understanding, there is continual movement between the parts and the whole of the text being analyzed. Gadamer (1975) stressed that, to interpret a text, researchers cannot separate themselves from the meanings of the text and must strive to understand possibilities that the text can reveal.

Ricoeur (1981) broadened this notion of text to include not just the written text but also any human action or situation.

Example of Gadamerian hermeneutics: Ryde and colleagues (2008) studied the significance of family members crying in a palliative home care context. Interviews were conducted with 14 family members. Guided by Gadamer's writings, the researchers maintained a dialogue between themselves and the transcribed text of the interviews. Questioning, reflecting, and validating were components of this process. Continuous movement between the whole and parts of the text occurred.

Diekelmann and colleagues (1989) proposed a seven-stage process of data analysis in hermeneutics that involves collaborative effort by a team of researchers. The goal of this process is to describe shared practices and common meanings. The seven stages include the following:

1. All the interviews or texts are read for an overall understanding.
2. Interpretive summaries of each interview are written.
3. A team of researchers analyzes selected transcribed interviews or texts.
4. Any disagreements on interpretation are resolved by going back to the text.
5. Common meanings are identified by comparing and contrasting the text.
6. Relationships among themes emerge.
7. A draft of the themes with exemplars from texts is presented to the team. Responses or suggestions are incorporated into the final draft.

According to Diekelmann and colleagues, the discovery in Step 6 of a **constitutive pattern**—a pattern that expresses the relationships among relational themes and is present in all the interviews or texts—forms the highest level of hermeneutical analysis. A situation is constitutive when it gives actual content to a person's self-understanding or to a person's way of being in the world.

Benner (1994) offered another analytic approach for hermeneutic phenomenology. Her interpretive analysis consists of three interrelated processes: the search for paradigm cases, thematic analysis, and analysis of exemplars. **Paradigm cases** are "strong instances of concerns or ways of being in the world" (Benner, 1994, p.113). Paradigm cases are used early in the analytic process as a strategy for gaining understanding. Thematic analysis is done to compare and contrast similarities across cases. Lastly, paradigm cases and thematic analysis can be enhanced by *exemplars* that illuminate aspects of a paradigm case or theme. The presentation of paradigm cases and exemplars in reports allows readers to play a role in consensual validation of the results by deciding whether the cases support the researchers' conclusions.

Grounded Theory Analysis

Grounded theory methods emerged in the 1960s in connection with Glaser and Strauss's (1967) research program on dying in hospitals. The two co-originators eventually split and developed divergent schools of thought, which have been called the "Glaserian" and "Straussian" versions of grounded theory (Walker & Myrick, 2006). The division

between the two mainly concerns the manner in which the data are analyzed.

Glaser and Strauss' Grounded Theory Method

Grounded theory in both systems of analysis uses the *constant comparative* method of analysis. This method involves a comparison of elements present in one data source (e.g., in one interview) with those in another to determine if they are similar. The process continues until the content of each source has been compared to the content in all sources. In this fashion, commonalities are identified.

The concept of fit is an important element in Glaserian grounded theory analysis. By **fit**, Glaser meant that the developing categories of the substantive theory must fit the data. Fit enables the researcher to determine if data can be placed in the same category or if they can be related to one another. However, Glaser (1992) warned qualitative researchers not to force an analytic fit, noting that "if you torture data enough it will give up!" (p. 123). Forcing a fit hinders the development of a relevant theory. *Fit* is also an important issue when a grounded theory is applied in new contexts: the theory must closely "fit" the substantive area where it will be used (Glaser & Strauss, 1967).

Coding in the Glaserian approach is used to conceptualize data into patterns. The substance of the topic under study is conceptualized through **substantive codes**, while **theoretical codes** provide insights into how substantive codes relate to each other. Substantive codes are either open or selective. **Open coding**, used in the first stage of the constant comparative analysis, captures what is going on in the data. Open codes may be the actual words used by the participants. Through open coding, data are broken down into incidents and their similarities and differences are examined. During open coding, researchers ask "What category or property of a category does this incident indicate?" (Glaser, 1978, p. 57).

There are three levels of open coding that vary in degree of abstraction. **Level I codes** (or *in vivo codes*) are derived directly from the language of

TABLE 23.2	Collapsing Level I Codes into the Level II Code of *"REAPING THE BLESSINGS"* (Beck, 2002)	

QUOTE	LEVEL I CODE
I enjoy just watching the twins interact so much. Especially now that they are mobile. They are not walking yet but they are crawling. I will tell you they are already playing. Like one will go around the corner and kind of peek around and they play hide and seek. They crawl after each other.	Enjoying Twins
With twins it's amazing. She was sick and she had a fever. He was the one acting sick. She didn't seem like she was sick at all. He was. We watched him for like 6–8 hours. We gave her the medicine and he started calming down. Like WOW! That is so weird. Cause you read about it but it's like, Oh come on! You know that doesn't really happen and it does. It's really neat to see.	Amazing
These days it's really neat cause you go to the store or you go out and people are like "Oh, they are twins, how nice." And I say, "Yeah they are. Look, look at my kids."	Getting Attention
I just feel blessed to have two. I just feel like I am twice as lucky as a mom who has one baby. I mean that's the best part. It's just that instead of having one baby to watch grow and change and develop and become a toddler and school-age child you have two.	Feeling Blessed
It's very exciting. It's interesting and it's fun to see them and how the twin bond really is. There really is a twin bond. You read about it and you hear about it but until you experience it, you just don't understand. One time they were both crying and they were fed. They were changed and burped. There was nothing wrong. I couldn't figure out what was wrong. So I said to myself, "I am just going to put them together and close the door." I put them in my bed together and they patty-caked their hands and put their noses together and just looked at each other and went right to sleep.	Twin Bonding

the substantive area and have vivid imagery. Table 23.2 presents five level I codes from Beck's (2002) grounded theory study on mothering twins, and interview excerpts associated with those codes. (A figure showing Beck's hierarchy of codes, from level I to one of her level III codes, is shown in the Toolkit of the accompanying *Resource Manual.* 🕸)

Researchers constantly compare new level I codes to previously identified ones, and then condense them into broader **level II codes**. For exam-

ple, in Table 23.2, Beck's five level I codes were collapsed into the level II code, "Reaping the Blessings." **Level III codes** (or theoretical constructs) are the most abstract. These constructs "add scope beyond local meanings" (Glaser, 1978, p. 70) to the generated theory. Collapsing level II codes aids in identifying constructs.

Open coding ends when the core category is discovered, and then selective coding begins. The **core category** is a pattern of behavior that is relevant and/or problematic for participants. In selective coding (which can also have three levels of abstraction), researchers code only those data that are related to the core variable. One kind of core variable is a **basic social process (BSP)** that evolves over time in two or more phases. All BSPs are core variables, but not all core variables have to be BSPs.

Glaser (1978) provided nine criteria to help researchers decide on a core category:

1. It must be central, meaning that it is related to many categories.
2. It must reoccur frequently in the data.
3. It takes more time to saturate than other categories.
4. It relates meaningfully and easily to other categories.
5. It has clear and grabbing implications for formal theory.
6. It has considerable carry-through.
7. It is completely variable.
8. It is a dimension of the problem.
9. It can be any kind of theoretical code.

Theoretical codes help grounded theorists to weave the broken pieces of data back together. Theoretical codes have the power "to grab," which Glaser (2005) called "theoretical code capture" (p. 74). Theoretical codes provide a grounded theory with greater explanatory power because they enhance the abstract meaning of the relationships among categories. Glaser (1978) first proposed 18 families of theoretical codes that researchers can use to conceptualize how substantive codes relate to each other (Box 23.2). Recently, Glaser (2005) identified many new possibilities for theoretical codes, offering examples from biochemistry (bias random walk), economics (amplifying causal looping), and political science (conjectural causation). The larger the array of theoretical codes available, the less tendency a researcher will have to force on the developing theory a pet or favorite theoretical code (Glaser, 2005).

Throughout coding and analysis, grounded theory analysts document their ideas about the data, categories, and emerging conceptual scheme in

---

BOX 23.2 Families of Theoretical Codes for Grounded Theory Analysis

1. The six C's: causes, contexts, contingencies, consequences, covariances, and conditions
2. Process: stages, phases, passages, transitions
3. Degree: intensity, range, grades, continuum
4. Dimension: elements, parts, sections
5. Type: kinds, styles, forms
6. Strategy: tactics, techniques, maneuverings
7. Interaction: mutual effects, interdependence, reciprocity
8. Identity–self: self-image, self-worth, self-concept
9. Cutting point: boundaries, critical junctures, turning points
10. Means–goal: purpose, end, products
11. Cultural: social values, beliefs
12. Consensus: agreements, uniformities, conformity
13. Mainline: socialization, recruiting, social order
14. Theoretical: density, integration, clarity, fit, relevance
15. Ordering/elaboration: structural ordering, temporal ordering, conceptual ordering
16. Unit: group, organization, collective
17. Reading: hypotheses, concepts, problems
18. Models: pictorial models of a theory

Adapted from Glaser, B. G. (1978). *Theoretical sensitivity*. Mill Valley, CA: Sociological Press.

memos. Memos preserve ideas that may initially not seem productive but may later prove valuable once further developed. Memos also encourage researchers to reflect on and describe patterns in the data, relationships between categories, and emergent conceptualizations.

➔ **TIP:** The Toolkit section of the *Resource Manual* includes an example of a memo from Beck's work. Glaser (1978) offered guidelines for preparing effective memos to generate substantive theory, including the following:

* Keep memos separate from data.
* Stop coding when an idea for a memo occurs, so as not to lose the thought.
* A memo can be brought on by forcing it, by beginning to write about a code.
* Memos can be modified as growth and realizations occur.
* In writing memos, do not focus on persons; talk conceptually about substantive codes.
* When you have two ideas, write each idea up as a separate memo to prevent confusion.
* Always remain flexible with memoing approaches.

Glaser's grounded theory method is concerned with the *generation* of categories and hypotheses rather than testing them. The product of the typical grounded theory analysis is a theoretical model that endeavors to generate "a theory of continually resolving the main concern, which explains most of the behavior in an area of interest" (Glaser, 2001, p.103). Once the basic problem or central concern emerges, the grounded theorist goes on to discover the process these participants experience in coping with or resolving this problem.

Example of Glaser and Strauss grounded theory analysis: Figure 23.3 presents Beck's (2002) model from a grounded theory study in which "Releasing the Pause Button" was conceptualized as the core category and process through which mothers of twins progressed as they attempted to resume their lives after giving birth. According to this model, the process involves four phases: Draining Power, Pausing own Life, Striving to Reset, and Resuming own Life. Beck used 10 coding families in her theoretical coding for the Releasing the Pause Button process. The family *cutting point* provides an illustration. Three months seemed to be the turning point for mothers, when life started to become more manageable. Here is an excerpt that Beck coded as a cutting point: "Three months came around and the twins sort of slept through the night and it made a huge, huge difference."

Although Glaser and Strauss cautioned against consulting the literature before a theoretical framework is stabilized, they also viewed grounded theory as an "ever modifying process" (Glaser, 1978, p. 5) that could benefit from scrutiny of other work. Glaser discussed the evolution of grounded theories through the process of **emergent fit**, to prevent individual

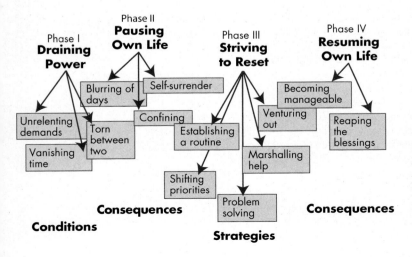

FIGURE 23.3 Beck's (2002) model of mothering twins. (Reprinted with permission from Beck, C. T. (2002). Releasing the pause button: Mothering twins during the first year of life. *Qualitative Health Research, 12*, 593–608.)

substantive theories from being "respected little islands of knowledge" (p. 148). As Glaser pointed out, generating grounded theory does not necessarily require discovering all new categories or ignoring ones previously identified in the literature: "The task is, rather, to develop an emergent fit between the data and a pre-existent category that might work. Therefore, as in the refitting of a generated category as data emerge, so must an extant category be carefully fitted as data emerge to be sure it works. In the bargain, like the generated category, it may be modified to fit and work. In this sense the extant category was not merely borrowed but earned its way into the emerging theory" (p. 4). Through constant comparison, researchers can compare concepts emerging from the data with similar concepts from existing theory or research to assess which parts have emergent fit with the theory being generated.

Example of emergent fit: Wuest (2000) described how she grappled with reconciling emergent fit with Glaser's warning to avoid reading the literature until a grounded theory is well on its way. She used examples from her grounded theory study on negotiating with helping systems (e.g., healthcare, religion) to illustrate how emergent fit with existing research on relationships in healthcare was used to support her emerging theory. Constant comparison provided the checks and balances on using preexisting knowledge.

Strauss and Corbin's Approach

The Strauss and Corbin approach to grounded theory analysis, most recently described in Corbin and Strauss (2008), differs from the original Glaser and Strauss method with regard to method, processes, and outcomes. Table 23.3 summarizes major analytic differences between these two grounded theory analysis methods.

Glaser (1978) stressed that to generate a grounded theory, the basic problem must emerge from the data—it must be discovered. The theory is, from the very start, grounded in the data, rather than starting with a preconceived problem. Strauss and Corbin, however, stated that the research itself is only one of four possible sources of a research problem. Research problems can, for example, come from the literature or a researcher's personal and professional experience. In the newest edition of their text, Corbin and Strauss (2008) defined grounded theory in a more general way. They stated that it "is used in a more generic sense to denote theoretical constructs derived from qualitative analysis of data" (p. 1).

The Corbin and Strauss method involves two types of coding: open and axial coding. In **open coding**, data are broken down into parts and concepts identified and their properties and dimensions are delineated. In **axial coding**, the analyst relates

TABLE 23.3	Comparison of Glaser's and Strauss/Corbin's Methods	
	GLASER	**STRAUSS & CORBIN**
Initial data analysis	Breaking down and conceptualizing data involves comparison of incident to incident so patterns emerge	Breaking down and conceptualizing data includes taking apart a single sentence, observation, and incident
Types of coding	Open, selective, theoretical	Open and axial
Connections between categories	18 coding families	Paradigm (conditions, interactions and emotions, and consequences) and the conditional/consequential matrix
Outcome	Emergent theory (discovery)	Conceptual description (verification)

concepts to each other. The *paradigm* is used as an analytic strategy to help integrate structure and process. The basic components of the paradigm include conditions, interactions and emotions, and consequences. Corbin and Strauss suggested the conditional/consequential matrix as an analytic strategy for considering the range of possible conditions and consequences that can enter into the context.

The first step in integrating the findings is to decide on the **central category** (sometimes called the *core category*), which is the main theme of the research. Recommended techniques to facilitate identifying the central category are writing the storyline, using diagrams, and reviewing and organizing memos. The outcome of the Strauss and Corbin approach is, as Glaser (1992) termed it, a full conceptual description. The original grounded theory method (Glaser & Strauss, 1967), by contrast, generates a theory that explains how a basic social problem that emerged from the data is processed in a social setting.

Example of Strauss and Corbin grounded theory analysis: Huang and colleagues (2009) studied processes in hospital-based home care for people with severe mental illness in Taiwan. Their data, which were collected through interviews with clients, family members, and healthcare professionals, were analyzed using Strauss and Corbin methods: "Data analysis consisted of three stages, open, axial, and selective coding. The first stage involved open coding and the development of substantive codes from a line-by-line examination of the data. Words, groups of words, or phrases were then categorized under a conceptual label. Subsequently, the categories and subcategories were connected according to their properties and dimensions in the axial coding process. This was done through a paradigm model, which included causal connections, context, intervening conditions, action/interaction strategies and consequences" (p. 2960).

Constructivist Grounded Theory Approach

The constructivist approach to grounded theory is not dissimilar to a Glaserian approach. According to Charmaz (2006), in constructivist grounded theory the "coding generates the bones of your analysis. Theoretical integration will assemble these

bones into a working skeleton" (p. 45). Charmaz offered guidelines for types of coding: word-by-word coding, line-by-line coding, and coding incident to incident.

Charmaz distinguished *initial coding* and *focused coding*. In initial coding, the pieces of data, such as words, lines, segments, and incidents, are studied so the researcher begins to learn what the participants view as problematic. In focused coding, the analysis is directed towards using the most significant codes from the initial coding. Decisions are made by the researcher on which codes are most important for further analysis, which are then theoretically coded.

Analysis of Focus Group Data

Focus group interviews yield rich and complex data that pose special analytic challenges. Indeed, there is little consensus about analyzing data from focus groups, despite their widespread use.

Focus group interviews are especially difficult to transcribe, partly because of technical problems. For example, it is difficult to place microphones so that the voices of all group members are picked up with equal clarity, particularly because participants tend to speak at different volumes. An additional issue is the inevitability that several participants will speak at once, making it impossible for transcriptionists to discern everything being said.

TIP: Scott and colleagues (2009) suggested that an alternative to postinterview transcription of focus group sessions is to use a court reporter. In their work, they found that use of court reporters resulted in increased accuracy, time savings, and less distraction for the moderators.

A controversial issue in the analysis of focus group data is whether the unit of analysis is the group or individual participants. Some writers (e.g., Morrison-Beedy et al., 2001) maintain that the group is the proper unit of analysis. Analysis of group-level data involves a scrutiny of themes, interactions, and sequences within and between groups. Others, however (e.g., Carey & Smith,

1994; Kidd & Parshall, 2000), have argued that analysis should occur at both the group and individual level. Those who insist on only group-level analysis argue that what individuals say in focus groups cannot be treated as personal disclosures because they are inevitably influenced by the dynamics of the group. However, even in personal interviews, individual responses are shaped by social processes, and analysis of individual-level data (independent of group) is thought by some analysts to add important insights.

Carey and Smith (1994) advocated a third level of analysis—namely, the analysis of individual responses *in relation* to group context (e.g., whether a participant's view is in accord with or in contrast to majority opinion). Duggleby (2005) observed that two methods for analyzing focus group interaction data have been suggested—first, describing interactions as a means of interpreting the findings, and second, incorporating the group interaction data directly into the transcripts. She proposed a third alternative: a *congruent methodologic approach* that analyzes interaction data in the same manner as group or individual data.

For those who wish to analyze data from individual participants, it is essential to maintain information about what each person said—a task that is not possible if researchers rely solely on audiotapes. Videotapes, as supplements to audiotapes, are sometimes used to identify who said what in focus group sessions. More frequently, however, researchers have members of the research team in attendance at the sessions, and their job is to take detailed field notes about the order of speakers and about significant nonverbal behavior, such as pounding or clenching of fists, crying, aggressive body language, and so on.

Transcription quality is especially important in focus group interviews: Emotional content as well as words must be faithfully recorded because participants are responding not only to the questions being posed, but also to the experience of being in a group. Field notes, debriefing notes, and verbatim transcripts ideally must be integrated to yield a comprehensive transcript for analysis.

Example of integrating focus group data:
Morrison-Beedy and colleagues (2001) provided several examples of integrating data across sources from their focus group research. For example, one verbatim quote was, "It was no big deal." This was supplemented with data from the field notes that the woman's eyes were cast downward as she said this, and that the words were delivered sarcastically. The complete transcript for this entry, which included researcher interpretation in brackets, was as follows: "'It was no big deal.' (said sarcastically, with eyes looking downward). [It really was a very big deal to her, but others had not acknowledged that.]" (p. 52).

Because of group dynamics, focus group analysts must be sensitive to both the thematic content of these interviews, and also to how, when, and why themes are developed. Some of the issues that could be central to focus group analysis are the following:

- Does an issue raised in a focus group constitute a *theme* or merely a strongly held viewpoint of one or two members?
- Do the same issues or themes arise in more than one group?
- If there are group differences, why might this be the case—were participants different in characteristics and experiences, or did group processes affect the discussions?
- Are some issues sufficiently salient that not only are they discussed in response to specific questions posed by the moderator, but also spontaneously emerge at multiple points in the session?
- Do group members find certain issues both interesting *and* important?

Some focus group analysts, such as Kidd and Parshall (2000), use quantitative methods as adjuncts to their qualitative analysis. Using qualitative analysis software, they conduct such analyses as assessing similarities and differences between groups, determining coding frequencies to aid pattern detection, examining codes in relation to participant characteristics, and examining how much dialogue individual members contributed. They use such methods not so that interpretation can be based on frequencies, but so that they can better understand context and identify issues that require further critical scrutiny and interpretation.

Also, **sociograms** can be used to understand the flow of conversation as it goes around the members of the focus group. In a sociogram, the structure of interpersonal relations in a focus group is plotted on a chart. Weighted arrows can illustrate the number of times the conversation goes from one person to another (Drahota & Dewey, 2008).

➲ **TIP:** Focus group data are sometimes analyzed according to the procedures of a formal research tradition, such as grounded theory.

INTERPRETATION OF QUALITATIVE FINDINGS

Interpretation and analysis of qualitative data occur virtually simultaneously, in an iterative process. That is, researchers interpret the data as they read and re-read them, categorize and code them, inductively develop a thematic analysis, and integrate the themes into a unified whole.

It is difficult to provide guidance about the process of interpretation in qualitative studies, but there is considerable agreement that the ability to "make meaning" from qualitative texts depends on researchers' immersion in and closeness to the data. **Incubation** is the process of *living* the data, a process in which researchers must try to understand their meanings, find their essential patterns, and draw legitimate, insightful conclusions. Another key ingredient in interpretation and meaning making is researchers' self-awareness and the ability to reflect on their own world view and perspectives—that is, reflexivity.

Creativity also plays an important role in uncovering meaning in the data. Chandler, in writing about the transition from *saturation* to *illumination* wrote that, "Strategies for creativity take time and require incubation for new ideas to percolate. Insight into the incubation of data is critical to the

final theoretical revelations" (Chandler in Hunter, et al., 2002, p. 396). Thus, researchers need to give themselves sufficient time to achieve the *aha* that comes with making meaning beyond the facts.

Efforts to validate the analysis are necessarily efforts to validate interpretations as well. Prudent qualitative researchers hold their interpretations up for closer scrutiny—self-scrutiny as well as review by peers and outside reviewers. For both qualitative and quantitative researchers, it is important to consider possible alternative explanations or meanings.

Example of seeking alternative explanations: James and colleagues (2009) studied family carers' experiences of hospital encounters between informal and professional care at the end of life. Their hermeneutic study followed Gadamer's analytic approach to identifying meanings and patterns in the data as a continuous movement between the whole and the parts. The researchers noted that "preliminary interpretations were called into question using counterarguments based on different theories" (p. 260).

In drawing conclusions, qualitative researchers are increasingly considering the transferability of the findings, and the potential uses to which the qualitative evidence can be put. Like quantitative researchers, qualitative researchers need to give thought to the implications of their study findings for future research and for nursing practice.

CRITIQUING QUALITATIVE ANALYSIS

Evaluating a qualitative analysis in a report is not easy to do, even for experienced researchers. The main problem is that readers do not have access to the information they would need to determine whether researchers exercised good judgment and critical insight in coding the narrative materials, developing a thematic analysis, and integrating materials into a meaningful whole. Researchers are seldom able to include more than a handful of examples of actual data in a journal article. Moreover, the process they used to abstract meaning from the data is difficult to describe and illustrate.

In a critique of qualitative analysis, a primary task usually is assessing whether researchers took sufficient steps to validate inferences and conclusions. A major focus of a critique, then, is whether the researchers adequately documented the analytic process. The report should provide information about the approach used to analyze the data. For example, a report for a grounded theory study should indicate whether the researchers used the Glaser and Strauss, Strauss and Corbin, or constructivist method.

Critiquing analytic decisions is substantially less clear-cut in a qualitative than in a quantitative study. For example, it would be inappropriate to critique a phenomenological analysis for following Giorgi's approach rather than Colaizzi's approach. Both are respected methods of conducting a phenomenological study—although phenomenologists themselves may have cogent reasons for preferring one approach over the other.

One aspect of a qualitative analysis that *can* be critiqued, however, is whether the researchers documented that they have used one approach consistently and have been faithful to the integrity of its procedures. Thus, for example, if researchers say they are using the Glaser and Strauss approach to grounded theory analysis, they should not also include elements from the Strauss and Corbin method. An even more serious problem occurs when, as sometimes happens, the researchers "muddle" traditions. For example, researchers who describe their study as a grounded theory study should not present *themes,* because grounded theory analysis does not yield themes. Furthermore, researchers who attempt to blend elements from two traditions may not have a clear grasp of the analytic precepts of either one. For example, a researcher who claims to have undertaken an ethnography using a grounded theory approach to analysis may not be well informed about the underlying goals and philosophies of these two traditions.

Some further guidelines that may be helpful in evaluating qualitative analyses are presented in Box 23.3. ✖

BOX 23.3 Guidelines for Critiquing Qualitative Analyses and Interpretations

1. Was the data analysis approach appropriate for the research design and nature of the data?
2. Is the category scheme described? If so, does the scheme appear logical and complete? Does there seem to be unnecessary overlap or redundancy in the categories?
3. Were manual methods used to index and organize the data, or was a computer program used?
4. Does the report adequately describe the process by which the actual analysis was performed? Does the report indicate whose approach to data analysis was used (e.g., Glaserian or Straussian or constructivist, in grounded theory studies)? Was this method consistently and appropriately applied?
5. What major themes or processes emerged? If excerpts from the data are provided, do the themes appear to capture the meaning of the narratives—that is, does it appear that the researcher adequately interpreted the data and conceptualized the themes or categories? Is the analysis parsimonious—could two or more themes be collapsed into a broader and perhaps more useful conceptualization?
6. What evidence does the report provide that the analysis is accurate and appropriate? Were data displayed in a manner that allows you to verify the researcher's conclusions?
7. Was a conceptual map, model, or diagram effectively displayed to communicate important processes?
8. Was a metaphor used to communicate key elements of the analysis? Did the metaphor offer an insightful view of the findings, or did it seem contrived?
9. Was the context of the phenomenon adequately described? Does the report give you a clear picture of the social or emotional world of study participants?
10. Did the analysis yield a meaningful and insightful picture of the phenomenon under study? Is the resulting theory or description trivial or obvious?

RESEARCH EXAMPLES

We have illustrated different analytic approaches through examples of studies throughout this chapter. Here, we present more detailed descriptions of two qualitative nursing studies.

Example of a Phenomenological Analysis

Study: The arm: There is no escaping the reality for mothers of children with obstetric brachial plexus injuries. (Beck, 2009). (This study appears in its entirety in Appendix E of the accompanying *Resource Manual*).

Statement of Purpose: The purpose of this study was to investigate mothers' experiences caring for their children who have an obstetric brachial plexus injury.

Method: Twenty-three mothers participated in this phenomenological study. Twelve women were interviewed in person and 11 mothers participated over the Internet. Each woman was asked to describe in as much detail as she wished her experiences caring for her child with an obstetric brachial plexus injury. All women were recruited through the United Brachial Plexus Network. Data were saturated before the final sample size of 23 mothers was attained.

Analysis: Transcripts of the 12 audiotaped face-to-face interviews were double checked for accuracy. Data were analyzed (manually) according to the steps described by Colaizzi (see Figure 23.2). (Beck also created several daily timelines that highlighted the demanding schedules of the study participants.) The first of Colaizzi's steps involved reading and re-reading each description provided by the mothers. In the next step, 252 significant statements were extracted. (*Significant statements* are phrases or sentences that are directly related to the experience being described). Next, meanings were formulated for each significant statement. All the formulated meanings were then clustered into repetitive patterns (themes). An exhaustive description of the results was written and condensed into a statement of the fundamental structure of mothers' experiences of caring for their children with obstetric brachial plexus injuries. Throughout data analysis, Beck continually referred back to her field notes to make sure she was remaining faithful to the mothers' descriptions. She also compared data obtained through Internet interviews with those from in-person interviews to assess whether they were providing a consistent picture of the mothers' experiences. Two participants were asked to review the study findings, and both agreed that the results captured their experiences.

Key Findings: Mothers' descriptions of their experiences caring for a child with an obstetric brachial plexus injury were categorized into 6 themes: (1) In an instant: Dreams shattered; (2) The arm: No escaping the reality; (3) Tormented: Agonizing worries and questions; (4) Therapy and surgeries: Consuming mothers' lives; (5) Anger: Simmering pot inside; and (6) So much to bear: Enduring heartbreak.

Example of a Grounded Theory Analysis

Study: The hope experience of older bereaved women who care for a spouse with terminal cancer (Holtslander & Duggleby, 2009)

Statement of Purpose: The purpose of this study was to explore the experience and processes of hope in older women who were bereaved after caring for a spouse with terminal cancer, and to develop a tenatative, emerging theory of their hope experiences.

Method: This study used constructivist grounded theory methods. The researchers conducted 30 in-depth, audiotaped interviews with a demographically diverse sample of 13 Canadian women, aged 60 or older, within the first year of their bereavement. Purposive and theoretical sampling was used to reach saturation. All but one participant was interviewed on two or more occasions. Interview questions were formulated to give the women opportunities to discuss their insights about hope. For example, two such questions were: What does hope mean for you right now? And, Have you noticed any changes in your hope? Also, each participant was asked to write in a diary over a 2-week period, guided by such questions as, "What did hope feel like or look like today?" Twelve women completed the diaries. Field notes were maintained regarding the setting and environment of the interviews, and memoing was used throughout to preserve ideas.

Analysis: Data management was handled using the NUD*IST software. Data were analyzed after each interview, using Charmaz's methods for initial, focused, and theoretical coding. Data were coded line by line, and categories and patterns of behavior were extracted using the participants' own words (in vivo coding) to ensure that findings were grounded in the data. During focused coding, the most frequent or significant codes were sorted, synthesized, and integrated. Constant comparison was used to develop and refine the focused codes. Theoretical coding involved specifying the relationships between the categories and concepts. The researchers integrated the focused codes into a coherent emerging theory of the bereaved palliative caregiver's experience of hope. The report provided a useful figure showing an example of the coding process. The figure illustrated how the researchers moved from the transcripts (e.g., "I hope I have a better day tomorrow"), to "incidents" (e.g., "Hope for tomorrow"), to categories (Losing hope, searching for hope), and finally to the overarching concept of searching for new hope.

Key Findings: The bereaved women defined hope as a gradual process of regaining inner strength. Their main, recurring concern was losing hope. The basic social process that the women used to deal with their concern was *searching for new hope* through such processes as finding balance, new perspectives, and new meaning and purpose. The researchers included a useful table that presented interview excerpts supporting their definition and conceptualized processes of hope, and a conceptual map displaying interrelationships in the basic social process of searching for new hope.

SUMMARY POINTS

- Qualitative analysis is a challenging, labor-intensive activity with few standardized rules.
- The first major step in analyzing qualitative data is to organize and index materials for easy retrieval, typically by coding the content of the data according to a category scheme.
- Traditionally, researchers organized their data by developing **conceptual files**—physical files in which coded excerpts of data relevant to specific categories are placed. Computer programs are now widely used to perform indexing functions and to facilitate analysis.
- The actual analysis of data usually begins with a search for categories or **themes**, which involves the discovery not only of commonalities across

participants, but also of natural variation and patterns in the data. Some qualitative analysts use **metaphors** or figurative comparisons to evoke a visual and symbolic analogy.

- The next analytic step often involves validating the thematic analysis. Some researchers use **quasi-statistics**, which involves a tabulation of the frequency with which certain themes or relations are supported by the data.
- In a final analytic step, analysts weave thematic strands together into an integrated picture of the phenomenon under investigation.
- Researchers whose focus is qualitative description may say that they used **qualitative content analysis** as their analytic method.
- In ethnographies, analysis begins as the researcher enters the field. Ethnographers continually search for *patterns* in the behavior and expressions of study participants.
- One approach to analyzing ethnographic data is Spradley's method, which involves four levels of data analysis: **domain analysis** (identifying *domains*, or units of cultural knowledge), **taxonomic analysis** (selecting key domains and constructing **taxonomies** or systems of classification), **componential analysis** (comparing and contrasting terms in a domain), and a **theme analysis** (uncovering cultural themes).
- Leininger's ethnonursing method involves four phases: collecting and recording data, categorizing descriptors, searching for repetitive patterns, and abstracting major themes.
- There are numerous approaches to phenomenological analysis, including the descriptive methods of Colaizzi, Giorgi, and Van Kaam, in which the goal is to find common patterns of experiences shared by particular instances.
- In Van Manen's approach, which involves efforts to grasp the essential meaning of the experience being studied, researchers search for themes, using either a **holistic approach** (viewing text as a whole), **selective approach** (pulling out key statements and phrases), or **detailed approach** (analyzing every sentence).
- Central to analyzing data in a hermeneutic study is the notion of the **hermeneutic circle**, which

signifies a methodologic process in which there is continual movement between the parts and the whole of the text under analysis.

- Hermeneutics has several choices for data analysis. Diekelmann's team approach calls for the discovery of a **constitutive pattern** that expresses the relationships among themes. Benner's approach consists of three processes: searching for **paradigm cases**, thematic analysis, and analysis of *exemplars.*

- Grounded theory uses the **constant comparative** method of data analysis, which involves identifying characteristics in one piece of data and comparing them with those of others to assess similarity. Developing categories in a substantive theory must **fit** the data and not be forced.

- One approach to grounded theory is the Glaser and Strauss (Glaserian) method, in which there are two broad types of codes: **substantive codes** (in which the empirical substance of the topic is conceptualized) and **theoretical codes** (in which relationships among the substantive codes are conceptualized).

- Substantive coding involves **open coding** to capture what is going on in the data and then **selective coding**, in which only variables relating to a core category are coded. The **core category**, a behavior pattern that has relevance for participants, is sometimes a **basic social process (BSP)** that involves an evolving process of coping or adaptation.

- In the Glaser and Strauss method, open codes begin with **level I (in vivo) codes**, which are collapsed into a higher level of abstraction in **level II codes**. Level II codes are then used to formulate **level III codes**, which are theoretical constructs.

- Through constant comparison, the researcher compares concepts emerging from the data with similar concepts from existing theory or research to determine which parts have **emergent fit** with the theory being generated.

- Strauss and Corbin's method is an alternative grounded theory method whose outcome is a full preconceived conceptual description. This approach to grounded theory analysis involves two types of coding: open (in which categories are generated) and **axial coding** (where categories are linked with subcategories and integrated).

- A controversy in the analysis of focus group data is whether the unit of analysis is the group or individual participants—some analysts examine the data at both levels. A third analytic option is the analysis of group interactions.

STUDY ACTIVITIES

Chapter 23 of the *Resource Manual for Nursing Research*: *Generating and Assessing Evidence for Nursing Practice*, *9th edition*, offers exercises and study suggestions for reinforcing concepts presented in this chapter. In addition, the following study questions can be addressed:

1. Read a qualitative nursing study. If a different investigator had gone into the field to study the same problem, how likely is it that the conclusions would have been the same? How transferable are the researcher's findings? What did the researcher learn that he or she would probably not have learned with a more structured and quantified approach?

2. Apply relevant questions in Box 23.3 to one of the two research examples at the end of the chapter, referring to the full journal article as necessary.

STUDIES CITED IN CHAPTER 23

Aga, F., Kylma, J., & Nikkonen, M. (2009). The conceptions of care among family caregivers of persons living with HIV/AIDS in Addis Ababa, Ethiopia. *Journal of Transcultural Nursing, 20*, 37–50.

Beck, C. T. (2002). Releasing the pause button: Mothering twins during the first year of life. *Qualitative Health Research, 12*, 593–608.

Beck, C. T. (2005). Benefits of participating in Internet interviews: Women helping women. *Qualitative Health Research, 15*, 411–422.

Beck, C. T. (2006). Anniversary of birth trauma: Failure to rescue. *Nursing Research*, 55, 381–390.

Beck, C. T. (2009). The arm: There is no escaping the reality for mothers of children with obstetric brachial plexus injuries. *Nursing Research, 58*, 237–245.

Beck, C. T., & Watson, S. (2008). Impact of birth trauma on breast-feeding: A tale of two pathways. *Nursing Research, 57*, 228–236.

Fraser, K., Estàbrooks, C., Allen, M., & Strang, V. (2009). Factors that influence case managers' resource allocation decisions in pediatric home care: An ethnographic study. *International Journal of Nursing Studies, 46*, 337–349.

Hawkins, Y., Ussher, J., Gilbert, E., Perz, J., Sandoval, M., & Sundquist, K. (2009). Changes in sexuality and intimacy after the diagnosis and treatment of cancer. *Cancer Nursing, 32*, 271–280.

Holtslander, L., & Duggleby, W. (2009). The hope experience of older bereaved women who cared for a spouse with terminal cancer. *Qualitative Health Research, 19*, 388–400.

Huang, X., Lin, M., Yang, T., & Sun, F. (2009). Hospital-based home care for people with severe mental illness in Taiwan: A substantive grounded theory. *Journal of Clinical Nursing, 18*, 2956–2968.

James, I., Andershed, B., & Ternestedt, B. (2009). The encounter between informal and professional care at the end of life. *Qualitative Health Research, 19*, 258–271.

Jessup, M., & Parkinson, C. (2010). "All at sea": The experience of living with cystic fibrosis. *Qualitative Health Research, 20*, 352–364.

Logsdon, M., & Hines-Martin, V. (2009). Barriers to depression treatment in low-income, unmarried, adolescent mothers in a Southern, urban area of the United States. *Issues in Mental Health Nursing, 30*, 451–455.

Morrison-Beedy, D., Côté-Arsenault, D., & Feinstein, N. (2001). Maximizing results with focus groups. *Applied Nursing Research, 14*, 48–53.

Nordfjaern, T., Rundmo, T., & Hole, R. (2010). Treatment and recovery as perceived by patients with substance addiction. *Journal of Psychiatric and Mental Health Nursing, 17*, 46–64.

Perry, C., Rosenfeld, A., Kendall, J. (2008). Rural women walking for health. *Western Journal of Nursing Research, 30*, 295–316.

Ryde, K., Strang, P., & Friedrichsen, M. (2008). Crying in solitude or with someone for support and consultation: Experiences from family members in palliative home care. *Cancer Nursing, 31*, 345–353.

Strang, V., Koop, P., Dupuis-Blanchard, S., Nordstrom, M., & Thompson, B. (2006). Family caregivers and transition to long-term care. *Clinical Nursing Research, 15*, 27–45.

Tzeng, W., Su, P., Chiang, H., Kuan, P., & Lee, J. (2010). A qualitative study of suicide survivors in Taiwan. *Western Journal of Nursing Research, 32*, 185–198.

Wuest, J. (2000). Negotiating with helping systems: An example of grounded theory evolving through emergent fit. *Qualitative Health Research, 10*, 51–70.

Yousefi, H., Abedi, H. A., Yarmohammadian, M. H., & Elliott, D. (2009). Comfort as a basic need in hospitalized patients in Iran: A hermeneutic phenomenology study. *Journal of Advanced Nursing, 65*, 1891–1898.

Methodologic and nonresearch references cited in this chapter can be found in a separate section at the end of the book.

24

Trustworthiness and Integrity in Qualitative Research

I ntegrity in qualitative research is an all-encompassing issue that begins as questions are formulated and continues through writing the report. The issues discussed in this chapter are critical for those learning to do qualitative research.

PERSPECTIVES ON QUALITY IN QUALITATIVE RESEARCH

Qualitative researchers agree on the importance of doing high-quality research, yet few issues in qualitative inquiry have generated more controversy than efforts to define what is meant by "high-quality." It is beyond the scope of this book to describe the debate in detail, but we provide an overview to help you identify a position that is compatible with your philosophical and methodologic views.

Debates about Rigor and Validity

One contentious issue in the debate about quality concerns the use of terms such as *rigor* and *validity*. These terms are shunned by some because of their association with the positivist paradigm—they are seen as inappropriate goals for research conducted in the constructivist or critical paradigms. Those

who advocate different criteria and terms for evaluating quality in qualitative research argue that the issues at stake in the various paradigms are fundamentally different in terms of philosophical underpinnings and goals and, therefore, require different terminology. For these critics, the concept of rigor does not fit into an interpretive approach that values insight and creativity (e.g., Denzin & Lincoln, 2000). As Sandelowski (1993a) put it, "We can preserve or kill the spirit of qualitative work; we can soften our notion of rigor to include the . . . soulfulness (and) imagination . . . we associate with more artistic endeavors, or we can further harden it by the uncritical application of rules. The choice is ours: rigor or rigor mortis" (p. 8).

Others defend using the term *validity*. Whittemore and colleagues (2001), for example, argued that validity is an appropriate term in all paradigms, noting that the dictionary definition of validity (the quality of being sound, just, and well-founded) lends itself equally to qualitative and quantitative research. Morse and colleagues (2002) posited that "the broad and abstract concepts of reliability and validity can be applied to all research because the goal of finding plausible and credible outcome explanations is central to all research" (p. 3). Another, more pragmatic, argument favoring the use of "mainstream" terms like validity and rigor is precisely that they *are* mainstream. In a world dominated by quantitative researchers whose quality criteria are used to make funding decisions, it may be useful to use recognizable and widely accepted terms and criteria.

Sparkes (2001) contended that the debate over validity is not a simple dichotomy and suggested that there are four possible perspectives on the issue. The first, which he called the *replication perspective*, is that validity is an appropriate criterion for assessing quality in both qualitative and quantitative studies, although qualitative researchers use different procedures to achieve it. Those who adopt a *parallel perspective* maintain that a separate set of evaluative criteria needs to be developed for qualitative inquiry. This perspective resulted in the development of standards for the **trustworthiness** of qualitative research that parallel the standards of reliability and validity in quantitative research (Lincoln & Guba, 1985). The third perspective in Sparke's typology is the *diversification of meanings perspective*, which is characterized by efforts to establish new forms of validity that do not have reference points in traditional quantitative research. As one example, Lather (1986) discussed *catalytic validity* in connection with critical and feminist research as the degree to which the research process energized study participants and altered their consciousness. The final perspective in Sparke's typology was what he called the *letting-go-of-validity perspective*, which involves a total abandonment of the concept of validity. Wolcott (1994), an ethnographer, represented this perspective in his discussion of the absurdity of validity. Yet, as Wolcott (1995) himself noted, validity can be dismissed, but the issue itself will not go away: "Qualitative researchers need to understand what the debate is about and *have* a position; they do not have to resolve the issue itself" (p. 170).

Generic versus Specific Standards

Another issue in the controversy about quality criteria for qualitative inquiry concerns whether there should be a generic set of standards, or whether specific standards are needed for different types of study—for example, for ethnographers and grounded theory researchers. Many writers have endorsed the notion that research conducted within different traditions must attend to different concerns, and that techniques for enhancing and demonstrating research integrity vary. Watson and Girard (2004), for example, proposed that quality standards must be "congruent with the philosophical underpinnings supporting the research tradition endorsed" (p. 875). Many writers have offered standards for specific forms of qualitative inquiry, such as grounded theory (Chiovitti & Piran, 2003), phenomenology and hermeneutics (Whitehead, 2004), ethnography (Hammersley, 1992; LeCompte & Goetz, 1982), descriptive qualitative research (Milne & Oberle, 2005), and critical research (Lather, 1986).

Some writers believe, however, that some quality criteria are fairly universal within the constructivist paradigm. In their synthesis of criteria for developing evidence of validity in qualitative studies, Whittemore and colleagues (2001) proposed four primary criteria that they viewed as essential to all qualitative inquiry.

Standards for Conduct versus Assessment of Qualitative Research

Yet another issue concerns whose point of view is being considered in the quality standards. Morse and colleagues (2002) contended that many of the established standards are relevant for *assessment* by readers rather than as guides to conducting high-quality qualitative research. They believe that Lincoln and Guba's criteria—often considered the gold standard—are best described as *post hoc* tools that reviewers can use to evaluate trustworthiness of a completed study: "While strategies of trustworthiness may be useful in attempting to *evaluate* rigor, they do not in themselves *ensure* rigor" (p. 9).

As an example of how the viewpoint of evaluators has been given prominence, one suggested indicator of integrity is **researcher credibility**—that is, the faith that can be put in the researcher (Patton, 1999, 2002). While such an indicator might affect readers' confidence in the integrity of the inquiry, it clearly is not a *strategy* that researchers can adopt to make their study more rigorous.

Morse and colleagues (2002) have emphasized the importance of verification strategies that researchers can use throughout the inquiry "so that reliability and validity are actively attained, rather than proclaimed by external reviewers on the completion of the project" (p. 9). In their view, responsibility for ensuring rigor should rest with researchers, not with external judges. They advocated a proactive stance involving self-scrutiny and verification. Morse (2006) noted that "good qualitative inquiry must be verified reflexively in each step of the analysis. This means that it is self-correcting" (p. 6).

From the point of view of qualitative researchers, the ongoing question must be: How can I be confident that my account is an accurate and insightful representation? From the point of view of a critical reader, the question is: How can I trust that the researcher has offered an accurate and insightful representation? The evidence and strategies needed for answering these questions overlap, but are not identical.

Terminology Proliferation and Confusion

The result of all these controversies is that there is no common vocabulary for quality criteria in qualitative research—or, for that matter, for quality goals. Terms such as *goodness, integrity, truth value, rigor,* and *trustworthiness* abound, and for each proposed descriptor, several critics refute the term as an appropriate name for an overall goal.

Establishing a consensus on what the quality criteria for qualitative inquiry should be, and what they should be named, remains elusive, and it is unlikely that a consensus will be achieved in the near future, if ever. Some feel that the ongoing debate is healthy, but others feel that "the situation is confusing and has resulted in a deteriorating ability to actually discern rigor" (Morse et al., 2002, p. 5). Given the lack of consensus, and the heated arguments supporting and contesting various frameworks, it is difficult to provide guidance about how qualitative researchers should proceed. We present information about *criteria* from two frameworks in

the section that follows, and then describe *strategies* for diminishing threats to integrity in qualitative research. We recommend that these frameworks and strategies be viewed as points of departure for explorations on how to make a qualitative study as rigorous/ trustworthy/insightful/valid as possible.

FRAMEWORKS OF QUALITY CRITERIA

Although not without critics, the quality criteria most often cited by qualitative researchers are those proposed by Lincoln and Guba (1985), and later augmented by Guba and Lincoln (1994). A second framework is a synthesis of 10 quality guidelines, as proposed by Whittemore and colleagues (2001).

In thinking about criteria for qualitative inquiry, attention needs to be paid to both "art" and "science" and to interpretation and description. Creativity and insightfulness need to be encouraged and sustained, but not at the expense of scientific excellence. And the quest for rigor cannot sacrifice inspiration and elegant abstractions, or else the results are likely to be "perfectly healthy but dead" (Morse, 2006, p. 6). Good qualitative work is both descriptively sound and explicit, and interpretively rich and innovative.

Lincoln and Guba's Framework

Lincoln and Guba (1985) suggested four criteria for developing the *trustworthiness* of a qualitative inquiry: credibility, dependability, confirmability, and transferability. These four criteria represent parallels to the positivists' criteria of internal validity, reliability, objectivity, and external validity, respectively. This framework provided the initial platform upon which much of the current controversy on rigor emerged. Responding to numerous criticisms and to their own evolving conceptualizations, a fifth criterion that is more distinctively within the constructivist paradigm was added: authenticity (Guba & Lincoln, 1994).

Credibility

Credibility is viewed by Lincoln and Guba as an overriding goal of qualitative research and is a criterion identified in several of the frameworks mentioned in the Whittemore and colleagues (2001) review. **Credibility** refers to confidence in the truth of the data and interpretations of them. Qualitative researchers must strive to establish confidence in the truth of the findings for the particular participants and contexts in the research. Lincoln and Guba pointed out that credibility involves two aspects: first, carrying out the study in a way that enhances the believability of the findings, and second, taking steps to *demonstrate* credibility in research reports.

Dependability

The second criterion in the Lincoln–Guba framework is **dependability**, which refers to the stability (reliability) of data over time and conditions. The dependability question is: Would the findings of an inquiry be repeated if it were replicated with the same (or similar) participants in the same (or similar) context? Credibility cannot be attained in the absence of dependability, just as validity in quantitative research cannot be achieved in the absence of reliability.

Confirmability

Confirmability refers to objectivity, that is, the potential for congruence between two or more independent people about the data's accuracy, relevance, or meaning. This criterion is concerned with establishing that the data represent the information participants provided, and that the interpretations of those data are not invented by the inquirer. For this criterion to be achieved, findings must reflect the participants' voice and the conditions of the inquiry, not the researcher's biases, motivations, or perspectives.

Transferability

Transferability refers to the potential for extrapolation, that is, the extent to which findings can be transferred to or have applicability in other settings or groups (See Chapter 21). As Lincoln and Guba noted, the investigator's responsibility is to provide sufficient descriptive data so that consumers can evaluate the applicability of the data to other contexts: "Thus the naturalist cannot specify the external validity of an inquiry; he or she can provide only the thick description necessary to enable someone interested in making a transfer to reach a conclusion about whether transfer can be contemplated as a possibility" (p. 316).

> **TIP:** You may run across the term *fittingness*, a term Guba and Lincoln used earlier to refer to the degree to which research findings have meaning to others in similar situations. In later work, however, they used the term *transferability*. Similarly, in their initial discussions of quality criteria, they used the term *auditability*, a concept that was later refined and called *dependability*.

Authenticity

Authenticity refers to the extent to which researchers fairly and faithfully show a range of realities. Authenticity emerges in a report when it conveys the feeling tone of participants' lives as they are lived. A text has authenticity if it invites readers into a vicarious experience of the lives being described, and enables readers to develop a heightened sensitivity to the issues being depicted. When a text achieves authenticity, readers are better able to understand the lives being portrayed "in the round," with some sense of the mood, feeling, experience, language, and context of those lives.

Whittemore and Colleagues' Framework

Whittemore and colleagues (2001), in their synthesis of quality criteria from 10 prominent systems (including that of Lincoln and Guba), used the term *validity* as the overarching goal. In their view, four primary criteria are essential to all qualitative inquiry, whereas six secondary criteria provide supplementary benchmarks of validity and are not relevant to every study. Researchers must decide, based on the goals of their research, the optimal weight that should be given to each criterion.

The primary criteria include credibility, authenticity, criticality, and integrity. Six secondary criteria include explicitness, vividness, creativity, thoroughness, and congruence. Thus, the terminology overlaps with that of Lincoln and Guba's framework regarding two criteria (credibility and authenticity), and the other eight concepts either are not captured in the Lincoln and Guba framework or are nuanced variations.

Criticality refers to the researcher's critical appraisal of every decision made throughout the research process. **Integrity** is demonstrated by ongoing self-reflection and self-scrutiny to ensure that interpretations are valid and grounded in the data. Criticality and integrity are strongly interrelated and are sometimes considered jointly (e.g., Milne & Oberle, 2005).

In terms of secondary criteria, **explicitness** (similar to auditability) is the ability to follow the researcher's decisions and interpretive efforts by means of carefully maintained records and explicitly presented results. **Vividness** involves the presentation of rich, vivid, faithful, and artful descriptions that highlight salient themes in the data. **Creativity** reflects challenges to traditional ways of thinking, as demonstrated through innovative approaches to collecting, analyzing, and interpreting data. **Thoroughness** refers to adequacy of the data as a result of sound sampling and data collection decisions (saturation), as well as the full development of ideas. **Congruence** refers to interconnectedness between methods and question, between the current study and earlier ones, and between theory and approach; it also refers to connections between study findings and contexts outside the study situation. Finally, **sensitivity** is the degree to which the research was done in a manner that reflects respectful sensitivity to and concern for the people, groups, and communities being studied.

Table 24.1 presents these 10 criteria, together with two sets of questions. The first set is intended as a guide to researchers in their thinking about quality issues during the conduct of a study. The second set is questions that are relevant after a study is completed. Researchers can use these questions as a means of self-evaluation, and those who scrutinize a study can apply them to evaluate both the process and the product of qualitative inquiry.

◗ TIP: The questions in Table 24.1, formatted onto worksheets, are available in a Word document in the Toolkit section of the accompanying *Resource Manual*.

STRATEGIES TO ENHANCE QUALITY IN QUALITATIVE INQUIRY

The criteria for establishing integrity in a qualitative study are challenging, regardless of the names people attach to them. Various strategies have been proposed to address these challenges, and this section describes many of them.

Some quality-enhancement strategies are linked to a specific criterion—for example, documenting methodologic decisions is a strategy that addresses the *explicitness* criterion in the Whittemore and colleagues framework. Many strategies, however, simultaneously address multiple criteria. For this reason, we have not organized strategies according to quality criteria—for example, identifying strategies specifically to enhance *credibility*. Instead, we have organized strategies according to different phases of an inquiry, namely data generation, coding and analysis, and report preparation. This organization is imperfect, due to the nonlinear and iterative nature of research activities in qualitative studies, so we acknowledge upfront that some activities described under one aspect of a study are likely to have relevance under another.

Table 24.2 suggests how various quality-enhancement strategies map onto the criteria in the Lincoln and Guba framework and the Whittemore framework.

Quality-Enhancement Strategies in Generating Data

Several strategies that qualitative researchers use to enrich and strengthen their studies have been mentioned in previous chapters and will not be elaborated here. For example, intensive listening during an interview, careful probing to obtain rich and comprehensive data, and audiotaping interviews for transcription are all strategies to enhance data quality, as are methods to gain people's trust during fieldwork (Chapter 22). In this section, we focus on additional strategies used primarily during the collection of qualitative data.

TABLE 24.1	Primary and Secondary Qualitative Validity Criteria: Whittemore et al. Framework*	
CRITERIA	**QUESTIONS FOR SELF-SCRUTINY DURING A STUDY**	**QUESTIONS FOR POST-HOC ASSESSMENTS OF A STUDY**
Primary Criteria		
Credibility	What steps can I take to have confidence that participants' experiences and context are represented in a believable way? What verification procedures can I use?	Do the research results reflect participants' experiences and context in a believable way? Were adequate verification procedures used?
Authenticity	What efforts can I make to adequately represent the multiple realities and voices of those being studied?	Has the researcher adequately represented the multiple realities of those being studied? Has an emic perspective been portrayed?
Criticality	What procedures can I use to support critical self-reflection and critical thinking about key decisions during the research? How can I cultivate responsiveness to the data?	Is there evidence that the inquiry involved critical appraisal of key decisions and self-reflection? Does the report demonstrate the researcher's responsiveness to the data?
Integrity	Have I put in place adequate checks on the validity of my interpretations? Have I grounded my interpretations in the data?	Does the research reflect ongoing, repetitive checks on the many aspects of validity? Are the findings humbly presented?
Secondary Criteria		
Explicitness	Have I maintained adequate records documenting decisions and interpretive processes? Have I taken steps to expose my own biases or perspectives?	Have methodologic decisions been explained and justified? Have biases been identified? Is evidence presented in support of conclusions and interpretations?
Vividness	Have I faithfully used the data to provide a rich, evocative, and compelling description, without using excessive detail?	Have rich, evocative, and compelling descriptions been presented?
Creativity	Have I sufficiently stretched my imagination and creative powers to develop insightful interpretations?	Do the findings illuminate the phenomenon in an insightful and original way? Are new perspectives and rich imagination brought to bear on the inquiry?
Thoroughness	Have I been sufficiently thorough in ensuring sampling and data adequacy? Have I explored the full scope of the phenomenon and convincingly answered the research question?	Has sufficient attention been paid to sampling adequacy, information richness, data saturation, and contextual completeness?
Congruence	Have I taken adequate steps to promote logical, philosophical, theoretic, and methodologic congruency? Have I made it possible for readers to identify congruence with other settings?	Is there congruity between the questions and methods, the methods and participants, the data and categories? Do themes fit together coherently? Is there adequate information for determining transferability to other contexts?
Sensitivity	Have my methods and questions reflected an ethical and sensitive respect for study participants and the groups, communities, and cultures to which they belong?	Has the research been undertaken in a way that is sensitive to the cultural, social, and political contexts of those being studied?

*Criteria are from Whittemore and colleagues' (2001) synthesis of qualitative validity criteria. Questions reflect the thinking of Whittemore et al., and other sources.

TABLE 24.2 Quality-Enhancement Strategies in Relation to Quality Criteria for Qualitative Inquiry

STRATEGY	CRITERIA: GUBA & LINCOLN[a]			SHARED CRITERIA		CRITERIA: WHITTEMORE et al.[b]							
Throughout the Inquiry	Dep.	Conf.	Trans.	Cred.	Auth.	Crit.	Integ.	Explic.	Viv.	Creat.	Thor.	Congr.	Sens.
Reflexivity/reflexive journaling				X	X		X					X	
Careful documentation, decision trail	X	X				X	X	X					
Data Generation													
Prolonged engagement				X	X						X		X
Persistent observation				X	X		X				X		X
Comprehensive field notes			X	X			X		X		X		
Theoretically driven sampling				X									
Audiotaping & verbatim transcription				X	X			X	X				
Triangulation (data, method)	X			X							X	X	
Saturation of data			X	X							X		
Member checking	X			X		X							
Data Coding/Analysis													
Transcription rigor				X		X							
Inter-coder checks; development of a codebook			X		X		X						
Quasi-statistics				X		X							
Triangulation (investigator, theory, analysis)		X		X		X						X	
Search for confirming evidence		X	X	X		X						X	
Search for disconfirming evidence/negative case analysis				X		X	X				X		
Peer review/debriefing		X		X		X							
Inquiry audit	X	X		X		X	X	X				X	
Presentation of Findings													
Documentation of quality-enhancement efforts			X	X	X		X				X		
Thick, vivid description			X	X	X		X		X			X	X
Impactful, evocative writing					X				X	X			X
Disclosure of researcher credentials, background				X				X			X		
Documentation of reflexivity				X			X	X			X		

[a]The criteria from the Lincoln and Guba (1985, 1996) framework include dependability (Dep.), confirmability (Conf.), transferability (Trans.), credibility (Cred.), and authenticity (Auth.); the last two criteria are identical to two primary criteria in the Whittemore et al. (2001) framework.

[b]The criteria from the Whittemore et al. (2001) framework include, in addition to credibility and authenticity, criticality (Crit.), integrity (Integ.), explicitness (Expl.), vividness (Viv.), creativity (Creat.), thoroughness (Thor.), congruence (Congr.), and sensitivity (Sens.)

Prolonged Engagement and Persistent Observation

An important step in establishing credibility is **prolonged engagement** (Lincoln & Guba, 1985)—the investment of sufficient time collecting data to have an in-depth understanding of the people under study, to test for misinformation and distortions, and to ensure saturation of key categories. Prolonged engagement is also essential for building trust and rapport with informants, which in turn makes it more likely that rich, accurate information will be obtained. In planning a qualitative study, researchers must ensure that they have adequate time and resources to stay engaged in fieldwork for a sufficiently long period.

➲ **TIP:** Thorne and Darbyshire (2005) have pointed out that *premature closure* can be a problem in qualitative research. Without a commitment to prolonged engagement, researchers sometimes make an inappropriate claim of saturation simply because they have reached a convenient stopping point.

Example of prolonged engagement: Mottram (2009) conducted a grounded theory study of therapeutic relationships in day-surgery settings. She interviewed 145 patients and 100 carers in day-surgery units in two hospitals in the United Kindgom. Data were gathered over a 2-year period, which involved "prolonged involvement of the researcher" (p. 2832).

High-quality data collection in constructivist inquiries also involves **persistent observation**, which concerns the salience of the data being gathered and recorded. Persistent observation refers to the researchers' focus on the characteristics or aspects of a situation or a conversation that are relevant to the phenomena being studied. As Lincoln and Guba (1985) noted, "If prolonged engagement provides scope, persistent observation provides depth" (p. 304).

Example of persistent observation: Denny (2009) explored women's experiences of living with endometriosis. She used a storytelling approach to solicit rich narratives from her sample of 30 women, who were interviewed on two separate occasions over a 1-year period. Several women also made entries into a diary, which contained full, extensive accounts.

Reflexivity Strategies

As noted in Chapter 8, reflexivity involves attending systematically and continually to the context of knowledge construction—and, in particular, to the researcher's effect on the collection, analysis, and interpretation of data. Reflexivity involves awareness that the researcher as an individual brings to the inquiry a unique background, set of values, and a social and professional identity that can affect the research process.

The most widely used strategy for maintaining reflexivity and delimiting subjectivity is to maintain a reflexive journal or diary, which we discussed in Chapter 20 in connection with bracketing in phenomenological inquiry. Reflexive notes can be used to record, from the outset of the study and in an ongoing fashion, thoughts about the impact of previous life experiences and previous readings about the phenomenon on the inquiry. Through self-interrogation and reflection, researchers seek to be well positioned to probe deeply and to grasp the experience, process, or culture under study through the lens of participants. Some argue that systematic efforts like maintaining a journal are not merely a means of constraining subjectivity—recognition of one's own perspectives can be exploited as an interpretive advantage because ultimately findings are co-created by participants and respondents (Jootun et al., 2009).

Additional reflexive strategies can be used. For example, researchers sometimes begin a study by being interviewed themselves with regard to the phenomenon under study. Of course, this approach only makes sense if the researcher has had experience with that phenomenon.

Example of a self-interview: Zinsli and Smythe (2009) explored the experience of humanitarian disaster nursing. Participants were New Zealand nurses who had been on international relief/disaster missions. The researchers wrote that the lead researcher "has himself been on several Red Cross missions. He was interviewed by a colleague early in the study for the purpose of revealing his own experiences and prejudices" (p. 235).

Other researchers ask a colleague to conduct a "bracketing interview." In such an interview, a person who is knowledgeable about reflexivity and perhaps about the study phenomenon queries the researcher about his or her a priori assumptions and perspectives.

Example of a bracketing interview: Champlin (2009) studied caretaking relationships between informal caretakers and mentally ill persons. An academic nurse with a background in phenomenology interviewed Champlin, asking such questions as "How do you expect that the participants will describe their experiences?" and "What have patients' families said to you in the past that made you interested in this experience?" (p. 1527). The interview was audiotaped and analyzed, and revealed several assumptions and expectations.

Reflexivity is typically discussed as an individual activity, engaged in by researchers working "solo" on a project. Barry and colleagues (1999) have argued, however, that when researchers collaborate in a qualitative study, both individual and group reflexivity are needed. They suggested mechanisms to promote reflexivity in studies conducted by teams of researchers, and implementation of their suggestions has been described by Canadian nurse researchers (Hall et al., 2005).

Further guidance with regard to reflexivity is available in an article by Bradbury-Jones (2007) and in an edited volume of papers by Finlay and Gough (2003).

⮞ TIP: Although reflexivity is usually considered a desirable attribute in qualitative inquiry, some writers have cautioned researchers not to become so reflexive that creativity is stifled (McGhee et al., 2007). Glaser (2001) also warned against "reflexivity paralysis," (p. 47) referring to a possibly damaging compulsion to locate the inquiry within a particular theoretical context.

Data and Method Triangulation

As previously noted, triangulation refers to the use of multiple referents to draw conclusions about what constitutes truth, and has been compared to convergent validation. The aim of triangulation is to "overcome the intrinsic bias that comes from single-method, single-observer, and single-theory studies" (Denzin, 1989, p. 313). Patton (1999) also advocated triangulation, arguing that "no single

method ever adequately solves the problem of rival explanation" (p. 1192). Triangulation can also help to capture a more complete and contextualized portrait of key phenomena. Denzin (1989) identified four types of triangulation (data triangulation, investigator triangulation, method triangulation, and theory triangulation), two of which we describe here because they relate to data collection.

Data triangulation involves the use of multiple data sources for the purpose of validating conclusions. There are three types of data triangulation: time, space, and person. **Time triangulation** involves collecting data on the same phenomenon multiple times. Time triangulation can involve gathering data at different times of the day or at different times in the year. This concept is similar to test–retest reliability assessment—the point is not to study a phenomenon longitudinally to assess change, but to assess congruence of the phenomenon across time. **Space triangulation** involves collecting data on the same phenomenon in multiple sites, to test for cross-site consistency. Finally, **person triangulation** involves collecting data from different types or levels of people (e.g., individuals; groups, such as families; and collectives, such as communities), with the aim of validating data through multiple perspectives on the phenomenon.

Example of time triangulation: Wongvatunyu and Porter (2008) conducted a phenomenological study of the maternal experience of helping young adult children who survived a traumatic brain injury. The 7 mothers were interviewed three times over a 2-month period. To verify the consistency of their data, the researchers asked several key questions at all three interviews.

Method triangulation involves using multiple methods of data collection about the same phenomenon. In qualitative studies, researchers often use a rich blend of unstructured data collection methods (e.g., interviews, observations, documents) to develop a comprehensive understanding of a phenomenon. Multiple data collection methods provide an opportunity to evaluate the extent to which a consistent and coherent picture of the phenomenon emerges.

Example of person and method triangulation: Gillespie and colleagues (2008), in their ethnographic study of operating theater culture, gathered data through participant observations and in-depth interviews with 27 staff, including surgeons, anesthetists, nurses, and support staff. The authors noted that "A triangulated approach using multiple sources of data enabled a broad range of issues to be cross-checked, thus achieving . . . confirmation of the data" (p. 266).

Comprehensive and Vivid Recording of Information

In addition to taking steps to record interview data accurately, researchers need to prepare thoughtful field notes that are rich with descriptions of what transpired in the field. Even if interviews are the primary data source, researchers should record descriptions of the participants' demeanor and behaviors during the interactions, and should thoroughly describe the interview context.

Other record-keeping activities are also important. A log of decisions needs to be maintained, and reflexive journals should be maintained regularly with rich detail. Thoroughness helps readers and reviewers to develop confidence in the data.

Researchers sometimes specifically develop an **audit trail**, that is, a systematic collection of materials and documentation that would allow an independent auditor to come to conclusions about the data. Six classes of records are useful in creating an adequate audit trail: (1) the raw data (e.g., interview transcripts), (2) data reduction and analysis products (e.g., theoretical notes, working hypotheses), (3) process notes (e.g., methodologic notes), (4) materials relating to researchers' intentions and dispositions (e.g., reflexive notes), (5) instrument development information (e.g., pilot forms), and (6) data reconstruction products (e.g., drafts of the final report).

⮕ **TIP:** As Morse and colleagues (2002) noted, diligence in maintaining information does not in and of itself ensure the validity of the inquiry. They pointed out that "audit trails may be kept as proof of the decisions made throughout the project, but they do not identify the quality of those decisions, the rationale behind those decisions, or the responsiveness and sensitivity of the investigator to data" (pp. 6–7).

Example of an audit trail: In their in-depth study of men undertaking surveillance for prostate cancer, Oliffe and colleagues (2009) maintained an audit trail "so that all procedures and decisions made were documented, including the origins and development of categories and patterns and the possible sources of bias" (p. 434).

Member Checking

Lincoln and Guba considered member checking a particularly important technique for establishing the credibility of qualitative data. In a **member check**, researchers provide feedback to participants about emerging interpretations, and obtain participants' reactions. The argument is that if researchers' interpretations are good representations of participants' realities, participants should be able to confirm their accuracy.

Member checking can be carried out in an ongoing way as data are being collected (e.g., through deliberate probing to ensure that participants' meanings were understood), and more formally after data have been fully analyzed. Member checking is sometimes done in writing. For example, researchers can ask participants to review and comment on case summaries, interpretive notes, thematic summaries, or drafts of the research report. Member checks are more typically done in face-to-face discussions with individual participants or small groups of participants.

⮕ **TIP:** For focus group studies, it is usually recommended that member checking occur *in situ*. That is, moderators develop a summary of major themes or viewpoints in real time, and present that summary to focus group participants at the end of the session for their feedback. Rich data often emerge from participants' reactions to those summaries.

Despite the potential contribution that member checking can make to a study's credibility, several issues need to be kept in mind. First, not all participants are willing to engage in this process. Some—especially if the topic is emotionally charged—may feel they have attained closure once they have shared their experiences. Further discussion might not be welcomed. Others may decline involvement in member checking because they are afraid it might arouse suspicions of their families.

> **TIP:** If member checking is used as a validation strategy, participants should be encouraged to provide critical feedback about factual errors or interpretive deficiencies. In writing about the study, it is important to be explicit about how member checking was done and what role it played as a validation strategy. Readers cannot develop much confidence in the study simply by learning that "member checking was done."

Another issue is that member checks can lead to misleading conclusions of credibility if participants "share some common myth or front, or conspire to mislead or cover up" (Lincoln & Guba, 1985, p. 315). Also, some participants might fail to disagree with researchers' interpretations either out of politeness or in the belief that researchers are "smarter" or more knowledgeable than they themselves are. Thorne and Darbyshire (2005), in fact, caution against what they irreverently called *Adulatory Validity*, which they described as "the epistemological pat on the back for a job well done, or just possibly it might be part of a mutual stroking ritual that satisfies the agendas of both researcher and researched" (p. 1110). They noted that member checking tends to privilege interpretations that place study participants in the most favorable light.

Thorne and Darbyshire are not alone in their concerns about member checking as a validation strategy. Indeed, few strategies for enhancing data quality are as controversial as member checking. Morse (1999), for example, disputed the idea that participants have more analytic and interpretive authority than the researcher. Giorgi (1989) also argued that asking participants to evaluate the researcher's psychological interpretation of their own descriptions exceeds the role of participants. Morse and colleagues (2002), as well as Sandelowski (1993b), have worried that because study results have been synthesized, decontextualized, and abstracted across various participants, individual participants may not recognize their own experiences or perspectives in a member check. Even more scathingly, some critics view member checking as antithetical to the epistemology of qualitative inquiry. Smith (1993), in particular, criticized the philosophical contradictions inherent in this strategy, arguing that it is inconsistent with inquiry that purports to reveal multiple realities and multiple ways of knowing.

> **TIP:** Researchers sometimes invite participants to review their own interview transcripts for accuracy and clarification. Hagens and colleagues (2009) carefully assessed this technique in terms of improvements to rigor among a study that involved interviews with 51 key informants. They found that the review added little to the accuracy of the transcript and in some cases resulted in biases when some participants wanted to remove valuable material.

Example of member checking: Adamshick (2010) studied the lived experience of girl-to-girl aggression among marginalized teenagers. Data were collected in alternative schools through several in-depth interviews with 6 girls, and through field notes. After a thematic analysis, the researcher met with 5 participants "to clarify whether the description accurately captured what the experience of girl-to-girl aggression was like" (p. 545).

Quality-Enhancement Strategies Relating to Coding and Analysis

Excellent qualitative inquiry is likely to involve the simultaneous collection and analysis of data, so several strategies described in the preceding section are also relevant to promoting analytic integrity. Member checking, for example, can occur in an ongoing fashion during data collection, but typically involves participants' review of preliminary findings. Also, we discussed some strategies for analytic validation in Chapter 23 (e.g., using quasi-statistics). In this section, we introduce a few other strategies that relate to the coding, analysis, and interpretation of qualitative data.

Investigator and Theory Triangulation

The overall purpose of triangulation is to converge on the truth. Triangulation offers opportunities to sort out "true" information from irrelevant or idiosyncratic information by using multiple perspectives. Several types of triangulation are pertinent during analysis. **Investigator triangulation** refers to the use of two or more researchers to make data collection, coding, and analytic decisions. The premise is that investigators can reduce the risk of biased decisions and idiosyncratic interpretations through collaboration.

Investigator triangulation, conceptually similar to interrater reliability in quantitative studies, is often used in coding qualitative data. Coding consistency, whether it be intra-coder or inter-coder, depends on having clearly defined categories and decision rules that are documented in a codebook or coding "dictionary." Researchers sometimes formally compare two or more independent category schemes or a subset of independent coding decisions. Some advice on developing a codebook and assessing coding reliability is offered by Fonteyn and colleagues (2008) and Burla and colleagues (2008).

Example of assessing intercoder reliability:
Dallas (2009) studied adolescent fathers' perceptions of their interactions with health professionals. Dallas developed a coding scheme and coded the interview transcripts. A colleague then used the coding scheme to code a random selection of excerpts. "Differences between the two coders were resolved by refining definitions and discussion until an inter-rater reliability of 90% on the codebook was reached" (p. 293).

Collaboration can also be used at the analysis stage. If investigators bring to the analysis task a complementary blend of methodologic, disciplinary, and clinical expertise, the analysis and interpretation can potentially benefit from divergent perspectives.

Example of investigator triangulation:
Peden-McAlpine and colleagues (2008) studied the experience of women living with and managing fecal incontinence. Ten women participated in in-depth interviews. The researchers wrote that "confirmability was achieved by using a three-member research team during the analysis phase who worked together to come to consensus on the interpretation and ensure the findings were grounded in the text" (p. 821).

➲ **TIP:** In focus group studies, immediate postsession debriefings are recommended. In such debriefings—which should be tape-recorded—team members who were present during the session meet to discuss issues and themes. They also should share their views about group dynamics, such as coercive group members, censoring of controversial opinions, individual conformity to group viewpoints, and discrepancies between verbal and nonverbal behavior.

With **theory triangulation**, researchers use competing theories or hypotheses in analyzing and interpreting the data. Qualitative researchers who develop alternative hypotheses while still in the field can test the validity of each because the flexible design of qualitative studies provides ongoing opportunities to direct the inquiry. Theory triangulation can help researchers to rule out rival hypotheses and to prevent premature conceptualizations.

Although Denzin's (1989) seminal work discussed four types of triangulation, other types have been suggested. For example, Kimchi and colleagues (1991) described **analysis triangulation** (i.e., using two or more analytic techniques to analyze the same set of data). This approach offers another opportunity to validate the meanings inherent in a qualitative data set. Analysis triangulation can also involve using multiple units of analysis (e.g., individuals, dyads, families).

➲ **TIP:** Farmer and colleagues (2006) provided a useful description of the triangulation protocol they used in the Canadian Heart Health Dissemination Project that illustrates how triangulation was operationalized.

Searching for Confirming Evidence

Member checking with participants, as already noted, is one approach to validating the findings. Another verification strategy is to seek external evidence from other studies or from sources such as artistic or literary representations of the phenomenon. Another possibility, and one that has implications for transferability, is to have people from other sites, or even other disciplines, review preliminary findings.

Example of external confirming evidence:
Norris and colleagues (2009) studied how nurses establish relationships with first-time pregnant teenagers. Grounded theory analysis revealed a core category of *partnering* that evolved over three phases. The investigators contacted nurses from other sites across the country and asked them to review the findings. Eight nurses confirmed that "the theory and exemplars were consistent with their own experiences in working with similar clients and provided a useful framework" (p. 314).

Searching for Disconfirming Evidence and Competing Explanations

A powerful verification procedure that occurs at the intersection of data collection and data analysis involves a systematic search for data that will challenge an emerging categorization or explanation. The search for disconfirming evidence occurs through purposive or theoretical sampling methods, as described in Chapter 21. Clearly, this strategy depends on concurrent data collection and data analysis: researchers cannot look for disconfirming data unless they have a sense of what they need to know.

Example of searching for disconfirming evidence: Enarsson and colleagues (2007) examined common staff approaches toward patients in long-term psychiatric care. The researchers found that all their initial categories were negative in nature. To assess the integrity of their categories, the researchers searched specifically for data on common staff approaches that related to positive experiences. No such positive episodes could be found either in interviews or observations.

Lincoln and Guba (1985) discussed the related activity of **negative case analysis**. This strategy is a process by which researchers revise their interpretations by including cases that appear to disconfirm earlier hypotheses. The goal of this procedure is to continuously refine a hypothesis or theory until it accounts for *all* cases.

Patton (1999) similarly encouraged a systematic exploration for rival themes and explanations during the analysis: Failure to find strong supporting evidence for alternative ways of presenting the data or contrary explanations helps increase confidence in the original, principal explanation generated by the analyst" (p. 1191). This strategy can be addressed both inductively and logically. Inductively, the strategy involves seeking other ways of organizing the data that might lead to different conclusions and interpretations. Logically, it means conceptualizing other logical possibilities and then searching for evidence that could support those competing explanations.

Example of a search for rival explanations: Fleury and Sedikides (2007) studied the role of self-knowledge as a factor in cardiovascular risk modification among patients undergoing cardiac rehabilitation. They analyzed data from interviews with 24 patients and explicitly explored alternative explanations for their emerging findings with cardiac rehabilitation staff and study participants.

Peer Review and Debriefing

Another quality-enhancement strategy involves external review. **Peer debriefing** involves sessions with peers to review and explore various aspects of the inquiry. Peer debriefing exposes researchers to the searching questions of others who are experienced in either the methods of constructivist inquiry, the phenomenon being studied, or both.

In a peer debriefing session, researchers might present written or oral summaries of the data, categories and themes that are emerging, and interpretations of the data. In some cases, taped interviews might be played or transcripts might be given to reviewers to read. Peer debriefers might be asked to address questions such as the following:

- Is there evidence of researcher bias? Have the researchers been sufficiently reflexive?
- Do the gathered data adequately portray the phenomenon?
- If there are important omissions, what strategies might remedy this problem?
- Are there any apparent errors of fact?
- Are there possible errors of interpretation? Are there competing interpretations? More comprehensive or parsimonious interpretations?
- Have all important themes been identified?
- Are the themes and interpretations knit together into a cogent and creative conceptualization of the phenomenon?

Example of peer review: Purtzer's (2010) grounded theory study focused on the process of decision making about mammography among rarely or never-screened rural women. Two peer reviewers reviewed the study design, procedures, and the data with an eye toward identifying areas of bias.

Inquiry Audits

A similar, but more formal, approach is to undertake an **inquiry audit**, which involves scrutiny of the data and supporting documents by an external reviewer. Such an audit requires careful documentation of all aspects of the inquiry, as previously discussed. Once the audit trail materials are assembled, the inquiry auditor proceeds to audit, in a fashion analogous to a financial audit, the trustworthiness of the data and the meanings attached to them. Although such auditing is complex, it can serve as a tool for persuading others that qualitative findings are worthy of confidence. Relatively few comprehensive inquiry audits have been reported in the literature, but some studies report partial audits or the assembling of auditable materials. Rodgers and Cowles (1993) and Erwin and colleagues (2005) provide useful information about inquiry audits.

Example of an inquiry audit: Vitale (2009) studied nurses' lived experiences of Reiki for self-care. In-depth interviews with 11 nurses were taped and transcribed. All study documents were independently reviewed in two separate audits by nurse researchers with expertise in phenomenology. The reviewers found the interpretations to be consistent with the data.

Quality-Enhancement Strategies Relating to Presentation

The strategies discussed thus far are steps that researchers can undertake to convince *themselves* that their study has integrity and credibility. This section describes some issues relating to convincing *others* of the high quality of the inquiry.

Disclosure of Quality-Enhancement Strategies

A large part of demonstrating integrity to others involves providing a good description of the quality-enhancement activities that were undertaken. Many research reports fail to include information that would give readers confidence in the integrity of the research. Some qualitative reports do not address the subject of rigor, integrity, or trustworthiness at all, while others pay lip service to such concerns, simply noting, for example, that member checking was done. Just as clinicians seek *evidence* supporting healthcare decisions, readers of reports need evidence that the findings are believable and true. Readers can draw their own conclusions about study quality only if they are provided with sufficient information about

quality-enhancement strategies. The research example at the end of this chapter is exemplary with regard to the information provided to readers.

> **TIP:** Avoid stating that your quality-enhancement strategies *ensured* validity or rigor. Strategies are used to *enhance* or *promote* rigor, but nothing ensures it. Rigor, like beauty, is in the eye of the beholder.

Thick and Contextualized Description

Thick description, as noted in previous chapters, refers to a rich, thorough, and vivid description of the research context, the people who participated in the study, and the experiences and processes observed during the inquiry. Transferability cannot occur unless investigators provide detailed information to permit judgments about contextual similarity. Lucid and textured descriptions, with the judicious inclusion of verbatim quotes from study participants, also contribute to the authenticity and vividness of a qualitative study.

> **TIP:** Sandelowski (2004) cautioned that " . . . the phrase *thick description* likely ought not to appear in write-ups of qualitative research at all, as it is among those qualitative research words that should be seen but not written" (p. 215).

In high-quality qualitative studies, descriptions typically need to go beyond a faithful and thorough rendering of information. Powerful description often has an evocative quality and the capacity for emotional impact. Qualitative researchers must be careful, however, not to misrepresent their findings by sharing only the most dramatic or poignant stories. Thorne and Darbyshire (2005) cautioned against "lachrymal validity," a criterion for evaluating research based on the extent to which the report can wring tears from its readers. At the same time, they noted that the opposite problem with some reports is that they are "bloodless." Bloodless findings are characterized by a tendency of some researchers to "play it safe in writing up the research, reporting the obvious (possibly in the most thinly 'salami-sliced' 'findings' articles), failing to apply any inductive analytic spin to the sequence, structure, or form of the findings" (p. 1109).

Researcher Credibility

In qualitative studies, researchers *are* the data collecting instruments—as well as creators of the analytic process. Therefore, researcher qualifications, experience, and reflexivity are relevant in establishing confidence in the findings. Patton (2002) argued that trustworthiness is enhanced if the report contains information about the researchers and their credentials. In addition, the report may need to make clear the personal connections researchers had to the people, topic, or community under study. For example, it is relevant for a reader of a report on AIDS patients' coping to know that the researcher is HIV positive. Patton recommended that researchers report "any personal and professional information that may have affected data collection, analysis and interpretation—either negatively or positively . . ." (p. 566).

Example of researcher credibility: Gabrielle and colleagues (2008) undertook a feminist study of older women nurses to explore their concerns about ageing and self-care strategies. The authors (three female nurses) wrote, "Motivation for this study came from the first author's concern for her own health as a practicing older nurse. This led to concern about other ageing working nurses . . . This shared view between participants and researcher added to the study's 'authenticity' and honesty" (p. 317).

Researcher credibility is also enhanced when research reports describe the researchers' efforts to be reflexive. During her study of the experience of Chronic Fatigue Syndrome, Whitehead (2004) used excerpts from her reflexive journal to illustrate how researcher credibility could be enhanced through this process.

DEVELOPMENT OF A QUALITY-MINDED OUTLOOK

Conducting high-quality qualitative research is not just about methods and strategies—that is, it is not just about what researchers *do*. It is also about who the researchers *are*—that is, about their outlook, self-demands, and ingenuity. As Morse and colleagues (2002) succinctly put it, "Research is only as good as the investigator" (p. 10). Attributes that good qualitative researchers must possess are difficult to teach, but it is nevertheless important to know what those attributes are so they can be cultivated. We express several important attributes as *commitments* to which researchers can aspire.

1. **Commitment to Transparency**. Good qualitative inquiry cannot be a secretive enterprise that masks decisions, biases, and limitations from outside scrutiny. Conscientious qualitative researchers maintain the records needed to document a decision trail and justify the decisions. A commitment to transparency also means seeking opportunities to have decisions reviewed by others. To the extent possible, researchers should seek opportunities to demonstrate transparency in their writing, including how themes and categories were formulated from the initial participant data.

2. **Commitment to Absorption and Diligence**. Meticulousness is essential to high-quality research. Researchers who are not thorough run the risk of having thin, unsaturated data that undermine rich description of phenomena. The concept of *replication* within the study is crucial: there must be sufficient, and redundant, data to account for all aspects of the phenomenon (Morse et al., 2002). In good qualitative research, investigators must commit to reading and re-reading their data, returning repeatedly to check whether their interpretations are true to their data. Thoroughness also implies that researchers will seek opportunities to challenge early conceptualizations, and to find sources of corroborating evidence both internally (i.e., within the study data) and externally (e.g., in the literature).

3. **Commitment to Verification**. Confidence in the data, and in the analysis and interpretation of those data, is possible only when researchers are committed to instituting verification and

self-correcting procedures throughout the study. Morse and colleagues (2002) wrote at length about the importance of verification, noting that verification is "the process of checking, confirming, making sure, and being certain" (p. 9). A strong commitment to verification strengthens methodologic coherence and helps to promote the likelihood that errors and missteps are corrected before they undermine the enterprise.

4. **Commitment to Reflexivity**. While there is not always agreement about the forms that self-reflection will assume, there is widespread agreement that qualitative researchers need to devote time and energy to analyzing and documenting their presuppositions, biases, and ongoing emotions. Reflexivity involves a continuous self-scrutiny and asking, How might my previous experiences, values, background, and prejudices be shaping my methods, my analysis, and my interpretations?

5. **Commitment to Participant-Driven Inquiry**. In good qualitative research, the inquiry is driven forward by the participants, not the researcher. Researchers must continuously remain responsive to the flow and content of interactions with, and observations of, their informants. Participants shape the scope and breadth of questioning, and they help to guide sampling decisions. The analysis and interpretation must give voice to those who participated in the inquiry.

6. **Commitment to Insightful Interpretation**. Morse (2006) has written that *insight* is a major process in qualitative inquiry but has been neglected and overlooked as a topic of discussion—perhaps because it is not an easily acquired commodity. Morse argued that insight requires researchers to be *ready* for insight—they must have considerable knowledge about their data and be able to link them meaningfully to relevant literature. Immersion in one's own data—and having good-quality data—are essential. Morse also noted, however, that qualitative researchers need to give themselves

"*permission* to use insight and the confidence to do it well" (p. 3). Relatedly, Morse and colleagues (2002) urged researchers to *think theoretically,* which "requires macro-micro perspectives, inching forward without making cognitive leaps, constantly checking and rechecking, and building a solid foundation" (p. 13).

CRITIQUING OVERALL QUALITY IN QUALITATIVE STUDIES

For qualitative research to be judged trustworthy, investigators must *earn* their readers' trust. Many qualitative reports do not provide much information about the researchers' efforts to enhance trustworthiness, but there appears to be a promising trend toward greater forthrightness about quality issues. In a world that is very conscious about the quality of research evidence, qualitative researchers need to be proactive in doing high-quality research and sharing their quality-enhancement strategies with readers.

Part of the difficulty that qualitative researchers face in demonstrating trustworthiness and authenticity is that page constraints in journals impose conflicting demands. It takes a precious amount of space to report quality-enhancement strategies adequately and convincingly. Using space for such documentation means that there is less space for the thick description of context and the rich verbatim accounts that are also necessary in high-quality qualitative research. As Pyett (2003) has noted, qualitative research is often characterized by the need for critical compromises. It is well to keep such compromises in mind in critiquing qualitative research reports.

Table 24.1 offered questions that are useful in considering whether researchers have attended to important quality criteria. As noted earlier, not all questions are equally relevant for all types of qualitative inquiry. Reports that explicitly state which criteria guided the inquiry demonstrate sensitivity to readers' needs. Some further guidelines that may be helpful in evaluating qualitative analyses are presented in Box 24.1.

BOX 24.1 Guidelines for Evaluating Quality and Integrity in Qualitative Studies

1. Does the report discuss efforts to enhance or evaluate the quality of the data and the overall inquiry? If so, is the description sufficiently detailed and clear? If not, is there other information that allows you to draw inferences about the quality of the data, the analysis, and the interpretations?
2. Which specific techniques (if any) did the researcher use to enhance the quality of the inquiry? Were these strategies used judiciously and to good effect?
3. What quality-enhancement strategies were *not* used? Would supplementary strategies have strengthened your confidence in the study and its evidence?
4. Given the efforts to enhance data quality, what can you conclude about the study's integrity, rigor, or trustworthiness?

RESEARCH EXAMPLE

Study: Family presence during resuscitation and invasive procedures: The nurse experience (Miller & Stiles, 2009).

Statement of Purpose: The purpose of this study was to understand nurses' experiences of family presence during a loved one's cardiopulmonary resuscitation or invasive procedures in the hospital.

Method: Data for this phenomenological study were collected through in-depth interviews with 17 nurses from several hospitals in the northeastern United States. All nurses had experienced family presence during a critical procedure or resuscitation. Participants were originally sampled by convenience and by snowballing, but purposive sampling was used later in the study to ensure more diverse representation. Transcripts were analyzed using Van Manen's approach.

Quality Enhancement Strategies: Miller and Stiles's report provided good detail about their efforts to enhance the integrity of their study. Indeed, they had a specific section labeled "Ensuring Methodologic Rigor." They stated that dependability was met through prolonged engagement, persistent observation, and member checking. Persistent observation was achieved primarily by continuing interviews beyond the point of data saturation. Prolonged engagement involved an intense period of participant recruitment through various organiza-

tions and websites, as well as the lead researcher's 25 years experience with emergency and critical care nursing. Member checking was accomplished by having most of the participants review their transcripts and by "sharing preliminary themes and clusters with each participant to verify interpretation and accurate description of their experiences" (p. 1433). Credibility was also enhanced by working with a peer reviewer. The researcher met three times with the peer reviewer, who independently read the transcripts and identified key themes. The researcher and reviewer continued to discuss thematic structure until agreement was obtained. Researcher credibility was fostered by presenting information about the clinical and research experience of the researcher and reviewer. For example, both "had participated with both patients and families during invasive procedures and resuscitation in the emergency department" (p. 1433). By sampling participants from multiple sites, including urban and suburban hospitals and adult and pediatric institutions, triangulation was accomplished and transferability was enhanced. The researchers maintained an audit trail. They also provided a good description of their sample members, and offered an abundance of rich excerpts in support of their thematic analysis. Their report included a useful table that identified the four major themes, theme clusters, and illustrative examples of raw data corresponding to each.

Key Findings: The researchers identified four main themes in nurses' experiences: forging a connection, engaging the family, transition to acceptance, and a cautious approach.

⊙⊙⊙⊙⊙⊙⊙⊙⊙⊙⊙⊙⊙⊙⊙⊙⊙⊙⊙⊙⊙⊙⊙⊙⊙⊙

SUMMARY POINTS

- Several controversies surround the issue of *quality* in qualitative studies, one of which involves terminology. Some have argued that terms such as *rigor* and *validity* are quantitative terms that are unsuitable goals in qualitative inquiry but others are adamant that these terms are appropriate.
- Other controversies involve what criteria to use as indicators of rigor or integrity, whether there should be generic or study-specific criteria, and what strategies to use to address the quality criteria.
- The most-often used framework of quality criteria is that of Lincoln and Guba, who identified five criteria for evaluating the **trustworthiness** of the inquiry: credibility, dependability, confirmability, transferability, and (added to their framework at a later date) authenticity.
- **Credibility**, which refers to confidence in the truth value of the findings, is sometimes said to be the qualitative equivalent of internal validity. **Dependability** refers to the stability of data over time and conditions and is somewhat analogous to reliability in quantitative studies. **Confirmability** refers to the objectivity or neutrality of the data. **Transferability**, the analog of external validity, is the extent to which findings from the data can be transferred to other settings or groups. **Authenticity** refers to the extent to which researchers fairly and faithfully show a range of different realities and convey the feeling tone of lives as they are lived.
- An alternative framework, representing a synthesis of 10 qualitative validity schemes (Whittemore et al., 2001), proposed four primary criteria (credibility, authenticity, criticality, and integrity) and six secondary criteria (explicitness, vividness, creativity, thoroughness, congruence, and sensitivity). The primary criteria can be applied to any

qualitative inquiry, but the secondary criteria can be given different weight depending on study goals.
- **Criticality** refers to the researcher's critical appraisal of every research decision. **Integrity** is demonstrated by ongoing self-scrutiny to enhance the likelihood that interpretations are valid and grounded in the data.
- **Explicitness** is the ability to follow the researcher's decisions through careful documentation. **Vividness** involves rich and vivid descriptions. **Creativity** reflects challenges to traditional ways of thinking. **Thoroughness** refers to comprehensive data and the full development of ideas. **Congruence** is interconnectedness between parts of the inquiry and the whole, and between study findings and external contexts. **Sensitivity**, the sixth secondary criterion in the Whittemore and colleagues framework, is the degree to which an inquiry reflects respect and compassion for those being studied.
- Strategies for enhancing the quality of qualitative data as they are being collected include **prolonged engagement**, which strives for adequate scope of data coverage; **persistent observation**, which is aimed at achieving adequate depth; reflexivity; comprehensive and vivid recording of information (including maintenance of an **audit trail** of key decisions); triangulation; and member checking.
- **Triangulation** is the process of using multiple referents to draw conclusions about what constitutes the truth. During data collection, key forms of triangulation include **data triangulation** (using multiple data sources to validate conclusions) and **method triangulation** (using multiple methods, such as interviews and observations, to collect data about the same phenomenon).
- **Member checks** involve asking participants to review and react to study data and emerging themes and conceptualizations. Member checking is among the most controversial methods of addressing quality issues in qualitative inquiry.
- Strategies for enhancing quality during the coding and analysis of qualitative data include **investigator triangulation** (independent coding and analysis of at least a portion of the data by two or

more researchers); **theory triangulation** (use of competing theories or hypotheses in the analysis and interpretation of data); searching for confirming and disconfirming evidence; searching for rival explanations and undertaking a **negative case analysis** (revising interpretations to account for cases that appear to disconfirm early conclusions); external validation through **peer debriefings** (exposing the inquiry to the searching questions of peers); and launching a formal **inquiry audit** (a formal scrutiny of the research process and audit trail documents by an independent external auditor).

- Strategies to convince qualitative report readers of high quality include disclosure of the quality-enhancement strategies the researcher adopted, using *thick description* to vividly portray contextualized information about participants and the central phenomenon, and making efforts to be transparent about researcher credentials and reflexivity so that **researcher credibility** can be established.

- Doing high-quality qualitative research is not just about *method* and what the researchers *do*—it is also about who they *are*. To become an outstanding qualitative researcher, there must be a commitment to transparency, thoroughness, verification, reflexivity, participant-driven inquiry, and insightful and artful interpretation.

STUDY ACTIVITIES

Chapter 24 of the *Resource Manual for Nursing Research: Generating and Assessing Evidence for Nursing Practice*, *9th edition*, offers exercises and study suggestions for reinforcing concepts presented in this chapter. In addition, the following study questions can be addressed:

1. You have been asked to be a peer reviewer for a team of nurse researchers who are conducting a phenomenological study of the experiences of physical abuse during pregnancy. What specific questions would you ask the team during debriefing, and what documents would you want the researchers to share?

2. Apply relevant questions in Table 24.1 and Box 24.1 to the research example at the end of the chapter, referring to the full journal article as necessary.

STUDIES CITED IN CHAPTER 24

Adamshick, P. Z. (2010). The lived experience of girl-to-girl aggression in marginalized girls. *Qualitative Health Research, 20*, 541–555.

Champlin, B. (2009). Being there for another with serious mental illness. *Qualitative Health Research, 19*, 1525–1535.

Dallas, C. M. (2009). Interactions between adolescent fathers and health care professionals during pregnancy, labor, and early postpartum. *Journal of Obstetric, Gynecologic, & Neonatal Nursing, 38*, 290–299.

Denny, E. (2009). "I never know from one day to another how I will feel": Pain and uncertainty in women with endometriosis. *Qualitative Health Research, 19*, 985–995.

Enarsson, P., Sandman, P-O., & Hellzen, O. (2007). The preservation of order: The use of common approaches among staff toward clients in long-term psychiatric care. *Qualitative Health Research, 17*, 718–729.

Fleury, J., & Sedikides, C. (2007). Wellness motivation in cardiac rehabilitation: The role of self-knowledge in cardiovascular risk modification. *Research in Nursing & Health, 30*, 373–384.

Gabrielle, S., Jackson, D., & Mannix, J. (2008). Older women nurses: Health, ageing concerns and self-care strategies. *Journal of Advanced Nursing, 61*, 316–325.

Gillespie, B., Wallis, M., & Chaboyer, W. (2008). Operating theater culture: Implications for nurse retention. *Western Journal of Nursing Research, 30*, 259–277.

Miller, J., & Stiles, A. (2009). Family presence during resuscitation and invasive procedures: The nurse experience. *Qualitative Health Research, 19*, 1431–1442.

Mottram, A. (2009). Therapeutic relationships in day surgery. *Journal of Clinical Nursing, 18*, 2830–2837.

Norris, J., Howell, E., Wydeven, M., & Kunes-Connell, M. (2009). Working with teen moms and babies at risk: The power of partnering. *MCN: The American Journal of Maternal/Child Nursing, 34*, 308–315.

Oliffe, J., Davison, B., Tickles, T., & Mroz, L. (2009). The self-management of uncertainty among men undertaking active surveillance for low-risk prostate cancer. *Qualitative Health Research, 19*, 432–443.

Peden-McAlpine, C., Bliss, D., & Hill, J. (2008). The experience of community-living women managing fecal incontinence. *Western Journal of Nursing Research, 30,* 817–835.

Purtzer, M. A. (2010). Processes inherent in mammography screening decisions of rarely or never-screened women. *Western Journal of Nursing Research, 32,* 199–217.

Vitale, A. (2009). Nurses' lived experience of Reiki for self-care. *Holistic Nursing Practice, 23,* 129–145.

Wongvatunyu, S., & Porter, E. (2008). Helping young adult children with traumatic brain injury: The lifeworld of mothers. *Qualitative Health Research, 18,* 1063–1074.

Zinsli, G., & Smythe, E. (2009). International humanitarian nursing work: Facing differences and embracing sameness. *Journal of Transcultural Nursing, 20,* 234–241.

Methodologic and nonresearch references cited in this chapter can be found in a separate section at the end of the book.

PART 5

DESIGNING AND CONDUCTING MIXED METHODS STUDIES TO GENERATE EVIDENCE FOR NURSING

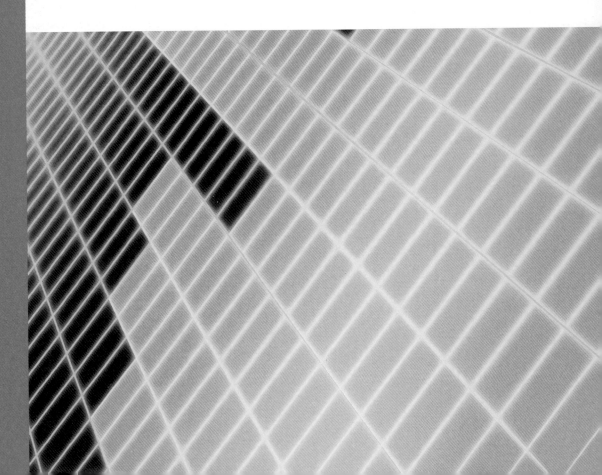

25 | Overview of Mixed Methods Research

OVERVIEW OF MIXED METHODS RESEARCH

A methodologic trend that has been gaining momentum is the planned integration of qualitative and quantitative data within single studies or a coordinated series of studies. **Mixed methods research** in the health sciences has been called "a quiet revolution" (O'Cathain, 2009). A decade ago, there was little guidance on conducting mixed methods research. Now there are abundant resources in the form of handbooks and textbooks (e.g., Andrew & Halcomb, 2009; Creswell & Plano Clark, 2007; Greene, 2007; Tashakkori & Teddlie, 2003; Teddlie & Tashakkori, 2009), as well as many examples of mixed methods studies in the nursing and healthcare literature.

This chapter presents basic information about mixed methods research in nursing, and the next discusses the use of mixed methods in developing and testing nursing interventions. To streamline these chapters, we will adopt Teddlie and Tashakkori's (2009) acronym in referring to mixed methods research as MM research.

Definition of MM Research

The concept of combining qualitative and quantitative data in a study is straightforward, but defini-

tions of MM research are not. This is partly because, in some sense, most studies could be considered MM if the definition is too broad. For example, if a grounded theory researcher asks structured demographic questions about age and education at the end of an in-depth interview, does that count as mixed methods? Or, if a survey asks a broad open-ended question at the end of a questionnaire (e.g., "Is there any thing else you would like to add?"), is that MM research? We do not consider such inquiries as MM research, although we would agree that this is a "gray area" (Creswell & Plano Clark, 2007, p. 11).

In this book, we use the definition offered in the first issue of the *Journal of Mixed Methods Research,* which is that MM research is "research in which the investigator collects and analyzes data, *integrates* the findings, and *draws inferences* using both qualitative and quantitative approaches or methods in a single study or program of inquiry" (Tashakkori & Creswell, 2007, p. 4, emphasis added). MM research at its best involves not only the collection of qualitative and quantitative data, but also the *integration* of the two at some stage of the research process, giving rise to meta-*inferences*. A **meta-inference** is a conclusion generated by integrating inferences obtained from the results of the qualitative and quantitative strands of an MM study (Teddlie & Tashakkori, 2009).

TIP: As mixed methods theory and methodology have evolved, so, too, has the terminology. There is widespread agreement that the term to use is *mixed methods research*, and not *multimethod research*, *triangulated research*, or *integrated research*, all terms that were used in the literature a decade ago.

Rationale for MM Studies

The dichotomy between quantitative and qualitative data represents a key methodologic distinction in the social, behavioral, and health sciences. Some have argued that the paradigms that underpin qualitative and quantitative research are fundamentally incompatible. Most people, however, now believe that many areas of inquiry can be enriched through the judicious triangulation of qualitative and quantitative data. The advantages of a mixed methods approach include the following:

- *Complementarity.* Qualitative and quantitative approaches are complementary; they represent words and numbers, the two fundamental languages of human communication. Researchers address problems with fallible methods. By using mixed methods, researchers can allow each to do what it does best, possibly avoiding the limitations of a single approach.
- *Practicality.* Given the complexity of phenomena, it is practical to use whatever methodologic tools are best suited to addressing pressing research questions, and to not have one's hands tied by rigid adherence to a single approach. MM researchers often answer questions that cannot be answered any other way.
- *Incrementality.* Progress on a topic tends to be incremental, relying on feedback loops. Qualitative findings can generate hypotheses to be tested quantitatively, and quantitative findings sometimes need clarification through in-depth probing. It can be productive to build such a loop into the design of a study, simultaneously addressing exploratory and confirmatory questions.
- *Enhanced validity.* When a hypothesis or model is supported by multiple and complementary types of data, researchers can be more confident about the validity of their results. The triangulation of methods can provide opportunities for testing alternative interpretations of the data, for examining the extent to which the context helped to shape the results, and for arriving at convergence in tapping a construct.
- *Collaboration.* Mixed methods research provides opportunity and encouragement for collaboration between qualitative and quantitative researchers working on similar problems.

Paradigm Issues and MM Studies

Although MM research has been around for decades, specific methodologic developments and widespread acceptance are recent phenomena. Mixed methods approaches emerged from the ashes of the so-called *paradigm wars* involving philosophical and methodologic debates between the post-positivist and constructivist camps that raged during the 1970s and 1980s. MM research gained momentum at the turn of the 21st century, in what some have called the *third methodological movement* (Tashakkori & Teddlie, 2003) or the *third research community* (Teddlie & Tashakkori, 2009).

Discussions about an appropriate paradigmatic stance for MM research have flourished. Viewpoints range from those claiming the irrelevance of paradigms, to those advocating multiple paradigms. The paradigm called **pragmatism** is most often associated with MM research. Pragmatism provides a basis for a stance that has been stated as the "dictatorship of the research question" (Tashakkori & Tedlie, 2003, p. 21). Pragmatist researchers consider that it is the research question that should drive the inquiry, and that the question is more important than the methods used. They reject a forced choice between the traditional post-positivists' and constructivists' modes of inquiry. In the pragmatist paradigm, both induction and deduction are important, theory generation and theory verification can be accomplished, and a pluralistic view is encouraged. Pragmatism is, as the name suggests, practical: whatever works best to arrive at good evidence is appropriate.

Practical Issues and MM Studies

Mixed methods studies have become attractive to graduate students and seasoned researchers alike, but the decision to pursue such a study should not be made lightly. The conduct of an MM study requires skills and resources that may not be available.

The researcher's skills should be critically evaluated in deciding whether to undertake an MM study because the researcher must be competent in both qualitative and quantitative methods. Although a team approach is a useful way to proceed because experts in both approaches can make contributions, all members of a team should be methodologically bilingual and have basic understanding of varied approaches.

➔ **TIP:** In dissertation MM research, the judicious selection of advisers with a mix of methodologic skills is imperative. Keep in mind, however, that advisers from different backgrounds may well have conflicting views about the merit of your strategies and the emphasis given to different aspects of your study.

Mixed methods research can be expensive. Although funding agencies increasingly are looking favorably on MM studies, it is obviously costly to collect, analyze, and integrate two or more types of data. Relatedly, mixed methods studies are often time consuming. Inevitably, the use of multiple methods will require more time to complete than if only a single method were used. It is wise to develop a realistic timeline before embarking on an MM inquiry.

GETTING STARTED ON A MIXED METHODS STUDY

In this chapter, we discuss many aspects of mixed methods research, with particular emphasis on research design and the analysis of MM data. We begin, however, by considering the kinds of problems and questions that lend themselves to MM research.

Purposes and Applications of MM Research

Creswell and Plano Clark (2007) identified four broad types of research situations that are especially well suited to MM research:

1. The concepts are new and poorly understood and there is a need for qualitative exploration before more formal, structured methods can be used.
2. The findings from one approach can be greatly enhanced with a second source of data.
3. Neither a qualitative nor a quantitative approach, by itself, is adequate in addressing the complexity of the research problem.
4. The quantitative results are puzzling and difficult to interpret, and qualitative data can help to explain the results.

As this list suggests, mixed methods research can be used in various situations. Some specific applications are noteworthy because MM research has made important contributions in these areas.

Instrumentation

Instrumentation is a good example of the first type of situation. Researchers sometimes collect qualitative data as a basis for developing structured instruments for use in research or clinical applications. The questions for a formal instrument are sometimes derived from clinical experience, theory, or prior research. When a construct is new, however, these mechanisms may be inadequate to capture its full dimensionality. Thus, researchers sometimes gather qualitative data as the basis for generating items for quantitative instruments that are subsequently subjected to rigorous testing, as described in Chapter 15.

Example of instrumentation: Beck and Gable (2000) developed the Postpartum Depression Screening Scale for screening new mothers. Scale items were based on in-depth interviews of mothers suffering from postpartum depression in three qualitative studies. As an example of how an item was developed from mothers' words, the quote "I was extremely obsessive with my thoughts. They would never stop. I could not control them" was developed into the item: I could not control the thoughts that kept coming into my mind (Beck & Gable, 2001).

Intervention Development

Qualitative research is playing an increasingly important role in the development of promising nursing interventions and in efforts to assess their efficacy. There is growing recognition that the development of effective interventions must take clients' perspective into account. Intervention research is increasingly likely to be MM research, a topic we address in the next chapter.

Example of intervention research: In developing an Internet coping skills training intervention for teenagers with Type I diabetes, Whittemore and colleagues (2010) used think-aloud and focus group methods to have teenagers and parents share their thoughts about a prototype of the intervention.

Hypothesis Generation and Testing

In-depth qualitative studies are often fertile with insights about constructs or relationships among them. These insights then can be tested and confirmed with larger samples in quantitative studies. This often happens in separate investigations. One problem, however, is that it usually takes years to do a study and publish results, which means that considerable time may elapse between the qualitative insights and the formal testing of hypotheses based on those insights. A researcher can undertake a coordinated set of MM studies that has hypothesis generation and testing as an explicit goal.

Example of hypothesis generation: Judith Wuest has developed a strong program of research focusing on women's caregiving. Her grounded theory research, which gave rise to a *theory of precarious ordering*, revealed that the basic social problem for caregiving women is multiple, competing, and changing demands. On the basis of her grounded theory, Wuest and colleagues (2007) developed hypotheses about how the nature and quality of relationship between the caregiver and a care recipient can predict health consequences for female caregivers. The hypotheses received support in a quantitative study of 236 female caregivers of adult family members.

Explication

Qualitative data are sometimes used to explicate the *meaning* of quantitative descriptions or relationships. Quantitative methods can demonstrate that variables are systematically related but may

fail to provide insights about *why* they are related. Such explications can corroborate statistical findings and guide the interpretation of results. Qualitative data can provide more global and dynamic views of the phenomena under study.

Example of explicating relationships with qualitative data: Manuel and colleagues (2007) undertook a mixed methods study of younger women's perceptions of coping with breast cancer. Results from the quantitative portion revealed that the most frequently used coping strategies were wishful thinking, making changes, and cognitive restructuring. Qualitative data suggested that the young women found different strategies particularly useful depending on the specific stressor.

Theory Building, Testing, and Refinement

An ambitious application of MM research is in the area of theory construction. A theory gains acceptance as it escapes disconfirmation, and the use of multiple methods provides good opportunity for potential disconfirmation of a theory. If the theory can survive these assaults, it can provide a stronger base for the organization of clinical and intellectual work.

Example of theory building: Gibbons (2009) conducted a theory-validating and theory-synthesizing mixed methods study of *self-neglect*. Qualitative and quantitative data were used to describe characteristics and behaviors of self-neglect among older adults in early stages of the phenomenon, and to explain the influence of several variables in the clinical evolution of self-neglect.

Research Questions for MM Research

In many mixed methods studies, the research questions are the driving force behind the scope of the inquiry. Investigators in MM studies typically pose questions that can *only* be addressed (or that can *best* be addressed) with more than one type of data. Within the pragmatist paradigm, the "dictatorship" of the research question underpins the inquiry.

In mixed methods research, there is typically an overarching goal, but there are inevitably at least two research questions, each of which requires a different type of data and approach. For example, MM researchers may simultaneously ask exploratory (qualitative) questions and confirmatory (quantitative) questions. In a mixed methods study, researchers can examine causal *effects* in a quantitative component, but can also shed light on causal *mechanisms* in a qualitative component.

Throughout this book, we have identified various designs and approaches, some qualitative and some quantitative. Table 25.1 has examples of questions that can be addressed in an MM study, according to a few of those design types. These examples illustrate that there are many opportunities for integrating multiple types of data in a study. As the questions in Table 25.1 suggest, research questions for an MM study will most often look like questions described in Chapter 4. Qualitative questions are likely to concern processes, experiences, and feelings. Quantitative questions will often involve descriptive prevalence, relationships among variables, and causal connections.

In addition to such questions, which are associated with particular strands of an inquiry, MM studies benefit from having a specific MM question relating to the mixing or linking of qualitative and quantitative data (Creswell & Plano Clark, 2007). Examples include such questions as, To what extent do the two types of data confirm each other? and How does one type of data help to explain the results from the other type?

> **TIP:** Creswell and Plano Clark's book included a table with a series of specific mixed methods questions (p. 106). An adapted version of this table is included in the Toolkit section of the accompanying *Resource Manual.*

TABLE 25.1	Examples of Mixed Methods Question Combinations	
TYPE OF RESEARCH	**EXAMPLE OF A QUANTITATIVE QUESTION**	**EXAMPLE OF A QUALITATIVE QUESTION**
Clinical trial	Are boomerang pillows more effective than straight pillows in improving the respiratory capacity of hospitalized patients?	Why did some patients complain about the boomerang pillows? How did the pillows feel?
Evaluation	How effective and cost-effective is a nurse-managed special care unit compared with traditional intensive care units?	How accepting were other healthcare workers of the special unit, and what problems of implementation ensued?
Outcomes research	What effect do alternative levels of nursing intensity have on the functional ability of elderly residents in long-term care facilities?	How do elderly long-term care residents interact with nurses in environments with different nursing intensity?
Survey	How prevalent is asthma among inner-city children, and what are the risk factors for this disease?	How is asthma experienced by inner-city children and their parents?
Ethnography	What percentage of women in rural Appalachia seek and obtain prenatal care, and what are their birth outcomes?	How do women in rural Appalachia view their pregnancies and how do they prepare for childbirth?
Case study	How have the demographic characteristics of the caseload of St. Jude's Homeless Shelter changed over a 10-year period?	How are social, health, and psychological services integrated in St. Jude's Homeless Shelter?

MIXED METHODS DESIGNS

Mixed methods designs have been developing over the past 2 decades and are likely to continue to evolve as greater thought is given to fruitful approaches—and as greater experience in conducting MM research occurs. At the moment, over a dozen design typologies have been developed by mixed methods scholars, so it is challenging to discuss this important topic.

We begin by describing some important design considerations, then present methods of portraying designs through a notation system and through diagrams, and finally present the design typology offered by Creswell and Plano Clark (2007). We note, however, that no typology will ever encompass every possible mixed methods design. This is because a hallmark of the MM approach is that it permits creativity and an emergent approach to design. Typologies and nomenclatures for designs are useful primarily because of their value in communicating an approach to others in proposals, IRB applications, and research articles. The specific designs we cover in this chapter are ones that have been adopted in many studies, but many other possibilities exist for structuring an MM study.

Key Decisions in MM Designs

In designing an MM study, researchers make several important decisions. One is whether to even *have* a fixed design at the outset. Students and novice researchers are likely to benefit by having a "roadmap" to follow, but seasoned researchers may profit from having the flexibility of allowing answers from an initial strand guide them in subsequent strands. Other key design decisions concern sequencing, prioritization, and integration.

Sequencing in MM Designs

There are three options for sequencing components of a mixed methods study: qualitative data are collected first, quantitative data are collected first, or both types are collected simultaneously (or at approximately the same time). When the two types of data are not collected at the same time, the approach is called **sequential**. When the data are collected at the same time, the approach usually is called **concurrent**, although the terms *simultaneous* and *parallel* have also been used. Concurrent designs occur in a single phase, whereas sequential designs unfold in two or more distinct phases. Creswell and Plano Clark (2007) noted that the timing decision encompasses more than the ordering of data collection—it concerns the ordering of the data analysis and interpretation. In well-conceived sequential designs, the analysis and interpretation in one phase informs the collection and analysis of data in the second.

Prioritization in MM Designs

Researchers usually decide which approach—qualitative or quantitative—to emphasize in an MM study. One option is that the two components are given equal, or roughly equal, weight. Often, however, one approach is given priority. The distinction is sometimes referred to as *equal status* versus *dominant status*.

Creswell and Plano Clark (2007) have identified several factors that may affect the priority decision. The first concerns the researcher's world view, an issue raised in Morse's (1991a) seminal paper. Researchers' philosophical orientation (positivist or constructivist) leads them to tackle research problems for which one approach is dominant, and the other is viewed as a useful supplementary data source. For example, in intervention research, qualitative data can be useful in developing the intervention and interpreting the dominant quantitative results. The dominant approach should be the one that is best suited to addressing the overall study goals.

Although giving equal priority to the qualitative and quantitative strands of a study may in some cases be attractive, practical considerations may influence the weighting decision. Creswell and Plano Clark (2007) have pointed out that if resources are limited, or if the researcher's skills are stronger in qualitative or quantitative methods, these issues will probably result in an MM study in which one approach has dominant status. The other factor to consider is the audience for the research. If the target audience—be that an adviser, funder, journal editor, or a broader research community—is unaccustomed to qualitative or quantitative research, then the prioritization decision may need to take that into account.

Integration in MM Designs

A third key design decision concerns how the qualitative and quantitative methods will be combined and integrated. Although it is apparent in looking at MM nursing studies that some researchers do little to integrate their data, it can be argued that MM research can only achieve its full potential for providing enhanced insights when integration occurs.

Creswell and Plano Clark (2007) have suggested that there are three basic strategies for integration decisions. First, the data types can be *merged* either during the analysis stage or during interpretation. Second, mixing can occur at the design level, through what is called an *embedding* strategy, a topic we discuss in the next section. Finally, researchers can *connect* the two data types. Integration strategies are addressed later in this chapter.

Notation and Diagramming in MM Designs

Morse (1991a), a prominent nurse researcher, made a critical contribution to the MM literature by proposing a notation system that has been adopted by virtually all writers across disciplines. Her notation system concerns the sequencing and prioritization decisions, and is thus useful in quickly summarizing major features of an MM design.

In Morse's notation system, priority is designated by upper case and lower case letters: QUAL/quan designate a mixed methods study in which the dominant approach is qualitative, while QUAN/qual designates the reverse. If neither approach is dominant (i.e., both are equal), the notation stipulates QUAL/QUAN. Sequencing in this system is indicated by the symbols + or →. The arrow designates a sequential approach. For example, QUAN → qual is the notation for a primarily quantitative MM study in which qualitative data collection occurs in Phase II. When both approaches occur concurrently, a plus sign is used (e.g., QUAL + quan).

Creswell and Plano Clark (2007) have suggested a modification of Morse's notation to include the use of parentheses, which designate an embedded design structure. The notation QUAN(qual) indicates a design in which the qualitative methods are embedded within a quantitative design. Figure 25.1 illustrates several possible permutations of design options that can be illustrated with the notation system. Several options have been named as specific designs by Creswell and Plano Clark and are discussed in the next section.

			SEQUENCE/TIMING	
			CONCURRENT	**SEQUENTIAL**
P R I O R I T Y	**EQUAL**		A1. QUAL + QUAN (Triangulation Design[a])	B1. QUAN → QUAL QUAL → QUAN
	DOMINANT	**Not Embedded**	A2. QUAN + qual QUAL + quan	B2. QUAN → qual quan → QUAL (Explanatory Design[a]) B3. QUAL → quan qual → QUAN (Exploratory Design[a])
		Embedded	A3. QUAN (qual) QUAL (quan) (Embedded Design[a])	B4. QUAN (qual) QUAL (quan) (Embedded Design[a])

[a]Design names are based on Creswell & Plano Clark, 2007.

FIGURE 25.1 Mixed methods design matrix.

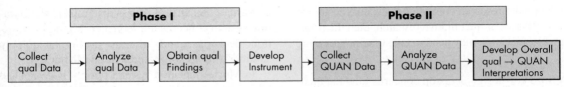

FIGURE 25.2 Visual diagram of a mixed methods instrument development study (Exploratory Design).

In addition to the notation system, MM designs can be visually diagrammed. Such diagrams can be useful in illustrating processes to advisors or reviewers, and can also provide guidance to researchers themselves. Figure 25.2 illustrates a basic diagram for an instrument development study in which qual data informed the development of QUAN instruments in a qual → QUAN design. Additional information can be added under the boxes in the diagram to provide richer detail. For example, under the first box (Collect qual Data), there might be greater detail, such as "Conduct focus group interviews."

The diagram in Figure 25.2 is a simplified version of what happens in MM instrument development research. In many carefully designed instrument development studies, there are more than two phases. For example, there is often a content validation effort involving the collection of data from a panel of experts (Chapter 15). Such a design might have the following notation: qual → qual+quan → QUAN. In this scheme, the middle term represents qualitative and quantitative feedback from content validity experts.

> ◑ **T I P :** Figure 3.1 of Creswell and Plano Clark's (2007) book offered 10 guidelines for drawing visual diagrams of MM studies. Their book also includes dozens of such visual diagrams that can be used as models.

Specific MM Designs

Although numerous design typologies have been developed by different MM methodologists, we focus on the typology developed by Creswell and Plano Clark (2007). As shown in Figure 25.1, they identified four designs that can be thought of as basic designs. Although these designs "are not complex enough to mirror actual practice" (Creswell, 2009), they are a good starting point for researchers undertaking their first MM study. We briefly describe some features of these designs. (Note that we have followed Creswell and Plano Clark in capitalizing the names of the designs).

Triangulation Designs

The purpose of the **Triangulation Design** is to obtain different, but complementary, data about the central phenomenon under study. In this design, qualitative and quantitative data are collected simultaneously and with equal priority. The notation for a Triangulation Design is QUAL + QUAN (Box A1, Figure 25.1). The goal of a Triangulation Design is to converge on "the truth" about a problem or phenomenon by allowing the weaknesses of one approach be offset by the strengths of the other. The researcher's job is to link the two datasets, often at the interpretation stage of the project.

> **Example of a Triangulation Design:** Hodges (2009) used a QUAL + QUAN Triangulation Design in her mixed methods study of factors that affect readmissions of older patients with heart failure. Data were collected concurrently by means of semi-structured interviews and standardized scales.

The Triangulation Design has several variants. The most conventional of these is called the *convergence model* (Creswell & Plano Clark, 2007). In this model, QUAN data are collected and analyzed in parallel with the collection and analysis of QUAL data. The results of the two separate analyses are compared and contrasted, leading to an overall interpretation of both sets of results. The goal of the convergence model is to develop internally confirmed conclusions about a single phenomenon.

Another variant is the *data transformation model*. This model also involves the separate but concurrent collection of QUAL and QUAN data, followed by QUAL and QUAN analysis. A novel step in this model involves the transformation of the QUAL data into quan data (or the QUAN data into qual data), and then comparing and interrelating the datasets. Data transformations are described later in this chapter.

An additional variant of a Triangulation Design is a *multilevel model* that is described at length in Teddlie and Tashakkori (2009). The multilevel model, which might be useful in many healthcare settings, involves using different methods at different levels of a complex system. For example, QUAL data could be collected at the top administrative level of nursing homes, followed by QUAN data at the staff level, and QUAL data at the client level. The findings from each level are then blended into one overall interpretation.

A major advantage of Triangulation Designs is that they are efficient because both types of data are collected simultaneously. A major drawback, however, is that these designs, which give equal weight to QUAL and QUAN data, are difficult for a single researcher working alone to do. Another potential problem can arise if the data from the two strands are not congruent.

Embedded Designs

In an **Embedded Design**, one type of data is used in a supportive capacity in a study based primarily on the other data type. Either qualitative or quantitative data can be dominant—although in most Embedded Designs, qual is supportive of QUAN data. The sequencing is often concurrent (A3 of Figure 25.1), but can also be sequential (B4 of Figure 25.1). The notation for Embedded Designs uses parentheses: QUAL(quan) or QUAN(qual).

➲ **TIP:** It is not always easy to distinguish Embedded Designs from other MM designs that have a dominant data type. The key is whether the second data type is really subservient. If the secondary data could not stand on their own merit in yielding interesting information about the phenomenon, then the design is likely an embedded one.

Many different Embedded Designs are possible, but Creswell and Plano Clark (2007) featured two models. The first is used in intervention research and is discussed in Chapter 26. The second is a *correlational model*. In such an MM study, QUAN data are collected to examine relationships among variables, often with the desire to predict important outcomes. For example, a correlational study might focus on factors that predict eating disorders in adolescent girls. An embedded qual component might explore comorbidities among those with an eating disorder, such as depression or sleep disturbances.

Although not specifically mentioned by Creswell and Plano Clark, ethnographic research sometimes involves an Embedded Design. For example, an ethnographic study of the healthcare practices of a particular cultural group (e.g., residents of a low-income housing project) would mostly involve participant observation and in-depth interviews with residents. A component of the study could also involve extraction of quantitative data from a sample of records in a neighborhood clinic, or a structured survey of the staff at the clinic.

Embedded Designs—especially the correlational model—are often a practical approach to doing MM research, especially when resources are limited. Creswell and Plano Clark (2007) noted that such designs might be appealing to graduate students because focused effort is needed primarily for one strand only. They also suggested that Embedded Designs might be appealing to audiences who are especially comfortable with one type of approach—such as funders who are more familiar with quantitative designs.

Example of an Embedded Design: Thomas (2009) used a concurrent QUAN(qual) Embedded Design to study effective dyspnea management strategies for elders with end-stage chronic obstructive pulmonary disease. Her primary means of data collection was quantitative, but participants were asked to elaborate on their experiences by answering the question: "What one thing seems to help the most when you have a severe attack of shortness of breath?" (p. 81). The data from both components were integrated in the study conclusions.

Explanatory Designs

Explanatory Designs are sequential designs with quantitative data collected in the first phase, followed by qualitative data collected in the second phase. Either the qualitative or the quantitative data can be given a stronger priority in Explanatory Designs. That is, the design can be either QUAN → qual or quan → QUAL (B2 in Figure 25.1).

In Explanatory Designs, qualitative data from the second phase are used to build on or explain the quantitative data from the initial phase. This design is especially suitable when the quantitative results are surprising (e.g., unanticipated nonsignificant results or significant serendipitous results), when results are complicated and tricky to interpret, or when the sample has numerous outliers that are difficult to explain.

Creswell and Plano Clark (2007) described two variants of the Explanatory Design. In the first, the *follow-up explanations model,* the researcher collects qual data that can best help to explain the initial QUAN findings. The primary emphasis is on the quantitative aspects of the study, and the analysis involves connecting data between the two phases. This model is one that is often very attractive to researchers who are primarily quantitative oriented, but who recognize that their study can be enriched by adding a qualitative component.

The second variant is the *participant selection model,* in which the first-stage quan data are in service of the second-phase QUAL component. In this model, information about the characteristics of a large group, as identified in the first phase, is used to purposefully select participants in the second dominant phase—for example, using extreme case sampling or stratified purposive sampling (Chapter 21).

⮕ TIP: In describing a design in a proposal or a report, it is probably best to combine words and notation. A citation should be provided for specifically named designs, given the diverse design typologies. For example, the following statement might summarize a design: "A sequential, qualitative-dominant (quan → QUAL) Explanatory Design, using a participant selection model (Creswell & Plano Clark, 2007), will be adopted in the proposed research." In proposals, a visual diagram ideally should be included as well.

Advantages of Explanatory Designs are that they are straightforward and easy to describe, and can be done by a single researcher. Another attractive feature, given page constraints in journals, is that the results can often be summarized in two separate papers. On the other hand, Explanatory Designs can be time consuming—the second phase cannot begin until data from the first phase are collected *and* analyzed. Another potential problem is that it may be difficult to secure upfront approval from ethical review boards for the second phase, because the details of the Phase II study design cannot be known in advance.

Example of an Explanatory Design: Sevelius (2009) used a QUAN → qual Explanatory Design to study HIV-related risk factors and protective behaviors among transgender men who have sex with nontransgender men. In the first phase, QUAN data were collected in structured interviews with 45 transgender men. In-depth interviews were conducted with 15 of those men in the second phase.

Exploratory Designs

Exploratory Designs are also sequential MM designs, but qualitative data are collected in the first phase. The design has as its central premise the need for initial in-depth exploration of a phenomenon. Findings from the initial phase are then used in a second, quantitative phase. Usually the first phase focuses on detailed exploration of a little-researched phenomenon, and the second phase is focused on measuring it or classifying it. In an Exploratory Design, either the qualitative phase can be dominant (QUAL → quan) or the quantitative phase can be dominant (qual → QUAN), as shown in B3 of Figure 25.1.

Creswell and Plano Clark (2007) described two models of an Exploratory Design. The first is the *instrument development model,* which is used when data from the qual phase are used in the development of QUAN instruments. This model, depicted graphically in Figure 25.2, has been used by many nurse researchers.

In the second model, the *taxonomy development model,* the researcher identifies important constructs and develops a taxonomy, classification system, or a theory grounded in the in-depth data gathered during the QUAL phase. Then, the quan phase is used to test or explore the taxonomy or theory with a broader group. This is the model used when formal hypotheses generated in the initial phase are tested in a subsequent phase.

The advantages and disadvantages of an Explanatory MM Design also apply to Exploratory MM Designs. Separate phases make the inquiry easy to explain, implement, and report. Yet such a project can be time-consuming, and it may be difficult to get upfront approval from ethics review committees because the second phase methods usually depend on what transpires in the first phase.

Example of an Exploratory Design: Kalisch and Williams (2009) used an Exploratory Design (qual → QUAN) to develop and test an instrument to measure *missed nursing care*. In the first phase of the study, 17 focus group interviews identified specific areas of missed nursing care and the reasons for missing care. In subsequent phases, items were generated and psychometric testing of the instrument was undertaken with more than 1,000 nurses.

Other MM Designs

Many MM designs do not have explicit names in the Creswell-Plano Clark (2007) system. In Figure 25.1 (A2), for example, we see that concurrent dominant QUAN + qual and qual + QUAN designs do not have names. Nor have sequential nondominant designs (QUAN → QUAL and QUAL → QUAN) been given a label (B1 in Figure 25.1). The truth is that many design options, including designs with three or more phases, are possible. Furthermore, each phase can have its own distinct design, which might be especially likely to occur in a program of research in which a series of interrelated studies might unfold as investigators pursue a topic.

Example of a QUAN + qual Design: Jurgens and colleagues (2009) used a QUAN + qual concurrent design to study why elders delay responding to heart failure symptoms. The most frequently reported symptoms were dyspnea and fatigue. Dyspnea duration ranged from 30 minutes to 90 days before action was taken. Data from the qualitative component shed light on some reasons for long delays.

⮕ **T I P :** Mixed methods designs are most often portrayed as being cross-sectional. The purpose of sequential designs as discussed thus far is not to track how a phenomenon unfolds over time (longitudinally), but rather to obtain different perspectives on a phenomenon using different approaches. Mixed methods can, however, be used in longitudinal studies. For example, concurrent triangulation (QUAL + QUAN) or embedding (QUAN[qual]) could occur multiple times. Specific notation for such designs has not been developed.

Selecting an MM Design

The most critical issue in selecting a design is its appropriateness for the research questions. Having a *name* for a design is far less important than having a solid rationale for structuring a study in a certain way. Yet practical issues are also relevant in designing a study. For example, few researchers are equally skillful in qualitative and quantitative methods. This suggests three possibilities: (1) selecting a design in which your methodologic strengths are dominant; (2) working as a team with researchers whose strengths are complementary; or (3) strengthening your skills in your nondominant area. In most cases, the first option is likely to be most realistic for students. As noted previously, practical concerns such as resource availability and time constraints also play a role in choosing a design. Concurrent designs often require shorter time commitments, and dominant designs can often be less resource-intensive.

Morse (2003b) advised researchers, in deciding on an MM design, to have a basic grasp of the project's *theoretical drive*. The theoretical drive may be *discovery*, which puts the main emphasis of a project on the inductive, QUAL aspects of the research. Alternatively, the theoretical drive can be *verification*, which would give priority to the deductive QUAN aspects of the inquiry.

It is advisable to learn the details of a particular MM design before making a selection. In addition to reading methodologic writings of MM scholars, it is useful to examine the methods section of reports that have used a design you are considering. Teddlie and Tashakkori (2009) also advised that "you should look for the most appropriate or single best available research design, rather than the 'perfect fit.' You may have to combine existing designs, or create new designs, for your study" (p. 163).

SAMPLING AND DATA COLLECTION IN MIXED METHODS STUDIES

When a study design has been selected, an MM researcher can proceed to plan how best to collect the needed qualitative and quantitative data by developing a sampling and data collection plan. Sampling and data collection in MM studies are often a blend of approaches that we described in earlier chapters. A few special sampling and data collection issues for an MM study merit brief discussion.

Sampling in an MM Study

Mixed methods researchers can combine sampling designs in various creative ways. The quantitative component is likely to rely on a sampling strategy that enhances the researcher's ability to generalize from the sample to a broader population. As noted in Chapter 12, probability samples are especially well suited to selecting a representative sample of participants, but researchers often must compromise, using such designs as consecutive samples or quota samples to enhance representativeness. For the qualitative strand of the project, MM researchers usually adopt purposive sampling methods (Chapter 21) to select information-rich cases who are good informants about the phenomenon of interest.

Sample sizes are also likely to be different in the qualitative and quantitative components in ways one might expect—that is, larger samples for the quantitative component. Ideally, MM researchers should use power analyses to guide sample size decisions for the quantitative component, to diminish the risk of Type II errors in their statistical analyses. The qualitative sample usually has fewer cases,

and saturation is the principle most often used to make decisions about when sampling can stop.

A unique sampling issue in MM studies concerns whether the same people will be in both the qualitative and quantitative strands. The best strategy depends on the study purpose and the research design, but using overlapping samples can be advantageous. Having the same people in both parts of an MM study offers opportunities for convergence and for comparison between the two datasets.

Onwuegbuzie and Collins (2007) have categorized mixed methods sampling designs according to the *relationship* between the qualitative and quantitative components. The four relationships are identical, parallel, nested, or multilevel. An **identical** relationship occurs when exactly the same people are in both components of the study. This approach might occur if everyone in a survey or intervention study was asked a series of probing, open-ended questions—or if everyone in a primarily QUAL study was administered a formal instrument, such as a self-efficacy scale.

Example of identical sampling: Beck and colleagues (2009) studied symptom experiences and quality of life of older cancer survivors 1 and 3 months after they completed initial treatment. All 52 participants provided quantitative data (obtained through hospital records and mailed questionnaires) and qualitative data (by means of in-depth telephone interviews) at both points in time.

In a **parallel** relationship, the samples in the two strands are completely different, although they are usually drawn from the same or a similar population. Like identical sampling, parallel sampling can occur in either concurrent or sequential designs, and with any of the prioritization schemes.

Example of parallel sampling: Reuter and colleagues (2009) reported qualitative results from Phase I of their MM sequential QUAL → QUAN study that focused on poverty stigma in two large Canadian cities. In the first phase, purposive sampling was used to select participants from 8 low-income neighborhoods for individual and focus group interviews. In Phase II, a representative sample of neighborhood residents was selected for a telephone interview.

In a **nested** relationship, the participants in the qualitative strand are a subset of the participants in the quantitative strand. Nested sampling is an especially common sampling approach in MM studies. Finally, a **multilevel** relationship involves selecting samples from different levels of a hierarchy—usually this means from different but related populations.

> **Example of nested sampling:** Grant and colleagues (2009) conducted a grounded theory study of the process of recovery following total hip replacement surgery, as part of a mixed method inquiry using an Explanatory Design. They purposively sampled 10 participants from the larger quantitative component who completed a structured questionnaire 3 months after surgery.

Explanatory and Embedded Designs are especially likely to involve samples with nested relationships. Indeed, as discussed in the previous section, one of the models of an Explanatory Design is specifically geared to participant selection from the first phase for in-depth scrutiny in the second. If the intent of a qualitative component is to offer detail and elaboration about phenomena and relationships captured quantitatively, then a nested sample is likely to enrich the researcher's understanding. Mixed methods studies with an Exploratory Design, by contrast, often use completely different people in the two study phases. For example, the people who are interviewed in depth about their experience with a phenomenon in an instrument development study are rarely used to test a new formal instrument in a later phase. In Triangulation Designs, the relationship is more variable; the decision should ultimately be based on which approach best addresses overall study aims.

Kemper and colleagues (2003) noted that the overall mixed method sample should be capable of generating a thorough dataset about the phenomenon under study. The sampling plan should allow for "credible explanations" (p. 276). Kemper and colleagues also pointed out that the sampling plan should be one that permits the conclusions from the study to be transferred/generalized to other settings or groups.

Data Collection in an MM Study

Mixed methods researchers, by definition, collect and analyze both qualitative and quantitative data. All of the data collection methods discussed in Chapters 13 (structured methods) and 22 (unstructured methods) can be creatively combined and triangulated in a mixed methods study. Thus, possible sources of data for MM studies include group and individual interviews, psychosocial scales, observations, biophysiologic measures, records, diaries, cognitive tests, Internet postings, photographs, and physical artifacts. Johnson and Turner (2003) noted that MM studies can involve both *intramethod mixing* (e.g., structured and unstructured self-reports), and *intermethod mixing* (e.g., biophyisologic measures and unstructured observation).

In selecting data collection methods for each strand of an MM study, a goal should be to use each method to address the research questions in a manner that enhances overall understanding of the problem. A fundamental consideration concerns the methods' complementarity—that is, having the limitations of one method be balanced and offset by the strengths of the other. This in turn means that when MM researchers are devising their data collection strategies, they need to be fully aware of the strengths and weaknesses of each approach. As we discussed in earlier chapters, there are advantages and disadvantages of unstructured versus structured methods, as well as of the different types of methods (self- report, observation, and so on).

➔ **TIP:** Self-reports are the most common data source in both qualitative and quantitative nursing studies, and blending unstructured and structured self-report data is the most usual approach in MM research as well.

In concurrent designs, decisions about the data collection methods must be made upfront. In sequential designs, however, MM researchers often have an emergent approach, with the types of data to be collected in the second phase shaped to some extent by findings in the first phase. Sequential designs have rich potential for incremental findings that build on one another.

In planning a data collection strategy, MM researchers may need to consider whether one method could introduce bias in the other method. For example, do closed-ended questions about a phenomenon have an effect on how participants might think about the phenomenon when asked in an unstructured fashion (or vice versa)? In other words, researchers should give some thought to whether one of the methods is an "intervention" that could influence people's behavior or their responses. Such bias clearly is not relevant when parallel sampling has been used.

Example of efforts to avoid bias: Wells and colleagues (2009) used a mixed methods approach in their study of burden, health, and mood in 34 female Mexican American cancer caregivers. Both qualitative and quantitative data were collected in two interviews, in a design that we might notate as QUAL(quan) → QUAL(quan). In the first interview, interviewers began by asking structured questions, but they avoided asking demographic questions about factors that could influence responses to open-ended questions about the caregiving experience—for example, questions about participants' employment status and health history. This information was obtained in the second interview, after all in-depth data had been gathered.

One final data collection issue concerns the possible need for additional data at the data analysis and interpretation stage of a project. If findings from the qualitative and quantitative strands conflict, it is sometimes useful to collect supplementary data to shed light on and possibly resolve contradictions or inconsistencies.

ANALYSIS OF MIXED METHODS DATA

One of the greatest challenges in doing mixed methods research concerns how best to analyze the qualitative and quantitative data in a manner that integrates the results and interpretation. It is not uncommon, unfortunately, for the two strands of data to be analyzed and reported separately, without attempts to integrate the findings. When this happens, it is more fitting to describe the endeavor as separate, linked studies than as MM research.

The real benefits of MM research cannot be realized if there is no attempt to merge results from the two strands and to develop interpretations and practice recommendations based on integrated understandings. A high-quality MM analysis merges measurement with meaning, graphs with graphical accounts, and tables with tableaux (Sandelowski, 2003).

Students often want specific guidance about how to analyze their data, but there are no formulas or sets of rules for MM data analysis and integration. Decisions about how to blend the datasets hinge on a number of factors. A particularly important factor is the study's sampling plan. Many of the techniques discussed in this section are only appropriate for identical and nested samples—that is, for sampling plans in which both qualitative and quantitative data are obtained from the same people. Research design, especially the sequencing decision, also affects analytic choices.

This section describes a few analysis options for MM studies, but it is far from comprehensive. Additional resources should be consulted, such as the work of Bazely (2009a, 2009b), Creswell and Plano Clark (2007), Greene (2007), Happ and colleagues (2006), and Onwuegbuzie and Teddlie (2003). Also, Mendlinger and Cwikel (2008) provided a useful illustration of how "spiraling" between qualitative and quantitative data contributed to an integration of their strands of data.

↪ TIP: We agree with Brewer and Hunter (2006), who recommended "a creative and at times even playful meshing of data-collecting methods to encourage serendipity and openness to new ideas" (p. 69). Because of the need for creativity, however, MM data analysis is difficult to describe in a proposal. It is probably best to identify a few strategies that seem fruitful a priori, but to pursue others that seem productive during the analysis process.

Decisions in Analyzing MM Data

Before pursuing a specific analytic strategy, MM researchers should make several broad preliminary decisions that will affect how they will proceed. Our list here is not exhaustive, but is meant to encourage preanalytic thinking about important issues.

1. *What is the overall goal of the study?* In selecting analytic strategies, the overall purpose of the study should be kept firmly in mind. For example, is the purpose primarily descriptive, exploratory, or explanatory? It is also important to consider the purpose in terms of evidence-based practice goals: How best can the data be analyzed to yield high-quality evidence for practicing nurses?

2. *Will integration occur at the analysis stage or the interpretation stage?* Sometimes interpretive integration is the only path possible—for example, when parallel sampling of different people in the two strands has been used—but in other cases researchers choose the point of integration. A frequent comment by those whose integration happens during analysis is that "this was the key to unfolding the complex relationships in the topic of the study" (Bazely, 2009b, p. 205).

3. *What will be the unit of analysis?* Often the unit is individual participants, but other options include events (Happ et al., 2006) or subgroups of people. If the MM design involves a multilevel model, the levels are usually the unit of primary interest.

4. *Is the focus of the study more case oriented or more construct oriented?* Case-oriented research, which is more common in QUAL-dominant research, is focused on the complexity of a phenomenon within its context and examines patterns within each case. Construct-oriented research is more conceptual and theory-centered and involves the exploration of a phenomenon with the goal of explicating key constructs and variables.

5. *Will either type of data be converted or transformed?* Sometimes researchers convert their qualitative data into quantitative data, and vice versa. We discuss such strategies later in this section.

6. *Will direct comparisons be made between the qualitative and quantitative data—and, if so, at what level will the comparisons be made?* In nested and identical sampling designs, comparisons can be made at the individual level—for example, comparing each participant's score on a health promotion scale with how he or she described lifestyle and activities in in-depth interviews. Comparisons can also be made between subgroups—for example, how high scorers on the health promotion scale differ from low scorers in terms of themes that emerge in the qualitative analysis. Finally, overall comparisons are possible—for example, is the picture of the salience of health promotion consistent in the qualitative and quantitative datasets? This latter type of comparison, at a minimum, is essential if the MM research question involves congruence or complementarity between the strands.

7. *Will integration involve the use of specialized software?* Tremendous advances have been made with regard to software for integration in MM studies. Bazely (2003, 2009a) has offered suggestions for how quantitative data can be transferred to a qualitative program and vice versa. Qualitative data analysis software such as NVivo and MaxQDA are especially useful, and statistical packages such as SPSS now have text analyses software that can categorize text responses and combine them with other quantitative variables. Even if specialized software for combining qualitative and quantitative data is not used, MM researchers can use basic spreadsheets to good advantage.

The next few sections describe a few of the many specific strategies that mixed methods researchers use to integrate their qualitative and quantitative strands of data. We begin with interpretive integration, followed by several strategies for analytic integration: data conversion, meta-matrixes, and mixed method displays. These strategies are not mutually exclusive and several can be effectively combined in an MM study.

Interpretive Integration

Many, and perhaps most, mixed methods researchers who make efforts to integrate the different strands do so at the point of interpretation rather than during analysis. Creswell and Plano Clark (2007) call this type of integration *merging*.

MM Designs and Interpretive Integration

Interpretive integration is especially common in concurrent MM designs—that is, Triangulation and Embedded Designs. In this approach, quantitative data are analyzed using statistical techniques and qualitative data are analyzed using qualitative analysis methods, both according to standards of excellence for each method. Findings from the two separate analyses are then drawn together in an effort to synthesize the results and to develop an overall interpretation. The focus is on *comparing* the two types of findings, which can involve data conversion or the creation of matrices—methods we describe in a later section. Often, however, the integration is simply at a narrative level and is summarized in the Discussion section of reports.

Interpretive integration can also occur in sequential designs—although such integration is often what Bazely (2009a) called "integration 'on the way'" (p. 92) rather than formal integration at the end of the study. That is, the analysis of one data strand is interpreted and used to inform the design and analysis of the second. An overall interpretive integration of the two strands may occur, but often does not—although opportunities for such global integration in sequential designs are especially rich in MM intervention research (Chapter 26).

Creswell and Plano Clark (2007) noted that in sequential designs, a focus of the first stage analysis is selecting results to use as a basis for scrutiny in the next phase. For example, in Explanatory Designs, the QUAN data are analyzed with an eye toward selecting cases or lines of questioning for the second qual phase. Options include selecting outliers or extreme cases, selecting negative cases, focusing on significant or nonsignificant results for more intensive follow-up, or identifying comparison groups based on key constructs. In Exploratory Designs, the QUAL results may suggest themes to examine (e.g., in an instrument development study) or hypotheses to test in the quan phase.

Bazely (2009a) has described what she called **iterative analysis**, which involves ongoing interpretive feedback loops. Iterative analysis involves "taking what is learned in one stage of a project into a further stage to inform that data collection or analysis, and then on again for refinement or development through one or more subsequent iterations" (p. 109). She offered as an example a study in which a researcher developed a formal instrument based on themes from in-depth phenomenological interviews. The factor analytic results from psychometric testing of the scale were then taken back to the phenomenological data for further thematic exploration.

Nature of Results from Interpretive Integration

Interpretive integration, which focuses on comparisons between the two strands, can result in convergent results, divergent results, or nuanced (qualifying) results. Most researchers consider that an ideal situation occurs when findings from each strand are consistent and shed complementary perspectives on the phenomenon of interest. Yet, many MM scholars have pointed out the critical role that divergent results can play in advancing knowledge. As Green (2007) noted, "Convergence, consistency, and corroboration are overrated in social inquiry. The interactive mixed methods analyst looks just as keenly for instances of divergence and dissonance, as these may represent important nodes for further and highly generative analytic work" (p. 144).

Moffatt and colleagues (2006) suggested possible steps to take when MM findings conflict. Their study involved quantitative data from 126 participants in a clinical trial, and in-depth data from a purposive sample of 25 of them. The quantitative results suggested that the intervention (which was designed to improve health and social outcomes for older people) was not successful, yet the qualitative data suggested wide-ranging improvements. The researchers suggested six ways of further exploring the discrepancy: (1) treating the methods as fundamentally different, (2) examining rigor in the respective strands, (3) exploring dataset comparability, (4) collecting additional data, (5) exploring intervention processes, and (6) exploring whether the outcomes of the two components were really matched. If data conversion has been done, as described next, a seventh strategy might be to re-examine the conversion rules.

Although many MM scholars discuss convergence-divergence of results as a dichotomy, in fact, it is often the case that interpretive integration leads to a nuanced portrayal of the phenomenon because results are neither precisely convergent nor divergent. Thus, although the MM research question often being addressed in interpretive integration is "To what extent do the quantitative and qualitative data converge?" (Creswell & Plano Clark, 2007, p. 106), another important question might be: How do the findings from one strand qualify, delimit, or temper findings from the other?

An example comes from an MM study of one of this book's authors, whose Triangulation Design involved a survey of 4,000 low-income women and ethnographic interviews with 67 women from a parallel sample (Polit et al., 2000). The analyses focused on hunger and food insecurity, and in both samples about half the women were food insecure—results that appeared convergent. Yet, the in-depth interviews revealed that the term "food secure" in low-income urban families may be a mis-leading label: Mothers in the qualitative sample had to *struggle* enormously to be food secure, piecing together with great effort "numerous strategies to make sure that there was an adequate amount of food for themselves and their children" (p. 22). This led the authors to hypothesize that *food security* is achieved in a different manner and is experienced differently among poor and middle-class families—and is perhaps a totally different phenomenon.

Example of interpretive integration: Carr (2008) used an Explanatory Design (QUAN → qual) to study anxiety in women undergoing gyneco-logic surgery. She measured anxiety using a formal scale six times prior to and following surgery. She found that anxiety rose steadily from admission to the point of having surgery. In the in-depth follow-up interviews, conducted with some of the participants a week after discharge, reasons for elevations in anxiety were explored. The integrated findings were used to make improvements to nursing care in the hospital where the study took place.

Converting Quantitative and Qualitative Data

A technique that can be used in analytic and interpretive integration in mixed methods research involves converting data of one type into data of another type. Qualitative data are sometimes converted into numeric codes that can be analyzed quantitatively. It is also possible to transform quantitative data into qualitative information.

➲ **TIP:** Although data conversion is most often described in connection with mixed methods research, it can be used as a technique in mono-method research as well. That is, even if only quantitative data are collected, conversion to qualitative data can occur, and vice versa. The use of quasi-statistics (Chapter 23), for example, involves using qualitative data quantitatively.

Using Quantitative Data Qualitatively

Most data that are analyzed quantitatively actually begin as qualitative data. If we ask participants if they have been severely depressed, moderately depressed, somewhat depressed, or not at all depressed in the previous week, the answers are words, not numbers. The words are transformed through coding into ordi-nal-level categories. Then, the codes are analyzed statistically to assess, for example, what percentage of participants was severely depressed in the prior week, or whether older people are more likely than younger ones to be depressed.

However, it is possible to go back to the data and "read" them qualitatively, a process that is called **qualitizing** data (Sandelowski, 2000; Tashakkori & Teddlie, 1998). For example, an entire survey interview can be read to get a glimpse of the circumstances, problems, and experiences of an individual participant. In such a situation, researchers can create a mini case study designed to "give life" to the patterns emerging in the quantitative analysis, to extract more information from the data, and to aid in interpreting them. A major purpose of qualitizing data, then, is for profiling.

As an example, Polit and colleagues (2001) studied single mothers who were receiving public cash assistance but who were subject to new requirements that compelled them to seek employment. Based on data from survey interviews with thousands of women, the researchers found that health problems of the women and their children were significant barriers to sustained employment. The researchers identified a survey respondent who typified the experiences of those who had employment problems, and prepared this profile:

Example of qualitizing survey data:
"Miranda, a 26-year-old Mexican-American woman from Los Angeles, had had a fairly steady work record until 4 months before we spoke with her, when she had left her job as a bank cashier because her son (age 4) had serious health problems. She also had a 2-year-old daughter and her husband, from whom she was separated, no longer lived nearby to help with child care. The bank job had paid her $210 a week before taxes, without health insurance, sick pay, or paid vacation. At the bank job, she had worked 36 hours a week, working daily from early afternoon until 8 p.m. Although at the time of the interview she was getting cash welfare assistance, food stamps, and SSI (disability) benefits on behalf of her son, her relatively high rent and utility costs (over $700 per month) without housing assistance made it difficult for her to make ends meet, and she reported that she sometimes couldn't afford to feed her children balanced meals" (Polit et al., 2001, p. 2).

The aggregate survey data in this study were used *quantitatively* to describe such things as the percentage of women who left work because of health-related problems. The data were used *qualitatively* (as in the preceding example) to translate statistical findings into what it was like in the lives of actual families.

When qualitizing of this type is done for illustrative purposes, researchers must be clear about what it is they wish to portray. Often, as in the example just cited, the intent is to illustrate a typical case. In such a situation, researchers look for an individual case whose quantitative values are near the average for the entire sample. However, researchers might also want to illustrate ways in which the averages fail to capture important aspects of a problem, in which case atypical (and often extreme) cases are identified to show the limitations of looking just at averages in the quantitative analysis.

➲ **TIP:** In creating such profiles, special care must be taken with regard to the issue of participant confidentiality. In small communities or with people recruited from a specific institution, the amount of detail provided in a profile could result in a confidentiality breach. Even though the data in our example were from a large urban community, a few of the details were slightly altered to minimize risk of identification without losing the flavor of the life stresses in the case.

Sometimes qualitizing is done for *all* cases in a sample, and the profiles are used in the next round of data collection. A good example of this is the study by Bowles and colleagues (2009), who used an array of quantitative data from hospital records and formal instruments (e.g., a depression and functional status scale) to create qualitized case profiles of 208 older hospitalized patients. The profiles were then read by a panel of discharge planning experts who categorized each case as needing or not needing post acute referral. Logistic regression was then used to predict factors affecting the need for such referral.

Using Qualitative Data Quantitatively

Quantitizing (Miles & Huberman, 1994) is the transformation of qualitative data into numerical values. Although some qualitative researchers believe that quantitizing is inappropriate, Sandelowski (2001) argued that some amount of quantitizing is almost inevitable. She noted that every time qualitative researchers use terms such as *a few, some, many,* or *most,* they are implicitly conveying quantitative information about the frequency of occurrence of a theme or pattern. In addition to being inevitable, quantification of qualitative data can sometimes offer distinct benefits. Sandelowski described how this strategy can be used to achieve two important goals:

- *Generating meaning from qualitative data.* If qualitative data are displayed in a quantitative fashion (e.g., by displaying frequencies of certain phenomena), *patterns* sometimes emerge with greater clarity than they might have had the researchers simply relied on their impressions. Tabular displays can also reveal unsuspected patterns that can help in the development of hypotheses.

- *Documenting and confirming conclusions.* The use of numbers can assure people that researchers' conclusions are valid. Researchers can be more confident that the data are fully accounted for if they can document the extent to which emerging patterns were observed—or *not* observed. Sandelowski noted that quantitizing can address some pitfalls of qualitative analysis, which include giving too much weight to dramatic or vivid accounts, giving too little weight to disconfirming cases, and smoothing out variation, to clean up some of the "messiness" of human experience.

In a more recent article, Sandelowski and her colleagues (2009) noted that quantitizing can also serve the critical function of encouraging researchers to think about and interact with their data. They noted that quantitizing, "when used creatively, critically, and reflexively, can show the complexity of qualitative data and, thereby the 'multivariate nature' of the experiential worlds researchers seek to understand" (p. 219). Such higher-level understanding of a phenomenon is an overarching goal of many MM studies.

The conversion of narrative information into quantitative codes can occur in various ways, but in most cases, the resulting quantitized data are nominal or ordinal. Often, for example, qualitative data are coded for presence (1) or absence (0) of a theme, code, or linguistic characteristic. Although this type of coding may seem straightforward, Sandelowski and colleagues (2009) highlighted the critical importance of having sound conceptualizations about what "it" is that is present or absent.

Categorization in a quantitization effort need not be dichotomous. For example, qualitative data could be read with an eye toward characterizing people in terms of three or four different coping styles. In this approach, an entire transcript may form the basis for the coding structure. Ordinal categories are also possible, and can be developed for codes, themes, or entire cases. For example, a theme could be coded as not present, moderately

present, or intensely present within a case. Chang and colleagues (2009) provide additional guidance on how to transform qualitative descriptive information into numbers.

➲ TIP: For many quantitizing procedures, it is important to establish intercoder reliability.

Software for qualitative analysis facilitates certain types of quantitization. The software Max-QDA, for example, allows researchers to weight each code on a scale of 1 to 100, to indicate its significance. Programs can also be used to *count*, which can result in ratio-level data. Many aspects of narrative data can be counted—for example, words, codes, themes, or lines of text. Counting can yield variables that can be used in subsequent MM analyses, and can form the basis for calculating *effect sizes* (Onwuegbuzie & Teddlie, 2003), which are methods of summarizing aspects of qualitative data. Several qualitative effect size indexes will be described in Chapter 27 because of their importance in metasyntheses of multiple qualitative studies.

These various quantitizing strategies can be extremely useful in mixed methods research, but it is important to have a clear rationale and a plan for how the quantitized data will be used analytically. There are many options, but many are only appropriate when identical sampling has been used.

When none of the participants in the qualitative and quantitative samples are the same people (parallel sampling), analytic options are limited primarily to profiling, illustration, or descriptive comparisons. For example, Polit and her colleagues (2000, 2001), in the previously mentioned food insecurity study, administered a structured food insecurity scale to the survey sample. Women in the nonoverlapping ethnographic sample were coded into the three ordinal food security categories (secure, insecure without hunger, and insecure with hunger) based on their detailed narratives about food and nutrition in the in-depth interviews. The researchers were then able to compare the percentage of women in both samples who were food insecure, which enhanced confidence that those in the small ethnographic sample were not atypical. It also allowed us to present rich illustrations of people in the different food security categories.

Example of an illustration using quantitized data: One participant in the ethnographic component was a woman with three small children who, despite receiving public food assistance (Food Stamps), was categorized as food insecure. Data from the ethnography illustrated how food insecurity was actually experienced and managed.

"It was hard, especially when you got kids at home saying, 'I'm hungry.'. . . I was doing very odd jobs that most people would not dare to do. I was making deliveries on pizza in bad neighborhoods where most people wouldn't go. I mean, I literally took my life in my own hands."
(Polit et al., 2001, p. 58).

When identical sampling is used in an MM study, the analytic options are almost limitless, because the quantitized qualitative information can be entered as variables into the database for fully integrated statistical analysis. All types of descriptive analyses can be performed. The quantitized variables can be used as independent variables (e.g., in *t*-tests and chi-square analyses), as covariates (e.g., in multiple regression), or as dependent variables (e.g., in logistic regression). Thus, with identical samples, quantitizing can serve directly in the testing of qualitatively derived hypotheses.

⮞ **TIP:** Bazely (2009a) described how quantitized data can be used in such advanced statistical techniques as factor analysis, cluster analysis, and multidimensional scaling to generate *metathemes* (p. 107).

When nested sampling is used—that is, when only some cases from the quantitative component are included in the qualitative component—researchers can use those cases for whom there is overlap in simple descriptive analyses, such as in a crosstabulation table. Another option is to use the quantitized data in matrices, which are widely used in the analysis of MM data. Both serve the important function of enhancing pattern recognition.

Example of quantitizing qualitative data: Altshuler and colleagues (2009) studied patients whose treatment for colorectal cancer involved a permanent ostomy. Patients completed a measure of quality of life in the survey portion of the study. A subsample of women was then interviewed in-depth about how having an ostomy affected their intimacy and sexuality. In analyzing the qualitative data, the researchers recognized distinct patterns in terms of the supportiveness of the women's husbands or partners, and women were categorized into one of three categories—those receiving positive emotional support, those whose partners withdrew support, and those with a mixture. The quantitized support variable was crosstabulated with quantitative quality of life scale scores, categorized into quartiles.

Constructing Meta-Matrices

A widely used approach to analytic integration involves the use of matrices, which is a good method for identifying patterns and making comparisons across data sources. Matrices are a method that has been advocated for qualitative data analysis (Miles & Huberman, 1994), and the concept has gained great popularity among MM researchers.

In a **meta-matrix**, researchers array information from qualitative and quantitative data sources. In a typical case-by-variable meta-matrix, the rows correspond to cases, that is, to individual participants. Then, for each participant, data from multiple data sources are entered in the columns, so that the analyst can see at a glance such information as scores on psychosocial, comments from open-ended dialogue with participants (e.g., verbatim narratives), hospital record data (e.g., physiologic information), and the researchers' own reflexive comments. A third dimension can be added if, for example, there are multiple sources of data relating to multiple constructs (e.g., depression, pain). A third dimension can also be used if the qualitative and quantitative data have been collected longitudinally.

Patterns of regularities, as well as anomalies, often come to light through detailed inspection of meta-matrices. Their strong advantage is that they allow for fuller exploration of all sources of data

Case	Pseudonym	Age	Sex	Average Hours of Sleep Daily	Current Fatigue Level (VAS score)[a]	Use of Sleep Medi-cation[b]	Fatigue Narrative
1	Anna	57	F	6.0	9	1	I *never* sleep through the night. I usually don't have much trouble falling asleep, but I just can't *stay* asleep. There is never a day when I don't wake up exhausted.
2	Jonathan	45	M	5.5	5	1	I've never really needed all that much sleep. Ever since I was in college, I get by with just a few hours and I feel just fine.
3	Claire	49	F	8.0	2	1	I'm a good sleeper, I can fall asleep anywhere, anytime. So, I get what I need.
4	Rosalind	51	F	7.0	7	2	I sleep just fine, but my husband is an insomniac, and a pain in my neck. When he's awake, he wants me awake, too!
5	Michael	54	M	7.5	6	3	I like my shut-eye. I can't concentrate if I don't get enough. I do what I have to, which usually means going to bed before anyone else and taking sleeping pills.

[a]VAS anchors: 0 = extremely energetic, 10 = extremely tired
[b]Use of medication codes: 1 = Never, 2 = Occasionally, 3 = Regularly

FIGURE 25.3 Fictitious example of a meta-matrix with raw qualitative data.

simultaneously. The construction of a meta-matrix also allows researchers to explore whether statistical conclusions are supported by the qualitative data for individual study participants, and vice versa.

A simplified example of a meta-matrix is presented in Figure 25.3. This example shows only five cases and a handful of variables/constructs, but it illustrates how diverse information can be displayed to facilitate inferences about patterns and relationships. It also suggests, however, that such meta-matrices may not be productive with large samples—although one strategy is to have separate matrices for distinct subgroups within a large sample, such as men and women, or (in this example) those with high or low levels of fatigue. Meta-matrices such as the one portrayed in Figure 25.3 can easily be entered into spreadsheet software, which has important advantages over manual methods—the most important of which is the ability to sort and re-sort the data in efforts to identify patterns.

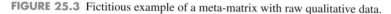 **TIP:** Some qualitative analysis software (e.g., NVivo) has matrix functions.

Meta-matrices can also be used to integrate data and findings after some level of analysis has been accomplished. For example, Figure 25.4 shows a meta-matrix summarizing themes identified from in-depth interviews, according to different subgroups defined on the basis of a response to a structured question.

Example of a study using a meta-matrix:
Wendler (2001) constructed a meta-matrix for her study of the impact of a therapeutic intervention, Tellington touch, on patient anxiety, pain, and physiologic status. She gathered quantitative data on such variables as blood pressure, state anxiety, pain, and nicotine and caffeine use. Participants also responded to open-ended questions. The clinician completed field notes on impressions and participant observers provided field notes on behaviors. The multiple data sources were analyzed quantitatively and qualitatively, and then arrayed in a meta-matrix, which yielded important insights.

Use of Sleep Medication	Themes from In-Depth Interviews		
	The Role of Others	**Health Issues**	**Patterns of Sleep**
Never (n = 12)	• No one in household with sleeping problems • No pets in household	• No special health problems • Avoids *all* medication	• Never a problem falling asleep • Lifelong history of being good sleeper • Despite problems, averse to sleeping aids
Occasionally (n = 13)	• Spouse sleeping problems • Teens coming home late • Pet disturbances	• Stressful job • On a diet causing jitters • Anxiety about upcoming medical procedures/tests	• Problem staying asleep, not falling asleep • Sleeping only a problem if under stress • Frequent napping
Regularly (n = 7)	• Spouse works late or irregular shift • Infant in household • Severely ill family member	• Recent hospitalization • Diagnosed with life-threatening illness • Severely depressed	• Problems arise if medications not taken • Daily battles with insomnia

FIGURE 25.4 Fictitious example of a summary meta-matrix.

Displaying Data in MM Analysis

Meta-matrixes are an important tool for displaying data from multiple sources, but other visual methods exist as well. These display techniques serve a similar function—helping MM analysts to recognize patterns and conceptualize higher-order constructs.

Happ and colleagues' (2006) article is a particularly useful resource for thinking about visual displays in mixed methods research. Their paper included examples of using bar charts to show frequencies of quantitized data, as well as a bar chart that involved showing frequencies of different challenges reported in in-depth interviews according to subgroups formed on the basis of scores from a structured scale.

Another type of display was what Happ and colleagues called a *modified stem leaf plot*. In their example from a study of health locus of control in lung transplant recipients, behaviors that were considered "internality behaviors" from unstructured data sources were listed on one side, and the identification numbers of the lung transplant recipients who exhibited those behaviors were listed on the right. The result was a re-presentation of the qualitative data in a quantitative manner that "provided a visual sense of the proportion of recipients who exhibited the internality behaviors" (p. S46). The display prompted further analyses about commonalities and differences among recipients' behaviors.

Another clever use of visualization involved the construction of a scatterplot. The values along the vertical axis were internality scores, those along the horizontal axis were externality scores. The scatterplot space was divided into quadrants (e.g., high internality, high externality) that corresponded to four profiles of health locus of control beliefs. The identification numbers of individual participants were then plotted in the two-dimensional space. This visual display allowed the researchers to more clearly identify clusterings and "outliers" that were difficult to identify from quantitative analysis alone.

Clearly, data analysis in mixed methods research is ripe with opportunities for creative blending and juxtaposition of data visually, verbally, and statistically.

Meta-Inferences in MM Research

It has been argued that the most important step in mixed methods studies is when the integrated findings from the qualitative and quantitative components are incorporated into an overall conceptualization that effectively answers the overarching mixed methods question (Teddlie & Tashakkori, 2009). To achieve this, *active* interpretation and exploration of the results are required.

In arriving at meta-inferences in an MM study, researchers must actively engage in meaning making. Teddlie and Tashakkori's (2009) suggested that researchers must consider the quality of the inputs (i.e., the quality of the design, the data, the analytic procedures), and the process of meaning making through systematic linking and interpreting of results. Interpretation can be enhanced by allowing the two strands of a study to "talk to each other" in a meaningful, reflexive, and thought-provoking way.

Teddlie and Tashokoori (2009) offered several guidelines for making appropriate inferences at the interpretive stage of an MM study. Their "golden rule" is especially noteworthy: "*Know thy participants*" (p. 289). Mixed methods research offers great potential for getting a rounded picture of the complex lives of human participants.

QUALITY CRITERIA IN MIXED METHODS RESEARCH

It can be argued that mixed methods research offers particularly good opportunities to assess the overall "goodness" of the data. As we noted in Chapter 24, triangulation is a technique that can be used to develop evidence about the trustworthiness and validity of the findings. Triangulation often occurs at the data, investigator, analysis, and theoretical level in MM research—and indeed is often a key reason why such research in undertaken.

Mixed methods scholars who have proposed standards for evaluating the quality of MM studies often avoid terms like *validity* (associated with quantitative quality criteria) and *trustworthiness* (associated with qualitative criteria). It is too early in the development of MM methodology to know what terms will be adopted, but one prominent team of scholars has proposed the terms *inference*

quality and *inference transferability* (Teddlie & Tashakkori, 2003, 2009).

Inference quality is an overarching criterion for evaluating the quality of conclusions and interpretations made on the basis of mixed methods findings. Inference quality incorporates notions of both *internal validity* and *statistical conclusion validity* within a quantitative framework, and *credibility* within a qualitative framework. Inference quality essentially refers to the believability and accuracy of the inductively and deductively derived conclusions from an MM study.

Inference transferability, another umbrella term, encompasses the quantitative term *external validity* and the qualitative term *transferability*. Inference transferability is the degree to which the mixed methods conclusions can be applied to other similar people, context, settings, time periods, and theoretical representations of the phenomenon.

Although mixed methods offers opportunities for triangulation and corroboration, it can be challenging to achieve and demonstrate strong inference quality in MM research because there are three sets of standards that apply: inferences derived from the quantitative component must be judged in terms of standard validity criteria, inferences from the qualitative component must be judged in terms of trustworthiness standards, and the meta-inferences from the two integrated strands must also be evaluated for their soundness. For the first two, methods of enhancing validity and trustworthiness that we have proposed in earlier chapters are relevant in strengthening the quality of MM research.

Teddlie and Tashakkori's (2009) have proposed an **integrative framework for inference quality**. This framework, which incorporates many of the standards from both qualitative and quantitative approaches, encompasses two broad families of criteria for evaluating quality: *design quality* and *interpretive rigor*. These criteria, which can serve as guides for MM researchers as well as for those evaluating an MM report, are briefly described in the next section. Those undertaking an MM study should review the detailed guidance that Teddlie and Tashakkori offer.

With regard to inference transferability, it can be argued that high-quality mixed methods research

BOX 25.1 Guidelines for Critiquing Mixed Methods Studies

1. Did the researcher state an overarching mixed methods (MM) objective that required the integration of qualitative and quantitative approaches? In addition to individual questions that formed the basis for the qualitative or quantitative components, was there an explicit MM question about how the findings of various strands relate to one another?
2. Did the researcher clearly identify the research design? Was MM design notation (or a visual diagram) used to communicate key aspects of the design? If a design was not specified, can you infer what the design was? Was it concurrent or sequential? Which strand (if either) was given priority?
3. Is the design appropriate for the research questions or study objective? Does the design for each component match the requirement for addressing its corresponding question? (*design suitability*)a
4. Do the components of the design fit together in a seamless manner? Are the strands linked logically? Were procedures implemented to enhance rigor and trustworthiness of the various components? (*within-design consistency*)
5. What sampling strategy was used (identical, parallel, nested, multilevel), and was this strategy appropriate? Are the setting, context, and participants adequately described, and are they appropriate for the research question?
6. How were study data gathered? Did the researcher take good advantage of opportunities to triangulate data sources? In sequential designs, did the second phase data collection (and sampling) flow appropriately from the analysis of data from the initial phase?
7. Overall, were the design components and sampling/data collection strategies implemented with the care and rigor needed to fully capture the complex nature of the target phenomenon? (*design fidelity*)
8. Did integration of the strands occur? Was integration at the interpretive or analytic level? Was adequate integration achieved? Do the combined findings suggest richly textured and comprehensive datasets from the respective strands?
9. What specific analytic techniques were used to achieve analytic integration (e.g., were data conversion or meta-matrices used)? Were these techniques adequate? Were visual displays of the data used effectively?
10. Were the analytic or interpretive steps appropriate and sufficient to answer the separate qualitative questions and to achieve integration? (*analytic adequacy*)
11. Are the researcher's meta-inferences consistent with the individual findings? Are the inferences consistent with each other? (*interpretive consistency*)
12. Are the researchers' interpretations consistent with the current state of evidence and theory? (*theoretical consistency*) What was done to assess agreement among team members, peers, or participants regarding the interpretations? Are the inferences consistent with participants' constructions? (*interpretive agreement*)
13. Are inferences and interpretations credible and more plausible than other possible interpretations of the findings? (*interpretive distinctiveness*)
14. Do the meta-inferences adequately encompass and integrate inferences from each strand? If the findings from each strand are conflicting or qualifying, are theoretical explanations for the discrepancies offered, and are they plausible? (*integrative efficacy*)
15. Do the meta-inferences adequately address the stated goals of the study? (*interpretive correspondence*)

---

aThe terms in parentheses correspond to criteria identified by Teddlie and Tashakkori (2009). The questions corresponding to the criteria were adapted from ones they included in their Table 12.5 (pp. 301–302).

has advantages over mono-method research because of its relative strengths in regard to the three models of generalizability discussed in Chapter 21: standard sample-to-population (statistical) generalizability, analytic generalization (conceptual power), and transferability (proximal similarity). Larger and more representative samples in the quantitative strand can promote confidence in the external validity of an MM study. Well-grounded meta-inference based on rich, complementary data sources can enhance analytic generalization. And, rich and diverse descriptive information can promote an understanding of proximal similarities and hence transferability.

CRITIQUING MIXED METHODS RESEARCH

Individual components of mixed methods studies can be critiqued using guidelines we have offered throughout this book. Key critiquing questions for quantitative studies (Box 5.2) and qualitative studies (Box 5.3) were presented in Chapter 5.

Box 25.1 ⊗ offers supplementary questions that are explicitly about the integration of methods in MM studies. Many of these questions were derived from Teddlie and Tashakkori's (2009) integrative framework for inference quality that encompasses design quality and interpretive rigor. Their criteria with regard to *design quality* are design suitability, design fidelity, within-design consistency, and analytic adequacy. Criteria with regard to *interpretive rigor* are interpretive consistency, theoretical consistency, interpretive agreement, interpretive distinctiveness, integrative efficacy, and interpretive correspondence. These criteria are shown in parentheses next to the relevant questions in Box 25.1. The overarching consideration in MM studies is whether true integration occurred and contributed to strong meta-inferences about the phenomenon under scrutiny.

⊃ **TIP:** In evaluating the strengths and weaknesses of mono-method (qualitative or quantitative) studies, it is worth asking whether a mixed methods approach would have enhanced the conclusions.

RESEARCH EXAMPLES OF MIXED METHODS STUDIES

In this section, we summarize two mixed methods studies, one using a concurrent design and the other using a sequential design.

Example of a Concurrent Design

Study: Adaptation, postpartum concerns, and learning needs in the first two weeks after caesarean birth (Weiss et al., 2009).

Statement of Purpose: The purpose of this study was to describe women's adaptation (physical, emotional, functional, and social), their postpartum concerns, and their learning needs in the first 2 weeks after cesarean birth, and to identify relevant nursing interventions. The qualitative portion of the study, which was guided by Roy's Adaptation Model, focused on the women's adaptation. The quantitative strand explored associations between type of cesarean birth (planned or unplanned) and ethnicity, and women's adaptation responses, postpartum concerns, and learning needs.

Methods: A concurrent Triangulation Design (QUAL + QUAN) was used. Qualitative and quantitative data were obtained from an identical sample of 233 culturally diverse women delivering by cesarean birth in two urban areas of the United States. Students who had been involved in the mothers' in-hospital care collected the study data either in a postdischarge home visit or by telephone. The interview included open-ended questions that focused on four modes of adaptation. For example, the physical adaptation question was: "How have you been feeling physically since you went home from the hospital?" (p. 2942). Responses were recorded verbatim. Participants also completed structured scales on maternal concerns and infant care knowledge and learning needs.

Data Analysis and Integration: Responses to the open-ended questions were categorized as either adaptive or ineffective, with words or phrases as the unit of analysis, and then further quantitized after intercoder reliability was established. For each of the four adaptation modes, adaptation scores were calculated by dividing the number of adaptive responses by the total of all responses (adaptive and ineffective) and multiplying by 100, to yield a score from 0 to 100 that represented the proportion of all adaptive responses. Also, based on the various qualitative and quantitative data sources, the nursing students identified priority areas of problems or needs, and then recommended a nursing intervention. The quantitative data from both the qualitative and quantitative strands of the study were tabulated, and subjected to various statistical analyses, such as *t*-tests and ANOVA, that compared adaptation and learning needs for different groups based on parity, ethnicity, and cesarean type.

Key Findings: Functional and social adaptation were found to be higher than physical or emotional adaptation. Adaptation was higher among the women with planned cesarean deliveries and among multiparas. There were also cultural differences with regard to adaptation, concerns, and learning needs. The nursing students identified a total of 676 actual and potential problems or needs.

Example of a Sequential Design

Study: Strategies used by rural women to stop, avoid, or escape from intimate partner violence (Riddell et al., 2009).

Statement of Purpose: The researchers stated three purposes: (a) to describe strategies, and their perceived effectiveness, that rural women use to stop, avoid, or escape from intimate partner violence (IPV); (b) to explore whether strategies vary by severity of abuse and women's background characteristics; and (c) to understand ways in which the rural culture affects the women's efforts to deal with IPV.

Methods: The researchers used a sequential Explanatory Design (QUAN → qual). The report included a helpful visual diagram that showed the design, data collection, and analytic procedures and products of each phase. Phase I involved the collection of structured self-report data from in-person interviews, as well as biophysical measures, from 43 women who had recently left abusive partners and who lived in a rural area. In Phase II, a parallel sample of 9 women who met the same inclusion criteria was recruited for in-depth interviews. The interviews, which lasted 60 to 90 minutes, probed the women's experiences with IPV.

Data Analysis and Integration: Data from Phase I were analyzed using descriptive and basic inferential statistics, with an eye to identifying the frequency and

helpfulness of various strategies that women experiencing IPV had used. Key findings were presented to women in the second phase, to elicit their interpretation of the findings. The in-depth interviews, which also explored the women's perceptions of the impact of the rural context and culture on efforts to stop or escape from their partners, were analyzed thematically. The researchers used the data from both phases to produce an interpretive description of rural women's experiences of dealing with IPV.

Key Findings: The most frequently used strategies, which involved placating and resistance, were rated as least helpful in dealing with IPV. Feelings of self-blame for causing the abuse were reinforced by others in their communities, whose patriarchal attitudes condoned men's domination of women. The rural location, with physical isolation and long distance from help, figured prominently in strategies of dealing with IPV.

SUMMARY POINTS

- **Mixed methods research** is research involving the collection, analysis, and integration of both qualitative and quantitative data within a study or series of studies, often with an overarching goal of achieving both discovery and verification.
- Mixed methods (MM) research has numerous advantages, including the complementarity of qualitative and quantitative data and the practicality of using methods that best address a question. MM research has many applications, including the development and testing of instruments, theories, and interventions.
- The paradigm most often associated with MM research is **pragmatism**, which has as a major tenet "the dictatorship of the research question."
- MM studies involve asking at least two questions that require different types of data, but high-quality MM research also asks integrative questions that focus on linking the two strands.
- Key decisions in designing an MM study involve how to sequence the components, which strand (if either) will be given priority, and how to integrate the two strands.
- In terms of sequencing, MM designs are either **concurrent designs** (both strands occurring in

one simultaneous phase) or **sequential designs** (one strand occurring prior to and informing the second strand).

- Notation for MM research often designates both priority—all capital letters for the dominant strand and all lower-case letters for the nondominant strand—and sequence. An arrow is used for sequential designs, and a "+" is used for concurrent designs. Parentheses can be used to show an embedded structure. QUAL → quan, for example, is a sequential, qualitative-dominant design; QUAN(qual) shows a qualitative component embedded within a quantitative study.
- Specific MM designs in the Creswell–Plano Clark taxonomy include the **Triangulation Design** (QUAL + QUAN), **Embedded Design** (QUAL[quan] or QUAN[qual]), **Explanatory Design** (QUAN → qual or quan → QUAL), and **Exploratory Design** (QUAL → quan or qual → QUAN). In reality, complex designs are often adopted in a creative, emergent fashion.
- Sampling strategies can be described as **identical** (the same participants are in both strands), **nested** (some of the participants from one strand are in the other strand); **parallel** (participants are either in one strand or the other, but drawn from a similar population), or **multilevel** (participants are not the same, and are drawn from different populations at different levels in a hierarchy).
- Data collection in MM research can involve all methods of structured and unstructured data. In sequential designs, decisions about data collection for the second phase are based on findings from the first phase.
- Data analysis in MM research should involve integration of the strands, to arrive at **meta-inferences** about the phenomenon under study. Integration often occurs at the interpretive level, after separate analyses have been completed. A focus in such integrations is often to assess congruence and to explore complementarity.
- Methods of integration of qualitative and quantitative data during analysis include *data conversions*, such as the **qualitizing** of quantitative data or the **quantitizing** of qualitative data, and

the use of **meta-matrices** in which both qualitative and quantitative data are arrayed in a spreadsheet-type matrix.

- Criteria that have been proposed for enhancing the integrity of MM studies include **inference quality** (the believability and accuracy of inductively and deductively derived conclusions) and **inference transferability** (the degree to which conclusions can be applied to other similar people or contexts).
- Two families of criteria in Teddlie and Tashakkori's **integrative framework for inference quality** are *design quality* and *interpretive rigor.*

STUDY ACTIVITIES

Chapter 25 of the *Resource Manual for Nursing Research: Generating and Assessing Evidence for Nursing Practice*, 9th edition, offers exercises and study suggestions for reinforcing concepts presented in this chapter. In addition, the following study questions can be addressed:

1. Look at the list of questions in Table 25.1. Add to the list of questions for several types of research design.
2. Use the criteria in Box 25.1 to assess one of the studies used at the end of the chapter, referring to the original article for full details.

STUDIES CITED IN CHAPTER 25

Altshuler, A., Ramirez, M., Grant, M., Wendel, C., Hornbrook, M., Herrinton, L., & Krouse, R. (2009). The influence of husbands' or male partners' support on women's psychosocial adjustment to having an ostomy resulting from colorectal cancer. *Journal of Wound, Ostomy, & Continence Nursing, 36*, 299–305.

Beck, C. T., & Gable, R. K. (2000). Postpartum Depression Screening Scale: Development and psychometric testing. *Nursing Research, 49*, 272–282.

Beck, C. T., & Gable, R. K. (2001). Ensuring content validity: An illustration of the process. *Journal of Nursing Measurement, 9*, 201–215.

Beck, S., Towsley, G., Caserta, M., Lindau, K., & Dudley, W. (2009). Symptom experiences and quality of life of rural and urban older adult cancer survivors. *Cancer Nursing, 32,* 359–369.

Bowles, K., Holmes, J., Ratcliffe, S., Liberatore, M., Nydick, R., & Nayloe, M. (2009). Factors identified by experts to support decision making for post acute referral. *Nursing Research, 58,* 115–122.

Carr, E. (2008). Understanding inadequate pain management in the clinical setting: The value of the sequential explanatory mixed methods study. *Journal of Clinical Nursing, 18,* 124–131.

Gibbons, S. W. (2009). Theory synthesis for self-neglect: A health and social phenomenon. *Nursing Research, 58,* 194–200.

Grant, S., St. John, W., & Patterson, E. (2009). Recovery from total hip replacement surgery: "It's not just physical." *Qualitative Health Research, 19,* 1612–1620.

Hodges, P. (2009). Factors impinging readmissions of older patients with heart failure. *Critical Care Nursing Quarterly, 32,* 33–43.

Jurgens, C., Hoke, L., Byrnes, J., & Riegel, B. (2009). Why do elders delay responding to heart failure symptoms? *Nursing Research, 58,* 274–282.

Kalisch, B., & Williams, R. (2009). Development and psychometric testing of a tool to measure missed nursing care. *Journal of Nursing Administration, 39,* 211–219.

Manuel, J., Burwell, S., Crawford, S., Lawrence, R., Farmer, D., Hege, A., Phillips, K., & Avis, N. E. (2007). Younger women's perceptions of coping with breast cancer. *Cancer Nursing, 30,* 85–94.

Polit, D. F., London, A. S., & Martinez, J. M. (2000). *Food security and hunger in poor, mother-headed families in four U. S. cities.* New York: MDRC (available at *www.mdrc.org*).

Polit, D. F., London, A. S., & Martinez, J. M. (2001). *The health of poor urban women.* New York: MDRC (available at *www.mdrc.org*).

Polit, D. F., Widom, R., & Edin, K. (2001). *Is work enough: Experiences of current and former welfare mothers who work.* New York: MDRC (available at *www.mdrc.org*).

Reutter, L., Stewart, M., Veenstra, G., Love, R., Raphael, D., & Makwarimba, E. (2009). "Who do they think we are, anyway?" Perceptions of and responses to poverty stigma. *Qualitative Health Research, 19,* 297–311.

Riddell, T., Ford-Gilboe, M., & Leipert, B. (2009). Strategies used by rural women to stop, avoid, or escape from intimate partner violence. *Health Care for Women International, 30,* 134–159.

Sevelius, J. (2009). "There's no pamphlet for the kind of sex I have": HIV-related risk factors and protective behaviors among transgender men who have sex with nontransgender men. *Journal of the Association of Nurses in AIDS Care, 20,* 398–410.

Thomas, L. A. (2009). Effective dyspnea management strategies identified by elders with end-stage chronic obstructive pulmonary disease. *Applied Nursing Research, 22,* 79–85.

Weiss, M., Fawcett, J., & Aber, C. (2009). Adaptation, postpartum concerns, and learning needs in the first two weeks after caesarean birth. *Journal of Clinical Nursing, 18,* 2938–2948.

Wells, J., Cagle, C., Marshall, D., & Hollen, M. (2009). Perceived mood, health, and burden in female Mexican American family cancer caregivers. *Health Care for Women International, 30,* 629–654.

Wendler, M. C. (2001). Triangulation using a meta-matrix. *Journal of Advanced Nursing, 35,* 521–525.

Whittemore, R., Grey, M., Lindemann, E., Ambrosino, J., & Jaser, S. (2010). Development of an Internet coping skills training program for teenagers with Type 1 diabetes. *Computers, Informatics, Nursing, 28,* 103–111.

Wuest, J., Hodgins, M., Malcolm, J., Merritt-Gray, M., & Seamon, P. (2007). The effects of past relationship and obligation on health and health promotion in women caregivers of adult family members. *Advances in Nursing Science, 30,* 206–220.

Methodologic and nonresearch references cited in this chapter can be found in a separate section at the end of the book.

26 Developing Complex Nursing Interventions Using Mixed Methods Research

T his chapter discusses research-based efforts to develop innovative nursing interventions. Historically, there has been considerably more guidance on how to test and evaluate interventions in clinical trials than on how to develop them, but that situation is changing. There is a growing recognition that new interventions should be based on solid research evidence and strong conceptualizations of the problem and potential solutions. There is also an emerging consensus that mixed methods research is required in such endeavors.

NURSING INTERVENTION RESEARCH

We have discussed interventions in many chapters of this book. Chapters 9 and 10 discussed designs and strategies for rigorously testing interventions. We described clinical trials and evaluations, both of which involve interventions, in Chapter 11. Yet, the term *intervention research* is increasingly being used by nurse researchers to describe a research approach distinguished not so much by its research methods as by a distinctive *process* of developing, implementing, testing, and disseminating interventions (e.g., Sidani & Braden, 1998; Whittemore & Grey, 2002). Naylor (2003)

defined **nursing intervention research** as "as studies either questioning existing care practices or testing innovations in care that are shaped by nursing's values and goals, guided by a strong theoretical basis, informed by recent advances in science, and designed to improve the quality of care and health of individuals, families, communities, and society" (p. 382).

Some nursing interventions are fairly simple and do not require extensive development. For example, Schultz and colleagues (2008) undertook a randomized controlled trial (RCT) to evaluate the effectiveness of using gel pillows, versus usual care on a standard mattress, for reducing bilateral head flattening in preterm infants. The intervention was "relatively simple" (p. 191), and the research team did not develop the product. Many nursing interventions that are currently being tested, however, are complex and designed by nurses themselves.

Complex Interventions

The term **complex intervention** has become a buzzword in research circles, and has been the topic of several articles in the nursing literature (e.g., Thompson, 2004; Seers, 2007; Blackwood, 2006). We begin, then, by discussing what the term means.

The Medical Research Council (MRC) in the United Kingdom proposed a highly influential framework for developing and testing complex interventions, and we describe that framework in the next section. According to the MRC report, complexity in an intervention can arise along several dimensions, including the following:

- The number of different components within the intervention ("bundling") and interactions between the components
- The number of different behaviors required by those delivering or receiving the intervention and the difficulty level of those behaviors
- The number of different groups or organizational levels targeted by the intervention
- The number and diversity of intervention outcomes targeted
- The degree to which the intervention can be tailored to individual patients (Craig et al., 2008a, 2008b).

Other dimensions can also contribute to complexity. For example, interventions that unfold over, say, 3 months are likely to be far more complex than those that can be administered in 30 minutes. Also, 10-session interventions are more complex than ones with a single session. Another complexity dimension concerns the number of different types of *intervention agents* needed to implement it (e.g., nurses, family members, other healthcare staff).

Complexity in interventions clearly exists along a continuum rather than as a dichotomy. There is no single point at which a simple intervention becomes complex. There is a wide range of possible complexities, and many nursing interventions are complex along more than one of the dimensions identified in the MRC model. The more complex the intervention, though, the stronger is the need for an intervention framework.

➲ **TIP:** Complex interventions are likely to be needed when complex problems are being treated, when a conceptual framework suggests multidimensional mediating forces, and when prior research suggests that simple interventions have little effect on reducing a problem.

Frameworks for Developing and Testing Complex Interventions

Proponents of using a framework to guide the intervention development and testing process are critical of the rather simplistic and atheoretical approach that has often been used with nursing interventions. The recommended process for intervention research involves an in-depth understanding of the problem and the people for whom the intervention is being developed; careful, collaborative planning with a diverse team; and the development of an intervention theory to guide the inquiry. These recommendations suggest a systematic and progressive sequence that requires a long investment of time to "get it right," and that places evidence-based developmental work at a premium.

Several intervention frameworks have been proposed, and they are similar in many respects. The most prominent to date is the original Medical Research Council framework, which appeared in the literature in 2000 (Campbell et al., 2000; Medical Research Council [MRC], 2000) and has been cited in hundreds of intervention reports in the healthcare literature.

Figure 26.1 shows that the original MRC framework was conceptualized as a 5-phase process in which a continuum of evidence is pursued. In Phase 0, which corresponds to what was called the *preclinical phase*, the focus is on developing a theoretical rationale for the intervention. Phase I, the *modeling phase*, involves achieving an understanding of the underlying mechanisms by which the components of the intervention will work in influencing the outcomes of interest. In practice, Phases 0 and I are often combined. In Phase II, the intervention protocol is piloted in an exploratory trial. Phase III corresponds to a full, rigorous test of the intervention's effects, most often using a randomized design. As noted in Chapter 11, this phase is often referred to as efficacy research, with a focus on understanding possible intervention effects under controlled conditions. Phase IV of the MRC framework involves tests of whether the intervention can be reliably replicated under more usual conditions (effectiveness research).

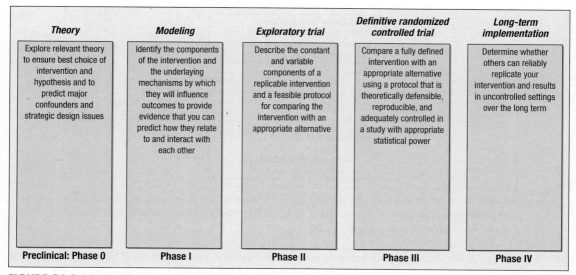

FIGURE 26.1 Medical Research Council's original framework for developing and testing complex healthcare interventions. (Adapted from Campbell, et al. [2000]. Framework for design and evaluation of complex interventions to improve health. *BMJ, 321.*)

The original MRC framework is similar in some regards to the four-phase sequence delineated by the National Institutes of Health for clinical trials, as we described in Chapter 11: (1) basic development, (2) pilot testing, (3) efficacy research, and (4) effectiveness research. Whittemore and Grey (2002) elaborated on the NIH model and proposed a fifth phase involving widespread implementation and efforts to document effects on public health. Another 4-phase model developed by nurses in the Netherlands emphasized the importance of strong development work and pilot testing (van Meijel et al., 2004).

In 2008, the MRC published a revised framework, which reflects suggestions made by many critics who thought the process outlined in the original was too linear. Figure 26.2 shows that the new MRC framework consists of a set of four interconnected "elements" of the intervention development and evaluation process: (1) development, (2) feasibility and piloting, (3) implementation, and (4) evaluation. Although these elements are not connected in a linear, nor even in a cyclical fashion,

Craig and colleagues (2008a) noted that it is often "useful to think in terms of stages" (p. 8).

Although we agree that intervention research does not always progress in a straight line, we think that an idealized, progressive framework of development (Phase 1), pilot testing (Phase 2), and rigorous testing (Phase 3) works reasonably well for describing broad processes in nursing intervention research. In both the old and new MRC framework, as well as in ones proposed by nurse researchers (Whittemore & Grey, 2002; van Meijel et al., 2004), there is consensus that mixed methods research is required.

Challenges in Developing Complex Interventions

Even with a good framework, those embarking on a path of intervention development and testing should recognize that the challenges are enormous—but that the work is vastly satisfying in the long run. Understanding some of the challenges might clarify the importance of thorough, creative,

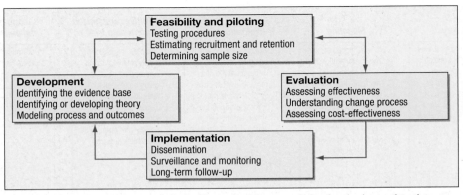

FIGURE 26.2 Medical Research Council's revised framework for developing and testing complex healthcare interventions. (From Craig, et al. [2008]. *Developing and evaluating complex interventions: New guidance.* London: MRC)

and collaborative work during the developmental phase.

A key reason that intervention development is challenging is that *human beings* are involved—as intervention agents, intervention beneficiaries, gatekeepers, and administrators and policy makers making decisions about adoption. Of special importance, clinical researchers have to address the needs, perspectives, and constraints of the people they are trying to help. Clients may not see the need for the intervention, may not like its content or format, may not want to participate in a study, may not want to be randomized, may not like or adhere to the intervention, may drop out of the study, and may not understand what is expected of them. Table 26.1 identifies some of the common "pitfalls" of intervention research, along with causes and contributors that have been found in several intervention studies.

Resistance to the intervention, or to a trial, might also come from other stakeholders, such as family members or advocates. Intervention agents or other healthcare staff also may undermine the intervention or the study. They may resist doing something differently, may disagree with the need to test an innovation, may not pay attention to the training, may make mistakes, may believe that everyone should get the intervention, may communicate their expectations to clients, and so on. Table 26.2 identifies some "pitfalls" associated with

intervention agents that have been found in development studies and pilot tests of interventions.

The point is not that intervention developers should give up their efforts to improve health outcomes. The point is that it is important to understand that a lot of things *can* go wrong, and so strategies should be designed to prevent them from happening to the extent possible.

TIP: Despite the challenges, in many ways the time is ripe for designing nursing interventions. Funders are increasingly sensitive to the need for strong development work, and evidence-based interventions are in high demand. A prominent nurse researcher asked her audience during a keynote address to a nursing research society: "If you are not doing nursing intervention research, why not? If not now, when?" (Conn, 2005, p. 249).

Ideal Features of a Nursing Intervention

Nursing interventions are developed to achieve beneficial effects and to lead to improvements in health outcomes. Before embarking on an intervention development project, nurse researchers should carefully consider the relative importance of achieving certain overall goals.

Box 26.1 identifies features that may be considered "ideal" for nursing interventions—although in any situation some features would be more important than others. In some cases, the desirable

TABLE 26.1	Common "Pitfalls" in Intervention Research: Clients and Study Participants[a]
PITFALL	**CAUSES/CONTRIBUTORS**
Clients who do not want to receive the intervention or participate in research	Lack of trust; language barriers; resistance by family gatekeepers; inadequate time; practical constraints (e.g., child care, transportation); health problems; lack of incentive; concerns about invasion of privacy; lack of "match" between clients' goals and researchers' goals
Clients who do not want to be randomized	Lack of trust; fear of experimentation; strong preference for one treatment condition or the other; resistance to not being "in control"
Clients who do not adhere to protocols (e.g., poor attendance, lack of attention)	Lack of incentive; lack of time or competing demands; concerns about the intervention; scheduling conflicts; material not engaging or understandable; agents not sufficiently persuasive; poor communication about scheduling
Participants who drop out of the study	Lack of incentive; lack of time or competing demands; health problems; transportation or child care problems; intervention material not engaging or understandable; boredom with treatment or with data collection; perceived irrelevance of assessment measures; inadequate attention or concerns about lack of special treatment (control group)
Inadequate enactment of intervention behaviors in real-life settings (e.g., at home)	Lack of incentive; lack of time or competing demands; lack of conviction about efficacy of intervention; inadequate support for continuation; inadequate "rehearsal" of behaviors; resistance to changing normal routines; family or peer opposition

[a]Pitfalls and contributing factors were compiled from various sources, including Pruit & Privette (2001); Rowlands et al. (2005); Whittemore & Grey (2002).

features compete with one another—for example, cost and efficacy often involve trade-offs. Indeed, most of the ideals could plausibly be achieved if cost were not an issue.

Yet, practical issues *are* always an important consideration. Especially in this time of heightened consciousness about healthcare costs, the intervention should be one that has potential to be cost effective. In designing new ways to address health needs, nurse researchers should give upfront thought to whether the intervention is feasible from a resource perspective in real-world settings. When resources are scarce, as they usually are, some of the ideals in Box 26.1 may need to be relaxed, but this should be a conscious decision and not left to serendipity.

One ideal feature that should never be relaxed, of course, is the first one on the list—having an intervention that addresses a pressing problem. When such problems arise in clinical settings, other ideals such as acceptability and feasibility are likely to be more easily attained.

PHASE 1: INTERVENTION DEVELOPMENT

The best current practice, according to the various intervention frameworks described earlier, is to develop interventions in a systematic fashion, using (or creating) good evidence and an appropriate theory of how the intervention would achieve

TABLE 26.2	Common "Pitfalls" in Intervention Research: Agents Delivering the Intervention[a]
PITFALL	**CAUSES/CONTRIBUTORS**
Staff who do not want to recruit participants	Inadequate time; lack of interest; low salience of problem; misgivings about the intervention or about research more generally; inadequate incentive to cooperate
Intervention agents who do not adhere to protocols (includes deliberate nonadherence, inadvertent nonadherence, and noncompetent delivery)	Inadequate time; lack of interest; low salience of problem; strong commitment to the status quo; inadequate training; inadequate incentive to change
Intervention agents who offer intervention to control group members ("contamination")	Commitment to or belief in efficacy of intervention; confusion or inadequate training; inability to "forget" intervention protocols when caring for nonintervention patients

[a]Pitfalls and contributing factors were compiled from various sources, including Kearney & Simonelli (2006); Mahoney et al. (2006); McGuire et al. (2000).

desired effects. In other words, interventions should be evidence-based from the start, and this can require extensive and diverse types of foundational work.

Each phase in the intervention development and testing process can be thought of as having three aspects: (1) key *issues* that must be addressed during this stage, (2) *actions* and strategies that can be brought to bear on those issues, and (3) the *products* that pave the way for movement onto the next phase. Table 26.3 summarizes Phase 1 issues, actions, and products.

BOX 26.1 Features of an "Ideal" Nursing Intervention

An ideal clinical intervention would be:

- **Salient**—addresses a pressing problem
- **Efficacious**—leads to improved client outcomes
- **Safe**—avoids any adverse outcomes, burdens, or stress
- **Conceptually sound**—has a theoretical underpinning
- **Cost effective**—is affordable and has economic benefits to clients or society
- **Feasible**—can be implemented in real-world settings and integrated into current models of care
- **Developmentally appropriate**—is suitable for the age group for whom it is intended
- **Culturally sensitive**—demonstrates sensitivity to various groups
- **Accessible**—can be easily accessed by the people for whom it is intended
- **Acceptable**—is viewed positively by clients and other stakeholders, including family members, nurses, physicians, administrators, policy makers
- **Adaptable**—can be tailored to local contexts
- **Readily disseminated**—can be sufficiently described and packaged for adoption in other locales

TABLE 26.3	Key Issues, Activities, and Products of Phase I Developmental Work for Nursing Interventions	
KEY ISSUES	**MAJOR ACTIVITIES**	**PRODUCTS AND OUTCOMES**
• Conceptualization of the problem • Conceptualization of solutions, strategies, and outcomes • Construct validity of the intervention • Articulation of an evidence base for the intervention • Identification of potential pitfalls within the implementation context • Cultivation of relationships	• Critical synthesis of the relevant literature • Concept and theory development • Exploratory and descriptive research • Consultation with experts • Brainstorming with colleagues, team building, partnerships with stakeholders • Building the intervention	• Delineation of an intervention theory • Preliminary development of the content, intensity, dose, timing, setting, and delivery method of the intervention • Preliminary identification of key outcomes • Strategies to overcome pitfalls in implementing and testing the intervention • A design for a pilot study • A plan for sponsorship of the pilot study

Key Issues in Intervention Development

Conceptualization and in-depth understanding of the problem are key issues during Phase 1. The starting point is the problem itself, which must be understood within the context where the intervention will be tested. In Chapter 5, we discussed how those doing a literature review must "own" the literature. When it comes to intervention development, researchers must "own" the problem. A thorough understanding of the target group—their needs, fears, preferences, constraints, and circumstances—is part of that ownership. It is only through such understanding that researchers can know whether the pitfalls shown in Table 26.1 are relevant in their own situation, and whether other pitfalls are likely to surface.

Thorough knowledge of the people for whom the intervention is intended can also clarify how far from the "ideal" (see Box 26.1) preliminary intervention ideas are likely to be. Awareness of patient preferences, for example, could provide insight into how acceptable an intervention would be (Sidani, et al., 2006). Moreover, patient preferences and needs are sometimes incorporated into the design of tailored or individualized interventions (Lauver et al., 2002).

Another development issue involves identifying key *stakeholders*—people who have a stake in the intervention—and getting them "on board." Interventions sometimes fail because researchers have not developed the relationships needed to ensure that the intervention will be given a fair test. Who the key stakeholders are varies from project to project. In addition to the target group, stakeholders might include family members, advocates, community leaders, service providers in multiple disciplines, intervention agents, healthcare administrators, support staff in intervention settings, and content experts. Buckwalter and colleagues (2009) advised that, "Investigators should think broadly about whose support could affect their ability to conduct the planned research" (p. 118).

Relationship building can contribute to the content of the intervention itself, because stakeholders can offer insight into the scope and depth of the problem. Relationships with stakeholders are also important because researchers must figure out not only *what* to deliver, but also *how* to deliver it in a manner that will gain the support of administrators and healthcare staff, appeal to the target group, enhance recruitment and retention of participants, and strengthen intervention fidelity in later phases.

Activities and Strategies in Intervention Development

Developmental issues can be addressed through a variety of activities, which may require several years before proceeding to a pilot test. We discuss several of them in this section. The vital importance of adequate development cannot be overemphasized.

Review of Relevant Literature

Developmental work often begins with intensive and extensive scrutiny of the literature. In intervention studies, the literature needs to be searched for guidance about the content and mechanisms of the intervention—for its active ingredients. Systematic reviews may be available for evidence about the efficacy of specific strategies, but it may also be necessary to undertake a new or updated review or meta-analysis (see Chapter 27).

Researchers' efforts to understand the problem and possible solutions are an important, but not exhaustive, part of a literature review effort. Table 26.4 provides examples of other questions that should be addressed through a scrutiny of existing evidence during the intervention development phase. When relevant literature is thin or cannot be located, other sources will need to be pursued.

Example of a literature review in nursing intervention research: Morrison-Beedy and colleagues (2009) did a pilot study of an HIV-prevention intervention for abstinent adolescent girls. They undertook extensive developmental work, including a detailed analysis of the "state of the science" in a systematic review (Morrison-Beedy & Nelson, 2004).

➲ **TIP:** Conn and colleagues (2001), in their useful article on intervention design, noted the importance of looking at both published and unpublished literature for guidance on how to design interventions. Strategies for searching the "grey literature" are discussed in Chapter 27.

Intervention Theory Development

A critical activity in the development phase is to delineate a strong conceptual basis for the intervention (Craig et al., 2008a, 2008b; MRC, 2000). The construct validity of the intervention is enhanced through efforts to develop an **intervention theory** that clearly articulates what must be done to achieve desired outcomes. In other words, the intervention theory provides a theoretical rationale for why an intervention should "work." The theory indicates, based on the best available knowledge, the nature of the clinical intervention and factors that would mediate the effects of clinical procedures on expected outcomes.

The intervention theory can be an existing one that has been well-validated. Examples of theories that have been used in many nursing intervention studies include Social Cognitive Theory, the Health Promotion Model, the Transtheoretical Model, the Health Belief Model, and the Theory of Planned Behavior (see Chapter 6). These theories provide guidance on how to fashion an intervention because they propose mechanisms to explain human behavior and behavioral change.

Intervention theories can also be developed from qualitatively derived theory, a point made most eloquently by Morse (2006a). Morse and colleagues (2000) also developed a strategy called qualitative outcome analysis (QOA), which is a process for extending the findings of a qualitative study by identifying intervention strategies related to the phenomenon of concern.

Researchers may find it most productive to develop their own evidence-based model that purports to explain the link between the causes of a problem and unfavorable outcomes. A fully worked out example concerning humor as an intervention was presented in Chapter 6. A conceptual map, such as the one we presented in Figure 6.2, can be a useful visual tool for articulating the intervention theory and can serve as a "road map" for designing and testing the intervention, as well as the counterfactual (control condition). Sidani and Braden (1998) have offered useful guidance about components of an intervention theory. Also, Keller and

TABLE 26.4	Examples of Literature Review Questions for Designing an Evidence-Based Intervention

ISSUE	QUESTIONS FOR WHICH EVIDENCE CAN BE SOUGHT IN A LITERATURE REVIEW
Conceptualizing the problem	What is known about the nature and causes of this problem and possible solutions? What theories help to explain the problem? What are key mediators in the pathway between the causes or contributing factors and the outcomes?
Focusing the target group	What have been the targets of efforts to address the problem—individuals? families? healthcare providers? healthcare systems? What populations appear to be most amenable to the intervention?
Developing intervention content and components	What is the content of other similar interventions? Is the presence of certain types of components linked to better outcomes? Are interventions general or individualized?
Selecting outcomes and assessment strategies	What behaviors or outcomes have been targeted by similar interventions? Have the interventions had significant effects on these outcomes? Have they affected key mediators? What assessment approaches and measures have been used with other similar interventions?
Making decisions about dose	How intense have other similar interventions been? Has dose been found to be related to outcomes?
Making decisions about timing of intervention	When are interventions of this type typically delivered? Is timing related to outcomes?
Making decision about mode of delivery	How have similar interventions been delivered? In face-to-face situations (group or individual delivery)? By telephone? Internet? Video? Is there evidence that different delivery modes are especially effective?
Making decisions about timing of outcome measurement	When have data for this type of intervention typically been collected? Does the literature suggest that effects deteriorate? Or, are there delayed effects?
Making decisions about settings and agents	Where (in what types of settings) have interventions of this type been delivered? Do impacts vary by type of setting? Who usually delivers them? Do outcomes vary by type of agent?
Assessing acceptability of the intervention	Is there evidence of strong (or weak) rates of participation in interventions of this type? Have recruitment or retention problems been reported?
Assessing cultural appropriateness	Is there evidence that cultural issues affect implementation of similar interventions? Is there cultural variation in outcomes?

colleagues (2009) have provided guidelines for assessing fidelity to theory in intervention studies.

> **Example of qualitatively derived intervention theory:** Harvey Chochinov and other researchers (including nurse researchers) developed a theory of dignity based on in-depth interviews with hospice patients. The theory formed the basis for a brief intervention (Dignity Therapy) to promote dignity and reduce stress at the end of life. Hall, Chochinov, and colleagues (2009) conducted a pilot test of the acceptability, feasibility, and potential effectiveness of the intervention.

Exploratory and Descriptive Research

Most researchers find that evidence from the literature is insufficient to satisfactorily address the questions suggested in Table 26.4. A literature review is particularly deficient for illuminating local contexts and specific target groups. Almost inevitably, the developmental phase involves exploratory and descriptive research, often using mixed methods. Qualitative studies are virtually essential to the success of well-founded intervention development efforts, a position articulated in all the intervention frameworks described earlier.

A widely endorsed view is that client groups are central to designing effective nursing interventions (e.g., Gamel et al., 2001; Gross & Fogg, 2001; Pruitt & Privette, 2001). Efforts to design acceptable and efficacious interventions require understanding people's perspective on the problem. Examples of the kinds of questions that could be pursued in exploratory research with clients include, What is it like to have this problem? Who is in greatest need of an intervention? What are clients' goals—what do *they* want as an intervention outcome? (Additional exploratory research questions are available in the Toolkit of the *Resource Manual.* 🔅) Answers to questions such as these could help to shape the intervention and make it more effective, tolerable, and appropriate for the group for whom the intervention is designed.

Exploratory research with other stakeholders can also be valuable. Many of the pitfalls of intervention research involve lack of cooperation, support, or trust among key stakeholders, including intervention

agents. During the developmental phase, stakeholders should be identified and engaged in the development process to the extent possible. Stakeholders who have had experience working with the target group can often contribute to the development of effective intervention strategies.

Exploratory work can also be undertaken to better understand the context within which an intervention would unfold (McGuire et al., 2000). For example, it may be important to understand issues such as staff turnover, staff morale, nurse workload, and nurse autonomy. An analysis of context may be especially important when introducing interventions into highly unstable environments (Buckwalter et al., 2009). Van Meijel and colleagues (2004) also recommended undertaking a "current practice analysis" to understand the status quo of how the problem under scrutiny is being addressed.

The nursing literature has hundreds of examples of descriptive or exploratory studies done as part of intervention development. Research strategies run the gamut of those discussed in this book, such as focus group interviews, needs assessment surveys, in-depth or critical-incident interviews, record reviews, and observations in clinical settings. It is not unusual for researchers to conduct three or four small descriptive studies during the development phase of an intervention project.

> **Example of exploratory research for a nursing intervention:** Blackwood (2006) developed a nurse-led intervention for weaning patients in intensive care units (ICUs) from mechanical ventilation. In the development phase, she conducted several small-scale studies to help in the design of her intervention protocol. One involved observation of the weaning process with 54 patients in the ICU where the intervention would be introduced. Another involved semistructured interviews with ICU anesthetists to explore their views on weaning. Also, ICU nurses were surveyed to explore their knowledge of weaning and their attitudes toward the use of a formal weaning protocol.

Consultation with Experts

Experts in the content area of the problem or with the target population can play a crucial role during

Phase 1 of an intervention project. Expert consultants are especially useful if the evidence base is thin and resources for undertaking exploratory research are limited. Experts can contribute to the intervention theory, components of the intervention, and protocols for its delivery. Many of the questions in Table 26.4 that are not answered in the research literature are good candidates for discussion with experts.

> **TIP:** In selecting expert consultants, think in an interdisciplinary fashion. For example, the use of a cultural consultant may be valuable to assess the cultural sensitivity and appropriateness of some interventions. A developmental psychologist could help assess developmental suitability.

Often, experts are asked to review preliminary intervention protocols, to corroborate their utility, and to solicit suggestions for strengthening them. Curiously, this process is less often formalized than the process for reviewing new measurement scales. Procedures used to assess the *content validity* of new instruments using an expert panel (Chapter 15) could easily be used to review draft intervention protocols. Indeed, if the intervention is ultimately intended for use in other settings or contexts, content validation is likely to be an extremely valuable approach.

> **Example of content validation of a nursing intervention:** Barkas and colleagues (2009) used a panel of 10 experts to assess the content validity of the Telephone Assessment and Skill-Building Kit (TASK), an 8-week intervention program based on individualized assessment of stroke caregiver needs.

Brainstorming and Team Building

Most intervention studies involve teams working collaboratively. Cross-fertilization of ideas can be productive, so it is often useful to build a team of researchers from different disciplines or specialty areas. As noted earlier, a part of the development work is interpersonal in nature and involves cultivation of relationships. At the team level, this involves putting together an enthusiastic and committed project team with diverse clinical, research,

and dissemination skills. (If development work is undertaken for a dissertation, the "team" includes the dissertation committee, so members of this committee should be chosen with care).

Ideally, frequent brainstorming sessions would occur during the development period to discuss literature review summaries, conceptual maps, descriptive findings, expert feedback, and preliminary protocols. Technological advances such as videoconferencing make it possible to include team members from different locations. The team may include ongoing involvement of key stakeholders as participating partners in the development and testing of an intervention.

> **TIP:** In addition to seeking information about the stakeholders' needs, concerns, and perspectives on the problem through in-depth research, it is wise to develop mechanisms for ongoing communication and collaboration. For example, it can be useful to form an advisory group of key stakeholders and to have a project-specific website.

Designing a Preliminary Intervention

After gathering evidence from various sources, the research team can proceed to put together the intervention components and strategies that will be used in a pilot study. Figure 26.3 depicts the synthesis of evidence from accumulated knowledge, experts, and research with key stakeholders, which can contribute to the development of an intervention that is as "ideal" as resources allow.

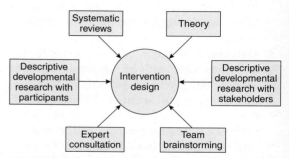

FIGURE 26.3 Synthesis of evidence sources for intervention development.

An evidence-based intervention theory will lay the groundwork for developing intervention components and their content. The theory might indicate, for example, that a skill-building or educational component is needed, and that a motivational component also must be included to effect behavior change. Intervention content can often be adapted from other similar interventions or from clinical practice guidelines. In addition to content, however, the research team needs to make many decisions about the intervention's ingredients. We have hinted at these decisions in Tables 26.4, but here, we offer more explicit information.

1. **Dose and intensity.** The treatment must be sufficiently powerful to achieve a desired, measurable effect on outcomes of interest, but cannot be so powerful that it is cost-prohibitive or burdensome to clients. Among the dose-related issues that need to be decided are the *potency* or *intensity* of the treatment (how much content is appropriate, and will it be given individually or in groups?), the *amount* of dose per session, the *frequency* of administering doses (number of sessions), and the *duration* of the intervention over time. It may be important to consider whether "boosters" are needed to maintain effects.

2. **Timing.** In some cases, it is important to decide when, relative to other events, the intervention will be delivered. The question is, When is the optimal point (in terms of an illness or recovery trajectory, individual development, or severity of a problem) to administer the intervention? Ideally, the intervention theory would suggest the most advantageous timing.

3. **Outcomes.** A major decision concerns the outcomes that will be targeted. Thought should be given to selecting outcomes that are nursing sensitive (Aranda, 2008; Sandelowski, 1996) and important to clients. One issue is whether the focus will be on proximal outcomes or more distal ones. *Proximal outcomes* are immediate and directly connected to the intervention—and thus, usually

most sensitive to intervention effects. For example, knowledge gains from a teaching component of an intervention are proximal. *Distal outcomes* are potentially more important ones, but more difficult to affect (e.g., behavior change). Consideration should also be given to the information needs of people making decisions about using the intervention—what outcomes would affect uptake by admin-istrators or policy makers? Timing of outcome measurement is also important. For example, do knowledge gains decay? Do behavior changes accumulate over time? The timing of measuring outcomes is important because effect size is not constant—the goal is to decide when the *peak response* to an intervention will occur. Finally, decisions must be made about how to measure the selected outcomes.

4. **Setting.** Another design decision involves the setting for the intervention. Settings can vary in terms of ease of implementation and costs. Conn et al. (2001) also noted that settings can influence intervention effectiveness. In deciding about settings (and sites), researchers need to think about the type of setting that will be acceptable and accessible to clients, offer good potential for impacts, provide needed resources or supports, and be cost-effective.

5. **Agents.** Researchers must decide who will deliver the intervention, and how intervention agents will be trained. In many cases, the agents will be nurses, but nurses are not necessarily the best choice. For example, some clients might feel more comfortable if the interventionists were peers, community members, or patients who have experienced a similar illness or problem.

6. **Delivery Mode.** With technological innovations occurring regularly, options for delivering interventions—or components of interventions—have broadened tremendously. Among the possibilities are face-to-face delivery, video or audio recordings, print materials, telephone contact, email transmissions, and

through social networking sites. Care should be taken to match any technological delivery methods to the needs of the clients and to the requirements of the content. The latest technology is not always the optimal. Conn et al. (2001) noted that there should be clarity about whether the intervention being tested is the content, the delivery mode, or both. When both the content and the delivery mode are new, a factorial design that varies mode on one dimension and receipt of content on the other might be a good design strategy for Phase 3 testing.

7. **Individualization.** Another decision concerns the extent to which the intervention will be tailored to the needs and circumstances of a particular group (e.g., the elderly), or individualized to particular clients. When individual information is used to guide content, the intervention is inherently more complex than a one-size-fits-all treatment, but may be more effective and attractive to participants (Lauver et al., 2002).

If adequate development work has been undertaken, these decisions can be evidence-based, using evidence from the synthesis from various sources (see Figure 26.3). The development work should provide the basis for preliminary testing of the intervention in the next phase. As noted by the authors of the MRC framework, "the intervention must be developed to the point where it can reasonably be expected to have a worthwhile effect" (Craig et al., 2008b, p. 980).

Outcomes of Phase 1 Development

Table 26.3 shows that there should be a number of products at the end of the development phase. These include an intervention theory and conceptual map, preliminary intervention components and protocols, and strategies for addressing potential implementation pitfalls. Hopefully, the research team will have documented the development work and major decisions in an ongoing fashion. Detailed written information about the theory,

the intervention components and strategies, and expected outcomes will be valuable for writing reports about the intervention and for funding requests.

> **TIP:** A matrix can often be useful in summarizing *key decisions* in one column, and *supporting evidence* for those decisions in another. Such a matrix is a good communication tool for discussing decisions with others. Another advantage of such a matrix is that you will be forced to think of a rationale for your decisions, and to identify evidence supporting them.

If the evidence synthesis provides support for moving forward with a pilot test of the intervention, another product of Phase 1 work will be a full design for a pilot study, usually in the form of a research proposal. Proposal development is discussed in Chapter 29.

PHASES 2 AND 3 OF INTERVENTION RESEARCH

Many aspects of Phase 2 (pilot testing) and Phase 3 (confirmatory testing for efficacy) have been discussed in several earlier chapters. Here, we mention only a few issues as they relate to an overall process of intervention development.

Phase 2: Pilot Testing an Intervention

The second phase of intervention research is a pilot test of the newly developed intervention, typically using simple quasi-experimental designs. A frequently used design in such pilot tests is a one-group pretest-posttest design, which can provide simple information about whether changes occurred among those exposed to the intervention.

Several *issues* are addressed in pilot testing, but one issue is central: feasibility. To what extent can the intervention be implemented as conceptualized, and is it plausible that there will be desired effects? Another important issue is corroboration—getting preliminary evidence that the conceptual efforts have yielded an intervention with potential to be beneficial. The third issue is refinement. During this stage, there are good opportunities to "tweak" the intervention (and the theory), based on data from the pilot study.

The central *activities* of Phase 2 are implementing the pilot study and analyzing pilot data. Chapter 8 described the types of assessments that should be made during a pilot study. The feasibility assessment should involve an analysis of factors that affected implementation, such as recruitment, retention, and adherence problems. The utility of the preliminary outcome measures—and the extent to which they were found burdensome to pilot participants—also should be evaluated. Participant experiences during the course of the intervention are also of interest for refining protocols. Thus, qualitative research can play an important role in gaining insight into the feasibility of a larger-scale RCT through efforts to understand the perspective of the intended beneficiaries of the intervention. Preliminary evidence of intervention effects is also useful, especially for guiding sample size decisions in the larger study.

An important *product* of a pilot study is documentation of the "lessons learned." These lessons should be carefully discussed in team meetings, and reviewed with expert consultants, stakeholders, or an advisory panel. Each pilot test yields its own context-specific and intervention-specific lessons. Yet, the research literature suggests that some "lessons" are recurrent. An overall lesson is that you should always expect the reality of the pilot to be different from what is on paper. The following are among the most frequently mentioned lessons from pilot intervention studies:

- Recruitment of participants will be more difficult and take longer than anticipated
- Materials intended for direct use by participants (e.g., pamphlets, educational materials) need to be simplified
- Participant burden, especially with regard to data collection, needs to be reduced

- Effect sizes tend to be larger in the pilot than in the main trial
- Key ingredients of the intervention should be front-loaded—that is, delivered early—because greater attention and attendance occur early
- If there is a control condition, diffusion is a recurrent problem
- Even expert interventionists need to be trained (and this includes the researchers themselves)
- Relationships with others need to be continuously nurtured.

Phase 2 outcomes and products usually include a formal intervention protocol for testing in a Phase 3 clinical trial, as well as ancillary products such as training and procedures manuals and finalized outcome measures. Another important product is a formal plan for a Phase 3 RCT—often in the form of a grant application—if the results of the feasibility assessment suggest that a full test is warranted.

Example of a mixed methods pilot intervention study: Stewart and colleagues (2009) developed a support intervention to promote health and coping among homeless youth, after doing developmental research with the youth and with service providers. A 20-week pilot intervention consisting of support groups, one-to-one support, and group recreational activities and meals. Both quantitative and qualitative data were collected to document intervention processes and outcomes. A major challenge during the pilot was attrition.

Phase 3: Controlled Trial of the Intervention

The third phase of an intervention study is to undertake a full experimental test of the intervention, typically using an experimental (or strong quasi-experimental) design. Many important issues of a Phase 3 trial were discussed at some length in Chapter 10, which outlined various threats to the validity of a rigorous quantitative study and presented some strategies to address those threats. Whereas construct validity is particularly salient in Phases 1 and 2 of an intervention project, internal validity and statistical conclusion validity are key issues during Phase 3. External validity, although important, is often not central to an efficacy clinical trial. (The RE-AIM framework described in Chapter 10 offers useful concepts for external validity.)

Although the central goal of Phase 3 intervention research is to assess the effects of the intervention, it is perhaps better to think of the RCT as ongoing development rather than as simply "confirmatory." Even with a strong pilot study, things will usually continue to go awry in the full experimental test. All of the problems should be documented and should lead to recommendations for how the intervention could be improved or how its implementation could be made smoother. It is advisable to collect both qualitative and quantitative data during this phase. Quantitative data are essential for providing evidence about effects, but many pressing questions simply cannot be answered with quantitative data alone. Some of the benefits of using a mixed methods approach during Phase 3 include the following:

1. **Intervention Fidelity.** Mixed methods research is often needed to inform judgments about whether the intervention was faithfully implemented and given a fair test. If intervention effects are weak, one possibility is that it was not implemented according to plan and might merit further scrutiny (see Chapter 10).
2. **Intervention Clarification.** A qualitative component in a clinical trial can help to clarify the nature and course of the intervention in its natural context. It is useful to understand how intervention recipients and other stakeholders, "actually experience the intervention in real time and in real life" (Sandelowski, 1996, p. 362).
3. **Variation in Effects.** Intervention effects represent averages. For individual participants, the effects may be much greater than the average, while for others the intervention could have no benefit. Sometimes subgroup analyses can be done quantitatively, but these are productive only if the dimension along which variation occurs is a measurable attribute. A

qualitative study of participants who experienced the intervention differently could illuminate how to target the intervention more effectively in the future, or how to improve it to reach a broader audience.

Example of exploring variation: Burke and colleagues (2009) conducted in-depth interviews with (and obtained diary data from) 15 people who completed a behavioral weight loss treatment. They explored variation in how people self-monitored their diet during the treatment. Three categories of self-monitoring were identified: well-disciplined (those with high adherence), those "missing the connection" (those with moderate adherence), and diminished support (those with poor adherence).

4. **Clinical Significance.** Quantitative results from an RCT indicate whether the results are statistically significant—that is, probably reliable and replicable with a new sample. Qualitative information could shed light on whether the results are also clinically significant. Moreover, clinically significant effects sometimes can be discerned even there are no statistically significant effects.
5. **Interpretation.** Quantitative results indicate *whether* an intervention had beneficial effects—but do not explain *why* effects occurred. A strong conceptual framework offers a theoretical rationale for explaining the results, but may not tell the whole story if the effects were weaker than expected, if they were observed for some outcomes but not for others, or even if they were consistent with expectations but represent *nonspecific effects*—that is, effects resulting from factors not specified in the intervention theory (Donovan et al., 2009). Moreover, even if there are specific theory-driven intervention effects, it is inevitable that people will ask "black box" questions when the intervention is complex (Conn, 2009). Some may ask, What is it that is *driving* the results? Which component or aspect of the intervention leads to observed benefits? Answers to such questions often stem from practical concerns, reflecting a desire to streamline successful interventions when resources are tight.

Example of interpreting results: Donovan and colleagues (2007) tested the effects of a web-based symptom management intervention, and included a qualitative component that involved a *manipulation check* to assess whether participants received the intervention as planned. The researchers analyzed the content of participants' Internet postings, and learned that the participants did in fact experience some (but not all) of the theoretically specified intervention factors, and that other nonspecific factors (e.g., emotional support) were part of the intervention experience.

6. **Visibility.** Quantitative results do not have much "sex appeal." As astutely pointed out by Sandelowski (1996), qualitative research embedded in intervention studies can enhance the communicability and power of the study findings: ". . . Storied accounts of scientific work are often the more compelling and culturally resonant way to communicate research results to diverse audiences, including patient groups and policy-makers" (p. 361).

The primary product of Phase 3 is a report summarizing intervention effects. Often, single papers are insufficient for providing the full range of information about the project, particularly if a mixed methods approach was used. Ideally, one report would integrate findings from the qualitative and quantitative components and offer recommendations for further adoption of the intervention.

➔ **TIP:** Several writers have observed recently that interventions are inadequately described in research reports (e.g., Conn, et al., 2008; Lindsay, 2004). Although journal constraints may limit a full elaboration of interventions, detailed descriptions should be prepared so they can be shared with others through correspondence.

MIXED METHODS DESIGNS FOR INTERVENTION RESEARCH

Creswell and Plano Clark (2007) identified one of the Embedded Designs in their mixed methods (MM) typology as an *embedded experimental model*, a model used to test interventions. They described this model as either a one-stage or two-stage QUAN-dominant approach, in which timing decisions reflect the overall purpose for including the qualitative data. Visual diagrams for two possible two-stage models as described by Creswell and Plano Clark are presented in Figure 26.4. The notation in the top panel would be qual → QUAN(qual), and that in the bottom panel would be QUAN(qual) → qual.

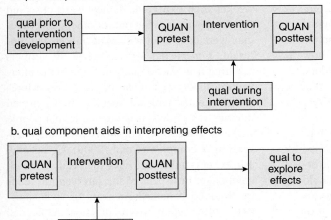

a. qual component informs intervention

b. qual component aids in interpreting effects

FIGURE 26.4 Embedded experimental mixed methods designs for a 2-phase intervention project. (Adapted from Creswell, J. W., & Plano Clark, V. L. [2007]. *Designing and conducting mixed methods research.* Thousand Oaks, CA: Sage.)

Models such as those shown in Figure 26.4 are likely to work reasonably well for interventions that are closer to the "simple" end of the simple → complex continuum. They might also be appropriate for a small-scale study (such as a dissertation project) in which the main QUAN component is essentially a pilot study.

For complex interventions such as those described in the MRC framework, it is better to think of a separate design structure for each phase, because each has its own purpose, design, sampling plan, and data collection strategy. For the project overall, it might be reasonable to think of QUAN as having priority and qual playing a subservient role. Yet, development work usually involves QUAL-dominant research.

Figure 26.5 shows some of the design possibilities for a three-phase intervention project, and many others are possible. For the project overall, the design is inherently sequential, but within each phase, the design could be either sequential or concurrent. Both qualitative and quantitative approaches are often used in each phase, although there may be no need to collect quantitative data during Phase 1 if there is a strong existing evidence base.

It is difficult to offer guidance on which of the myriad design possibilities to adopt because many factors influence which is most appropriate. Fewer design components may be required for simpler interventions, for "mainstream" target populations, for studies in a familiar site, and for studies of adaptations to well-tested interventions, for example. Also, resources may force researchers to forego

components they would have liked to include. The design for the Phase 3 trial is also likely to be affected by which of the six goals described in the previous section is most salient. For example, if the researchers want to understand variation in intervention effects, the design likely would be a QUAN → qual sequential one. If the desire to monitor intervention fidelity is the primary objective of including a qualitative component, a QUAN(qual) embedded design would be needed.

Sampling designs, as discussed in Chapter 25, are also likely to differ in the three phases. During Phase 1, a multilevel sampling approach is often used to gather in-depth QUAL data from different populations—for example, from patients, family members, and healthcare staff. In Phases 2 and 3, by contrast, sampling is likely to be either identical or nested—although multilevel sampling is also a possibility for understanding intervention fidelity.

In summary, researchers can be creative in developing an overall design that matches their needs, circumstances, and budgets. Inevitably, however, strong research for developing and testing complex interventions will rely on a mixed methods design.

CRITIQUING INTERVENTION RESEARCH

Many chapters of this book offer guidelines for evaluating methodologic aspects of the studies that

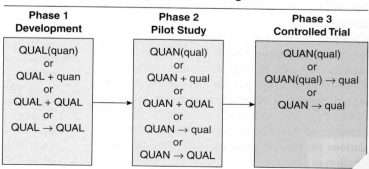

FIGURE 26.5 Possible mixed methods designs for a 3-phase nursing intervention program.

BOX 26.2 Guidelines for Critiquing Aspects of Intervention Projects

1. On the simple-to-complex continuum, where would you locate the intervention? If the intervention is complex, along which dimensions is complexity found (e.g., number of components, complexity of behaviors required, number of intervention sessions, time required, and so on)?
2. Is there an intervention theory, and is it adequate? Is there an explanation of how the theory was selected, adapted, or developed?
3. What strategies were used to identify and create evidence in support of intervention development? Was a systematic review performed? Were expert consultants involved? Were descriptive or exploratory studies undertaken? Overall, was developmental work adequate?
4. What efforts were made to validate the intervention and its protocols?
5. Was there a pilot study? Did it attend to feasibility issues? Did it explore how the intervention was received by clients or other stakeholders? Were recruitment and retention adequate? Overall, was pilot work sufficient for a decision to move forward with a full clinical trial?
6. For the overall project and for individual phases, was a mixed methods approach used? Which design was adopted, and is the design appropriate for the goals of different phases of the project?
7. What *was* the intervention? Was it described in sufficient detail in terms of content, target population, dose, outcomes, timing, individualization, intervention agents, and so on?
8. Does the final report integrate the key findings from the various strands of research? Does the report offer recommendations for replication, extension, or adaptation of the intervention, or for use in different settings or with different populations?

would be included in an intervention project. For example, guidelines in Chapters 9 and 10 would be useful for critiquing the Phase 3 design. Qualitative components could be evaluated using guidelines in Chapters 20 through 24. Additionally, the previous chapter included critiquing suggestions for mixed methods research.

Box 26.2 offers a few additional questions on intervention issues, with many of them focusing on intervention development. An overarching question might be: How close did the researchers get to an "ideal" intervention, in terms of criteria identified in Box 26.1? Of course, being able to answer this overall question and many of the questions in Box 26.2 will depend on the care taken in documenting the full effort. Most often, aspects of the development and testing are reported in separate articles, but ideally the team would prepare a summary report that integrates qualitative and quantitative findings from all phases, and that offers evidence-based recommen how to proceed with using the inter practice.

EXAMPLE OF MIXED METHODS INTERVENTION RESEARCH

Key Articles: Symptom-focused management for African American women with type 2 diabetes: A pilot study (Skelly et al., 2005); Conceptual model of symptom-focused diabetes care for African Americans (Skelly et al., 2008); Tailoring a diabetes self-care intervention for use with older, rural African American women (Leeman et al., 2008); Controlled trial of nursing interventions to improve health outcomes of older African American women with type 2 diabetes (Skelly et al., 2009).

Statement of Purpose: The overall purpose of this research was to develop a theory-based intervention to improve the health outcomes of older African American women with type 2 diabetes. The intervention was specifically tailored to a population that faces distinct challenges in managing diabetes self-care. Thus, the project goals were to develop and refine an intervention theory, develop an evidence-based intervention consistent with the theory, and to test the intervention with a community sample.

Phase 1: The developmental work for this project unfolded over a number of years. The study team, which included professionals with many years of clinical experience in diabetes care, reviewed the literature. Exploratory research, which included both qualitative and quantitative studies (QUAN + QUAL), was undertaken to understand the experiences of diabetes self-care and symptom management among older, rural African American women. In their quantitative survey of 75 older women with type 2 diabetes, they found that although women with diabetes experienced multiple symptoms, they did not often relate the symptoms to their diabetes. The specific symptoms guided the focus of the intervention's modules. A qualitative study, which involved focus group interviews with 70 participants, revealed high levels of stress that created barriers to self-care. The results highlighted the importance of including stress-management strategies in the intervention and further informed the training of interventionists. The conceptual model for the intervention was the Symptom Management Model, which provided "an ideal vehicle for individualizing self-care education to the distinct needs of each participant" (Leeman et al., 2008, p. 314). The synthesis of evidence, theory, and clinical experience formed the basis for a culturally sensitive symptom-focused intervention involving four intervention modules delivered in four 1-hour bimonthly visits to participants' homes by trained nurses. Intervention materials were refined through review by a community advisory board.

Phase 2: The intervention was pilot tested using a QUAN(qual) design that involved random assignment of 41 participants to the intervention or a control group. The quantitative results encouraged ongoing testing of the intervention, and identified a few areas of needed refinement. Participants in the intervention group showed significant improvement in their medication, diet, home glucose monitoring practices, and distress from symptoms. Data from in-depth interviews and field observations were used to understand participants' experience and satisfaction with the intervention (Skelly et al., 2005).

Phase 3: The efficacy of the intervention was tested in a full clinical QUAN(qual) trial with 180 women using a 3-arm experimental design. Participants were randomly assigned to either an attention control group that received a weight and diet program, a symptom-focused intervention group, or a symptom-focused intervention group that also received a telephone "booster" 3 months after the end of the regular intervention. Field observations were undertaken to assess intervention fidelity, and in-depth interviews with participants were conducted. Retention in the study was high (91% over 9 months). Over the 9-month study period, self-care practices, metabolic control, symptom distress, and quality of life improved for the entire sample. The researchers speculated that the absence of group differences in improvement could reflect the fact that all interventions were tailored to the particular population of older African American women, as well as individualized to each person (Skelly et al., 2009).

SUMMARY POINTS

- **Nursing intervention research** refers to a distinctive *process* of developing, implementing, testing, and disseminating nursing interventions—particularly complex interventions.

- In a **complex intervention**, complexity can arise along several dimensions, including number of components, number of outcomes targeted, number and complexity of behaviors required, and the time needed for the full intervention to be delivered.

- Several frameworks for developing and testing complex interventions have been proposed. The most widely cited one is the **Medical Research Council framework** (United Kingdom) that was published in 2000; a revised framework was released in 2008.

- Most frameworks emphasize the critical importance of strong development efforts at the outset (Phase 1), followed by pilot tests of the intervention (Phase 2), and then a controlled trial to assess efficacy (Phase 3). Studies to assess effectiveness of interventions in real-world clinical settings (Phase 4) are rare in nursing. The frameworks are idealized models; the process is rarely linear. Virtually all frameworks for intervention development call for mixed methods (MM) research.

- Conceptualization and in-depth understanding of the problem and the target population are key issues during Phase 1 development work. An important product during Phase 1 is a carefully conceived **intervention theory** from which the design of the intervention flows. The theory indicates what inputs are needed to effect improvements on specific outcomes.
- In addition to theory, resources for developing an evidence-based intervention and intervention strategies during Phase 1 include systematic reviews, descriptive research with the target population or key stakeholders, consultation with experts, and discussions with a dedicated and diverse team.
- In developing an intervention, researchers must make decisions about not only the *content* of the intervention, but also about dose and intensity, timing of the intervention, outcomes to target and when to measure them, intervention setting, intervention agents, mode of delivery, and individualization.
- In Phase 2, the preliminary intervention is tested, usually using a simple quasi-experimental design. Pilots often include supplementary qualitative components to understand the experience of being in the intervention and problems with recruitment and retention.
- The primary focus of the pilot study is on the feasibility of more rigorous testing. The pilot study typically yields a number of "lessons" about how to refine the intervention, improve its acceptance and appeal, and enhance its delivery.
- A mixed methods approach can strengthen the test of the intervention during the Phase 3 controlled trial. The inclusion of qualitative components can shed light on intervention fidelity, variation in effects, clinical significance, and interpretive ambiguities.
- Mixed methods are appropriate (and beneficial) in all phases of an intervention project. Broadly speaking, the design is sequential, but each phase can involve the use of various mixed methods designs. In Phase 1, QUAL often has priority, while in Phases 2 and 3, QUAN is usually dominant.

STUDY ACTIVITIES

Chapter 26 of the *Resource Manual for Nursing Research: Generating and Assessing Evidence for Nursing Practice, 9th edition*, offers various exercises and study suggestions for reinforcing concepts presented in this chapter. In addition, the following study questions can be addressed:

1. Review the research example of a randomized controlled trial described at the end of Chapter 10 ("Effects of abdominal massage in management of constipation," Lämås et al., 2009). Suggest how the study could potentially be enhanced using a QUAN(qual) or QUAN → qual design. What mixed methods questions would be addressed by your proposed enhancement?
2. For the same study as in Question 1 (Lämås et al., 2009), would you describe the intervention as complex? Why or why not?

STUDIES CITED IN CHAPTER 26

Barkas, T., Farran, C., Austin, J., Given, B., Johnson, E., & Williams, L. (2009). Content validity and satisfaction with a stroke caregiver intervention program. *Journal of Nursing Scholarship, 41*, 368–375.

Blackwood, B. (2006). Methodologic issues in evaluating complex interventions. *Journal of Advanced Nursing, 54*, 612–622.

Burke, L., Swigart, V., Turk, M., Derro, N., & Ewing, L. (2009). Experiences of self-monitoring: Successes and struggles during treatment for weight loss. *Qualitative Health Research, 19*, 815–828.

Donovan, H., Ward, S., Song, M., Heidrich, S., Gunnarsdottir, S., & Phillips, C. (2007). An update on the representational approach to patient education. *Journal of Nursing Scholarship, 39*, 259–265.

Hall, S., Chochinov, H., Harding, R., Murray, S., Richardson, A., & Higginson, I. (2009). A phase II randomised controlled trial assessing the feasibility, acceptability and potential effectiveness of Dignity Therapy for older people in care homes. *BMC Geriatrics, 9*, 9.

Leeman, J., Skelly, A., Burns, D., Carlson, J., & Soward, A. (2008). Tailoring a diabetes self-care intervention for use with older, rural African American women. *The Diabetes Educator, 34*, 310–317.

Morrison-Beedy, D., Carey, M., Seibold-Simpson, S., Xia, Y., & Tu, X. (2009). Preliminary efficacy of a comprehensive HIV prevention intervention for abstinent girls. *Research in Nursing & Health, 32*, 569–581.

Morrison-Beedy, D., & Nelson, L. (2004). HIV prevention interventions I adolescent girls: What is the state of the science? *Worldviews of Evidence-Based Nursing, 1*, 165–175.

Schultz, A., Goodwin, P., Jesseman, C., Toews, H., Lane, M., & Smith, C. (2008). Evaluating the effectiveness of gel pillows for reducing bilateral head flattening in preterm infants. *Applied Nursing Research, 21*, 191–198.

Skelly, A., Carlson, J., Leeman, J., Holditch-Davis, D., & Soward, A. (2005). Symptom-focused management for African American women with type 2 diabetes: A pilot study. *Applied Nursing Research, 18*, 213–220.

Skelly, A., Carlson, J., Leeman, J., Soward, A., & Burns, D. (2009). Controlled trial of nursing interventions to improve health outcomes of older African American women with type 2 diabetes. *Nursing Research, 58*, 410–418.

Skelly, A., Leeman, J., Carlson, J., Soward, A., & Burns, D. (2008). Conceptual model of symptom-focused diabetes care for African Americans. *Journal of Nursing Scholarship, 40*, 261–267.

Stewart, M., Reutter, L, Letourneau, N., & Makwarimba, E. (2009). A support intervention to promote health and coping among homeless youth. *Canadian Journal of Nursing Research, 41*, 55–77.

Methodologic and nonresearch references cited in this chapter can be found in a separate section at the end of the book.

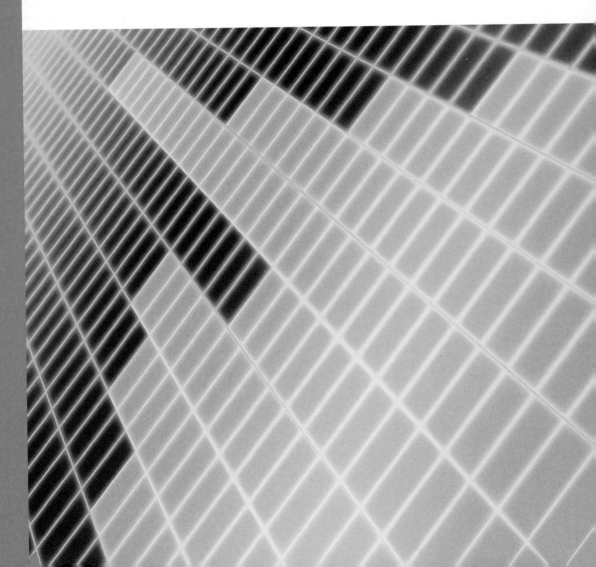

PART 6

BUILDING AN EVIDENCE BASE FOR NURSING PRACTICE

27 | Systematic Reviews of Research Evidence: Meta-Analysis, Metasynthesis, and Mixed Studies Review

I n Chapter 5, we described major steps in conducting a literature review as an early step in designing and conducting a new study. This chapter also discusses reviews of existing evidence, but focuses on the conduct and evaluation of systematic reviews, which in themselves are considered research.

RESEARCH INTEGRATION AND SYNTHESIS

A **systematic review** is a review that methodically integrates research evidence about a specific research question using carefully developed sampling and data collection procedures that are spelled out in advanced in a protocol. In a systematic review, reviewers use methodical procedures that are, for the most part, reproducible and verifiable. Although subjectivity cannot be totally removed in a systematic review, or in any research endeavor (Sandelowski, 2008a), the review process is disciplined and largely transparent, so that readers of the systematic review can assess the conclusions. Systematic reviews explicitly aim to avoid reaching incorrect or misleading conclusions that

could arise from a biased review process or from a biased selection of studies included in the review.

Evidence-based practice relies on meticulous integration of research evidence. Indeed, many consider systematic reviews a cornerstone of EBP. The type of integrative activities we discuss in this chapter are not just literature reviews, but rather systematic inquiries that follow many of the same rules as those described in this book for **primary studies**, that is, original research investigations.

Literature reviews, such as those often done by students or those done by researchers in preparing a proposal for a new study, do not necessarily yield different conclusions about a body of evidence than are found in a systematic review. What is distinctive about a systematic review is the process of developing, testing, and adhering to a protocol with explicit rules for gathering the data—the research evidence—from studies that address a particular question.

Systematic reviews that integrate research evidence can take various forms and result in different products. Systematic reviews of evidence from quantitative studies—especially those that assess the effects of an intervention—are likely to use meta-analytic techniques. In a meta-analysis, reviewers use a common metric for combining evidence statistically. Most of the reviews in the Cochrane Collaboration, for example, are meta-analyses. As we shall see, however, statistical integration is sometimes inappropriate. When evidence cannot be integrated statistically, a systematic review usually involves narrative integration.

Qualitative researchers also are developing techniques to integrate findings across studies. Many terms exist for such endeavors (e.g., metastudy, metamethod, metasummary, metaethnography, qualitative meta-analysis, formal grounded theory), but the one that appears to be emerging as the leading term among nurses researchers is *metasynthesis.*

A recent development involves systematic reviews that integrate findings from qualitative *and* quantitative studies, and from mixed methods studies. *Mixed studies reviews* are relatively new, and many different strategies are being pursued. In the years ahead, methodologic developments will likely lead to enhancements and greater clarity on how best to undertake such reviews.

In this chapter, we focus primarily on meta-analysis for synthesizing quantitative findings and meta-synthesis for integrating qualitative findings, but we offer a few suggestions with regard to mixed methods reviews. The field of research integration is expanding at a rapid pace, both in terms of the number of integration studies being conducted and in the techniques used to perform them. This chapter provides a brief introduction to this extremely important and complex topic. Our advice for those embarking on a review project is to keep abreast of developments in this emerging field and to seek more detailed information in books devoted to the topic. Particularly good resources for further guidance on meta-analysis include the *Cochrane Handbook for Systematic Reviews of Interventions* (Higgins & Green, 2008) and books by Cooper (2010) and Lipsey and Wilson (2001). For qualitative integration, we recommend Noblit and Hare (1988), Paterson and colleagues (2001), and Sandelowski and Barroso (2007).

META-ANALYSIS

In evidence hierarchies relating to cause-probing questions, meta-analyses of RCTs are at the pinna-

cle (see Figure 2.1). The essence of a meta-analysis is that information from various studies is used to develop a common metric, the *effect size.* Effect sizes are averaged across studies, yielding aggregated information about not only the *existence* of a relationship between variables, but also an estimate of its *magnitude.*

Advantages of Meta-Analyses

For systematic integration of quantitative evidence, meta-analysis offers a simple advantage: *objectivity.* In a narrative review, reviewers almost inevitably use unidentified or subconscious criteria in integrating disparate results. For example, narrative reviewers make subjective decisions about how much weight to give findings from different studies, and so different reviewers could come to different conclusions about the evidence. Meta-analysts also make decisions—sometimes based on personal preferences—but in a meta-analysis most decisions are made explicit. Moreover, the integration itself is objective because it is statistical. Calculating the average efficacy of nurse-led interventions for smoking cessation across 20 studies is analogous to calculating the average efficacy of a single smoking cessation trial across 20 participants. Readers of a meta-analysis can be confident that another analyst using the same data set would reach the same conclusions.

Another advantage of meta-analysis concerns *power,* a statistical concept described in Chapter 17. Power, it may be recalled, is the probability of detecting a true relationship between the independent and dependent variables. By combining results across multiple studies, power is increased. Indeed, in a meta-analysis it is possible to conclude, with a given probability, that a relationship is real (e.g., an intervention is effective), even when several small studies yielded nonsignificant findings. In a narrative review, 10 nonsignificant findings would almost surely be interpreted as lack of evidence of a true relationship, which could be an erroneous conclusion.

Another benefit concerns precision. Meta-analysts can draw conclusions about how big an effect an intervention has, with a specified probability that the results are accurate. Estimates of effect size across multiple studies yield smaller confidence intervals than individual studies, and thus precision is enhanced. Both power and precision are enticing qualities in evidence-based practice, as suggested by the EBP questions for appraising evidence described in Chapter 2 (see Table 2.1).

Despite these strengths, meta-analysis is not always appropriate. Indiscriminate use has led critics to warn against potential abuses, and so reviewers must carefully assess whether meta-analysis is justified.

Criteria for Using Meta-Analytic Techniques in a Systematic Review

In deciding whether statistical integration of effects is sensible, a basic criterion is that the research question being addressed or the hypothesis being tested across studies is similar, if not identical. This essentially means that the independent and the dependent variables, and the study populations, are sufficiently similar to merit integration. The variables may be operationalized differently, to be sure. Interventions to promote exercise among diabetics could take the form of a 4-week clinic-based program in one study and an 8-week web-based intervention in another, for example. The dependent variable (exercise) also could be operationalized differently across studies. Yet, a study of the effects of a 1-hour lecture to improve *attitudes* toward exercise among overweight adolescents would be a poor candidate to include in this meta-analysis. This is frequently called the "apples and oranges" or "fruit" problem. A meta-analysis should not be about *fruit*—that is, a broad and encompassing category—but rather about a specific question that has been addressed in multiple studies—that is, "apples," or, even better, "Granny Smith apples."

A second criterion concerns whether there is a sufficient base of knowledge for statistical integration. If there are only a few studies, or if all of the studies are weakly designed and harbor extensive bias, it usually is not sensible to compute an "average" effect.

A final issue concerns consistency of the evidence. When the same hypothesis has been tested in multiple studies and results are highly conflicting, meta-analysis is not appropriate. As an extreme example, if half the studies testing an intervention found benefits for those in the intervention group, but the other half found benefits for the controls, it would be misleading to compute an average effect. A more appropriate strategy would be to do an in-depth narrative analysis of why results are conflicting.

Example of inability to conduct a meta-analysis: Oeseburg and colleagues (2009) did a systematic review of research on the effects of patient advocacy case management on service use and healthcare costs for community-dwelling older people or adults with a chronic illness. They noted as a limitation "the impracticability of statistical pooling of the data across studies" (p. 208) due to such problems as missing data.

Steps in a Meta-Analysis

A systematic review, like a primary study, requires considerable upfront planning, including an evaluation of whether there are sufficient resources and personnel to complete the project. In this section, we describe seven major steps in the conduct of a meta-analysis: formulating the research problem, designing the meta-analysis, searching for data, evaluating study quality, extracting and encoding the data, calculating effects, analyzing the data, and reporting results.

Formulating the Problem

Like any study, a systematic review begins with a problem statement and a research question or hypothesis. Data cannot be meaningfully collected and integrated until there is a clear sense of what question is being addressed. Question templates such as those provided in Chapters 2 or 4 serve as a good starting place. ✪

As described in Chapter 4, a broad question form for a quantitative study is: "In (population), what is the effect of (independent variable) on (outcome)?" This serves as an adequate starting place for many meta-analyses, but variations described in Chapter 4 may be preferred. As with a primary study, care should be taken to develop a problem statement and questions that are clearly worded and specific. Key constructs should be conceptually defined, and the definitions should indicate the boundaries of the inquiry. The definitions will serve as an indispensable tool for deciding whether a primary study qualifies for the synthesis, and for extracting appropriate information from the studies.

> **Example of a question from a systematic review:** Cortes and colleagues (2009) conducted a meta-analysis that addressed the following question: "Is there an impact on mortality and re-infarction rates among patients receiving early mobilization after an AMI (acute myocardial infarction)" (p. 1497). Early mobilization, the independent variable, was "defined as programmed changes of position from bed to chair, bed to standing, or bed to walking added to conventional care" (p. 1497).

As indicated previously, questions for a meta-analysis are usually narrow, focusing, for example, on a particular type of intervention and specific outcomes. The broader the question, the more complex (and costly) the meta-analysis becomes—and sometimes broad questions make it impossible to integrate studies through meta-analysis.

A strategy that is gaining momentum is to undertake a **scoping review** (or *scoping study*) as a means of refining the specific question for the systematic review. Although scoping studies have been defined in many ways (Davis et al., 2009), we refer here to scoping as a preliminary investigation that clarifies the range and nature of the evidence base. Unlike a systematic review, a scoping review addresses broad questions and uses flexible procedures, and typically does not formally evaluate the quality of evidence. Such scoping reviews can provide background and suggest refinements and strategies for a full systematic review and can also indicate whether statistical integration (a meta-analysis) is feasible. Arksey and O'Malley (2005) have written an often-cited paper on the conduct of scoping reviews.

> **Example of a scoping review:** Griffiths and colleagues (2009) conducted a scoping review of the size, extent, and nature of learning disability nursing. They found that few studies evaluated the clinical impact or patient experiences of nurse-led interventions.

Designing the Meta-Analysis Study

Meta-analysts, like other researchers, make many decisions that affect the rigor and validity of their conclusions. Most decisions should be made in a conscious, planful manner *before the study is underway*, and should be fully documented so they can be communicated to readers of the review. We identify a few major design decisions in this section. Some design options of a technical nature, however, can best be explained in our discussion of analytic procedures.

One upfront decision involves project organization. Systematic reviews are sometimes done by individuals, but it is preferable to have at least two reviewers. Multiple reviewers help not only in sharing the workload but also in minimizing subjectivity. Reviewers should have both substantive and clinical knowledge of the problem, and sufficiently strong methodologic skills to evaluate study quality and undertake the analysis. Even with a knowledgeable team, clear guidelines and training in the use of the guidelines are essential, just as they are in the collection of data for a primary study.

Sampling must also be planned. In a systematic review, the sample consists of the primary studies that have addressed the research question. Reviewers make many decisions about the sample, including a specification of the exclusion or inclusion criteria for the search. Sampling criteria typically cover substantive, methodologic, and practical elements. Substantively, the criteria must stipulate specific variables. For example, if the review concerns the effectiveness of a nursing intervention, what outcomes (dependent variables) must the researchers have studied, and what types of intervention are of specific interest? Another substantive issue concerns the study population—for example, will certain age groups of participants (e.g., children, the elderly) be excluded? Methodologically, the criteria might specify that (for example) only studies that used a true experimental design will be included. From a practical standpoint, the criteria might exclude reports written in a language other than English, or reports published before a certain date. Of particular importance is the decision about whether both published and unpublished reports will be included in the review, a topic we discuss in the next section.

Example of sampling criteria: Pate (2009) did a meta-analysis that compared e-based versus provider interventions to promote breastfeeding. Studies were eligible if they compared intervention delivery methods, reported breastfeeding initiation or duration as an outcome, were conducted in a developed country, were published between 2004 and 2008, and used a concurrent control group design. Studies were excluded if they contained insufficient information for calculating effects.

A related issue concerns the quality of the primary studies, a topic that has stirred debate. Researchers sometimes use quality as a sampling criterion, either directly or indirectly. Indirect screening can occur if, for example, a meta-analyst excludes studies that did not use a randomized design, or studies that were not published in a peer-reviewed journal. More directly, potential primary studies can be rated for quality, and excluded if the quality score falls below a threshold. Alternatives to handling study quality are discussed in a later section. Suffice it to say, however, that evaluations of study quality are inevitably part of the review process. Thus, analysts need to decide how quality assessments will be made, and what will be done with assessment information.

Another design issue concerns the **statistical heterogeneity** of results in primary studies. For each study, meta-analysts compute an index to summarize the strength and direction of relationship between an independent variable and a dependent variable. Just as there is inevitably variation *within* studies (not all people in a study have identical scores on outcome measures), so there is inevitably variation in effects *across* studies. If results are highly variable (e.g., results are conflicting across studies), a meta-analysis may be inappropriate. But if the results are modestly variable, an important design decision concerns steps that will be taken to explore the source of the variation. For example, the effects of an intervention might be systematically different for men and women (*clinical heterogeneity*). Or, the effects may be different if the period of follow-up is 6 months

rather than 3 months (*methodologic heterogeneity*). If such effects are hypothesized, it is important to plan for subgroup analyses during the design phase of the project.

Design decisions are incorporated into a formal protocol that articulates the sampling criteria that will be applied, the search methods that will be used, and the information that will be extracted from the studies. The protocol and aspects of it (e.g., the search strategy) should be pilot tested before it is finalized.

Searching the Literature for Data

In Chapter 5, we discussed the importance of *owning* the research literature before preparing a written review. Ownership—becoming a leading authority on the research question under review—is even more important in a systematic review because of the pivotal role that such reviews play in EBP. Traditional strategies of searching for relevant studies, using electronic databases and ancestry/descendancy approaches that were described in Chapter 5, are rarely adequate without further retrieval efforts.

A decision that should be made before a search begins is whether the review will cover both published and unpublished results. There is some disagreement about whether reviewers should limit their sample to published studies, or should cast as wide a net as possible and include **grey literature**—that is, studies with a more limited distribution, such as dissertations, unpublished reports, and so on. Some people restrict their sample to published reports in peer-reviewed journals, arguing that the peer review system is an important, tried-and-true screen for findings worthy of consideration as evidence.

The limitations of excluding nonpublished findings, however, have been noted in the literature on systematic reviews (e.g., Ciliska & Guyatt, 2005; Conn et al., 2003). The primary issue is **publication bias**—the tendency for published studies to over-represent statistically significant findings (this bias is sometimes called the *bias against the null hypothesis*). Explorations of this bias have revealed that the bias is widespread: Authors tend to refrain from submitting reports with negative findings, reviewers and editors tend to reject such reports when they are submitted, and users of evidence tend to ignore the findings when they are published. Studies have found that the exclusion of grey literature in a systematic review can lead to bias, particularly the overestimation of effects (Conn et al., 2003; Dwan et al., 2008).

We advocate retrieving as many relevant studies as possible, because methodologic weaknesses in unpublished reports can be dealt with later. Aggressive search strategies are essential and may include, in addition to methods noted in Chapter 5, the following:

- *Handsearching* journals known to publish relevant content—that is, doing a manual search of the tables of contents of key journals; handsearching of the literature more than a decade old is especially valuable because computerized indexing systems were less sophisticated before the mid 1990s.
- Identifying and contacting key researchers in the field to see if they have done studies that have not (yet) been published, and asking them about other members of the *"invisible college"* and about their participation in relevant listservs or newsgroups.
- Doing an "author search" of key researchers in the field in bibliographical databases and on the Internet.
- Reviewing abstracts from conference proceedings, and networking with researchers at conferences; conference abstracts are often available on the websites of the professional organizations sponsoring the conference.
- Searching for unpublished reports, such as dissertations and theses, government reports (e.g. in the U.S., *www.access.gpo.gov*), and registries of studies in progress (e.g., in the U.S., through Computer Retrieval of Information on Scientific Projects or CRISP, *http://crisp.cit.nih.gov*).
- Contacting foundations, government agencies, or corporate sponsors of the type of research under study to get leads on work in progress or recently completed.

Once relevant studies are identified, they must be retrieved, which can be a labor-intensive and expensive process. Retrieved studies need to be carefully screened to determine if they do, in fact, meet the inclusion criteria. All decisions relating to exclusions (preferably made by at least two reviewers to ensure objectivity) should be well documented and justified.

Example of a search strategy from a systematic review: Davenport (2004) did a systematic review to examine whether a standard (25 gauge 16 mm) needle is more effective than a wider or longer needle in reducing local reactions in children receiving immunizations. Davenport's comprehensive search strategy included a search of electronic databases, handsearching of journals, reference and citation searching, contacting researchers, and looking for unpublished reports. Screening to assess whether an identified study met the sampling criteria was independently completed by two people.

➲ **T I P :** The reports of studies that meet the sampling criteria do not always contain sufficient information for computing effect sizes. Be prepared to devote time and resources to communicating with researchers to obtain supplementary information.

Evaluating Study Quality

In systematic reviews, the evidence from primary studies should be evaluated to determine how much confidence to place in the findings, using criteria similar to those we have presented throughout this book. Strong studies should be given more weight than weaker ones in coming to conclusions about a body of evidence.

Evaluations of study quality sometimes involve quantitative ratings of each study in terms of the strength of evidence it yields. Literally dozens of quality assessment scales that yield summary scores have been developed (Agency for Healthcare Research and Quality [AHRQ], 2002). Despite the availability of many quality assessment instruments, overall scales are becoming less popular in meta-analyses. Quality criteria vary from instrument to instrument, and the result is that study quality can be rated differently with different assessment tools—or by different raters using the same tool. Moreover, there is a decided lack of transparency to users of the review when an overall scale score is used.

Because of these problems, the Cochrane *Handbook* (Higgins & Greene, 2008) recommends against using a global scale. They recommend a *domain-based evaluation*, that is, a *component approach*, as opposed to a *scale approach*. Individual features are given a separate rating or code for each study, and the relationship between these features and effect size estimates can be analyzed. So, for example, a researcher might code for such design elements as whether randomization was used, whether subjects were blinded, the extent of attrition from the study, and so on. Decisions about such features need to be articulated in the review protocol so that the relevant information can be systematically extracted from reports. Cooper (2010) offers an excellent discussion about quality assessment in meta-analyses.

⮕ **T I P :** For systematic reviews of interventions, the Cochrane *Handbook* (Higgins & Greene, 2008) includes a tool for assessing the risk of bias in six domains (Table 8.5).

Coding for quality elements in primary studies should be done by at least two qualified individuals. If there are disagreements between the coders, there should be a discussion until a consensus has been reached or, if necessary, a third person should be asked to help resolve the difference. Intercoder reliability should be calculated to demonstrate to readers that rater agreement on study quality elements was adequate.

Example of quality assessments: Bryanton and Beck (2010) completed a Cochrane review of RCTs testing the effects of structured postnatal education for parents. They used the Cochrane domain approach to capture elements of trial quality. Both reviewers completed assessments, and disagreements were resolved by discussion.

Extracting and Encoding Data for Analysis

The next step in a systematic review is to extract relevant information about study characteristics, methods, and findings from each report. A data

extraction form (either paper-and-pencil or computerized) must be developed, along with a coding manual to guide those who will be extracting and encoding information.

Basic data source information should be recorded for all studies. This includes such features as year of publication, country where data were collected, type of report (journal article, dissertation, etc.), and language in which the report was published. Supplementary information that may also be of interest includes whether the report was peer-reviewed, the impact factor of the journal (see Chapter 28), whether the study was funded (and by whom), and the year in which data were collected.

In terms of methodologic information that should be encoded, a critical element across all studies is sample size. Measurement issues may also be important. For example, there could be codes to designate the specific instruments used to operationalize outcome variables, and scale reliability could be recorded. Other attributes that should be recorded vary by study question. In longitudinal studies, length of time between waves of data collection is important, as well as rates of attrition. In intervention studies, codes for the assessment of biases should be recorded (e.g., whether there was randomization and blinding, whether selection bias was discerned, whether intention-to-treat analysis was used). Features of the intervention also should be recorded, such as type of setting, length of intervention, and primary modality of the intervention. If an assessment scale was used to rate methodologic quality, the scale score should be recorded.

Characteristics of the study participants must be encoded as well. A useful strategy is to record characteristics as percentages. For example, it is almost always possible to determine the percentage of the sample that was female. Other categorical characteristics that could be represented as percentages include race/ethnicity, educational level, and illness/treatment information (e.g., percentages of participants in different stages of cancer). Age should be recorded as mean age of sample members.

Finally, the findings must be encoded. Either effect sizes (discussed in the next section) need to be calculated and entered, or the data extraction form needs to record sufficient statistical information that the computer program can compute the indexes. Effect size information is often recorded for multiple outcomes, and may also be recorded for different subgroups of study participants (e.g., effects for males versus females on the various outcomes).

Extraction and coding of information should be completed by two or more people, at least for a portion of the studies. This allows for an assessment of interrater agreement, which should be sufficiently high to persuade readers of the review that the recorded information is accurate.

Example of intercoder agreement: In Yarcheski and colleagues' (2009) meta-analysis of predictors of maternal–fetal attachment, all 72 primary studies were coded by two researchers. The initial interrater agreement was 97% to 100%. All disagreements were discussed until there was 100% consensus.

A basic data extraction form is provided in the Toolkit section of the accompanying *Resource Manual* as a Word document that can be adapted for use in simple meta-analyses. ✴ A paper-and-pencil form such as this one should be developed and pretested, but moving to a computerized platform is often attractive because data can be entered using pull-down menus and error-detection is usually possible by establishing out-of-range values (e.g., it would be impossible to enter a publication date of 1011 in lieu of 2011). Guidance on developing coding forms is offered by Brown and colleagues (2003) and by Higgins and Green (2008).

Calculating Effects

Meta-analyses depend on the calculation of an index that encapsulates the relationship between the independent and dependent variable in each study. Because effects are captured differently depending on the variables' level of measurement, there is no single formula for calculating an effect size. In nursing, the most common scenarios for meta-analysis involve comparisons of two groups on a continuous outcome (e.g., the body mass index or BMI), comparisons of two groups on a dichotomous outcome (e.g., continued smoking versus stopped smoking), or correlations between two continuous variables (e.g., the correlation between BMI and scores on a depression scale). Other scenarios are described in the Cochrane *Handbook* (Higgins & Greene, 2008).

The first scenario, comparison of group means, is especially common in nursing studies; for simplicity, most of our discussion focuses on this situation. When the outcomes across studies are on identical scales (e.g., all outcomes are measures of weight in pounds), the effect is captured by simply subtracting the mean for one group from the mean for the other. For example, if the mean weight in an intervention group were 182.0 pounds and that for a control group were 194.0 pounds, the effect would be −8.0. More typically, outcomes are measured on different scales. For example, postpartum depression might be measured by Beck's Postpartum Depression Screening Scale in one study and by the CES-D in another. In such situations, mean differences across studies cannot be combined and averaged—we need an index that is neutral to the original metric used in the primary study. Cohen's *d*, described in Chapter 17, is the effect size index most often used. It may be recalled that the formula for *d* is the group difference in means, divided by the pooled standard deviation, or:

$$d = \frac{\overline{X}_1 - \overline{X}_2}{SD_p}$$

This effect size index transforms all effects to standard deviation units. That is, if *d* were .50, it means that the mean for one group was one-half a standard deviation higher than that for the other group—regardless of the original measurement scale.

➤ **TIP:** The preferred term for the effect size *d* in Cochrane reviews is **standardized mean difference** or SMD. Lipsey and Wilson (2001) refer to *d*, as described here, as ES_{SM}, that is, the effect size for standardized means. Cooper (2010) uses both *d* and SMD interchangeably.

If meta-analysis software is used in the meta-analysis—as it often is—there is no need to calculate effect sizes manually. The relevant means and SDs would be entered. But what if this information is absent from the report, as is all too often the case? Fortunately, there are alternative formulas for calculating *d* from information in the primary study reports. For example, it is possible to derive the value of *d* when the report gives such information as the value of *t* or *F*, an exact probability value, or a 95% confidence interval around the mean group difference. (The Toolkit in the *Resource Manual* includes alternative formulas for computing *d*. ⊗) If none of this information is available in a report, the authors could be contacted for additional information.

When the outcomes in the primary studies are expressed as dichotomies, meta-analysts have a choice of effect index, but the most usual are ones we discussed in earlier chapters—the relative risk (RR) index, the odds ratio (OR), and absolute risk reduction (ARR). Details for how to compute these indexes were provided in Table 16.6. The selection of a summary effect index depends on several criteria such as mathematical properties, ease of interpretation, and consistency. As noted in the Cochrane *Handbook* (Higgins & Greene, 2008), no single index is uniformly best. The odds ratio is, unfortunately, difficult for many users of systematic reviews to interpret. Nevertheless, it appears to be the most frequently used effect size index for dichotomous outcomes in the nursing literature.

Sometimes, especially for nonexperimental studies, the most common statistic used to express the relationship between independent and dependent variables in Pearson's *r*. If the primary studies in a meta-analysis provide statistical information in the form of a correlation coefficient, the *r* itself serves as the indicator of the magnitude and direction of effect.

Meta-analysts sometimes face a situation in which findings are not all reported using the same level of measurement. For example, if the variable *weight* (a continuous variable) was our key outcome variable, some studies might present findings for weight as a dichotomous outcome (e.g., *obese* versus *not obese*). One approach is to do separate meta-analyses for differently expressed effects.

Another is to re-express some of the effect indicators so that all effects can be pooled. For example, an odds ratio can be converted to *d*, as can a value of *r*—and vice versa. A large number of formulas for converting effect size information is presented in Appendix B of Lipsey and Wilson (2001).

➔ **TIP:** Our discussion of calculating effects sizes glosses over a number of complexities. Alternative methods may be needed when, for some studies, the unit of analysis is not individual people, cross-over designs were used, data were severely skewed, and so on. Those embarking on a meta-analysis project should seek additional guidance from books on meta-analysis or from statisticians.

Analyzing the Data

Meta-analysis is often described as a two-step analytic process. In the first step, a summary statistic that captures an effect is computed for each study, as just described. In the second step, a pooled effect estimate is computed as a **weighted average** of the effects for individual primary studies. A weighted average is defined as follows, with ES representing effect size estimates from each study:

$$\text{weighted average} = \frac{\text{sum of (ES} \times \text{weight for that ES)}}{\text{sum of the weights}}$$

The bigger the weight given to any study, the more that study will contribute to the weighted average. Thus, weights should reflect the amount of information that each study provides. One widely used approach is the **inverse variance method**, which uses the inverse of the variance of the effect size estimate (i.e., one divided by the square of its standard error) as the weight. Thus, larger studies, which have smaller standard errors, are given greater weight than smaller ones. The basic data needed for this type of analysis is the estimate of the effect size and its standard error, for each study.

Meta-analysts make many decisions at the point of analysis. In this brief overview, we present some basic information about the following analytic issues: identifying heterogeneity, deciding whether to use a fixed effects or random effects meta-analysis, incorporating clinical and methodologic diversity into the analysis, handling study quality, and addressing possible publication biases.

> ➡ **T I P :** The Cochrane Collaboration has developed its own software, the Review Manager (RevMan) software, which is currently distributed as copyrighted freeware. Macros are also available for doing meta-analyses within major software packages such as SPSS and SAS. Links to websites for other meta-analysis software are included in the Toolkit.

Identifying Heterogeneity. Heterogeneity across studies may rule out the possibility that a meta-analysis can be done, but it also remains an issue for the analyst even when statistical pooling is justifiable. Unless it is obvious that effects are consistent in magnitude and direction based on a casual perusal, heterogeneity should be formally tested.

Visual inspection of heterogeneity can most readily be accomplished by constructing a **forest plot**, which can be generated using meta-analytic software. A forest plot graphs the estimated effect size for each study, together with the 95% CI around each estimate. Figure 27.1 illustrates two forest plots for situations in which there is low heterogeneity (A) and high heterogeneity (B) for five studies in which the odds ratio was the effect size index. In Panel A, all effect size estimates favor the intervention group and are statistically significant for three of them

(studies 2, 4, and 5), according to the 95% CI information. In Panel B, by contrast, results are "all over the map," with two studies favoring controls at significant levels (studies 1 and 5) and two favoring the treatment group (studies 2 and 4). A meta-analysis is not appropriate for the five studies in B.

Heterogeneity can be evaluated using statistical procedures that test the null hypothesis that heterogeneity across studies represents random fluctuations. The test—often a chi-squared test—yields a p value that indicates the probability of obtaining effect size differences as large as those observed if the null hypothesis were true. A p value of .05 is usually used to determine significance but, because the test is underpowered when the meta-analysis involves a small number of studies, a p of .10 is sometimes considered an acceptable criterion.

Deciding on a Fixed Effect versus Random Effects Analysis. Two basic statistical models can be used in a meta-analysis, and the choice relates to heterogeneity. In a **fixed effects model**, the underlying assumption is that a single true effect size underlies all study results and that observed estimates vary only as a function of chance. The error term in a fixed effects model represents only within-study variation, and between-study variation is ignored.

A **random effects model**, by contrast, assumes that each study estimates *different*, yet related, true effects and that the various effects are normally

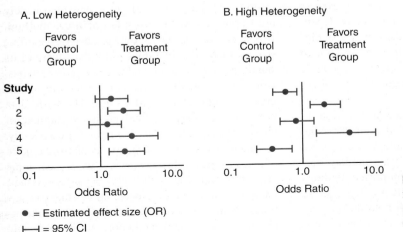

A. Low Heterogeneity

B. High Heterogeneity

FIGURE 27.1 Two forest plots for five studies with low (**A**) and high (**B**) heterogeneity of effect size estimates.

distributed around a mean effect size value. A random effects model takes both within- and between-study variation into account.

When there is little heterogeneity, both models yield nearly identical results. With extensive heterogeneity, however, the analyses yield different estimates of the average effect size. Moreover, when there is heterogeneity, the random effects model yields wider confidence intervals than the fixed effects model and is thus usually more conservative. But, it is precisely when there *is* heterogeneity that the random effects model should be used.

Some argue that a random effects model is needed only when the test for heterogeneity is statistically significant, and others argue that a random effects model is almost always more tenable. A recommended approach is to perform a *sensitivity analysis*—a test of how sensitive the results of an analysis are to changes in the way the analysis was done. In this case, it would involve using both models to assess how the results are affected. If the results differ substantially, it is more prudent to use estimates from the random effects model.

⮞ **TIP:** In a set of studies with heterogeneous effects, a random effects model will award relatively more weight to small studies than such studies would receive in a fixed effects model. If effects from small studies are systematically different from those in larger ones, a random effects meta-analysis could yield biased results. One strategy is to perform another sensitivity analysis, running the analysis with and without small studies to see if results vary.

Examining Factors Affecting Heterogeneity. A random effects meta-analysis incorporates heterogeneity into the analysis, but is intended primarily to address variation that cannot be explained. Many meta-analysts seek to understand determinants of effect size heterogeneity through formal analyses. Such analyses should always be considered exploratory because they are inherently nonexperimental (observational). Consequently, causal interpretations are necessarily speculative. To be considered scientifically appropriate, explorations of heterogeneity should be specified before doing the review, to minimize the risk of finding spurious associations.

Heterogeneity across studies could reflect systematic differences with regard to clinical characteristics or methodologic characteristics, and both can be explored. Clinical heterogeneity can result from differences in study groups (e.g., men and women) or in the way that the independent variable was operationalized. For example, in intervention studies, variation in effects could reflect who the agents were (e.g., nurses versus others), what the setting or delivery mode was, or how long the intervention lasted.

Methodologic heterogeneity could involve any number of study characteristics. Some could represent research design decisions, such as when the measurements were made (e.g., 3 months versus 6 months after an intervention), whether a randomized design was used, or whether other design features (e.g., blinding) were in place. Other methodologic variables could be after-the-fact "outcomes," such as a high versus low attrition rates.

Explorations of methodologic diversity focus primarily on the possibility that the studies suffer from different types or degrees of bias. Explorations of clinical diversity are more substantively relevant, in that they examine the possibility that effects differ because of factors that could affect clinical practice (e.g., are effects larger for certain types of people?).

Two types of strategy can be used to explore moderating effects on effect size: subgroup analysis and meta-regression. **Subgroup analyses** involve splitting the effect size information from studies into distinct categorical groups—for example, gender. Effects for studies with all-male (or predominantly male) samples could be compared to those for studies with all or predominantly female samples, using some threshold for "predominance" (e.g., 75% or more of participants). Of course, if it is possible to derive separate effect size estimates for males and females directly from study data, it is advantageous to do so, but this is seldom possible without contacting the researchers. The most straightforward procedure for comparing effects for different subgroups is to see whether there is any overlap in the confidence intervals around the effect size estimates for the groups.

Example of a subgroup analysis: Kim and colleagues (2009) did a meta-analysis of the effects of aerobic exercise interventions for women with breast cancer in terms of cardiopulmonary function and body composition. Significant aggregate effects were observed for several outcomes. The researchers also tested effects for subgroups of studies based on timing of intervention (during versus after adjuvant therapy), length of intervention (less than 12 weeks versus longer), and high versus low quality studies.

When variables thought to influence study heterogeneity are continuous (e.g., "dose" of the intervention), or when there is a mix of continuous and categorical factors, then meta-regression might be appropriate. **Meta-regression** involves predicting the effect size based on possible explanatory factors. As in ordinary regression, the statistical significance of regression coefficients indicates a nonrandom linear relationship between effect sizes and the associated explanatory variable.

⇨ **TIP:** Not all software can do meta-regression, but it can be done by a macro in the Stata statistical package and in Comprehensive Meta-Analysis (CMA) software.

Handling Study Quality. There are four basic strategies for dealing with the issue of study quality in a meta-analysis. One is to set a quality threshold for study inclusion. Exclusions could reflect requirements for certain methodologic features (e.g., only randomized studies) or for a sufficiently high score on a quality assessment scale. We prefer other alternatives that allow reviewers to summarize the full range of evidence in an area, but quality exclusions might in some cases be justified.

Example of excluding low-quality studies: DeNiet and colleagues (2009) did a meta-analysis of the effects of music-assisted relaxation interventions to improve sleep quality in adults with sleep complaints. They used a 9-item quality assessment list, and only studies with a score of at least 5 were included in the review.

A second strategy is to undertake sensitivity analyses to determine whether the exclusion of lower-quality studies changes the results of analyses based only on the most rigorous studies. Conn and colleagues (2003) have described as one option beginning the meta-analysis with high-quality studies and then sequentially adding studies of progressively lower quality to evaluate how robust the effect size estimates are to variation in quality.

Another approach is to consider quality as the basis for exploring heterogeneity of effects, the issue discussed in the previous section. For example, do randomized designs yield different average effect size estimates than quasi-experimental designs? Do effects vary as a function of the study's score on a quality assessment scale? Both individual study components and overall study quality can be used in subgroup analyses and meta-regressions.

A fourth strategy is to weight studies according to quality criteria. Most meta-analyses routinely give more weight to larger studies, but effect sizes can also be weighted by quality scores, thereby placing more weight on the estimates from rigorous studies. One persistent problem, however, is the previously mentioned issue of the validity of quality assessment scales and the unreliability of ratings. A mix of strategies, together with appropriate sensitivity analyses, is probably the most prudent approach to dealing with variation in study quality.

⇨ **TIP:** Quality information, using either a formal scale approach or a component approach, is important descriptively and should be reported in the review. For example, with a 25-point quality scale, the reviewers should report the mean scale score across primary studies, or the percent scoring above a threshold (e.g., 20 or higher).

Addressing Publication Bias. Even a comprehensive search for reports on a research question is unlikely to identify all relevant studies. Some researchers, therefore, use strategies to assess publication bias and to make adjustments for them.

The most usual way to examine the possibility of publication bias among studies in the meta-analysis is to construct a **funnel plot**. In a funnel plot, effects from individual studies are plotted on the horizontal axis and precision (e.g., the inverse of the standard

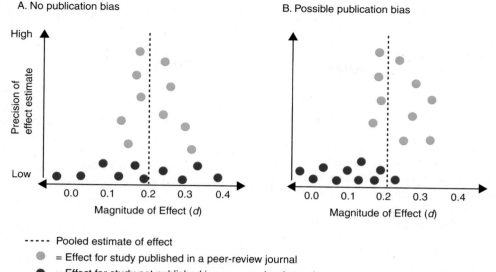

FIGURE 27.2 Two funnel plots for studies suggesting no publication bias (**A**) or possible publication bias (**B**).

error) is plotted on the vertical axis. Figure 27.2 illustrates two hypothetical funnel plots for a meta-analysis of a nursing intervention in which the pooled effect size estimate (*d*) for 20 studies (10 published and 10 unpublished) is 0.2. In the funnel plot on the left (A), the effects are fairly symmetric around the pooled effect size for both published and unpublished studies. In the asymmetric plot on the right (B), however, unpublished studies appear to have consistently lower effect size estimates, suggesting the possibility that the pooled effect size has been overestimated. More detailed guidance on detecting publication bias can be found in Soeken and Sripusanapan (2003) and in the Cochrane *Handbook* (Higgins & Greene, 2008).

> **TIP:** Funnel plots can be created within many of the meta-analytic software packages. Often, sample size rather than type of publication is used to dichotomize studies in the plot—that is, small versus large study, with some cutoff point used to distinguish the two. Biases and issues other than publication bias could be the cause of asymmetry in funnel plots, and this can often be explored in analyses of heterogeneity.

Strategies for *addressing* publication bias have been proposed in the meta-analytic literature. One is to compute a **fail-safe number** that estimates the number of studies reporting nonsignificant results that would be needed to reverse the conclusion of a significant effect in a meta-analysis. The fail-safe number is compared with a *tolerance level* (5k + 10), where *k* is the number of studies included in the analysis (Rosenthal, 1991). Although fail-safe information is sometimes reported in meta-analyses, the Cochrane *Handbook* noted several problems with this approach and does not recommend its use.

Writing a Meta-Analytic Report

The final step in a systematic review project is to prepare a report to disseminate the findings. Typically, such reports follow much the same format as for a research report for a primary study, with an Introduction, Method section, Results section, and Discussion (see Chapter 28).

Particular care should be taken in preparing the Method section. Readers of the review need to be able to assess the validity of the review, so methodologic and statistical decisions, and their rationales, should be described. If the reviewers decided that a meta-analysis was not justified, the rationale for this decision must be made clear. The Cochrane *Handbook* (Higgins & Greene, 2008) offers excellent suggestions for preparing reports for a systematic review. There is also an explicit reporting guideline for meta-analyses of RCTS called **PRISMA** or Preferred Reporting Items for Systematic reviews and Meta-Analyses (Liberati et al., 2009; Moher et al., 2009) and another for meta-analyses of observational studies called **MOOSE** (Meta-analysis of Observational Studies in Epidemiology, Stroup et al., 2000). Our critiquing guidelines later in this chapter also suggest the types of information to include.

A thorough discussion section is also crucial in systematic reviews. The Discussion should include an overall summary of the findings, noting the magnitude of effects and the numbers of studies and participants involved. The discussion should present an assessment of the overall quality of the body of evidence and the consistency of findings across studies—as well as an interpretation of why there might be inconsistencies. Implications of the review should also be described, including a discussion of further research needed to improve the evidence base and the clinical implications of the review. It is important in reports of meta-analyses of interventions to emphasize that "insufficient evidence of effectiveness" is not the same as "evidence of no effectiveness" (Stoltz et al., 2009).

Tables and figures typically play a key role in reports of systematic reviews. Forest plots are often presented, showing effect size and 95% CI information for each study, as well as for the overall pooled result. Typically, there is also a table showing the characteristics of studies included in the review. A template for such a table is included in the Toolkit of the accompanying *Resource Manual.* 😣 Also, the PRISMA guidelines call for the inclusion of a flow chart, analogous to a CONSORT flow chart (Chapter 28), that documents the identification, screening, and inclusion of studies in a systematic review. 😣

Finally, full citations for the entire sample of studies should be included in the bibliography of the review. Often these are identified separately from other citations—for example, by noting them with asterisks.

METASYNTHESIS

The systematic integration of qualitative findings is a burgeoning field. As several commentators have noted, metasynthesis holds exciting promise for those concerned about the generalizability and transferability of findings from individual studies (Finfgeld-Connett, 2010; Polit & Beck, 2010). Metasyntheses, like meta-analyses, can play an important role in evidence-based practice.

Approaches to systematic qualitative integration are rapidly evolving, so there are no standard procedures. Indeed, five leading thinkers on qualitative integration noted the "terminological landmines" (p. 1343) that complicate the field, "the creeping use of the term *metasynthesis* to represent something more akin to 'metasoup'" (p. 1347), and the challenges of working in "an era of metamadness" (p. 1357) (Thorne et al., 2004).

Metasynthesis: Definition and Types

Terminology and approaches to qualitative synthesis are diverse and complex. Thorne and colleagues (2004), acknowledging the diversity, used the term metasynthesis as an umbrella term, with metasynthesis broadly representing "a family of methodologic approaches to developing new knowledge based on rigorous analysis of existing qualitative research findings" (p. 1343).

Like other types of systematic reviews, metasyntheses are a systematic approach to reviewing and integrating findings from completed studies. Yet, just as there are many different approaches to doing qualitative research, there are diverse approaches to doing a metasynthesis and to defining what it is. There is more agreement on what a metasynthesis is *not* than on what it *is*. Metasynthesis is not a literature review—that is, not the collating of research findings—nor is it a concept analysis. Many writers have followed the definition of metasynthesis offered by Schreiber and colleagues (1997): ". . . the bringing together and breaking down of findings, examining them, discovering the essential features and, in some way, combining phenomena into a transformed whole" (p. 314). Sandelowski (in Thorne et al., 2004) suggested that "metasyntheses are integrations that are more than the sum of parts, in that they offer novel interpretations of findings" (p. 1358). Most, but not all, methods of qualitative synthesis involve a transformational process.

Barnett-Page and Thomas (2009) identified 12 different approaches for synthesizing qualitative research. The approaches that are arguably of greatest utility to nurse researchers are:

- Meta-ethnography (Noblit & Hare, 1988)
- Meta-study (Paterson et al., 2001)
- Qualitative metasummary (Sandelowski & Barroso, 2007)
- Critical interpretive synthesis or CIS (Dixon-Woods et al., 2006)
- Grounded formal theory (Eaves, 2001)
- Thematic synthesis (Thomas & Harden, 2008)

As a means of characterizing and comparing the various approaches, Barnett-Page and Thomas (2009) used a system called *dimensions of difference* to distinguish them. One dimension concerned underlying epistemological assumptions, which they felt explained the rationale for different approaches. Both Patterson's metastudy method and critical interpretive synthesis (CIS) were categorized as exemplars of *subjective idealism* in which "there is no shared reality independent of multiple alternative human constructions." Meta-ethnography and grounded formal theory were viewed as having an epistemological stance described as *objective idealism*, in which "there is a world of collectively shared understandings." Thematic synthesis was categorized as *critical realism*, "knowledge of reality is mediated by our perceptions and beliefs" (p. 5).

Other dimensions of difference in the Barnett-Page and Thomas system were the degree of iteration, the type and degree of quality assessment in the process, the degree of focus on comparisons among primary studies, and the extent to which the aim is to "go beyond" the primary studies. With respect to the latter, all of the approaches most closely allied with nursing seek to push beyond the data in the original primary studies to a fresh interpretation of the phenomenon under review—although they go about this in different ways.

Different typologies of metasynthesis have been proposed. For example, Schreiber and colleagues (1997) suggested a typology that puts the role of theory at center stage. Their categorization includes three types linked to the purpose of the synthesis—theory building, theory explication, and description. *Theory-building metasyntheses* are inquiries that extend the level of theory beyond what could be achieved in individual studies. Both grounded formal theory and metastudy methods fall in this category. In *theory explication metasyntheses*, researchers "flesh out" and reconceptualize abstract concepts. Finally, *descriptive metasynthesis* involves a comprehensive analysis of a phenomenon based on a synthesis of qualitative findings; findings are not typically deconstructed and then reconstructed as they are in theory-related reviews.

The decision on which approach to use is likely to depend on several factors, including the nature of the problem and the philosophical leanings of the reviewers. For students, the decision is likely to be affected by the skills and preferences of their advisers.

Steps in a Metasynthesis

Many of the steps in a metasynthesis are similar to ones we described in connection with a meta-analysis, so some details will not be repeated here. However, we point out a few distinctive issues relating to qualitative integration that are relevant in the various steps.

Formulating the Problem

In metasynthesis, researchers begin with a research question or a focus of investigation, and a key issue concerns the scope of the inquiry. Finfgeld (2003) recommended a strategy that balances breadth and utility. She advised that the scope be broad enough to fully capture the phenomenon of interest, but sufficiently focused to yield findings that are meaningful to clinicians, other researchers, and public policy makers. Reviewers sometimes state a specific research question guiding the synthesis, but often declare their overall study purpose.

> **Example of a statement of purpose in a meta-ethnography:** Purc-Stephenson and Thrasher (2010) stated that the aim of their synthesis "was to explore nurses' experiences with telephone triage and advice within the primary care sector and to understand the factors that facilitate or impede their decision-making process" (p. 483).

Designing a Metasynthesis

Like a quantitative systematic review, a metasynthesis requires advance planning. Having a team of at least two researchers to design and implement the study is often advantageous, perhaps to an even greater extent than for a quantitative systematic review because of the subjective nature of interpretive efforts. Just as in a primary study, the design of a qualitative metasynthesis should involve efforts to enhance integrity and rigor, and investigator triangulation is one such strategy.

> ➲ **TIP:** Meta-analyses often are undertaken by researchers who did not do one of the primary studies in the review. Metasyntheses, by contrast, are often completed by researchers whose area of interest has led them to do both original studies and metasyntheses on the same topic. Prior work in an area offers advantages in terms of researchers' ability to grasp subtle nuances and to think abstractly about a topic, but a disadvantage may be a certain degree of partiality about one's own work.

Metasynthesists, like meta-analysts, must also make upfront decisions about sampling, and they face the same issue of deciding whether to include findings only from peer-reviewed journals in the analysis. One advantage of including alternative sources, in addition to wanting a more comprehensive analysis, is that journal articles are constrained in what can be reported because of space limitations. Finfgeld (2003) noted that in her metasynthesis on *courage,* she used dissertations even when a peer-reviewed journal article was available from

the same study because the dissertation offered richer information.

An aspect of sampling that has been controversial in metasyntheses concerns whether to integrate studies based on different research traditions and methods. Some researchers have argued against combining studies from different epistemological perspectives, and have recommended separate analyses for different traditions. Others, however, advocate combining findings across traditions and methodologies. Which path to follow is likely to depend on the focus of the inquiry, its intent vis-à-vis theory development, and the nature of the available evidence.

> **Example of sampling decisions:** Nelson (2002) conducted a metasynthesis of qualitative studies related to mothering other-than-normal children. She explained that, "I made a deliberate decision to include studies that used various qualitative methodologies and represented a wide variety of children because I was unable to locate a sufficient number of studies using the same qualitative methodology and focusing on one group of children. . . . I believed that the potential significance of synthesizing qualitative knowledge in the broad area of mothering other-than-normal children outweighed the limitations of the endeavor and was philosophically consistent with the qualitative paradigm" (p. 517).

Another sampling issue concerns decisions about the *type* of findings to include. Sandelowski and Barroso (2003a, 2007) describe a continuum of qualitative findings that involves how close the analysis was to the original data—that is, the extent to which the researcher *transformed* the data to yield findings. The continuum ranges from a category closest to the data that they called "no finding" (meaning that the data themselves are presented, without judgments or integrated discoveries) to a category farthest from the data that they called "interpretive explanation." The category scheme is intended to be neutral to the underlying method and research tradition. Sandelowski and Barroso argued that "no finding" studies are not research, so metasynthesists may choose not to include them.

Searching the Literature for Data

It is generally more difficult to find qualitative than quantitative studies using mainstream approaches, such as searching electronic databases. One factor contributing to this difficulty is that some databases do not index studies by methodology—although there have been many improvements in recent years. For example, "qualitative research" was added as a MeSH (medical subject heading) term in MEDLINE in 2003. "Qualitative studies" is also used in the controlled vocabulary of CINAHL. Still, it is risky to rely totally on proper coding of studies for a metasynthesis. It may be wise to search for many different terms (e.g., "grounded theory," phenomenolog*, ethnograph*, "case study," and so on). Strategies for searching the grey literature, such as those suggested earlier, may also yield important sources. Barroso and colleagues (2003) have discussed strategies for finding qualitative primary studies for integration purposes. Further search guidance is offered by Wilczynski and colleagues (2007) and in a document on the website of the Cochrane Qualitative Review Methods Group of the Joanna Briggs Institute (*http://www.joannabriggs.edu.au/cqrmg/tools.html*).

⏩ **TIP:** Sample sizes in nursing metasyntheses are highly variable, ranging from a very small number—for example, three primary studies in the meta-ethnography of Varcoe and colleagues (2003)—to nearly 300 in Paterson's (2001) synthesis of qualitative studies on chronic illness. Sample size is likely to vary as a function of scope of the inquiry and the extent of prior research. As with primary studies, one guideline for sampling adequacy is whether categories in the metasynthesis are saturated (Finfgeld, 2003).

Evaluating Study Quality

Formal evaluations of primary study quality are not as common in metasynthesis as in meta-analysis. Yet, it is often useful to perform some type of quality assessment of primary studies, if for no other purpose than to be able to describe the sample of studies in the review.

Many nurse researchers use the 10-question assessment tool from the Critical Appraisal Skills Programme (CASP) of the Centre for Evidence-Based Medicine in the United Kingdom (*http://www.phru.nhs.uk/Pages/PHD/CASP.htm*). Sandelowski and Barroso (2007) offered a "reading guide" that can be used for a more detailed appraisal.

The Primary Research Appraisal Tool developed by Paterson and colleagues (2001), was designed to be used to screen primary studies for inclusion in a metasynthesis—although metastudy in its most recent form includes all relevant studies except those deemed not to be qualitative (Paterson, 2007).

There is some disagreement about whether quality ought to be a criterion for eliminating studies for a metasynthesis. Sandelowski and Barroso (2003c), for example, advocated inclusiveness: "Excluding reports of qualitative studies because of inadequacies in reporting . . ., or because of what some reviewers might perceive as methodologic mistakes, will result in the exclusion of reports with findings valuable to practice that are not necessarily invalidated by these errors" (p. 155). Finfgeld (2003) suggested that, at a minimum, studies included in the review must have used accepted qualitative methods and must have findings that are well supported by raw data—that is, quotes from participants.

Noblit and Hare (1988) advocated including all relevant studies, but also suggested giving more weight to higher-quality studies. A more systematic application of assessments in a metasynthesis is to use quality information in a sensitivity analysis that explores whether interpretations are altered when low-quality studies are removed (Thomas & Hardin, 2008).

Example of a sensitivity analysis: Bridges and colleagues (2010) synthesized studies on the experiences of older people and relatives in acute care settings, using a thematic synthesis approach. Primary studies were appraised using the CASP criteria. A total of 42 primary studies and a previous synthesis were included in the review. A sensitivity analysis revealed that the findings and interpretations were robust to the removal of the nine low-quality studies.

Extracting and Encoding Data for Analysis

Information about various features of the study need to be abstracted and coded as part of the project. Just as in quantitative integration, the metasynthesist should abstract and record features of the data source (e.g., year of publication, country), characteristics of the sample (e.g., age, gender, number of participants), and methodologic features (e.g., research tradition).

Most important, of course, information about the study findings must be extracted and recorded. Sandelowski and Barroso (2003b) have defined *findings* as the "data-based and integrated discoveries, conclusions, judgments, or pronouncements researchers offered regarding the events, experiences, or cases under investigation (i.e., their interpretations, no matter the extent of the data transformation involved)" (p. 228). Others characterize findings as the key themes, metaphors, categories, concepts, or phrases from each study.

As Sandelowski and Barroso (2002, 2003a) have noted, however, *finding* the findings is not always easy. For example, qualitative researchers intermingle data with interpretation, and findings from other studies with their own. Noblit and Hare (1988) advised that, just as primary study researchers must read and re-read their data before they can proceed with a meaningful analysis, metasynthesists must read the primary studies multiple times to fully grasp the categories or metaphors being explicated. In essence, a metasynthesis becomes "another 'reading' of data, an opportunity to reflect on the data in new ways" (McCormick et al., 2003, p. 936).

Analyzing and Interpreting the Data

Strategies for metasynthesis diverge most markedly at the analysis stage. We briefly describe three approaches, and advise you to consult more advanced resources for further guidance. No matter which approach researchers use, they need to understand that metasynthesis is a complex interpretive task that involves "carefully peeling away the surface layers of studies to find their hearts and souls in a way that does the least damage to them" (Sandelowski et al., 1997, p. 370).

> ➲ **TIP:** The approach called *thematic synthesis* (Thomas & Harden, 2008) was developed at the EPPI-Centre (Evidence for Policy and Practice Information Centre, London), and involves the use of software (EPPI-Reviewer) that has a component designed to support thematic synthesis.

The Noblit and Hare Approach. Noblit and Hare's (1988) methods of integration, which they called **meta-ethnography**, have been influential among nurse researchers. Noblit and Hare argued that a meta-ethnography should be interpretive and not aggregative—that is, that the synthesis should focus on constructing interpretations rather than analyses. Their approach for synthesizing qualitative studies included seven phases that overlap and repeat as the metasynthesis progresses, the first three of which are pre-analytic: (1) deciding on the phenomenon, (2) deciding which studies are relevant for the synthesis, and (3) reading and re-reading each study. Phase 7 involves writing up the synthesis, but Phases 4 through 6 concern the analysis:

Phase 4: Deciding how the studies are related to each other. In this phase, the researcher makes a list of the key metaphors in each study and their relationship to each other. Noblit and Hare used the term "metaphor" to refer to themes, perspectives, and/or concepts that emerged from the primary studies. Studies can be related in three ways: *reciprocal* (directly comparable), *refutational* (in opposition to each other), and in a line of argument other than either reciprocal or refutational.

Phase 5: Translating the qualitative studies into one another. Noblit and Hare noted that "translations are especially unique syntheses because they protect the particular, respect holism, and enable comparison. An adequate translation maintains the central metaphors and/or concepts of each account in their relation to other key metaphors or concepts in that account" (p. 28). *Reciprocal translation analysis* (RTA) involves exploring and explaining similarities and contradictions between studies, and is not unlike a constant comparative process.

Phase 6: Synthesizing translations. Here the challenge for the researcher is to make a whole into more than the individual parts imply. *Line-of-argument* (LOA) *synthesis* involves building up a new picture of the whole (e.g., a whole culture or phenomenon) from a scrutiny of its parts.

Atkins and colleagues (2008), noting that some aspects of meta-ethnography were not well defined, have offered further guidance on the process.

Example of Noblit and Hare's approach:
Beck (2002) used Noblit and Hare's approach in her metasynthesis of 18 qualitative studies on postpartum depression. As part of the analysis, key metaphors were listed and organized under four overarching themes, one being "spiraling downward." For instance, in one of the primary studies, the key metaphors listed under this theme included "total isolation; façade of normalcy; obsessive thoughts; pervasive guilt; panic/overanxious/feels trapped; completely overwhelmed by infant demands; anger" (p. 459). Beck's paper presented an excellent table illustrating how the individual metaphors mapped onto the four themes.

The Paterson, Thorne, Canam, and Jillings Approach. Paterson and colleagues' (2001) **metastudy** method of metasynthesis involves three components: metadata analysis, metamethod, and metatheory. These components often are conducted concurrently, and the metasynthesis results from the integration of findings from these 3 analytic components. Paterson and colleagues define **metadata analysis** as the study of results of reported research in a specific substantive area of investigation by means of analyzing the "processed data." **Metamethod** is the study of the methodologic rigor of the studies included in the metasynthesis. Lastly, **metatheory** refers to the analysis of the theoretical underpinnings on which the studies are grounded. Metastudy uses metatheory to describe and deconstruct theories that shape a body of inquiry. The end product of a metastudy is a metasynthesis that results from bringing back together the findings of these three components.

Example of Paterson's approach: Bench and Day (2010) used the Paterson framework in their metasynthesis focusing on the specific problems faced by patients and relatives immediately following discharge from a critical care unit to another hospital unit.

The Sandelowski and Barroso Approach. The strategies developed by Sandelowski and Barroso (2007) are likely to inspire metasynthesists in the years ahead. In their multiyear methodologic project, they developed the previously described continuum relating to how much data transformation had occurred in a primary study. Further, they

dichotomized studies based on level of synthesis and interpretation. Reports are described as *summaries* if the findings are descriptive synopses of the qualitative data, usually with lists and frequencies of topics and themes, without conceptual reframing. *Syntheses* are findings that are more interpretive and explanatory and that involve conceptual or metaphorical reframing. Sandelowski and Barroso have argued that only syntheses should be used in a metasynthesis.

Both summaries and syntheses can, however, be used in a **metasummary**, which can lay a good foundation for a metasynthesis. Sandelowski and Barroso (2003b) provided an example of a metasummary in which they used studies (including both summaries and syntheses) of mothering within the context of HIV infection. The first step, extracting findings, resulted in almost 800 complete sentences from the 45 reports they identified. The 800 sentences were then reduced to 93 thematic statements, or abstracted findings.

The next step in the metasummary was to calculate **manifest effect sizes**, that is, effect sizes calculated from the manifest content pertaining to motherhood within the context of HIV as represented in the 93 abstracted findings. Qualitative effect sizes are not to be confused with treatment effects: the ". . . calculation of effect sizes constitutes a quantitative transformation of qualitative data in the service of extracting more meaning from those data and verifying the presence of a pattern or theme" (Sandelowski & Barroso, 2003b, p. 231). They argued that by calculating effect sizes, integration can avoid the possibility of over- or underweighting findings.

Two types of effect size can be created from the abstracted findings. A **frequency effect size**, which indicates the magnitude of the findings, is the number of reports with unduplicated information that contain a given finding, divided by all unduplicated reports. For example, Sandelowski and Barroso (2003b) calculated an overall frequency effect size of 60% for the finding about a mother's struggle about whether or not to disclose her HIV status to her children. In other words, 60% of the 45 reports had a finding of this nature. Such effect size information can be calculated for subgroups of reports—for example, for published versus unpublished reports, for reports from different research traditions, and so on.

An **intensity effect size** indicates the concentration of findings *within* each report. It is calculated by dividing the number of different findings in a given report, divided by the total number of findings in all reports. As an example, one primary study reported in a book had 29 out of the 93 total findings, for an intensity effect size of 31% (Sandelowski & Barroso, 2003b).

Metasyntheses can build upon metasummaries, but require findings that are more interpretive, that is, from reports that are characterized as syntheses. The purpose of a metasynthesis is not to summarize, but to offer novel interpretations of interpretive findings. Such interpretive integrations require metasynthesists to piece the individual syntheses together to craft a new coherent description or explanation of a target event or experience. An array of quantitative analytic methods can be used to achieve this goal, including, ". . . for example, constant comparison, taxonomic analysis, the reciprocal translation of in vivo concepts, and the use of imported concepts to frame data" (Sandelowski in Thorne et al., 2004, p. 1358).

➔ **T I P :** Rigor and integrity are important in metasyntheses, as in all research. Sandelowski and Barroso (2007) offered useful advice on how to optimize the validity of metasyntheses (Chapter 8).

Example of Sandelowski and Barroso's approach: Draucker and colleagues (2009) conducted a metasynthesis to identify the essence of healing from sexual violence, as described by adults who experienced it as children or as adults. Metasummary techniques were used to aggregate findings from 51 reports, and metasynthesis techniques were used to interpret the findings. A total of 11 meta-findings with frequency effect sizes over 15% were abstracted and summarized in a table.

Writing a Metasynthesis Report
Metanythesis reports are similar in many respects to meta-analytic reports—except that the Results section contains the new interpretations rather than the quantitative findings. When a metasummary has been done, meta-findings would typically be presented in a table, a template for which is available in the Toolkit of the accompanying *Resource Manual.* ✖

The method section of a metasynthesis report should contain a detailed description of the sampling criteria, the search procedures, and efforts made to enhance the integrity and rigor of the integration. The sample of selected studies should also be described. Key features of the sample of studies are often summarized in a table. A PRISMA-type flowchart highlighting sampling decisions and outcomes ideally should be included.

As with primary studies, alternatives to written metasyntheses have been proposed. Noblit and Hare (1988) noted, for example, that when the qualitative synthesis' purpose is to inform clinicians or practitioners, other forms of expressing the synthesis may be preferred, such as through music, artwork, plays, or videos.

SYSTEMATIC MIXED STUDIES REVIEWS

The emergence of mixed methods research as a "third research community" (Chapter 25) has given rise to interest in systematic reviews that integrate findings from a broad methodologic array of studies. Such reviews are a relatively new endeavor, and so both terminology and approaches are still evolving. Pluye and colleagues (2009) used the term mixed studies review (MSR), but noted that many other names have been used, such as *mixed methods review* (Harden & Thomas, 2005) and *mixed research synthesis* (Sandelowski et al., 2006). We use the term **systematic mixed studies review** to refer to a systematic review that uses disciplined and auditable procedures to integrate and synthesize findings from qualitative, quantitative, and mixed methods studies.

As in mixed methods research, the "dictatorship of the research question" is a driving force behind mixed studies reviews. Harden and Thomas (2005), whose work at the EPPI-Centre in London focused on health promotion interventions, noted that their reviews "were beginning to answer multiple questions" and that their reviews increasingly involved "more than one section in which the results of studies are brought together" (p. 261). As a result, they began to develop strategies for doing systematic mixed study reviews.

Margarete Sandelowski has been in the forefront of such development in the United States. She and her colleagues (2007) astutely noted that "the research synthesis enterprise, in general, and the mixed research synthesis, in particular, entail *comparability work* whereby reviewers impose similarity and difference on the studies to be reviewed" (p. 236, emphasis added). In other words, part of the reviewers' job in any synthesis project is to manage difference, and this takes on particular prominence when there are major difference in goals, epistemological assumptions, and methodologic approaches. Comparability work is what allows "the previously incompatible and uncommon to be compared" (p. 238).

Sandelowski and colleagues (2006) described three models of mixed studies review that vary in terms of both approach and goals. In a *segregated design*, two separate syntheses are undertaken, one of qualitative findings and the other of quantitative findings, and then the mixed methods synthesis integrates the two. They viewed this approach as appropriate when qualitative and quantitative findings are viewed as complementing each other, as opposed to confirming or refuting each other. Complementarity is observed when the qualitative and quantitative research has addressed different but connected questions.

The segregated design model characterizes many mixed studies reviews and is similar to the approach described by Harden and Thomas (2005), who noted that this model "preserves the integrity of findings of different types of studies" (p. 268). This design has been found to be especially useful in integrating information about both effectiveness and context in intervention research. Harden and Thomas provided a good example of their integration of findings on interventions to promote fruit and vegetables in children's diets. They combined findings from a meta-analysis of intervention effects with those from a metasynthesis of findings about barriers to and facilitators of children's healthy eating to address such questions as

these: "Which interventions match recommendations derived from children's views and experiences? Which recommendations have yet to be addressed by soundly evaluated interventions? and Do those interventions that match recommendations show bigger effect sizes and/or explain heterogeneity?" (p. 264).

The second model is an *integrated design* (Sandelowski et al., 2007), which can be used when qualitative and quantitative findings in an area of inquiry are perceived as able to confirm, extend, or refute each other. In an integrated design, studies are grouped not by method but by findings viewed as answering the same research question. The analytic approach may involve transforming the findings (qualitizing quantitative findings or quantitizing qualitative findings) to enable them to be combined. A particularly sophisticated variant of this model is to use a *Bayesian synthesis*, as exemplified in a study in which Sandelowski participated (Voils et al., 2009).

A third model is a *contingent design* (Sandelowski et al., 2007) that involves a coordinated and sequential series of syntheses. In such a design, the findings from the systematic synthesis to address one research question is used to address a second research question—which may lead to yet another synthesis addressing a different question. Some of the mixed studies reviews as described in the Cochrane *Handbook* (Higgins & Greene, 2008) might use such a design. For example, a qualitative synthesis can precede a meta-analysis and may help to define key outcomes or key variables for an analysis of heterogeneity for the meta-analysis.

As with all types of systematic review, mixed studies reviews face several issues of contention. One issue concerns how best to evaluate quality (see Pluye et al., 2009), and what role appraisals should play in the reviews. Another concerns the specific analytic approaches that are likely to be productive. Techniques such as textual narrative, thematic synthesis, and critical interpretive synthesis (an adaptation of meta-ethnography) have been described (Lucas et al., 2007; Flemming, 2010). It seems likely that guidance (and debate) on how best to conduct mixed studies reviews will continue in the years ahead, and that such reviews will play an important role in evidence-based practice.

BOX 27.1 Guidelines for Critiquing Systematic Reviews

THE PROBLEM

- Did the report clearly state the research problem and/or research questions? Is the scope of the project appropriate?
- Is the topic of the review important for nursing?
- Were concepts, variables, or phenomena adequately defined?
- Was the integration approach adequately described, and was the approach appropriate?

SEARCH STRATEGY

- Did the report clearly describe criteria for selecting primary studies, and are those criteria reasonable?
- Were the bibliographic databases used by the reviewers identified, and are they appropriate and comprehensive? Were key words identified, and are they exhaustive?
- Did the reviewers use adequate supplementary efforts to identify relevant studies?
- Was a PRISMA-type flow chart included to summarize the search strategy and results?

THE SAMPLE

- Were inclusion and exclusion criteria clearly articulated, and were they defensible?
- Did the search strategy yield a strong and comprehensive sample of studies? Were strengths and limitations of the sample identified?
- If an original report was lacking key information, did reviewers attempt to contact the original researchers for additional information—or did the study have to be excluded?
- If studies were excluded for reasons other than insufficient information, did the reviewers provide a rationale for the decision?

QUALITY APPRAISAL

- Did the reviewers appraise the quality of the primary studies? Did they use a defensible and well-defined set of criteria, or a respected quality appraisal scale?
- Did two or more people do the appraisals, and was inter-rater agreement reported?
- Was the appraisal information used in a well-defined and defensible manner in the selection of studies, or in the analysis of results?

DATA EXTRACTION

- Was adequate information extracted about methodologic and administrative aspects of the study? Was adequate information about sample characteristics extracted?
- Was sufficient information extracted about study findings?
- Were steps taken to enhance the integrity of the dataset (e.g., were two or more people used to extract and record information for analysis)?

DATA ANALYSIS—GENERAL

- Did the reviewers explain their method of pooling and integrating the data?
- Was the analysis of data thorough and credible?
- Were tables, figures, and text used effectively to summarize findings?

(continued)

BOX 27.1 Guidelines for Critiquing Systematic Reviews (continued)

DATA ANALYSIS—QUANTITATIVE

- If a meta-analysis was not performed, was there adequate justification for using a narrative integration method? If a meta-analysis *was* performed, was this justifiable?
- For meta-analyses, were appropriate procedures followed for computing effect size estimates for all relevant outcomes?
- Was heterogeneity of effects adequately dealt with? Was the decision to use a random effects model or a fixed effects model sound? Were appropriate subgroup analyses undertaken—or was the absence of subgroup analyses justified?
- Was the issue of publication bias adequately addressed?

DATA ANALYSIS—QUALITATIVE

- In a metasynthesis, did the reviewers describe the techniques they used to compare the findings of each study, and did they explain their method of interpreting their data?
- If a metasummary was undertaken, did the abstracted findings seem appropriate and convincing? Were appropriate methods used to compute effect sizes? Was information presented effectively?
- In a metasynthesis, did the synthesis achieve a fuller understanding of the phenomenon to advance knowledge? Do the interpretations seem well grounded? Was there a sufficient amount of data included to support the interpretations?

CONCLUSIONS

- Did the reviewers draw reasonable conclusions about the quality, quantity, and consistency of evidence relating to the research question?
- Were limitations of the review/synthesis noted?
- Were implications for nursing practice and further research clearly stated?

☐ All systematic reviews
▨ Systematic reviews of quantitative studies
☐ Metasyntheses

Example of a systematic mixed studies review: Roberts and Noyes (2009) used the EPPI-Centre segregated design model in their mixed study review of factors that are barriers to, and facilitators of, the contraceptive decisions of women over 40 years old.

CRITIQUING SYSTEMATIC REVIEWS

Like all studies, systematic reviews should be thoroughly critiqued before the findings are deemed trustworthy and relevant to clinicians. ⊗ Box 27.1 offers guidelines for evaluating systematic reviews. Although these guidelines are fairly broad, not all questions apply equally well to all types of systematic reviews. In particular, we have distinguished ques-

tions about analysis separately for meta-analyses and metasyntheses. The list of questions in Box 27.1 is not necessarily comprehensive. Supplementary questions might be needed for particular types of review—for example, for mixed studies reviews. The PRISMA guidelines are an additional resource for checking on whether a review included sufficient information.

In drawing conclusions about a research synthesis, a major issue concerns the nature of the decisions the researcher made. Sampling decisions, approaches to handling quality of the primary studies, and analytic approaches should be carefully evaluated to assess the soundness of the reviewers' conclusions. Another aspect, however, is drawing inferences about how you might use the evidence in clinical practice. It is not the reviewers' job, for example, to consider such issues as barriers to making use of the evidence, acceptability of an innovation, costs and benefits of change in various settings, and so on. These are issues for practicing nurses seeking to maximize the effectiveness of their actions and decisions.

●●●●●●●●●●●●●●●●●●●●●●●●

RESEARCH EXAMPLES

We conclude this chapter with a description of two systematic reviews. Two integration reports (a meta-analysis and a metasynthesis) appear in their entirety in the accompanying *Resource Manual.*

Example 1: A Meta-Analysis

Study: Meta-analysis of quality-of-life outcomes from physical activity interventions (Conn et al., 2009).

Purpose: The purpose of the meta-analysis was to integrate research evidence on the effects of physical activity (PA) on quality of life (QOL) outcomes among adults with chronic illness. Two of the specific research questions addressed were: (a) What is the overall mean difference effect size (ES) in QOL scores between treatment and control subjects after interventions to increase PA? (b) Do the effects of PA interventions on QOL outcomes vary depending on the characteristics of participants, methodology, or interventions?

Eligibility Criteria: Criteria for study inclusion were spelled out in Table 1 of the report, together with an explicit rationale for each criterion. A study was included if it examined the effects of a PA intervention on QOL for people with a chronic illness and if it: (a) was an English-language study, (b) was published in a report after 1970, (c) involved a sample of at least 5 subjects, and (d) included measures designed specifically to assess QOL (not, for example, QOL-related constructs such as mood). Both published and unpublished reports were eligible, and diverse research designs were permitted (not just RCTs).

Search Strategy: A reference librarian performed searches, using well-specified search terms, in 11 databases (e.g., MEDLINE, CINAHL, Dissertation Abstracts, Scopus, PsycINFO). The National Institutes of Health database of funded studies was also searched. Ancestry searching was conducted, as well as a search of all authors on eligible studies. Hand searches of 42 journals were performed, and several methods were used to identify studies in the grey literature.

Sample: This analysis was part of a larger project that examined PA in relation to various health outcomes. For the overall project, over 12,000 reports were reviewed. In the analysis that focused on QOL, there were 66 studies in which 7,291 subjects participated (sample sizes ranged from 9 to 927). Ten of the 66 reports were unpublished. The most common chronic illnesses were cardiac, cancer, diabetes, and arthritis. Intervention duration ranged from 1 to 52 weeks.

Data Extraction: A formal extraction protocol was developed, pilot tested, and revised. A wide array of information about participants, interventions, and methods was extracted from the studies. Key attributes of methodologic quality such as random assignment and attrition were coded. Two well-trained coders extracted the data. Discrepancies were resolved by the senior author.

Effect Size Calculation: The standardized mean difference (d) was used as the effect size for QOL outcomes. Each ES was weighted by the inverse of within-study variance.

Statistical Analyses: Both fixed effects and random effects models were used to estimate pooled effect size. Random effects results were reported because of heterogeneity of effects. Moderator analyses (including meta-regression) were conducted to assess whether the overall ES was related to methods, participant characteristics, or intervention characteristics. Publication bias was also assessed.

Key Findings: The overall average weighted ES (d) for 2-group designs was 0.11, with a 95% CI of .05 to .17, indicating that across studies, PA interventions have had positive, but modest, effects on QOL. Most design (e.g., randomized design or not), sample (e.g., age), and intervention (e.g., group versus individualized) attributes were unrelated to ES. Funnel plots suggested no publication bias.

Discussion: The researchers noted that the interventions were not specifically designed to improve QOL, and that "even a small change in QOL might be important because QOL is a complex phenomenon likely affected by diverse factors" (p. 180).

Example 2: A Metasynthesis

Study: A systematic review and meta-ethnography of the qualitative literature: Experiences of the menarche (Chang et al., 2010).

Purpose: The purpose of the meta-ethnography was to synthesize qualitative studies on women's lived experience of the menarche.

Eligibility Criteria: A study was included if it used a qualitative approach, was published in English, and described women's experiences of menarche. No limitation on publication date was used.

Search Strategy: An expert panel guided the review process. The authors searched 9 databases (e.g., MEDLINE, CINAHL, EMBASE, Web of Science), using a broad range of keywords, which they listed in a table of their report. An ancestry search was also conducted, using the reference lists of eligible studies.

Sample: The report presented a PRISMA-type flow chart showing the researchers' sampling decisions. Of the 2,377 studies initially identified by title, 125 abstracts were screened, and then 22 full papers were examined for eligibility. Some were rejected after full reading or as a result of critical appraisal. In all, 14 papers were included in the analysis. The combined sample of participants included 483 women, mostly adolescents, from the United States, United Kingdom, and Zimbabwe. Most existing research was descriptive qualitative studies.

Data Extraction and Analysis: Two reviewers independently assessed and extracted studies. Quality assessment was performed using the CASP critical appraisal criteria. Four studies were deemed to be of insufficient quality and were excluded. Data were extracted using an extraction protocol. Disagreements between reviewers were resolved by consensus. Noblit and Hare's approach, as elaborated by Atkins and colleagues (2008), was used to analyze, compare, and synthesize study findings.

Key Findings: The 5 cross-cutting themes were: (1) Preparing for menarche, (2) the response of significant others, (3) the physical experience of menarche, (4) the psychological experience of menarche, and (5) sociocultural perspectives.

Discussion: The reviewers concluded that the menarche experience had a major impact on women. They felt their findings were of particular importance to school nurses, and could provide a framework for interventions aimed at helping adolescents to better accept the transition to womanhood.

SUMMARY POINTS

- Evidence-based practice relies on rigorous integration of research evidence on a topic through systematic reviews. A **systematic review** methodically integrates research evidence about a specific research question using carefully developed sampling and data collection procedures that are spelled out in advanced in a protocol.

- Systematic reviews of quantitative studies often involve statistical integration of findings through **meta-analysis**, a procedure whose advantages include objectivity, enhanced power, and precision; meta-analysis is not appropriate, however, for broad questions or when there is substantial inconsistency of findings.

- The steps in both quantitative and qualitative integration are similar and involve: formulating the problem, designing the study (including establishing sampling criteria), searching the literature for a sample of **primary studies**, evaluating study quality, extracting and encoding data for analysis, analyzing the data, and reporting the findings.

- There is no consensus on whether systematic reviews should include the **grey literature**—that is, unpublished reports. In quantitative studies, a concern is that there is a *bias against the null hypothesis*, a **publication bias** stemming from the underrepresentation of nonsignificant findings in the published literature. Publication bias can be examined by constructing a **funnel plot**.

- In meta-analysis, findings from primary studies are represented by an **effect size** index that quantifies the magnitude and direction of relationship between variables (e.g., an intervention and its outcomes). Two common effect size indexes in nursing are *d* (the **standardized mean difference**) and the odds ratio.

- Effects from individual studies are pooled to yield an estimate of the population effect size by calculating a **weighted average** of effects, often using the **inverse variance** as the weight—which gives greater weight to larger studies.

- **Statistical heterogeneity** (diversity in effects across studies) is an issue in meta-analysis, and affects decisions about using a **fixed effects model** (which assumes a single true effect size) or a **random effects model** (which assumes a distribution of effects). Heterogeneity can be examined using a **forest plot**.

- Nonrandom heterogeneity (moderating effects) can be explored through **subgroup analyses** or **meta-regression**, in which the purpose is to identify clinical or methodologic features systematically related to variation in effects.
- Quality assessments (which may involve formal ratings of overall methodologic rigor) are sometimes used to exclude weak studies from reviews, but they can also be used to differentially weight studies or in *sensitivity analyses* to test whether including or excluding weaker studies changes conclusions.
- **Metasyntheses** are more than just summaries of prior qualitative findings. They involve a discovery of essential features of a body of findings and, typically, a transformation that yields new insights and interpretations.
- Numerous approaches to metasynthesis (and many terms related to qualitative integration) have been proposed.
- Approaches to metasynthesis that have been used by nurse researchers include meta-ethnography, metastudy, metasummary, critical interpretive synthesis (CIS), grounded formal theory, and thematic synthesis.
- The various metasynthesis approaches have been classified on various *dimensions of difference*, including epistemological stance, extent of iteration, and degree of "going beyond" the primary studies. Another system classifies approaches according to the degree to which theory building and theory explication are achieved.
- One approach to qualitative integration, **meta-ethnography** as proposed by Noblit and Hare, involves listing key themes or metaphors across studies and then reciprocally translating them into each other, followed by a *line-of-argument synthesis*.
- Paterson and colleagues' metastudy method integrates three components: (1) **metadata analysis**, the study of results in a specific substantive area through analysis of the "processed data;" (2) **metamethod**, the study of the studies' methodologic rigor; and (3) **metatheory**, the analysis of the theoretical underpinnings on which the studies are grounded.

- Sandelowski and Barroso distinguish qualitative findings in terms of whether they are *summaries* (descriptive synopses) or *syntheses* (interpretive explanations of the data). Both summaries and syntheses can be used in a **metasummary**, which can lay the foundation for a metasynthesis.
- A metasummary involves developing a list of abstracted findings from the primary studies and calculating **manifest effect sizes**. A **frequency effect size** is the percentage of studies that contain a given findings. An **intensity effect size** indicates the percentage of all findings that are contained in any given report.
- In the Sandelowski and Barroso approach, only studies described as *syntheses* can be used in a metasynthesis, which can use a variety of qualitative approaches to analysis and interpretations (e.g., constant comparison).
- Mixed methods research has contributed to the emergence of **systematic mixed studies reviews**, which refer to systematic reviews that use disciplined and auditable procedures to integrate and synthesize findings from qualitative, quantitative, and mixed methods studies.
- An explicit reporting guideline called **PRISMA** (Preferred Reporting Items for Systematic reviews and Meta-Analyses) is useful for writing up a systematic review of RCTs, and another called **MOOSE** (Meta-analysis of Observational Studies in Epidemiology) guides reporting of meta-analyses of observational studies.

STUDY ACTIVITIES

Chapter 27 of the *Resource Manual for Nursing Research: Generating and Assessing Evidence for Nursing Practice, 9th ed.*, offers various exercises and study suggestions for reinforcing the concepts taught in this chapter. In addition, the following study questions can be addressed:

1. Discuss the similarities and differences between the term "effect size" in qualitative and quantitative integration.

2. Apply relevant questions in Box 27.1 to one of the research examples at the end of the chapter, referring to the full journal article as necessary.

⬤⬤⬤⬤⬤⬤⬤⬤⬤⬤⬤⬤⬤⬤⬤⬤⬤⬤

STUDIES CITED IN CHAPTER 27

Beck, C. T. (2002). Postpartum depression: A metasynthesis. *Qualitative Health Research, 12*, 453–472.

Bench, S., & Day, T. (2010). The user experience of critical care discharge: A meta-synthesis of qualitative research. *International Journal of Nursing Studies, 47*, 487–499.

Bridges, J., Flatley, M., & Meyer, J. (2010). Older people's and relatives' experiences in acute care settings: Systematic review and synthesis of qualitative studies. *International Journal of Nursing Studies, 47*, 89–107.

Bryanton, J., & Beck, C. T. (2010). Postnatal parental education for optimizing infant general health and parent-infant relationships. *Cochrane Database of Systematic Reviews,* Issue 1, Article CD004068.

Chang, Y., Hayter, M., & Wu, S. (2010). A systematic review and meta-ethnography of the qualitative literature: Experiences of the menarche. *Journal of Clinical Nursing, 19*, 447–460.

Conn, V., Hafdahl, A., & Brown, L. (2009). Meta-analysis of quality of life outcomes from physical activity interventions. *Nursing Research, 58*, 175–183.

Cortes, O., Villar, J., Devereaux, P., & DiCenso, A. (2009). Early mobilization for patients following acute myocardial infarction: A systematic review and meta-analysis of experimental studies. *International Journal of Nursing Studies, 46*, 1496–1504.

Davenport, J. (2004). A systematic review to ascertain whether the standard needle is more effective than a longer or wider needle in reducing the incidence of local reaction in children receiving primary immunization. *Journal of Advanced Nursing, 46*, 66–77.

DeNiet, G., Tiemens, B., Lendemeijer, B., & Hutschemaekers, G. (2009). Music-assisted relaxation to improve sleep quality: Meta-analysis. *Journal of Advanced Nursing, 65*, 1356–1364.

Draucker, C., Martsolf, D., Ross, R., Cook, C., Stidham, A., & Mweemba, P. (2009). The essence of healing from sexual violence. *Research in Nursing & Health, 32*, 366–378.

Griffiths, P., Bennett, J., & Smith, E. (2009). The size, extent and nature of the learning disability nursing research base: a systematic scoping review. *International Journal of Nursing Studies, 46*, 490–507.

Kim, C., Kang, D., & Park, J. (2009). A meta-analysis of aerobic exercise interventions for women with breast cancer. *Western Journal of Nursing Research, 31*, 437–461.

Nelson, A. M. (2002). A metasynthesis: Mothering other-than-normal children. *Qualitative Health Research, 12*, 515–530.

Oeseburg, B., Wynia, K., Middel, B., & Reijneveld, S. (2009). Effects of case management for frail older people or those with chronic illness: A systematic review. *Nursing Research, 58*, 201–210.

Pate, B. (2009). A systematic review of the effectiveness of breastfeeding intervention delivery methods. *Journal of Obstetric, Gynecologic, & Neonatal Nursing, 38*, 642–653.

Paterson, B. (2001). The shifting perspectives model of chronic illness. *Journal of Nursing Scholarship, 33*, 57–62.

Paterson, B. (2007). Coming out as will: Understanding self-disclosure in chronic illness from a meta-synthesis of qualitative research. In C. Webb, & B. Roe (Eds.), *Reviewing research evidence for nursing practice* (pp. 73–83). Oxford: Blackwell Publishing.

Purc-Stephenson, R., & Thrasher, C. (2010). Nurses' experiences with telephone triage and advice: A meta-ethnography. *Journal of Advanced Nursing, 66*, 482–494.

Roberts, A., & Noyes, J. (2009). Contraception and women over 40 years of age: Mixed-method systematic review. *Journal of Advanced Nursing, 65*, 1155–1170.

Stoltz, P., Skärsäter, I., & Willman, A. (2009). "Insufficient evidence of effectiveness" is not "evidence of no effectiveness": Evaluating computer-based education for patients with severe mental illness. *Worldviews of Evidence-Based Nursing, 6*, 190–199.

Thorpe, G., McArthur, M., & Richardson, B. (2009). Bodily changes following faecal stoma formation: Qualitative interpretive synthesis. *Journal of Advanced Nursing, 65*, 1778–1789.

Varcoe, C., Rodney, P., & McCormick, J. (2003). Health care relationships in context: An analysis of three ethnographies. *Qualitative Health Research, 13*, 957–973.

Voils, C., Hasselblad, V., Crandell, J., Chang, Y., Lee, E., & Sandelowski, M. (2009). A Bayesian method for the synthesis of evidence from qualitative and quantitative reports: The example of antiretroviral medication adherence. *Journal of Health Services Research & Policy, 14*, 226–233.

Yarcheski, A., Mahon, N., Yarcheski, T., Hanks, M., & Cannella, B. (2009). A meta-analytic study of predictors of maternal-fetal attachment. *International Journal of Nursing Studies, 46*, 708–715.

Methodologic and nonresearch references cited in this chapter can be found in a separate section at the end of the book.

28

Disseminating Evidence: Reporting Research Findings

N o study is complete until the findings have been shared. This chapter offers assistance on disseminating research results.

GETTING STARTED ON DISSEMINATION

Researchers sort out various issues in developing a dissemination plan, as we discuss in this section.

Selecting a Communication Outlet

Researchers who want to communicate their findings to others can present them orally or in writing. Oral presentations (typically at professional conferences) can be a formal talk in front of an audience or integrated with written material in a **poster session**. Major advantages of conference presentations are that they typically can be done soon after study completion, and offer opportunities for dialogue among people interested in the same topic. Written reports, in addition to theses or dissertations, can take the form of journal articles published in traditional professional journals, or in Internet outlets. A major advantage of journal articles is worldwide accessibility. Much of our advice in this chapter is relevant for most types of dissemination.

Knowing the Audience

Good research communication depends on providing information that can be understood, so researchers should think about the audience they are hoping to reach. Here are some questions to consider:

1. Will the audience be nurses only, or will it include professionals from other disciplines (e.g., physicians, psychologists)?
2. Will the audience be researchers, or will it include other professionals (clinicians, healthcare policy makers)?
3. Are clients (lay people) a possible audience?
4. Will the audience include people whose native language is not English?
5. Will reviewers, editors, and readers be experts in the field?

Researchers often have to write with multiple audiences in mind, which means writing clearly and avoiding technical jargon to the extent possible. It also means that researchers sometimes must develop a multipronged strategy—for example, publishing a report for nurse researchers in a journal such as *Nursing Research*, and then publishing a summary for clinicians in a hospital newsletter.

➲ **TIP:** Oermann and colleagues (2006) provide some suggestions about presenting research results to clinical audiences.

Although writing for a broad audience may be an important goal, it is also important to keep in mind the needs of the *main* intended audience. If consumers of a report are mostly clinical nurses, it is important to emphasize what the findings mean for practice. If the audience is administrators or policy makers, explicit information should be included about how the findings relate to such outcomes as *cost* and *accessibility*. If other researchers are the primary audience, explicit information about methods, study limitations, and implications for future research is important.

Developing a Plan

Before preparing a report, researchers should have a plan. Part of that plan involves how best to coordinate the actual tasks of preparing a **manuscript** (i.e., an unpublished paper).

Deciding on Authorship

When a study has been completed by a team, division of labor and authorship must be addressed. The International Committee of Medical Journal Editors (ICMJE, 2009) advised that authorship credit should be based on (1) having made a substantial contribution to the study's conception and design, to data acquisition, or to analysis and interpretation; (2) drafting or revising the manuscript; and (3) approving the final version of the manuscript.

The **lead author**, usually the first-named author, has overall responsibility for the report. The lead author and coauthors should reach an agreement in advance about responsibilities for producing the manuscript. To avoid possible subsequent conflicts, they should also decide beforehand the order of authors' names. Ethically, it is most appropriate to list names in the order of authors' contribution to the work, not according to status. When contributions of coauthors are comparable, an alphabetical listing is appropriate.

Deciding on Content

In many studies, more data are collected than can be presented in one report, and multiple publications are thus possible. In such situations, an early decision involves what part of the findings to

present in a given paper. If there are multiple research questions, more than one paper may be required to communicate results adequately. In mixed methods research, separate reports are sometime needed to summarize qualitative and quantitative findings.

It is, however, inappropriate and even unethical to write several papers when one would suffice, a practice that has been called "salami slicing" (Baggs, 2008). Each paper from a study should independently make a contribution. Editors, reviewers, and readers expect original work, so unnecessary overlap should be avoided. It is also unethical to submit essentially the same or similar paper to two journals simultaneously. Oermann and Hays (2010) offer guidelines regarding duplicate and redundant publications.

Assembling Materials

Planning also involves assembling materials needed to begin a draft, including information about manuscript requirements. Traditional and online journals issue guidelines for authors, and these guidelines should be retrieved and understood.

Other materials also need to be assembled, including the relevant literature, instruments used in the study, descriptions of the study sample, output of computer analyses, relevant analytic memos or reflexive notes, figures or photographs that illustrate some aspect of the study, and permissions to use copyrighted materials. Other important tools are style manuals that provide information about both grammar and language use (e.g., Strunk, et al., 2000), as well as more specific information about writing professional and scientific papers (e.g., American Psychological Association [APA], 2010; ICMJE, 2009).

Finally, a written outline and a timeline should be developed, especially if there are multiple coauthors who have responsibility for different sections of the paper. The overall outline and individual assignments, together with due dates, should be developed collaboratively.

Writing Effectively

Many people have a hard time putting their ideas down on paper. It is beyond the scope of this book to teach good writing skills, but we can offer a few suggestions. One suggestion, quite simply is: *do it*. Get in the habit of writing, even if it is only 15 minutes a day. *Writer's block* is probably responsible for thousands of unfinished (or never-started) manuscripts each year. So, just begin somewhere, and keep at it regularly—writing gets easier with practice.

Writing *well* is, of course, important, and several resources offer suggestions on how to write compelling sentences, select good words, and organize your ideas effectively (e.g., Wager, 2010; Zinsser, 2006). It is usually better to write a draft in its entirety, and then go back later to rewrite awkward sentences, correct errors, reorganize, and generally polish it up.

In a recent survey of 63 nursing journal editors, Northam and colleagues (2010) found that the single most common reason for rejecting a manuscript was that it was poorly written. A frequently mentioned suggestion by these editors was to have others review the manuscript—and even to read it out loud to someone to see if it is understood.

CONTENT OF RESEARCH REPORTS

Research reports vary in terms of audience, purpose, and length. Theses or dissertations not only communicate research results, but they also document students' ability to perform scholarly work and, therefore, tend to be long. Journal articles, by contrast, are short because they compete for limited journal space and are read by busy professionals. Nevertheless, the general form and content of research reports are often similar. Chapter 3 summarized the content of major sections of research reports, and here we offer a few additional tips. Distinctions among various kinds of reports are described later in the chapter.

Quantitative Research Reports

Quantitative reports typically follow the **IMRAD format**, which involves organizing content into four sections—the **I**ntroduction, **M**ethod, **R**esults,

and **D**iscussion. These sections, respectively, address the following questions:

- Why was the study done? (I)
- How was the study done? (M)
- What was learned? (R)
- What does it mean? (D)

The Introduction

The introduction acquaints readers with the research problem, its significance, and the context in which it was developed. The introduction sets the stage by describing the existing literature, the study's conceptual framework, the problem, research questions or hypotheses, and the study rationale. Although the introduction includes multiple components, it should be concise. A common critique of research manuscripts by reviewers is that the introduction is too long.

Introductions are often written in a funnel-shaped structure, beginning broadly to establish a framework for understanding the study, and then narrowing to the specifics of what researchers sought to learn. The end point of the introduction should be a concise delineation of the research questions or hypotheses, which provides a good transition to the method section.

> ➲ **TIP:** An up-front, clearly stated problem statement is of immense value in communicating the study's context. The first paragraph should be written with special care, because the goal is to grab the readers' attention.

The introduction typically includes a summary of related research to provide a pertinent context. Except for dissertations, the literature review should be a brief summary, not an exhaustive review. The review should make clear what is already known, and what the deficiencies are, thus helping to clarify the contribution of the new study.

The introduction also should describe the study's theoretical or conceptual framework. The framework should be sufficiently explained so that readers who are unfamiliar with it can understand its main thrust. The introduction should include conceptual definitions of the concepts under investigation.

The various background strands need to be convincingly and cogently interwoven to persuade readers that, in fact, the new study holds promise for adding to evidence for nursing.

➡ **TIP:** Many journals articles begin without an explicit heading labeled *Introduction*. In general, all the material before the method section is considered to be the introduction. Some introductions include subheadings such as *Literature Review* or *Hypotheses*.

The Method Section

To evaluate the quality of a study's evidence, readers need to know exactly what methods were used to address the research problem. In traditional dissertations, the method section should provide sufficient detail that another researcher could replicate the study. In journal articles and conference presentations, the method section is condensed, but the degree of detail should permit readers to draw conclusions about the validity of the findings. Faulty method sections are a leading cause of manuscript rejection by research journals. Your job in writing the method section of a quantitative report is to persuade readers that evidence from your study has sufficient validity to merit consideration.

➡ **TIP:** The method section is often subdivided into several parts, which helps readers to locate vital information. As an example, the method section might contain the following subsections: Research Design, Sample and Setting, Data Collection Instruments, Procedures, Data Analysis.

The method section usually begins with the description of the research design and its rationale. The design is often given detailed coverage in experimental studies, with information about what specific design was adopted, how subjects were assigned to groups, and whether (and with whom) blinding was used. Reports for studies with multiple points of data collection should indicate the number of times data were collected and the amount of time elapsed between those points. In all types of quantitative studies, it is important to identify steps taken to control the research situation in general and confounding variables in particular. The method section also addresses steps taken to protect the rights of study participants.

Readers also need to know about study participants. This subsection (which may be labeled *Research Sample*, *Subjects*, or *Study Participants*) normally includes a list of eligibility criteria, to clarify the group to whom results can be generalized. The method of sample selection and its rationale, recruitment techniques, and sample size should be indicated so readers can determine how representative subjects are of the target population. If a power analysis was undertaken to estimate sample size needs, this should be described. There should also be information about response rates and, if possible, about response bias (or attrition bias, if this is relevant). Basic characteristics of study participants (e.g., age, gender, health status) should also be described.

Data collection methods are another critical component of the method section and may be presented in a subsection labeled *Instruments*, *Measures*, or *Data Collection*. A description of study instruments, and a rationale for their use, should be provided. If instruments were constructed specifically for the project, the report should describe their development. Any special equipment that was used (e.g., to gather biophysiologic or observational data) should be described, including information about the manufacturer. The report should also indicate who collected the data (e.g., the authors, research assistants, nurses) and how they were trained. The report must also convince readers that the data collection methods were sound. Any information relating to data quality, and the procedures used to evaluate that quality, should be described.

In intervention research, there is usually a procedures subsection that includes information about the actual intervention. What exactly did the intervention entail? How was the intervention theory translated into components? How and by whom was the treatment administered, and how were they trained? What was done with subjects in the control group? How much time elapsed between the intervention and the measurement of the dependent variable? How was intervention fidelity monitored?

➲ **TIP:** There is growing evidence and commentary about the insufficient amount of description about interventions themselves in reports of nursing clinical trials (Conn et al., 2008; Leeman et al., 2006), making it difficult for clinicians to translate evidence into practice improvements. Key elements of an intervention should always be summarized in a report of a trial, but a separate article describing the intervention in greater detail might be needed.

Analytic procedures are described either in the method or results section. It is usually sufficient to identify the statistical tests used; formulas or references for commonly used statistics such as analysis of variance are not necessary. For unusual procedures, or unusual applications of a common procedure, a technical reference justifying the approach should be noted. If confounding variables were controlled statistically, the specific variables controlled should be mentioned. The level of significance is typically set at .05 for two-tailed tests, which may or may not be explicitly stated; however, if a different significance level or one-tailed tests were used, this must be specified.

A recent development is that there are now explicit guidelines for reporting methodologic information for various types of studies, as shown in Table 28.1. The most well known is the Consolidated Standards of Reporting Trials or **CONSORT guidelines**. These guidelines focus on reporting information about RCTs, and extensions have been developed for particular types of research design, such as cluster randomized trials. The CONSORT guidelines have been adopted by most major medical and nursing journals. The 2010 CONSORT guidelines contain a checklist of 25 items to include in reports of RCTs.

The CONSORT guidelines, as well as other guidelines, recommend inclusion of a flow chart to track participants through a study, from eligibility assessment through analysis of outcomes. Flow charts should be as detailed as possible, within space constraints, about reasons for loss of subjects during the study. Figure 28.1 provides an example of such a flow chart for a randomized controlled trial (RCT). This chart summarizes withdrawals from the intervention, as well as loss of participants during follow-up. It also shows that data for all subjects were analyzed in an intention-to-treat analysis, which is recommended in CONSORT (Polit & Gillespie, 2010).

Guidelines for various types of studies are regularly being updated or expanded. The EQUATOR Network (*www.equator-network.org*) is a useful resource for information on reporting guidelines and for tips on good reporting in health studies.

➲ **TIP:** The CONSORT checklist is included in the Toolkit of the *Resource Manual* that accompanies this book. Further information about the CONSORT guidelines is available at *www.consort-statement.org*, which includes an interactive checklist with detailed information about components in the checklist.

The Results Section

Readers scrutinize the method section to know if the study was done with rigor, but the results section is the heart of the report. In a quantitative study, the results of the statistical analyses are summarized in a factual manner. Descriptive statistics are ordinarily presented first, to provide an overview of study variables. If key research questions involve comparing groups with regard to dependent variables (e.g., in an experimental or case–control study), the results section often begins with information about the groups' comparability on baseline variables, so readers can evaluate selection bias.

Research results are usually ordered in terms of overall importance. If, however, research questions or hypotheses have been numbered in the introduction, the analyses addressing them should be ordered in the same sequence.

When reporting results of hypothesis-testing statistical tests, three pieces of information are typically reported: the value of the calculated statistic, degrees of freedom, and the exact probability level. For instance, it might be stated, "Patients who were

TABLE 28.1	Reporting Guidelines for Various Types of Papers
TYPE OF STUDY	**GUIDELINE**
Parallel group randomized controlled trials (RCTs)	CONSORT: Consolidated Standards of Reporting Trials (Moher et al., 2010)
Pragmatic trials	CONSORT extension for pragmatic trials (Zwarenstein et al., 2008)
Trials of nonpharmacalogic interventions	CONSORT extension for nonpharmacologic treatments (Boutron et al., 2008)
Cluster randomized trials	CONSORT extension for cluster randomized trials (Campbell et al., 2004)
Noninferiority and equivalence trials	CONSORT extension for noninferiority and equivalence trials (Piaggio et al., 2006)
Nonexperimental (observational) studies	STROBE: Strengthening the Reporting of Observational Studies in Epidemiology (von Elm et al., 2008)
Qualitative studies (focus groups and interview studies)	COREQ: Consolidated Criteria for Reporting Qualitative Research (Tong et al., 2007)
Meta-analyses of RCTs	PRISMA: Preferred Reporting Items for Systematic Reviews and Meta-Analyses (Moher et al., 2009)
Meta-analyses of non-RCTs	MOOSE: Meta-analysis of Observational Studies in Epidemiology (Stroup et al., 2000)
Diagnostic accuracy studies	STARD: Standards for Reporting of Diagnostic Accuracy (Bossuyt et al., 2003)
Healthcare quality improvement studies	SQUIRE: Standards for Quality Improvement Reporting Excellence (Ogrinc et al., 2008)
Evaluations of interventions using quasi-experimental designs	TREND: Transparent Reporting of Evaluations with Nonrandomized Designs (Des Jarlais et al., 2004)

exposed to the intervention were significantly less likely to develop decubitus ulcers than patients in the control group ($\chi^2 = 8.23$, $df = 1$, $p = .008$)." However, the recent publication manual of the American Psychological Association (2010) urges authors to report confidence intervals: "Because confidence intervals combine information on location and precision and can often be directly used to infer significance levels, they are, in general, the best reporting strategy" (p. 34). The manual also

strongly encourages reporting effect sizes, which can facilitate meta-analyses.

When results from several statistical analyses are reported, they should be summarized in a **table**. Good tables, with precise headings and titles, are an important way to avoid dull, repetitious statements. When tables are used, the text should refer to the table by number (e.g., "As shown in Table 2, patients in the intervention group . . ."). Box 28.1 ✪ presents some suggestions regarding the construction of

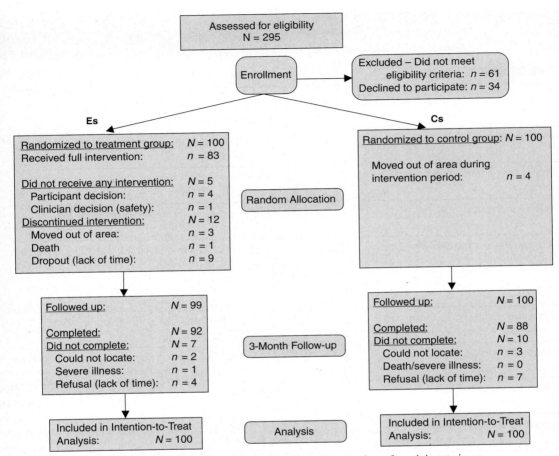

FIGURE 28.1 Example of CONSORT guidelines flowchart: Progression of participants in an intervention study.

effective statistical tables, and the table templates in the Toolkit (Chapters 16 through 18) can help you create clear and concise tables. ✴

➡ **TIP:** Do not repeat statistical information in text and tables. Tables should present information that would be monotonous to present in the text, and display it in such a way that patterns among the numbers are more evident. The text can be used to highlight major findings.

Figures may also be used to summarize results. Figures that display the results in graphic form are used less as an economy than as a means of dramatizing important findings and relationships. Figures are especially helpful for displaying information on

some phenomenon over time or for portraying conceptual or empirical models.

➡ **TIP:** Research evidence does not constitute *proof* of anything, so the report should never claim that the data proved, verified, confirmed, or demonstrated that hypotheses were correct or incorrect. Hypotheses are supported or unsupported, accepted or rejected.

The Discussion Section
The meaning that researchers give to the results plays an important role in reports. The discussion section is devoted to a thoughtful (and, it is hoped, insightful) analysis of the findings, leading to a discussion of their clinical and theoretical utility. A typical discussion section addresses the following questions: What

BOX 28.1 Guidelines for Preparing Statistical Tables

1. Number tables so they can be referenced in the text.
2. Give tables a brief but clear explanatory title.
3. Avoid both overly simple tables with information more efficiently presented in the text, and overly complex tables that intimidate and confuse readers.
4. Arrange data in such a way that patterns are obvious at a glance; take care to organize information in an intelligible way.
5. Give each column and row of data a heading that is succinct but clear; table headings should establish the logic of the table structure.
6. Express data values to the number of decimal places justified by the precision of the measurement. In general, it is preferable to report numbers to one decimal place (or to two decimal places for correlation coefficients) because rounded values are easier to absorb than more precise ones. Report all values in a table to the same level of precision.
7. Make each table a "stand-alone" presentation, capable of being understood without reference to the text.
8. Indicate probability levels, either as actual p values or with confidence intervals. In correlation matrixes, use the system of asterisks and a probability level footnote. The usual convention is to use one asterisk when $p < 05$, two when p, .01, and three when $p < .001$.
9. Indicate units of measurement for numbers in the table whenever appropriate (e.g., pounds, milligrams).
10. Use footnotes to explain abbreviations or special symbols used in the table, except commonly understood abbreviations such as N.

were the main findings? What do the findings mean? What evidence is there that the results and the interpretations are valid? What limitations might threaten validity? How do the results compare with prior knowledge on the topic? What are the implications of the findings for future research? What are the implications for nursing practice?

⊃ **TIP:** The discussion is typically the most challenging section to write. It deserves your most intense intellectual and creative effort—and careful review by peers. The peers should be asked to comment on how persuasive your arguments are, how well organized the section is, and whether it is too long, which is a common flaw.

Typically, the discussion section begins with a summary of key findings. The summary should be brief, however, because the focus of the discussion is on making sense of (and not merely repeating) the results.

Interpretation of results is a global process, encompassing findings themselves, methods and methodologic limitations, sample characteristics, related research findings, clinical dimensions, and theoretical issues. Researchers should justify their interpretations, explicitly stating why alternative explanations have been ruled out. Unsupported conclusions are among the most common problems in discussion sections. If the findings conflict with those of earlier studies, tentative explanations should be offered. A discussion of the generalizability of study findings should also be included.

Implications of study findings are speculative and so should be couched in tentative terms, as in the following example: "The results *suggest* that nurses' communication about advanced directives is inconsistent and that nurses' years of experience affect the nature and amount of communication." The interpretation is, in essence, a hypothesis that can be tested in another study. The discussion should include recommendations for studies that would help to test this hypothesis.

Finally, and importantly, implications of the findings for nursing practice need to be discussed. What aspects of the evidence are clinically significant, and how might the evidence be put to use by nurses? The importance of adequately addressing nursing implications has been discussed by the editors of several nursing journals (Becker, 2009; Gennaro, 2008).

Other Aspects of the Report

The materials covered in the four major IMRAD sections are found, in some form, in most quantitative research reports, although the organization might differ slightly. In addition to these major divisions, other aspects of the report deserve mention.

Title. Every research report needs a title indicating the nature of the study. Insofar as possible, the dependent and independent variables (or central constructs under study) should be named in the title. It is also desirable to indicate the study population. Yet, the title should be brief (no more than about 15 words), so writers must balance clarity with brevity. The length of titles can often be reduced by omitting unnecessary terms such as "A Study of . . .," "Report of . . ." or "An Investigation to Examine the Effects of . . .," and so forth. The title should communicate concisely what was studied and stimulate interest in the research. A few journals, however, such as the *International Journal of Nursing Studies,* require that the basic method be stated in the title. For example, Kottner and colleagues (2010) wrote a paper titled "Prevalence of deep tissue injuries in hospitals and nursing homes: two cross-sectional studies." Thus, it is always important to review journal guidelines and requirements before finalizing a manuscript.

Abstract. Research reports usually include an abstract, that is, brief descriptions of the problem, methods, and findings of the study, written so readers can decide whether to read the entire report. As noted in Chapter 3, journal abstracts are sometimes written as an unstructured paragraph of 100 to 200 words, or in a structured form with subheadings.

⬤ T I P : Take the time to write a compelling abstract, which is your first main point of contact with reviewers and readers. It should demonstrate that your study is important clinically and that it was done with conceptual and methodologic rigor. It should also contain words that will help people find your paper if they search for articles on your topic.

Keywords. It is often necessary to include key words that will be used in indexes to help others locate your study. Sometimes authors are given a list of keywords from which to chose (often Medical Subject Headings or MeSH terms), but additional keywords can often be added. Substantive, methodologic, and theoretical terms can be used as keywords.

References. Each report concludes with a list of references cited in the text, using a reference style specified by those reviewing the manuscript. References can be cumbersome to prepare, but software programs are available to facilitate the preparation of reference lists (e.g., EndNote, ProCite, Reference Manager, Format Ease). Some journal editors, however, prohibit use of reference citation managers (Northam et al., 2010).

Acknowledgments. People who helped with the research but whose contribution does not qualify them for authorship are sometimes acknowledged in the report. This might include statistical consultants, data collectors, or people who reviewed the manuscript. Acknowledgments should also give credit to organizations that made the project possible, such as funding agencies or organizations that helped with subject recruitment.

Checklist. A few journals, such as the *International Journal of Nursing Studies,* require the completion of an author checklist that requires authors to state their compliance with various requirements, such as total word count, declaration of keywords, and so on.

Qualitative Research Reports

There is no single style for reporting qualitative findings, but qualitative research reports do often follow the IMRAD format, or something akin to it. Thus, we present some issues of particular relevance for writing qualitative reports within the IMRAD structure.

Introduction

Qualitative reports usually begin with a problem statement, in a similar fashion to quantitative reports, but the focus is squarely on the phenomenon under study. The way in which the problem is expressed and the types of questions the researchers sought to answer are usually tied to the research tradition underlying the study (e.g., grounded theory, ethnography), which is usually explicitly stated in the introduction. Prior research on the phenomenon under study may be summarized in the introduction, but is sometimes described in the discussion section.

In many qualitative studies, but especially in ethnographic ones, it is critical to explain the study's cultural context. For studies with an ideological orientation (e.g., critical theory or feminist research), it is also important to describe the sociopolitical context. For studies using phenomenological or grounded theory designs, the philosophy of phenomenology or symbolic interaction, respectively, may be described.

As another aspect of explaining the study's background, qualitative researchers sometimes provide information about relevant personal experiences or qualifications. If a researcher who is studying decisions about long-term care placements is caring for two elderly parents and participates in a caregiver support group, this is relevant for readers' understanding of the study. In descriptive phenomenological studies, researchers may discuss their personal experiences in relation to the phenomenon being studied to communicate what they bracketed.

The concluding paragraph of the introduction usually offers a succinct summary of the purpose of the study or the research questions.

Method

Although the research tradition of the study is often noted in the introduction, the method section usually elaborates on specific methods used in conjunction with that tradition. Design features such as whether the study was longitudinal should also be noted.

The method section should provide a good description of the research setting, so that readers can assess transferability of findings. Study participants and methods by which they were selected should also be described. Even when samples are small, it is often useful to provide a table summa-

rizing participants' key characteristics. If researchers have a personal connection to participants or to groups with which they are affiliated, this connection should be noted. At times, to disguise a group or institution, it may be necessary to omit or modify potentially identifying information.

Qualitative reports usually cannot provide much specific information about data collection, but some researchers provide a sample of questions, especially if a topic guide was used. The description of data collection methods should include how data were collected (e.g., interview or observation), who collected the data, how data collectors were trained, and what methods were used to record the data.

Information about quality and integrity is particularly important in qualitative studies. The more information included in the report about steps researchers took to ensure the trustworthiness of the data, the more confident readers can be that the findings are credible.

Quantitative reports typically have only brief descriptions of data analysis techniques because standard statistical procedures are widely understood. By contrast, analytic procedures are often described in some detail in qualitative reports because readers need to understand how researchers organized, synthesized, and made sense of their data.

Results

In their results sections, qualitative researchers summarize their themes, categories, taxonomic structure, or the theory that emerged. This section can be organized in a number of ways. For example, if a process is being described, results may be presented chronologically, corresponding to the unfolding of the process. Key themes, metaphors, or domains are often used as subheadings, organized in order of salience to participants or to a theory.

Example of organization of qualitative results: O'Donnell and colleagues (2010) did a grounded theory study to explain sickness absence among women who experienced workplace bullying. They found that the problem was addressed through a process they called *discerning a path*. The three phases of the process—*gaining space, making sense,* and *moving forward*—were used as subheadings to organize the results.

Sandelowski (1998) emphasized the importance of developing a story line before beginning to write the findings. Because of the richness of qualitative data, researchers have to decide which story, or how much of it, they want to tell. They must also decide how best to balance description and interpretation. The results section in a qualitative paper, unlike that in a quantitative one, intertwines data and interpretations of those data. It is important, however, to give sufficient emphasis to the voices, actions, and experiences of participants themselves so that readers can gain an appreciation of their lives and their worlds. Most often, this occurs through the inclusion of direct quotes to illustrate important points. Because of space constraints in journals, quotes cannot be extensive, and great care must be exercised in selecting the best possible exemplars. Gilgun (2005) offered guidance in writing up the results of qualitative research in a manner that has "grab."

> ⊃ **TIP:** Using quotes is not only a skill but also a complex process. When inserting quotes in the results section, pay attention to how the quote is introduced and how it is put in context. Quotes should not be used haphazardly or listed one after the other in a string.

Figures, diagrams, and word tables that organize concepts are often useful in summarizing an overall conceptualization of the phenomena under study. Grounded theory studies are especially likely to benefit from a schematic presentation of the basic social process. Ethnographic and ethnoscience studies often present taxonomies in tabular form.

Discussion

In qualitative studies, findings and interpretation are typically interwoven in the results section because the task of integrating qualitative materials is essentially interpretive. The discussion section of a qualitative report, therefore, is not so much designed to give meaning to the results, but to summarize them, link them to other research, and suggest their implications for theory, research, or nursing practice.

Other Aspects of a Qualitative Report

Qualitative reports, like quantitative ones, include abstracts, keywords, references, and acknowledgments. Abstracts for journals that feature qualitative reports (e.g., *Qualitative Health Research*) tend to be the traditional (single-paragraph) type, rather than structured abstracts.

The titles of qualitative reports usually state the central phenomenon under scrutiny. Phenomenological studies often have titles that include such words as "the lived experience of . . ." or "the meaning of. . . ." Grounded theory studies often indicate something about the *findings* in the title—for example, mentioning the core category or basic social process. Ethnographic titles usually indicate the culture being studied. Two-part titles are not uncommon, with substance and method, research tradition and findings, or theme and meaning, separated by a colon.

> ⊃ **TIP:** Preparing a report for a mixed methods (MM) study has challenges of its own. Creswell and Plano Clark (2007) offer useful guidance for writing up integrated MM reports.

THE STYLE OF RESEARCH REPORTS

Research reports, especially for quantitative studies, are written in a distinctive style. Some style issues were discussed previously, but additional points are elaborated here.

A research report is not an essay. It is an account of how and why a problem was studied, and what was discovered as a result. The report should not include overtly subjective statements, emotionally laden statements, or exaggerations. This is not to say that the research story should be told in a dreary manner. Indeed, in qualitative reports there are ample opportunities to enliven the narration with rich description, direct quotes, and insightful interpretation. Authors of quantitative reports, although somewhat constrained by structure and the need to include numeric information, should strive to keep the presentation lively.

Quantitative researchers often avoid personal pronouns such as "I," "my," and "we" because impersonal pronouns, and use of the passive voice, suggest greater impartiality. Qualitative reports, by contrast, are often written in the first person and in an active voice. Even among quantitative researchers, however, there is a trend toward striking a greater balance between active and passive voice and first-person and third-person narration. If a direct presentation can be made without suggesting bias, a more readable product usually results.

It is not easy to write simply and clearly, but these are important goals of scientific writing. The use of technical jargon does little to enhance the communicative value of the report, and should especially be avoided in communicating findings to practicing nurses. The style should be concise and straightforward. If writers can add elegance to their reports without interfering with clarity and accuracy, so much the better, but the product is not expected to be a literary achievement.

A common flaw in reports of novice researchers is inadequate organization. The overall structure is fairly standard, but organization within sections and subsections also needs attention. Sequences should be in an orderly progression with appropriate transitions. Continuity and logical thematic development are critical to good communication.

It may seem a trivial point, but methods and results should be described in the past tense. For example, it is inappropriate to say, "Nurses who receive special training perform triage functions significantly better than those without training." In this sentence, "receive" and "perform" should be changed to "received" and "performed" to reflect the fact that the statement pertains only to a particular sample whose behavior was observed in the past.

TYPES OF RESEARCH REPORTS

This section describes features of four major kinds of research reports: theses and dissertations, traditional journal articles, online reports, and presentations at professional meetings. Reports for class projects are excluded—not because they are unimportant but rather because they so closely resemble theses on a smaller scale.

Theses and Dissertations

Most doctoral degrees, and some master's degrees, are granted on the successful completion of an empirical project. Most universities have a preferred format for their dissertations. Until recently, most schools used a traditional IMRAD format. The following organization for a traditional dissertation is typical:

- Front Matter: Title Page, Abstract, Copyright Page, Approval Page, Acknowledgment Page, Table of Contents, List of Tables, List of Figures, List of Appendices
- Main Body: Chapter I. Introduction; Chapter II. Review of the Literature; Chapter III. Methods; Chapter IV. Results; Chapter V. Discussion and Summary
- Supplementary Pages: Bibliography, Appendices, Curriculum vitae

The **front matter** (preliminary pages) for dissertations is much the same as those for a scholarly book. The title page indicates such information as the title of the study, the author's name, the degree requirement being fulfilled, and the name of the university awarding the degree. The acknowledgment page gives writers the opportunity to thank those who contributed to the project. The table of contents outlines major sections and subsections of the report, indicating on which page readers will find sections of interest. The lists of tables and figures identify by number, title, and page the tabular and graphic material in the text.

The main body of a traditionally formatted dissertation incorporates the IMRAD sections described earlier. The literature review often is so extensive that a separate chapter may be devoted to it. When a short review is sufficient, the first two chapters may be combined. In some cases, a separate chapter may also be required to elaborate the study's conceptual framework.

➡ **T I P :** In some traditional dissertations, the early chapters describe students' intellectual journey, including a description of the paths they took and decisions they made in selecting their final research question and methodology.

The supplementary pages include a bibliography or list of references used to prepare the report and one or more appendixes. An appendix contains materials relevant to the study that are either too lengthy or too tangential to be incorporated into the body of the report. Data collection instruments, scoring instructions, codebooks, cover letters, permission letters, IRB approval, category schemes, and peripheral statistical tables are examples of materials included in the appendix. Some universities also require a *curriculum vitae* of the author.

A growing number of universities offer a new formatting option, what has been called the **paper format thesis** or **publication option** (Robinson & Dracup, 2008). In a typical paper format thesis, there is an introduction, two or more publishable papers, and then a conclusion. Such a format permits students to move directly from dissertation to journal submission, but can be more demanding than the traditional format on both students and their advisers. Formats for the paper format thesis vary, and are typically decided by the dissertation committee. Some universities require that a certain number of the publishable papers (e.g., two out of three) be data-based—that is, reports of original research. Other papers within the dissertation, however, might be publishable systematic reviews, concept analyses, or methodologic papers (e.g., describing the development of an instrument). Some universities require that the papers be under review or *in press* (that is, accepted and awaiting publication), but other universities require that the papers be ready to submit.

If an academic institution does not accept paper format theses, students need to adapt their dissertations before submission to a journal. Several writers have provided guidance on converting a traditional dissertation into a manuscript, including Johnson (1996), Heyman and Cronin (2005), and, for qualitative dissertations, Boyle (1997).

Journal Articles

Progress in evidence-based practice depends on researchers' efforts to share their work. Traditional dissertations, which are too lengthy and inaccessible for widespread use, are read only by a handful of people. Publication in a professional journal ensures broad circulation of research findings, and it is professionally advantageous—or even necessary—to publish. This section discusses issues relating to publication in journals.

➡ **T I P :** A valuable resource for nurse authors is the Nurse Author & Editor website at *http://www.nurseauthoreditor.com/*. This website offers helpful information for writing and publishing, and a listing of many nursing journals with links to author guidelines.

Selecting a Journal

Before writing begins, there should be a clear idea of the journal to which a manuscript will be submitted. Journals differ in their goals, types of manuscript sought, and readership; these factors need to be matched against personal interests and preferences. All journals issue goal statements, as well as guidelines for preparing and submitting a manuscript. This information is published in journals themselves and on their websites.

Example of statement of journal goal: *Qualitative Health Research* is an international, interdisciplinary, refereed journal for the enhancement of healthcare and to further the development and understanding of qualitative research methods in healthcare settings. We welcome manuscripts in the following areas: the description and analysis of the illness experience, health and health-seeking behaviors, the experiences of caregivers, the sociocultural organization of healthcare, healthcare policy, and related topics. We also seek critical reviews and commentaries addressing conceptual, theoretical, methodological, and ethical issues pertaining to qualitative enquiry.

More than 500 nursing journals are indexed in CINAHL. In addition to variation in focus, journals differ in prestige, acceptance rates, issues per year, word limits, and reference styles. Several of these characteristics are usually taken into account in selecting a journal.

Prestige is often assessed in terms of a journal's **impact factor** (IF), which is a measure of citation frequency for an average article in a journal. Specifically, a journal's IF for, say, 2010 is the number of times in 2010 that articles published in the journal in the two prior years (2008 and 2009) were cited in journals, divided by the number of the journal's articles in those two years that *could* have been cited (i.e., actual citations divided by potentially citable articles). As examples, the 2009 IF for *Worldviews on Evidence-Based Nursing*, the highest-ranking nursing journal in 2009, was 1.94, while that for *Journal of Nursing Scholarship,* ranked 12th, was 1.46. Impact factor information can be found in *Journal Citation Reports.* Impact factor information for 2009 for select journals with a high concentration of research articles is shown in Table 28.2. Not all nursing journals are included in the rankings, but the number included continues to grow (Polit & Northam, in press, a).

Northam and colleagues (2010) reported information on the focus, word limit, reference style, and article review time for 63 nursing journals, although only a handful of the editors surveyed stated that research was their primary focus. The analysis revealed great variation across many dimensions, including article word limit (ranging from 1,200 to 9,000 words), number of issues (ranging from 2 to 26), and length of time from submission to acceptance or rejection decision (ranging from 3 to 45 weeks). Editors' reasons for rejection also varied, but among the research-focused articles, the primary reasons were poor writing and methodologic problems.

In an article written a decade earlier, Northam and colleagues (2000) offered information on the acceptance rate for 83 journals in nursing and related health fields. They found that some journals were far more competitive than others. For example, *Nursing Research* accepted only 20% of submitted manuscripts, whereas acceptance rates for many specialty journals was greater than 50%. Competition for journal publication likely became even keener in the years since that article was written.

> ➲ **TIP:** Nurses publish in many health-related journals, not just in nursing journals. Publishing opportunities for nurses in nonnursing journals have been discussed by Polit and Northam (in press, b).

It is sometimes useful to send a **query letter** to a journal to ask the editor whether there is interest in a manuscript. The query letter should briefly describe the topic and methods, title, and a tentative submission date. Query letters are not essential if you have done a lot of homework about the journal's goals, but they might help to avoid problems that arise if editors have recently accepted several papers on a similar topic and do not wish to consider another. Query letters can be submitted by traditional mail or by email using contact information provided at the journal's website. In Northam and colleagues' 2010 survey, editors had different views about query letters, ranging from those who said they were not important (e.g., *Research in Nursing & Health*), somewhat important (*International Journal of Nursing Studies*), or very important (*Canadian Journal of Nursing Research*).

Query letters can be sent to multiple journals simultaneously, but ultimately, the manuscript can be submitted only to one—or rather, to one at a time. If several editors express interest in reviewing a manuscript, journals can be prioritized according to criteria previously described. The priority list should not be discarded, because the manuscript can be resubmitted to the next journal on the list if the journal of first choice rejects it.

> ➲ **TIP:** A useful strategy in selecting a journal is to peruse your citation list. Journals that appear in your list have shown an interest in your topic and are strong candidates for publishing new studies on that topic.

Preparing the Manuscript

Once a journal has been selected, the information included in the journal's **Instructions to Authors**

TABLE 28.2

Impact Factor of Peer-Reviewed Nursing Journals with High Concentration of Research Articles

NAME OF JOURNAL	IMPACT FACTOR IN 2009[a]	JOURNAL RANK, 2009[b]
Advances in Nursing Science	1.41	13
American Journal of Critical Care	1.66	7
Applied Nursing Research	0.87	41
Archives of Psychiatric Nursing	0.90	40
Australian Journal of Advanced Nursing	0.59	60
Biological Research for Nursing	0.93	36
Birth	1.92	2
Cancer Nursing	1.88	5
CIN: Computers, Informatics, Nursing	0.95	31
Critical Care Nursing	1.03	27
European Journal of Oncology Nursing	1.13	22
Heart & Lung	1.04	26
International Journal of Nursing Studies	1.91	33
Journal of Advanced Nursing	1.52	10
Journal American Academy of Nurse Practitioners	0.91	38
Journal of the Association of Nurses in AIDS Care	0.96	31
Journal of Cardiovascular Nursing	1.53	9
Journal of Clinical Nursing	1.19	17
Journal of Family Nursing	1.25	15
Journal of Gerontologic Nursing	0.82	45
Journal of Nursing Administration	1.15	20
Journal of Nursing Care Quality	0.94	35
Journal of Nursing Scholarship	1.46	12
Journal of Obstetric, Gynecologic, & Neonatal Nursing	0.95	34
Journal of Psychiatric & Mental Health Nursing	1.06	25
Journal of Transcultural Nursing	0.95	32
Journal of Wound, Ostomy & Continence Nursing	1.17	18
MCN: American Journal of Maternal/Child Nursing	0.79	48
Midwifery	1.16	19
Nursing Outlook	1.54	8
Nursing Research	1.80	6
Nursing Science Quarterly	1.22	16
Oncology Nursing Forum	1.91	4
Pain Management Nursing	1.31	14
Perspectives in Psychiatric Care	1.00	30
Public Health Nursing	0.81	46
Qualitative Health Research	1.92	
Research in Nursing & Health	1.51	11
Scandinavian Journal of Caring Sciences	0.69	
Western Journal of Nursing Research	1.09	23
Worldviews on Evidence-Based Nursing	1.94	1

[a]Impact factor information is from the *Journal Citation Reports*. Nursing journals are not listed if they are not primarily research-focused (e.g., *American Journal of Nursing*, impact factor = 0.69 in 2009).

[b]Ranks are for journals within the Nursing category of the JCR Science Edition, which ranked 72 nursing journals in 2009. *Qualitative Health Research* ranked 16th in the Health Policy & Services category of the Social Science Edition. The *Scandinavian Journal of Caring Sciences* is listed in the Nursing category of the Social Science Edition of JCR; it was ranked 53rd out of 70 in 2009.

should be carefully reviewed. These instructions typically give authors such information as maximum page length, what font and margins are permissible, what type of abstract is desired, what reference style should be used, and how to submit the manuscript. In most cases, manuscripts now must be submitted online rather than mailing hard copies to the journal. It is important to adhere to the journal's guidelines to avoid rejection for a nonsubstantive reason. In an informal survey of journal editors, Froman (2008) found that the most aggravating author behavior was "disregard for journal format or mission" (p. 399).

> ➲ **TIP:** Don't begin to write until you have identified a research article that you can use as a model. Select a journal article on a topic similar to your own, or one that used similar methods, in the journal you have selected as first choice. When you have written a draft, a review by colleagues or advisers can be invaluable in improving its quality.

Typically, a manuscript for journals must be no more than 15 to 20 pages, double-spaced, not counting references and tables. In a typical article, the greatest space should be allocated to methods and results. A frequent complaint of journal editors is that submitted manuscripts are too long (Northam et al., 2010).

Care should be taken in using and preparing citations. Some nursing journals suggest that there be not more than 15 references, or no more than three citations supporting a single point. In general, only published work can be cited (e.g., not papers at a conference or manuscripts submitted but not accepted for publication). The reference style of the American Psychological Association (2010) is the style used by many nursing journals.

> ➲ **TIP:** There is a wealth of resources to assist you with the APA style, including an APA "cribsheet" (*http://www.docstyles.com*) and tutorials at university libraries. Several websites are listed in the Toolkit for you to click on directly. There is also software (e.g. StyleEase for APA Style) that helps with formatting manuscripts.

Submission of a Manuscript

When the manuscript is ready for journal submission, a cover letter should be drafted. The cover letter should state the title of the paper, name and contact information of the **corresponding author** (the author with whom the journal communicates—usually, but not always, the lead author). The letter may include assurances that (1) the paper is original and has not been published or submitted elsewhere, (2) all authors have read and approved the manuscript, and (3) there are no conflicts of interest. Many journals also require a signed copyright transfer form, which transfers all copyright ownership of the manuscript to the journal and warrants that all authors signing the form participated sufficiently in the research to justify authorship.

In submitting an article online, it is usually necessary to upload several files with different parts of your manuscript. The title page, which has identifying information, should be in the first file. The next file usually contains the abstract, main text, and the reference list. Tables and figures are submitted separately, one file at a time. In other words, if there are two tables and one figure, these would be submitted in three files. At the end of the submission process, a PDF file that contains all the various elements is created for your review prior to submission. The entire process often takes a fair amount of time, but fortunately, it is usually possible to begin the process and return to it later if you need to track down information, such as the addresses of all coauthors.

Manuscript Review

Most nursing journals that include research reports—including those listed in Table 28.2—have a policy of independent, anonymous (**blind**) **peer reviews** by two or more experts in the field. In a blind review, reviewers do not know the identity of the authors, and authors do not learn the identity of reviewers. Journals that have such a policy are **refereed journals**, and are in general more prestigious than nonrefereed journals. When submitting a manuscript to a refereed journal, authors' names should not appear anywhere except on the title page.

Peer reviewers make recommendations to the editors about whether to accept the manuscript for publication, accept it contingent on revisions, or reject it. Relatively few papers are accepted outright—both substantive and editorial revisions are the norm. Jennings (2010) has described how the review process works at *Research in Nursing & Health*.

Example of reviewer recommendation categories: The journal *Research in Nursing & Health* asks reviewers to make one of six recommendations: (1) Highly recommend; few revisions needed; (2) Publish if suggested revisions are satisfactorily completed; (3) Major revisions needed; revised version should be re-reviewed; (4) May have potential; encourage resubmission as a new manuscript; (5) Reject; do not encourage resubmission; and (6) Not appropriate for journal; send to another type of journal.

Authors are sent information about the editors' decision together with reviewers' comments. When resubmitting a revised manuscript to the same journal, each reviewer recommendation should be addressed, either by making the requested change, or by explaining in the cover letter accompanying the resubmission the rationale for not revising (Bearinger et al., 2010). Defending some aspect of a paper against a reviewer's recommendation often requires a strong supporting argument and a citation. Typically, many months go by between submission of the original manuscript and the publication of a journal article, especially if there are revisions, as there usually are.

Example of journal timeline: Beck and Watson (2010) published a paper in the journal *Nursing Research* entitled "Subsequent childbirth after a previous traumatic birth." The timeline for acceptance and publication of this manuscript, which was relatively fast, is as follows:

August 17, 2009	Manuscript submitted to *Nursing Research* for review
October 13, 2009	Letter from editor informing of a revise-and-resubmit decision
December 18, 2009	Revised manuscript resubmitted
January 27, 2010	Revised manuscript accepted for publication
July, 2010	Publication in *Nursing Research*

Many manuscripts, including many worthy and publishable ones, are rejected because of keen competition. If a manuscript is rejected, the reviewers' comments should be taken into consideration before submitting it to another journal. Manuscripts may need to be reviewed by several journals before final acceptance. Northam and colleagues (2010) offered this useful advice: "Resubmit to a different journal as soon as possible" (p. 35).

➔ **TIP:** For some articles, the journal *Nursing Research* posts supplementary information on its website, including information documenting the review process (e.g., Polit and Gillespie's 2009 study of intention-to-treat in nursing RCTs). These are posted at *http://www.nursing-research-editor.com*.

Electronic Publication

Computers and the Internet have changed forever how information of all types is disseminated. Many nurse researchers are exploring opportunities to share their research findings through electronic publication. Most journals that publish in hard copy format (e.g., *Nursing Research*) now also have online capabilities. Such mechanisms, which serve as a document delivery system, expand a journal's circulation and make findings accessible worldwide, but they have few implications for authors. Such electronic publication is just a method of distributing reports already available in hard copy.

There are, however, other ways to disseminate research findings on the Internet. For example, some researchers or research teams develop their own web page with information about their studies. When there are hyperlinks embedded in the websites, consumers can navigate between files and websites to retrieve relevant information on a topic of interest. At the other extreme are peer-reviewed electronic journals (**ejournals**) that are exclusively in online format, such as the *Online Journal of Issues in Nursing*. In between are a variety of outlets of research communication, such as websites of nursing organizations and electronic magazines.

Electronic publication is advantageous in that dissemination can occur more rapidly, cutting down on publication lag time. Electronic research reports are accessible to a worldwide audience of potential consumers, typically without page limitations, thus enabling researchers to describe and discuss complex studies more fully. Qualitative researchers are able to use more extensive quotes from their raw data, for example. Research reports on the Internet can incorporate a variety of graphic material, including audio and video supplements not possible in hard copy journals. Raw data can also be appended to reports on the Internet for secondary analysis by other researchers.

Still, there are some potential drawbacks, one of which concerns peer review. Although many online journals perform peer reviews (in some cases postpublication review), there are many opportunities to "publish" results on the Internet without a peer review process. While there are also non–peer-reviewed traditional journals, nonrefereed journal articles are not as accessible worldwide as nonreviewed information on the Internet. There is a greater risk of having a glut of low-quality research available for consumption via the Internet than there was previously. Researchers who want their evidence to have an impact on nursing practice should seek publication in outlets that subject manuscripts to external review.

Presentations at Professional Conferences

Numerous international, national, and regional professional organizations sponsor meetings at which nursing studies are presented, either through an oral presentation or through visual display in a poster session. Professional conferences are particularly good forums for presenting results to clinical audiences. Researchers also can take advantage of meeting and talking with other conference attendees who are working on similar problems in different geographic regions.

The mechanism for submitting a presentation to a conference is simpler than for journal submission. The association sponsoring the conference ordinarily publishes an announcement or **Call for Abstracts** in its website or journal, or by email to its members, 6 to 9 months before the meeting date. The notice indicates topics of interest, submission requirements, and deadlines for submitting a proposed paper or poster. Most universities and major healthcare agencies receive and post Call for Abstracts notices. Sigma Theta Tau International also posts a schedule of nursing conferences on its website (*http://www.nursingsociety.org*).

Oral Reports

Most conferences require prospective presenters to submit abstracts of 250 to 1,000 words. Abstracts are usually submitted online. Each conference has its own guidelines for abstract content and form. Abstracts are sometimes submitted to the organizer of a particular session; in other cases, conference sessions are organized after-the-fact, with related papers grouped together. Abstracts are evaluated based on the quality and originality of the research and the appropriateness of the paper for the conference audience. If abstracts are accepted, researchers are committed to appear at the conference to make a presentation.

Oral reports at meetings usually follow the IMRAD format. The time allotted for presentation usually is about 10 to 15 minutes, with 5 minutes or so for audience questions. Thus, only the most important aspects of the study, with emphasis on the results, can be included. It is especially challenging to condense a qualitative report to a brief oral summary without losing the rich, in-depth character of the data. A handy rule of thumb is that a page of double-spaced text requires 2½ to 3 minutes to read aloud. Although presenters often prepare a written paper or a script, presentations are most effective if they are delivered informally or conversationally, rather than if they are read verbatim. The presentation should be rehearsed to gain comfort with the script and to ensure that time limits are not exceeded.

⮕ **T I P :** Most conference presentations include visual materials, notably, PowerPoint slides. Visual materials should be kept simple for maximum impact. Tables are difficult to read on a slide but can be distributed to members of the audience in hard copy form. Make sure a sufficient number of copies is available.

The question-and-answer period can be a good opportunity to expand on aspects of the research and to get early feedback. Audience comments can be helpful in turning the conference presentation into a manuscript for journal submission.

Poster Presentations

Researchers sometimes present their findings or their study designs in poster sessions. Abstracts, often similar to those required for oral presentations, must be submitted to conference organizers according to specific guidelines. In poster sessions, several researchers simultaneously present visual displays summarizing study highlights, and conference attendees circulate around the exhibit area perusing displays. Those interested in a particular topic can devote time to discussing the study with the researcher and bypass posters dealing with topics of less interest. Poster sessions are efficient and encourage one-on-one discussions. Poster sessions are typically 1 to 2 hours in length. Researchers are expected to stand near their posters throughout the session to ensure effective communication.

It is challenging to design an effective poster. The poster must convey essential information about the background, design, and results of a study, in a format that can be perused in minutes. Bullet points, graphs, and photos are useful for communicating a lot of information quickly. Large,

bold fonts are essential, because posters are often read from a distance of several feet. Posters must be sturdily constructed for transport to the conference site. It is important to follow conference guidelines in determining such matters as poster size (often 4 ft high $\times$ 6 or 8 ft wide), format, allowable display materials, and so on.

Several authors have offered advice on preparing for poster sessions (e.g., Hardicre et al., 2007; Keely, 2004; Miller, 2007; Nicol & Pexman, 2010). Russell and colleagues (1996) alerted qualitative researchers to the special challenges that await them in designing a poster. Software is available for producing posters (*www.postersw.com*).

CRITIQUING RESEARCH REPORTS

Although various aspects of study methodology can be evaluated using guidelines presented throughout this book, the manner in which study information is communicated in the research report can also be critiqued in a comprehensive critical appraisal. Box 28.2 ✸ summarizes major points to consider in evaluating the presentation of a research report.

An important issue is whether the report provided sufficient information for a thoughtful critique of

---

BOX 28.2 Guidelines for Critiquing the Presentation of a Research Report

1. Does the report include a sufficient amount of detail to permit a thorough critique of the study's purpose, conceptual framework, design and methods, handling of ethical issues, analysis of data, and interpretation?
2. Is the report well written and grammatical? Are pretentious words or jargon used when a simpler wording would have been possible?
3. Is the report well organized? Is there an orderly, logical presentation of ideas? Is the report characterized by continuity of thought and expression?
4. Does the report effectively combine text with tables or figures?
5. Does the report suggest overt biases, exaggerations, or distortions?
6. Is the report written using appropriately tentative language?
7. Is sexist language avoided?
8. Does the title of the report adequately capture the key concepts and the population under investigation? Does the abstract (if any) adequately summarize the research problem, study methods, and important findings?

other dimensions. When vital pieces of information are missing, researchers leave readers little choice but to assume the worst because this would lead to the most cautious interpretation of the results. For example, if there is no mention of blinding, then the safest conclusion is that blinding was not used.

Styles of writing differ for qualitative and quantitative reports, and it is unreasonable to apply the standards considered appropriate for one paradigm to the other. Regardless of style, however, you should, in critiquing a report, be alert to indications of overt biases, unwarranted exaggerations, or melodramatic language.

In summary, the research report is meant to be an account of how and why a problem was studied and what results were obtained. The report should be clearly written, cogent, and concise and written in a manner that piques readers' interest and curiosity.

SUMMARY POINTS

- In developing a dissemination plan, researchers select a communication outlet (e.g., journal article versus conference presentation), identify the audience they wish to reach, and decide on the content that can be effectively communicated.
- In the planning stage, researchers need to decide authorship credits (if there are multiple authors), who the **lead author** and **corresponding author** will be, and in what order authors' names will be listed.
- Quantitative reports (and many qualitative reports) follow the **IMRAD format**, with the following sections: introduction, method, results, and discussion.
- The *introduction* acquaints readers with the research problem. It includes the problem statement and study purpose, the research hypotheses or questions, a brief literature review, and description of a framework. In qualitative reports, the introduction indicates the research tradition and, if relevant, the researchers' connection to the problem.

- The *method section* describes what researchers did to solve the research problem. It includes a description of the study design (or an elaboration of the research tradition), the sampling approach and a description of study participants, instruments and procedures used to collect and evaluate the data, and methods used to analyze the data.
- Standards for reporting methodologic elements are increasingly used. Researchers reporting an RCT follow **CONSORT guidelines** (Consolidated Standards of Reporting Trials), which includes use of a flow chart to show the flow of subjects in the study. Other guidelines include **STROBE** for observational studies, and **TREND** for nonrandomized evaluations of interventions.
- In the *results section*, findings from the analyses are summarized. Results sections in qualitative reports necessarily intertwine description and interpretation. Quotes from transcripts are essential for giving voice to study participants.
- Both qualitative and quantitative researchers include **figures** and **tables** that dramatize or succinctly summarize major findings or conceptual schema.
- The *discussion section* presents the interpretation of results, how the findings relate to earlier research, study limitations, and implications of the findings for nursing practice and future research.
- The major types of research reports are theses and dissertations, journal articles, online publications, and presentations at professional meetings.
- Theses and dissertations normally follow a standard IMRAD format, but some schools now accept **paper format theses**, which include an introduction, two or more publishable papers, and a conclusion.
- In selecting a journal for publication, researchers consider the journal's goals and audience, its prestige and acceptance rates, and how often it publishes. One proxy for a journal's prestige is its **impact factor**, the ratio between citations to a journal and recent citable items published.
- Before beginning to prepare a **manuscript** for submission to a journal, researchers must

carefully review the journal's **Instructions to Authors**.

- Most nursing journals that publish research reports are **refereed journals** with a policy of basing publication decisions on **peer reviews** that are usually **blind reviews** (identities of authors and reviewers are not divulged).
- Nurse researchers can explore new opportunities for electronic publishing, such as in **ejournals**. An advantage of electronic publishing is speedy, worldwide dissemination.
- Nurse researchers can also present their research at professional conferences, either through a 10- to 15-minute oral report to a seated audience, or in a **poster session** in which the "audience" moves around a room perusing research summaries attached to posters. Sponsoring organizations usually issue a **Call for Abstracts** for the conference 6 to 9 months before it is held.

STUDY ACTIVITIES

Chapter 28 of the *Resource Manual for Nursing Research: Generating and Assessing Evidence for Nursing Practice, 9th ed.*, offers various exercises and study suggestions for reinforcing the concepts presented in this chapter. In addition, the following questions can be addressed:

1. Skim a qualitative and a quantitative research report. Make a bullet-point list of differences in style and organization between the two.
2. Read a research report. Now, write a two- to three-page summary of the report that communicates the major points of the report to a clinical audience with minimal research skills.

STUDIES CITED IN CHAPTER 28

Beck, C. T., & Watson, S. (2010). Subsequent childbirth after a previous traumatic birth. *Nursing Research, 59*, 241–249.

Kottner, J., Dassen, T., & Lahmann, N. (2010). Prevalence of deep tissue injuries in hospitals and nursing homes: Two cross-sectional studies. *International Journal of Nursing Studies, 47*, 665–670.

O'Donnell, S., MacIntosh, J., & Wuest, J. (2010). A theoretical understanding of sickness absence among women who have experienced workplace bullying. *Qualitative Health Research, 20*, 439–452.

Methodologic and nonresearch references cited in this chapter can be found in a separate section at the end of the book.

29

Writing Proposals to Generate Evidence

Research **proposals** communicate a research problem and proposed methods of solving it to an interested party. Research proposals are written both by students seeking faculty approval for studies and by researchers seeking financial support. In this chapter, we offer tips on how to improve the quality of research proposals and how to develop proficiency in **grantsmanship**—the set of skills involved in securing research funding.

OVERVIEW OF RESEARCH PROPOSALS

In this section, we provide some general information regarding research proposals. Most of the information applies equally to dissertation proposals and grant applications.

Functions of a Proposal

Proposals are a means of opening communication between researchers and other parties. Those parties typically are either funding agencies or faculty advisers, whose job it is to accept or reject the proposed plan or to request modifications. An accepted proposal is a two-way contract: those accepting the proposal are effectively saying, "We are willing to offer our (emotional or financial) support, for a study

that proceeds as proposed," and those writing the proposal are saying, "If you offer support, then we will conduct the study as proposed."

Proposals often serve as the basis for negotiating with other parties as well. For example, a proposal may be shared with administrators when seeking institutional approval to conduct a study (e.g., for gaining access to participants). Proposals are often incorporated into submissions to human subjects committees or Institutional Review Boards.

Proposals help researchers to clarify their own thinking. By committing ideas to writing, ambiguities can be addressed at an early stage. Proposal reviewers also offer suggestions for conceptual and methodologic improvements. When studies are undertaken collaboratively, proposals can help ensure that all researchers are "on the same page" about how the study is to proceed and can thus minimize the possibility of friction.

Proposal Content

Proposal reviewers want a clear idea of what the researcher plans to study, why the study is needed, what methods will be used to achieve study goals, how and when tasks are to be accomplished, and whether the researcher has the skills to complete the project successfully. Proposals are evaluated on a number of criteria, including the importance of the question, the adequacy of the methods, and, if money is being requested, the reasonableness of the budget.

Proposal authors are usually given instructions about how to structure proposals. Funding agencies often supply an application kit that includes forms to be completed and specifies the format for organizing proposal contents. Universities issue guidelines for dissertation proposals.

The content and organization of most proposals are broadly similar to that for a research report, but proposals are written in the future tense (i.e., indicating what the researcher *will* do) and obviously do not include results and conclusions. The description of proposed methods—what the researchers propose to do to develop evidence that is valid and trustworthy—is critically important to the success of the proposal.

Proposals for Qualitative Studies

Preparing proposals for qualitative research entails special challenges. Methodologic decisions typically evolve in the field; therefore, it is seldom possible to provide detailed or in-depth information about such matters as sample size or data collection strategies. Sufficient detail needs to be provided, however, so that reviewers will have confidence that the researcher will assemble strong data and do justice to the data collected.

Qualitative researchers must persuade reviewers that the topic is important and worth studying, that they are sufficiently knowledgeable about the challenges of field work and adequately skillful in eliciting rich data, and, in short, that the project would be a very good risk. Knafl and Deatrick (2005) offered 10 tips for successful qualitative proposals. The first tip was to make the case for the *idea*, not the method. Qualitative researchers were also advised to avoid methodologic tutorials, to use examples to clarify the research design, and to write for both the experts and the skeptics.

Resources are available to help qualitative researchers with proposal development. For example, an entire issue of the journal *Qualitative Health Research* was devoted to proposal writing—the July 2003 issue (volume 13, issue 6). Useful advice is also available in Morse and Richards (2002), Sandelowski and colleagues (1989), and Padgett and Henwood (2009).

Proposals for Theses and Dissertations

Dissertation proposals are sometimes a bigger hurdle than dissertations themselves. Many doctoral candidates founder at the proposal development stage rather than when writing or defending the dissertation. Much of our advice—especially in our "Tips" section later in the chapter—applies equally to proposals for theses and dissertations as for grant applications, but some additional advice might prove helpful.

The Dissertation Committee

Choosing the right adviser (if an adviser is chosen rather than appointed) is almost as important as choosing the right research topic. The ideal adviser is one who is a mentor, an expert with a strong reputation in the field, a good teacher, a patient and supportive coach and critic, and an advocate. The ideal adviser is also a person who has sufficient time and interest to devote to your research and who is likely to stick with your project until its completion. This means that it might matter whether the prospective adviser has plans for a sabbatical leave, or is nearing retirement.

Dissertation committees often involve three or more members. If the adviser lacks certain "ideal" characteristics, those characteristics can be balanced across committee members by seeking people with complementary talents. Putting together a group who will work well together and who have no personal antagonism toward each other can, however, be tricky. Advisers can usually make good suggestions about other committee members.

Once a committee has been formed, it is important to develop a good working relationship with members and to learn about their viewpoints before and during the proposal development stage. This means, at a minimum, becoming familiar with their research and the methodologic strategies they have favored. It also means meeting with them and sounding them out with ideas about topics and methods. If the suggestions from two or more members are at odds, it is prudent to seek your adviser's counsel on how to resolve this.

➲ TIP: When meeting with your adviser and committee members, take notes about their suggestions, and write them out in more detail after the meeting while they are still fresh in your mind. The notes should be reviewed while developing the proposal.

Practices vary from one institution to another and from adviser to adviser, but some faculty require a prospectus before giving the go-ahead to prepare a full proposal. The prospectus is usually a three- to four-page paper outlining the research questions and proposed methods.

Content of Dissertation Proposals

Specific requirements regarding the length and format of dissertation proposals vary in different settings, and it is important to know at the outset what is expected. Typically, dissertation proposals are 20 to 40 pages in length. In some cases, however, committees prefer "mini-dissertations," that is, a document with fully developed sections that can be inserted with minor adaptation into the dissertation itself. For example, the review of the literature, theoretical framework, hypothesis formulation, and the bibliography may be sufficiently refined at the proposal stage that they can be incorporated into the final product.

Literature reviews are often the most important section of a dissertation proposal (at least for quantitative studies). Committees may not desire lengthy literature reviews, but they want to be assured that students are in command of knowledge in their field of inquiry.

Dissertation proposals sometimes include elements not normally found in proposals to funding agencies. One such element may be table shells (see Chapter 19), which can demonstrate that the student knows how to analyze data and present results effectively. Another element is a table of contents for the dissertation. The table of contents serves as an outline for the final product, and shows that the student knows how to organize material.

Several books provide additional advice on writing a dissertation proposal, including Locke and colleagues (2007) and Rudestam and Newton (2007).

FUNDING FOR RESEARCH PROPOSALS

Funding for research projects is becoming increasingly difficult to obtain because of keen and growing competition. As more nurses gain research skills, and as the push for evidence-based practice grows, so too are applications for research funding increasing. Successful proposal writers need to have good research and proposal-writing skills, and they must also know from whom funding is available.

Federal Funding in the United States

The largest funder of research activities in the United States is the federal government. For healthcare researchers, the National Institutes of Health (NIH) and the Agency for Healthcare Research and Quality (AHRQ) are leading agencies. Two major types of federal disbursements are grants and contracts. **Grants** are awarded for studies conceived by researchers themselves, whereas **contracts** are for studies desired by the government.

There are several mechanisms for NIH grants, which can be awarded to researchers in both domestic and foreign institutions. Most grant applications are unsolicited, and reflect the research interests of individual researchers. Unsolicited applications should be consistent with the broad objectives of an NIH funding agency, such as NINR. Investigator-initiated applications are submitted in response to **Parent Announcements**, which are covered under omnibus Funding Opportunity Announcements (FOAs).

NIH also issues periodic **Program Announcements** (PA) that describe new, continuing, or expanded program interests. For example, in March 2010, NINR issued a joint program announcement with 16 other NIH institutes titled "Behavioral and Social Science Research on Understanding and Reducing Health Disparities" (PA-10-136). The purpose of this PA, which expires in 2013, is "to encourage behavioral and social science research on the causes and solutions to health and disabilities disparities in the U.S. population."

Another grant mechanism allows federal agencies to identify a *specific* topic area in which they are interested in receiving proposals by a **Request for Applications** (**RFA**). RFAs are one-time opportunities with a single submission date. As an example, NINR issued an RFA titled "Chronic Co-Morbid Conditions in HIV+ U.S. Adults on Highly-Effective Anti-Retroviral Therapy" in February 2010, with grant applications due in May 2010. The RFA states general guidelines and goals for the competition, but researchers can develop the specific research problem within the topic area. A weekly electronic publication, the *NIH Guide for Grants and Contracts,* contains announcements about RFAs, PAs, and Parent Announcements.

In addition to grants, some government agencies award contracts to do *specific* studies. Contract offers are announced in a **Request for Proposals** (**RFP**), which details the *exact* study that the government wants. Contracts, which are typically awarded to only one competitor, constrain researchers' activities and so most nurse researchers compete for grants rather than contracts. A summary of federal RFPs is published in the *Commerce Business Daily* (*http://cbdnet.gpo.gov*).

Government funding for nursing research is, of course, also available in other countries. In Canada, for example, various types of health research are sponsored by the Canadian Institutes of Health Research (CIHR). Information about CIHR's program of grants, training awards, and other funding opportunities is available at its website (*http://www.cihr.ca*).

Private Funds

Healthcare research is supported by numerous philanthropic foundations, professional organizations, and corporations. Many researchers prefer private funding to government support because there is less "red tape" and fewer requirements.

Information about philanthropic foundations that support research is available through the Foundation Center (*http://www.fdncenter.org*). A comprehensive resource for identifying funding opportunities is the Center's *The Foundation Directory*, now available online for a fee. The directory lists the purposes and activities of the foundations and information for contacting them. The Foundation Center also offers seminars and training on grant writing and funding opportunities in locations around the United States. Another resource for information on funding is the Community of Science, which maintains a database on funding opportunities (*http://www.cos.com*).

Professional associations (e.g., the American Nurses' Foundation, Sigma Theta Tau) offer funds for conducting research. Health organizations, such as the American Heart Association and the American Cancer Society, also support research activities.

Finally, research funding is sometimes donated by private corporations, particularly those dealing with healthcare products. The Foundation Center publishes a directory of corporate grantmakers and provides links through its website to a number of corporate philanthropic programs. Additional information concerning corporate requirements and interests should be obtained either from the organization directly or from staff in the research administration offices of the institution with which you are affiliated.

GRANT APPLICATIONS TO NIH

NIH funds many nursing studies through NINR and through other institutes. Because of the importance of NINR as a funding source for nurse researchers, this section describes the process of proposal submission and review at NIH. AHRQ, which also funds nurse-initiated studies, uses the same application kit and similar procedures.

Types of NIH Grants and Awards

NIH awards different types of research grants, and each has its own objectives and review criteria. The basic grant program—and the primary funding mechanism for independent research—is the traditional **Research Project Grant** (R01). The objective of R01 grants is to support specific research projects in areas reflecting the interests and competencies of a Principal Investigator (PI).

Beside the R01 grant program, three others that are available through NINR are worth noting. A special program (R15) has been established for researchers working in institutions that have not been major participants in NIH programs. These **Academic Research Enhancement Awards (AREA)** are designed to stimulate research in institutions that provide baccalaureate training for many individuals who go on to do health-related research. There is also a **Small Grant** Program (R03) that provides support for pilot, feasibility, and methodology development studies. R03 grants provide a maximum of $50,000 of direct support for up to 2 years. Finally, the R21 grant mechanism—the **Exploratory/Developmental Research Grant Award**—is intended to encourage new, exploratory, and developmental research projects by providing support for early stages of research.

NIH and other agencies also offer individual and institutional predoctoral and postdoctoral fellowships, as well as career development awards. Examples of individual fellowship mechanisms available through the National Research Service Award (NRSA) program within NINR include the following:

- F31, Ruth Kirshstein Individual Predoctoral NRSA Fellowships, support nurses in a supervised training leading to a doctoral degree in areas related to the NINR mission
- F32, Ruth Kirshstein Individual Postdoctoral NRSA Fellowships, support postdoctoral training to nurses to broaden their scientific background
- F33, Senior NRSA Fellowships, support doctorally trained researchers with at least 7 years of research in pursuing opportunities to change the direction of their research careers.

> ⟩ T I P : Advice on developing a proposal for an NRSA fellowship has been offered in a paper by Parker and Steeves (2005).

Four important Career Development Awards offered through NINR are as follows:

- K01, Mentored Research Scientist Development Award, available to doctorally prepared scientists who would benefit from a mentored research experience with an expert sponsor

- K22, NINR's Career Transition Awards, offers support to postdoctoral fellows in transition to a faculty position
- K23, Mentored Patient-Oriented Research Career Development Award, supports the career development of investigators who are committed to focusing on patient-oriented research
- K99, Pathways to Independence Awards, provide for postdoctoral research activity leading to the submission of an independent research project application.

> ⟩ T I P : If you have an idea for a study and are not sure which type of grant program is suitable—or you are unsure whether NINR or another NIH institute might be interested—you should contact NINR directly (telephone number: 301-594-6906). NINR staff can provide feedback about whether your proposed study matches NINR's program interests. Information about NINR's ongoing priorities and areas of opportunity is available at *http://www.nih.gov/ninr*. A one- to two-page concept paper can also be e-mailed to the address listed on the NINR website.

NIH Forms and Schedule

In 2007, NIH transitioned from hard-copy application submissions to electronic submissions using the SF424 (R&R) application, most recently revised in early 2010, through *www.grants.gov*. The SF424 is used for all the types of grants and awards described in the previous section, although there are supplemental components needed for some of them. Researchers use Adobe Reader (version 8.1.6 or later) to "fill in" and complete this new application. There is abundant information online about the new application process, and NIH offers training sessions on how to submit applications electronically. The application kit can be accessed from the NIH website at *http:// www.nih.gov* under their "Grants and Opportunities" section.

New grant applications are usually processed in three cycles annually. Different deadlines apply to different types of grants, as shown in Table 29.1. For most new applications, except fellowships in the F series and AIDS-related research, the deadline for

TABLE 29.1	Schedule for Selected New Research Applications, National Institutes of Health*				
Application Deadline	**MECHANISM OF SUPPORT (TYPE OF AWARD)**				
	R01	**R03, R21**	**R15**	**K Series**	**F Series**
Cycle I a	February 5	February 16	February 25	February 12	April 8
Cycle II b	June 5	June 16	June 25	June 12	August 8
Cycle III c	October 5	October 16	October 25	October 12	December 8

a Cycle I: Scientific Review: June–July; Earliest start date: December
b Cycle II: Scientific Review: October–November; Earliest start date: April
c Cycle III: Scientific Review: February–March; Earliest start date: July
*AIDS-related applications are on a different schedule; consult the NIH website for information.

receipt is in February, June, and October. The scientific merit review dates are about 4 to 5 months after each submission date. For example, applications submitted for the February cycle are reviewed in June or July; the earliest project start date for applications funded in that cycle would be in December. Applicants should begin a registration process through the Electronic Research Administration (eRA) Commons at least 2 weeks prior to the submission date.

Preparing a Grant Application for NIH

Although many substantive aspects of the NIH grant application have remained stable, the forms and procedures for NIH grant applications have been changing. It is crucial to carefully review up-to-date instructions for grant application submission rather than relying on information in this chapter.

Forms: Screens and Uploaded Attachments

The SF424 form set has numerous components. The "front matter" of SF424 consists of various forms that appear on a series of fillable screens. These forms help in processing the application and provide administrative information. Careful attention to detail with these forms is very important. Major forms include the following:

- *Cover Component.* On the cover form, researchers state a brief, descriptive title of the project (not to

exceed 81 characters), the name and affiliation of the PI, and other administrative information.

TIP: The project title should be given careful thought. It is the first thing that reviewers see, and should be crafted to create a good impression. The title should be concise and informative, but should also be compelling.

- *Project/Performance Site Location Component.* The next screen requests information about the primary site where the work will be performed.
- *Other Project Information Component.* This screen is the mechanism for submitting key information. The form begins with questions about human subjects, and the last few items require attachments to be uploaded, including a project summary, a project narrative, bibliography, and facilities and equipment information. Attachments, which must be in PDF format, have strict size limitations. The *Project Summary* serves as a succinct description of aims and methods of the proposed study and must be no longer than 30 lines. The *Project Narrative* is a brief (two to three sentences) description of the relevance of the research to public health. The *Bibliography* is a list of references cited in the research plan; any reference style is acceptable.

The *Facilities* attachment is used to describe needed and available resources (e.g., laboratories).

- *Senior/Key Person Profile(s) Component.* For each key person, the form requests basic identifying information and calls for an attachment, a Biographical Sketch. The sketch must list education and training, as well as the following: (a) a personal statement describing the qualifications that make the person well suited for his or her role, (b) positions and honors, (c) selected peer-reviewed publications or manuscripts in press, and (d) recently completed and ongoing research support. A maximum of four pages is permitted for each person.
- *Budget Component.* For NIH applications, researchers must chose between two budget options—the R&R Budget Component or the PHS398 Modular Budget Component. Detailed R&R budgets showing specific projected expenses are required if annual direct project costs exceed $250,000, but for smaller projects, budget information is obtained in another section. (Modular budgets are only appropriate for R-type grants.)

For grant applications to NIH and other public health service agencies, additional forms referred to as PHS398 components are required and include the following:

- *Cover Letter Component.* Cover letters to the funding agency are strongly encouraged. Information in the cover letter should include the application title, the name and number of the funding opportunity, and any request to be assigned to a particular review group.
- *Cover Page Supplement Component.* This form supplements the SF424 cover page and requests mainly administrative information.
- *Modular Budget Component.* **Modular budgets**, paid in modules of $25,000, are appropriate for R-series applications (e.g., R01s) requesting $250,000 or less per year of direct costs. (**Direct costs** include specific project-related costs such as staff and supplies; **indirect costs** are institutional **overhead** costs.) This form provides budget fields for annual summaries of projected costs for up to 5 years of support. There are also fields for cumulative summaries

across all project years. A *budget justification* attachment, detailing primarily personnel costs, must be uploaded.

➲ **TIP:** Even though modular budget forms ask only for summaries of the funds needed to complete a study, you should prepare a more detailed budget to arrive at a reasonable projection of needed funds. Beginning researchers are likely to need the assistance of a research administrator or an experienced, funded researcher in preparing their first budget. Higdon and Topp (2004) have offered some advice on developing a budget.

- *Research Plan Component.* The PHS398 Research Plan form asks about application type (e.g., new, resubmission) and then requires information, in the form of attachments, about the proposed study and the research plan. Research plan requirements are described in the next section.
- *Checklist Component.* The checklist includes various miscellaneous items, including organizational assurances and certifications.

➲ **TIP:** Examples of selected forms for SF424 are presented in the Toolkit of the *Resource Manual* in nonfillable form—that is, they are included simply as illustrations, not to be used for submitting a grant application.

The Research Plan Component

The research plan component consists of 16 items, not all of which are relevant to every application—for example, item 1 is for revised applications or resubmissions. Each item involves uploading separate PDF attachments. In this section, we briefly describe guidelines for items 2 through 16, with emphasis on items 2 and 3. We also present some advice based on a study (Inouye & Fiellin, 2005) in which the researchers content-analyzed the criticisms in the review sheets of 66 R01 applications submitted to a clinical research review group (not NINR). Thus, the advice relating to specific pitfalls is "evidence-based," that is, based on identified problems in actual applications.

⟶ **T I P :** Based on their analysis, Inouye and Fiellin (2005) created a grant-writing checklist designed as a self-assessment tool for proposal developers. We have included an adapted and expanded checklist in the Toolkit that is part of the accompanying *Resource Manual*.

Specific Aims (Item 2). In this section, which is restricted to a single page, researchers must provide a succinct summary of the research problem and the specific objectives of the study, including any hypotheses to be tested. The aims statement should indicate the scope and importance of the problem. Care should be taken to be precise and to identify a problem of manageable proportions—a broad and complex problem is unlikely to be solvable.

Inouye and Fiellin (2005) found that the most frequent critique of the Specific Aims section was that the goals were overstated, overly ambitious, or unrealistic (18% of the review sheets). Other complaints were that the project was poorly conceptualized (15%) or that hypotheses were not clearly articulated (12%).

Research Strategy (Item 3). In the new application forms released in 2010, several sections from earlier forms (Background, Preliminary Studies, and Research Design and Methods) were combined and page restrictions were severely tightened. Unless otherwise specified in a Funding Opportunity Announcement (FOA), the Research Strategy section is now restricted to 12 pages for R01 and R15 applications, and to 6 pages for R03, R21, and F-series applications. For other funding mechanisms, page restrictions are specified in the FOA.

⟶ **T I P :** Career Development Awards (K-series) involve completion of a special form, requiring attachments that include a description of the applicant's background, a statement of career goals and objectives, career development or training activities during the award period, and training in the responsible conduct of research. These items plus the Research Strategy section must, in combination, be no more than 12 pages. The applicant's institution must also submit a letter describing its commitment to the candidate and to his or her development.

The Research Strategy section is organized into three subsections: Significance, Innovation, and Approach. In the Significance section, researchers must convince reviewers that the proposed study idea has clinical or theoretical relevance and that the study will make a contribution to scientific knowledge or clinical practice. Researchers describe the study context in this section through a brief analysis of existing knowledge and gaps on the topic. Researchers should demonstrate command of current knowledge in a field, but this section must be very tightly written. Inouye and Fiellin (2005) found that a frequent critique expressed by reviewers about this section was that the need for the study was not adequately justified (29%). In the Innovation section, researchers should describe how the proposed study challenges, refines, or improves current research or clinical practice paradigms.

The proposed design and methods for the study are described in the third subsection, Approach. This section, which is the heart of the application, should be written with extreme care and reviewed with a self-critical eye. The Approach section needs to be concise, but with sufficient detail to persuade reviewers that methodologic decisions are sound and that the study will yield important and reliable evidence.

A thorough Approach section typically describes the following: (1) the research design, including a discussion of comparison group strategies and methods of controlling confounding variables (for qualitative studies, the research tradition should be described); (2) the experimental intervention, if applicable, including a description of the treatment and control group conditions; (3) procedures, such as what equipment will be used, how participants will be assigned to groups, and what type of blinding, if any, will be achieved; (4) the sampling plan, including eligibility criteria and sample size; (5) data collection methods and information about reliability and validity of measures; and (6) data analysis strategies. The Approach should identify potential methodologic problems and intended strategies for handling such problems. In proposals for qualitative studies, special care should be given to steps that will be taken to enhance the integrity and trustworthiness of the study.

Inouye and Fiellin (2005) found that *all* of the reviews they analyzed had one or more criticism of this section, the most general of which was that the description of methods was underdeveloped (15%). A few of the most persistent criticisms were as follows:

- Inadequate blinding for outcome assessment (36%)
- Sample was flawed—biased or unrepresentative (36%)
- Important confounding variables inadequately controlled (32%)
- Inadequate sample size or inadequate power calculations (26%)
- Insufficient description of the approach to data analysis (24%)
- Outcome measures inadequately specified or described (23%)

Although some of these concerns relate to clinical trials (e.g., blinding), many have broad relevance—small sample size, sample biases, uncontrolled variables, and poorly described data collection and analysis plans can be problematic in any type of study.

The Approach section must also include information on Preliminary Studies. In new applications, researchers must describe the PI's preliminary or developmental studies and any experience pertinent to the application. This section must persuade reviewers that you have the skills and background needed to do the research. Any pilot work that has served as a foundation for the proposed project should be described. Inouye and Fiellin's (2005) analysis is especially illuminating with regard to Preliminary Studies. They found that the single biggest criticism across the 66 review sheets was that more pilot work was needed, mentioned in 41% of the reviews.

➲ **TIP:** For applications submitted by Early Stage Investigators (a person within 10 years of completing their terminal degree and who has not yet been awarded an R01 grant), reviewers are instructed to place less emphasis on the applicant's Preliminary Studies.

Human Subjects Sections (Items 6–9). Researchers who plan to collect data from human subjects must complete items relating to the protection of subjects. An entire section of the application kit ("Part II, Supplemental Instructions for Preparing the Human Subjects Section of the Research Plan") provides guidance on the attachments needed for these items. Applicants must either address the involvement of human subjects and describe protections from research risks or provide a justification for exemption with enough information that reviewers can determine the appropriateness of requests for exemption. If no exemption is sought, the section must address various issues, as outlined in the application kit. The application must also include various types of information regarding the inclusion of women, minorities, and children. These sections often serve as the cornerstone of the document submitted to Institutional Review Boards.

Other Research Plan Sections (Items 10–15). Most remaining sections in the research plan component are not relevant universally. These include such items as a description and justification of the use of vertebrate animals and a leadership plan if there are multiple principal investigators. One item, however, has relevance to many applications: Letters of support (Item 14). This item requires you to attach letters from individuals agreeing to provide services to the project, such as consultants.

Appendices (Item 16). Grant applications often include appended materials. A maximum of 10 PDF attachments is allowed, and a summary sheet listing all appended items is encouraged. Examples of appended materials include data collection instruments, clinical protocols, detailed sample size calculations, complex statistical models, and other supplementary materials in support of the application. Researchers can no longer submit publications or manuscripts, except under restricted circumstances. Essential information should never be relegated to an appendix because only primary reviewers receive appendices. The guidelines warn that appendices should not be used to circumvent the page limitations of the Research Strategy section.

➲ **TIP:** In terms of content, the research plan for NIH applications is similar to what is required in most research proposals — although emphases and page restrictions may vary, and supplementary information may be required.

The Review Process

Grant applications submitted to NIH are reviewed for completeness and relevance by the NIH Center for Scientific Review. Acceptable applications are assigned to an appropriate Institute or Center, and to a peer review group.

NIH uses a sequential, dual review system for informing decisions about its grant applications. The first level involves a panel of peer reviewers (not NIH employees), who evaluate applications for their scientific merit. These review panels are called **scientific review groups** (SRGs) or, more commonly, **study sections**. Each panel consists of about 20 researchers with backgrounds appropriate to the specific study section for which they have been selected. Appointments to the review panels are usually for 4-year terms and are staggered so that about one-fourth of each panel is new each year.

➲ **TIP:** Applications by nurse researchers usually are assigned to one of two Nursing Science study sections. One is the "Nursing Science: Adults and Older Adults Study Section" (NSAA) and the other is the "Nursing Science: Children and Families Study Section" (NSCF). Fellowship applications in the F series are reviewed in a separate study section, often with K-series applications.

The second level of review is by a National Advisory Council, which includes scientific and lay representatives. The Advisory Council considers not only the scientific merit of an application but also the relevance of the proposed study to the programs and priorities of the Center or Institute to which the application has been submitted, as well as budgetary considerations.

Applications are assigned to primary and secondary (and sometimes tertiary) reviewers for detailed analysis. Each assigned reviewer prepares comments and assigns scores according to five core review criteria.

1. *Significance.* Does the proposed study address an important problem? If the aims of the application are achieved, how will scientific knowledge or clinical practice be advanced? What will be the effect of the study on the concepts or methods that drive this field?
2. *Investigator.* Is the investigator appropriately trained and well suited to carry out this work? Is the proposed work appropriate to the experience level of the PI and other researchers? Do Early Stage Investigators have appropriate training and experience?
3. *Innovation.* Does the project employ novel concepts, approaches, or methods? Are the aims original and innovative? Does the project challenge existing paradigms or develop new methods or technologies?
4. *Approach.* Are the overall strategy, design, methods, and analyses adequately developed and appropriate to the aims of the project? Does the applicant acknowledge potential problem areas and consider alternative tactics?
5. *Environment.* Does the scientific environment in which the work will be done contribute to the probability of success? Do the proposed experiments take advantage of unique features of the scientific environment or employ useful collaborative arrangements? Is there evidence of institutional support?

In addition to these five criteria, other factors are relevant in evaluating proposals, including the reasonableness of the proposed budget, the adequacy of protections for human or animal subjects, and the appropriateness of the sampling plan in terms of including women, minorities, and children as participants. These factors are not, however, formally scored.

Scoring of applications changed in 2010. In the current system, each of the five core criteria is scored on a scale from 1 (exceptional) to 9 (poor). Assigned reviewers score applications and submit their scores before attending a study section meeting, and also submit a preliminary overall **impact score** (also called a **priority score**) on the same 1 to 9 scale. An impact score reflects a reviewer's assessment of the extent to which the study will exert a powerful influence in an area of research. Based on preliminary impact scores, applications with unfavorable scores (usually those in the lower half) are not discussed or scored by the entire study section in its meeting. This streamlined process was instituted so that study section members could focus their discussion on the most worthy applications.

For applications that *are* discussed in the meeting, each study section member (not just those who were assigned as reviewers) designates an impact score, based on their own critique of the application and the committee's discussion. Individual impact scores from all committee members are averaged, and the mean is then multiplied by 10 to arrive at a final score. Thus, final impact scores for applications that are discussed can range from 10 (the best possible score) to 90 (the lowest possible score). Final scores tend to cluster in the 10 to 50 range, however, inasmuch as the least meritorious applications were previously screened out and not scored by the full study section. Among all scored applications, only those with the best priority scores actually obtain funding. Cut-off scores for funding vary from agency to agency and year to year, but a score of 20 or lower may be needed to secure funding.

Within a few days after the study section meeting, applicants are able to learn their priority score and percentile ranking online via the NIH eRA Commons (*https://commons.era. nih.gov/commons*). Within about 30 days, applicants can access a summary of the study section's evaluation. These **summary sheets** include critiques written by the assigned reviewers, a summary of the study section's discussion, study section recommendations, and administrative notes of special consideration (e.g., human subjects issues). All applicants receive a summary sheet, even if their applications were unscored. (Applicants of unscored applications also learn how the assigned reviewers scored the five core criteria).

> ▶ **TIP:** Unless an unfunded proposal is criticized in some fundamental way (e.g., the problem area was not judged to be significant), applications often should be resubmitted, with revisions that reflect the concerns of the peer reviewers. When a proposal is resubmitted, the next review panel members are given a copy of the original application and the summary sheet so that they can evaluate the degree to which initial reviewers' concerns have been addressed. Applications can be resubmitted up to two times.

TIPS ON PROPOSAL DEVELOPMENT

Although it is impossible to tell you exactly what steps to follow to produce a successful proposal, we conclude this chapter with some advice that might help to improve the process and the product. Many of these tips are especially relevant for those preparing proposals for funding. Further suggestions for writing effective grant applications may be found in Beitz and Bliss (2005), Grey (2000), Lusk (2004), and Inouye and Fiellin (2005).

Things to Do before Writing Begins

Advance planning is essential to the development of a successful proposal. This section offers suggestions for things you can do to prepare for the actual writing.

Start Early

Writing a proposal, and attending to all of the details of a formal submission process, is time consuming and almost always takes longer than originally envisioned. Be sure to build in enough time that the product can be reviewed and re-reviewed by members of the team (including any faculty mentors) and by willing colleagues. Make sure there is adequate time for administrative issues such as securing permissions and getting budgets approved.

Having a proposal timeline is a good way to impose discipline on the proposal development process. Figure 29.1 presents one example, but the list of tasks is merely suggestive. Ask an experienced person to review your timeline, and try to adhere to the timeline once you start.

Task	Timeline (Months Before Submission)												
	12+	12	11	10	9	8	7	6	5	4	3	2	1
Identify/conceptualize the problem	X												
Undertake a literature review	X												
Identify and approach possible data collection sites	X												
Initiate descriptive or pilot work	X												
Analyze pilot data, assess feasibility	XXXXX												
Develop a "brief," outlining significance & preliminary thoughts about overall study design		XX											
Identify methodologic and content experts; solicit input and possible collaboration			XXX										
Begin building a team of co-investigators and consultants		XXXX											
Identify contact funder/program officer (as needed)		XX											
Obtain all application forms and instructions			XX										
Review funding agencies' priorities; review recently funded grants			XXX										
Develop research plan, identify instruments, etc.; consult with statisticians, psychometricians, etc., as needed					XXXXXXX								
Collect site data for describing site, staff, clients					XXX								
Obtain written letters of agreement and/or support from data collection sites					XXX								
Prepare an outline of the proposal; develop writing assignments							XX						
Write draft of proposal							XXXXXXX						
Draft a budget									XX				
Draft other ancillary components (bio sketches, etc.)									XX				
Internal review by team members										XXX			
Make revisions based on review											XXX		
External review by colleagues/experts											XXX		
Team review of comments, make final revisions												XXX	
Write abstract/summary												XX	
Finalize budget and other ancillary components													X
Prepare all final documents, get needed signatures													X

FIGURE 29.1 Example of a grant-writing timeline.

TIP: It is advantageous to build pilot or preliminary work into your proposal development timeline. As noted earlier, NIH reviewers frequently criticize the absence of adequate pilot work. Incremental knowledge building is attractive to reviewers. When you apply for funding, you are asking funders to make an *investment* in you; they will have the sense of being offered a better investment opportunity if some groundwork for a study has already been completed.

Select an Important Problem

A factor that is critical to the success of a proposal is selecting a problem that has clinical or theoretical significance and that is viewed in a positive light by reviewers. The proposal must make a persuasive argument that the research could make a noteworthy contribution to evidence on a topic that is important and appealing to those making recommendations.

Kuzel (2002), who shared some lessons about securing funding for a qualitative study, noted that researchers could profit by taking advantage of certain "hot topics" that have the special attention of the public and government officials. Proposals can sometimes be cast in a way that links them to topics of national concern, and such a linkage can contribute to a favorable review. Kuzel used as an example his funded study of quality of care and medical errors in primary care practices, with emphasis on patient perspectives. The proposal was submitted at a time when the U.S. government was putting resources into research to enhance patient safety and noted that "the reframing of 'quality' under the name of 'patient safety' has captured the stage and is likely to have an enduring effect on what work receives funding" (p. 141). Both qualitative and quantitative researchers should be sensitive to political realities.

Know Your Audience

Learn as much as possible about the audience for your proposal. For dissertations, this means getting to know your committee members and learning about their expectations, interests, and schedules. If you are writing a proposal for funding, you should obtain information about the funding organization's priorities. It is also wise to examine recently funded projects. Funding agencies often publish the criteria that reviewers use to make funding decisions—such as the ones we described for NIH—and these criteria should be studied carefully.

Grey (2000), in her tips on grantsmanship, urged researchers to "talk it up" (p. 91), that is, to call program staff in agencies and foundations, or to send letters of inquiry about possible interest in a project. Grey also noted the importance of *listening* to what these people say and following their recommendations.

Another aspect to "knowing your audience" concerns appreciating reviewers' perspectives. Reviewers for funding agencies are busy professionals who are taking time away from their own work to consider the merits of proposed new studies. They are likely to be methodologically sophisticated and experts in *their* field—but they may have limited knowledge of your own area of research. It is, therefore, imperative to help time-pressured reviewers to grasp the merits of your proposed study, without relying on jargon or specialized terminology.

Review a Successful Proposal

Although there is no substitute for actually writing a proposal as a learning experience, novice proposal writers can profit by examining a successful proposal. It is likely that some of your colleagues or fellow students have written a proposal that has been accepted (either by a funding sponsor or by a dissertation committee), and many people are glad to share their successful efforts with others. Also,

proposals funded by the government are usually in the public domain—that is, you can ask for a copy of funded proposals. To obtain a funded NIH project, for example, you can contact the NIH Freedom of Information Coordinator for the appropriate institute.

Several journals have published entire proposals, except for administrative and budgetary information. An early example was a proposal for a study of comprehensive discharge planning for the elderly (Naylor, 1990). More recently, a proposal for a qualitative study of adolescent fathers was published, together with reviewers' comments (Dallas et al., 2005a, 2005b).

> **➲ TIP:** The accompanying *Resource Manual* includes the entire successful grant application to NINR by Deborah Dillon McDonald entitled "Older adults response to healthcare practitioner pain communication," together with reviewers' comments and McDonald's response.

Create a Strong Research Team

For funded research, it is important to think strategically in putting together a team because reviewers often give considerable weight to researchers' qualifications. It is not enough to have a team of competent people; it is necessary to have the right *mix* of competence. Gaps and weaknesses can often be compensated for by the judicious use of consultants.

Another shortcoming of some project teams is that there are too many researchers with small time commitments. It is unwise to propose a staff with five or more top-level professionals who are able to contribute only 5% to 10% of their time to the project. Such projects often run into management problems because no one is in control of the workflow. Although collaborative work is commendable, you should be able to justify the inclusion of every person.

Things to Do as You Write

If you have planned well and drafted a realistic schedule, the next step is to move forward with the development of the proposal. Some suggestions for the writing stage follow.

Build a Persuasive Case

In a proposal, whether or not funding is sought, you need to persuade reviewers that you are asking the right questions, that you are the right person to ask those questions, and that you will get valid and credible answers. You must also convince them that the answers will make a difference to nursing and its clients.

Beginning proposal writers sometimes forget that they are *selling* a product: themselves and their ideas. It is appropriate, therefore, to think of the proposal as a marketing opportunity. It is not enough to have a good idea and sound methods—you must have a persuasive presentation. When funding is at stake, the challenge is greater because *everyone is trying to persuade reviewers that their proposal is more meritorious than yours.*

Reviewers know that most applications they review will *not* get funded. For example, in fiscal year 2009, fewer than one out of five R01 applications got NIH support. The reviewers' job is to identify the most scientifically worthy applications. In writing the proposal, you must consciously include features that will put your application in a positive light. That is, you should think of ways to gain a competitive edge. Be sure to give thought to issues persistently identified as problematic by reviewers (Inouye & Fiellin, 2005), and use a well-conceived checklist to ensure that you have not missed an opportunity to strengthen your study design and your proposal.

The proposal should be written in a positive, confident tone. If you do not sound convinced that the proposed study is important and will be rigorously done, then reviewers will not be persuaded either. It is unwise to promise what cannot be achieved, but you should think about ways to put the proposed project in a positive light.

Justify Methodologic Decisions

Many proposals fail because they do not instill confidence that key decisions have a good rationale. Methodologic decisions should be made carefully, keeping in mind the benefits and drawbacks of alternatives, and a compelling—if brief—justification should be provided. To the extent possible, make your decisions evidence-based and *defend* the proposed methods with citations demonstrating their utility. Insufficient detail and scanty explanation of methodologic choices can be perilous, although page constraints often make full elaboration impossible.

Begin and End with a Flourish

The abstract or summary to the proposal should be crafted with extreme care. Because it is one of the first things that reviewers read, you need to be sure that it will create a favorable impression. (For NIH applications, nonassigned reviewers may read *only* the summary and not the entire application). The ideal abstract is one that generates excitement and inspires confidence in the proposed study's rigor. Although abstracts appear at the beginning of a proposal, they are often written last.

Proposals typically conclude with material that is somewhat unexciting, such as a data analysis plan. A brief, upbeat concluding paragraph that summarizes the significance and innovativeness of the proposed project can help to remind reviewers of its potential to contribute to nursing practice and nursing science.

Adhere to Instructions

Funding agencies (and universities) provide instructions on what is required in a research proposal. It is crucial to read these instructions carefully and to follow them precisely. Proposals are sometimes rejected without review if they do not adhere to such guidelines as minimum font size or page limitations.

Pay Attention to Presentation

Reviewers are put in a better frame of mind if the proposals they are reading are attractive, well organized, grammatical, and easy to read. Glitzy figures are not needed, but the presentation should be professional and show respect for weary reviewers. In Inouye and Fiellin's (2005) study, 20% of the grant applications were criticized for such presentation issues as typographical or grammatical errors, poor layout, inconsistencies, and omitted tables.

Have the Proposal Critiqued

Before formal submission of a proposal, a draft should be reviewed by others. Reviewers should be selected for both substantive and methodologic expertise. If the proposal is being submitted for funding, one reviewer ideally would have first-hand knowledge of the funding source. If a consultant has been proposed because of specialized expertise that you believe will strengthen the study, he or she should be asked to participate by reviewing the draft and making recommendations for its improvement.

In universities, mock review panels are often held before submitting a proposal to a funding agency. Faculty and students are invited to these mock reviews and provide valuable feedback for enhancing a proposal.

RESEARCH EXAMPLES

NIH makes available the abstracts of all funded projects through its Research Portfolio Online Reporting Tools (RePORT). Abstracts can be searched by subject, researcher, study section, type of funding mechanism, year of support, and so on. Abstracts for two projects funded through NINR are presented here.

Example of a Funded Quantitative (R01) Project

Elizabeth Schlenk of the University of Pittsburgh prepared the following abstract for a project entitled "Promoting Physical Activity in Older Adults with Comorbidity." The application was reviewed by the Adults and Older Adults Study Section (NSAA), and received NINR funding in March 2010. The project is scheduled for completion in January 2014.

Project Summary: Over 9 million Americans have symptomatic osteoarthritis (OA) of the knee, a chronic disease associated with frequent joint pain, functional limitations, and quadriceps weakness that intrude on everyday life. At least half of those with OA of the knee are diagnosed with hypertension or high blood pressure (HBP), one of the most prevalent risk factors for cardiovascular disease. Many other individuals with OA of the knee unknowingly have HBP and remain untreated. Our own work and that of others suggest that persons with OA of the knee experience reductions in BP when they participate in a regular regimen of physical activity. Even small decreases in systolic and diastolic BP found with physical activity are clinically significant, e.g., a 2 mm Hg decrease reduces the risk of stroke by 14%–17%, and the risk of coronary heart disease is reduced by 6%–9%. Yet, only 15% of persons with OA and 47% with HBP engage in regular physical activity. The purpose of this study is to investigate how the individually delivered, home-based, 6-month modified Staying Active with Arthritis (STAR) intervention, guided by self-efficacy theory and modified to address comorbid HBP, affects lower extremity exercise (flexibility, strengthening, and balance), fitness walking, functional status, BP, quadriceps strength, pain, and health-related quality of life (HRQoL) in a convenience sample of 224 adults age 50 years or older with OA of the knee and HBP. Using a randomized controlled, 2-group design, we (1) hypothesize that at the end of the 6-month intervention period and 6 months after the intervention period ends, those who receive the modified STAR intervention will be more likely to perform lower extremity exercise, participate in fitness walking, show improvements in objective functional status, and demonstrate reductions in BP than those who receive attention-control. Secondarily, we will (2) evaluate the impact of the modified STAR intervention, compared to attention-control, on subjective functional status, quadriceps strength, pain, and HRQoL at both time points; (3) explore the impact of the modified STAR intervention, compared to attention-control, on self-efficacy and outcome expectancy at both time points; (4) explore the relationship between self-efficacy and outcome expectancy; and (5) explore the extent to which self-efficacy and outcome expectancy mediate the relationship between the modified STAR intervention and performance of lower extremity exercise and participation in fitness walking. Data will be analyzed using repeated measures modeling. PUBLIC HEALTH RELEVANCE: The proposed study is relevant to public health because it examines the modified Staying Active with Arthritis (STAR) program to improve leg exercise, fitness walking, and clinical outcomes (function, blood pressure, leg strength, pain, and health-related quality of life) in older Americans with osteoarthritis of the knee and high blood pressure. The modified STAR program addresses the barriers to physical activity from osteoarthritis of the knee as well as high blood pressure–related physical activity concerns. The modified STAR program has the potential to reduce the risk of heart disease in the 5 million older adults who have both osteoarthritis of the knee and high blood pressure and who do not engage in the recommended amount of physical activity.

Example of a Funded Qualitative Training (F31) Project

Maureen Metzger, a doctoral student at the University of Rochester, submitted a successful application for a NRSA predoctoral (F31) fellowship. The project was funded by NINR in March 2010 and is scheduled to end in March 2012. She prepared the following abstract for a descriptive qualitative study, which was titled "Patients' Perceptions of the Role of Palliative Care in Late-Stage Heart Failure":

Project Summary: Cardiovascular (CV) disease is the leading cause of death in the US, with heart failure (HF) accounting for the majority of deaths from CV disease. Heart failure, which affects more than 5 million people in the US, is a life-limiting condition associated with markedly decreased function and quality of life and high mortality rates. The National Institutes of Health have indicated that a more thorough understanding of the experiences of people confronting life-limiting conditions, including those with non-cancer diagnoses, is warranted. There is consensus that communication with healthcare providers, specifically about prognosis and treatment decisions, is not well managed in late-stage HF, and this is associated with adverse consequences. Many clinicians and researchers have recently been advocating for an increased role of palliative care (PC) consultation in HF and there has been a subsequent trend toward increased referrals to PC services for patients with HF, for goals of care discussions. Despite this trend, the perspectives of HF patients and their family members of PC remain unknown. We do not know what patients and families expect from PC consultations, what their experience of these consultations is, and their perceptions of whether and how PC goals of care discussions affect their treatment planning and decision-making. The proposed qualitative descriptive study will describe the perspectives of 25 HF patient-family member dyads. The specific aims include: 1) To describe the experience of patients with later stage HF and their family members referred to an acute care based PC consultation service for goals of care; and 2) To articulate patients' and family members' perceptions of the role of PC in the care of the patient's disease.

Increasing our understanding of the experiences of HF patients and their family members referred for PC consultations would add substantively to the existing body of knowledge in PC and inform the development of future interventions. PUBLIC HEALTH RELEVANCE: Heart failure is a life-limiting and debilitating condition affecting a large number of people in this country. In an attempt to improve the care of patients with later-stage HF, clinicians have been calling for an expanded role of PC in HF. However, in order to design and implement interventions that will appropriately serve patients with HF and the people who love them, we need a better understanding of the experience of HF patients and their family members referred for PC consultations.

SUMMARY POINTS

- A **research proposal** is a written document specifying what a researcher intends to study; proposals are written by students seeking approval for dissertations and theses and by researchers seeking financial or institutional support. The set of skills associated with developing proposals that can be funded is referred to as **grantsmanship**.

- Preparing proposals for qualitative studies is especially challenging because methodologic decisions are made in the field; qualitative proposals need to persuade reviewers that the proposed study is important and a good risk.

- Students preparing a proposal for a dissertation or thesis need to work closely with a well-chosen committee and adviser. Dissertation proposals are often "mini-dissertations" that include sections that can be incorporated into the dissertation.

- The federal government is the largest source of research funds for health researchers in the United States. In addition to regular grant programs through **Parent Announcements**, federal agencies such as the National Institutes of Health (NIH) announce special opportunities in the form of **Program Announcements (PAs)** and **Requests for Applications (RFAs)** for **grants** and **Requests for Proposals (RFPs)** for **contracts**.

- Nurses can apply for a variety of grants from NIH, the most common being **Research Project Grants** (R01 grants), **AREA Grants** (R15), **Small Grants** (R03), or **Exploratory/Developmental Grants** (R21). NIH also awards training fellowships through the National Research Service Award (NRSA) program as F-series awards and Career Development Awards (K-series awards).
- Grant applications to NIH are submitted online using the SF424, which has a series of special forms (fillable screens) that require uploaded PDF attachments.
- The heart of an NIH grant application is the **research plan component**, which includes two major sections: Specific Aims and Research Strategy. The latter, which is restricted to 12 pages for R01 applications and 6 pages for training fellowships, includes subsections called Significance, Innovation, and Approach.
- NIH grant applications also require a budget, which can be an abbreviated **modular budget** if requested funds for R01 grants do not exceed $250,000 in direct costs per year.
- Grant applications to NIH are reviewed three times a year in a dual review process. The first phase involves a review by a peer review panel (or **study section**) that evaluates each proposal's scientific merit; the second phase is a review by an Advisory Council.
- In NIH's review procedure, the study section assigns **priority** (**impact**) **scores** only to applications judged to be in the top half of proposals based on a preliminary appraisal by assigned reviewers. A score of 10 is the most meritorious ranking, and a score of 90 is the lowest possible score.
- All applicants for NIH grants are sent a summary statement, which offers a critique of the proposal. Applicants of scored proposals also receive information on the priority score and percentile ranking.

- Some suggestions for writing a strong proposal include several for the planning stage (e.g., starting early, selecting an important topic, learning about the audience, reviewing a successful proposal, and creating a strong team) and several for the writing stage (building a persuasive case, justifying methodologic decisions, beginning and ending with a flourish, adhering to proposal instructions, and having the draft proposal critiqued by reviewers).

STUDY ACTIVITIES

Chapter 29 of the *Resource Manual for Nursing Research: Generating and Assessing Evidence for Nursing Practice, 9th ed.*, offers various exercises and study suggestions for reinforcing the concepts taught in this chapter. In addition, the following study questions can be addressed:

1. Suppose that you were planning to study the self-care behaviors of aging AIDS patients.
   a. Outline the methods you would recommend adopting.
   b. Develop a project timeline.
2. Suppose you were interested in studying separation anxiety in hospitalized children. Using references cited in this chapter, identify potential funding sources for your project.

STUDIES CITED IN CHAPTER 29

All references cited in this chapter can be found in a separate section at the end of the book.

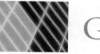

Glossary

Absolute risk (AR) The proportion of people in a group who experienced an undesirable outcome.

Absolute risk reduction (ARR) The difference between the absolute risk in one group (e.g., those exposed to an intervention) and the absolute risk in another group (e.g., those not exposed); sometimes called the *risk difference* or *RD*.

abstract A brief description of a completed or proposed study, usually located at the beginning of a report or proposal.

accessible population The population of people available for a particular study; often a nonrandom subset of the target population.

acquiescence response set A bias in self-report instruments, especially in psychosocial scales, created when participants characteristically agree with statements ("yea-say") independent of content.

adherence to treatment The degree to which those in an intervention group adhere to protocols or continue getting the treatment.

adjusted mean The mean group value for the dependent variable, after statistically removing the effect of covariates.

after-only design An experimental design in which data are collected from subjects only after an intervention has been introduced.

AGREE instrument A widely used instrument (Appraisal of Guidelines Research and Evaluation) for systematically assessing clinical practice guidelines.

allocation concealment The process used to ensure that the people enrolling subjects into a clinical trial are unaware of upcoming assignments, that is, of the treatment group to which new enrollees will be assigned.

alpha (α) (1) In tests of statistical significance, the significance criterion—the risk the researcher is willing to accept of making a Type I error; (2) in assessments of internal consistency reliability, a reliability coefficient, Cronbach's alpha.

alternative hypothesis In hypothesis testing, a hypothesis different from the one actually being tested—usually, different from the null hypothesis.

analysis The process of organizing and synthesizing data so as to answer research questions and test hypotheses.

analysis of covariance (ANCOVA) A statistical procedure used to test mean group differences on a dependent variable, while controlling for one or more covariate.

analysis of variance (ANOVA) A statistical procedure for testing mean differences among three or more groups by comparing variability between groups to variability within groups, yielding an *F*-ratio statistic.

analysis triangulation The use of two or more analytic approaches to analyze the same set of data.

analytic generalization One of three models of generalization that concerns researchers' efforts to generalize from particulars to broader conceptualizations and theories.

ancestry approach In literature searches, using citations from relevant studies to track down earlier research upon which the studies are based (the "ancestors").

anonymity Protection of participants' confidentiality such that even the researcher cannot link individuals with information provided.

applied research Research designed to find a solution to an immediate practical problem.

arm A group of participants allocated a particular treatment (e.g., the control *arm* or treatment *arm*).

ascertainment bias Systematic differences between groups being compared in how outcome variables are measured, verified, or recorded when data collectors have not been blinded; also called *detection bias*.

assent The affirmative agreement of a subject (e.g., a child) to participate in a study, typically to supplement formal consent by a parent or guardian.

associative relationship An association between two variables that cannot be described as causal.

assumption A principle that is accepted as being true based on logic or custom, without proof.

asymmetric distribution A skewed distribution of data values, with two halves that are not mirror images of each other.

attention control group A control group that gets a similar amount of attention as those in the intervention group, without the "active ingredients" of the treatment.

attribute variables Preexisting characteristics of study participants, which the researcher simply observes or measures.

attrition The loss of participants over the course of a study, which can create bias by changing the composition of the sample initially drawn.

audio-CASI (computer assisted self-interview) An approach to collecting self-report data in which respondents listen to questions being read over headphones, and respond by entering information directly onto a computer.

audit trail The systematic documentation of material that allows an independent auditor of a qualitative study to draw conclusions about trustworthiness.

authenticity The extent to which qualitative researchers fairly and faithfully show a range of different realities in the collection, analysis, and interpretation of data.

auto-ethnography Ethnographic studies in which researchers study their own culture or group.

axial coding The second level of coding in a grounded theory study using the Strauss and Corbin approach, involving the process of categorizing, recategorizing, and condensing first level codes by connecting a category and its subcategories.

back-translation The translation of a translated text back into the original language, so that original and back-translated versions can be compared as a means of enhancing semantic equivalence.

baseline data Data collected prior to an intervention, including pretreatment measures of the dependent variables.

basic research Research designed to extend the base of knowledge in a discipline for the sake of knowledge production or theory construction, rather than for solving an immediate problem.

basic social process (BSP) The central social process emerging through an analysis of grounded theory data.

before–after design A design in which data are collected from subjects both before and after the introduction of an intervention.

beneficence A fundamental ethical principle that seeks to maximize benefits for study participants and prevent harm.

beta (β) (1) In multiple regression, the standardized coefficients indicating the relative weights of the predictor variables in the equation; (2) in statistical testing, the probability of a Type II error.

between-subjects design A research design in which separate groups of people are compared (e.g., smokers and nonsmokers).

bias Any influence that distorts the results of a study and undermines validity.

bibliographic database Data files containing bibliographic (reference) information that can be accessed electronically (e.g., for conducting a literature review).

bimodal distribution A distribution of data values with two peaks (high frequencies).

binomial distribution A statistical distribution with known properties describing the number of occurrences of an event in a series of observations; forms the basis for analyzing dichotomous data.

bivariate statistics Statistics derived from analyzing two variables simultaneously to assess the empirical relationship between them.

blind review The review of a manuscript or proposal such that neither the author nor the reviewer is identified to the other party.

blinding The process of preventing those involved in a study (subjects, intervention agents, data collectors, or healthcare providers) from having information that could lead to a bias, particularly information about which treatment group a subject is in; also called *masking*.

Bonferroni correction An adjustment made to establish a more conservative alpha level when multiple statistical tests are being run from the same data set;

the correction is computed by dividing the desired α by the number of tests—for example, $.05/3 = .017$.

borrowed theory A theory, borrowed from another discipline, that has utility for nursing practice or research.

bracketing In phenomenological inquiries, the process of identifying and holding in abeyance any preconceived beliefs and opinions about the phenomena under study.

bricolage The tendency in qualitative research to derive a complex array of data from a variety of sources, using a variety of methods.

calendar question A question used to obtain retrospective information about the chronology of events and activities in people's lives.

carry-over effect The influence that one treatment can have on subsequent treatments, notably in a crossover design.

case-control design A nonexperimental research design involving the comparison of a "case" (i.e., a person with the condition under scrutiny, such as lung cancer) and a matched control (a similar person without the condition).

case mean substitution An approach to imputation of missing values that involves imputing a missing value with the mean of other relevant variables from the case with the missing value (e.g., using the mean of nine nonmissing items on a scale to impute the value of the 10th item, which is missing).

case study A research method involving a thorough, in-depth analysis of an individual, group, or other social unit.

categorical variable A variable with discrete values (e.g., gender) rather than values along a continuum (e.g., weight).

category system In studies involving observation, the prespecified plan for recording the behaviors and events under observation; in qualitative studies, the system used to sort and organize the data.

causal modeling The development and statistical testing of an explanatory model of hypothesized causal relationships among phenomena.

causal (cause-and-effect) relationship A relationship between two variables such that the presence or absence of one variable (the "cause") determines the presence or absence (or value) of the other (the "effect").

cause-probing research Research designed to illuminate the underlying causes of phenomena.

ceiling effect The effect of having scores at or near the highest possible value, which can constrain the amount of upward change possible and also tends to reduce variability in a variable.

cell (1) The intersection of a row and column in a table with two or more dimensions; (2) in an experimental design, the representation of an experimental condition in a schematic diagram.

census A survey covering an entire population.

central (core) category The main category or pattern of behavior in grounded theory analysis using the Strauss and Corbin approach.

central limit theorem A statistical principle stipulating that the larger the sample, the more closely the sampling distribution of the mean will approximate a normal distribution, and that the mean of a sampling distribution equals the population mean.

central tendency A statistical index of what is "typical" in a set of scores, derived from the center of the score distribution; indices of central tendency include the mode, median, and mean.

Certificate of Confidentiality A certificate issued by the National Institutes of Health in the United States to protect researchers against forced disclosure of confidential research information

chi-square test A statistical test used in various contexts, often to assess differences in proportions; symbolized as χ^2.

classical measurement theory (CMT) A measurement perspective underlying most scales in the affective domain; in CMT, items on a scale are roughly equivalent indicators of the same underlying phenomenon that gain strength through aggregation in a scale.

clinical practice guidelines Practice guidelines that are evidence based, combining a synthesis and appraisal of research evidence with specific recommendations for clinical decisions.

clinical relevance The degree to which a study addresses a problem of significance to clinical practice.

clinical research Research designed to generate knowledge to guide practice in nursing and healthcare fields.

clinical trial A study designed to assess the safety, efficacy, and effectiveness of a new clinical intervention, sometimes involving several phases (e.g., Phase III typically is a *randomized controlled trial* using an experimental design).

closed-ended question A question that offers respondents a set of specific response options.

cluster randomization The random assignment of intact groups or sites—rather than individual subjects—to treatment conditions.

cluster sampling A form of sampling in which large groupings ("clusters") are selected first (e.g., nursing schools), typically with successive subsampling of smaller units (e.g., nursing students) in a multistage approach.

Cochrane Collaboration An international organization that aims to facilitate well-informed decisions about healthcare by preparing and disseminating systematic reviews of the effects of healthcare interventions.

code of ethics The fundamental ethical principles established by a discipline or institution to guide researchers' conduct in research with human (or animal) subjects.

codebook A record documenting categorization and coding decisions.

coding The process of transforming raw data into standardized form for data processing and analysis; in quantitative research, the process of attaching numbers to categories; in qualitative research, the process of identifying and indexing recurring words, themes, or concepts within the data.

coefficient alpha (Cronbach's alpha) A reliability index that estimates the internal consistency or homogeneity of a composite measure composed of several items or subparts.

coercion In a research context, the explicit or implicit use of threats (or excessive rewards) to gain people's cooperation in a study.

cognitive questioning A method sometimes used during a pretest of an instrument in which respondents are asked to verbalize what comes to mind when they hear a question.

cognitive test An instrument designed to assess cognitive skills or cognitive functioning (e.g., an IQ test).

Cohen's *d* An effect size for comparing two group means, computed by subtracting one mean from the other and dividing by the pooled standard deviation; also called *standardized mean difference* or *SMD*.

cohort design A nonexperimental design in which a defined group of people (a cohort) is followed over time to study outcomes for subsets of the cohorts; also called a *prospective design*.

comparison group A group of subjects whose scores on a dependent variable are used to evaluate the outcomes of the group of primary interest (e.g., nonsmokers as a comparison group for smokers); term often used in lieu of control group when the study design is not a true experiment.

compensatory equalization A potential threat to construct validity that can occur if healthcare staff try to compensate for the control group members' failure to receive a perceived beneficial treatment.

compensatory rivalry A potential threat to construct validity that can arise from the control group members' desire to demonstrate that they can do as well as those receiving a special treatment.

complex intervention An intervention in which complexity exists along one or more dimensions, including number of components, number of targeted outcomes, and the time needed for the full intervention to be delivered.

computer-assisted personal interviewing (CAPI) In-person interviewing in which the interviewer reads questions from, and enters responses onto, a laptop computer.

computer-assisted telephone interviewing (CATI) Interviewing done over the telephone in which the interviewer reads questions from, and enters responses onto, a computer.

concealment A tactic involving the unobtrusive collection of research data without participants' knowledge or consent, used to obtain an accurate view of naturalistic behavior when the known presence of an observer would distort the behavior of interest.

concept An abstraction inferred from observation of behaviors, situations, or characteristics (e.g., stress, pain).

conceptual definition The abstract or theoretical meaning of the concept being studied.

conceptual file A manual method of organizing qualitative data, by creating file folders for each category in the coding scheme, and inserting relevant excerpts from the data.

conceptual map A schematic representation of a theory or conceptual model that graphically represents key concepts and linkages among them.

conceptual model Interrelated concepts or abstractions assembled in a rational and often explanatory scheme to illuminate relationships among them; sometimes called *conceptual framework*.

conceptual utilization The use of research findings in a general, conceptual way to broaden one's thinking about an issue, without putting the knowledge to any specific, documentable use.

concurrent design A study design for a mixed methods study in which the qualitative and quantitative strands of data collection occur simultaneously; symbolically designated with a plus sign, as in QUAL + QUAN.

concurrent validity The degree to which scores on an instrument are correlated with an external criterion, measured at the same time.

confidence interval (CI) The range of values within which a population parameter is estimated to lie, at a specified probability (e.g., 95% CI).

confidence limit The upper (or lower) boundary of a confidence interval.

confidentiality Protection of study participants so that identifying information is never publicly divulged.

confirmability A criterion for integrity in a qualitative inquiry, referring to the objectivity or neutrality of the data and interpretations.

confirmatory factor analysis (CFA) A factor analysis designed to confirm a hypothesized measurement model, using maximum likelihood estimation.

confounding variable A variable that is extraneous to the research question and that confounds the relationship between the independent and dependent variables; confounding variables need to be controlled either in the research design or through statistical procedures.

consecutive sampling Involves recruiting *all* of the people from an accessible population who meet the eligibility criteria over a specific time interval, or for a specified sample size.

consent form A written agreement signed by a study participant and a researcher concerning the terms and conditions of voluntary participation in a study.

consistency check A procedure performed in cleaning a set of data to ensure that the data are internally consistent.

CONSORT guidelines Widely adopted guidelines (Consolidated Standards of Reporting Trials) for reporting information for a randomized controlled trial, including a checklist and flow chart for tracking participants through the trial, from recruitment through data analysis.

constant comparison A procedure used in a grounded theory analysis wherein newly collected data are compared in an ongoing fashion with data obtained earlier, to refine theoretically relevant categories.

constitutive pattern In hermeneutic analysis, a pattern that expresses the relationships among relational themes and is present in all the interviews or texts.

construct An abstraction or concept that is deliberately invented (constructed) by researchers for a scientific purpose (e.g., health locus of control).

construct validity The validity of inferences from *observed* persons, settings, and interventions in a study to the constructs that these instances might represent; with an instrument, the degree to which it measures the construct under investigation.

constructivist grounded theory An approach to grounded theory, developed by Charmaz, in which the grounded theory is constructed from shared experiences and relationships between the researcher and study participants and interpretive aspects are emphasized.

constructivist paradigm An alternative paradigm (also called *naturalistic paradigm*) to the traditional positivist paradigm that holds that there are multiple interpretations of reality, and that the goal of research is to understand how individuals construct reality within their context; often associated with qualitative research.

consumer An individual who reads, reviews, and critiques research findings and who attempts to use and apply the findings in his or her practice.

contact information Information obtained from study participants in longitudinal studies, to facilitate their relocation at a future date.

contamination The inadvertent, undesirable influence of one treatment condition on another treatment condition, as when members of the control group receive the intervention; sometimes called *treatment diffusion*.

content analysis The process of organizing and integrating material from documents, often narrative information from a qualitative study, according to key concepts and themes.

content validity The degree to which the items in an instrument adequately represent the universe of content for the concept being measured.

content validity index (CVI) An index of the degree to which an instrument is content valid, based on aggregated ratings of a panel of experts; both item content validity (I-CVI) and the overall scale content validity (S-CVI) can be assessed.

contingency table A two-dimensional table in which the frequencies of two categorical variables are cross-tabulated.

continuous variable A variable that can take on an infinite range of values along a specified continuum (e.g., height).

contrast validity An aspect of construct validity, often assessed using the known groups technique, which involves contrasting the scores on the instrument being assessed for groups expected to differ.

control The process of holding constant extraneous influences on the dependent variable under study.

control group Subjects in an experiment who do not receive the experimental treatment and whose performance provides a baseline against which the effects of the treatment can be measured (see also *comparison group*).

controlled trial A trial that has a control group, with or without randomization.

convenience sampling Selection of the most readily available persons as participants in a study; sometimes called *accidental sampling.*

convergent validity An approach to construct validation that involves assessing the degree to which two methods of measuring a construct yield similar information (i.e., converge).

core variable (category) In a grounded theory study, the central phenomenon that is used to integrate all categories of the data.

correlation An association or bond between variables, with variation in one variable systematically related to variation in another.

correlation coefficient An index summarizing the degree of relationship between variables, typically ranging from +1.00 (for a perfect positive relationship) through 0.0 (for no relationship) to –1.00 (for a perfect negative relationship).

correlation matrix A two-dimensional display showing the correlation coefficients between all pairs of a set of several variables.

correlational research Research that explores the interrelationships among variables of interest without researcher intervention.

cost–benefit analysis An economic analysis in which both costs and outcomes of a program or intervention are expressed in monetary terms and compared.

cost-effectiveness analysis An economic analysis in which costs of an intervention are measured in monetary terms, but outcomes are expressed in natural units (e.g., the costs per added year of life).

cost-utility analysis An economic analysis that expresses the effects of an intervention as overall health improvement and describes costs for some additional utility gain—usually in relation to gains in quality-adjusted life years (QALY).

counterbalancing The process of systematically varying the order of presentation of stimuli or treatments to control for ordering effects, especially in a crossover design.

counterfactual The condition or group used as a basis of comparison in a study, embodying what would have happened *to the same people* exposed to a causal factor if they *simultaneously* were *not* exposed to the causal factor.

covariate A variable that is statistically controlled (held constant) in certain multivariate analyses (e.g., ANCOVA), typically an extraneous influence on, or a preintervention measure of, the dependent variable.

covert data collection The collection of information in a study without participants' knowledge.

Cox regression A regression analysis in which independent variables are used to model the risk (or hazard) of experiencing an event at a given point in time, given that one has not experienced the event before that time.

Cramér's V An index describing the magnitude of relationship between nominal-level data, used when the contingency table to which it is applied is larger than 2×2.

credibility A criterion for evaluating integrity and quality in qualitative studies, referring to confidence in the truth of the data; analogous to internal validity in quantitative research.

criterion-related validity The degree to which scores on an instrument are correlated with some external criterion.

criterion sampling A purposive sampling approach used by qualitative researchers that involves selecting cases that meet a predetermined criterion of importance.

critical case sampling A sampling approach used by qualitative researchers involving the purposeful selection of cases that are especially important or illustrative.

critical ethnography An ethnography that focuses on raising consciousness in the group or culture under study in the hope of effecting social change.

critical incident technique A method of obtaining data from study participants by in-depth exploration of specific incidents and behaviors related to the topic under study.

critical region The area in the sampling distribution representing values that are "improbable" if the null hypothesis is true.

critical theory An approach to viewing the world that involves a critique of society, with the goal of envisioning new possibilities and effecting social change.

critique A critical appraisal—ideally one that analyzes both weaknesses and strengths—of a research report or proposal.

Cronbach's alpha A widely used reliability index that estimates the internal consistency of a composite measure composed of several subparts; also called *coefficient alpha.*

crossover design An experimental design in which one group of subjects is exposed to more than one condition or treatment, preferably in random order.

cross-sectional design A study design in which data are collected at one point in time; sometimes used to infer change over time when data are collected from different age or developmental groups.

crosstabulation A calculation of frequencies for two variables considered simultaneously—for example, gender (male/female) crosstabulated with smoking status (smoker/nonsmoker).

cutoff point The score on a screening or diagnostic instrument used to distinguish cases and noncases.

d A widely used effect size index for comparing two group means, computed by subtracting one mean from the other and dividing by the pooled standard deviation; also called *Cohen's d* or *standardized mean difference.*

data The pieces of information obtained in a study (singular is *datum*).

data analysis The systematic organization and synthesis of research data and, in quantitative studies, the testing of hypotheses using those data.

data cleaning The preparation of data for analysis by performing checks to ensure that the data are consistent and accurate.

data collection The gathering of information to address a research problem.

data collection protocols The formal procedures researchers develop to guide the collection of data in a standardized fashion.

data entry The process of entering data onto an input medium for computer analysis.

data saturation See *saturation.*

data set The total collection of data on all variables for all study participants.

data transformation A step often undertaken before data analysis, to put the data in a form that can be meaningfully analyzed (e.g., recoding of values).

data triangulation The use of multiple data sources for the purpose of validating conclusions.

debriefing Communication with study participants after participation is complete regarding aspects of the study.

deception The deliberate withholding of information, or the provision of false information, to study participants, usually to reduce potential biases.

deductive reasoning The process of developing specific predictions from general principles (see also *inductive reasoning*).

degrees of freedom (*df*) A statistical concept referring to the number of sample values free to vary (e.g., with a given sample mean, all but one value would be free to vary).

de-identification The removal of identifying information from records and datasets to protect the privacy of individuals.

delayed treatment design A design for an intervention study that involves putting control group members on a waiting list for the intervention until follow-up data have been collected; also called a *wait-list design.*

Delphi survey A technique for obtaining judgments from an expert panel about an issue of concern; experts are questioned individually in several rounds, with a summary of the panel's views circulated between rounds, to achieve some consensus.

dependability A criterion for evaluating integrity in qualitative studies, referring to the stability of data over time and over conditions; analogous to reliability in quantitative research.

dependent variable The variable hypothesized to depend on or be caused by another variable (the *independent variable*); the outcome variable of interest.

descendancy approach In literature searches, finding a pivotal early study and searching forward in citation indexes to find more recent studies ("descendants") that cited the key study.

descriptive research Research that typically has as its main objective the accurate portrayal of people's characteristics or circumstances and/or the frequency with which certain phenomena occur.

descriptive statistics Statistics used to describe and summarize data (e.g., means, percentages).

descriptive theory A broad characterization that thoroughly accounts for a phenomenon.

detection bias Systematic differences between groups being compared in how outcome variables are measured, verified, or recorded; a bias that can result when data collectors are not blinded.

determinism The belief that phenomena are not haphazard or random, but rather have antecedent causes; an assumption in the positivist paradigm.

deviation score A score computed by subtracting an individual score from the mean of all scores.

dichotomous variable A variable having only two values or categories (e.g., gender).

direct costs Specific project-related costs incurred during a study (e.g., for supplies, salaries, subject stipends, and so on).

directional hypothesis A hypothesis that makes a specific prediction about the direction of the relationship between two variables.

disconfirming case A concept used in qualitative research that concerns a case that challenges the researchers' conceptualizations; sometimes used in a sampling strategy.

discourse analysis A qualitative tradition, from the discipline of sociolinguistics, that seeks to understand the rules, mechanisms, and structure of conversations.

discrete variable A variable with a finite number of values between two points.

discriminant function analysis A statistical procedure used to predict group membership or status on a categorical (nominal level) variable on the basis of two or more independent variables.

discriminant validity An aspect of construct validity that involves assessing the degree to which a single method of measuring two constructs yields different results (i.e., discriminates the two).

disproportionate sample A sample in which the researcher samples subjects disproportionately from different population strata to ensure adequate representation from smaller strata.

domain In ethnographic analysis, a unit or broad category of cultural knowledge.

domain analysis One of Spradley's levels of ethnographic analysis, focusing on the identification of domains, or units of cultural knowledge.

domain sampling model The model used in developing a scale in the classical measurement theory framework, which involves the random sampling of a homogeneous set of items from a hypothetical universe of items relating to the construct

dose-response analysis An analysis to assess whether larger doses of an intervention are associated with greater benefits, usually in a quasi-experimental framework.

double-blind study A study (usually a clinical trial) in which two groups are blinded with respect to the group that a study participant is in; often a situation in which neither the subjects nor those who administer the treatment know who is in the experimental or control group.

dummy variable Dichotomous variables created for use in many multivariate statistical analyses, typically using codes of 0 and 1 (e.g., female = 1, male = 0).

economic analysis An analysis of the relationship between costs and outcomes of alternative healthcare interventions.

ecological psychology A qualitative tradition that focuses on the environment's influence on human behavior and attempts to identify principles that explain the interdependence of humans and their environmental context.

ecological validity The extent to which study designs and findings have relevance and meaning in a variety of real-world contexts.

efficacy study A tightly controlled trial designed to establish the efficacy of an intervention under ideal conditions, using a design that maximizes internal validity.

effect size A statistical expression of the magnitude of the relationship between two variables, or the magnitude of the difference between groups on an attribute of interest; also used in metasynthesis to characterize the salience of a theme or category.

effectiveness study A clinical trial designed to shed light on effectiveness of an intervention under ordinary conditions, often with an intervention already found to be efficacious in an efficacy study.

egocentric network analysis An ethnographic method that focuses on the pattern of relationships and networks of individuals; researchers develop lists of a person's network members (called *alters*) and seek to understand the scope and nature of interrelationships and social supports.

eigenvalue In factor analysis, the value equal to the sum of the squared weights for each factor.

element The most basic unit of a population for sampling purposes, typically a human being.

eligibility criteria The criteria designating the specific attributes of the target population, by which people are selected for inclusion in a study.

embedded design A particular mixed methods design in which one strand is primarily in a supportive role to the other strand; symbolized with parentheses, as in QUAL(quan).

emergent design A design that unfolds in the course of a qualitative study as the researcher makes ongoing design decisions reflecting what has already been learned.

emergent fit A concept in grounded theory that involves comparing new data and new categories with previously existing conceptualizations.

emic perspective A ethnographic term referring to the way members of a culture themselves view their world; the "insider's view."

empirical evidence Evidence rooted in objective reality and gathered using one's senses as the basis for generating knowledge.

endogenous variable In path analysis, a variable whose variation is determined by other variables within the model.

equivalence The degree of similarity between alternate forms of a measuring instrument.

equivalence trial A trial designed to assess whether the outcomes of two or more treatments do *not* differ, by a prespecified amount judged to be clinically unimportant.

error of measurement The deviation between true scores and obtained scores of a measured characteristic.

error term The mathematic expression (e.g., in a regression analysis) that represents all unknown or unmeasurable attributes that can affect the dependent variable.

estimation procedures Statistical procedures that estimate population parameters based on sample statistics.

eta squared In ANOVA, a statistic calculated to indicate the proportion of variance in the dependent variable explained by the independent variables, analogous to R^2 in multiple regression.

ethics A system of moral values that is concerned with the degree to which research procedures adhere to professional, legal, and social obligations to the study participants.

ethnography A branch of human inquiry, associated with anthropology, that focuses on the culture of a group of people, with an effort to understand the world view of those under study.

ethnomethodology A branch of human inquiry, associated with sociology, that focuses on the way in which people make sense of their everyday activities and come to behave in socially acceptable ways.

ethnonursing research The study of human cultures, with a focus on a group's beliefs and practices relating to nursing care and related health behaviors.

etic perspective An ethnographic term referring to the "outsider's" view of the experiences of a cultural group.

evaluation research Research that assesses how well a program, practice, or policy is working.

event history calendar A data collection matrix that plots time on one dimension and events or activities of interest on the other.

event sampling A sampling plan that involves the selection of integral behaviors or events to be observed.

evidence-based practice A clinical problem-solving strategy that emphasizes the integration of best available evidence from disciplined research with clinical expertise and patient preferences.

evidence hierarchy A ranked arrangement of the validity and dependability of evidence based on the rigor of the method that produced it; the traditional evidence hierarchy is appropriate primarily for cause-probing research.

exclusion criteria Sampling criteria specifying characteristics that a population does *not* have.

exogenous variable In path analysis, a variable whose determinants lie outside the model.

expectation maximization (EM) imputation A sophisticated single-imputation process that generates an estimated value for missing data in two steps (an expectation or E-step and a maximization or M-step), using maximum likelihood estimation.

experiment A study using a design in which the researcher controls (manipulates) the independent variable by randomly assigning subjects to different treatment conditions; randomized controlled trials use experimental designs.

experimental group The subjects who receive the experimental treatment or intervention.

explanatory design A sequential mixed methods design in which quantitative data are collected in the first phase and qualitative data are collected in the second phase to build on or explain quantitative findings; symbolized as QUAN → qual or quan → QUAL.

exploratory design A sequential mixed methods design in which qualitative data are collected in the first phase and quantitative data are collected in the second phase based on the initial in-depth exploration; symbolized as QUAL → quan or qual → QUAN.

exploratory factor analysis (EFA) A factor analysis undertaken to explore the underlying dimensionality of a set of variables.

exploratory research A study that explores the dimensions of a phenomenon or that develops or refines hypotheses about relationships between phenomena.

external criticism In historical research, the systematic evaluation of the authenticity and genuineness of data.

external validity The degree to which study results can be generalized to settings or samples other than the one studied.

extraneous variable A variable that confounds the relationship between the independent and dependent variables and that needs to be controlled either in the research design or through statistical procedures; often called *confounding variable*.

extreme case sampling A sampling approach used by qualitative researchers that involves the purposeful selection of the most extreme or unusual cases.

extreme response set A bias in psychosocial scales created when participants select extreme response alternatives (e.g., "strongly agree"), independent of the item's content.

F-ratio The statistic obtained in several statistical tests (e.g., ANOVA) in which variation attributable to different sources (e.g., between-group variation and within-group variation) is contrasted.

face validity The extent to which a measuring instrument looks as though it is measuring what it purports to measure.

factor analysis A statistical procedure for reducing a large set of variables into a smaller set of variables with common underlying dimensions.

factor extraction The first phase of a factor analysis, which involves the extraction of as much variance as possible through the successive creation of linear combinations of the variables in the data set.

factor rotation The second phase of factor analysis, during which the reference axes for the factors are moved to more clearly align variables with a factor.

factor score A person's score on a latent variable (factor).

factor loading In factor analysis, the weight associated with a variable on a given factor.

factorial design An experimental design in which two or more independent variables are simultaneously manipulated, permitting a separate analysis of the main effects of the independent variables and their interaction.

fail-safe number In meta-analysis, an estimate of the number of studies with nonsignificant results that would be needed to reverse the conclusion of a significant effect.

feasibility study A small-scale test to assess the viability of a larger study (often called a *pilot study*).

feminist research Research that seeks to understand, typically through qualitative approaches, how gender and a gendered social order shape women's lives and their consciousness.

field diary A daily record of events and conversations in the field; also called a log.

field notes The notes taken by researchers to record the unstructured observations made in the field, and the interpretation of those observations.

field research Research in which the data are collected "in the field" from people in their normal roles, with the aim of understanding the practices, behaviors, and beliefs of individuals or groups as they normally function in real life.

fieldwork The activities undertaken by qualitative researchers to collect data out in the field, that is, in natural settings.

findings The results of the analysis of research data.

Fisher's exact test A statistical procedure for testing the significance of differences in proportions, used when the sample size is small or cells in the contingency table have no observations.

fit An element in Glaserian grounded theory analysis in which the researcher develops categories of a substantive theory that fit the data.

fittingness The degree of congruence between a sample of people in a qualitative study and another group or setting of interest.

fixed alternative question A question that offers respondents a set of prespecified response options.

fixed effects model In meta-analysis, a model in which studies are assumed to be measuring the same overall effect; a pooled effect estimate is calculated under the assumption that observed variation between studies is attributable to chance.

floor effect The effect of having scores at or near the lowest possible value, which can constrain the amount of downward change possible and also tends to reduce variability in a variable.

focus group interview An interview with a group of individuals assembled to answer questions on a given topic.

focused interview A loosely structured interview in which an interviewer guides the respondent through a set of questions using a topic guide.

follow-up study A study undertaken to ascertain the outcomes of individuals who have a specified condition or who received a specified treatment.

forced-choice question A question requiring respondents to choose between two statements that represent polar positions.

forest plot A graphic representation of effects across studies in a meta-analysis, permitting a visual assessment of heterogeneity.

formal grounded theory A theory of a substantive grounded theory's core category that is extended by sampling widely in a range of substantive areas.

formative evaluation An ongoing assessment of a product or program as it is being developed, to optimize its quality and effectiveness.

framework The conceptual underpinnings of a study—for example, a *theoretical framework* in theory-based studies, or *conceptual framework* in studies based on a specific conceptual model.

frequency distribution A systematic array of numeric values from the lowest to the highest, together with a count of the number of times each value was obtained.

frequency effect size In a metasynthesis, the percentage of reports that contain a given thematic finding.

frequency polygon Graphic display of a frequency distribution, in which dots connected by a straight line indicate the number of times score values occur in a data set.

Friedman test A nonparametric analog of ANOVA, used with paired-groups or repeated measures situations.

full disclosure The communication of complete information about a study to potential study participants.

functional relationship A relationship between two variables in which it cannot be assumed that one variable caused the other.

funnel plot A graphical display that plots a measure of study precision (e.g., sample size) against effect size, to explore the possibility of publication bias.

gaining entrée The process of gaining access to study participants through the cooperation of key gatekeepers in the selected community or site.

generalizability The degree to which the research methods justify the inference that the findings are true for a broader group than study participants; usually, the inference that the findings can be generalized from the sample to the population.

"going native" A pitfall in ethnographic research wherein a researcher becomes emotionally involved with participants and therefore loses the ability to observe objectively.

grand theory A broad theory aimed at describing large segments of the physical, social, or behavioral world; also called a *macrotheory*.

grand tour question A broad question asked in an unstructured interview to gain a general overview of a phenomenon, on the basis of which more focused questions are subsequently asked.

grant A financial award made to a researcher to conduct a proposed study.

grantsmanship The combined set of skills and knowledge needed to secure financial support for a research idea.

graphic rating scale A scale in which respondents are asked to rate a concept along an ordered, numbered continuum, typically on a bipolar dimension (e.g., "excellent" to "very poor").

grey literature Unpublished, and thus less readily accessible, papers or research reports.

grounded theory An approach to collecting and analyzing qualitative data that aims to develop theories grounded in real-world observations.

hand searching The planned searching of a journal article by article (i.e. by hand), to identify relevant reports that might be missed by electronic searching.

Hawthorne effect The effect on the dependent variable resulting from subjects' awareness that they are participants under study.

hermeneutic circle In hermeneutics, a methodologic and interpretive process in which, to reach understanding, there is continual movement between the parts and the whole of the text that are being analyzed.

hermeneutics A qualitative research tradition, drawing on interpretive phenomenology, that focuses on the lived experiences of humans, and on how they interpret those experiences.

heterogeneity The degree to which objects are dissimilar (i.e., characterized by variability) on some attribute.

hierarchical multiple regression A multiple regression analysis in which predictor variables are entered into the equation in a series of prespecified steps.

histogram A graphic presentation of frequency distribution data.

historical research Systematic studies designed to discover facts and relationships about past events.

history threat The occurrence of events external to an intervention, but concurrent with it, that can affect the dependent variable and threaten the study's internal validity.

homogeneity (1) In terms of the reliability of an instrument, the degree to which its subparts are internally consistent (i.e., are measuring the same critical attribute). (2) More generally, the degree to which objects are similar (i.e., characterized by low variability).

homogenous sampling A purposive sampling approach used by qualitative researchers involving the deliberate selection of cases with limited variation.

Hosmer-Lemeshow test A test used in logistic regression to evaluate the degree to which observed frequencies of predicted probabilities correspond to expected frequencies in an ideal model over the range of probability values; a good fit is indicated by lack of statistical significance.

hypothesis A statement of predicted population parameters or relationships between variables.

identical sampling An approach to sampling in mixed methods studies in which all of the participants are included in both the qualitative and quantitative strands of the study.

impact analysis An evaluation of the effects of a program or intervention on outcomes of interest, net of other factors influencing those outcomes.

impact factor An annual measure of citation frequency for an average article in a given journal, that is, the ratio between citations and citable items published in the journal in a specified period.

implementation analysis In evaluations, a descriptive analysis of the process by which a program or intervention was implemented in practice.

implementation potential The extent to which an innovation is amenable to implementation in a new setting, an assessment of which is usually made in an evidence-based practice project.

implied consent Consent to participate in a study that a researcher assumes has been given based on participants' actions, such as returning a completed questionnaire.

imputation methods A broad class of methods used to address missing data problems by estimating (imputing) the missing values.

IMRAD format The organization of a research report into four sections: the Introduction, Method, Results, and Discussion sections.

incidence rate The rate of new cases with a specified condition, computed by dividing the number of new cases over a given period of time by the number at risk of becoming a new case (i.e., free of the condition at the outset of the time period).

independent variable The variable that is believed to cause or influence the dependent variable; in experimental research, the manipulated (treatment) variable.

indirect costs Administrative costs, over and above the specific direct costs of conducting the study; also called *overhead*.

inductive reasoning The process of reasoning from specific observations to more general rules (see also *deductive reasoning*).

inference In research, a conclusion drawn from the study evidence, taking into account the methods used to generate that evidence.

inference quality An overarching criterion for the integrity of mixed methods studies, referring to the believability and accuracy of inductively and deductively derived conclusions.

inferential statistics Statistics that permit inferences about whether results observed in a sample are likely to be found in the larger population.

informant An individual who provides information to researchers about a phenomenon under study, usually in qualitative studies.

informed consent An ethical principle that requires researchers to obtain the voluntary participation of subjects, after informing them of possible risks and benefits.

inquiry audit An independent scrutiny of qualitative data and relevant supporting documents by an external reviewer, to evaluate the dependability and confirmability of qualitative data.

insider research Research on a group or culture—usually in an ethnography—by a member of the group or culture.

Institutional Review Board (IRB) A term used primarily in the United States to refer to the institutional group that convenes to review proposed and ongoing studies with respect to ethical considerations.

instrument The device used to collect data (e.g., a questionnaire, test, observation schedule, and so on).

instrumental utilization Clearly identifiable attempts to base some specific action or intervention on the results of research findings.

instrumentation threat The threat to the internal validity of the study that can arise if the researcher changes the measuring instrument between two points of data collection.

intensity effect size In a metasynthesis, the percentage of all thematic findings that are contained in any given report.

intensity sampling A sampling approach used by qualitative researchers involving the purposeful selection of intense (but not extreme) cases.

intention-to-treat A strategy for analyzing data in a randomized controlled trial that includes all randomized participants in the group to which they were assigned, whether or not they received or completed the treatment associated with the group, and whether or not their outcome data were missing.

interaction effect The effect of two or more independent variables acting in combination (interactively) on a dependent variable.

intercoder reliability The degree to which two coders, operating independently, agree on coding decisions.

internal consistency The degree to which the subparts of a composite scale are all measuring the same attribute or dimension, as a measure of the scale's reliability.

internal criticism In historical research, an evaluation of the worth of the historical evidence.

internal validity The degree to which it can be inferred that the experimental intervention (independent variable), rather than uncontrolled, extraneous factors, is responsible for observed effects.

interpretation The process of making sense of the results of a study and examining their implications.

interquartile range (*IQR*) A measure of variability, indicating the difference between Q_3 (the third quartile or 75th percentile) and Q_1 (the first quartile or 25th percentile).

interrater (interobserver) reliability The degree to which two raters or observers, operating independently, assign the same ratings or values for an attribute being measured or observed.

interrupted time series design. *See* time series design.

interval estimation A statistical estimation approach in which the researcher establishes a range of values that are likely, within a given level of confidence, to contain the true population parameter.

interval measurement A measurement level in which an attribute of a variable is rank ordered on a scale that has equal distances between points on that scale (e.g., Fahrenheit degrees).

intervention In experimental research (clinical trials), the treatment being tested.

intervention fidelity The extent to which the implementation of a treatment is faithful to its plan.

intervention protocol The specification of exactly what the intervention and alternative (or control) treatment conditions are, and how they should be administered.

intervention research Research involving the development, implementation, and testing of an intervention.

intervention theory The conceptual underpinning of a healthcare intervention, which articulates the theoretical basis for what must be done to achieve desired outcomes.

interview A data collection method in which an interviewer asks questions of a respondent, either face-to-face or by telephone.

interview schedule The formal instrument that specifies the wording of all questions to be asked of respondents in structured self-report studies.

intuiting The second step in descriptive phenomenology, which occurs when researchers remain open to the meaning attributed to the phenomenon by those who experienced it.

inverse relationship A relationship characterized by the tendency of high values on one variable to be associated with low values on the second variable; also called a *negative relationship.*

inverse variance method In meta-analysis, a method that uses the inverse of the variance of the effect estimate (one divided by the square of its standard error) as the weight to calculate a weighted average of effects.

investigator triangulation The use of two or more researchers to analyze and interpret a data set, to enhance rigor.

Iowa Model of Evidence-Based Practice A widely used framework that can be used to guide the development and implementation of a project to promote evidence-based practice.

item A single question on an instrument, or a single statement on a scale.

item analysis A type of analysis used to assess whether items on a scale are tapping the same construct and are sufficiently discriminating.

item difficulty The amount of an attribute (such as knowledge) that a respondent must possess in order to "pass" the item.

item response theory (IRT) A measurement perspective, also referred to as *latent trait theory,* that is increasingly adopted in lieu of classical measurement theory in developing cognitive measures (e.g., achievement tests); in IRT, the focus is on the item rather than the overall scale or tests, and procedures involve examining a person's response to each item.

joint interview An interview where two or more people are interviewed simultaneously, typically in either a semi-structured or unstructured interview.

jottings Short notes jotted down quickly while engaged in fieldwork so as to not distract researchers from their observations or their role as participating members of a group.

journal article A report appearing in a professional journal such as *Nursing Research* or *International Journal of Nursing Studies.*

journal club A group that meets in clinical settings to discuss and critique research reports appearing in journals.

kappa An index, used to measure interrater agreement, that summarizes the extent of agreement beyond the level expected to occur by chance.

Kendall's tau A correlation coefficient used to indicate the magnitude of a relationship between ordinal-level variables.

key informant A person knowledgeable about the phenomenon of research interest and who is willing to share information and insights with the researcher (often an ethnographer).

keyword An important term used to search for references on a topic in a bibliographic database, and used by authors to enhance the likelihood that their report will be found.

known-groups technique A technique for estimating the construct validity of an instrument through an analysis of the degree to which the instrument separates groups predicted to differ based on known characteristics or theory.

Kruskal-Wallis test A nonparametric test used to test the difference between three or more independent groups, based on ranked scores.

last observation carried forward (LOCF) A method of imputing a missing outcome using the person's previous value for that same outcome.

latent trait scale A scale developed within an *item response theory* framework, an alternative psychometric theory to *classical measurement theory*.

latent variable An unmeasured variable that represents an underlying, abstract construct (usually in the context of a structural equations analysis).

least-squares estimation A method of statistical estimation in which the solution minimizes the sums of squares of error terms; also called OLS (ordinary least squares).

level of measurement A system of classifying measurements according to the nature of the measurement and the type of permissible mathematical operations; the levels are nominal, ordinal, interval, and ratio.

level of significance The risk of making a Type I error in a statistical analysis, with the criterion (alpha) established by the researcher beforehand (e.g., $\alpha = .05$).

life history A narrative self-report about a person's life experiences vis-à-vis a theme of interest.

life table analysis A statistical procedure used when the dependent variable represents a time interval between an initial event (e.g., onset of a disease) and an end event (e.g., death); also called *survival analysis*.

likelihood ratio (LR) For a screening or diagnostic instrument, the relative likelihood that a given result is expected in a person with (as opposed to one without) the target attribute; LR indexes summarize the relationship between specificity and sensitivity in a single number.

likelihood ratio test A test for evaluating the overall model in logistic regression, or to test improvement between models when predictors are added; computed by subtracting -2LL for the larger model from -2LL for the reduced model, resulting in a statistic distributed as a chi-square; also called a *goodness-of-fit test*.

Likert scale A composite measure of attitudes involving the summation of scores on a set of items that respondents rate for their degree of agreement or disagreement.

linear regression An analysis for predicting the value of a dependent variable from one or more predictors by determining a straight-line fit to the data that minimizes deviations from the line.

LISREL An acronym for linear structural relation analysis, used for testing causal models.

listwise deletion A method of dealing with missing values in a data set that involves the elimination of cases with missing data.

literature review A critical summary of research on a topic of interest, often prepared to put a research problem in context.

log In participant observation studies, the observer's daily record of events and conversations.

logical positivism The philosophy underlying the traditional scientific approach; see also *positivist paradigm*.

logistic regression A regression procedure that analyzes relationships between one or more independent variables and a categorical dependent variable; also called *logit analysis*.

logit The natural log of the odds, used as the dependent variable in logistic regression; short for logistic probability unit.

longitudinal study A study designed to collect data at more than one point in time, in contrast to a cross-sectional study.

macrotheory A broad theory aimed at describing large segments of the physical, social, or behavioral world; also called a *grand theory*.

main effects In a study with multiple independent variables, the effects of a single independent variable on the dependent variable.

manifest variable An observed, measured variable that serves as an indicator of an underlying construct, that is, a latent variable.

manipulation An intervention or treatment introduced by the researcher in an experimental or quasi-experimental study to assess its impact on the dependent variable.

manipulation check In experimental studies, a test to assess whether the manipulation was implemented or experienced as intended.

Mann-Whitney *U* test A nonparametric statistic used to test the difference between two independent groups, based on ranked scores.

MANOVA See *multivariate analysis of variance.*

masking See *Blinding*

matching The pairing of subjects in one group with those in another group based on their similarity on one or more dimension, to enhance the overall comparability of groups.

maturation threat A threat to the internal validity of a study that results when changes to the outcome measure (dependent variable) result from the passage of time.

maximum likelihood estimation An estimation approach in which the estimators are ones that estimate the parameters most likely to have generated the observed measurements.

maximum variation sampling A sampling approach used by qualitative researchers involving the purposeful selection of cases with a wide range of variation.

McNemar test A statistical test for comparing differences in proportions when values are derived from paired (nonindependent) groups.

mean A measure of central tendency, computed by summing all scores and dividing by the total number of cases.

mean substitution A relatively weak technique for addressing missing data problems that involves substituting missing values on a variable with the sample mean for that variable.

measurement The assignment of numbers to objects according to specified rules to characterize quantities of some attribute.

measurement model In structural equations modeling, the model that stipulates the hypothesized relationships among the manifest and latent variables.

median test A nonparametric statistical test involving the comparison of median values of two independent groups to test whether the groups are from populations with different medians.

mediating variable A variable that mediates or acts like a "go-between" in a causal chain linking two other variables; also called a *mediator.*

Medical Research Council framework A framework developed in the U.K. for developing and testing complex interventions.

member check A method of validating the credibility of qualitative data through debriefings and discussions with informants.

MeSH Medical Subject Headings, used to index articles in MEDLINE and also used by several nursing journals to help authors identify keywords for their articles.

meta-analysis A technique for quantitatively integrating the results of multiple similar studies addressing the same research question.

meta-inference A higher-order inference that can be gleaned in a mixed methods study when findings from the two strands (qualitative and quantitative) are integrated and interpreted.

metamatrix A two-dimensional device used in a mixed methods study that permits researchers to recognize important patterns and themes across data sources.

metaphor A figurative comparison used by some qualitative analysts to evoke a visual or symbolic analogy.

meta-regression In meta-analyses, an analytic approach for exploring clinical and methodologic factors contributing to heterogeneity of effects.

meta-summary A type of analysis that lays the foundation for a metasynthesis, involving the development of a list of abstracted findings from primary studies and calculating manifest effect sizes (frequency and intensity effect size).

metasynthesis The interpretive translations produced from the integration or comparison of findings from qualitative studies on a specific topic.

method triangulation The use of multiple methods of data collection about the same phenomenon, to enhance rigor or validity.

methodologic notes In observational field studies, the researcher's notes about the methods used in collecting data.

methodologic research Research designed to develop or refine methods of obtaining, organizing, or analyzing data.

methods (research) The steps, procedures, and strategies for gathering and analyzing data in a study.

middle-range theory A theory that focuses on only a portion of reality or human experience, involving a selected number of concepts (e.g., a theory of stress).

minimal risk Anticipated risks that are no greater than those ordinarily encountered in daily life or during the performance of routine tests or procedures.

missing at random (MAR) Values that are missing from a data set in such a manner that missingness is unrelated to the value of the missing data, after controlling for another variable; missingness is unrelated to the value of the missing data, but *is* related to values of other variables.

missing completely at random (MCAR) Values that are missing from a data set in such a manner that missingness is unrelated either to the value of the missing data, or to the value of any other variable; the subsample with missing values is a totally random subset of the original sample.

missing not at random (MNAR) Values that are missing from a data set in such a manner that missingness *is* related to the value of the missing data and, usually, to values of other variables as well.

missing values Values missing from a data set for some participants as a result of such factors as refusals, withdrawals from the study, failure to complete forms, or researcher error.

mixed design A design that lends itself to comparisons both within groups over time (within subjects) and between different groups of participants (between subjects).

mixed methods (MM) research Research in which both qualitative and quantitative data are collected and analyzed, to address different but related questions.

mixed studies review A systematic review that integrates and synthesizes findings from qualitative, quantitative, and mixed methods studies on a topic.

modality A characteristic of a frequency distribution describing the number of peaks, that is, values with high frequencies.

mode A measure of central tendency; the score value that occurs most frequently in a distribution of scores.

model A symbolic representation of concepts or variables, and interrelationships among them.

moderator variable A variable that affects (moderates) the strength or direction of a relationship between the independent and dependant variables.

MOOSE guidelines Guidelines for reporting meta-analyses of observational (nonexperimental) primary studies.

mortality threat A threat to the internal validity of a study, referring to differential attrition (loss of participants) from different groups.

multicollinearity A problem that can occur in multiple regression when predictor variables are too highly intercorrelated, which can lead to unstable estimates of the regression coefficients.

multilevel sampling An approach to sampling in mixed methods studies in which participants in the two strands are not the same, and are drawn from different populations at different levels of a hierarchy (e.g., nurses, nurse administrators).

multimodal distribution A distribution of values with more than one peak (high frequency).

multiple comparison procedures Statistical tests, normally applied after an ANOVA indicates statistically significant group differences, that compare different pairs of groups; also called *post hoc tests*.

multiple correlation coefficient An index that summarizes the degree of relationship between two or more independent variables and a dependent variable; symbolized as R.

multiple imputation (MI) The gold standard approach for dealing with missing values, involving the imputation of multiple (m) estimates of the missing value, which are later pooled and averaged in estimating parameters.

multiple regression analysis A statistical procedure for understanding the effects of two or more independent (predictor) variables on a dependent variable.

multistage sampling A sampling strategy that proceeds through a set of stages from larger to smaller sampling units (e.g., from states, to census tracts, to households).

multitrait–multimethod matrix method A method of assessing an instrument's construct validity using multiple measures for a set of subjects; the target instrument is valid to the extent that there is a strong relationship between it and other measures of the same attribute (convergence) and a weak relationship between it and measures purporting to measure a different attribute (discriminability).

multivariate analysis of variance (MANOVA) A statistical procedure used to test the significance of differences between the means of two or more groups on two or more dependent variables, considered simultaneously.

multivariate statistics Statistical procedures designed to analyze the relationships among three or more variables (e.g., multiple regression, ANCOVA).

N The symbol designating the total number of subjects (e.g., "the total N was 500").

n The symbol designating the number of subjects in a subgroup or cell of a study (e.g., "each of the four groups had an n of 125, for a total N of 500").

Nagelkerke R^2 A pseudo R^2 statistic used as an overall effect size index in logistic regression, analogous to R^2 in least-squares multiple regression, but lacking the ability to truly capture the proportion of variance explained in the outcome variable.

narrative analysis A qualitative approach that focuses on stories as the object of the inquiry.

natural experiment A nonexperimental study that takes advantage of a naturally occurring event (e.g., an earthquake) that is explored for its effect on people's behavior or condition, typically by comparing people exposed to the event with those not exposed.

naturalistic paradigm An alternative paradigm (also called *constructivist paradigm*) to the traditional positivist paradigm that holds that there are multiple interpretations of reality, and that the goal of research is to understand how individuals construct reality within their context; often associated with qualitative research.

naturalistic setting A setting for the collection of research data that is natural to those being studied (e.g., homes, places of work, and so on).

needs assessment A study designed to describe the needs of a group, community, or organization, usually as a guide to policy planning and resource allocation.

negative case analysis The refinement of a theory or description in a qualitative study through the inclusion of cases that appear to disconfirm earlier hypotheses.

negative predictive value (NPV) A measure of the usefulness of a screening/diagnostic test that can be interpreted as the probability that a negative test result is correct; calculated by dividing the number with a negative test who do not have disease by the number with a negative test.

negative relationship A relationship between two variables in which there is a tendency for high values on one variable to be associated with low values on the other (e.g., as stress increases, emotional well-being decreases); also called an *inverse relationship*.

negative results Results that fail to support the researcher's hypotheses.

negatively skewed distribution An asymmetric distribution of data values with a disproportionately high number of cases at the upper end; when displayed graphically, the tail points to the left.

nested sampling An approach to sampling in mixed methods studies in which some, but not all, of the participants from one strand are included in the sample for the other strand.

net effect The effect of an independent variable on a dependent variable, after controlling for the effect of one or more covariates through multiple regression or ANCOVA.

network sampling The sampling of participants based on referrals from others already in the sample; also called *snowball sampling*.

nominal measurement The lowest level of measurement involving the assignment of characteristics into categories (e.g., males, category 1; females, category 2).

nominated sampling A sampling method in which researchers ask early informants to make referrals to other potential participants.

nondirectional hypothesis A research hypothesis that does not stipulate the expected direction of the relationship between variables.

nonequivalent control group design A quasi-experimental design involving a comparison group that was not created through random assignment.

nonexperimental research Studies in which the researcher collects data without introducing an intervention; also called *observational research*.

noninferiority trial A trial designed to assess whether the effect of a new treatment is not worse than a standard treatment, by no more than a prespecified, clinically important amount.

nonparametric tests A class of statistical tests that do not involve stringent assumptions about the distribution of critical variables.

nonprobability sampling The selection of sampling units (e.g., participants) from a population using non-random procedures (e.g., convenience and quota sampling).

nonrecursive model A causal model that predicts reciprocal effects (i.e., a variable can be both the cause of and an effect of another variable).

nonresponse bias A bias that can result when a non-random subset of people invited to participate in a study fail to participate.

nonsignificant result The result of a statistical test indicating that group differences or an observed relationship could have occurred by chance, at a given probability level; sometimes abbreviated as NS.

normal distribution A theoretical distribution that is bell-shaped and symmetrical; also called a *normal curve* or a *Gaussian distribution*.

norms Performance standards, based on test or scale score information from a large, representative sample.

novelty effect A potential threat to construct validity that can occur when participants or research agents alter their behavior because an intervention is new or different, not because of its inherent qualities.

null hypothesis A hypothesis predicting no relationship between the variables under study; used primarily in statistical testing as the hypothesis to be rejected.

number needed to treat (NNT) An estimate of how many people would need to receive an intervention to prevent one undesirable outcome, computed by dividing 1 by the value of the absolute risk reduction.

nursing research Systematic inquiry designed to develop knowledge about issues of importance to the nursing profession.

objectivity The extent to which independent researchers would arrive at similar judgments or conclusions (i.e., judgments not biased by personal values or beliefs).

oblique rotation In factor analysis, a rotation of factors such that the reference axes are allowed to move to acute or oblique angles and hence the factors are allowed to be correlated.

observational notes An observer's in-depth descriptions about events and conversations observed in naturalistic settings.

observational research Studies that do not involve an experimental intervention—that is, nonexperimental research in which phenomena are merely observed.

observed (obtained) score The actual score or numerical value assigned to a person on a measure.

odds A way of expressing the chance of an event—the probability of an event occurring to the probability that it will not occur, calculated by dividing the number of people who experienced an event by the number for whom it did not occur.

odds ratio (OR) The ratio of one odds to another odds, for example, the ratio of the odds of an event in one group to the odds of an event in another group; an odds ratio of 1.0 indicates no difference between groups.

on-protocol analysis A principle for analyzing data that includes data only from those members of a treatment group who actually received the treatment; often called a *per protocol analysis.*

one-tailed test A statistical test in which only values in one tail of a distribution are considered in determining significance; sometimes used when the researcher states a directional hypothesis.

open-ended question A question in an interview or questionnaire that does not restrict respondents' answers to preestablished alternatives.

open coding The first level of coding in a grounded theory study, referring to the basic descriptive coding of the content of narrative materials.

operational definition The definition of a concept or variable in terms of the procedures by which it is to be measured.

operationalization The process of translating research concepts into measurable phenomena.

opportunistic sampling An approach to sampling in qualitative studies that involves adding new cases based on changes in research circumstances or in response to new leads that develop in the field.

oral history An unstructured self-report technique used to gather personal recollections of events and their perceived causes and consequences.

ordinal measurement A measurement level that rank orders phenomena along some dimension.

ordinary least squares (OLS) regression Regression analysis that uses the least-squares criterion for estimating the parameters in the regression equation.

orthogonal rotation In factor analysis, a rotation of factors such that the reference axes are kept at right angles, and hence the factors remain uncorrelated.

outcome analysis An evaluation of what happens to outcomes of interest after implementing a program or intervention, typically using a one group before-after design.

outcome measure A term often used to refer to the dependent variable, that is, the measure that captures the outcome of an intervention.

outcomes research Research designed to document the effectiveness of healthcare services and the end results of patient care.

outliers Values that lie outside the normal range of values for other cases in a data set.

p value In statistical testing, the probability that the obtained results are due to chance alone; the probability of a Type I error.

pair matching See *matching.*

pairwise deletion A method of dealing with missing values in a data set involving the deletion of cases with missing data selectively (i.e., on a variable by variable basis).

panel study A longitudinal survey study in which data are collected from the same people (*a panel*) at two or more points in time.

paradigm A way of looking at natural phenomena—a world view—that encompasses a set of philosophical assumptions and that guides one's approach to inquiry.

paradigm case In a hermeneutic analysis following the precepts of Benner, a strong examplar of the phenomenon under study, often used early in the analysis to gain understanding of the phenomenon.

parallel sampling An approach to sampling in mixed methods studies in which the participants in one strand are not included in the sample for the other strand, but sampling for both strands is from the same or a similar population.

parameter A characteristic of a population (e.g., the mean age of all U.S. citizens).

parametric tests A class of statistical tests that involve assumptions about the distribution of the variables and the estimation of a parameter.

participant See *study participant.*

partially randomized patient preference (PRPP) design A design that involves randomizing only patients without a strong preference for a treatment condition.

participant observation A method of collecting data through the participation in and observation of a group or culture.

participatory action research (PAR) A collaborative research approach between researchers and participants based on the premise that the production of knowledge can be political and used to exert power.

path analysis A regression-based procedure for testing causal models, typically using correlational data.

path coefficient The weight representing the impact of one variable on another in a path analytic model.

path diagram A graphic representation of the hypothesized interrelationships and causal flow among variables.

patient-centered intervention (PCI) An intervention tailored to meet individual needs or characteristics.

Pearson's *r* A correlation coefficient designating the magnitude of relationship between two variables measured on at least an interval scale; also called *the product-moment correlation.*

peer debriefing Sessions with peers to review and explore various aspects of a study, sometimes used to enhance trustworthiness in a qualitative study.

peer reviewer A researcher who reviews and critiques a research report or proposal of another researcher, and who makes a recommendation about publishing or funding the research.

pentadic dramatism An approach for analyzing narratives, developed by Burke, that focus on five key elements of a story: act (what was done), scene (when and where it was done), agent (who did it), agency (how it was done), and purpose (why it was done).

per protocol analysis Analysis of data from a randomized controlled trial that excludes participants who did not obtain the protocol to which they were assigned (or who received an insufficient dose of the intervention); sometimes called an *on-protocol analysis.*

perfect relationship A correlation between two variables such that the values of one variable permit perfect prediction of the values of the other; designated as 1.00 or –1.00.

performance bias In clinical trials, systematic differences in the care provided to (or care received by) members of different groups of participants, apart from the intervention that is the focus of the inquiry, which can occur when there is no blinding.

performance ethnography A scripted, staged reenactment of ethnographically derived findings that reflect an interpretation of the culture.

permuted block randomization Randomization that occurs for blocks of subjects (e.g., 6 or 8 at a time), to ensure a balanced allocation to groups within cohorts of participants; the size of the blocks is varied (permuted).

persistent observation A qualitative researcher's intense focus on the aspects of a situation that are relevant to the phenomena being studied.

person triangulation The collection of data from different levels of persons, with the aim of validating data through multiple perspectives on the phenomenon.

personal interview A face-to-face interview between an interviewer and a respondent.

personal notes In field studies, written comments about the observer's own feelings during the research process.

phenomenon The abstract concept under study, often used by qualitative researchers in lieu of the term *variable.*

phenomenology A qualitative research tradition, with roots in philosophy and psychology, that focuses on the lived experience of humans.

phi coefficient A statistical index describing the magnitude of relationship between two dichotomous variables.

photo elicitation An interview stimulated and guided by photographic images.

pilot study A small scale version, or trial run, done in preparation for a major study; sometimes called a *feasibility study.*

placebo A sham or pseudo intervention, often used as a control group condition.

placebo effect Changes in the dependant variable attributable to the placebo condition.

point estimation A statistical procedure in which information from a sample (a statistic) is used to estimate the single value that best represents the population parameter.

point prevalence rate The number of people with a condition or disease divided by the total number at risk, multiplied by the total number for whom the rate is being established (e.g., per 1,000 population).

population The entire set of individuals or objects having some common characteristics (e.g., all RNs in Canada); sometimes called *universe*.

positive predictive value (PPV) A measure of the usefulness of a screening/diagnostic test that can be interpreted as the probability that a positive test result is correct; calculated by dividing the number with a positive test who have the disease by the number with a positive test.

positive relationship A relationship between two variables in which high values on one variable tend to be associated with high values on the other (e.g., as physical activity increases, heart rate increases).

positive results Research results that are consistent with the researcher's hypotheses.

positively skewed distribution An asymmetric distribution of values with a disproportionately high number of cases at the lower end; when displayed graphically, the tail points to the right.

positivist paradigm The paradigm underlying the traditional scientific approach, which assumes that there is an orderly reality that can be objectively studied; often associated with quantitative research.

post hoc test A test for comparing all possible pairs of groups following a significant test of overall group differences (e.g., in an ANOVA).

poster session A session at a professional conference in which several researchers simultaneously present visual displays summarizing their studies, while conference attendees circulate around the room perusing the displays.

posttest The collection of data after introducing an intervention.

posttest-only design An experimental design in which data are collected from subjects only after the intervention has been introduced; also called an *after-only design*.

power The ability of a design or analysis strategy to detect true relationships that exist among variables.

power analysis A procedure used to estimate (1) sample size requirements prior to undertaking a study, or (2) the likelihood of committing a Type II error.

practical (pragmatic) clinical trial Trials that address practical questions about the benefits, risks, and costs of an intervention as they would unfold in routine clinical practice, using designs that yield information needed for making clinical decisions.

pragmatism A paradigm on which mixed methods research is often said to be based, in that it acknowl-

edges the practical imperative of the "dictatorship of the research question."

precision In statistics, the extent to which random errors have been reduced, usually expressed in terms of the width of the confidence interval around an estimate.

prediction The use of empirical evidence to make forecasts about how variables will behave, sometimes in a new setting or with different individuals.

predictive validity The degree to which an instrument can predict a criterion observed at a future time.

pretest (1) The collection of data prior to the experimental intervention; sometimes called baseline data. (2) The trial administration of a newly developed instrument to identify problems or assess time requirements.

pretest–posttest design An experimental design in which data are collected from subjects both before and after introducing an intervention; also called a *before–after design*.

prevalence study A cross-sectional study undertaken to estimate the proportion of a population having a particular condition (e.g., multiple sclerosis) at a given point in time.

primary source First-hand reports of facts or findings; in research, the original report prepared by the investigator who conducted the study.

primary study In a systematic review, an original study with findings that are used in the review.

principal investigator (PI) The person who is the lead researcher and who will have primary responsibility for overseeing a study.

priority A key issue in mixed methods research, concerning which strand (qualitative or quantitative) will be given more emphasis; symbolically, the dominant strand is in all capital letters, as QUAL or QUAN, and the nondominant strand is in lower case, as qual or quan.

PRISMA guidelines Guidelines for reporting meta-analyses of randomized controlled trials

probability sampling The selection of sampling units (e.g., participants) from a population using random procedures (e.g., simple random sampling).

probing Eliciting more useful or detailed information from a respondent in an interview than was volunteered in the first reply.

problem statement An expression of a dilemma or disturbing situation that needs investigation.

process analysis A descriptive analysis of the process by which a program or intervention gets implemented and used in practice.

process consent In a qualitative study, an ongoing, transactional process of negotiating consent with study participants, allowing them to play a collaborative role in the decision making regarding their continued participation.

product moment correlation coefficient (*r*) A correlation coefficient designating the magnitude of relationship between two variables measured on at least an interval scale; also called *Pearson's r*.

prolonged engagement In qualitative research, the investment of sufficient time during data collection to have an in-depth understanding of the group or phenomenon under study, thereby enhancing credibility.

propensity score A score that captures the conditional probability of exposure to a treatment, given various preintervention characteristics; can be used to match comparison groups or as a statistical control variable to enhance internal validity.

proportional hazards model A model in which independent variables are used to predict the risk (hazard) of experiencing an event at a given point in time.

proportionate sample A sample that results when the researcher samples from different strata of the population in direct proportion to their representation in the population.

proposal A document communicating a research problem, its significance, proposed procedures for solving the problem, and, when funding is sought, how much the study will cost.

prospective design A study design that begins with an examination of presumed causes (e.g., cigarette smoking) and then goes forward in time to observe presumed effects (e.g., lung cancer); also called a *cohort design.*

proximal similarity model A conceptualization relating to generalization that concerns the contexts that are more or less like the one in a study in terms of a *gradient of similarity* for people, settings, times, and contexts.

pseudo *R*² A type of statistic used to evaluate overall effect size in logistic regression, analogous to R^2 in least-squares multiple regression; the statistic does not, strictly speaking, indicate the proportion of variance explained in the outcome variable.

psychometric assessment An evaluation of the quality of an instrument, based primarily on evidence of its reliability and validity.

psychometrics The theory underlying principles of measurement and the application of the theory in the development of measuring tools.

publication bias The tendency for published studies to systematically over-represent statistically significant findings, reflecting the tendency of researchers, reviewers, and editors to not publish negative results; also called a *bias against the null hypothesis.*

purposive (purposeful) sampling A nonprobability sampling method in which the researcher selects participants based on personal judgment about which ones will be most informative; sometimes called *judgmental sampling.*

Q sort A data collection method in which participants sort statements into a number of piles (usually 9 or 11) according to some bipolar dimension (e.g., most helpful/least helpful).

qualitative analysis The organization and interpretation of narrative data for the purpose of discovering important underlying themes, categories, and patterns of relationships.

qualitative data Information collected in narrative (nonnumeric) form, such as the dialog from a transcript of an unstructured interview.

qualitative research The investigation of phenomena, typically in an in-depth and holistic fashion, through the collection of rich narrative materials using a flexible research design.

qualitizing The process of reading and interpreting quantitative data in a qualitative manner.

quantitative analysis The manipulation of numeric data through statistical procedures for the purpose of describing phenomena or assessing the magnitude and reliability of relationships among them.

quantitative data Information collected in a numeric (quantified) form.

quantitative research The investigation of phenomena that lend themselves to precise measurement and quantification, often involving a rigorous and controlled design.

quantitizing The process of coding and analyzing qualitative data quantitatively.

quasi-experimental design A design for an intervention study in which subjects are not randomly assigned to treatment conditions; also called a *nonrandomized trial* or a *controlled trial without randomization.*

quasi-statistics An "accounting" system used to assess the validity of conclusions derived from qualitative analysis.

query letter A letter written to a journal editor to ask whether there is interest in a proposed manuscript, or to a funding source to ask if there is interest in a proposed study.

questionnaire A document used to gather self-report data via self-administration of questions.

quota sampling A nonrandom sampling method in which "quotas" for certain sample characteristics are established to increase the representativeness of the sample.

r The symbol for a bivariate correlation coefficient (*Pearson's r*), summarizing the magnitude and direction of a relationship between two variables measured on an interval or ratio scale.

R The symbol for the multiple correlation coefficient, indicating the magnitude (but not direction) of the relationship between the dependent variable and multiple independent variables, taken together.

R² The squared multiple correlation coefficient, indicating the proportion of variance in the dependent variable explained by a group of independent variables.

random assignment The assignment of subjects to treatment conditions in a random manner (i.e., in a manner determined by chance alone); also called *randomization*.

random effects model In meta-analysis, a model in which studies are not assumed to be measuring the same overall effect, but rather a distribution of effects; often preferred to a fixed effect model when there is extensive heterogeneity of effects.

random number table A table displaying hundreds of digits (from 0 to 9) in random order; each number is equally likely to follow any other.

random sampling The selection of a sample such that each member of a population has an equal probability of being included.

randomization The assignment of subjects to treatment conditions in a random manner (i.e., in a manner determined by chance alone); also called *random assignment*.

randomized block design An experimental design involving two or more factors (independent variables), with one or more factors experimentally manipulated and one or more factors not manipulated.

randomized controlled trial (RCT) A full experimental test of an intervention, involving random assignment to treatment groups; sometimes, phase III of a full clinical trial.

randomized consent design An experimental design in which subjects are randomized prior to informed consent; also called a *Zelen design*.

randomness An important concept in quantitative research, involving having certain features of the study established by chance rather than by design or personal preference.

range A measure of variability, computed by subtracting the lowest value from the highest value in a distribution of scores.

Rasch model In measures developed using item-response theory, the model that considers item difficulty in assessing items for the scale.

rating scale A scale that requires ratings of an object or concept along a continuum.

ratio measurement A measurement level with equal distances between scores and a true meaningful zero point (e.g., weight).

raw data Data in the form in which they were collected, without being coded or analyzed.

reactivity A measurement distortion arising from the study participant's awareness of being observed, or, more generally, from the effect of the measurement procedure itself.

readability The ease with which materials (e.g., a questionnaire) can be read by people with varying reading skills, often empirically evaluated through readability formulas.

RE-AIM framework (*Reach, Efficacy, Adoption, Implementation,* and *Maintenance*) A model for designing and evaluating intervention research that is strong on multiple forms of study validity, including external validity.

receiver operating characteristic curve (ROC curve) A method used in developing and refining a screening instrument to determine the best cutoff point for "caseness."

rectangular matrix A matrix of data (variables × subjects) that is complete and contains no missing values.

recursive model A path model in which the causal flow is unidirectional, without any feedback loops; opposite of a nonrecursive model.

refereed journal A journal in which decisions about the acceptance of manuscripts are made based on recommendations from peer reviewers.

reflexive notes Notes that document a qualitative researcher's personal experiences, reflections, and progress in the field.

reflexivity In qualitative studies, critical self-reflection about one's own biases, preferences, and preconceptions.

regression analysis A statistical procedure for predicting values of a dependent variable based on one or more independent variables.

regression discontinuity design A quasi-experimental design that involves *systematic* assignment of subjects to groups based on cut-off scores on a preintervention measure.

relationship A bond or a connection between two or more variables.

relative risk (RR) An estimate of risk of "caseness" in one group compared to another, computed by dividing the absolute risk for one group (e.g., an exposed group) by the absolute risk for another (e.g., the nonexposed); also called the *risk ratio*.

relative risk reduction (RRR) The estimated proportion of baseline (untreated) risk that is reduced through exposure to the intervention, computed by dividing the absolute risk reduction (ARR) by the absolute risk for the control group.

reliability The degree of consistency or dependability with which an instrument measures an attribute.

reliability coefficient A quantitative index, usually ranging in value from .00 to 1.00, that provides an estimate of how reliable an instrument is (e.g., Cronbach's alpha).

repeated-measures ANOVA An analysis of variance used when there are multiple measures of the dependent variable over time (e.g., in a crossover design).

repeated measures design A design that involves the collection of data multiple points in time, usually to track changes in an intervention study.

replication The deliberate repetition of research procedures in a second investigation for the purpose of assessing whether earlier results can be confirmed.

representative sample A sample whose characteristics are comparable to those of the population from which it is drawn.

reputational case sampling A variant of purposive sampling used in qualitative studies that involves selecting cases based on a recommendation of an expert or key informant.

research Systematic inquiry that uses orderly, disciplined methods to answer questions or solve problems.

research control See *control*.

research design The overall plan for addressing a research question, including specifications for enhancing the study's integrity.

research hypothesis The actual hypothesis a researcher wishes to test (as opposed to the *null hypothesis*), stating the anticipated relationship between two or more variables.

research methods The techniques used to structure a study and to gather and analyze information in a systematic fashion.

research misconduct Fabrication, falsification, plagiarism, or other practices that seriously deviate from those that are commonly accepted within the scientific community for conducting or reporting research.

research problem An enigmatic or perplexing condition that can be investigated through disciplined inquiry.

research proposal See *proposal*.

research question A statement of the specific query the researcher wants to answer to address a research problem.

research report A document (often a journal article) summarizing the main features of a study, including the research question, the methods used to address it, the findings, and the interpretation of the findings.

research utilization The use of some aspect of a study in an application unrelated to the original research.

researcher expectancies The expectations that a researcher has, usually regarding treatment effectiveness, that can be communicated to subjects and can alter or bias their behavior or responses.

researcher credibility The faith that can be put in a researcher, based on his or her training, qualifications, and experience.

residuals In multiple regression, the error term, that is, unexplained variance.

respondent In a self-report study, the person responding to questions posed by the researcher.

response rate The rate of participation in a study, calculated by dividing the number of people participating by the number of people sampled.

response set bias The measurement error resulting from the tendency of some individuals to respond to items in characteristic ways (e.g., always agreeing), independently of item content.

results The answers to research questions, obtained through an analysis of the collected data.

retrospective design A study design that begins with the manifestation of the dependent variable in the present (e.g., lung cancer), followed by a search for a presumed cause occurring in the past (e.g., cigarette smoking).

revelatory case sampling An approach to sampling in a case study that involves identifying and gaining access to a case representing a phenomenon that was previously inaccessible to research scrutiny.

risk–benefit ratio The relative costs and benefits, to an individual subject and to society at large, of participation in a study; also, the relative costs and benefits of implementing an innovation.

risk ratio *See* Relative risk

rival hypothesis An alternative explanation, competing with the researcher's hypothesis, for interpreting the results of a study.

sample A subset of a population comprising those selected to participate in a study.

sample size The number of people who participate in a study; an important factor in the *power* of the analysis and in statistical conclusion validity.

sampling The process of selecting a portion of the population to represent the entire population.

sampling bias Distortions that arise when a sample is not representative of the population from which it was drawn.

sampling distribution A theoretical distribution of a statistic, using the values of the statistic (e.g., the means) computed from an infinite number of samples as the data points in the distribution.

sampling error The fluctuation of the value of a statistic from one sample to another drawn from the same population.

sampling frame A list of all the elements in the population, from which the sample is drawn.

sampling plan The formal plan specifying a sampling method, a sample size, and procedures for recruiting subjects.

saturation The collection of qualitative data to the point where a sense of closure is attained because new data yield redundant information.

scale A composite measure of an attribute, involving the combination of several items that have a logical and empirical relationship to each other, resulting in the assignment of a score to place people on a continuum with respect to the attribute.

scatter plot A graphic representation of the relationship between two variables.

scientific method A set of orderly, systematic, controlled procedures for acquiring dependable, empirical—and typically quantitative—information; the methodologic approach associated with the positivist paradigm.

scientific merit The degree to which a study is methodologically and conceptually sound.

scoping review A preliminary review of research findings designed to refine the questions and protocols for a systematic review.

screening instrument An instrument used to ascertain whether potential subjects for a study meet eligibility criteria, or for determining whether a person tests positive for a specified condition.

secondary analysis A form of research in which the data collected by one researcher are reanalyzed by another investigator to answer new questions.

secondary source Second-hand accounts of events or facts; in research, a description of a study prepared by someone other than the original researcher.

selection threat (self-selection) A threat to the internal validity of the study resulting from preexisting differences between groups under study; the differences affect the dependent variable in ways extraneous to the effect of the independent variable.

selective coding A level of coding in a grounded theory study that involves selecting the core category, systematically integrating relationships between the core category and other categories, and validating those relationships.

selective deposit A bias that can result when records and documents that are stored are not a complete set of records, but rather are selectively retained based on criteria that could bias the set.

selective survival A bias that can result when records and documents that are available are not a complete set of records because of a nonrandom mechanism of maintaining them.

self-determination A person's ability to voluntarily decide whether or not to participate in a study.

self-report A method of collecting data that involves a direct verbal report of information by the person who is being studied (e.g., by interview or questionnaire).

semantic differential A technique used to measure attitudes in which respondents rate concepts of interest on a series of bipolar rating scales.

semi-structured interview An interview in which the researcher has a list of topics to cover rather than a specific series of questions to ask.

sensitivity The ability of screening instruments to correctly identify a "case," that is, to correctly diagnose a condition.

sensitivity analysis An effort to test how sensitive the results of a statistical analysis are to changes in assumptions or in the way the analysis was done (e.g., in a meta-analysis, used to assess whether conclusions are sensitive to the quality of the studies included).

sequential design A mixed methods design in which one strand of data collection (qualitative or quantitative) occurs prior to the other, informing the design of the second strand; symbolically shown with an arrow, as QUAL → QUAN.

sequential clinical trial   A trial in which data are continuously analyzed, and *stopping rules* are used to decide when the evidence about treatment efficacy is sufficiently strong that the trial can be stopped.

setting   The physical location and conditions in which data collection takes place in a study.

significance level   The probability that an observed relationship could be the result of chance; significance at the .05 level indicates the probability that a relationship of the observed magnitude would be found by chance only 5 times out of 100.

simple random sampling   Basic probability sampling involving the selection of sample members from a sampling frame through completely random procedures.

simultaneous multiple regression   A multiple regression analysis in which all predictor variables are entered into the equation simultaneously.

single-blind study   A study in which only one group (e.g., the subjects or data collectors) know the status of participants in terms of the group to which they have been assigned.

single-subject experiment   An intervention study that tests the effectiveness of an intervention with a single subject, typically using a time series design; sometimes called an *N-of-1 experiment*.

site   The overall location where a study is undertaken.

skewed distribution   The asymmetric distribution of a set of data values around a central point.

snowball sampling   The selection of participants through referrals from earlier participants; also called *network sampling.*

social desirability response set   A bias in self-report instruments created when participants have a tendency to misrepresent their opinions in the direction of answers consistent with prevailing social norms.

space triangulation   The collection of data on the same phenomenon in multiple sites, to enhance the validity of the findings.

Spearman's rank-order correlation (Spearman's rho)   A correlation coefficient indicating the magnitude of a relationship between variables measured on the ordinal scale.

specificity   The ability of a screening instrument to correctly identify noncases.

standard deviation   The most frequently used statistic for measuring the degree of variability in a set of scores.

standard error   The standard deviation of a sampling distribution, such as the sampling distribution of the mean.

standard scores   Scores expressed in terms of standard deviations from the mean, with raw scores typically transformed to have a mean of zero and a standard deviation of one; sometimes called *z* scores.

standardized mean difference (SMD)   In meta-analysis, the effect size for comparing two group means, computed by subtracting one mean from the other and dividing by the pooled standard deviation; also called Cohen's *d*.

statement of purpose   A broad declarative statement of the overall goals of a study.

statistic   An estimate of a parameter, calculated from sample data.

statistical analysis   The organization and analysis of quantitative data using statistical procedures, including both descriptive and inferential statistics.

statistical conclusion validity   The degree to which inferences about relationships from a statistical analysis of the data are correct.

statistical control   The use of statistical procedures to control confounding influences on the dependent variable.

statistical heterogeneity   Diversity of effects across primary studies included in a meta-analysis.

statistical inference   The process of drawing inferences about the population based on information from a sample, using laws of probability.

statistical power   The ability of the research design to detect true relationships among variables.

statistical significance   A term indicating that the results from an analysis of sample data are unlikely to have been caused by chance, at a specified level of probability.

statistical test   An analytic tool that estimates the probability that results obtained from a sample reflect true population values.

stepwise multiple regression   A multiple regression analysis in which predictor variables are entered into the equation in steps, in the order in which the increment to R is greatest.

stipend   A monetary payment to individuals participating in a study to serve as an incentive for participation and/or to compensate for time and expenses.

strata   Subdivisions of the population according to some characteristic (e.g., males and females); singular is *stratum.*

stratification The division of a sample of a population into smaller units (e.g., males and females), typically to enhance representativeness or to explore results for subgroups of people; used in both sampling and in allocation to treatment groups.

stratified random sampling The random selection of study participants from two or more strata of the population independently.

STROBE guidelines Guidelines for reporting observational studies.

structural equations Equations representing the magnitude of hypothesized relations among sets of variables in a theory, typically used to test a model or theory.

structured data collection An approach to collecting data from participants, either through self-report or observations, in which categories of information (e.g., response options) are specified in advance.

study section Within the National Institutes of Health, a group of peer reviewers that evaluates grant applications in the first phase of the review process.

study participant An individual who participates and provides information in a study.

subgroup effect The differential effect of the independent variable on the dependent variable for subsets of the sample.

subject An individual who participates and provides data in a study; term used primarily in quantitative research.

summated rating scale A scale consisting of multiple items that are added together to yield an overall, continuous measure of an attribute (e.g., a Likert scale).

survey research Nonexperimental research obtains information about people's activities, beliefs, preferences, and attitudes via direct questioning.

survival analysis A statistical procedure used when the dependent variable represents a time interval between an initial event (e.g., onset of a disease) and an end event (e.g., death).

symmetric distribution A distribution of values with two halves that are mirror images of each other.

systematic review A rigorous synthesis of research findings on a particular research question, using systematic sampling and data collection procedures and a formal protocol.

systematic sampling The selection of sample members such that every *kth* (e.g., every tenth) person or element in a sampling frame is chosen.

table shell A table without any numeric values, prepared in advance of data analysis as a guide to the analyses to be performed.

tacit knowledge Information about a culture that is so deeply embedded that members do not talk about it or may not even be consciously aware of it.

target population The entire population in which a researcher is interested and to which he or she would like to generalize the study results.

taxonomy In an ethnographic analysis, a system of classifying and organizing terms and concepts, developed to illuminate the internal organization of a domain and the relationship among the subcategories of the domain

test statistic A statistic used to test for the statistical reliability of relationships between variables (e.g., chi-squared, *t*); the sampling distributions of test statistics are known for circumstances in which the null hypothesis is true.

test–retest reliability Assessment of the stability of an instrument by correlating the scores obtained on two administrations.

testing threat A threat to a study's internal validity that occurs when the administration of a pretest or baseline measure of a dependent variable results in changes on the variable, apart from the effect of the independent variable.

theme A recurring regularity emerging from an analysis of qualitative data.

theoretical notes In field studies, notes detailing the researcher's interpretations of observed behavior and events.

theoretical sampling In qualitative studies, especially in a grounded theory study, the selection of sample members based on emerging findings to ensure adequate representation of important theoretical categories.

theory An abstract generalization that presents a systematic explanation about the relationships among phenomena.

theory triangulation The use of competing theories or hypotheses in the analysis and interpretation of data.

thick description A rich and thorough description of the research context in a qualitative study.

think aloud method A qualitative method used to collect data about cognitive processes (e.g., decision making), in which people's reflections on decisions or problem solving are captured as they are being made.

time sampling In structured observations, the sampling of time periods during which observations will take place.

time series design A quasi-experimental design involving the collection of data over an extended time period, with multiple data collection points both prior to and after an intervention.

time triangulation   The collection of data on the same phenomenon or about the same people at different points in time, to enhance validity.

topic guide   A list of broad question areas to be covered in a semistructured interview or focus group interview.

tracing   Procedures used to relocate subjects to avoid attrition in a longitudinal study.

transferability   The extent to which qualitative findings can be transferred to other settings or groups; one of several models of generalizability.

treatment   The experimental intervention under study; the condition being manipulated.

treatment group   The group receiving the intervention being tested; the experimental group.

TREND guidelines   Guidelines (Transparent Reporting of Evaluations with Non-randomized Designs) for reporting non-RCT intervention studies.

trend study   A form of longitudinal study in which different samples from a population are studied over time with respect to some phenomenon (e.g., annual national polls on abortion attitudes).

triangulation   The use of multiple methods to collect and interpret data about a phenomenon, so as to converge on an accurate representation of reality.

triangulation design   A concurrent, equal-priority mixed methods design in which different, but complementary data, qualitative and quantitative, are gathered about a central phenomenon under study; symbolized as QUAL + QUAN.

true score   A hypothetical score that would be obtained if a measure were infallible.

trustworthiness   The degree of confidence qualitative researchers have in their data, assessed using the criteria of credibility, transferability, dependability, confirmability, and authenticity.

t-**test**   A parametric statistical test for analyzing the difference between two means.

Type I error   An error created by rejecting the null hypothesis when it is true (i.e., the researcher concludes that a relationship exists when in fact it does not—a false positive).

Type II error   An error created by accepting the null hypothesis when it is false (i.e., the researcher concludes that *no* relationship exists when in fact it does—a false negative).

two-tailed tests   Statistical tests in which both ends of the sampling distribution are used to determine improbable values.

unimodal distribution   A distribution of values with one peak (high frequency).

unit of analysis   The basic unit or focus of a researcher's analysis—typically individual study participants.

univariate descriptive study   A study that gathers information on the occurrence, frequency of occurrence, or average value of the variables of interest, one variable at a time, without focusing on interrelationships among variables.

univariate statistics   Statistical analysis of a single variable for purposes of description (e.g., computing a mean).

unstructured interview   An interview in which the researcher asks respondents questions without having a predetermined plan regarding the content or flow of information to be gathered.

unstructured observation   The collection of descriptive data through direct observation that is not guided by a formal, prespecified plan for observing, enumerating, or recording the information.

utilization   See *research utilization*.

validity   A quality criterion referring to the degree to which inferences made in a study are accurate and well-founded; in measurement, the degree to which an instrument measures what it is intended to measure.

validity coefficient   An index, usually ranging from .00 to 1.00, yielding an estimate of how valid an instrument is.

variability   The degree to which values on a set of scores are dispersed.

variable   An attribute that varies, that is, takes on different values (e.g., body temperature, heart rate).

variance   A measure of variability or dispersion, equal to the standard deviation squared.

vignette   A brief description of an event, person, or situation to which respondents are asked to express their reactions.

visual analog scale (VAS)   A scaling procedure used to measure certain clinical symptoms (e.g., pain, fatigue) by having people indicate on a straight line the intensity of the symptom.

vulnerable groups   Special groups of people whose rights in studies need special protection because of their inability to provide meaningful informed consent or because their circumstances place them at higher-than-average risk of adverse effects (e.g., children, unconscious patients).

wait-list design   A design for an experimental study that involves putting control group members on a waiting list for the intervention until follow-up data have been collected; also called a *delayed treatment design*.

Wald statistic A statistic, distributed as a chi-square, used to evaluate the significance of individual predictors in a logistic regression equation.

web-based survey The administration of a self-administered questionnaire over the Internet on a dedicated survey website.

weighting A correction procedure used to estimate population values when a disproportionate sampling design has been used.

Wilcoxon signed ranks test A nonparametric statistical test for comparing two paired groups, based on the relative ranking of values between the pairs.

wild code A coded value that is not legitimate within the coding scheme for that data set.

Wilk's lambda An index used in discriminant function analysis to indicate the proportion of variance in the dependent variable *un*accounted for by predictors; $(\lambda) = 1 - R^2$.

within-subjects design A research design in which a single group of subjects is compared under different conditions or at different points in time (e.g., before and after surgery).

z score A standard score, expressed in terms of standard deviations from the mean; raw scores are transformed such that the mean equals zero and the standard deviation equals 1.

Zelen design An experimental design in which subjects are randomized prior to informed consent; also called *randomized consent design*.

Check out these online glossaries:
http://ktclearinghouse.ca/cebm/glossary
http://www.unc.edu/~jssumpte/ebm/Glossary.htm
http://www2.cochrane.org/software/Documentation/
  glossary.pdf

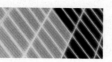

Appendix:
Statistical Tables of Theoretical Probability Distributions

| TABLE A.1 | Critical Values for the t Distribution |

df	α, 2-tailed test: α, 1-tailed test:	.10 .05	.05 .025	.02 .01	.01 .005	.001 .0005
1		6.314	12.706	31.821	63.657	636.619
2		2.920	4.303	6.965	9.925	31.598
3		2.353	3.182	4.541	5.841	12.941
4		2.132	2.776	3.747	4.604	8.610
5		2.015	2.571	3.376	4.032	6.859
6		1.953	2.447	3.143	3.707	5.959
7		1.895	2.365	2.998	3.449	5.405
8		1.860	2.306	2.896	3.355	5.041
9		1.833	2.262	2.821	3.250	4.781
10		1.812	2.228	2.765	3.169	4.587
11		1.796	2.201	2.718	3.106	4.437
12		1.782	2.179	2.681	3.055	4.318
13		1.771	2.160	2.650	3.012	4.221
14		1.761	2.145	2.624	2.977	4.140
15		1.753	2.131	2.602	2.947	4.073
16		1.746	2.120	2.583	2.921	4.015
17		1.740	2.110	2.567	2.898	3.965
18		1.734	2.101	2.552	2.878	3.922
19		1.729	2.093	2.539	2.861	3.883
20		1.725	2.086	2.528	2.845	3.850
21		1.721	2.080	2.518	2.831	3.819
22		1.717	2.074	2.508	2.819	3.792
23		1.714	2.069	2.500	2.807	3.767
24		1.711	2.064	2.492	2.797	3.745
25		1.708	2.060	2.485	2.787	3.725
26		1.706	2.056	2.479	2.779	3.707
27		1.703	2.052	2.473	2.771	3.690
28		1.701	2.048	2.467	2.763	3.674
29		1.699	2.045	2.462	2.756	3.659
30		1.697	2.042	2.457	2.750	3.646
40		1.684	2.021	2.423	2.704	3.551
60		1.671	2.000	2.390	2.660	3.460
120		1.658	1.980	2.358	2.617	3.373
∞		1.645	1.960	2.326	2.576	3.291

TABLE A.2	Critical Values for the F Distribution $\alpha = .05$ (Two-Tailed)								$\alpha = .025$ (One-Tailed)	

df_B / df_W	1	2	3	4	5	6	8	12	24	∞
1	161.4	199.5	215.7	224.6	230.2	234.0	238.9	243.9	249.0	254.3
2	18.51	19.00	19.16	19.25	19.30	19.33	19.37	19.41	19.45	19.50
3	10.13	9.55	9.28	9.12	9.01	8.94	8.84	8.74	8.64	8.53
4	7.71	6.94	6.59	6.39	6.26	6.16	6.04	5.91	5.77	5.63
5	6.61	5.79	5.41	5.19	5.05	4.95	4.82	4.68	4.53	4.36
6	5.99	5.14	4.76	4.53	4.39	4.28	4.15	4.00	3.84	3.67
7	5.59	4.74	4.35	4.12	3.97	3.87	3.73	3.57	3.41	3.23
8	5.32	4.46	4.07	3.84	3.69	3.58	3.44	3.28	3.12	2.93
9	5.12	4.26	3.86	3.63	3.48	3.37	3.23	3.07	2.90	2.71
10	4.96	4.10	3.71	3.48	3.33	3.22	3.07	2.91	2.74	2.54
11	4.84	3.98	3.59	3.36	3.20	3.09	2.95	2.79	2.61	2.40
12	4.75	3.88	3.49	3.26	3.11	3.00	2.85	2.69	2.50	2.30
13	4.67	3.80	3.41	3.18	3.02	2.92	2.77	2.60	2.42	2.21
14	4.60	3.74	3.34	3.11	2.96	2.85	2.70	2.53	2.35	2.13
15	4.54	3.68	3.29	3.06	2.90	2.79	2.64	2.48	2.29	2.07
16	4.49	3.63	3.24	3.01	2.85	2.74	2.59	2.42	2.24	2.01
17	4.45	3.59	3.20	2.96	2.81	2.70	2.55	2.38	2.19	1.96
18	4.41	3.55	3.16	2.93	2.77	2.66	2.51	2.34	2.15	1.92
19	4.38	3.52	3.13	2.90	2.74	2.63	2.48	2.31	2.11	1.88
20	4.35	3.49	3.10	2.87	2.71	2.60	2.45	2.28	2.08	1.84
21	4.32	3.47	3.07	2.84	2.68	2.57	2.42	2.25	2.05	1.81
22	4.30	3.44	3.05	2.82	2.66	2.55	2.40	2.23	2.03	1.78
23	4.28	3.42	3.03	2.80	2.64	2.53	2.38	2.20	2.00	1.76
24	4.26	3.40	3.01	2.78	2.62	2.51	2.36	2.18	1.98	1.73
25	4.24	3.38	2.99	2.76	2.60	2.49	2.34	2.16	1.96	1.71
26	4.22	3.37	2.98	2.74	2.59	2.47	2.32	2.15	1.95	1.69
27	4.21	3.35	2.96	2.73	2.57	2.46	2.30	2.13	1.93	1.67
28	4.20	3.34	2.95	2.71	2.56	2.44	2.29	2.12	1.91	1.65
29	4.18	3.33	2.93	2.70	2.54	2.43	2.28	2.10	1.90	1.64
30	4.17	3.32	2.92	2.69	2.53	2.42	2.27	2.09	1.89	1.62
40	4.08	3.23	2.84	2.61	2.45	2.34	2.18	2.00	1.79	1.51
60	4.00	3.15	2.76	2.52	2.37	2.25	2.10	1.92	1.70	1.39
120	3.92	3.07	2.68	2.45	2.29	2.17	2.02	1.83	1.61	1.25
∞	3.84	2.99	2.60	2.37	2.21	2.09	1.94	1.75	1.52	1.00

(continued)

| TABLE A.2 | Critical Values for the *F* Distribution (continued) $\alpha = .01$ (Two-Tailed) | | | | | | | | $\alpha = .005$ (One-Tailed) |

df_B df_W	1	2	3	4	5	6	8	12	24	∞
1	4052	4999	5403	5625	5764	5859	5981	6106	6234	6366
2	98.49	99.00	99.17	99.25	99.30	99.33	99.36	99.42	99.46	99.50
3	34.12	30.81	29.46	28.71	28.24	27.91	27.49	27.05	26.60	26.12
4	21.20	18.00	16.69	15.98	15.52	15.21	14.80	14.37	13.93	13.46
5	16.26	13.27	12.06	11.39	10.97	10.67	10.29	9.89	9.47	9.02
6	13.74	10.92	9.78	9.15	8.75	8.47	8.10	7.72	7.31	6.88
7	12.25	9.55	8.45	7.85	7.46	7.19	6.84	6.47	6.07	5.65
8	11.26	8.65	7.59	7.01	6.63	6.37	6.03	5.67	5.28	4.86
9	10.56	8.02	6.99	6.42	6.06	5.80	5.47	5.11	4.73	4.31
10	10.04	7.56	6.55	5.99	5.64	5.39	5.06	4.71	4.33	3.91
11	9.65	7.20	6.22	5.67	5.32	5.07	4.74	4.40	4.02	3.60
12	9.33	6.93	5.95	5.41	5.06	4.82	4.50	4.16	3.78	3.36
13	9.07	6.70	5.74	5.20	4.86	4.62	4.30	3.96	3.59	3.16
14	8.86	6.51	5.56	5.03	4.69	4.46	4.14	3.80	3.43	3.00
15	8.68	6.36	5.42	4.89	4.56	4.32	4.00	3.67	3.29	2.87
16	8.53	6.23	5.29	4.77	4.44	4.20	3.89	3.55	3.18	2.75
17	8.40	6.11	5.18	4.67	4.34	4.10	3.78	3.45	3.08	2.65
18	8.28	6.01	5.09	4.58	4.29	4.01	3.71	3.37	3.00	2.57
19	8.18	5.93	5.01	4.50	4.17	3.94	3.63	3.30	2.92	2.49
20	8.10	5.85	4.94	4.43	4.10	3.87	3.56	3.23	2.86	2.42
21	8.02	5.78	4.87	4.37	4.04	3.81	3.51	3.17	2.80	2.36
22	7.94	5.72	4.82	4.31	3.99	3.76	3.45	3.12	2.75	2.31
23	7.88	5.66	4.76	4.26	3.94	3.71	3.41	3.07	2.70	2.26
24	7.82	5.61	4.72	4.22	3.90	3.67	3.36	3.03	2.66	2.21
25	7.77	5.57	4.68	4.18	3.86	3.63	3.32	2.99	2.62	2.17
26	7.72	5.53	4.64	4.14	3.82	3.59	3.29	2.96	2.58	2.13
27	7.68	5.49	4.60	4.11	3.78	3.56	3.26	2.93	2.55	2.10
28	7.64	5.45	4.57	4.07	3.75	3.53	3.23	2.90	2.52	2.06
29	7.60	5.42	4.54	4.04	3.73	3.50	3.20	2.87	2.49	2.03
30	7.56	5.39	4.51	4.02	3.70	3.47	3.17	2.84	2.47	2.01
40	7.31	5.18	4.31	3.83	3.51	3.29	2.99	2.66	2.29	1.80
60	7.08	4.98	4.13	3.65	3.34	3.12	2.82	2.50	2.12	1.60
120	6.85	4.79	3.95	3.48	3.17	2.96	2.66	2.34	1.95	1.38
∞	6.64	4.60	3.78	3.32	3.02	2.80	2.51	2.18	1.79	1.00

(table continues on page 750)

TABLE A.2	Critical Values for the F Distribution (continued) α = .001 (Two-Tailed)						α = .0005 (One-Tailed)			

df_B / df_W	1	2	3	4	5	6	8	12	24	∞
1	405284	500000	540379	562500	576405	585937	598144	610667	623497	636619
2	998.5	999.0	999.2	999.2	999.3	999.3	999.4	999.4	999.5	999.5
3	167.5	148.5	141.1	137.1	134.6	132.8	130.6	128.3	125.9	123.5
4	74.14	61.25	56.18	53.44	51.71	50.53	49.00	47.41	45.77	44.05
5	47.04	36.61	33.20	31.09	29.75	28.84	27.64	26.42	25.14	23.78
6	35.51	27.00	23.70	21.90	20.81	20.03	19.03	17.99	16.89	15.75
7	29.22	21.69	18.77	17.19	16.21	15.52	14.63	13.71	12.73	11.69
8	25.42	18.49	15.83	14.39	13.49	12.86	17.04	11.19	10.30	9.34
9	22.86	16.39	13.90	12.56	11.71	11.13	10.37	9.57	8.72	7.81
10	21.04	14.91	12.55	11.28	10.48	9.92	9.20	8.45	7.64	6.76
11	19.69	13.81	11.56	10.35	9.58	9.05	8.35	7.63	6.85	6.00
12	18.64	12.97	10.80	9.63	8.89	8.38	7.71	7.00	6.25	5.42
13	17.81	12.31	10.21	9.07	8.35	7.86	7.21	6.52	5.78	4.97
14	17.14	11.78	9.73	8.62	7.92	7.43	6.80	6.13	5.41	4.60
15	16.59	11.34	9.34	8.25	7.57	7.09	6.47	5.81	5.10	4.31
16	16.12	10.97	9.00	7.94	7.27	6.81	6.19	5.55	4.85	4.06
17	15.72	10.66	8.73	7.68	7.02	6.56	5.96	5.32	4.63	3.85
18	15.38	10.39	8.49	7.46	6.81	6.35	5.76	5.13	4.45	3.67
19	15.08	10.16	8.28	7.26	6.61	6.18	5.59	4.97	4.29	3.52
20	14.82	9.95	8.10	7.10	6.46	6.02	5.44	4.82	4.15	3.38
21	14.59	9.77	7.94	6.95	6.32	5.88	5.31	4.70	4.03	3.26
22	14.38	9.61	7.80	6.81	6.19	5.76	5.19	4.58	3.92	3.15
23	14.19	9.47	7.67	6.69	6.08	5.65	5.09	4.48	3.82	3.05
24	14.03	9.34	7.55	6.59	5.98	5.55	4.99	4.39	3.74	2.97
25	13.88	9.22	7.45	6.49	5.88	5.46	4.91	4.31	3.66	2.89
26	13.74	9.12	7.36	6.41	5.80	5.38	4.83	4.24	3.59	2.82
27	13.61	9.02	7.27	6.33	5.73	5.31	4.76	4.17	3.52	2.75
28	13.50	8.93	7.19	6.25	5.66	5.24	4.69	4.11	3.46	2.70
29	13.39	8.85	7.12	6.19	5.59	5.18	4.64	4.05	3.41	2.64
30	13.29	8.77	7.05	6.12	5.53	5.12	4.58	4.00	3.36	2.59
40	12.61	8.25	6.60	5.70	5.13	4.73	4.21	3.64	3.01	2.23
60	11.97	7.76	6.17	5.31	4.76	4.37	3.87	3.31	2.69	1.90
120	11.38	7.31	5.79	4.95	4.42	4.04	3.55	3.02	2.40	1.56
∞	10.83	6.91	5.42	4.62	4.10	3.74	3.27	2.74	2.13	1.00

TABLE A.3 — Critical Values for the χ^2 Distribution

LEVEL OF SIGNIFICANCE

df	.10	.05	.02	.01	.001
1	2.71	3.84	5.41	6.63	10.83
2	4.61	5.99	7.82	9.21	13.82
3	6.25	7.82	9.84	11.34	16.27
4	7.78	9.49	11.67	13.28	18.46
5	9.24	11.07	13.39	15.09	20.52
6	10.64	12.59	15.03	16.81	22.46
7	12.02	14.07	16.62	18.48	24.32
8	13.36	15.51	18.17	20.09	26.12
9	14.68	16.92	19.68	21.67	27.88
10	15.99	18.31	21.16	23.21	29.59
11	17.28	19.68	22.62	24.72	31.26
12	18.55	21.03	24.05	26.22	32.91
13	19.81	22.36	25.47	27.69	34.53
14	21.06	23.68	26.87	29.14	36.12
15	22.31	25.00	28.26	30.58	37.70
16	23.54	26.30	29.63	32.00	39.25
17	24.77	27.59	31.00	33.41	40.79
18	25.99	28.87	32.35	34.81	42.31
19	27.20	30.14	33.69	36.19	43.82
20	28.41	31.41	35.02	37.57	45.32
21	29.62	32.67	36.34	38.93	46.80
22	30.81	33.92	37.66	40.29	48.27
23	32.01	35.17	38.97	41.64	49.73
24	33.20	36.42	40.27	42.98	51.18
25	34.38	37.65	41.57	44.31	52.62
26	35.56	38.89	42.86	45.64	54.05
27	36.74	40.11	44.14	46.96	55.48
28	37.92	41.34	45.42	48.28	56.89
29	39.09	42.56	46.69	49.59	58.30
30	40.26	43.77	47.96	50.89	59.70

TABLE A.4 Critical Values of the r Distribution

	LEVEL OF SIGNIFICANCE FOR ONE-TAILED TEST				
	.05	.025	.01	.005	.0005
	LEVEL OF SIGNIFICANCE FOR TWO-TAILED TEST				
df	.10	.05	.02	.01	.001
1	.98769	.99692	.999507	.999877	.9999988
2	.90000	.95000	.98000	.990000	.99900
3	.8054	.8783	.93433	.95873	.99116
4	.7293	.8114	.8822	.91720	.97406
5	.6694	.7545	.8329	.8745	.95074
6	.6215	.7067	.7887	.8343	.92493
7	.5822	.6664	.7498	.7977	.8982
8	.5494	.6319	.7155	.7646	.8721
9	.5214	.6021	.6851	.7348	.8471
10	.4973	.5760	.6581	.7079	.8233
11	.4762	.5529	.6339	.6835	.8010
12	.4575	.5324	.6120	.6614	.7800
13	.4409	.5139	.5923	.5411	.7603
14	.4259	.4973	.5742	.6226	.7420
15	.4124	.4821	.5577	.6055	.7246
16	.4000	.4683	.5425	.5897	.7084
17	.3887	.4555	.5285	.5751	.6932
18	.3783	.4438	.5155	.5614	.5687
19	.3687	.4329	.5034	.5487	.6652
20	.3598	.4227	.4921	.5368	.6524
25	.3233	.3809	.4451	.5869	.5974
30	.2960	.3494	.4093	.4487	.5541
35	.2746	.3246	.3810	.4182	.5189
40	.2573	.3044	.3578	.3932	.4896
45	.2428	.2875	.3384	.3721	.4648
50	.2306	.2732	.3218	.3541	.4433
60	.2108	.2500	.2948	.3248	.4078
70	.1954	.2319	.2737	.3017	.3799
80	.1829	.2172	.2565	.2830	.3568
90	.1726	.2050	.2422	.2673	.3375
100	.1638	.1946	.2301	.2540	.3211

Methodologic and Nonresearch References

Academic Center for Evidence-Based Practice. (2009). ACE Star Model of Knowledge Transformation. Retrieved October 8, 2009, from http://www.acestar.uthscsa.edu.

AERA, APA, & NCME Joint Committee. (1999). *Standards for educational and psychological testing.* Washington: American Psychological Association.

Agency for Healthcare Research and Quality. (2002). *Systems to rate the strength of scientific evidence.* Washington, DC: AHRQ.

AGREE Collaboration. (2001). *Appraisal of guidelines for research and evaluation (AGREE) instrument.* Retrieved May 2009, from www.agreecollaboration.org.

Ahern, K. J. (1999). Ten tips for reflexive bracketing. *Qualitative Health Research, 9,* 407–411.

Ajzen, I. (2005). *Attitudes, personality, and behavior* (2nd ed.). Milton Keynes, United Kingdom: Open University Press/McGraw Hill.

Akhtar-Danesh, N., Baumann, A., & Cordingly, L. (2008). Q-methodology in nursing research. *Western Journal of Nursing Research, 30,* 759–773.

Allen, F. M., & Warner, M. (2002). A developmental model of health and nursing. *Journal of Family Issues, 8,* 96–135.

American Nurses' Association. (2001). *Code for nurses with interpretive statements.* Kansas City, MO: Author.

American Psychological Association. (2010). *Publication manual of the American Psychological Association* (6th ed.). Washington, DC: Author.

Andrew, S., & Halcomb, E. (Eds.). (2009). *Mixed methods research for nursing and the health sciences.* Oxford: Blackwell-Wiley.

Aranda, S. (2008). Designing nursing interventions. *Collegian, 15,* 19–25.

Arksey, H., & O'Malley, L. (2005). Scoping studies: Toward a methodologic framework. *International Journal of Social Research Methodology, 8,* 19–32.

Artinian, N., Froelicher, E., & Wal, J. (2004). Data and safety monitoring during randomized controlled trials of nursing interventions. *Nursing Research, 53,* 414–418.

Atkins, S., Lewin, S., Smith, H., Engel, M., Fretheim, A., & Volminck, J. (2008). Conducting a meta-ethnography of qualitative literature: Lessons learned. *BMC Medical Research Methodology, 8,* 21.

Atkinson, P., Coffey, A., Delamount, S., Lofland, J., & Lofland, L. (2001). *Handbook of ethnography.* Thousand Oaks, CA: Sage Publications.

Atwood, J. R., & Taylor, W. (1991). Regression discontinuity design: Alternative for nursing research. *Nursing Research, 40,* 312–315.

Australian Nursing & Midwifery Council. (2008). *Code of ethics for nurses in Australia.* Dickson, Australia: Author.

Ayres, L., Kavanagh, K., & Knafl, K. (2003). Within-case and across-case approaches to qualitative data analysis. *Qualitative Health Research, 13,* 871–883.

Bader, G., & Rossi, C. (2002). *Focus groups: A step-by-step guide* (3rd ed.). San Diego, CA: The Bader Group.

Baggs, J. G. (2008). Issues and rules for authors concerning authorship versus acknowledgements, dual publication, self-plagiarism, and salami publishing. *Research in Nursing & Health, 31,* 295–297.

Baker, C., Wuest, J., & Stern, P. N. (1992). Method slurring: The grounded theory/phenomenology example. *Journal of Advanced Nursing, 17,* 1355–1360.

Bandura, A. (1985). *Social foundations of thought and action: A social cognitive theory.* Englewood Cliffs, NJ: Prentice Hall.

Bandura, A. (1997). *Self-efficacy: The exercise of control.* New York: W. H. Freeman.

Bandura, A. (2001). Social cognitive theory: An agentic perspective. *Annual Review of Psychology, 52,* 1–26.

Barkauskas, V. H., Lusk, S. L., Eakin, B. L. (2005). Selecting control interventions for clinical outcome studies. *Western Journal of Nursing Research, 27*(3), 346–363.

Barnett-Page, E., & Thomas, J. (2009). Methods for the synthesis of qualitative research: A critical review. *BMC Medical Research Methodology, 9,* 59.

Barnum, B. S. (1998). *Nursing theory: Analysis, application, evaluation* (5th ed.). Philadelphia: Lippincott Williams & Wilkins.

Barratt, A. (2008). Evidence-based medicine and shared decision making: The challenge of getting both evidence and preferences into health care. *Patient Education and Counseling, 73,* 407–412.

Barroso, J., Gollop, C., Sandelowski, M., Meynell, J., Pearce, P., & Collins, L. (2003). The challenges of searching for and retrieving qualitative studies. *Western Journal of Nursing Research, 25,* 153–178.

Barry, C. A., Britten, N., Barber, N., Bradley, C., & Stevenson, F. (1999). Using reflexivity to optimize teamwork in qualitative research. *Qualitative Health Research, 9,* 26–44.

Bazely, P. (2003). Computerized data analysis for mixed methods research. In A. Tashakkori & C. Teddlie (Eds.), *Handbook of mixed methods in social and behavioral research* (pp. 385–422). Thousand Oaks, CA: Sage.

Bazely, P. (2009a). Analysing mixed methods data. In S. Andrew & E. Halcom (Eds.), *Mixed methods research for nursing and the health sciences* (pp. 84–117). Oxford: Blackwell-Wiley.

Bazely, P. (2009b). Integrating data analyses in mixed methods research. *Journal of Mixed Methods Research, 3,* 203–207.

Bearinger, L., Taliaferro, L., & Given, B. (2010). When R & R is not rest and recovery but revise and resubmit. *Research in Nursing & Health, 33,* 381–385.

Beck, C. T. (1994). Replication strategies for nursing research. *Image: The Journal of Nursing Scholarship, 26,* 191–194.

Beck, C. T. (2005). Benefits of participating in internet interviews: Women helping women. *Qualitative Health Research, 15,* 411–422.

Beck, C. T. (2007). Exemplar: Teetering on the edge: A continually emerging theory of postpartum depression. In P.L. Munhall (Ed.). *Nursing research: A qualitative perspective* (4th ed.) (pp. 27–292). Sudbury, MA: Jones & Bartlett.

Beck, C. T. (2009). Metasynthesis: A goldmine for evidence-based practice. *AORN Journal, 90,* 701–702.

Beck, C. T. (2012). Exemplar: Teetering on the edge: A second grounded theory modification. In P. L. Munhall (Ed.). *Nursing research: A qualitative perspective* (5th ed.) (pp. 225–256). Sudbury, MA: Jones & Bartlett Publishers.

Beck, C. T., Bernal, H., & Froman, R. D. (2003). Methods to document semantic equivalence of a translated scale. *Research in Nursing & Health, 26,* 64–73.

Beck, C. T., & Gable, R. K. (2001). Ensuring content validity: An illustration of the process. *Journal of Nursing Measurement, 9,* 201–215.

Becker, H. S. (1970). *Sociological work.* Chicago: Aldine.

Becker, M. (1976). *Health Belief Model and personal health behavior.* Thorofare, NJ: Slack, Inc.

Becker, M. (1978). The Health Belief Model and sick role behavior. *Nursing Digest, 6,* 35–40.

Becker, P. (2004). What happens to my manuscript when I send it to… *Research in Nursing & Health? Research in Nursing & Health, 27,* 379–381.

Becker, P. T. (2009). Thoughts on the end of the article: The implications for nursing practice. *Research in Nursing & Health, 32,* 241–242.

Beitz, J. M., & Bliss, D. Z. (2005). Preparing a successful grant application—Part I. *Journal of Wound Ostomy & Continence Nursing, 32*(1), 16–18.

Bellg., A., Borrelli, B., Resnick, B., Hecht, J., Minicucci, D., Ory, M., Ogedegbe, G., Orwig, D., Ernst, D., Czajkowski, S.; Treatment Fidelity Workgroup of the NIH Behavior Change Consortium. (2004). Enhancing treatment fidelity in health behavior change studies: Best practices and recommendations from the NIH Behavior Change Consortium. *Health Psychology, 23,* 443–451.

Benner, P. (1994). The tradition and skill of interpretive phenomenology in studying health, illness, and caring practices. In P. Benner (Ed), *Interpretive phenomenology* (pp. 99–127). Thousand Oaks, CA: Sage.

Bennett, J. A. (2000). Mediator and moderator variables in nursing research: Conceptual and statistical differences. *Research in Nursing & Health, 23,* 415–420.

Berger, A., Neumark, D., & Chamberlain, J. (2007). Enhancing recruitment and retention in randomized clinical trials of cancer symptom management. *Oncology Nursing Forum, 34,* E17–22.

Berk, R. A. (1990). Importance of expert judgment in content-related validity evidence. *Western Journal of Nursing Research, 12,* 659–671.

Bernard, H. R. (2006). *Research methods in anthropology: Qualitative and quantitative approaches* (4th ed.). Lanham, MD: AltaMira Press.

Best, S. J., & Krueger, B. S. (2004). *Internet data collection.* Thousand Oaks, CA: Sage.

Bibb, S. C. G. (2007). Issues associated with secondary analysis of population health data. *Applied Nursing Research, 20,* 94–99.

Blackwood, B. (2006). Methodologic issues in evaluating complex interventions. *Journal of Advanced Nursing, 54,* 612–622.

Blumer, H. (1986). *Symbolic interactionism: Perspective and method.* Berkeley: University of California Press.

Bossuyt, P., Reitsma, J., Bruns, D., Gatsonis, C., Glasziou, P., Irwig, L., Moher, D., Rennie, D., de Vet, H. C., Lijmer, J. G.; Standards for Reporting of Diagnostic Accuracy. (2003). The STARD statement for reporting studies of diagnostic accuracy: explanation and elaboration. *Annals of Internal Medicine, 138,* W1–12.

Boutron, I., Moher, D., Altman, D., Schulz, K., Ravaud, P., for the CONSORT group. Extending the CONSORT. (2008) Statement to randomized trials of nonpharmacologic treatment: explanation and elaboration. *Annals of Internal Medicine,148,* 295–309.

Boyle, J. S. (1997). Writing up: Dissecting the dissertation. In J. M. Morse (Ed.), *Completing a qualitative project: Details and dialogue* (pp. 9–37). Thousand Oaks, CA: Sage.

Bradburn, N., Sudman, S., & Wansink, B. (2004). *Asking questions: The definitive guide for questionnaire design.* San Francisco: Jossey Bass.

Bradbury-Jones, C. (2007). Enhancing rigour in qualitative health research: Exploring subjectivity through Peshkin's I's. *Journal of Advanced Nursing, 59,* 290–298.

Bradford-Hill, A. (1971). *Principles of medical statistics* (9th ed.). New York: Oxford University Press.

Braitman, L. (1991). Confidence intervals assess both clinical significance and statistical significance. *Annals of Internal Medicine, 114,* 515–517.

Brewer, J., & Hunter, A. (2006). *Foundations of multimethod research: Synthesizing styles.* Thousand Oaks, CA: Sage.

Bringer, J. D., Johnston, L. H., & Brackenridge, C. H. (2004). Maximizing transparency in a doctoral thesis: the complexities of writing about the use of QRS*NVIVO within a grounded theory study. *Qualitative Research, 4,* 247–265.

Brislin, R. W. (1970). Back-translation for cross-cultural research. *Journal of Cross-Cultural Psychology, 1,* 185–216.

Broome, M. E. (2008). The "truth, the whole truth and nothing but the truth . . ." *Nursing Outlook, 56,* 282–282.

Brown, C. A., & Lilford, R. (2006). The stepped wedge trial design: A systematic review. *BMC Medical Research Methodology, 6,* 54.

Brown, C. H., Wyman, P., Guo, J., & Peña, J. (2006). Dynamic wait-list designs for randomized trials: New designs for prevention of youth suicide. *Clinical Trials, 3,* 259–271.

Brown, E. L. (1948). *Nursing for the future.* New York: Russell Sage.

Brown, S. J. (2009). *Evidence-based nursing: The research-practice connection.* Boston: Jones and Bartlett.

Brown, S., Upchurch, S., & Acton, G. (2003). A framework for developing a coding scheme for meta-analyses. *Western Journal of Nursing Research, 25,* 205–222.

Brown, T. (2006). *Confirmatory factor analysis for applied research.* New York: Guilford Press.

Bruner, J. (1991). *Acts of meaning.* Cambridge, MA: Harvard University Press.

Buck, J. (2008). Using frameworks in historical research (pp. 45–62) in S. B. Lewenson & E. K. Herrmann (Eds.). *Capturing nursing history.* New York: Springer.

Buckwalter, K., Grey, M., Bowers, B., McCarthy, A., Gross, D., Funk, M., & Beck, C. (2009). Intervention research in highly unstable environments. *Research in Nursing & Health, 32,* 110–121.

Bulechek, G., Butcher, H., & Dochterman, J. M. (2008). *Nursing interventions classification (NIC)* (5th ed.). St. Louis: Mosby.

Burke, K. (1969). *A grammer of motives.* Berkley, CA: University of California Press.

Burla, L., Knierim, B., Barth, J., Liewald, K., Duetz, M., & Abel, T. (2008). From text to codings: Intercoder reliability assessment in qualitative content analysis. *Nursing Research, 57,* 113–117.

Buros Institute, Spies, R., Plake, B., Geisinger, K., & Carlson, J. (Eds.). (2007). *The 17th mental measurements yearbook.* Lincoln, NE: The Buros Institute.

Campbell, D. T., & Stanley, J. C. (1963). *Experimental and quasi-experimental designs for research.* Chicago: Rand McNally.

Campbell, D. T. (1986). Relabeling internal and external validity for the applied social sciences. In W. Trochim (Ed.), *Advances in quasi-experimental design and analysis* (pp. 67–77). San Francisco: Jossey-Bass.

Campbell, D. T., & Fiske, D. W. (1959). Convergent and discriminant validation by the multitrait-multimethod matrix. *Psychological Bulletin, 56,* 81–105.

Campbell, D. T., & Stanley, J. C. (1963). *Experimental and quasi-experimental designs for research.* Chicago: Rand McNally.

Campbell, M., Elbourne, D., & Altman, D. (2004). CONSORT statement: extension to cluster randomised trials. *BMJ, 328,* 702–708.

Campbell, M., Fitzpatrick, R., Haines, A., Kinmonth, A., Sandercrock, P., Spiegelhalter, D., & Tryer, P. (2000). Framework for design and evaluation of complex interventions to improve health. *BMJ, 321.*

Canadian Nurses Association. (2002). *Ethical research guidelines for registered nurses.* Ottawa, ON: Author.

Cantrell, M. A., & Luopinacci, P. (2007). Methodological issues in online data collection. *Journal of Advanced Nursing, 60,* 544–549.

Carey, M. A., & Smith, M. W. (1994). Capturing the group effect in focus groups: A special concern in analysis. *Qualitative Health Research, 4,* 123–127.

Carpenter, J. (2008). Metaphors in qualitative research: Shedding light or casting shadows? *Research in Nursing & Health, 31,* 274–282.

Carroll, K., & Rounsaville, B. (2003). Bridging the gap: A hybrid model to link efficacy and effectiveness research in substance abuse treatment. *Psychiatric Services, 54,* 333–339.

Carspecken, P. F. (1996). *Critical ethnography in educational research.* New York: Routledge.

Chang, W., & Henry, B. M. (1999). Methodologic principles of cost analyses in the nursing, medical, and health services literature, 1990–1996. *Nursing Research, 48,* 94–104.

Chang, Y. K., Voils, C., Sandelowski, M., Hasselblad, V., & Crandell, J. (2009). Transforming verbal counts in reports of qualitative description studies into numbers. *Western Journal of Nursing Research, 31,* 837–852.

Charmaz, K. (2000). Constructivist and objectivist grounded theory. In N. K. Denzin & Y. Lincoln (Ed.), *Handbook of qualitative research* (pp. 509–535). Thousand Oaks, CA: Sage.

Charmaz, K. (2006). *Constructing grounded theory: A practical guide through qualitative analysis.* Thousand Oaks, CA: Sage Publications.

Chinn, P. L., & Kramer, M. K. (2004). *Theory and nursing: Integrated knowledge development* (6th ed.). St. Louis: C. V. Mosby.

Chiovitti, R., & Piran, N. (2003). Rigour and grounded theory research. *Journal of Advanced Nursing, 44,* 427–435.

Christensen, E. (2007). Methodology of superiority vs. equivalence trials and non-inferiority trials. *Journal of Hepatology, 46,* 947–954.

Christie, J., O'Halloran, P., & Stevenson, M. (2009). Planning a cluster randomized trial. *Nursing Research, 58,* 128–134.

Ciliska, D., & Guyatt, G. (2005). Publication bias. In A. DiCenso, G. Guyatt, & D. Ciliska. *Evidence-based nursing: A guide to clinical practice.* St. Louis, Mo: Elsevier Mosby.

Code of Federal Regulations. (2005). *Protection of human subjects: 45CFR46* (revised as of June 23, 2005. Washington, DC: U.S. Department of Health and Human Services.

Cohen, J. (1988). *Statistical power analysis for the behavioral sciences* (2nd ed.). Hillsdale, NJ: Lawrence Erlbaum Associates.

Cohen, M. Z., Kahn, D., & Steeves, R. (2000). Hermeneutic phenomenological research: A practical guide for nurse researchers. Thousand Oaks, CA: Sage.

Colaizzi, P. F. (1973). *Reflection and research in psychology.* Dubuque, IA: Kendall/Hunt.

Colaizzi, P. F. (1978). Psychological research as the phenomenologist views it. In R. Valle & M. King (Eds.), *Existential phenomenological alternative for psychology.* New York: Oxford University Press.

Conn, V. (2004). Buidling a research trajectory. *Western Journal of Nursing Research, 26,* 592–594.

Conn, V. (2005). Nursing intervention research. *Western Journal of Nursing Research, 27,* 249–251.

Conn, V. (2009). Identifying effective components of interventions. *Western Journal of Nursing Research, 31,* 981–982.

Conn, V. S., Cooper, P., Ruppar, T., & Russell, C. (2008). Searching for the intervention in intervention research reports. *Journal of Nursing Scholarship, 40,* 52–59.

Conn, V. S., Rantz, M. J., Wipke-Tevis, D. D., & Maas, M. L. (2001). Designing effective nursing interventions. *Research in Nursing & Health, 24,* 433–442.

Conn, V., Valentine, J., Cooper, H., & Rantz, M. (2003). Grey literature in meta-analyses. *Nursing Research, 52,* 256–261.

Cook, K. E. (2005). Using critical ethnography to explore issues in health promotion. *Qualitative Health Research, 15*(1), 129–138.

Cooper, H. (2010). *Research synthesis and meta-analysis* (4th ed.). Thousand Oaks, CA: Sage.

Corbin, J., & Strauss, A. (2008). *Basics of qualitative research: Techniques and procedures for developing grounded theory.* Los Angeles: Sage.

Côté-Arsenault, D., & Morrison-Beedy, D. (1999). Practical advice for planning and conducting focus groups. *Nursing Research, 48,* 280–283.

Côté-Arsenault, D., & Morrison-Beedy, D. (2005). Maintaining your focus in focus groups: Avoiding common mistakes. *Research in Nursing & Health, 28,* 172–179.

Courtney, K., & Craven, C. (2005). Factors to weigh when considering electronic data collection. *Canadian Journal of Nursing Research, 37*(3), 150–159.

Cowling, W. R. (2004). Pattern, participation, praxis, and power in unitary appreciative inquiry. *Advances in Nursing Science, 27*(3), 202–214.

Craig, J., & Smyth, R. (2007). *The evidence-based practice manual for nurses* (2nd ed.). Edinburgh: Elsevier.

Craig, P., Dieppe, P., Macintyre, S., Michie, S., Nazareth, I., & Petticrew, M. (2008a). *Developing and evaluating complex interventions: New guidance.* London: MRC. Available at www.mrc.ac.uk/complexinterventionsguidance.

Craig, P., Dieppe, P., Macintyre, S., Michie, S., Nazareth, I., & Petticrew, M. (2008b). Developing and evaluating complex interventions: The new Medical Research Council guidance. *BMJ, 337,* 979–983.

Creswell, J. (2003). *Research design: Qualitative, quantitative, and mixed method approaches.* Thousand Oaks, CA: Sage.

Creswell, J. (2009). Mapping the field of mixed methods research. *Journal of Mixed Methods Research, 3,* 95–108.

Creswell, J. W. (2006). *Qualitative inquiry and research design: Choosing among five traditions* (2nd ed.). Thousand Oaks, CA: Sage.

Creswell, J. W., & Plano Clark, V. L. (2007). *Designing and conducting mixed methods research.* Thousand Oaks, CA: Sage.

Cronbach, L. (1975). Beyond the two disciplines of scientific psychology. *American Psychologist, 30,* 116–127.

Cronbach, L. (1990). *Essentials of psychological testing* (5th ed.). New York: Harper & Row.

Curtis, S., Gesler, W., Smith, G., & Washburn, S. (2000). Approaches to sampling and case selection in qualitative research. *Social Science & Medicine, 50,* 1001–1014.

da Silva, G. T., Logan, B., & Klein, J. (2009). Methods for equivalence and noninferiority testing. *Biology of Blood and Marrow Transplantation, 15,* 120–127.

Dallas, C., Norr, K., Dancy, B., Kavanagh, K., & Cassata, L. (2005a). An example of a successful research proposal: Part I. *Western Journal of Nursing Research, 27,* 50–72.

Dallas, C., Norr, K., Dancy, B., Kavanagh, K., & Cassata, L. (2005b). An example of a successful research proposal: Part II. *Western Journal of Nursing Research, 27,* 210–231.

Davies, B., Larson, J., Contro, N., Reyes-Hailey, C., Ablin, A., Chesla, C., Sourkes, B., & Cohen, H. (2009). Conducting a qualitative culture study of pediatric palliative care. *Qualitative Health Research, 19,* 5–16.

Davis, G., & Parker, C. (1997). *Writing the doctoral dissertation: A systematic approach* (2nd ed.). New York: Barron's.

Davis, K., Drey, N., & Gould, D. (2009). What are scoping studies? A review of the nursing literature. *International Journal of Nursing Studies, 46,* 1386–1400.

Denzin, N. K. (1989). *The research act* (3rd ed.). New York: McGraw-Hill.

Denzin, N. K. (1997). *Interpretive ethnography: Ethnographic practices for the 21st century.* Thousand Oaks, CA: Sage.

Denzin, N. K. (2000). The practices and politics of interpretation. In N. K. Denzin, & Y. S. Lincoln, (Eds.). *Handbook of qualitative research* (2nd ed.) (pp. 897–922). Thousand Oaks, CA: Sage.

Denzin, N. K., & Lincoln, Y. S. (Eds.). (2000). *Handbook of qualitative research* (2nd ed.). Thousand Oaks, CA: Sage.

Des Jarlais, D., Lyles, C., Crepaz, N., The TREND group. (2004). Improving the reporting quality of nonrandomized evaluations of behavioral and public health interventions: the TREND statement. *American Journal of Public Health, 94,* 361–366.

DeSantis, L., & Ugarriza, D. N. (2000). The concept of theme as used in qualitative nursing research. *Western Journal of Nursing Research, 22,* 351–372.

DeVellis, R. F. (2003). *Scale development: Theory and application* (2nd ed.). Thousand Oaks, CA: Sage.

DeVon, H., Block, M., Moyle-Wright, P., Ernst, D., Hayden, S., Lazzara, D., Savoy, S. M., & Kostas-Polston, E. (2007). A psychometric toolbox for testing validity and reliability. *Journal of Nursing Scholarship, 39,* 155–164.

DiCenso, A., Guyatt, G., & Ciliska, D. (2005). *Evidence-based nursing: A guide to clinical practice.* St. Louis, MO: Elsevier Mosby.

DiCenso, A., Virano, T., Bajnok, I. Borycki, E., Davies, B., Graham, I., Harrison, M., Logan, J., McCleary, L., Power, M., & Scott, J. (2002). A toolkit to facilitate the implementation of clinical practice guidelines in healthcare settings. *Hospital Quarterly, 5,* 55–60.

Diekelmann, N. L., Allen, D., & Tanner, C. (1989). *The NLN criteria for appraisal of baccalaureate programs: A critical hermeneutic analysis.* New York: NLN Press.

Dillman, D., Smyth, J., & Christian, L. M. (2009). *Internet, mail, and mixed-mode surveys: The tailored design method* (3rd ed.). New York: John Wiley & Sons.

Dixon-Woods, M., Cavers, D., Agarwal, S., Annandale, E., Arthur, A., Harvey, J., Hsu, R., Katbamma, S., Olsen, R., Smith, L., Riley, R., & Sutton, A. J. (2006). Conducting a critical interpretive synthesis of the literature on access to healthcare by vulnerable groups. *BMC Medical Research Methodology, 6,* 35.

Dodd, M., Janson, S., Facione, N., Fawcett, J., Froelicher, E.S., Humphreys, J., Lee, K., Miaskowski, C., Puntillo, K., Rankin, S., & Taylor, D. (2001). Advancing the science of symptom management. *Journal of Advanced Nursing, 33,* 668–676.

Doig, G., & Simpson, F. (2005). Randomization and allocation concealment: A practical guide for researchers. *Journal of Critical Care, 20,* 187–191.

Donabedian, A. (1987). Some basic issues in evaluating the quality of health care. In L. T. Rinke (Ed.), *Outcome measures in home care* (Vol. I, pp. 3–28). New York: National League for Nursing.

Donaldson, S. K. (2000). Breakthroughs in scientific research: The discipline of nursing, 1960–1999. *Annual Review of Nursing Research, 18,* 247–311.

Donner, A., & Klar, N. (2004). Pitfalls and controversies in cluster randomization trials. *American Journal of Public Health, 94,* 416–422.

Donovan, H., Kwekkeboom, K., Rosenzweig, M., & Ward, S. (2009). Nonspecific effects in psychoeducational intervention research. *Western Journal of Nursing Research, 31,* 983–998.

Doran, D. M., & Sidani, S. (2007). Outcomes-Focused Knowledge Translation: A framework for knowledge translation and patient outcomes improvement. *Worldview of Evidence-Based Nursing, 4,* 3–13.

Drahota, A., & Dewey, A. (2008). The sociogram: A useful tool in the analysis of focus groups. *Nursing Research, 57,* 293–297.

Draucker, C., Martsoff, D., Ross, R., & Rusk, T. (2007). Theoretical sampling and category development in grounded theory. *Qualitative Health Research, 17,* 1137–1148.

Drummond, M., O'Brien, B., Stoddart, G., & Torrance, G. (2005). *Methods for the economic evaluation of health care programs* (3rd ed.). Oxford: Oxford Medical Publications.

Duggleby, W. (2005). What about focus group interaction data? *Qualitative Health Research, 15,* 832–840.

Duren-Winfield, V., Berry, M. J., Jones, S. A., Clark, D. H., & Sevick, M. A. (2000). Cost-effectiveness analysis methods for the REACT study. *Western Journal of Nursing Research, 22*, 460–474.

Dwan, K., Altman, D., Arnaiz, J., Bloom, J., Chan, A., Cronin, E., Decullier, E., Easterbrook, P. J., Von Elm, E., Gamble, C., Ghersi, D., Ioannidis, J. P., Simes, J., & Williamson, P. R. (2008). Systematic review of the empirical evidence of study publication bias and outcome reporting bias. *PLoS ONE, 3*, e3081.

Eaves, Y. D. (2001). A synthesis technique for grounded theory data analysis. *Journal of Advanced Nursing, 35*, 654–663.

Eder, C., Fullerton, J., Benroth, R., & Lindsay, S. (2005). Pragmatic strategies that enhance the reliability of data abstracted from medical records. *Applied Nursing Research, 18*, 50–54.

Edwards, P., Roberts, I., Clark, M., Diguiseppi, C., Wentz, R., Kwan, I., Cooper, R., Felix, L. M., & Prarap, S. (2009). Methods to increase response to postal and electronic questionnaires. *Cochrane Database of Systematic Reviews*, No. MR000008.

Eide, P., & Kahn, D. (2008). Ethical issues in the qualitative researcher-participant relationship. *Nursing Ethics, 15*, 199–207.

Ellett, M., Lane, L., & Keffer, J. (2004). Ethical and legal issues of conducting nursing research via the Internet. *Journal of Professional Nursing, 20*, 68–74.

Ellis, C., & Bochner, A. P. (2000). Autoethnography, personal narrative, reflexivity. In N. K. Denzin & Y. S. Lincoln (Eds.). *Handbook of qualitative research*, (2nd ed., pp. 733–768). Thousand Oaks, CA: Sage.

Embretson, S. E., & Reise, S. P. (2000). *Item response theory for psychologists*. Mahwah, NJ: Lawrence Erlbaum.

Erlandson, D.A., Harris, E. L., Skipper, B. L., & Allen, S. (1993). *Doing naturalistic inquiry: A guide to methods*. Thousand Oaks, CA: Sage.

Erwin, E., Meyer, A., & McClain, N. (2005). Use of an audit in violence prevention research. *Qualitative Health Research, 15*, 707–718.

Fahs, P., Morgan, L., & Kalman, M. (2003). A call for replication. *Journal of Nursing Scholarship, 35*, 67–72.

Farmer, T., Robinson, K., Elliott, S., & Eyles, J. (2006). Developing and implementing a triangulation protocol for qualitative health research. *Qualitative Health Research, 16*, 377–394.

Fawcett, J. (2005). *Contemporary nursing knowledge: Analysis and evaluation of nursing models and theories* (2nd ed.). Philadelphia: F.A. Davis Company.

Ferketich, S. (1991). Focus on psychometrics: Aspects of item analysis. *Research in Nursing & Health, 14*, 165–168.

Ferketich, S. L., Figueredo, A., & Knapp, T. R. (1991). The multitrait-multimethod approach to construct validity. *Research in Nursing & Health, 14*, 315–319.

Fetterman, D. M. (2010). *Ethnography: Step by step* (3rd ed.). Thousand Oaks, CA: Sage.

Findorff, M., Wyman, J., Croghan, C., & Nyman, J. (2005). Use of time studies for determining intervention costs. *Nursing Research, 54* 280–285.

Fineout-Overholt, E., & Johnston, L. (2005). Teaching EBP: Asking searchable, answerable clinical questions. *Worldviews on Evidence-Based Nursing, 2*(3), 157–160.

Finfgeld, D. (2003). Metasynthesis: The state of the art—so far. *Qualitative Health Research, 13*, 893–904.

Finfgeld-Connett, D. (2010). Generalizability and transferability of meta-synthesis research findings. *Journal of Advanced Nursing, 66*, 246–254.

Fink, A. (2009). *Conducting research literature reviews: From paper to the Internet* (3rd ed.). Thousand Oaks, CA: Sage.

Finlay, L., & Gough, B. (Eds.). (2003). *Reflexivity: A practical guide for researchers in health and social sciences*. Oxford: Blackwell Science.

Firestone, W. A. (1993). Alternative arguments for generalizing from data as applied to qualitative research. *Educational Researcher, 22*, 16–23.

Fishbein, M., & Ajzen, I. (2009). *Predicting and changing behavior: The reasoned action approach*. St. Helier, NJ: Psychology Press.

Fitzpatrick, J. J., & Montgomery, K. S. (2004). *Internet for nursing research: A guide to strategies, skills, and resources*. New York: Springer.

Flanagan, J. C. (1954). The critical-incident technique. *Psychological Bulletin, 51*, 327–358.

Flemming, K., & Briggs, M. (2006). Electronic searching to locate qualitative research: Evaluation of three strategies. *Journal of Advanced Nursing, 57*, 95–100.

Flemming, K. (2010). Synthesis of quantitative and qualitative research: An example using Critical Interpretive Synthesis. *Journal of Advanced Nursing, 66*, 201–217.

Flesch, R. (1948). New readability yardstick. *Journal of Applied Psychology, 32*, 221–223.

Fletcher, R. H., Fletcher, S. W., & Wagner, E. H. (2005). *Clinical epidemiology: The essentials* (4th ed.). Philadelphia: Lippincott Williams & Wilkins.

Flicker, S., Haans, D., & Skinner, H. (2004). Ethical dilemmas in research on Internet communities. *Qualitative Health Research, 14*, 124–134.

Fogg, T., Wightman, C. W. (2000). Improving transcription of qualitative research interviews with speech recognition technology. Paper presented at Annual Meeting of American Educational Research Association, New Orleans, April, 2000.

Fontana, A., & Frey, J. H. (2003). The interview: From structured questions to negotiated text. In N. K. Denzin & Y. S. Lincoln (Eds.), *Collecting and interpreting qualitative materials* (pp.61–106). Thousand Oaks, CA: Sage.

Fonteyn, M. E., Kuipers, B., & Grober, S. J. (1993). A description of the think-aloud method and protocol analysis. *Qualitative Health Research, 3*, 430–441.

Fonteyn, M., Vettese, M., Lancaster, D., & Bauer-Wu, S. (2008). Developing a codebook to guide content analysis of expressive writing transcripts. *Applied Nursing Research, 21,* 165–168.

Forbat, L., & Henderson, J. (2003). "Stuck in the middle with you": The ethics and process of qualitative research with two people in an intimate relationship. *Qualitative Health Research, 13,* 1453–1462.

Fowler, F. J. (1995). *Improving survey questions.* Thousand Oaks, CA: Sage.

Fowler, F. J. (2009). *Survey research methods* (4th ed.). Thousand Oaks, CA: Sage.

Fowler, F. J., & Mangione, T. W. (1990). *Standardized survey interviewing: Minimizing interviewer-related error.* Thousand Oaks, CA: Sage.

Fox-Wasylyshyn, S., & El-Masri, M. (2005). Handling missing data in self-report measures. *Research in Nursing & Health, 28*(6), 488–495.

Frank-Stromberg, M., & Olsen, S. J. (Eds.). (2004). *Instruments for clinical health-care research* (3rd ed.). Sudbury, MA: Jones and Bartlett.

Frith, H., & Harcourt, D. (2007). Using photographs to capture women's experiences with chemotherapy: Reflecting on the method. *Qualitative Health Research, 17,* 1340–1350.

Froman, R. (2008). Hitting the bull's eye rather than shooting yourself between the eyes. *Research in Nursing & Health, 31,* 399–401.

Froman, R., & Schmitt, M. H. (2003). Thinking both inside and outside the box on measurement articles. *Research in Nursing & Health, 26,* 335–336.

Gable, R. K., & Wolf, M. B. (1993). *Instrument development in the affective domain* (2nd ed.). Boston: Kluwer Academic.

Gadamer, H. G. (1975). *Truth and method.* (G. Borden & J. Cumming Trans.). London: Sheed and Ward.

Gadamer, H. G. (1976). *Philosophical hermeneutics.* (D. E. Linge, Ed. & Trans.). Berkeley: University of California Press.

Gaglio, B., Nelson, C., & King, D. (2006). The role of rapport: Lessons learned from conducting research in a primary care setting. *Qualitative Health Research, 16,* 723–734.

Galvan, J. L. (2009). *Writing literature reviews: A guide for students of the social and behavioral sciences* (4th ed.). Los Angeles: Pyrczak.

Gamel, C., Grypdonck, M., Hengevels, M., & Davis, B. (2001). A method to develop a nursing intervention: The contribution of qualitative studies to the process. *Journal of Advanced Nursing, 33,* 806–819.

Garrard, J. (2006). *Health sciences literature review made easy: The matrix method* (2nd ed.) Boston: Jones and Bartlett.

Gawlinski, A. & Rutledge, D. (2008). Selecting a model for evidence-based practice changes. *AACN Advanced Critical Care, 19,* 291–300.

Gearing, R. E. (2004). Bracketing in research: A typology. *Qualitative Health Research, 14*(10), 1429–1452.

Gee, J. P. (1996). *Social linguistics and literacies: Ideology in discourses* (2nd ed.). London: Taylor & Francis.

Gennaro, S. (2008). Sing of significance. *Journal of Nursing Scholarship, 40,* 99.

Gilgun, J. F. (2004). Qualitative methods and the development of clinical assessment tools. *Qualitative Health Research, 14,* 1008–1019.

Gilgun, J. (2005). "Grab" and good science: Writing up the results of qualitative research. *Qualitative Health Research, 15,* 256–262.

Giorgi, A. (1985). *Phenomenology and psychological research.* Pittsburgh, PA: Duquesne University Press.

Giorgi, A. (1989). Some theoretical and practical issues regarding the psychological and phenomenological method. *Saybrook Review, 7,* 71–85.

Giorgi, A. (2005). The phenomenologicql movement and research in the human sciences. *Nursing Science Quarterly, 18,* 75–82.

Glaser, B. (1978). *Theoretical sensitivity.* Mill Valley, CA: Sociology Press.

Glaser, B. (1992). *Emergence versus forcing: Basics of grounded theory analysis.* Mill Valley, CA: Sociology Press.

Glaser, B. (1998). *Doing grounded theory: Issues and discussions.* Mill Valley, CA: Sociology Press.

Glaser, B. (2001). *The grounded theory perspective: Conceptualization contrasted with description.* Mill Valley, CA: Sociology Press.

Glaser, B. (2002). Conceptualisation: On theory and theorizing using grounded theory. In A. Bron & M. Schemmenn (Eds.), *Social science theories and adult education research* (pp. 313–335). Munster: Lit Verlag.

Glaser, B. (2003). *The grounded theory perspective II: Description's remodeling of grounded theory methodology.* Mill Valley, CA: Sociology Press.

Glaser, B. (2005). *The grounded theory perspective III: Theoretical coding.* Mill Valley, CA: Sociology Press.

Glaser, B. (2007). *Doing formal grounded theory: A proposal.* Mill Valley, CA: Sociology Press.

Glaser, B. G., & Strauss, A. (1967). *The discovery of grounded theory: Strategies for qualitative research.* New York: Aldine de Gruyter.

Glasgow, R. E. (2006). RE-AIMing research for application: Ways to improve evidence for family medicine. *Journal of the American Board of Family Medicine, 19,* 11–19.

Glasgow, R. E., Magid, D., Beck, A., Ritzwoller, D., & Estabrooks, P. (2005). Practical clinical trials for translating research to practice: Design and measurement recommendations. *Medical Care, 43,* 551–557.

Gobo, G. (2008). *Doing ethnography.* Thousand Oaks, CA: Sage.

Godwin, M., Ruhland, L., Casson, I., MacDonald, S., Delva, D., Birtwhistle, R., Lam, M., & Seguin, R. (2003).

Pragmatic controlled clinical trials in primary care: The struggle between external and internal validity. *BMC Medical Research Methodology, 3,* 28.

Grant, J. S., & Davis, L. T. (1997). Selection and use of content experts in instrument development. *Research in Nursing & Health, 20,* 269–274.

Gravetter, F., & Wallnau, L. (2007). *Statistics for the behavioral sciences* (7th ed.). Belmont, CA: Wadsworth.

Greene, J. C. (2007). *Mixing methods in social inquiry.* San Francisco: Jossey-Bass.

Grey, M. (2000). Top 10 tips for successful grantsmanship. *Research in Nursing & Health, 23,* 91–92.

Groleau, D., Zelkowitz, P., & Cabral, I. (2009). Enhancing generazability: Moving from an intimate to a political voice. *Qualitative Health Research, 19,* 416–426.

Gross, D. (2005). On the merits of attention control groups. *Research in Nursing & Health, 28*(2), 93–94.

Gross, D., & Fogg, L. (2001). Clinical trials in the 21st century: The case for participant-centered research. *Research in Nursing & Health, 24,* 530–539.

Guadagno, L., VandeWeerd, C., Stevens, D., Abraham, I., Paveza, G., & Fulmer, T. (2004). Using PDAs in data collection. *Applied Nursing Research, 17,* 283–291.

Guba, E. (1978). *Toward a methodology of naturalistic inquiry in educational evaluations.* Los Angeles: University of California, Center for the Study of Evaluation.

Guba, E., & Lincoln, Y. (1994). Competing paradigms in qualitative research. In N. Denzin & Y. Lincoln (Eds.). *Handbook of qualitative research* (pp. 105–117). Thousand Oaks, CA: Sage.

Gubrium, J. F., & Holstein, J. A. (Eds.). (2001). *Handbook of interview research: Context and method* (2nd ed.). Thousand Oaks, CA: Sage.

Gul, R. B., & Ali, P. (2010). Clinical trials: The challenge of recruitment and retention of participants. *Journal of Clinical Nursing, 19,* 227–233.

Gunning, R. (1968). *The technique of clear writing* (Rev. ed.). New York: McGraw-Hill.

Guyatt, G., & Rennie, D., Meade, M., & Cook, D. (2008). *Users' guide to the medical literature: Essentials of evidence-based clinical practice* (2nd ed.). New York: McGraw Hill.

Hagens, C., Dobrow, M., & Chafe, R. (2009). Interviewee transcript review: Assessing the impact on qualitative research. *BMC Medical Research Methodology, 9,* 47.

Haidet, K. K., Tate, J., Divirgilio-Thomas, D., Kolanowski, A., & Happ, M. (2009). Methods to improve reliability of video-recorded behavioral data. *Research in Nursing & Health, 32,* 465–474.

Hair, J., Black, W., Babin, B., Anderson, R., & Tatham, R. (2009). *Multivariate data analysis* (7th ed.). Upper Saddle River, NJ: Prentice-Hall.

Hall, W. A., Long, B., Bermbach, N., Jordan, S., & Patterson, K. (2005). Qualitative teamwork issues and strategies: Coordination through mutual adjustment. *Qualitative Health Research, 15,* 394–410.

Hambleton, R. K., Swaminathan, H., & Rogers, H. J. (1991). *Fundamentals of item response theory.* Newbury Park, CA: Sage Publications.

Hammersley, M. (1992). *What's wrong with ethnography? Methodological explorations.* London: Routledge.

Happ, M., Dabbs, A., Tate, J., Hricik, A., & Erlen, J. (2006). Exemplars of mixed methods data combination and analysis. *Nursing Research, 55,* S43–S49.

Harden, A., & Thomas, J. (2005). Methodologic issues in combining diverse study types in systematic reviews. *International Journal of Social Research Methodology, 8,* 257–271.

Hardicre, J., Devitt, P., & Coad, J. (2007). Ten steps to successful poster presentation. *British Journal of Nursing, 16,* 398–401.

Harrington, D. (2008). *Confirmatory factor analysis.* New York: Oxford University Press.

Harris, M., Vanderboom, C., & Hughes, R. (2009). Nursing-sensitive safety and quality outcomes: The taming of a wicked problem. *Applied Nursing Research, 22,* 146–151.

Heath, H., & Cowley, S. (2004). Developing a grounded theory approach: A comparison of Glaser and Strauss. *International Journal of Nursing Studies, 41,* 141–150.

Heidegger, M. (1962). *Being and time.* New York: Harper & Row.

Heidegger, M. (1971). *Poetry, language, thought.* New York: Harper & Row.

Hertzog, M. (2008). Consideration in determining sample size for pilot studies. *Research in Nursing & Health, 31,* 180–191.

Hesse-Biber, S., (Ed.). (2007). *Handbook of feminist research: Theory and praxis.* Thousand Oaks, CA: Sage Publications.

Heyman, B., & Cronin, P. (2005). Writing for publication: Adapting academic work into articles. *British Journal of Nursing, 14,* 400–403.

Higdon, J., & Topp, R. (2004). How to develop a budget for a research proposal. *Western Journal of Nursing Research, 26,* 922–929.

Higgins, P. A., & Daly, B. J. (1999). Research methodology issues related to interviewing the mechanically ventilated patient. *Western Journal of Nursing Research, 21,* 773–784.

Higgins, J., & Green, S. (Eds.). (2008). *Cochrane handbook for systematic reviews of interventions.* Chichester, England: Wiley-Blackwell.

Hilton, A., & Skrutkowski, M. (2002). Translating instruments into other language: Development and testing processes. *Cancer Nursing, 25,* 1–7.

Holmes, S. (2009). Methodological and ethical considerations in designing an Internet study of quality of life. *International Journal of Nursing Studies, 46,* 394–405.

Holtzclaw, B. J., & Hanneman, S. K. (2002). Use of non-human biobehavioral models in critical care nursing research. *Critical Care Nursing Quarterly, 24*(4), 30–40.

Homer, C. S. (2002). Using the Zelen design in randomized controlled trials: Debates and controversies. *Journal of Advanced Nursing, 38,* 200–207.

Horsley, J. A., Crane, J., & Bingle, J. D. (1978). Research utilization as an organizational process. *Journal of Nursing Administration, 8,* 4–6.

Hosmer, D., & Lemeshow, S. (2000). *Applied logistic regression.* New York: John Wiley.

Hosmer, D., Lemeshow, S., & May, S. (2008). *Applied survival analysis: regression modeling of time to event data* (2nd ed.). New York: John Wiley.

Houser, J., & Bokovoy, J. (2006). *Clinical research in practice: A guide for the bedside scientist.* Boston: Jones & Bartlett.

Hsieh, H., & Shannon, S. (2005). Three approaches to qualitative content analysis. *Qualitative Health Research, 15,* 1277–1288.

Huberman, A. M., & Miles, M. (1994). Data management and analysis methods. In N. K. Denzin & Y. S. Lincoln (Eds.). *Handbook of qualitative research* (1st ed.). Thousand Oaks, CA: Sage.

Hunter, A., Lusardi, P., Zucker, D., Jacelon, C., & Chandler, G. (2002). Making meaning: The creative component in qualitative research. *Qualitative Health Research, 12,* 388–398.

Husserl, E. (1962). *Ideas: General introduction to pure phenomenology.* New York: Macmillan.

Ingersoll, G. L. (2005). Generating evidence through outcomes management. In B. Melnyk & E. Fineout-Overholt (Eds.). *Evidence-based practice in nursing and healthcare.* Philadelphia: Lippincott Williams & Wilkins.

Inouye, S. K., & Fiellin, D. A. (2005). An evidence-based guide to writing grant proposals for clinical research. *Annals of Internal Medicine, 142,* 274–282.

International Committee of Medical Journal Editors. (2009). *Uniform requirements for manuscripts submitted to biomedical journals.* Retrieved May 5, 2010, from www.icmje.org.

Jacobson, G. A. (2005). Vulnerable research participants: Anyone may qualify. *Nursing Science Quarterly, 18,* 359–363.

Jack, S. (2008). Guidelines to support nurse-researchers' reflect on role conflict in qualitative interviewing. *The Open Nursing Journal, 2,* 58–62.

Jeffers, B. & Whittemore, R. (2005). Research environments that promote integrity. *Nursing Research, 54,* 63–70.

Jennings, B. M. (2010). It takes a village to publish a manuscript in *Research in Nursing & Health, 33,* 175–178.

Johnson, B., & Turner, L. (2003). Data collection strategies in mixed methods research. In A. Tashakkori & C. Teddlie (Eds.), *Handbook of mixed methods in social and behavioral research* (pp. 297–319). Thousand Oaks, CA: Sage.

Johnson, J. E. (1999). Self-Regulation Theory and coping with physical illness. *Research in Nursing & Health, 22,* 435–448.

Johnson, S. H. (1996). Adapting a thesis to publication style: Meeting editor's expectations. *Dimensions of Critical Care Nursing, 15,* 160–167.

Jones, R. (2003). Survey data collection using audio computer assisted self-interview. *Western Journal of Nursing Research, 25,* 349–358.

Jootun, D., McGhee, G., & Marland, G. (2009). Reflexivity: Promoting rigour in qualitative research. *Nursing Standard, 23,* 42–46.

Junker, B. H. (1960). *Field work: An introduction to the social sciences.* Chicago: University of Chicago Press.

Kahn, D. L. (2000). How to conduct research. In M. Z. Cohen, D. L. Kahn, & R. H. Steeves (Eds.), *Hermeneutic phenomenological research* (pp. 57–70). Thousand Oaks, CA: Sage.

Kang, D., Davis, L., Huberman, B., Rice, M., & Broome, M. (2005). Hiring the right people and management of research staff. *Western Journal of Nursing Research, 27,* 1059–1066.

Kanner, S., Langerman, S., & Grey, M. (2004). Ethical considerations for a child's participation in research. *Journal for Specialists in Pediatric Nursing, 9,* 15–23.

Kearney, M. H. (1998). Ready-to-wear: Discovering grounded formal theory. *Research in Nursing & Health, 21,* 179–186.

Kearney, M., & Simonelli, M. (2006). Intervention fidelity: Lessons learned from an unsuccessful pilot study. *Applied Nursing Research, 19,* 163–166.

Keely, B. (2004). Planning and creating effective scientific posters. *Journal of Continuing Education in Nursing, 35,* 182–185.

Keeney, S., Hasson, F., & McKenna, H. (2006). Consulting the oracle: Ten lessons from using the Delphi technique in nursing research. *Journal of Advanced Nursing, 53,* 205–212.

Keller, C., Fleury, J., Sidano, S., & Ainsworth, B. (2009). Fidelity to theory in PA intervention research. *Western Journal of Nursing Research, 31,* 289–311.

Kemper, E., Stringfield, S., & Teddlie, C. (2003). Mixed methods sampling strategies in social science research. In A. Tashakkori & C. Teddlie (Eds.), *Handbook of mixed methods in social and behavioral research* (pp. 273–296). Thousand Oaks, CA: Sage.

Kennedy, H. P. (2004). Enhancing Delphi research: Methods and results. *Journal of Advanced Nursing, 45,* 504–511.

Kerig, P., & Baucom, D. (2004). *Couple observational coding systems.* Mahwah, NJ: Lawrence Erlbaum.

Kerig, P., & Lindahl, K. (2001). *Family observational coding systems: Resources for systematic research.* Mahwah, NJ: Lawrence Erlbaum.

Kerlinger, F. N., & Lee, H. B. (2000). *Foundations of behavioral research* (4th ed.). Orlando, FL: Harcourt College.

Kidd, P. S., & Parshall, M. B. (2000). Getting the focus and the group: Enhancing analytic rigor in focus group research. *Qualitative Health Research, 10*, 293–308.

Kimchi, J., Polivka, B., & Stevenson, J. S. (1991). Triangulation: Operational definitions. *Nursing Research, 40*, 364–366.

Kline, R. (2005). *Principles and practice of structural equation modeling* (2nd ed.). New York: Guilford Press.

Knafl, K., & Deatrick, J. (2005). Top 10 tips for successful qualitative grantsmanship. *Research in Nursing & Health, 28*, 441–443.

Knapp, T. R. (1970). N vs. N − 1. *American Educational Research Journal, 7*, 625–626.

Knapp, T. R. (1994). Regression analysis: What to report. *Nursing Research, 43*, 187–189.

Koch, T., & Kralik, D. (2006). *Participatory action research in health care.* Oxford: Blackwell.

Kolcaba, K. (2003). *Comfort theory and practice.* New York: Springer.

Kralik, D., Proce, K., Warren, J., & Koch, T. (2006). Issues in data generation using email group conversations for nursing research. *Journal of Advanced Nursing, 53(2)*, 213–220.

Krippendorff, K. (2005). *Content analysis: An introduction to its methodology.* Thousand Oaks, CA: Sage.

Krueger, R., & Casey, M. (2008). *Focus groups: A practical guide for applied research* (4th ed.). Thousand Oaks, CA: Sage.

Kuzel, A. J. (2002). Some lessons from the story of a funded project. *Qualitative Health Research, 12*, 140–142.

Kwak, C., & Clayton-Matthews, A. (2002). Multinomial logistic regression. *Nursing Research, 51*, 404–409.

Labov, W., & Waletzky, J. (1967). Narrative analysis: Oral versions of personal experience. In J. Helm (Ed.), *Essays on the verbal and visual arts* (pp. 12–44). Seattle: University of Washington Press.

Lalor, J. G., Begley, C. M., & Devane, D. (2006). Exploring painful experiences: Impact of emotional narratives on members of a qualitative research team. *Journal of Advanced Nursing, 56*, 607–616.

Lambert, M. F., & Wood, J. (2000). Incorporating patient preferences into randomized trials. *Journal of Clinical Epidemiology, 53*, 163–166.

Lange, J. W. (2002). Methodological concerns for non-Hispanic investigators conducting research with Hispanic Americans. *Research in Nursing & Health, 25*, 411–419.

Lapadat, J. C. (2000). Problematizing transcription: Purpose, paradigm and quality. International *Journal of Social Research Methodology, 3*, 203–219.

Lather, P. (1986). Issues of validity in openly ideological research: Between a rock and a hard place. *Interchange, 17*, 63–84.

Lather, P. (1991). Getting smart: Feminist research and pedagogy with/in the postmodern. New York: Routledge.

Lauver, D. R., Ward, S. E., Heidrich, S. M., Keller, M. L., Bowers, B. J., Brennan, P. F., Kirchhoff, K. T., & Wells, T. J. (2002). Patient-centered interventions. *Research in Nursing & Health, 25*, 246–255.

Lazarsfeld, P. (1955). Foreword. In H. Hyman (Ed.), *Survey design and analysis.* New York: The Free Press.

Lazarus, R. (2006). *Stress and emotion: A new synthesis.* New York: Springer.

Lazarus, R., & Folkman, S. (1984). *Stress, appraisal, and coping.* New York: Springer.

Leathem, C., Cupples, M., Byrne, M., O'Malley, M., Houlihan, A., Murphy, A., & Smith, S. (2009). Identifying strategies to maximize recruitment and retention of practices and patients in a multicentre randomized controlled trial of an intervention to optimize secondary prevention for coronary heart disease in primary care. *BMC Medical Research Methodology, 9,* 40.

LeCompte, M., & Goetz, J. (1982). Problems of reliability and validity in ethnographic research. *Review of Educational Research, 52,* 31–60.

Leeman, J., Jackson, B., & Sandelowski, M. (2006). An evaluation of how well research reports facilitate the use of findings in practice. *Journal of Nursing Scholarship, 38,* 171–177.

Leininger, M. M. (1985). Life-health-care history: Purposes, methods and techniques. In M. M. Leininger (Ed.), *Qualitative research methods in nursing* (pp. 119–132). New York: Grune & Stratton.

Leininger, M. M. (Ed.). (1985). *Qualitative research methods in nursing.* New York: Grune and Stratton.

Leininger, M. M., & McFarland, M. (2006). *Culture care diversity and universality: A worldwide nursing theory* (2nd ed.). Sudbury, MA: Jones & Bartlett.

Lenz, E. R., Pugh, L. C., Milligan, R. A., Gift, A., & Suppe, F. (1997). The middle-range theory of unpleasant symptoms. *Advances in Nursing Science, 19,* 14–27.

Lesaffre, E. (2008). Superiority, equivalence, and non-inferiority trials. *Bulletin of the NYU Hospital for Joint Diseases, 66,* 150–154.

Levine, M. E. (1996). The conservation principles: A retrospective. *Nursing Science Quarterly, 9,* 38–41.

Levy, P., & Lemeshow, S. (2009). *Sampling of populations: Methods and applications* (4th ed.) New York: John Wiley & Sons.

Lewenson, S. B. (2003). Historical research approach. In H. J. Speziale & D. R. Carpenter (Eds.), *Qualitative research in nursing: Advancing the humanistic perspective* (pp. 207–233). Philadelphia: Lippincott Williams & Wilkins.

Lewins, A., & Silver, C. (2007). *Using software in qualitative research.* Thousand Oaks, CA: Sage.

Liberati, A., Altman, D., Tetzlaff, J., Mulrow, C., Gotzsche, P., Ioannidis, J., Clarke, M., Devereaux, P. J., Kleijnen, J., &

Moher, D. (2009). The PRISMA statement for reporting systematic reviews and meta-analyses of studies that evaluate health care interventions: Explanation and elaboration. *Journal of Clinical Epidemiology, 62,* e1–e34.

Lincoln, Y. S., & Guba, E. G. (1985). *Naturalistic inquiry.* Newbury Park, CA: Sage.

Lindsay, B. (2004). Randomized controlled trials of socially complex nursing interventions: Creating bias and unreliability? *Journal of Advanced Nursing, 45,* 84–94.

Lindeke, L., Hauck, M. R., & Tanner, M. (2000). Practical issues in obtaining child assent for research. *Journal of Pediatric Nursing, 15,* 99–104.

Lipsey, M. W. (1990). *Design sensitivity: Statistical power for experimental research.* Newbury Park, CA: Sage.

Lipsey, M. W., & Wilson, D. B. (2001). *Practical meta-analysis.* Thousand Oaks, CA: Sage.

Lipson, J. G. (1991). The use of self in ethnographic research. In J. M. Morse (Ed.). *Qualitative nursing research: A contemporary dialogue* (pp. 73–89). Newbury Park, CA: Sage.

Locke, L., Spirduso, W., & Silverman, S. (2007). *Proposals that work: A guide for planning dissertations and grant proposals* (5th ed.). Thousand Oaks, CA: Sage.

Loehlin, J. C. (2003). *Latent variable models: An introduction to factor, path, and structural equation analysis.* (4th ed.). Mahwah, NJ: Lawrence Erlbaum Associates.

Logan, J., & Graham, I. (1998). Toward a comprehensive interdisciplinary model of health care research use. *Science Communication, 20,* 227–246.

Lopez, K. A., & Willis, D. G. (2004). Descriptive versus interpretive phenomenology: Their contributions to nursing knowledge. *Qualitative Health Research, 14,* 726–735.

Lowe, N. K., & Ryan-Wenger, N. M. (1992). Beyond Campbell and Fiske: Assessment of convergent and discriminant validity. *Research in Nursing & Health, 15,* 67–75.

Lucas, P., Barid, J., Arai, L., Law, C., & Roberts, H. (2007). Worked examples of alternative methods for the synthesis of qualitative and quantitative research in systematic reviews. *BMC Medical Research Methodology, 7,* 4.

Lundy, K. S. (2012). Historical research. In P. L. Munhall (Ed.). *Nursing research: A qualitative perspective* (5th ed.) (pp. 381–398). Sudbury, MA: Jones & Bartlett.

Lusk, B., & Sacharski, S. (2005). Dead or alive: HIPAA's impact on nursing historical research. *Nursing History Review, 13,* 189–197.

Lusk, S. L. (2004). Developing an outstanding grant application. *Western Journal of Nursing Research, 26,* 367–373.

Lutz, K. F., Shelton, K. C., Robrecht, L. C., Hatton, D. C., & Beckett, A. K. (2000). Use of Certificates of Confidentiality in nursing research. *Journal of Nursing Scholarship, 32,* 185–188.

MacDonald, K., & Greggans, A. (2008). Dealing with chaos and complexity: The reality of interviewing children and families in their own homes. *Journal of Clinical Nursing, 17,* 3123–3130.

MacDonald, S., Newburn-Cook, C., Schopflocher, D., & Richter, S. (2009). Addressing nonresponse bias in postal surveys. *Public Health Nursing, 26,* 95–105.

Mackey, S. (2005). Phenomenological nursing research: Methodologic insights derived from Heidigger's interpretive phenomenology. *International Journal of Nursing Studies, 42,* 179–186.

MacLean, L., Meyer, M., & Estable, A. (2004). Improving accuracy of transcripts in qualitative research. *Qualitative Health Research, 14*(1), 113–123.

Magee, T., Lee, S., Giuliano, K., & Munro, B. (2006). Generating new knowledge from existing data. *Nursing Research, 55,* S50–S56.

Magnani, R., Sabin, K., Saidel, T., & Heckathorn, D. (2005). Review of sampling hard-to-reach and hidden populations for HIV surveillance. *AIDS, 19,* S67–72.

Mahoney, E., Trudeau, S., Penyack, S., & MacLeod, C. (2006). Challenges to intervention implementation: Lessons learned in the Bathing Persons with Alzheimer's Disease at Home study. *Nursing Research, 55,* S10–16.

Manderson, L., Kelaher, M., & Woelz-Sirling, N. (2001). Developing qualitative databases for multiple users. *Qualitative Health research, 11,* 149–160.

Mann, C., & Stewart, F. (2001). Internet interviewing. In J. F. Gubrium & J. A. Holstein. *Handbook of interview research: Context and method* (pp. 603–627). Thousand Oaks, CA: Sage.

Martyn, K., & Belli, R. (2002). Retrospective data collection using event history calendars. *Nursing Research, 51,* 270–274.

McCain, N. L., Gray, D. P., Walter, J. M., & Robins, J. (2005). Implementing a comprehensive approach to the study of health dynamics using the psychoimmunology paradigm. *Advances in Nursing Science, 28*(4), 320–332.

McCleary, L. (2002). Using multiple imputation for analysis of incomplete data in clinical research. *Nursing Research, 51,* 339–343.

McConnell, E. A. (2000). Publishing opportunities outside the United States. *Journal of Nursing Scholarship, 32,* 87–92.

McCormick, J., Rodney, P., & Varcoe, C. (2003). Reinterpretations across studies: An approach to meta-analysis. *Qualitative Health Research, 13,* 933–944.

McEwen, M., & Wills, E. (2006). *Theoretical basis for nursing* (2nd ed.). Philadelphia: Lippincott Williams & Wilkins.

McGhee, G., Marland, G., & Atkinson, J. (2007). Grounded theory research: Literature reviewing and reflexivity. *Journal of Advanced Nursing, 60,* 334–342.

McGuire, D., DeLoney, V., Yeager, K., Owen, D., Peterson, D., Lin, L., & Webster, J. (2000). Maintaining study validity in a changing clinical environment. *Nursing Research, 49,* 231–235.

McKnight, P., McKnight, K., Sidani, S., & Figueredo, A. (2007). *Missing data: A gentle introduction.* New York: Guilford Press.

McNeill, P. (1993). *The ethics and politics of human experimentation.* Cambridge, UK: Cambridge University Press.

Medical Research Council (2000). *A framework for development and evaluation of RCTs for complex interventions to improve health.* London: MRC. Available at: http://www.mrc.ac.uk.

Meleis, A. I., Sawyer, L. M., Im, E., Hilfinger Messias, D., & Schumacher, K. (2000). Experiencing transitions: An emerging middle-range theory. *Advances in Nursing Science, 23,* 12–28.

Melnyk, B. M., & Fineout-Overholt, E. (2011). *Evidence-based practice in nursing and healthcare* (2nd ed.). Philadelphia: Lippincott Williams & Wilkins.

Mendlinger, S., & Cwikel, J. (2008). Spiraling between qualitative and quantitative data on women's health behaviors: A double helix model for mixed methods. *Quantitative Health Research, 18,* 280–293.

Mertens, D. M. (2007). Transformative paradigm: Mixed methods and social justice. *Journal of Mixed Methods Research, 1,* 212–225.

Miles, M., & Huberman, M. (1994). *Qualitative data analysis: An expanded sourcebook* (2nd ed.). Thousand Oaks, CA: Sage.

Miller, F., & Alvarado, K. (2005). Incorporating documents into qualitative nursing research. *Journal of Nursing Scholarship, 37,* 348–353.

Miller, J. E. (2007). Preparing and presenting effective research posters. *Health Services Research, 42,* 311–328.

Milne, J., & Oberle, K. (2005). Enhancing rigor in qualitative description. *Journal of Wound, Ostomy, & Continence Nursing, 32,* 413–420.

Misco, T. (2007). The frustrations of reader generalizability and grounded theory: Alternative considerations for transferability. *Journal of Research Practice, 3,* 1–11.

Mishel, M. H. (1990). Reconceptualization of the Uncertainty in Illness Theory. *Image: Journal of Nursing Scholarship, 22,* 256–262.

Mitchell, P., & Lang, N. (2004). Framing the problem of measuring and improving healthcare quality: Has the quality health outcomes model been useful? *Medical Care, 42,* II4–11.

Mitchell, P., Ferketich, S., & Jennings, B. (1998). Quality health outcomes model. *Image: The Journal of Nursing Scholarship, 30,* 43–46.

Moffatt, S., White, M., Mackintosh, J., & Howel, D. (2006). Using quantitative and qualitative data in health services research—what happens when mixed method findings conflict? *BMC Health Services Research, 6,* 28.

Moher, D., Hopewell, S., Schulz, K. F., Montori, V., Gotzsche, P., Devereaux, P., Elbourne, D., Egger, M., Altman, D. G., & Consolidated Standards of Reporting Trials Group. (2010). CONSORT 2010 explanation and elaboration: Updated guidelines for reporting parallel-group randomised trials. *BMJ, 340,* c869.

Moher, D., Liberati, A., Tetzlaff, J., Altman, D., & The PRISMA Group (2009). Preferred reporting items for systematic reviews and meta-analyses: The PRISMA statement. *Journal of Clinical Epidemiology, 62,* 1006–1012.

Moloney, M., Dietrich, A., Strickland, O., & Myerburg, S. (2003). Using Internet discussion boards as virtual focus groups. *Advances in Nursing Science, 26,* 274–286.

Montgomery, P., & Bailey, P. (2007). Field notes and theoretical memos in grounded theory. *Western Journal of Nursing Research, 29,* 65–79.

Moore, L. W., Augspurger, P., King, M. O., & Proffitt, C. (2001). Insights on the poster presentation and presentation process. *Applied Nursing Research, 14,* 100–104.

Morgan, D. L. (2001). Focus group interviewing in J. F. Gubrium & J. A. Holstein (Eds.). *Handbook of interview research: Context and method* (2nd ed., pp. 141–159). Thousand Oaks, CA: Sage.

Morris, S. M. (2001). Joint and individual interviewing in the context of cancer. *Qualitative Health Research, 11,* 553–567.

Morrison-Beedy, D., Côté-Arsenault, D., & Feinstein, N. (2001). Maximizing results with focus groups. *Applied Nursing Research, 14,* 48–53.

Morrow, R. A., & Brown, D. D. (1994). *Critical theory and methodology.* Thousand Oaks, CA: Sage.

Morse, J. M. (1991a). Approaches to qualitative-quantitative methodological triangulation. *Nursing Research, 40,* 120–123.

Morse, J. M. (1991b). Strategies for sampling. In J. M. Morse (Ed.), *Qualitative nursing research: A contemporary dialogue.* Newbury Park, CA: Sage.

Morse, J. M. (1999). Myth # 93: Reliability and validity are not relevant to qualitative inquiry. *Qualitative Health Research, 9,* 717–718.

Morse, J. M. (2000). Determining sample size. *Qualitative Health Research, 10,* 3–5.

Morse, J. M. (2002). Theory innocent or theory smart? *Qualitative Health Research, 12,* 295–296.

Morse, J. M. (2003a). Biasphobia. *Qualitative Health Research, 13,* 891–892.

Morse, J. M. (2003b). Principles of mixed methods and multimethod research design. In A. Tashakkori & C. Teddlie (Eds.), *Handbook of mixed methods in social and behavioral research* (pp. 189–208). Thousand Oaks, CA: Sage.

Morse, J. M. (2004a). Constructing qualitatively derived theory. *Qualitative Health Research, 14,* 1387–1395.

Morse, J. M. (2004b). Qualitative comparison: Appropriateness, equivalence, and fit. *Qualitative Health Research, 14,* 1323–1325.

Morse, J. M. (2005). Beyond the clinical trial: Expanding criteria for evidence. *Qualitative Health Resaerch, 15,* 3–4.

Morse, J. M. (2006a). The scope of qualitative derived clinical interventions. *Qualitative Health Research, 16,* 591–593.

Morse, J. M. (2006b). Insight, inference, evidence, and verification: Creating a legitimate discipline. *International Journal of Qualitative Methods, 5*(1), Article 8. Retrieved November 4, 2010, from http://ejournals.library.ualberta.ca/index.php/IJQM/issue/ view/362.

Morse, J. M. (2009). Mixing qualitative methods. *Qualitative Health Research, 19,* 1523.

Morse, J. M., Barrett, M., Mayan, M., Olson, K., & Spiers, J. (2002). Verification strategies for establishing reliability and validity in qualitative research. *International Journal of Qualitative Methods, 1*(2), Article 2. Retrieved November 4, 2010, from http:// ejournals.library.ualberta.ca/index.php/IJQM/issue/ view/384.

Morse, J. M., & Field, P. A. (1995). *Qualitative research methods for health professionals* (2nd ed.). Thousand Oaks, CA: Sage.

Morse, J., Hupcey, J., Mitcham, C., & Lenz, E. (1996). Concept analysis in nursing research: A critical appraisal. *Scholarly Inquiry for Nursing Practice, 10,* 253–277.

Morse, J., Penrod, J., & Hupcey, J. (2000). Qualitative outcome analysis: Evaluating nursing interventions for complex clinical phenomena. *Journal of Nursing Scholarship, 32,* 125–130.

Morse, J. M., & Richards, L. (2002). *Read me first for a user's guide to qualitative methods.* Thousand Oaks, CA: Sage.

Morse, J. M., Solberg, S. M., Neander, W. L., Bottorff, J. L., & Johnson, J. L. (1990). Concepts of caring and caring as a concept. *Advances in Nursing Science, 13,* 1–14.

Motulsky, H. (1995). *Intuitive biostatistics.* New York: Oxford University Press.

Munhall, P. L. (2012). *Nursing research: A qualitative perspective* (5th ed.). Sudbury, MA: Jones & Bartlett.

NANDA International. (2009). *Nursing diagnoses: definitions and classification,* 2009–2011. Philadelphia: Author.

National Commission for the Protection of Human Subjects of Biomedical and Behavioral Research. (1978). *Belmont report: Ethical principles and guidelines for research involving human subjects.* Washington, DC: U.S. Government Printing Office.

National Institute for Nursing Research (2006). *NINR strategic plan, 2006–2010.* Bethesda, MD: NINR. Retrieved January 22, 2010, from http://www.ninr.nih.gov/NR/rdonlyres/9021E5EB-B2BA-47EA-B5DB-1E4DB11B1289/4894/NINR_StrategicPlanWebsite.pdf.

Naylor, M. D. (1990). An example of a research grant application: Comprehensive discharge planning for the elderly. *Research in Nursing & Health, 13,* 327–347.

Naylor, M. D. (2003). Nursing intervention research and quality of care. *Nursing Research, 52,* 380–385.

Nelson, L., & Morrison-Beedy, D. (2008). Research team training: Moving beyond job descriptions. *Applied Nursing Research, 21,* 159–164.

Nepal, V. (2010). On mixing qualitative methods. *Qualitative Health Research, 20,* 281.

Neuman, B., & Fawcett. J. (2001). *The Neuman Systems Model* (4th ed.). Englewood, NJ: Prentice Hall.

Newhouse, R., Dearholt, S., Poe, S., Pugh, L. C., & White, K. M. (2005). Evidence-based practice: A practical approach to implementation. *Journal of Nursing Administration, 35,* 35–40.

Newman, M. (1994). *Health as expanding consciousness* (2nd ed.). New York: National League for Nursing.

Newman, M. A. (1997). Evolution of the theory of health as expanding consciousness. *Nursing Science Quarterly, 10,* 22–25.

Nicol, A., & Pexham, P. (2010). *Displaying your findings: A practical guide for creating figures, posters, and presentations* (6th ed.). Washington, DC: American Psychological Association.

Nightingale, F. (1859). *Notes on nursing: What it is, and what it is not.* Philadelphia: J. B. Lippincott.

Noblit, G., & Hare, R. D. (1988). *Meta-ethnography: Synthesizing qualitative studies.* Newbury Park, CA: Sage.

Northam, S., Trubenbach, M., & Bentov, L. (2000). Nursing journal survey: Information to help you publish. *Nurse Educator, 25,* 227–236.

Northam, S., Yarbrough, S., Haas, B., & Duke, G. (2010). Journal editor survey: Information to help authors publish. *Nurse Educator, 35,* 29–36.

Norušis, M. J. (2008). *SPSS 16.0: Statistical procedures companion.* Upper Saddle River, NJ: Prentice Hall.

Novak, J., & Canas, A. (2006). *The theory underlying concept maps and how to construct them.* (IHMC CmapTools Technical Report 2006-01: Pensacola, FL: Institute for Human and Machine Cognition.

Novick, G. (2008). Is there a bias against telephone interviews in qualitative research? *Research in Nursing & Health, 31,* 391–398.

Nunnally, J., & Bernstein, I. H. (1994). *Psychometric theory* (3rd ed.). New York: McGraw-Hill.

O'Cathain, A. (2009). Mixed methods research in the health sciences: A quiet revolution. *Journal of Mixed Methods Research, 3,* 3–6.

O'Quigley, J. (2008). *Proportional hazards regression.* New York: Springer.

Oermann, M., & Hays, J. (2010). *Writing for publication in nursing* (2nd ed.). Philadelphia: Lippincott Williams & Wilkins.

Oermann, M., Galvin, E., Floyd, J., & Roop, J. (2006). Presenting research to clinicians: Strategies for writing about research findings. *Nurse Researcher, 13,* 66–74.

Ogrinc, G., Mooney, S., Estrada, C., Foster, T., Goldmann, D., Hall, L., Huizinga, M. M., Liu, S. K., Millis, P., Neily, J., Nelson, W., Pronovost, P. J., Provost, L., RubenStein, L. V., Speroff, T., Splaine, M., Thompson, R., Tomolo, A. M., & Watts, B. (2008). The SQUIRE (Standards for QUality Improvement Reporting Excellence) guidelines for quality improvement reporting:

explanation and elaboration. *Quality & Safety in Health Care, 17,* Suppl, 13–32.

Olesen, V. (2000). Feminisms and qualitative research at and into the millennium. In N. K. Denzin & Y. S. Lincoln (Eds.), *Handbook of qualitative research* (2nd ed., pp. 215–255). Thousand Oaks, CA: Sage.

Oliffe, J., Bottorff, J., Kelly, M., & Halpin, M. (2008). Analyzing participant produced photographs from an ethnographic study of fatherhood and smoking. *Research in Nursing & Health, 31,* 529–539.

Olobatuyi, M. (2006). *A user's guide to path analysis.* Lanham, MD: University Press of America.

Olsen, D. P. (2003). HIPAA privacy regulations and nursing research. *Nursing Research, 52,* 344–348.

Onwuegbuzie, A., & Collins, K. (2007). A typology of mixed methods sampling designs in social science research. *The Qualitative Report,* 281–316.

Onwuegbuzie, A., & Leech, N. (2007). Sampling designs in qualitative research: Making the sampling process more public. *The Qualitative Report, 12,* 238–254.

Onwuegbuzie, A., & Teddlie, C. (2003). A framework for analyzing data in mixed methods research. In A. Tashakkori & C. Teddlie (Eds.), *Handbook of mixed methods in social and behavioral research* (pp. 351–384). Thousand Oaks, CA: Sage.

Orem, D. E.. Taylor, S. G., Renpenning, K.M., & Eisenhandler, S. A. (2003). *Self-care theory in nursing: Selected papers of Dorothea Orem.* New York: Springer.

Padgett, D., & Henwood, B. (2009). Obtaining large-scale funding for empowerment-oriented qualitative research: A report from personal experience. *Qualitative Health Research, 19,* 868–874.

Padhye, N., Cron, S., Gusick, G., Hamlin, S., & Hanneman, S. (2009). Randomization for clinical research: An easy-to-use spreadsheet method. *Research in Nursing & Health, 32,* 561–566.

Parker, B., & Steeves, R. (2005). The National Research Service Award: Strategies for developing a successful proposal. *Journal of Professional Nursing, 21,* 23–31.

Parker, M. E. (2006). *Nursing theories and nursing practice.* Philadelphia: F.A. Davis.

Parse, R. R. (1999). *Illuminations: The human becoming theory in practice and research.* Sudbury, MA: Jones & Bartlett.

Parse, R. R. (2001). *Qualitative inquiry. The path of sciencing.* Sudbury, MA: Jones & Bartlett.

Paterson, B. L., Thorne, S. E., Canam, C., & Jillings, C. (2001). *Meta-study of qualitative health research.* Thousand Oaks, CA: Sage.

Patrician, P. (2004). Single-item graphic representational scales. *Nursing Research, 53,* 347–352.

Patrician, P. A. (2002). Multiple imputation for missing data. *Research in Nursing & Health, 25,* 76–84.

Patton, M. (1999). Enhancing the quality and credibility of qualitative analysis. *Health Services Research, 34,* 1189–1208.

Patton, M. Q. (2002). *Qualitative evaluation and research methods* (3rd ed.). Thousand Oaks, CA: Sage.

Patton, M. Q. (2008). *Utilization focused evaluation* (4th ed.). Thousand Oaks, CA: Sage.

Pender, N. J., Murdaugh, C., & Parsons, M. A. (2006). *Health promotion in nursing practice* (5th ed.). Upper Saddle River, NJ: Prentice Hall.

Peplau, H. E. (1997). Peplau's theory of interpersonal relations. *Nursing Science Quarterly, 10,* 162–167.

Peterson, S. J., & Bredow, T. S. (2009). *Middle range theories: Applications to nursing research* (2nd ed.). Philadelphia: Lippincott Williams & Wilkins.

Pett, M., Lackey, N., & Sullivan, J. (2003). *Making sense of factor analysis: The use of factor analysis for instrument development in health care research.* Thousand Oaks, CA: Sage Publications.

Piaggio, G., Elbourne, D., Altman, D., Pocock, S., & Evans S. (2006). Reporting of noninferiority and equivalence randomized trials: An extension of the CONSORT statement. *Journal of the American Medical Association, 295,* 1152–1160.

Plummer, M., & Young, L. (2010). Grounded theory and feminist inquiry: Revitalizing links to the past. *Western Journal of Nursing Research, 32,* 305–321.

Pluye, P., Gagnon, M., Griffiths, F., & Johnson-Lafleur, J. (2009). A scoring system for appraising mixed methods research, and concomitantly appraising qualitative, quantitative and mixed methods primary studies in Mixed Studies Review. *International Journal of Nursing Studies, 46,* 529–546.

Poland, B. D. (1995). Transcription quality as an aspect of rigor in qualitative research. *Qualitative Inquiry, 1,* 190–310.

Polit, D. F. (2010). *Statistics and data analysis for nursing research* (2nd ed.). Upper Saddle River, NJ: Pearson.

Polit, D., & Beck, C. (2006). The content validity index: Are you sure you know what's being reported? *Research in Nursing & Health, 29,* 489–497.

Polit, D. F., & Beck, C. T. (2010). Generalization in qualitative and quantitative research: Myths and strategies. *International Journal of Nursing Studies, 47,* 1451–1458.

Polit, D., Beck, C., & Owen, S. (2007). Is the CVI an acceptable indicator of content validity? Appraisal and recommendations. *Research in Nursing & Health, 30,* 459–467.

Polit, D. F., & Chaboyer, W. (in review). Statistical process control in nursing research.

Polit, D. F., & Gillespie, B. (2009). The use of the intention-to-treat principle in nursing clinical trials. *Nursing Research, 58,* 391–399.

Polit, D. F. & Gillespie, B. (2010). Intention-to-treat in randomized controlled trials: Recommendations for a total trial strategy. *Research in Nursing & Health, 33,* 355–368.

Polit, D., & Gillespie, B., & Griffin, R. (in press). Deliberate ignorance: A systematic review of the use of blinding in nursing clinical trials. *Nursing Research.*

Polit, D. F., & Northam, S. (in press, a). Impact factors in nursing journals. *Nursing Outlook.*

Polit, D. F., & Northam, S. (in press, b). Publishing opportunities for nurse authors in non-nursing journals. *Nurse Educator.*

Polit, D. F., & Sherman, R. (1990). Statistical power in nursing research. *Nursing Research, 39,* 365–369.

Porter, E. J. (1999). Defining the eligible, accessible population for a phenomenological study. *Western Journal of Nursing Research, 21,* 796–804.

Portney, L. G., & Watkins, M. (2000). *Foundations of clinical research: Applications to practice* (2nd ed.). Upper Saddle River, NJ: Prentice-Hall Heath.

Prochaska, J. O., & Velicer, W. F. (1997). The Transtheoretical Model of health behavior change. *American Journal of Health Promotion, 12,* 38–48.

Prochaska, J. O., Redding, C. A., & Evers, K. E. (2002). The Transtheoretical Model and stages of changes. In F. M. Lewis (Ed), *Health behavior and health education: Theory, research and practice* (pp. 99–120). San Francisco: Jossey Bass.

Pruitt, R. H., & Privette, A.B. (2001). Planning strategies for the avoidance of pitfalls in intervention research. *Journal of Advanced Nursing, 35,* 514–520.

Punch, M. (1994). Politics and ethics in qualitative research. In N. K. Denzin, & Y. S. Lincoln (Eds.), *Handbook of qualitative research.* Thousand Oaks, CA: Sage.

Pyett, P. M. (2003). Validation of qualitative research "in the real world." *Qualitative Health Research, 13,* 1170–1179.

Qin, R., Titler, M., Shever, L., & Kim, T. (2008). Estimating effects of nursing intervention via propensity score analysis. *Nursing Research, 57,* 444–452.

Reed, P. G. (1991). Toward a nursing theory of self-transcendence. *Advances in Nursing Science, 13*(4), 64–77.

Reynolds, W. (1982). Development of reliable and valid short forms of the Marlow-Crowne social desirability scale. *Journal of Clinical Psychology, 38,* 119–125.

Ricoeur, P. (1981). *Hermeneutics and the social sciences.* (J. Thompson, trans. & Ed). New York: Cambridge University Press.

Riessman, C. K. (1991). Beyond reductionism: Narrative genres in divorce accounts. *Journal of Narrative and Life History, 1,* 41–68.

Riessman, C. K. (2008). *Narrative methods for the human sciences.* Thousand Oaks, CA: Sage.

Reverby, S. M. (in press). "Normal exposure" and inoculation syphilis: A PHS "Tuskegee" doctor in Guatemala, 1946-1948. *Journal of Policy History.*

Robinson, K. A., Dennison, C., Wayman, D., Pronovost, P., & Needham, D. (2007). Systematic review identifies number of strategies important for retaining study participants. *Journal of Clinical Epidemiology, 60,* 757–765.

Robinson, K. M. (2001). Unsolicited narratives from the Internet: A rich source of qualitative data. *Qualitative Health Research, 11,* 706–714.

Robinson, S., & Dracup, K. (2008). Innovative options for the doctoral dissertation in nursing. *Nursing Outlook, 56,* 174–178.

Rodgers, B. L., & Cowles, K. V. (1993). The qualitative research audit trail: A complex collection of documentation. *Research in Nursing and Health, 16,* 219–226.

Rogers, E. M. (1995). *Diffusion of innovations* (4th ed.). New York: Free Press.

Rogers, M. E. (1990). Nursing: A science for unitary, irreducible human beings: Update 1990. In E. Barrett (Ed.), *Visions of Rogers' science-based nursing.* New York: National League for Nursing.

Rogers, M. E. (1994). The science of unitary human beings: Current perspectives. *Nursing Science Quarterly, 7,* 33–35.

Romazanoglu, C., & Holland, J. (2002). *Feminist methodology: Challenges and choices.* Thousand Oaks, CA: Sage.

Rosenthal, R. (1991). *Meta-analytic procedures for social research.* Newbury Park, CA: Sage.

Rossi, P., Lipsey, M., & Freeman, H. (2004). *Evaluation: A systematic approach* (7th ed.). Thousand Oaks, CA: Sage.

Rosswurm, M. A., & Larrabee, J. H. (1999). A model for change to evidence-based practice. *Image: The Journal of Nursing Scholarship, 31,* 317–322.

Rowlands, G., Sims, J., & Kerry, S. (2005). A lesson learned: The importance of modeling in randomized controlled trials for complex interventions in primary care. *Family Practice, 22,* 132–139.

Roy, C. Sr., & Andrews, H. (2009). *The Roy Adaptation Model* (3rd ed.). Upper Saddle River, NJ: Prentice Hall.

Rubin, H., & Rubin, I. S. (2005). *Qualitative interviewing: The art of hearing data* (2nd ed.). Thousand Oaks, CA: Sage.

Rudestam, K., & Newton, R. (2007). *Surviving your dissertation: A comprehensive guide to content and process* (3rd ed.). Thousand Oaks, CA: Sage.

Russell, C. K., Gregory, D. M., & Gates, M. F. (1996). Aesthetics and substance in qualitative research posters. *Qualitative Health Research, 6,* 542–553.

Russell, K., Maraj, M., Wilson, L., Shedd-Steele, R., & Champion, V. (2008). Barriers to recruiting urban African American women into research studies in community settings. *Applied Nursing Research, 21,* 90–97.

Rycroft-Malone, J., Seers, K., Titchen, A., Harvey, G., Kitson, A., & McCormack, B. (2002). Getting evidence into practice: Ingredients for change. *Nursing Standard, 16*(37), 38–43.

Sackett, D. L., Straus, S. E., Richardson, W. S., Rosenberg, W., & Haynes, R. B. (2000). *Evidence-based medicine:*

How to practice and teach EBM (2nd ed.). Edinburgh: Churchill Livingstone.

Saldaña, J. (2009). *The coding manual for qualitative researchers.* Thousand Oaks, CA: Sage.

Sandelowski, M. (1993a). Rigor or rigor mortis: The problem of rigor in qualitative research revisited. *Advances in Nursing Science, 16,* 1–8.

Sandelowski, M. (1993b). Theory unmasked: The uses and guises of theory in qualitative research. *Research in Nursing & Health, 16,* 213–218.

Sandelowski, M. (1996). Using qualitative methods in intervention studies. *Research in Nursing & Health, 19,* 359–365.

Sandelowski, M. (1997). "Making the best of things": Technology in American nursing 1870–1940. *Nursing History Review, 8,* 3–22.

Sandelowski, M. (1998). Writing a good read: Strategies for re-presenting qualitative data. *Research in Nursing & Health, 21,* 375–382.

Sandelowski, M. (2000a). Combining qualitative and quantitative sampling, data collection, and analysis techniques in mixed-method studies. *Research in Nursing & Health, 23,* 246–255.

Sandelowski, M. (2000b). Whatever happened to qualitative description? *Research in Nursing & Health, 23,* 334–340.

Sandelowski, M. (2001). Real qualitative researchers do not count: The use of numbers in qualitative research. *Research in Nursing & Health, 24,* 230–240.

Sandelowski, M. (2003). Tables or tableaux? The challenges of writing and reading mixed methods studies. In A. Tashakkori & C. Teddlie (Eds.), *Handbook of mixed methods in social and behavioral research* (pp. 321–350). Thousand Oaks, CA: Sage.

Sandelowski, M. (2004). Counting cats in Zanzibar. *Research in Nursing & Health, 27,* 215–216.

Sandelowski, M. (2008). Reading, writing and systematic review. *Journal of Advanced Nursing, 64,* 104–110.

Sandelowski, M. (2010). What's in a name? Qualitative description revisited. *Research in Nursing & Health, 33,* 77–84.

Sandelowski, M., & Barroso, J. (2002). Finding the findings in qualitative studies. *Journal of Nursing Scholarship, 34,* 213–219.

Sandelowski, M., & Barroso, J. (2003a). Classifying the findings in qualitative studies. *Qualitative Health Research, 13*(7), 905–923.

Sandelowski, M., & Barroso, J. (2003b). Creating metasummaries of qualitative findings. *Nursing Research, 52,* 226–233.

Sandelowski, M., & Barroso, J. (2003c). Toward a metasynthesis of qualitative findings on motherhood in HIV-positive women. *Research in Nursing & Health, 26,* 153–170.

Sandelowski, M., & Barroso, J. (2007). *Handbook for synthesizing qualitative research.* New York: Springer.

Sandelowski, M., Davis, D., & Harris, B. (1989). Artful design: Writing the proposal for research in the naturalist paradigm. *Research in Nursing & Health, 12,* 77–84.

Sandelowski, M., Docherty, S., & Emden, C. (1997). Qualitative metasynthesis: Issues and techniques. *Research in Nursing & Health, 20,* 365–377.

Sandelowski, M., Voils, C., & Barroso, J. (2006). Defining and designing mixed research synthesis studies. *Research in the Schools, 13,* 29.

Sandelowski, M., Voils, C., & Barroso, J. (2007). Comparability work and the management of difference in research synthesis studies. *Social Science and Medicine, 64,* 236–247.

Sandelowski, M., Voils, C., & Knafl, G. (2009). On quantitizing. *Journal of Mixed Methods Research, 3,* 208–222.

Schreiber, R., Crooks, D., & Stern, P. N. (1997). Qualitative meta-analysis. In J. M. Morse (Ed.), *Completing a qualitative project* (pp. 311–326). Thousand Oaks, CA: Sage.

Schultz, A. (2005). Clinical scholars at the bedside. An EBP mentorship model for how nurses work today. Nursing Knowledge International, Sigma Theta Tau International. Retrieved April 6, 2009, from http://www.nursingknowledge.org.

Schulz, K. F., Chalmers, I., & Altman, D. G. (2002). The landscape and lexicon of blinding in randomized trials. *Annals of Internal Medicine, 136,* 254–259.

Schwandt, T. (2007). *The Sage dictionary of qualitative inquiry* (3rd ed.). Thousand Oaks, CA: Sage.

Schwartz-Barcott, D., & Kim, H. S. (2000). An expansion and elaborating of hybrid model of concept development. In B. L. Rodgers & K. A. Knafl (Eds.), *Concept development in nursing* (pp. 107–133). Philadelphia: Saunders.

Scott, K. & McSherry, R. (2008). Evidence-based nursing: Clarifying the concepts for nurses in practice. *Journal of Clinical Nursing, 18,* 1085–1095.

Scott, S., Sharpe, H., O'Leary, K., Dehaeck, U., Hindmarsh, K., Moore, J., & Osmond, M. (2009). Court reporters: A viable solution for the challenges of focus group data collection. *Qualitative Health Research, 19,* 140–146.

Seers, K. (2007). Evaluating complex interventions. *Worldviews on Evidence-Based Nursing, 4,* 67.

Shadish, W. R., Cook, T. D., & Campbell, D. T. (2002). *Experimental and quasi-experimental designs for generalized causal inference.* Boston: Houghton Mifflin.

Shapiro, S. E. (2005). Evaluating clinical decision rules. *Western Journal of Nursing Research, 27,* 655–664.

Shapiro, S. E., & Driever, M. (2004). Clinical decision rules as tools for evidence-based nursing. *Western Journal of Nursing Research, 26,* 930–937.

Shin, J. H. (2009). Application of repeated-measures analysis of variance and hierarchical linear model in nursing research. *Nursing Research, 58,* 211–217.

Shrout, P., & Fleiss, J. (1979). Intraclass correlations: Uses in assessing rater reliability. *Psychological Bulletin, 86,* 420–428.

Sidani, S., & Braden, C. J. (1998). *Evaluating nursing interventions: A theory driven approach*. Thousand Oaks, CA: Sage.

Sidani, S., Epstein, D., & Miranda, J. (2006). Eliciting patient treatment preferences: A strategy to integrate evidence-based and patient-centered care. *Worldviews of Evidence-Based Nursing, 3,* 116–123.

Sigma Theta Tau International. (2008). Sigma Theta Tau International position statement on evidence-based practice, February 2007 summary. *Worldviews of Evidence-Based Nursing, 5,* 57–59.

Silva, M. C. (1986). Research testing nursing theory: State of the art. *Advances in Nursing Science, 9,* 1–11.

Silva, M. C. (1995). *Ethical guidelines in the conduct, dissemination, and implementation of nursing research*. Washington, DC: American Nurses' Association.

Silverman, D. (2001). *Interpreting qualitative data: Methods for analyzing talk, text, and interaction* (2nd ed.). London: Sage.

Smith, D. E. (1999). *Writing the social: Critique, theory, and investigation*. Toronto: University of Toronto Press.

Smith, J. (1993). *After the demise of empiricism: The problem of judging social and educational inquiry*. Norwood, NJ: Ablex.

Smith, J. A., Flowers, P., & Larkin, M. (2009). *Interpetive phenomenological analysis: Theory, method and research*. Los Angeles: Sage.

Smith, M. J., & Liehr, P. (2003). *Middle-range theory for nursing*. New York: Springer Publishing Co.

Soeken, K., & Sripusanapan, A. (2003). Assessing publication bias in meta-analysis. *Nursing Research, 52*(1), 57–60.

Sousa, V., Zauszieewski, J., & Musil, C. (2004). How to determine whether a convenience sample represents the population. *Applied Nursing Research, 17,* 130–133.

Sparkes, A. (2001). Myth 94: Qualitative health researchers will agree about validity. *Qualitative Health Research, 11,* 538–552.

Spillane, V., Byrne, M., Byrne, M. Leathen, C., O'Malley, M., & Cupples, M. (2007). Monitoring treatment fidelity in a randomized controlled trial of a complex intervention. *Journal of Advanced Nursing, 60,* 343–352.

Spradley, J. (1979). *The ethnographic interview*. New York: Holt Rinehart & Winston.

Spradley, J. P. (1980). *Participant observation*. New York: Holt, Rinehart & Wilson.

Stake, R. (1995). *The art of case study research*. Thousand Oaks, CA: Sage.

Stake, R. E. (2005). Qualitative case studies. In N. Denzin & Y. Lincoln (Eds.), *The Sage handbook of qualitative research* (3rd ed., pp. 443–466). Thousand Oaks, CA: Sage.

Stein, K., Sargent, J., & Rafaels, N. (2007). Intervention research: Establishing fidelity of the independent variable in nursing clinical trials. *Nursing Research, 56,* 54–62.

Stemler, S. (2004). A comparison of consensus, consistency, and measurement approaches to estimating interrater reliability. *Practical Assessment, Research, and Evaluation, 9*(4). Retrieved May 16, 2006, from http://pareonline.net/getvn.asp?v=9&n=4.

Stetler, C. B. (2001). Updating the Stetler model of research utilization to facilitate evidence-based practice. *Nursing Outlook, 49,* 272–279.

Stetler, C. B., & Marram, G. (1976). Evaluating research findings for applicability in practice. *Nursing Outlook, 24,* 559–563.

Strahan, R., & Gerbasi, K. (1972). Short, homogeneous version of the Marlowe-Crowne Social Desirability Scale. *Journal of Clinical Psychology, 28,* 191–193.

Strauss, A., & Corbin, J. (1990). *Basics of qualitative research: Grounded theory procedures and techniques*. Newbury Park, CA: Sage.

Strauss, A., & Corbin, J. (1998). *Basics of qualitative research: Grounded theory procedures and techniques* (2nd ed.). Thousand Oaks, CA: Sage.

Streiner, D. L., & Norman, G. R. (2008). *Health measurement scales: A practical guide to their development and use* (4th ed.). Oxford: Oxford University Press.

Strickland, O. L., & DiIorio, C. (Eds.). (2003a). *Measurement of nursing outcomes: Vol. II, Client outcomes and quality of care* (2nd ed.). New York: Springer.

Strickland, O. L., & DiIorio, C. (Eds.). (2003b). *Measurement of nursing outcomes: Volume III, Self-care and coping* (2nd ed.). New York: Springer.

Stroup, D. F., Berlin, J., Morton, S., Olkin, I., Williamson, G., Rennie, D., & Thacker, S. (2000). Meta-analysis of observational studies in epidemiology: A proposal for reporting. Meta-analysis Of Observation Studies in Epidemiology (MOOSE) group. *Journal of the American Medical Association, 283,* 2008–2012.

Strunk, W., Jr., White, E. B., & Angell, R. (2000). *The elements of style* (4th ed). Boston: Allyn & Bacon.

Subcommittee on Measuring and Reporting the Quality of Survey Data. (2001). *Statistical working paper 31: Measuring and reporting sources of error in surveys*. Washington, DC: Office of Management and Budget. Retrieved September, 2005, from http://www.fcsm.gov/01papers/SPWP31_final.pdf.

Swanson, E., Moorhead, S., Johnson, M., & Maas, M. (2008). *Nursing Outcomes Classification (NOC)* (4th ed.). St. Louis: Mosby.

Tabachnick, B. G., & Fidell, L. S. (2007). *Using multivariate statistics* (5th ed.). New York: Harper Collins College.

Tashakkori, A., & Teddlie, C. (1998). *Mixed methodology: Combining the qualitative and quantitative approaches*. Thousand Oaks, CA: Sage.

Tashakkori, A., & Teddlie, C., Eds. (2003). *Handbook of mixed methods in social and behavioral research*. Thousand Oaks, CA: Sage.

Tashkorri, A., & Creswell, J. (2007). The new era of mixed methods. *Journal of Mixed Methods Research, 1,* 3–7.

Taylor, C. (2005). What packages are available? Retrieved October 6, 2006, from http://caqdas.soc. surrey.ac.uk/.

Teddlie, C., & Tashkkori, A. (2003). Major issues and controversies in the use of mixed methods in the social and behavioral sciences. In A. Tashakkori & C. Teddlie (Eds.), *Handbook of mixed methods in social and behavioral research* (pp. 3–50). Thousand Oaks, CA: Sage.

Teddlie, C., & Tashkkori, A. (2009). *Foundations of mixed methods research.* Thousand Oaks, CA: Sage Publications.

Thomas, J., & Harden, A. (2008). Methods for the thematic synthesis of qualitative research in systematic reviews. *BMC Medical Research Methodology, 8,* 45.

Thompson, A., Pickler, R., & Reyna, B. (2005). Clinical coordination of research. *Applied Nursing Research, 18,* 102–105.

Thompson, C. (2004). Fortuitous phenomena: On complexity, pragmatic randomised controlled trials, and knowledge for evidence-based practice. *Worldviews on Evidence-Based Nursing, 1,* 9–17.

Thorne, S. (1994). Secondary analysis in qualitative research. In J. M. Morse (Ed.), *Critical issues in qualitative research methods.* Thousand Oaks, CA: Sage Publications.

Thorne, S. (2008). *Interpretive description.* Walnut Creek, CA: Left Coast Press.

Thorne, S. (2009). The role of qualitative research within an evidence-based context. *International Journal of Nursing Studies, 46,* 569–575.

Thorne, S., & Darbyshire, P. (2005). Land mines in the field: A modest proposal for improving the craft of qualitative health research. *Qualitative Health Research, 15,* 1105–1113.

Thorne, S., Jensen, L., Kearney, M., Noblit, G., & Sandelowski, M. (2004). Qualitative metasynthesis: Reflections on methodologic orientation and ideological agenda. *Qualitative Health Research, 14,* 1342–1365.

Tilden, V. P., Nelson, C. A., & May, B. A. (1990). Use of qualitative methods to enhance content validity. *Nursing Research, 39,* 172–175.

Titler, M. G., & Everett, L. Q. (2001). Translating research into practice. Considerations for critical care investigators. *Critical Care Nursing Clinics of North America, 13,* 587–604.

Titler, M. G., Kleiber, C., Steelman, V., Rakel, B., Budreau, G., Everett, L., & Goode, C. (2001). The Iowa model of evidence-based practice to promote quality care. *Critical Care Nursing Clinics of North America, 13,* 497–509.

Tomey, A. M., & Alligood, M. R. (2006). *Nurse theorists and their work* (6th ed.). St. Louis, MO: Mosby Elsevier.

Tong, A., Sainsbury, P., & Craig, J. (2007). Consolidated criteria for reporting qualitative research (COREQ): A 32-item checklist for interviews and focus groups. *International Journal of Qualitative Health Care Research, 19,* 349–357.

Topp, R., Newman, J., & Jones, V. (2008). Including African Americans in health care research. *Western Journal of Nursing Research, 30,* 197–203.

Tuchman, G. (1994). Historical social science: Methodologies, methods, and meanings. In N. K. Denzin & Y. S. Lincoln (Eds.), *Handbook of qualitative research* (pp. 306–323). Thousand Oaks, CA: Sage.

Tunis, S. R., Stryer, D., & Clancy, C. (2003). Practical clinical trials: Increasing the value of clinical research for decision making in clinical and health policy. *Journal of the American Medical Association, 290,* 1624–1632.

Turkel, M. C., Reidinger, G., Ferket, K., & Reno, K. (2005). An essential component of the magnet journey: Fostering an environment for evidence-based practice and nursing research. *Nursing Administration Quarterly, 29,* 254–262.

Turner, T., Misso, M., Harris, C., & Green, S. (2008). Development of evidence-based clinical practice guidelines (CPGs): Comparing approaches. *Implementation Science, 3,* 45.

Urbina, S. (2004). *Essentials of psychological testing.* New York: John Wiley & Sons.

UyBico, S., Pavel, S., & Gross, C. (2007). Recruiting vulnerable populations into research: Systematic review of recruitment interventions. *Journal of General Internal Medicine, 22,* 852–863.

Van den Hoonaard, W. C. (2002). *Walking the tightrope: Ethical issues for qualitative researchers.* Toronto: University of Toronto Press.

Van Kaam, A. (1966). *Existential foundations of psychology.* Pittsburgh, PA: Duquesne University Press.

Van Manen, M. (1990). *Researching lived experience: Human science for an action sensitive pedagogy.* London, Ontario: Althouse Press.

Van Manen, M. (1997). From meaning to method. *Qualitative Health Research, 7,* 345–369.

Van Manen, M. (2002). *Writing in the dark: Phenomenological studies in interpretive inquiry.* Ontario, Canada: Althouse Press.

Van Manen, M. (2006). Writing qualitatively or the demands of writing. *Qualtiative Health Research, 16,* 713–722.

Van Meijel, B., Gamel. C., van Swieten-Duijfjes, B., & Grypdonck, M. (2004). The development of evidence-based nursing interventions. *Journal of Advanced Nursing, 48,* 84–92.

Vessey, J., & Gennarao, S. (1994). The ghost of Tuskegee. *Nursing Research, 43,* 67–68.

Vickers, A. J. (2006). How to randomize. *Journal of the Society for Integrative Oncology, 4,* 194–198.

von Elm, E., Altman, D., Egger, M., Pocock, S., Gotzsche, P., & Vandenbroucke, J. (2008). The Strengthening the Reporting of Observational Studies in Epidemiology (STROBE) statement: guidelines for reporting observational studies. *Journal of Clinical Epidemiology, 61,* 344–349.

Wager, E. (2010). *Getting research published: An A-Z of publication strategy* (2nd ed.). London: Radcliffe Books.

Walker, D., & Myrick, F. (2006). Grounded theory: An exploration of process and procedure. *Qualitative Health Research, 16*, 547–559.

Walker, L. O., & Avant, K. C. (2005). *Strategies for theory construction in nursing* (4th ed.). Upper Saddle River, NJ: Prentice Hall.

Walters, L. A., Wilczynski, N. L., & Haynes, R. B. (2006). Developing optimal search strategies for retrieving relevant qualitative studies in EMBASE. *Qualitative Health Research, 16*, 162–168.

Waltz, C. F., Strickland, O. L., & Lenz, E. R. (2010). *Measurement in nursing and health research* (4th ed.). New York: Springer.

Wang, W., Lee, H., & Fetzer, S. (2006). Challenges and strategies of instrument translation. *Western Journal of Nursing Research, 28*, 310–321.

Warnock, F. F., & Allen, M. (2003). Ethological methods to develop nursing knowledge. *Research in Nursing & Health, 26*, 74–84.

Watson, J. (2005). *Caring science as sacred science.* Philadelphia: F. A. Davis.

Watson, L., & Girard, F. (2004). Establishing integrity and avoiding methodological misunderstanding. *Qualitative Health Research, 14*, 875–881.

Weaver, K., Mitcham, C. (2008). Nursing concept analysis in North America: State of the art. *Nursing Philosophy, 9*, 180–194.

Webb, M., Seigers, D., & Wood, E. (2009). Recruiting African American smokers into intervention research. *Research in Nursing & Health, 32*, 86–95.

Weber, B., Yarandi, H., Rowe, M., & Weber, J. (2005). A comparison study: Paper-based versus web-based data collection and management. *Applied Nursing Research, 18*, 182–185.

Wheeler, M. M. (2009). APACHE: An evaluation. *Critical Care Nursing Quarterly, 32*, 46–48.

Whitehead, L. (2004). Enhancing the quality of hermeneutic research. *Journal of Advanced Nursing, 45*, 512–518.

Whitmer, K., Sweeney, C., Slivjak, A., Sumner, C., & Barsevick, A. (2005). Strategies for maintaining integrity of a behavioral intervention. *Western Journal of Nursing Research, 27*, 338–345.

Whittemore, R., & Grey, M. (2002). The systematic development of nursing interventions. *Journal of Nursing Scholarship, 34*, 115–120.

Whittemore, R., Chase, S. K., & Mandle, C. L. (2001). Validity in qualitative research. *Qualitative Health Research, 11*, 522–537.

Wilczynski, N., Marks, S., & Haynes, R. (2007). Search strategies for identifying qualitative studies in CINAHL. *Qualitative Health Research, 17*, 705– 710.

Wimpenny, P., Johnson, N., Walter, I., & Wilkinson, J. (2008). Tracing and identifying the impact of evidence—use of a modified pipeline model. *Worldviews of Evidence-Based Nursing, 5*, 3–12.

Wipke-Tevis, D., & Pickett, M. (2008). Impact of the Health Insurance Portability and Accountability Act on participant recruitment and retention. *Western Journal of Nursing Research, 30*, 39–53.

Wolcott, H. (1994). *Transforming qualitative data.* London: Sage Ltd.

Wolcott, H. (1995). *The art of fieldwork.* London: Sage Ltd.

Wood, M. J. (2000). Influencing health policy through research. *Clinical Nursing Research, 9*, 213–216.

Yates, B., Dodendorf, D., Lane, J., LaFramboise, L., Pozehl, B., Duncan, K., et al. (2009). Testing an alternate informed consent process. *Nursing Research, 58*, 135–139.

Yen, M., & Lo, L. (2002). Examining test–retest reliability: An intraclass correlation approach. *Nursing Research, 51*, 59–62.

Yin, R. (2009). *Case study research: Design and methods* (4th ed.). Thousand Oaks, CA: Sage.

Zelen, M. (1979). A new design for randomized controlled trials. *New England Journal of Medicine, 300*, 1242–1245.

Zeni, M., & Kogan, M. (2007). Existing population-based health databases: Useful resources for nursing research. *Nursing Outlook, 55*, 20–30.

Zinsser, W. (2006). *On writing well* (7th ed.). New York: Harper Collins.

Zwarenstein, M., Treweek, S., Gagnier, J., Altman, D., Tunis, S., Haynes, B., Oxman, A. D., & Moher, D. (2008). Improving reporting of pragmatic trials: Extensions of the CONSORT statement. *BMJ, 337*, 1–8.

Index

Page numbers in bold type indicate glossary entries.